THE APhA
COMPLETE REVIEW
FOR PHARMACY 13th EDITION

THE APhA COMPLETE REVIEW FOR PHARMACY 13th EDITION

Andrea S. Franks, PharmD, BCPS
Editor-in-Chief
Professor and Vice Chair for Education
Department of Clinical Pharmacy and Translational Science
The University of Tennessee Health Science Center College of Pharmacy
Knoxville, Tennessee

J. Aubrey Waddell, BS Pharm, MA, PharmD, FAPhA, BCOP
Associate Editor
Clinical Specialist Pharmacist – Oncology
Thompson Infusion Services – Oak Ridge, Tennessee
Professor, Department of Clinical Pharmacy and Translational Science
The University of Tennessee Health Science Center College of Pharmacy
Knoxville, Tennessee

Bradley A. Boucher, PharmD, FCCP, FNAP, MCCM, BCPS
Associate Editor
Professor, Department of Clinical Pharmacy and Translational Science
Associate Dean for Strategic Initiatives and Operations
The University of Tennessee Health Science Center College of Pharmacy
Memphis, Tennessee

Nancy D. Borja-Hart, PharmD, FCCP, BCPS
Associate Editor
Associate Professor, Department of Clinical Pharmacy and Translational Science
The University of Tennessee Health Science Center College of Pharmacy
Nashville, Tennessee

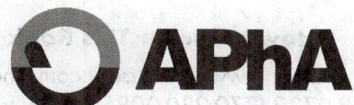

American Pharmacists Association
Washington, D.C.

Senior Director, Books and Digital Publishing: Eleanore Tapscott
Editorial Director: Jesse Vineyard
Production Editor: Brittany Williams
Editorial Services: Circle Graphics, Inc.
Cover Design: Michelle I. Powell, APhA Integrated Design and Production
Indexer: Arc Indexing, Inc.

©2022 by the American Pharmacists Association
APhA was founded in 1852 as the American Pharmaceutical Association.

Published by the American Pharmacists Association
2215 Constitution Avenue, NW
Washington, DC 20037-2985
www.pharmacist.com
www.pharmacylibrary.com

To comment on this book by e-mail, send your message to the publisher at aphabooks@aphanet.org.

Library of Congress Cataloging-in-Publication Data

Names: Franks, Andrea S., editor. | Boucher, Bradley A., editor. |
  Borja-Hart, Nancy D., editor. | Waddell, J. Aubrey, editor. |
  American Pharmacists Association, issuing body.
Title: The APhA complete review for pharmacy / Andrea S. Franks,
  editor-in-chief ; Bradley A. Boucher, Nancy D. Borja-Hart, J. Aubrey Waddell,
  associate editor[s].
Other titles: Complete review for pharmacy
Description: 13th edition. | Washington, D.C. : American Pharmacists Association, [2022] |
  Includes bibliographical references and index. | Summary: "The North American Pharmacist Licensure
  Examination® (NAPLEX®) is the licensing exam that each U.S. college or school of pharmacy graduate
  must pass in order to practice as a pharmacist. This comprehensive yet concise review prepares the reader
  to succeed on the NAPLEX by focusing on the information most pertinent to the exam. The APhA Complete
  Review for Pharmacy is in an easy-to-read format with icons, key points, study guide checklists, figures, tables,
  and boxes to organize information. The best way to prepare for an exam is with practice questions. This book
  provides more than 900 practice questions that include an answer key and explanations of the answer options.
  In addition to being a valuable resource for individuals preparing for the NAPLEX®, The APhA Complete
  Review for Pharmacy is a useful resource for busy pharmacists seeking to stay current"—Provided by publisher.
Identifiers: LCCN 2021049561 | ISBN 9781582123615 (paperback)
Subjects: MESH: Pharmacy | Pharmaceutical Preparations | Examination Questions
Classification: LCC RM301.13 | NLM QV 18.2 | DDC 615.1076—dc23/eng/20211015
  LC record available at https://lccn.loc.gov/2021049561

How to Order This Book

Online: www.pharmacist.com/shop
By phone: 800-878-0729 (770-280-0085 from outside the United States)
VISA®, MasterCard®, and American Express® cards accepted.

Dedication

We dedicate this book to our mentors, colleagues, residents, and students, who have shaped our pharmacy path, along with our family and friends who nurtured our souls and supported us along the way.

ANDREA, BRAD, NANCY, AND AUBREY

"The beautiful thing about learning is that no one can take it away from you." —B.B. King

Contents

Preface

The 13th edition of *The APhA Complete Review for Pharmacy* introduces several new features. All chapters have been reviewed and revised by the authors and editorial team to provide up-to-date information and concepts. The information in the chapters focuses on the depth expected for a practice-ready, newly graduated pharmacist. Self-assessment questions contain "mark all that apply" responses, as well as other NAPLEX question formats. The authors and editors are aware of the new NAPLEX competencies and exam details effective January 2021 and have been mindful to incorporate these changes in their work. One example is the emphasis on FDA boxed warnings, a component of the 2021 NAPLEX competency statements.

This edition also retains many of the features from the 12th edition. The tables that list medications have the top 100 drugs indicated in bold to alert the reader of medicines in frequent use. A summary of a chapter's concepts, Key Points, should give the reader a quick and ready snapshot of some important points discussed in the chapter. The Key Points section is followed by the Study Guide Checklist that should serve as a guide in preparation for the NAPLEX as part of a self-assessment. The Checklist covers broad areas of information, including concepts and skills that are not necessarily covered fully in *The APhA Complete Review for Pharmacy* but should be considered in the overall preparation for the exam. This information can be found in comprehensive textbooks and references that are typically used in a pharmacy curriculum and can be easily retrieved, and many are listed at the end of each chapter in the Additional Resources section. Although *The APhA Complete Review for Pharmacy* is complete in covering key topics, no single reference can fully condense the entire curriculum and body of knowledge into a review. The items in the Checklist should stimulate the reader to seek supplemental information to fill in any gaps in a self-assessment.

These enhancements would not have been possible without the talents and cooperation of the authors. The 13th edition includes the work of 13 new and 34 returning authors. All authors have a strong pharmacy tie to the College of Pharmacy at The University of Tennessee Health Science Center at its locations in Knoxville, Memphis, and Nashville. They are past or present faculty members, alumni, fellows, or residents of the College, and many have more than one of those University of Tennessee ties. A common core of education and training at the University of Tennessee that has been diversified and complemented through experiences in clinical care, teaching, community outreach, professional service, and research has served as a strong foundation for this publication.

The editorial team is aware of the responsibility to bring relevant and contemporary information to readers in their preparation for the NAPLEX. We bring a combined 124 years of experience as educators, clinicians, and scholars to the editorial process. Our efforts have been supported by the staff at the American Pharmacists Association (APhA), to whom we owe much gratitude.

Although this edition includes changes, it also is a product of the longstanding support of APhA. The guidance, ideas, and encouragement of Janan Sarwar, PharmD, and Jesse Vineyard, Editorial Director, Books and Digital Publishing, have been invaluable in contributing to this work. The copyeditors and proofreaders of Circle Graphics also have been involved with this publication for several years and bring important items to the attention of authors and editors from their unique point of view.

We, the editorial team for *The APhA Complete Review for Pharmacy,* hope you find this publication, either print or digital, to be an asset to your successful preparation for and passing of the NAPLEX. We often have found that by globally reviewing a topic, we gain new insights and understanding that reinforce and build on previous knowledge. As a health care professional in your role as a pharmacist, you will be challenged out of necessity to continue your education as a life-long learner for the benefit of your patients and profession. We look forward to you joining the profession of pharmacists and making contributions throughout your career.

Andrea S. Franks, PharmD, BCPS
Editor-in-Chief

J. Aubrey Waddell, BS Pharm, MA, PharmD, FAPhA, BCOP
Associate Editor

Bradley A. Boucher, PharmD, FCCP, FNAP, MCCM, BCPS
Associate Editor

Nancy D. Borja-Hart, PharmD, FCCP, BCPS
Associate Editor

Contributors

Hassan Almoazen, PhD (4)
Director, PhD Program—Pharmaceutical Sciences
Associate Professor, Department of Pharmaceutical
    Sciences
The University of Tennessee Health Science Center
    College of Pharmacy
Memphis, Tennessee

Drew L. Armstrong, PharmD, BCACP (35)
Ambulatory Care Clinical Pharmacist
Regional One Health
Memphis, Tennessee

Gillian C. Bell, PharmD (8)
Pharmacogenomics Service Lead
Genome Medical
South San Francisco, California

Nancy D. Borja-Hart, PharmD, FCCP, BCPS (16)
Associate Professor, Department of Clinical Pharmacy
    and Translational Science
The University of Tennessee Health Science Center
    College of Pharmacy
Nashville, Tennessee

Bradley A. Boucher, PharmD, FCCP, FNAP, MCCM, BCPS (10)
Professor, Department of Clinical Pharmacy and
    Translational Science
Associate Dean for Strategic Initiatives and Operations
The University of Tennessee Health Science Center
    College of Pharmacy
Memphis, Tennessee

Joyce E. Broyles, MS, MHA, PharmD, BCNSP (18)
Pharmacy Manager, Department of Pharmacy
Methodist University Hospital
Memphis, Tennessee

Michael L. Christensen, PharmD (3)
Professor, Departments of Clinical Pharmacy and
    Translational Science and Pediatrics
The University of Tennessee Health Science Center
    College of Pharmacy
Memphis, Tennessee

Peter A. Chyka, BSPharm, PharmD, DABAT, FAACT (43)
Professor Emeritus
The University of Tennessee Health Science Center
    College of Pharmacy
Knoxville, Tennessee

Catherine M. Crill, PharmD, FCCP, BCNSP (31)
Associate Professor, Departments of Clinical Pharmacy
    and Translational Science and Pediatrics
Director, Experiential Learning and International
    Programs, College of Pharmacy
The University of Tennessee Health Science Center
    College of Pharmacy
Memphis, Tennessee

Benjamin T. Duhart, Jr., MS, PharmD (42)
Associate Professor, Department of Clinical Pharmacy
    and Translational Science
The University of Tennessee Health Science Center
    College of Pharmacy
Memphis, Tennessee

Henry M. Dunnenberger, PharmD, BCPS (8)
Director of Personalized Medicine and
    Pharmacogenomics
Mark R. Neaman Center for Personalized Medicine
NorthShore University HealthSystem
Evanston, Illinois

Michelle Z. Farland, PharmD, BCPS, CDCES (17)
Clinical Associate Professor and Division Head
   Community-Based Pharmacotherapy
The University of Florida College of Pharmacy
Gainesville, Florida

Glen E. Farr, PharmD, JAPhA (2)
Professor Emeritus
The University of Tennessee Health Science Center
   College of Pharmacy
Knoxville, Tennessee

Christopher K. Finch, PharmD, FCCM, FCCP (32)
Professor and Chair, Department of Clinical Pharmacy
   and Translational Science
The University of Tennessee Health Science Center
   College of Pharmacy
Memphis, Tennessee

**Shannon W. Finks, PharmD, FCCP, BCPS, BCCP,
   ASHCP-CHC (15)**
Professor, Department of Clinical Pharmacy and
   Translational Science
The University of Tennessee Health Science Center
   College of Pharmacy
Memphis, Tennessee

Andrea S. Franks, PharmD, BCPS (1, 37)
Professor and Vice Chair for Education, Department
   of Clinical Pharmacy and Translational Science
The University of Tennessee Health Science Center
   College of Pharmacy
Knoxville, Tennessee

Wesley Geminn, PharmD, BCPP (29)
Chief Pharmacist, State Opioid Treatment Authority
Assistant Professor, Department of Clinical Pharmacy
   and Translational Science
The University of Tennessee Health Science Center
   College of Pharmacy
Nashville, Tennessee

Christa M. George, PharmD, CDCES, BCACP (25)
Associate Professor, Department of Clinical Pharmacy
   and Translational Science
The University of Tennessee Health Science Center
   College of Pharmacy
Memphis, Tennessee

**Benjamin N. Gross, PharmD, FCCP, MBA, BCPS, BCACP,
   CDCES, ASH-CHC, BC-ADM (12)**
Associate Professor, Department of Pharmacy Practice
Director of Assessment
Lipscomb University College of Pharmacy and Health
   Sciences
Nashville, Tennessee

Tracy M. Hagemann, PharmD, FCCP, FPPA (38)
Associate Dean, Nashville Campus
Professor, Department of Clinical Pharmacy and
   Translational Science
The University of Tennessee Health Science Center
   College of Pharmacy
Nashville, Tennessee

Gale L. Hamann, PharmD, BCPS, CDCES (30)
Professor, Department of Clinical Pharmacy and
   Translational Science
The University of Tennessee Health Science Center
   College of Pharmacy
Clinical Pharmacist, Ambulatory Care
Regional One Health
Memphis, Tennessee

Leslie A. Hamilton, PharmD, FCCP, FCCM, BCPS, BCCCP (28)
Associate Professor, Department of Clinical Pharmacy
   and Translational Science
The University of Tennessee Health Science Center
   College of Pharmacy
Knoxville, Tennessee

Jessica N. Hodge, PharmD (24)
Director of Oncology Pharmacy Services
Covenant Health
Knoxville, Tennessee

Kenneth C. Hohmeier, PharmD (40)
Associate Professor, Department of Pharmaceutical
   Sciences
Director of Community Affairs
The University of Tennessee Health Science Center
   College of Pharmacy
Nashville, Tennessee

Joanna Q. Hudson, PharmD, BCPS, FASN, FCCP, FNKF (20)
Professor, Department of Clinical Pharmacy and
   Translational Science
The University of Tennessee Health Science Center
   College of Pharmacy
Memphis, Tennessee

Tyler M. Kiles, PharmD, BC-ADM (40)
Assistant Professor, Department of Clinical Pharmacy
and Translational Science
The University of Tennessee Health Science Center
College of Pharmacy
Memphis, Tennessee

S. Casey Laizure, PharmD, FCCP (7)
Professor, Department of Clinical Pharmacy and
Translational Science
The University of Tennessee Health Science Center
College of Pharmacy
Memphis, Tennessee

Daniel R. Malcom, PharmD, BCPS, BCCCP (41)
Associate Professor and Chair, Department of Pharmacy
Practice
Sullivan University College of Pharmacy and Health
Sciences
Louisville, Kentucky

Lance Morgan, PharmD, BCPP (29)
Pharmacy Director, Middle Tennessee Mental Health
Institute
Assistant Professor, Department of Clinical Pharmacy
and Translational Science
The University of Tennessee Health Science Center
College of Pharmacy
Nashville, Tennessee

Susan H. Morgan, PharmD, MBA, BCNP (6)
Assistant Dean and Director of Nuclear Pharmacy
Programs
The University of Tennessee Health Science Center
College of Pharmacy
Memphis, Tennessee

Michelle Moseley, PharmD, BCPS, BCGP (39)
Pharmacy Section Chief and Clinical Pharmacist
Practitioner
Veterans Integrated Service Network (VISN 9) Clinical
Resource Hub
Veterans Administration MidSouth Healthcare Network
Nashville, Tennessee

Robert B. Parker, PharmD, FCCP (13, 14)
Professor, Department of Clinical Pharmacy and
Translational Science
The University of Tennessee Health Science Center
College of Pharmacy
Memphis, Tennessee

Chelsea P. Renfro, PharmD, CHSE (2)
Assistant Professor, Department of Clinical Pharmacy
and Translational Science
The University of Tennessee Health Science Center
College of Pharmacy
Memphis, Tennessee

Kelly C. Rogers, PharmD, BCCP, FCCP, FACC (15)
Professor, Department of Clinical Pharmacy and
Translational Science
The University of Tennessee Health Science Center
College of Pharmacy
Memphis, Tennessee

A. Shaun Rowe, MS, PharmD, BCCCP, FNCS (11)
Associate Professor, Department of Clinical Pharmacy
and Translational Science
The University of Tennessee Health Science Center
College of Pharmacy
Knoxville, Tennessee

Chasity M. Shelton, BS, PharmD, FCCP, BCPS, BCPPS (36)
Associate Professor, Department of Clinical Pharmacy
and Translational Science
Assistant Dean for Student Success
The University of Tennessee Health Science Center
College of Pharmacy
Memphis, Tennessee

Gregory T. Sneed, PharmD, BCOP (23)
Assistant Professor, Department of Clinical Pharmacy
and Translational Science
The University of Tennessee Health Science Center
College of Pharmacy
Memphis, Tennessee

Shannon L. Stewart, PharmD (19)
Clinical Pharmacy Specialist—Geriatrics/Palliative Care
Veterans Affairs Medical Center
Memphis, Tennessee

Joseph M. Swanson, PharmD, FCCM, FCCP (22)
Professor, Department of Clinical Pharmacy and
Translational Science
Assistant Director, Experiential Learning and
International Programs
The University of Tennessee Health Science Center
College of Pharmacy
Memphis, Tennessee

Melanie P. Swims, PharmD, BCPS (26)
Clinical Pharmacy Specialist, Ambulatory Care
Veterans Affairs Medical Center
Associate Professor, Department of Clinical Pharmacy
    and Translational Science
The University of Tennessee Health Science Center
    College of Pharmacy
Memphis, Tennessee

James W. Torr, MS, PharmD (5)
Associate Professor, Department of Pharmacy Practice
Lipscomb University College of Pharmacy and Health
    Sciences
Nashville, Tennessee

Edward T. Van Matre, PharmD, MS, BCCCP (22)
Assistant Professor, Department of Clinical Pharmacy
    and Translational Science
The University of Tennessee Health Science Center
    College of Pharmacy
Memphis, Tennessee

Michael P. Veve, PharmD, MPH (33, 34)
Clinical Assistant Professor, Department of Pharmacy
    Practice
Eugene Applebaum College of Pharmacy and Health
    Sciences, Wayne State University
Clinical Pharmacy Specialist, Division of Infectious
    Diseases
Henry Ford Hospital
Detroit, Michigan

Junling Wang, MS, PhD (9)
Professor and Vice Chair for Research, Department
    of Clinical Pharmacy and Translational Science
The University of Tennessee Health Science Center
    College of Pharmacy
Memphis, Tennessee

James S. Wheeler, PharmD, BCPS (27)
Associate Professor, Department of Clinical Pharmacy
    and Translational Science
Associate Dean, Knoxville Campus
The University of Tennessee Health Science Center
    College of Pharmacy
Knoxville, Tennessee

Brian L. Winbigler, PharmD, MBA (43)
Assistant Professor, Department of Clinical Pharmacy
    and Translational Science
The University of Tennessee Health Science Center
    College of Pharmacy
Knoxville, Tennessee

G. Christopher Wood, PharmD, FCCP, FCCM, BCPS (21)
Professor, Department of Clinical Pharmacy and
    Translational Science
The University of Tennessee Health Science Center
    College of Pharmacy
Memphis, Tennessee

You + APhA
Stronger Together

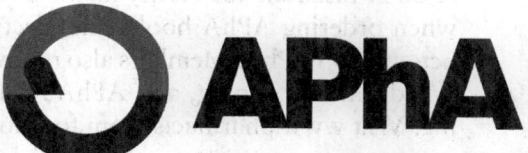

APhA

American Pharmacists Association

For Every Pharmacist. For All of Pharmacy.

At every stage of your career or practice, membership in the American Pharmacists Association is a wise investment!

Membership in the American Pharmacists Association (APhA) is the simplest way to gain access to a solid support system to help you meet even the toughest career challenges. For more than 150 years, APhA has supported tens of thousands of pharmacists in their professional goals. Whether you're a current member or thinking of joining, we're here to support you today, so you'll be prepared for tomorrow!

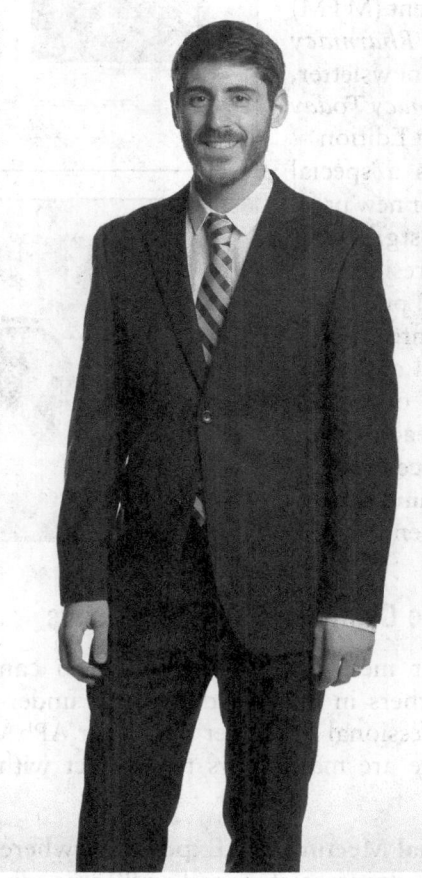

"Being a member of APhA has given me the chance to network with peers across the country who share common interests. I have been able to have numerous conversations with pharmacists regarding how to establish services and have been able to utilize their stories and advice to elevate and advance the care I can offer patients."

—Frank Fanizza, PharmD, BCACP, AAHIVP
Ambulatory Care Clinical Pharmacist
LMH Health
APhA Member Since 2012

APhA has all the resources you need to succeed!

APhA supports you every step of the way as you begin your career in pharmacy. From programs and benefits to help you find the perfect job and become more marketable to potential employers to management and leadership information, training programs, and the latest in pharmacy news, APhA wants to be your primary resource!

Look to APhA to help you with the issues you face every day: new perspectives on drug therapy and disease state management, changing laws and regulations, and pressing decisions related to clinical and practice management. Membership in APhA gives you easy access to the tools you need to connect with like-minded pharmacists from across the country—working to improve medication use and advance patient care.

Strengthen Your Career

Through the **New Practitioners Network**, pharmacists in their first five years of practice enjoy discounted dues and special programming and information to help them get started in their careers. APhA members enjoy opportunities designed to increase professional knowledge and keep up with the latest information. You can take advantage of extensive benefits—to name just a few:

- APhA provides a variety of **Career Development Tools** to help you navigate your career—the **Pathway Program**; career development publications; and access to **APhA's Career Center**, an online resource featuring hundreds of job listings.
- **APhA Community-based Pharmacy Residency Program** fosters the development of formal postgraduate education and training experiences for pharmacists in innovative pharmacy practice to meet the challenges presented by the rapidly changing health care system, the implementation of pharmaceutical care, the explosion of drug and therapeutics information, and the needs of society for improving patient care and monitoring therapeutic outcomes.
- **APhA's Educational Library** links you to more than 80 CPE opportunities, all free to members. **Advanced training programs** include Pharmacy-Based Travel Health Services and APhA Advanced Preceptor Training, publications, drug information resources, and more.
- **Suite of financial education webinars.** APhA understands that as a new practitioner, one of the biggest challenges you face is managing your finances. That's why we've partnered with **Your Financial Pharmacist** to deliver financial education webinars . . . exclusively for APhA members.
- **Student loan refinancing through Credible.** Get instant offers for student loan refinancing from top lenders. Members receive an $86 credit toward APhA membership when they activate a loan through Credible.
- **APhA Certificate Training Programs**, such as Delivering Medication Therapy Management Services, Pharmacy-Based Cardiovascular Disease Risk Management, and more, provide nationally and regionally conducted practice-based educa-

tion and training sessions designed to promote quality pharmaceutical care services and expand the pharmacist's role as a health care provider.

- A 20% discount for APhA members is available when ordering APhA books and electronic products at **Shop APhA**. Members also receive discounts on education training, and APhA's Annual Meeting. Visit www.pharmacist.com for more details!

Advance Patient Care

The more you learn about drug and treatment updates, the better equipped you are to help your patients. APhA is a vital source of information, delivering resources to you in a variety of convenient ways:

- **Pharmacist.com**, the one-stop online resource, fulfills your information needs
- *Journal of the American Pharmacists Association (JAPhA)* in print or online AND the online *Journal of Pharmaceutical Sciences (JPharmSci)*
- *Pharmacy Today*, the monthly medication therapy management (MTM) magazine, *Pharmacy Today* daily newsletter, or select *Pharmacy Today* Health System Edition

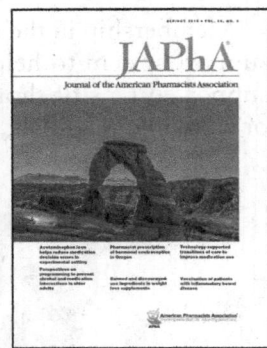

- *Transitions* is a special e-newsletter for new practitioners, postgraduate students, and residents
- **MTM Central** puts comprehensive information on the clinical and business aspects of MTM within easy reach online and allows access to our **MTM e-Community**, as a benefit of membership

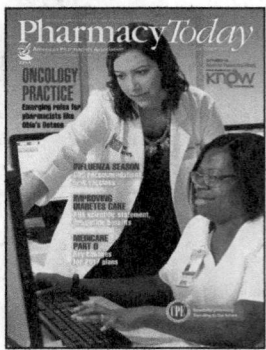

Engage With the Community of Pharmacists

Through your membership in APhA, you can network with others in your field. No one understands your professional life better than your APhA colleagues. There are many ways to connect with your peers:

- **APhA's Annual Meeting and Exposition**, where attendees take advantage of more than 80 core edu-

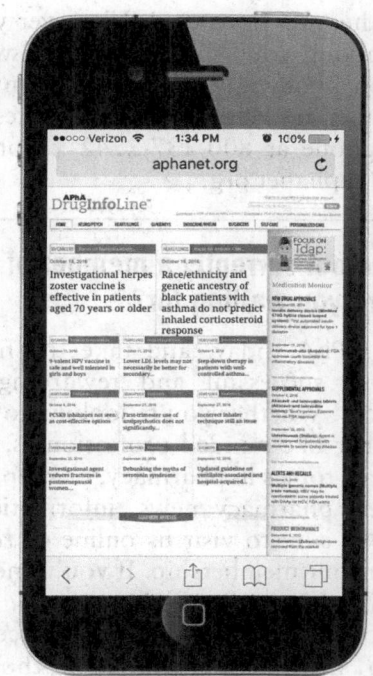

cation sessions, a state-of-the-art exposition, and the opportunity to network with 7,000 of your peers. Join us annually at our Annual Meeting and Exposition; visit aphameeting.org for more information.

- APhA's networking sites on **LinkedIn, Facebook,** and **Pharmacist.com** to meet members online from your state or from across the country. ENGAGE, a members' exclusive online community featuring the APhA New Practitioner Network Community and nine **APhA Academy of Pharmacy Practice and Management (APhA-APPM)** Special Interest Groups (SIGs).

- **APhA's Academies** provide invigorating networking opportunities through the **APhA-APPM** and the **APhA Academy of Pharmaceutical Research and Science (APhA-APRS)**. Most likely you are currently or have been a member of APhA's **Academy of Student Pharmacists (APhA-ASP)** and are acquainted with the many valuable benefits of belonging to a like-minded group of dedicated professionals.

Advocate for Your Profession

APhA serves as the unified voice of pharmacists and is the only organization representing pharmacists in all practice settings. APhA works to do the following:

- Through the **APhA Pharmacists Provide Care** initiative, APhA promotes patient access to pharmacists'

services. Achieving "provider status" recognition is crucial to the pharmacy profession and the key to expanding professional opportunities for pharmacists. Visit PharmacistsProvideCare.com for more details.

- Keep pharmacists informed of new developments in health care legislation and regulation including the steps necessary to implement recognition and reform through the **Advocacy Issues** section of pharmacist.com and the members-only newsletter *APhA Legislative and Regulatory Update.*

- Enhance pharmacists' professional development through the **APhA Advocacy Key Contact Network.** To ensure our voices are heard, APhA provides support to volunteer leaders to help spread the word on pharmacy issues and get the attention of legislators.

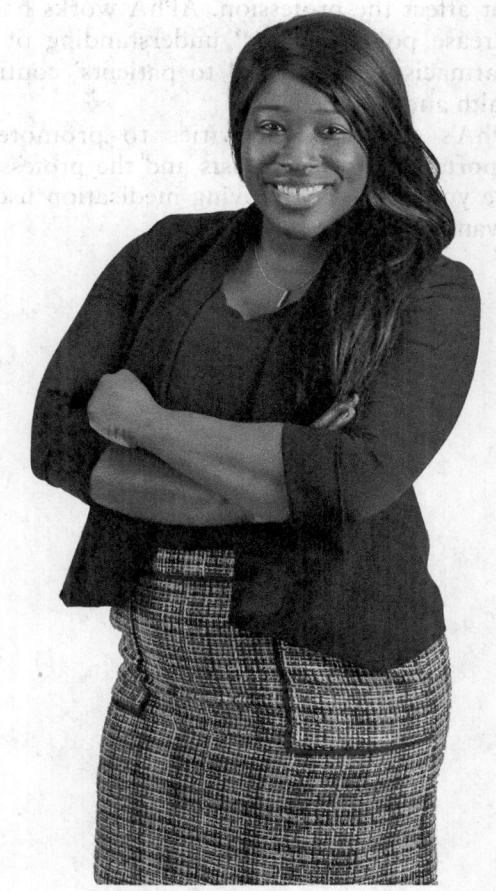

"Being a member of APhA has had a profound impact on every step of my pharmacy journey. My experiences in APhA have cultivated my leadership skills, empowered me to become a confident patient care provider, and given me an overwhelming sense of fulfillment in my professional life. My time in

APhA has allowed me to meet incredible leaders in our profession and ultimately led me to a career that I'm extremely passionate about."

—Tola Adebanjo, PharmD
Clinical Pharmacist
The University of Kansas Cancer Center
APhA Member Since 2015

Proclaim Your Professionalism

As a member of APhA, you'll join more than 60,000 pharmacy professionals, declaring your pride in pharmacy's activities and achievements. Your membership dues help to support work that benefits the entire profession such as:

- APhA's **advocacy efforts** on health care reform and other pending legislation and regulations that affect the profession. APhA works hard to increase policy makers' understanding of how pharmacists are integral to patients' continued health and well-being.
- APhA's concerted activities to promote the **importance of pharmacists** and the professional role you play in improving medication use and advancing patient care.

We are here to serve you! Whenever you have a question about your membership or want more information about any of APhA's many benefits, please contact an APhA Member Services representative by phone at 800-237-2742 x2 or e-mail at infocenter@aphanet.org.

If you're not currently a member of APhA, what are you waiting for?

Join APhA today, and take the first step toward a successful and rewarding career tomorrow! Whether you're looking to interact with other like-minded professionals, explore additional topics in pharmacy, or keep up with the latest pharmacy news, information, and trends, be sure to visit us online to *renew or activate* your membership. If you've never had a membership with APhA, *join now* so that you, too, can have the quality resources necessary to stay competitive with those who already enjoy being a part of APhA.

Become an APhA member today!

pharmacist.com/join

Study Guide for the NAPLEX

1

ANDREA S. FRANKS

 1-1 KEY POINTS

- The NAPLEX is a comprehensive exam that is based on competencies for general practice knowledge established by the National Association of Boards of Pharmacy (NABP) for licensure to practice as a pharmacist.
- Establish a routine of a positive attitude, steady preparation, and adequate practice in studying for the exam during a period of several months before the exam date.
- Take the Pre-NAPLEX exam to become familiar with navigating in the computerized format, experience the type of questions, and assess your stamina and ability to focus for a 6-hour exam.
- In reviewing the chapters of *The APhA Complete Review for Pharmacy*, perform a self-assessment of your knowledge using the questions at the end of each chapter.
- The majority of questions require referring to a patient medication profile or medical record. Practice identifying key information from patient profiles as well as answering stand-alone questions.
- Be mindful of distractions and stress, and maintain your focus on the NAPLEX.

 1-2 STUDY GUIDE CHECKLIST

The following topics may guide your study of this subject area:

- ☐ Create and begin a routine studying schedule several months before the exam.
- ☐ Review NAPLEX guidance and rules in the current *NAPLEX/ MPJE Candidate Application Bulletin* (https://nabp.pharmacy/ programs/examinations/naplex/).
- ☐ Practice answering sample questions to answer easier questions quickly and allow more time for challenging questions. (The 6-hour NAPLEX has 225 questions.)
- ☐ Review NAPLEX competencies (*The NAPLEX Competency Statements* in the *Candidate Application Bulletin*) to identify strengths and weaknesses.
- ☐ Review generic and trade names of commonly used prescription drugs and active ingredients of commonly used over-the-counter medications.
- ☐ Study pharmacy calculations thoroughly to answer confidently and conserve time for other questions.
- ☐ Review medications in commonly used drug classes and different characteristics within a drug class.
- ☐ Review counseling points for commonly used drug classes and the need for warning labels.
- ☐ Review basic pathophysiology of common chronic diseases.
- ☐ Know normal values of basic laboratory tests.
- ☐ Review exam-taking strategies a few weeks before exam day.
- ☐ Visit the testing center location before exam day, and plan to arrive at least 30 minutes before your exam appointment.

1-3   Introduction

Think of yourself as an elite athlete or an accomplished musician for a moment. Would you wait until the week before a competition or a performance to begin training or practicing? Would you focus only on your mind and not include your body? Would you neglect knowing the rule book or the sheet music? Would you check your smartphone periodically while practicing? Would you rely only on what you remember to do without the benefit of a coach or a trainer? Successful athletes and musicians train for months, focus on mind and body, avoid distractions, and look to coaches to find strengths and weaknesses. You might still be competitive and accomplished with your natural abilities, but the odds are working against you without a proper conditioning and training period. This same attitude should translate to your preparation for the NAPLEX. Throughout your pharmacy curriculum, you have already been road tested and have not only learned facts and skills but also should have developed learning and study habits that were successful for you. Now is the time to apply what you have learned about yourself to pass the NAPLEX by considering attitude, preparation, and practice.

1-4   Attitude

Begin with and maintain a positive attitude. The majority of first-time test takers pass the NAPLEX, but they don't just show up and pass. Unlike most tests in a single course that are like sprints of a discrete collection of knowledge, the NAPLEX is like a marathon covering years of a large body of knowledge. Adjust your attitude and habits accordingly. Consider creating a schedule for study at least 4 to 5 months before the exam date. If possible, prioritize some of your best time of the day to studying. Do not just fit your studying in whenever. Like an athlete or a musician, focus on the material during your study time, because studying is more efficient and effective without distractions or multitasking. Distractions and lack of focus make it easy to procrastinate. Develop a personal system and a routine leading up to the exam. There is no doubt that the months leading up to the NAPLEX will be stressful at times for all sorts of reasons. Be sure to routinely take breaks and use relaxation techniques that you find helpful, such as exercising or yoga, listening to music, playing a musical instrument, working on a hobby, or socializing. Write down your goal for the next study session the night before; this practice may help relieve anxiety and allow you to relax. Positively look forward to reviewing material for the NAPLEX. You might be surprised by what you remember from your curriculum that just needs reinforcement. Your self-confidence will also be reinforced to move on to the next topic. Admittedly, the scope and breadth of information and skills are broad and deep, but these are things that you will need to know in varying degrees as you start your career as a pharmacist. Your study session can also be a time of discovery of things that were not quite clear the first time; but now you have an opportunity to put the pieces of the puzzle together. By keeping to a schedule to review 3 to 4 chapters a week and by maintaining a list of things to go over again, you will have time to address problem areas. Adequate preparation is key for successfully passing the NAPLEX. If self-study isn't sufficient to clear up a concept, ask a friend, colleague, or instructor for advice. Consider the Key Points, Study Guide Checklist, and practice questions as a self-assessment and guide to focus your follow-up of the material.

1-5   Preparation

The Rule Book

Before you start studying, take time to review the guidance, rules, and description of the NAPLEX provided by the organization conducting the exam—the National Association of Boards of Pharmacy (NABP). The NABP website's section on its programs (https://nabp.pharmacy/programs/) has critical information about exam procedures and policies, content areas, question format, and other important information. Each year, NABP produces the *NAPLEX/MPJE Candidate Application Bulletin*, which is essential for you to download (https://nabp.pharmacy/programs/examinations/naplex/) and review. This publication will help you focus your attention on the exam and describe essential procedures from start to finish. Be sure to know the rules and follow the guidance provided by the NABP. With a metaphor to an athletic competition, an athlete may be the fastest and strongest, but if he or she fails to know and follow the rules, then that athlete will not successfully finish or even compete.

The Playing Field

Only 200 of the 225 questions on the NAPLEX are used for exam scoring. The remaining 25 questions are being evaluated for future use, distributed throughout the exam, and not used in exam scoring. The exam is administered as a linear form exam, which means the questions are assembled before the start of the exam. Each exam offering is unique and comprises questions of varying levels of difficulty. The majority are scenario-based, and you will refer to a patient's medical record or medication profile in order to answer the question. The exam lasts 6 hours, which averages about 1.6 minutes per question. Some questions will take more or less time, but the time period is sufficient for you to answer all questions. Preparation and practice will allow you to answer the easier questions in less time so you may devote more time to the more challenging ones.

There are several question formats on the NAPLEX. *You cannot skip a question or return to it later.*

1. Multiple-choice question with a single answer out of 4 to 5 possible responses, for example:

   Which of the following is the agent of choice for the initial treatment of contact dermatitis, whether irritant or allergic?
   A. Topical antihistamine
   B. Oral antihistamine
   C. Topical corticosteroid
   D. Local anesthetic
   E. Coal tar product

2. Multiple-response question, which is followed by the phrase "Select all that apply," for which there is no partial credit, for example:

   Isotretinoin adverse effects may include which of the following? (Select all that apply.)
   A. Cheilitis
   B. Hypertriglyceridemia
   C. Photosensitivity
   D. Muscle and joint pain
   E. Cardiac arrhythmias

3. Constructed-response question, where a value is typically entered, for example:

   How much dextrose is required to prepare 500 mL of an aqueous 10% solution? (Answer must be numeric: Round the final answer to the nearest WHOLE number.)

4. Ordered-response question, where the choices are ranked by dragging an option to the appropriate rank position, for example:

   Rank the following β-blockers from shortest to longest half-life. (ALL options must be used.)

Unordered options	Ordered response
Betaxolol	
Carteolol	
Bisoprolol	
Acebutolol	

5. Hot-spot question, where the response is marked on a location of a diagram using the cursor to mark the spot following the directions for doing so, for example:

Using the diagram below, identify the site of action of **furosemide** in the nephron.

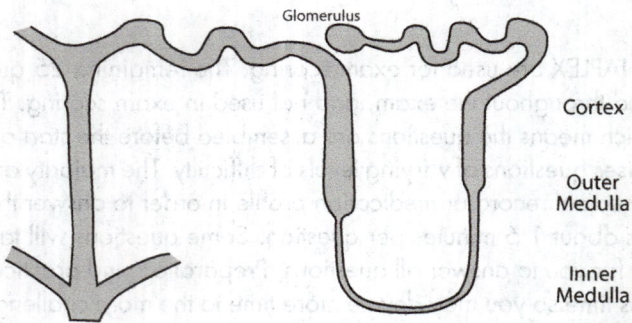

6. Scenario-based questions are typically associated with a patient profile or medical record. The scenario will be in a separate window on the same screen. The questions refer to the scenario or are stand-alone questions related to the scenario. Because the entire scenario may not be fully displayed in the window, you may be prompted to navigate within the profile or medical record to review the complete scenario. Use the erasable note board and pen provided at the testing site to write down significant points from the scenario, such as allergies, age, medical history and co-morbidities, pregnancy, breast-feeding. Review the scenario first to look for the potential of a drug allergy, duplicate therapy, contraindication, or adverse drug effect. Medications may appear with trade or generic names.

The Play Book

The NAPLEX tests for two general domains of competency, referred to as *The NAPLEX Competency Statements*, which is included in the *NAPLEX/MPJE Candidate Application Bulletin* (https://nabp.pharmacy/programs/examinations/naplex/). The 2021 *Candidate Application Bulletin* describes the competency domains as follows:

- **AREA 1:** Obtain, interpret, or assess data, medical, or patient information (approximately 18% of test)
- **AREA 2:** Identify drug characteristics (approximately 14% of test)
- **AREA 3:** Develop or manage treatment plans (approximately 35% of test)
- **AREA 4:** Perform calculations (approximately 14% of test)
- **AREA 5:** Compound, dispense, or administer drugs, or manage delivery systems (approximately 11% of test)
- **AREA 6:** Develop or manage practice or medication-use systems to ensure safety and quality (approximately 7% of test)

Priorities for Review

The following suggested strategies provide some guidance on priorities for review. Several areas are not high priorities for review because they are not emphasized in the current NAPLEX, such as the manufacturer of a drug product, chemical structures, and identification or physical descriptions (e.g., color, shape) of the drug product. The emphasis is greater on patient-oriented competencies.

Generic and trade names: Although generic products are widely used, there are many drugs with trade names in practice and in the NAPLEX. Generic or trade names can appear in the scenarios, questions, and response options for the different question formats. Reviewing the generic and trade names for commonly used or unique medications is critical. If you are not familiar with these names, you may be unable to comprehend the question or responses.

Calculations: Pharmacy math is another critical area to review. Key information includes conversion factors among the systems of measurement; calculations for compounding typical dosage forms such as topical, solution, and intravenous preparations; and basic elements of statistics. Be careful to take notice of the units of measure and decimal points in any math problem and calculations. By making this area a high priority for study, the questions can be answered confidently and efficiently, conserving time for more complicated questions.

Dosage schedules: The frequency of use has greater emphasis in the competencies than specific dosages. Be able to recognize that a medication is administered in a divided schedule during the day, once a day, or at greater intervals such as monthly or yearly.

Classes of drugs: Focus on a review of medications within a class of drugs, such as β-adrenergic blockers, calcium channel blockers, angiotensin-converting enzyme inhibitors and angiotensin II receptor blockers, benzodiazepines, antibiotics, nonsteroidal anti-inflammatory drugs, histamine-2 blockers, protease inhibitors, diabetes medications, and statins. Be able to recognize drugs within these categories, the general indications, contraindications, adverse effects, and drug interactions for the class, as well as the different characteristics of a drug within the category, such as duration of action, dosage schedules, unique adverse effects, and preference for certain diseases.

Patient counseling and warning labels: In the review of drug classes, recognize specific points for patient counseling, particularly about possible untoward effects, duration of therapy, and special handling, in addition to the general counseling advice. Also consider if warning labels may be necessary, such as refrigerate, avoid hazardous activities, or shake well. Be sure to know a medication's FDA-required boxed warnings and/or Risk Evaluation and Mitigation Strategy (REMS) as well as safety in pregnancy and lactation.

Chronic and common diseases: Focus on the more common and chronic diseases and their management. A general knowledge of the disease process is important, but avoid focusing the majority of study time on detailed disease characteristics, such as etiology, pathophysiology, diagnosis, staging, and signs and symptoms at the expense of drug and nondrug therapy. To evaluate a patient scenario, having knowledge of basic laboratory tests and their normal values is important. Although the NAPLEX leans strongly toward drug therapy as indicated by the competencies, be aware of the effects of healthy lifestyle habits on disease prevention and management.

General guidance on content: The NAPLEX is heavily weighted toward drug therapy as indicated by the competencies. As a general guide, you should be familiar with the following information regarding drug therapy and should focus your study time on areas of weakness or unfamiliarity:

- What is the therapeutic category or categories of this drug?
- What is the basic mechanism of action?
- What type of patient counseling information should be provided?
- What are the major adverse effects (side effects and toxic effects)?
- What is the dosage schedule (frequency)?
- What are the major drug interactions, contraindications, precautions, and warnings?

Exam-Taking Advice

The following list contains suggestions for test taking that should be second nature after years of college and professional education:

1. Read directions carefully, and read questions at least twice to be sure of the nature of the question. Note any modifying terms such as *always, all, never, most,* or *usually;* any double negatives; and anything else about the way the question is worded that may change the meaning of the question and your response.

2. Review the case scenario first (briefly, but fully), and then refer back to the scenario for specific facts for each question associated with the scenario.

3. Read all the answer options thoroughly and eliminate the obvious distractors or incorrect answers. Typically, two to three options can be eliminated for one or more reasons, and the final choice is between two answers. Select the *single best answer* for the multiple-choice format. Be cautious about reading multiple possibilities into questions, because most questions should be straightforward. If you simply do not know the answer, eliminate any distractors and guess intelligently from the remaining options.

4. Pace yourself, but do not rush through the exam. The 6 hours scheduled for the NAPLEX should be more than adequate to complete the exam. Proceed at a reasonable pace, and answer approximately 35 to 40 questions per hour to finish comfortably in the time available. A timer is displayed on the computer screen for your information. If only 25 to 30 questions are completed in the first hour, you should increase your speed.

5. If you feel that you have made a mistake on a previous question, don't dwell on it, and move on to the next question. As it relates to the musician metaphor, all musicians make mistakes in a performance, but they don't stop. They continue to the end of the song. A performance is not judged by a few errors; the same can be said for your performance on the NAPLEX. Because the NAPLEX contains 25 unscored questions being tested for suitability on a future exam and 200 scored questions, there is no way to determine if you made a mistake on a scored or unscored question.

The Venue

Testing center location: If you are not familiar with or have never been to the exact location of the testing center, locate it (better to actually visit it) at least the day before the exam. You are advised by NABP to arrive at the testing site at least 30 minutes before the scheduled time so you can comfortably register and get settled. You do not want to be caught in traffic or get lost on the way to the testing center and panic before taking the exam.

Hours before the exam: Avoid studying the day and evening before the exam—last-minute cramming may cause anxiety and affect your performance. On the evening before the exam, do something relaxing. Like an athlete, keep to your regular sleeping schedule and eating habits. On the day of the exam, eat a healthy breakfast. If your exam is scheduled in the afternoon, be on guard against fatigue by having a light lunch and adequate, but not excessive, hydration. (Hint: If you find that you are becoming tired during the exam, take some long, deep breaths. Check your posture to assure that you are sitting up straight—you may become more alert as your lungs can more effectively ventilate and oxygenate when you are not slouching.) Then go to the testing center like a prepared athlete or musician, and perform at your best.

1-6   Practice

As any athlete or musician will tell you, "practice, practice, practice leads to good performance." The same is true for the NAPLEX. Early observance of general practices, such as devote your best time, start early, create a routine, avoid distractions, keep a steady pace of studying, and self-assess your weaknesses and strengths in the competencies tested, will serve you well.

Weekly Review

In *The APhA Complete Review for Pharmacy*, review the tables of the major categories of drugs. Look for the generic and trade names, commonly available dosage forms, and frequency of use. Develop a method to review generic and trade names. If you work in a pharmacy or are on a pharmacy rotation, ask the pharmacist or pharmacy technician to quiz you on the generic or trade name of medications in a section of the pharmacy stock of medications. Perhaps even reverse the roles and be the quizzer. Look at the container before and after the quiz. On a computer, smartphone, or tablet, perform a Web or app search with an expression like *generic and brand name drug quiz* to find a program that allows you to quiz yourself during a spare moment throughout the day and week. Be sure you are using a U.S. site that is relatively current, because trade names may change (often for drug safety reasons) and can be different in another country.

Pre-NAPLEX and Tutorial

The NABP offers a tremendous opportunity to take a practice exam that uses past questions to simulate the NAPLEX testing experience (https://nabp.pharmacy/programs/naplex/pre-naplex/). The small fee is very worthwhile to take the 100-question, 140-minute practice exam to become familiar with navigating in the computerized format, experience the type of questions, and assess your stamina to be able to sit in front of a computer for 2 hours for test taking. The content is not in the current version of the NAPLEX, so the score is not particularly relevant to success in the NAPLEX. The Pre-NAPLEX can be taken on any computer with an Internet connection. You may take the exam twice. Take the practice exam early in your preparation for the NAPLEX, and consider taking it again a month before the NAPLEX exam date.

On the day of the exam after check-in at the testing site, a tutorial is available on how to respond to the types of questions in the NAPLEX. Take the tutorial so you are familiar with the mechanics of the computerized exam on the computer you will be using for the NAPLEX.

Self-assessment

As you review each chapter of *The APhA Complete Review for Pharmacy*, perform a self-assessment of your knowledge by responding to the questions at the end of each chapter. These questions can be supplemented by additional questions found in the NAPLEX review section of the APhA PharmacyLibrary (https://pharmacylibrary.com/self-assessments). To make your learning experience more effective, study the explanations for the correct responses. Also note the distractors, and learn why they are incorrect.

1-7   Conclusion

The NAPLEX is comprehensive in scope and is not an easy exam. By adopting and maintaining a positive attitude, steady preparation, and adequate practice, taking the exam will be less stressful and the likelihood of your success on first attempt will be improved. Consider some principles about how your brain works from John Medina's book, *Brain Rules*:

Rule #1: Exercise boosts brain power.
Rule #3: Every brain is wired differently.
Rule #5: Repeat to remember (short-term memory).
Rule #6: Remember to repeat (long-term memory).
Rule #7: Sleep well, think well.
Rule #8: Stressed brains don't learn the same way.
Rule #9: Stimulate more of the senses at the same time (sensory integration).

Review all 12 of the principles on the *Brain Rules* website (http://brainrules.net/about-brain-rules).

In conclusion, the contributors to *The APhA Complete Review for Pharmacy* hope that this publication will assist you in your preparation for and your successful completion of the licensure exams to practice as a pharmacist. By imagining yourself as an elite athlete or an accomplished musician preparing for a competition or a performance, you will become an accomplished professional—a pharmacist ready to perform at the highest level of practice.

1-8   Additional Resources

Barker E. Most productive people: 6 things they do every day. Barking Up the Wrong Tree (blog), June 1, 2014. Available at: http://www.bakadesuyo.com/2014/06/most-productive-people. Accessed February 12, 2021.

Medina J. *Brain Rules: 12 Principles for Surviving and Thriving at Work, Home, and School.* Seattle, WA: Pear Press; 2014.

National Association of Boards of Pharmacy. *NAPLEX/MPJE 2021 Candidate Application Bulletin.* Mount Prospect, IL: National Association of Boards of Pharmacy; 2020. Available at: https://nabp.pharmacy/wp-content/uploads/2019/03/NAPLEX-MPJE-Bulletin-2021.pdf. Accessed February 12, 2021.

Fundamentals of Pharmacy Practice

2

GLEN E. FARR   CHELSEA P. RENFRO

 ## 2-1 KEY POINTS

- The Pharmacists' Patient Care Process is applicable to any practice setting where pharmacists provide patient care. It includes collecting, assessing, planning, implementing, and following up (monitoring and evaluating) the delivery of patient care.
- Characteristics of tertiary, secondary, and primary literature resources differ and are sources of evidence-based drug information.
- Accurate, up-to-date, and unbiased drug information from various sources, particularly the Internet, should be determined by assessment of the reliability of the source before its use.
- The U.S. Food and Drug Administration (FDA) has programs on medication safety, which include a system to manage medication risk through Risk Evaluation and Mitigation Strategies (REMS) and the issuance of boxed warnings in drug package inserts.
- Three price measures are typically used for the payment system for prescription drugs in the retail pharmacy market: average manufacturer price, average wholesale price, and wholesale acquisition cost.
- The Institute for Safe Medication Practices has resources and notices to help health care practitioners prevent errors and ensure that medications are used safely.
- Adverse drug effects and medication errors should be reported to the FDA MedWatch website; after clinical review, these adverse drug effects and medication errors become part of the FDA Adverse Event Reporting System.
- All medications that are out-of-date or no longer needed should be safely disposed of as described by the Drug Enforcement Administration.
- Because three of four patients do not adhere to medication instructions, pharmacists should counsel patients on ways to remember to take a prescribed medication and to fill a prescription. In addition, pharmacists should counsel patients to avoid both taking more or less than the recommended dosage and substituting an over-the-counter medication or dietary supplement for the prescribed medication.
- Pharmacists function as managers of the pharmacy team members, general operations, and the medication use system. In this managerial role, having communication and problem-solving skills will allow pharmacists to maximize productivity and foster a positive workplace.

Patient safety and medication management are key components of pharmacists' providing quality patient care. Therefore, pharmacists' participation in quality and performance improvement is vital to the overall success of the health care system.

 ## 2-2 STUDY GUIDE CHECKLIST

The following topics may guide your study of this subject area:

- [ ] Familiarity with the delivery of patient care as described in the *Pharmacists' Patient Care Process*.
- [ ] The characteristics of literature sources for drug information and the hierarchy of evidence.
- [ ] Factors to consider when responding to drug information requests from health care providers or patients.
- [ ] Awareness of "sound alike, look alike" drugs and confusing abbreviations.
- [ ] Medications that have REMS or boxed warnings.
- [ ] The way to report an adverse drug effect or a medication error to the FDA's MedWatch.
- [ ] Procedure for the disposal of out-of-date or unused drugs versus controlled substances.
- [ ] Factors leading to medication nonadherence and counseling points to minimize its negative consequences.
- [ ] General drug supply chain and the flow of drug costs.
- [ ] Principles of management and quality improvement in pharmacy practice.
- [ ] Successful strategies for effective communication with patients, health care professionals, coworkers, and supervisors.

2-3   Pharmacists' Patient Care Process

Pharmacy practice encompasses a plethora of different knowledge, skills, and attitudes. There are numerous fundamentals necessary for good pharmacy practice. Many of these principles will be addressed in subsequent chapters of this text. However, some of the more general fundamentals are discussed in this chapter.

Recognizing the need for a consistent process in the delivery of patient care across the profession, in 2014 the Joint Commission of Pharmacy Practitioners released the Pharmacists' Patient Care Process. The process is applicable to any practice setting where pharmacists provide patient care and any patient care service provided by pharmacists. Using principles of evidence-based practice, pharmacists practicing patient-centered care should perform the following processes: collect, assess, plan, implement, and follow up (monitor and evaluate). To optimize pharmacist-provided patient care, pharmacists should incorporate these 5 fundamental elements into practice (Figure 2-1). Throughout the process, pharmacists should continuously collaborate and communicate with other health care providers as well as properly document any patient care services provided.

Collect necessary subjective and objective information about patients to understand their relevant medical and medication history and clinical status. Pharmacists can use multiple sources, including existing patient records (i.e., prescription fill history, electronic health records), the patient, and other health care providers. This process includes collecting the following:

- A current medication list and medication use history for prescription and nonprescription (over-the-counter [OTC]) medications, herbals, and other dietary supplements
- Relevant health data, which may include medical history, health and wellness information, biometric test results, and physical assessment findings
- Patient lifestyle habits, preferences and beliefs, overall health goals, and socioeconomic factors that affect access to medications and care

FIGURE 2-1. Model of the Pharmacists' Patient Care Process

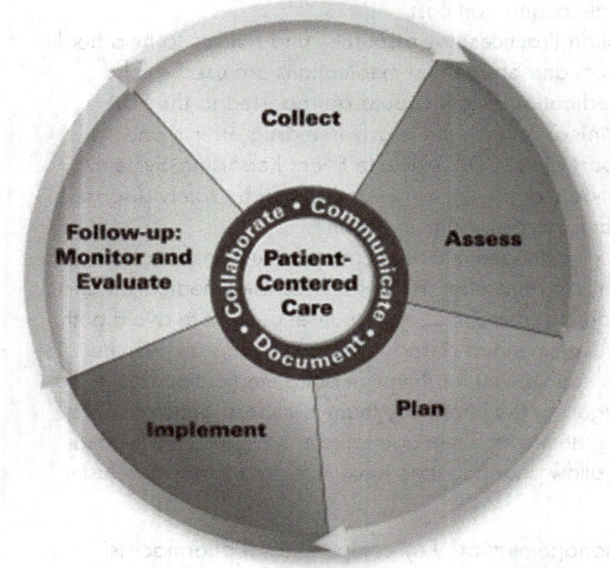

Joint Commission of Pharmacy Practitioners, 2014.

Assess the information collected and analyze the clinical effects of the patient's therapy in the context of their overall health goals. This information should be used to identify and prioritize medication therapy problems to achieve optimal care for the patient. This process includes assessing all medications for appropriateness, effectiveness, safety, and adherence. Identified medication therapy problems can be related, but not limited, to: drug interactions, allergic reactions, duplication of therapy, or need for additional therapy. When appropriate, a pharmacist should assess the need for immunizations, preventive care, and other health care services.

In collaboration with other health care professionals and the patient or caregiver, the pharmacy should develop an individualized care **plan** that is evidence-based, patient-centered, and cost-effective. It should address medication therapy problems and optimize medication use. The plan should engage the patient or caregiver and set goals of therapy for achieving clinical outcomes in the context of the patient's overall health goals and access to care. As appropriate, the plan should support care continuity, including follow-up and transitions of care.

Implement the care plan in collaboration with other health care providers and the patient or caregiver. This process should address health-related and medication therapy problems and engage in preventive care strategies, including vaccine administration. Implementation includes initiation, modification, discontinuation, or administration of medication therapy as authorized. When necessary, the pharmacist should refer the patient to another health care professional to provide appropriate care.

Follow up (monitor and evaluate) on the effectiveness of the care plan and modify, as needed, the plan in collaboration with other health care providers and the patient or caregiver. This critical process includes the continuous monitoring and evaluation of clinical endpoints that contribute to the patient's overall health and outcomes. Medication appropriateness, effectiveness, safety, and adherence should continuously be monitored and evaluated to track progress toward or the achievement of therapeutic goals.

2-4 Fundamentals of Drug Information

Drug information is printed, electronic, or verbal information pertaining to prescription and nonprescription medications and dietary supplements. The term *medication information* is also used and pertains to the use of information to influence medication therapy outcomes. Providing drug information to health care providers and the patient is at the core of all types of pharmacy practice. Drug information can be a simple verbal response to a patient's question, or it can be an involved, researched monograph presented to a hospital's pharmacy and therapeutics committee to aid in the decision of whether or not a drug is added to the formulary.

Biomedical and pharmaceutical literature is generally categorized as primary, secondary, and tertiary sources. Primary sources are original research publications and are usually published in peer-reviewed journals such as *American Journal of Health-System Pharmacy, Annals of Pharmacotherapy, Journal of the American Medical Association, Journal of the American Pharmacists Association, New England Journal of Medicine,* and *Pharmacotherapy.* Secondary literature consists of interpretations and reviews of primary sources and abstracting/indexing services. Examples include review articles; meta-analyses; and systematic reviews, practice guidelines, and indexing programs such as PubMed, Scopus, Embase, CINAHL, Cochrane Library, and Web of Science. Tertiary literature distills a collection of primary and secondary sources to create textbooks, encyclopedic articles, guidebooks, handbooks, and electronic information databases (e.g., UpToDate, Micromedex, *AHFS Drug Information* online). The resources provide an overview of key research findings, practice guidelines, and an introduction to the principles and practices for a discipline or topic.

Biomedical literature is further classified by clinical levels of evidence that are based on the quality of the design, validity, and applicability to patient care and provide a grade (or strength) of recommendation (Table 2-1).

TABLE 2-1. Example of Clinical Levels of Evidence Hierarchy

Level	Description
I	Evidence obtained from a systematic review or meta-analysis of all relevant randomized controlled trials (RCTs) or evidence-based clinical practice guidelines based on systematic reviews of RCTs or three or more RCTs of good quality that have similar results
II	Evidence obtained from at least one well-designed RCT (e.g., large multisite RCT)
III	Evidence obtained from well-designed controlled trials without randomization
IV	Evidence obtained from well-designed case-control or cohort studies
V	Evidence obtained from systematic reviews of descriptive and qualitative studies (meta-synthesis)
VI	Evidence obtained from a single descriptive or qualitative study
VII	Evidence obtained from the opinion of authorities or from the reports of expert committees

For some topics, few high-level studies are available for a clinical question. The level of evidence descends in the following order:

- **Meta-analysis:** A systematic review that uses quantitative methods to summarize the results
- **Systematic review:** A systematic search, appraisal, and summary of all of the literature for a specific topic
- **Randomized controlled trials (RCTs):** A study of a randomized group of specified patients in an experimental group and a control group with specific variables and outcomes of interest
- **Cohort study:** Identification of two groups (cohorts) of patients, one that received a treatment and one that did not, and studies of these cohorts going forward for the outcome
- **Case-control study:** Identification of patients who have the outcome of interest (cases) and control patients without the same outcome and studies of the outcome of an exposure or treatment of interest
- **Background information and expert opinion:** Handbooks, textbooks, electronic information databases, and editorials and commentaries that provide a foundation and a summary of generalized information about a treatment and condition
- **Animal research and laboratory studies:** Research studies that are at the bottom of clinical evidence but generate critical scientific ideas and foundational knowledge, which ultimately may lead to therapies, diagnostic tools, and an understanding of disease pathogenesis and treatment mechanisms of action

Major compendia contain drug monographs and are commonly used by pharmacists in a variety of practice settings. Many major compendia of drug information, such as *AHFS Drug Information* (https://www.ahfsdruginformation.com), Micromedex (https://micromedexsolutions.com), Lexicomp (https://www.wolterskluwer.com/en/solutions/lexicomp), UpToDate (https://www.uptodate.com/home), and *Drug Facts and Comparisons* (https://fco.factsandcomparisons.com), provide many different aspects of drug information, including information on pediatrics and neonates, intravenous incompatibilities, toxicology, and patient education materials. Some compendia include documented off-label (non–U.S. Food and Drug Administration [FDA] approved) indications. The *Prescribers' Digital Reference* (PDR), however, contains only FDA-approved medication uses (https://pdr.net). As of 2017, PDR is no longer printed and all drug information is now available using "mobilePDR." However, most health care providers still use the hardcover editions.

The FDA's *Orange Book: Approved Drug Products with Therapeutic Equivalence Evaluations* (or *Orange Book*) can be accessed on the FDA website (https://www.fda.gov). (*Note:* https://www.fda.com is not the official FDA website.) This reference provides bioequivalence data on chemical entities. The FDA's *Purple Book: Database of Licensed Biological Products* contains biological products, including any biosimilar and interchangeable biological products, licensed by the FDA (https://purplebooksearch.fda.gov). "Biosimilars" is defined by the FDA as biologic agents developed to be "highly similar" to approved drugs with expired patent protection. The term is used to describe officially approved subsequent versions of innovator biopharmaceutical or biological products made by a different sponsor following patent and exclusivity expiry on the innovator product.

The IBM Micromedex's *Red Book* contains information regarding availability and pricing for prescription and OTC medications, as well as information regarding dosage form, size, strength, and routes of administration. This reference also includes the product's National Drug Code numbers and average wholesale price (AWP). Lists of sugar-free, lactose-free, and alcohol-free preparations also can be found in the *Red Book* (https://ibm.com/products/micromedex-red-book).

Information from government agencies can be identified through the websites of the FDA, the Drug Enforcement Administration (DEA) (https://www.dea.gov), and the Centers for Disease Control and Prevention (CDC) (https://www.cdc.gov). These websites also include clinical information and information about new drug approvals, drugs of abuse, and FDA-required information on the drug product label. A product package insert can be obtained from the website of the pharmaceutical company or the official provider of FDA label information (https://dailymed.nlm.nih.gov/).

The National Institutes of Health (NIH) operates PubMed (https://www.ncbi.nlm.nih.gov/pubmed), which comprises more than 26 million citations for biomedical literature from MEDLINE, life science journals, and online books. Citations may include links to full-text content from PubMed Central and publisher websites.

The website of the American Pharmacists Association (https://www.pharmacist.com) provides drug news updates and drug information, and the website of the American Society of Health-System Pharmacists (https://www.ashp.org) provides timely information on drug shortages and other drug information. The FDA has a mobile device app to speed public access to information about drug shortages, such as current drug shortages, resolved shortages, and discontinuations of drug products.

Several proprietary sources provide general reviews and reports that are searchable and provide an excellent resource for many questions pharmacists receive from patients and practitioners. For example, *Pharmacist's Letter* (https://pharmacist.therapeuticresearch.com/Home/PL/) and *Prescriber's Letter* (https://prescriber.therapeuticresearch.com/Home/PRL/) offer print and online access to practical information, including patient information materials for subscribers. *Natural Medicines* (https://naturalmedicines. therapeuticresearch.com) provides well-researched and useful information on dietary supplements.

Medscape (https://www.medscape.com) is a general drug information database that may be freely accessed through the Internet and mobile devices. The drug information contained in this reference is considered broad in scope and depth and relies on authoritative sources of drug information.

Clinical decision support systems (CDSSs) are used to support decision making in a variety of clinical settings. These systems are computer-based programs designed to provide information support for health professionals making clinical decisions typically at the point of care and to provide drug information and are integrated in pharmacy computer systems. These systems have emerged as an important part of any clinical information system, particularly for computerized prescriber order entry (CPOE) systems that allow the direct entry of orders and instructions for the treatment of patients. The orders are communicated through a computer network to the appropriate hospital department responsible for fulfilling an order, which includes pharmacy, radiology, or laboratory. Used properly, CPOE decreases delays in order completion, reduces errors related to handwriting or transcriptions, allows order entry at the point of care or off site, provides error checking for duplicate or incorrect doses or tests, and simplifies inventory and posting of charges. Similar CDSSs are used in many community pharmacy computer programs to support monitoring for appropriate doses, drug interactions, and safety warnings.

Wikipedia (https://www.wikipedia.org) is a free Internet resource that is edited by its worldwide users. It may be a useful source for providing information supplementary to other more reliable sources, but its recognized shortcomings include errors in information, lack of referenced documentation, and omissions of information. Pharmacists should be cautious of user-edited sites and blogs as definitive sources of drug information and advise patients of the shortcomings of information contained in Wikipedia.

2-5   Pharmaceutical Supply Chain and Costs

As pharmaceuticals move from manufacturers to consumers, a complex set of market transactions involving prices, discounts, and rebates occurs along the supply chain (Figure 2-2). Although the drugs themselves move in a relatively straightforward path from manufacturers to wholesalers to retail pharmacies or nonretail providers (such as hospitals and clinics) to final consumers, the flow of costs and payments is more complicated.

In 2007, the Congressional Budget Office examined the process by which payments are determined and provided estimates of the relative prices that retail pharmacies and nonretail providers pay for prescription drugs. Several factors determine the price that consumers and health plans ultimately pay for prescription drugs, and interactions often become complicated and confusing (Figure 2-3).

The price that a purchaser pays depends on both the degree of competition in a marketplace and the purchaser's bargaining power. In the pharmaceutical marketplace, competition depends on whether a brand-name drug has patent protection or whether brand-name and generic versions of the drug are available. In addition, even brand-name drugs under patent protection can face competition from other brand-name drugs that are considered to be therapeutic substitutes. A purchaser's bargaining power depends on both the volume purchased and the purchaser's ability to choose which drug to purchase from a set of competing drugs.

A chain pharmacy or a community pharmacy that is a member of a buying group usually dispenses prescriptions as written by the prescriber for brand-name drugs under patent protection. Although a chain pharmacy or a buying group may buy a large volume of brand-name drugs under patent protection, it generally cannot significantly negotiate prices as effectively as a health plan that can choose to cover only one or two brand-name drugs from a set of drugs considered to be therapeutic substitutes. A health plan can negotiate lower prices from manufacturers in the form of rebates by buying large volumes of

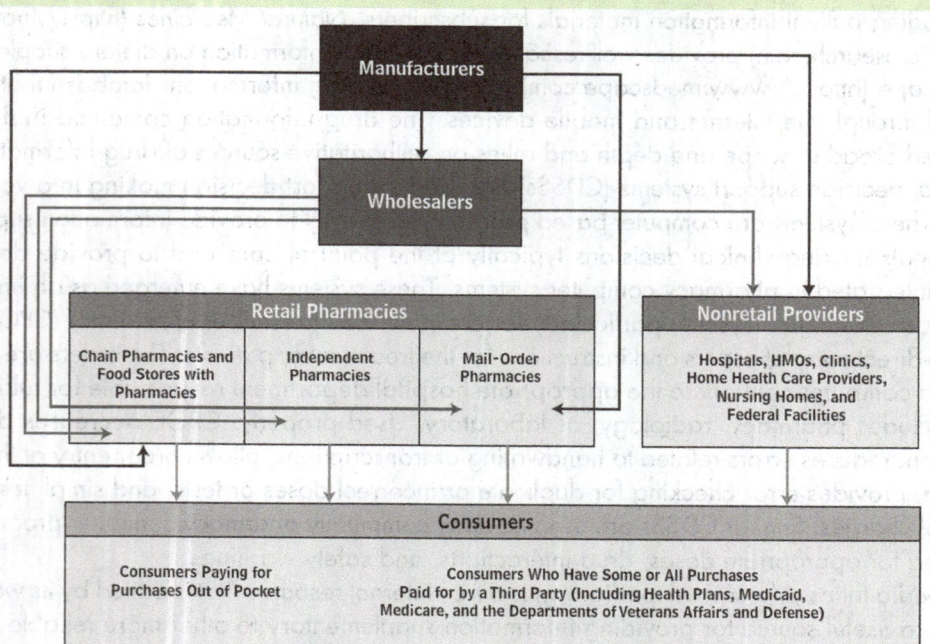

FIGURE 2-2. Example of the Drug Supply Chain from Manufacturer to Consumer

Congressional Budget Office, 2007.
HMO, health maintenance organization.

FIGURE 2-3. **Example of the Flow of Funds for Brand-Name Drugs Purchased at a Retail Pharmacy and Managed by a Pharmacy Benefit Manager**

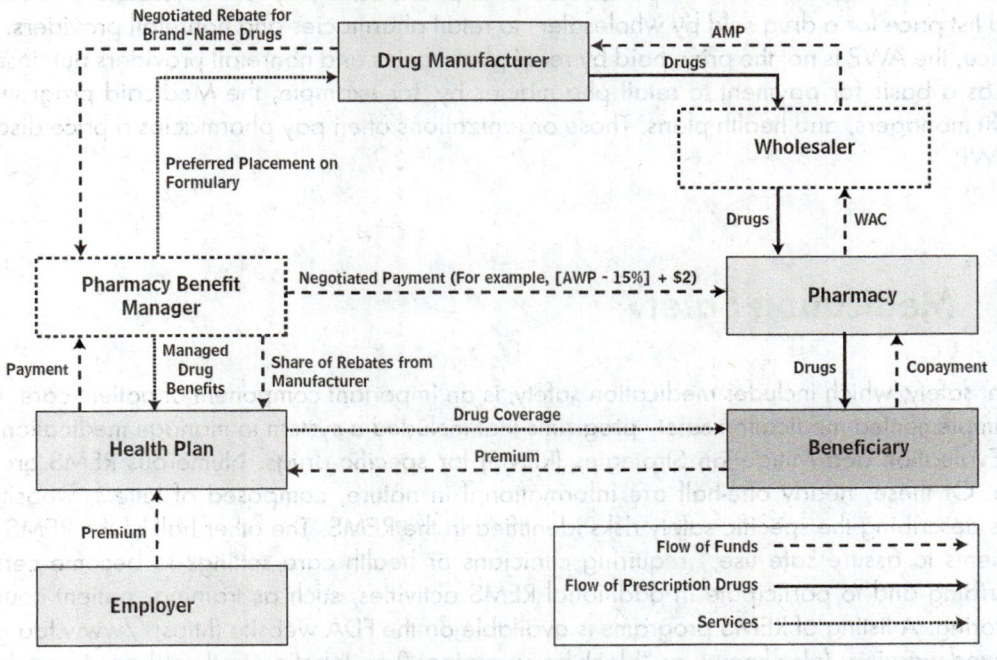

Congressional Budget Office, 2007.
AMP, average manufacturer price; AWP, average wholesale price; WAC, wholesale acquisition cost.

the brand-name drugs of the plan's choice. For generic drugs, the chain pharmacy or buying group has greater negotiating leverage compared to a health plan. Chain pharmacies and buying groups can choose which of several generic drugs to stock, and by purchasing large volumes of those drugs, they can negotiate lower prices from manufacturers. In contrast, a health plan does not choose which generic drugs to dispense. Instead, the health plan's beneficiaries go to their pharmacies to fill prescriptions, and the pharmacies dispense the generic drugs that they have chosen to stock. Manufacturers have no incentive to negotiate price terms with a health plan for generic drugs even if the health plan buys a large volume.

Three price measures are important in understanding the payment system for prescription drugs in the retail pharmacy market:

1. Average manufacturer price (AMP)
2. Average wholesale price (AWP)
3. Wholesale acquisition cost (WAC)

The AMP is an average of actual transaction prices. In contrast, the AWP and WAC are list prices, like a "sticker price" in the automobile industry. The AMP is the average price paid by wholesalers to manufacturers or by retail pharmacies that buy directly from manufacturers for drugs distributed through those pharmacies. It reflects all rebates paid by manufacturers to wholesalers and retail pharmacies. It does not include rebates paid by manufacturers to pharmacy benefit managers, Medicaid, or other third-party payers. Manufacturers are required to report the AMP to the Department of Health and Human Services Centers for Medicare and Medicaid Services, which uses it to calculate the rebates that manufacturers are required to pay state Medicaid programs for sales to Medicaid beneficiaries. For manufacturers, such rebates are a cost of participating in the Medicaid market.

The WAC represents manufacturers' published catalog, or list, price for sales of a drug (brand name or generic) to wholesalers. However, in practice, the WAC is not the price paid by wholesalers. To the extent that the WAC is meaningful in conveying information about actual transaction costs, the utility is limited to single-source drugs (that is, brand-name drugs still under patent protection). For those drugs, the WAC often approximates the prices that retail pharmacies pay to wholesalers. The AWP is a published list price for a drug sold by wholesalers to retail pharmacies and nonretail providers. However, in practice, the AWP is not the price paid by retail pharmacies and nonretail providers but, instead, is often used as a basis for payment to retail pharmacies by, for example, the Medicaid program, pharmacy benefit managers, and health plans. Those organizations often pay pharmacies a price discounted from the AWP.

2-6 Medication Safety

Patient safety, which includes medication safety, is an important component of patient care. In 2010, the FDA implemented medication safety programs that included a system to manage medication risk through Risk Evaluation and Mitigation Strategies (REMS) for specific drugs. Numerous REMS are currently in place. Of these, nearly one-half are informational in nature, composed of letters, websites, and fact sheets describing the specific safety risks identified in the REMS. The other half of the REMS also include "elements to assure safe use," requiring clinicians or health care settings to become certified before prescribing and to participate in additional REMS activities, such as training, patient counseling, and monitoring. A listing of REMS programs is available on the FDA website (https://www.fda.gov).

Boxed warnings (also known as "black box warnings") on labeling and package inserts are designed to call attention to serious or life-threatening risks. These warnings and other safety issues are discussed with individual drugs throughout this text. These safety warnings are available on the FDA website (https://www.fda.gov/drugs/drug-safety-and-availability). Package inserts also contain these warnings and approved indications.

A nonprofit organization that focuses on medication safety is the Institute for Safe Medication Practices (ISMP) (https://www.ismp.org). The ISMP offers a wide range of resources and information to help health care providers in a variety of health care settings prevent errors and ensure that medications are used safely. Some of the tools, all of which are free and downloadable, include the following:

- "Do Not Crush" list
- FDA boxed warnings
- Information for consumers on medication misuse
- Error-prone abbreviations list
- FDA patient safety news, videos, and alerts
- High-alert medications consumer leaflets
- Reports on medication errors and the root cause analysis workbook
- SALAD (sound-alike, look-alike drugs) listing, including "Tall Man" lettering

There are more than 10,000 generic drug names and 40,000 trademarked brand names in use in the United States—but still only 26 letters in the alphabet! Examples of SALAD drugs leading to injury cited by the FDA:

- An 8-year-old child died after receiving methadone instead of **methylphenidate**.
- A 19-year-old man showed signs of potentially fatal complications after he was given clozapine instead of olanzapine.
- A 50-year-old woman was hospitalized after taking Flomax, instead of Volmax.

Some drug products are branded with a sales-leading product's name but contain different active ingredients. For example, Dulcolax enteric-coated tablets and suppositories contain bisacodyl, a stimulant laxative. Other Dulcolax products include Dulcolax Stool Softener (docusate sodium), Dulcolax Milk of

Magnesia (magnesium hydroxide), and Dulcolax Balance (polyethylene glycol 3350). Product names that previously contained unique active ingredients include Pepto Bismol, Maalox Total Stomach Relief, and Kaopectate; these products now all have bismuth subsalicylate as the active ingredient.

2-7 Adverse Drug Effect and Medication Errors Reporting

Patients should report adverse drug effects or medication errors to both the prescriber and the pharmacist. If the reaction or error is serious or unusual in the clinical judgment of the prescriber or the pharmacist, it should be reported to the FDA via the MedWatch website (https://www.fda.gov/safety /medwatch-fda-safety-information-and-adverse-event-reporting-program/reporting-serious-problems-fda).

The FDA Adverse Event Reporting System (FAERS) is a database (https://www.fda.gov/drugs /surveillance/questions-and-answers-fdas-adverse-event-reporting-system-faers) that contains information on adverse events and medication error reports submitted to the FDA. The database is designed to support the FDA's postmarketing safety surveillance program for drug and therapeutic biological products

Reporting of adverse events and medication errors by health care providers and consumers is voluntary in the United States. The FDA receives some adverse event and medication error reports directly from health care providers and consumers (such as patients, family members, and lawyers). However, health care providers and consumers may also report adverse events and medication errors to a product's manufacturer. If a manufacturer receives an adverse event report, it is required to send the report to the FDA. The reports received directly by the FDA and those from manufacturers are entered into FAERS after clinical review and are made available to the public.

The FDA uses FAERS to identify new safety concerns that might be related to a marketed product, evaluate a manufacturer's compliance to reporting regulations, and respond to outside requests for information. The reports in FAERS are evaluated by clinical reviewers in the Center for Drug Evaluation and Research and the Center for Biologics Evaluation and Research to monitor the safety of products after they are approved by the FDA. If a potential safety concern is identified in FAERS, further evaluation is performed. Further evaluation might include conducting studies using other large databases, such as those available in the FDA's Sentinel Initiative (https://www.fda.gov/safety/fdas-sentinel-initiative). Based on an evaluation of the potential safety concern, the FDA may take regulatory action(s) to improve product safety and protect the public health, such as updating a product's labeling and package insert information, restricting the use of the drug, communicating new safety information to the public, or, in rare cases, removing a product from the market.

There are limitations to the interpretation and application of FAERS data. There is no certainty that the reported event (adverse event or medication error) was actually due to the product. The FDA does not require that a causal relationship between a product and an event be proven, and reports do not always contain enough detail to properly evaluate an event. Further, the FDA does not receive reports for every adverse event or medication error that occurs with a product. Many factors can influence whether or not an event will be reported, such as the time a product has been marketed and publicity about an event. Therefore, FAERS data cannot be used to calculate the incidence of an adverse event or medication error in the U.S. population.

2-8 Disposal of Drugs

Drugs that are out-of-date or no longer needed should be disposed of safely. Almost all medications can be safely disposed of by using medication take-back programs or DEA-authorized collectors. DEA-authorized collectors safely and securely collect and dispose of pharmaceutical controlled substances and other prescription drugs. Authorized collection sites may be community pharmacies, hospital or clinic pharmacies, and law enforcement locations. Some pharmacies may also offer mail-back envelopes and drop boxes to facilitate consumers' safely disposing of their unused medications.

If a take-back, mail-back, or drop-box program is not available, most unused or expired medications can be disposed of in household trash. First, mix the medications (do not crush tablets or capsules) with an unpalatable substance such as dirt, cat litter, or used coffee grounds. Then place the mixture in a container such as a sealable plastic bag, and discard the container in household trash. Before discarding an empty bottle or other empty medication packaging, remove all personal information on the prescription label.

Medications that contain controlled substances are especially harmful if taken accidentally by someone other than the patient. Thus, these medications should not be discarded in the trash because this method may still provide an opportunity for a child or pet to accidentally take the medication. If a DEA-authorized collector or drug take-back program is not available, the FDA recommends that these medications be disposed of by flushing them down the toilet. For safety reasons to fish, wildlife, and drinking water, the FDA recommends that only these few, select medications that contain controlled substances be disposed of in wastewater.

2-9   Medication Nonadherence or Misuse

Nearly three of four consumers admit they do not always take their prescribed medications as directed. Forms of nonadherent behavior include forgetting to take a prescribed medication, not filling a prescription, taking less than the recommended dosage, or substituting an OTC medication or dietary supplement. In some studies, almost one-third of all initial drug prescriptions were not filled within 9 months, with nonadherence highest for expensive drugs and chronic preventive therapies.

Medication nonadherence can have negative consequences for the patient, the prescriber, the pharmacist, and health care researchers all seeking to establish the value of the medication for a patient or target population. Medication adherence presents a particularly complex issue for older adults. For these patients, medication issues and abuses may also result in accidents, such as a fall that causes a hip fracture. In addition, older adults could forget that they have already taken the prescribed amount of medication and unwittingly overdose.

Many factors are involved in patient nonadherence, including factors related to the disease, medication side effects, duration of drug therapy, frequency and complexity of treatment, dosage form, and cost. For example, patients are less likely to continue their medication regimen over long periods and are less likely to be adherent when the daily doses increase from 1 tablet to 4 tablets. To help prevent this problem of nonadherence in a multi-dosage regimen, medications to be taken once a day should be prescribed for ingestion in the morning or at bedtime, those prescribed twice a day can be scheduled to be given in the morning and bedtime, and those prescribed 3 times a day can be taken after each meal. Schedules calling for medication to be taken four or more times a day create an unnatural division of the day for most people, increasing the possibility of nonadherence. Studies reported that 40% to 60% of patients could not correctly report their physicians' expectations of them 10 to 80 minutes after they were provided the information. One study reported that more than 60% of the patients interviewed immediately after their medical visit had misunderstood the directions regarding prescribed medications.

Health care providers generally overestimate adherence rates. Asking patients themselves is a more valid procedure, but it has many difficulties. Patients may not be truthful to avoid displeasing their health care providers, or they may simply not know their rate of adherence. Patients not only under-report poor adherence but also over-report good adherence.

Gender, personality, and cultural factors also may influence adherence rates. Women are generally better than men at adhering to their medication regimens, particularly for drugs that treat behavioral health conditions, such as antidepressant medication. Cultural traditions are important factors in determining who is and who is not likely to adhere to medication regimens.

To help improve adherence, patients should be encouraged to indicate to their prescriber and pharmacist verbally or in writing that they understand the choice of medication and its requirements. Patients are more likely to adhere to medication regimens when they are convinced that the medication they are taking is clearly linked to future health and wellness and when they are made an active participant in the decision-making process regarding the medication. Patient interpretation of instructions also varies widely. For example, instructions for a diuretic that is ordered "as needed for water retention" may be interpreted to mean that the drug would be used to cause water retention.

Patient nonadherence to medication has many facets. The seriousness of the illness, the cost of treatment, and treatment side effects can all affect adherence. The patient's age, mental status, and memory capacity are also important factors. The complexity of the recommendation, the duration of the regimen, the type of medical advice, the clarity of the written instructions based on the person's health literacy, and the amount of instruction provided are examples of these factors.

2-10   Basic Principles of Management and Quality Improvement

Whether planned or not, most pharmacists will become managers in title or actions. Management is the art of maximizing productivity by using and developing people's talents, while providing them self-enrichment and opportunities for growth. Classical management descriptions involve the skills of leadership, decision making, and communication.

The most effective managers are those who understand the context in which their organization exists, the organization's culture, and industry- and organization-specific knowledge to get things done. By understanding their environment, managers are able to understand organizational decisions and pharmacy-related changes, anticipate emerging needs, and help employees make sense of new directions.

Effective managers surround themselves with talented people and develop these individuals into high-performing team members who can translate vision into reality. Managing human resources involves establishing goals and performance standards and providing feedback. Employees look to managers to establish clear expectations and outcome measures. Communication is a critical skill to good management as well as overall patient care. Several strategies can be used to successfully communicate with patients (Box 2-1), their caregivers and other interdisciplinary health care providers (Box 2-2).

Another primary role for a manager is problem solving; to optimally solve problems and issues that arise, a manager must be adept at many aspects of problem solving (Box 2-3). Pharmacists are well positioned to assist the health care system by problem solving and implementing quality improvement strategies to improve patient care. One of the most common tools used for quality improvement is the Plan-Do-Study-Act (PDSA) Cycle (Figure 2-4). By incorporating quality improvement tools into daily practice, pharmacists can help improve medication use and patient care.

BOX 2-1. Strategies for Communicating with Patients and Caregivers

- Actively listen and allow the patient to tell his or her story.
- Use paraphrased summaries to indicate your understanding.
- Use questions appropriately. Open-ended questions are useful to begin a topic, while closed-ended questions can help screen for other pertinent positives/negatives.

- Consider your body language.
- Monitor your tone, volume, and rate of speech.
- Avoid using medical jargon.

BOX 2-2. Elements of Interprofessional Communication

- Choose an effective communication tool that enhances team function.
- Avoid discipline-specific terminology when possible.
- Express one's knowledge and opinions with confidence, clarity, and respect.

- Actively listen and encourage opinions and ideas from other team members.
- Give timely, instructive, and sensitive feedback to others about their performance.
- Use respectful language appropriate for a given crucial conversation, difficult situation, or conflict.

BOX 2-3. Strategies for Problem Solving

- Define the problem.
- Analyze the problem.
- Develop possible solutions to the problem.
- Analyze proposed solutions.

- Select the best solution given the environment, resources, and parties involved.
- Plan the next course of action (how a solution will be implemented).
- Involve others in the process.

FIGURE 2-4. Plan-Do-Study-Act Cycle

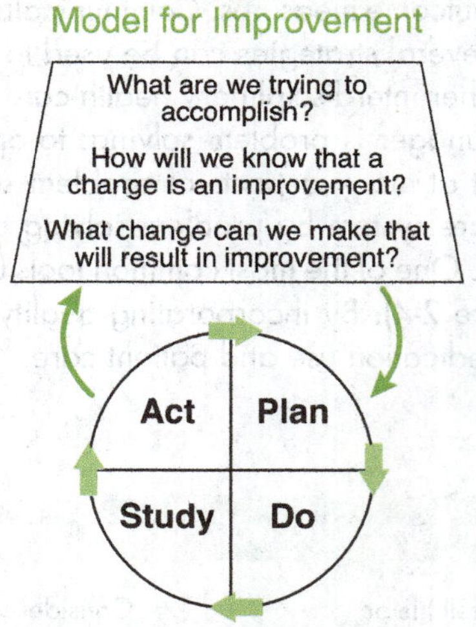

Model for Improvement

What are we trying to accomplish?

How will we know that a change is an improvement?

What change can we make that will result in improvement?

Act | Plan

Study | Do

2-11   Pharmacist's Role

Pharmacists are an integral part of the patient care process. Pharmacists should be collecting, assessing, planning, implementing, and following up (monitoring and evaluating) the delivery of patient care in any patient setting. Part of the patient care process is providing evidence-based drug information from reliable sources and ensuring adherence to medication instructions. Pharmacists are managers with or without a managerial title and should strive to communicate effectively, use sound and effective management principles, and surround themselves with talented, motivated people. Quality improvement tools, such as the PDSA Cycle, can help pharmacists improve medication-use and patient care.

NAPLEX Competency Statements

The questions in this chapter cover the following 2021 NAPLEX Competency Statements: **AREA 1:** 1.2; 1.3; 1.4; 1.7 **AREA 2:** 2.3 **AREA 3:** 3.11 **AREA 5:** 5.6 **AREA 6:** 6.1; 6.4; 6.5.

2-12   Questions

1. Which actions are described in the Pharmacists' Patient Care Process as outlined by the Joint Commission of Pharmacy Practitioners in the delivery of patient care across the profession of pharmacy? (Mark all that apply.)

   A. Assessing
   B. Planning
   C. Implementing
   D. Judging
   E. Following up

2. Which elements apply to the pharmacist's collection of necessary subjective and objective information about patients to understand their relevant medical and medication history and clinical status? (Mark all that apply.)

   A. Current prescription medications and medication use history, including OTC medications, herbals, and other dietary supplements
   B. Medical history, health and wellness information, biometric test results, and physical assessment findings
   C. Marital status and birth order, if they have siblings
   D. Patient lifestyle habits, preferences and beliefs, health and functional goals
   E. Socioeconomic factors that affect access to medications

3. Which of the following references would be the best source to identify drug information regarding whether a medication is lactose free?

   A. *AHFS Drug Information*
   B. FDA *Orange Book*
   C. *Red Book*
   D. *Martindale: The Complete Drug Reference*
   E. FDA *Purple Book*

4. Which of the following drug information resources would provide information on biosimilars?

   A. *AHFS Drug Information*
   B. FDA *Orange Book*
   C. FDA *Purple Book*
   D. CDC website
   E. *Red Book*

5. Which element of medication use does the FDA's REMS program target for reduction?

   A. Cost
   B. Risk
   C. Nonadherence
   D. Error
   E. Storage

6. For which of the following aspects of appropriate medication use does the Institute for Safe Medication Practices provide tools? (Mark all that apply.)

A. Cost of medication
B. Error-prone abbreviations list
C. High-alert medications
D. "Do Not Crush" list
E. FDA boxed warnings

7. Which of the following is true about the FAERS database? (Mark all that apply.)

A. It is a database designed to support the FDA's post-marketing safety surveillance program.
B. Reporting of adverse events and medication errors by pharmacists is required by the FDA.
C. If a manufacturer receives an adverse event report, it is required to send the report to the FDA.
D. Reports in FAERS have been evaluated by clinical reviewers in the FDA's Center for Drug Evaluation and Research and the Center for Biologics Evaluation and Research.
E. Patients are not allowed to report adverse medication events and medication errors to FAERS.

8. What are the proper methods to dispose of medications? (Mark all that apply.)

A. Pharmacies that are approved as DEA-authorized collectors may accept out-of-date drugs or drugs no longer needed by patients.
B. Controlled substances should be flushed down a toilet because they are not acceptable for drug take-back programs.
C. Only licensed pharmacies may be approved as a medication take-back site.
D. If a take-back program is not available, non-controlled medications can be mixed with an unpalatable substance and placed in the trash.
E. Medications can only be disposed of in person as mail-back envelopes and drop boxes are not considered safe.

9. What is the approximate percentage of patients who do not take their prescription medications as directed?

A. 25%
B. 50%
C. 75%
D. 90%
E. 100%

10. Which of the following describes aspects of adherence to medications? (Mark all that apply.)

A. Patients are more likely to adhere to once-a-day or twice-a-day dosing than four-times-a-day dosing.
B. Prescribers generally overestimate adherence rates of their patients.
C. Men are generally better at adhering to their medication regimen than women.
D. Older adults are at a greater risk from nonadherence to medications.
E. Patients are more likely to adhere to a medication when they are active participants in the decision-making process.

11. Which of the following concepts comprise inter-professional communications? (Mark all that apply.)

A. Choose a communication tool that works best for your discipline.
B. Avoid discipline-specific terminology when possible.
C. Actively listen and encourage opinions and ideas from other team members.
D. Use respectful language appropriate for a given crucial conversation or difficult situation.
E. Feedback should only be given to others once a year.

12. Which of the following price measures reflects all rebates paid by manufacturers to wholesalers and retail pharmacies but does not include rebates paid by manufacturers to pharmacy benefit managers, Medicaid, or other third-party payers?

A. Average manufacturer price
B. Wholesale acquisition cost
C. Average wholesale price
D. List price
E. Average acquisition cost

13. A regular patient of yours comes to the community pharmacy with a new prescription. She says, "I am having to get another prescription today because the one I spent $300 on last week does not work! I can't believe this!" What response is appropriate to demonstrate active listening?

A. I can only fill half of the prescription so you can see if it works for you.

B. It must be very frustrating to have to try a new prescription after the previous one didn't work.

C. I am sure your doctor is just trying to do what is best for you.

D. I am sorry we don't do refunds for prescriptions we have already filled.

E. Would it help if I loaned you a couple of pills from the new prescription to see if it works for you?

14. Which of the following factors play a role in a patient's medication adherence? (Mark all that apply.)

A. Duration of the regimen

B. Clarity of the written instructions based on the person's health literacy

C. Patient's mental status

D. Amount of instruction provided

E. Patient's socioeconomic status

15. Which source would you use if a patient has a question about drug interactions with ginkgo?

A. DEA's website

B. *Prescriber's Letter*

C. *Red Book*

D. *Purple Book*

E. *Natural Medicines*

16. A patient with hypertension is prescribed a medication with several contraindications. The pharmacist identifies that the patient has one of these contraindications and determines that the patient should not take this medication. This is an assessment of _____.

A. safety

B. cost

C. effectiveness

D. adherence

E. appropriateness

17. What is the first step that should be conducted as part of the PDSA Cycle?

A. Carry out the test or change.

B. Determine what is to be accomplished.

C. Act by planning the next change cycle.

D. Develop a plan for change by defining the objective, questions, predictions, and data collection.

E. Carry out the plan.

18. Which of the following would be classified as a secondary reference? (Mark all that apply.)

A. Micromedex

B. An original research publication published in the *New England Journal of Medicine*

C. A systematic review published in the *Journal of the American Pharmacists Association*

D. American Diabetes Association *Standards of Medical Care in Diabetes*

E. *AHFS Drug Information* online

19. Which clinical level is evidence obtained from one large multisite randomized controlled trial (RCT)?

A. I

B. II

C. III

D. IV

E. V

20. What strategies should be used when communicating with a patient or caregiver? (Mark all that apply.)

A. Make regular eye contact.

B. Use paraphrased summaries to indicate your understanding.

C. Use close-ended questions to begin a topic.

D. Interrupt the patient when they are talking to gather needed information.

E. Avoid use of medical jargon.

 **2-13   Answers**

1. **A, B, C, E.** Judging is not one of the elements of the Pharmacists' Patient Care Process, which includes collecting, assessing, planning, implementing, monitoring, and evaluating a consistent process in the delivery of patient care across the profession.

2. **A, B, D, E.** A pharmacist does not need to know patients' marital status and birth order to understand their relevant health care, medication history, and clinical status.

3. **C.** Of the choices provided, the *Red Book* would be the best source to identify information regarding whether a medication is lactose free.

4. **C.** The FDA *Purple Book* contains information on biosimilars; chemical bioequivalence is found in the FDA *Orange Book*.

5. **B.** The risk evaluation and mitigation strategies are targeted toward mitigating medication risks.

6. **B, C, D, E.** Cost of a medication is not found on the ISMP website.

7. **A, C, D.** Reporting adverse events and medication errors by pharmacists is voluntary. Patients are also allowed to report any adverse events or medication errors experienced.

8. **A, D.** Controlled substances are acceptable for take-back programs. In addition to pharmacists who are approved, law enforcement sites can serve as a take-back site. Also some pharmacies offer mail-back envelopes and drop boxes to facilitate consumers' safely disposing of their unused medications.

9. **C.** Nearly three of four patients are nonadherent.

10. **A, B, D, E.** Women are generally more adherent than men.

11. **B, C, D.** Effective communication tools should be chosen that enhances team function. Also, feedback about others' performance should be timely, instructive, and sensitive.

12. **A.** The average manufacturer price (AMP) is the average price paid by wholesalers to manufacturers or by retail pharmacies that buy directly from manufacturers for drugs distributed through such pharmacies. It reflects all rebates paid by manufacturers to wholesalers and retail pharmacies but does not include rebates paid by manufacturers to pharmacy benefit managers, Medicaid, or other third-party payers.

13. **B.** It is important to acknowledge the patient's feelings when actively listening to a patient.

14. **A, B, C, D, E.** All factors listed play a role in a patient's medication adherence.

15. **E.** *Natural Medicines* provides well-researched and useful information on dietary supplements, such as ginkgo.

16. **A.** By assessing this medication and the patient's current medical conditions, the pharmacist identified a safety issue and prevented the patient from experiencing a potential adverse event from the medication.

17. **B.** Before you are able to develop a plan to be implemented for change, you first have to identify what you are trying to accomplish. This includes setting clear and focused goals with measurable targets.

18. **C, D.** Original research publications are classified as primary sources, and electronic databases (e.g., Micromedex and *AHFS Drug Information* online) are classified as tertiary sources.

19. **B.** Evidence from at least one well-designed RCT (e.g., large multisite RCT) is classified as level II evidence.

20. **A, B, E.** Open-ended questions should be used to begin a topic while close-ended questions should be used to screen for pertinent positives/negatives (e.g., "Did you have any stomach pain?"). Follow-up questions should be asked after the patient finished talking.

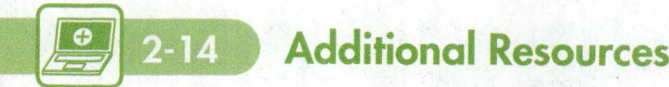

2-14 Additional Resources

American Society of Health-System Pharmacists. *The Pharmacist's Role in Quality Improvement.* Available at: https:// www.ashp.org/-/media/assets/pharmacy-practice/resource-centers/leadership/leadership-of-profession-pharmacists -role-quality-improvement-guide. Accessed June 15, 2020.

Congressional Budget Office. *Prescription Drug Pricing in the Private Sector.* Washington, DC: Congress of the United States; 2007. Available at https://www.cbo.gov/sites/default/files/110th-congress-2007-2008/reports/01-03 -prescriptiondrug.pdf. Accessed June 15, 2020.

IBM Micromedex. *Red Book.* Available at: https://ibm.com/products/micromedex-red-book.

Joint Commission of Pharmacy Practitioners. Pharmacists' patient care process. 2014. Available at: https://jcpp.net /wp-content/uploads/2016/03/PatientCareProcess-with-supporting-organizations.pdf.

McEvoy GK, ed. *AHFS Drug Information 2020.* Bethesda, MD: American Society of Health-System Pharmacists; 2020.

PDR Network. mobilePDR. Available at: https://www.pdr.net/resources/mobilePDR/.

U.S. Food and Drug Administration. *Orange Book: Approved Drug Products with Therapeutic Equivalence Evaluations.* 40th ed. Silver Spring, MD: U.S. Food and Drug Administration; 2020.

U.S. Food and Drug Administration. *Purple Book: Database of Licensed Biological Products.* Available at: https:// purplebooksearch.fda.gov.

Wolters Kluwer Health. *Drug Facts and Comparisons 2017.* Philadelphia, PA: Lippincott Williams and Wilkins; 2016.

Pharmacy Math

3

MICHAEL L. CHRISTENSEN

3-1 KEY POINTS

- Pharmacy math is used daily for the preparation of prescriptions, determining required doses, measuring the weight or volume of a drug, and determining a patient's nutritional needs and the content of nutrient sources.
- Many pharmacy math problems are based on ratio and proportion.
- Paying close attention to units is important; the dose of a drug may be in mcg/kg/min, the drug concentration in mg/mL, and the infusion rate in mL/h.
- A pharmacist should know the relationship of common measurement units to metric equivalents as shown below.

Avoirdupois or household	Exact metric equivalent	Approximate metric equivalent
Liquids		
1 teaspoon	5 mL	5 mL
1 tablespoon	15 mL	15 mL
1 fluid ounce (1 fl oz)	29.57 mL	30 mL
16 fluid ounces (1 pint)	473 mL	480 mL
2 pints (1 quart)	946 mL	960 mL
1 gallon (4 quarts)	3784 mL	3840 mL
Solids		
2.2 pounds	1 kg	1 kg
5 grains	325 mg	325 mg
1 pound	453.59 g	454 g

3-2 STUDY GUIDE CHECKLIST

The following topics may guide your study of this subject area:

- ☐ Math calculations include ratio/ proportion, enlarging, reducing, alligation, dilution, and concentration.
- ☐ Dosing can be calculated on the basis of body weight or body surface area, especially in children.
- ☐ Know how to calculate the quantity of medication to be dispensed, compounded, or administered.
- ☐ Know how to calculate the minimum weighable quantity of a prescription balance.
- ☐ Conversion of drug concentrations may be among percentage strength, ratio strength, and weight per volume (e.g., mg/mL or mcg/dL).
- ☐ Know how to use specific gravity to measure volume by weighing a solution.
- ☐ Know how to calculate doses and preparations using various systems of measure, such as the International System of Units (SI or metric), avoirdupois, apothecaries', and household measurements, and their relationships for conversion.
- ☐ Be able to perform calculations of milliequivalents, millimoles, osmolarity, and isotonicity. Know how to calculate patients' nutritional needs and the content of nutrient sources.

TABLE 3-1. Metric System Prefixes

Prefix	Meaning
tera-	one trillion times the base unit (10^{12})
giga-	one billion times the base unit (10^9)
mega-	one million times the base unit (10^6)
kilo-	one thousand times the base unit (10^3)
deci-	one-tenth the base unit (10^{-1})
centi-	one-hundredth the base unit (10^{-2})
milli-	one-thousandth the base unit (10^{-3})
micro-	one-millionth the base unit (10^{-6})
nano-	one-billionth the base unit (10^{-9})
pico-	one-trillionth the base unit (10^{-12})

3-3   Units of Measure

Calculations in pharmacy may involve four different systems of measure: the metric system, the apothecaries' system, the avoirdupois system, and the household system.

Metric System

The fundamental units of the *metric system* are the gram, the liter, and the meter. Prefixes are used extensively to express quantities much greater and much less than the fundamental units. Some of the most commonly used prefixes are provided in Table 3-1.

Apothecaries' System

Although the metric system is the official system of measure for pharmacy today, the *apothecaries' system* is the traditional system, and some elements might still be found in prescriptions. Units of the apothecaries' system are presented in Table 3-2.

Avoirdupois System

The *avoirdupois system* of measure for weight is used in ordinary commerce. Here, the ounce corresponds to 437.5 grains. The avoirdupois grain unit is equal to the apothecaries' grain unit. Sixteen ounces (7000 grains) correspond to 1 pound. Note that the avoirdupois ounce (437.5 grains) and

TABLE 3-2. Apothecaries' System of Measure

Weight	Volume
1 pound = 12 ounces	1 pint = 16 fluid ounces
1 ounce = 8 drams	1 fluid ounce = 8 fluid drams
1 dram = 3 scruples	1 fluid dram = 3 fluid scruples
1 scruple = 20 grains	1 fluid scruple = 20 minim

Common Measures

1 gallon = 4 quarts	1 cup = 8 fluid ounces
1 quart = 2 pints	1 fluid ounce (fl oz) = 2 tablespoonfuls
1 pint = 2 cups	1 tablespoonful (tbsp) = 3 teaspoonfuls (tsp)

Conversion Factors

A short list of convenient conversion factors follows:

Length Equivalents

1 in = 2.54 cm

1 meter = 39.37 in

Weight Equivalents

1 g = 15.4 grains

1 kg = 2.20 lb (avoirdupois)

1 lb (avoirdupois) = 454 g

1 oz = 28.4 g

1 grain = 64.8 mg

Volume Equivalents

1 gallon (U.S.) = 3785 mL

1 pint = 473 mL

1 fl oz = 29.57 mL

1 tbsp = 15 mL

1 tsp = 5 mL

pound (7000 grains) measures are not equal to the apothecaries' ounce (480 grains) and pound (5760 grains, 12 ounces) measures.

3-4   Ratios and Proportions

Most calculations in pharmacy use ratios and proportions for dosage calculations. A *ratio* is used to convey the relationship between two quantities and a proportion is a comparison where two ratios are equal. You can always solve for one of those quantities when the other three are known. If the ratio x/y is equal to the ratio a/b, then the proportion $x/y = a/b$ exists, and x can be obtained by algebraic manipulation ($x = ay/b$, etc.). Such problems frequently are encountered when calculating doses.

Example: If 300 mL of a preparation contains 250 mg of drug, what weight of drug (x) is contained in 1800 mL of the preparation?

Equate the ratios x:250 mg and 1800 mL:300 mL to solve for x:

$$\frac{x}{250\,\text{mg}} = \frac{1800\,\text{mL}}{300\,\text{mL}}$$

$$x = \frac{250\,\text{mg} \times 1800\,\text{mL}}{300\,\text{mL}} = 1500\,\text{mg}$$

Note that because the new volume is six times greater, the new weight should be six times greater as well.

3-5   Specific Gravity and Density

To convert a volume measure to a weight measure, or vice versa, you will need to use either the specific gravity or the density of the ingredient. This process is used by parenteral nutrition compounding devices that prepare multicomponent intravenous (IV) solutions. *Specific gravity* (SpGr) is a ratio of the weight of the ingredient to the weight of the same volume of standard substance. For liquids, the standard substance is water, which has an SpGr of 1. Specific gravity is unitless. *Density* is determined by dividing a substance's weight by its volume. The units must be explicitly expressed (e.g., g/mL, lb/gal). When density is expressed in g/mL, it is numerically equal to specific gravity.

Example: What is the weight of 750 mL of 70% dextrose (D70) (SpGr = 1.24) required to prepare a parenteral nutrition solution that contains 210 g of dextrose?

$$\text{volume D70} = 210 \text{ g}/0.7 \text{ g/mL} = 300 \text{ mL}$$

$$\text{weight D70} = 300 \text{ mL} \times 1.24 = 372 \text{ g}$$

Thus, the parenteral nutrition compounder would weigh 372 g D70 to add 300 mL of D70 to provide 210 g of dextrose.

3-6   Percentage of Error

Because all measurements are approximations, one must characterize the extent of error involved, or *percentage of error,* which is defined as

$$\% \text{ error} = \frac{(\text{error} \times 100\%)}{(\text{quantity desired})}$$

The term *error* in the numerator indicates the maximum potential error in the measurement (error = larger quantity – smaller quantity), while the term *quantity desired* in the denominator represents the total amount measured. Percentage of error may be calculated for either a weight or a volume measurement.

Example: A quantity of material weighs 5.81 g on a prescription balance. When one uses a much more accurate analytical balance, the quantity weighs 5.893 g. What is the percentage of error for the original weighing?

$$\text{error} = 5.893 \text{ g} - 5.810 \text{ g} = 0.083 \text{ g}$$

The quantity desired is 5.81 g. Thus,

$$\% \text{ error} = 0.083 \text{ g} \times \frac{100\%}{5.81} = 1.4\%$$

Example: You intend to weigh out 75 mg of an ingredient but mistakenly weigh out 65 mg instead. Based on the quantity desired, what is the percentage of error?

$$\% \text{ error} = \frac{(\text{error} \times 100\%)}{(\text{quantity desired})}$$

$$= \frac{(10 \text{ mg} \times 100\%)}{75 \text{ mg}} = 13\%$$

3-7   Minimum Measurable

According to United States Pharmacopeial Convention (USP) Standard 1176, Prescription Balances and Volumetric Apparatus, weighing by a pharmacist cannot exceed an error greater than 5%, which requires that the sensitivity of the balance be known and limits the smallest quantity that can be weighed. Balance sensitivity is defined in terms of the *sensitivity requirement* (SR), which is the weight of material that will move the indicator one marked unit on the index plate of the balance. For a class A prescription balance, SR = 6 mg. The minimum weighable quantity (MWQ) for a given balance can be calculated by dividing SR by the acceptable error as a fraction. Thus, for an SR = 6 mg and error = 5% or 0.05 (as a fraction):

$$MWQ = \frac{SR}{error}$$

$$MWQ = \frac{6 \text{ mg}}{0.05} = 120 \text{ mg}$$

Example: For a balance that has an SR of 4 mg, what is the minimum weighable quantity to ensure a percentage of error no greater than 2%?

$$MWQ = \frac{4 \text{ mg}}{0.02} = 200 \text{ mg}$$

Example: What is the SR for a balance with a percentage of error of 5% when weighing 120 mg?

$$SR = MWQ \times error$$
$$SR = 120 \text{ mg} \times 0.05 = 6 \text{ mg}$$

3-8   Patient-Specific Dosage Calculations

Drugs with a narrow therapeutic range often are dosed on the basis of patient weight or body surface area. For patients with renal impairment, some drugs are dosed on the basis of creatinine clearance.

Dosing Based on Body Weight

Weight-based dosing might involve using the patient's total body weight (TBW), ideal body weight (IBW), or perhaps an adjusted body weight (ABW) that is a function of IBW and TBW. Those weights are invariably expressed in kilograms.

Example: A patient weighing 180 lb is to receive 0.25 mg/kg/day amphotericin B (reconstituted and diluted to 0.1 mg/mL) by IV infusion. What volume of solution is required to deliver the daily dose?

$$weight \text{ (kg)} = \frac{180 \text{ lb}}{2.2 \text{ lb/kg}} = 82 \text{ kg}$$

$$daily \text{ dose} = 82 \text{ kg} \times 0.25 \text{ mg/kg} = 20.5 \text{ mg}$$

$$volume = \frac{20.5 \text{ mg}}{0.1 \text{mg/mL}} = 205 \text{ mL}$$

A commonly used equation for calculating IBW is

$$IBW\,(kg) = (sex\,factor) + (2.3 \times height\,[in > 5\,ft])$$

where the sex factor for males is 50 and the sex factor for females is 45.5.

Example: The recommended adult daily dosage for patients with normal renal function for tobramycin is 3 mg/kg/day ABW divided every 8 hours. The formula for ABW for tobramycin is: ABW = IBW + 0.4(TBW − IBW). What would each dose be for a male patient who weighs 185 lb and is 5 ft 9 in tall?

$$TBW = \frac{185\,lb}{2.2\,lb/kg} = 84.1\,kg$$

$$IBW = 50\,kg + (2.3\,kg/in \times 9\,in) = 50\,kg + 20.7\,kg = 70.7\,kg$$

$$ABW = 70.7\,kg + 0.4(84.1\,kg - 70.7\,kg) = 70.7\,kg + 5.4\,kg = 76.1\,kg$$

$$Each\,dose = 1\,mg/kg \times 76.1\,kg = 76.1\,mg$$

When there are no pediatric dosing guidelines, the dose can be estimated on the basis of 70 kg. An adjusted dosage for a child is obtained by multiplying the usual dose by the ratio of child's weight to 70 kg (Clark's rule).

Example: If the adult dose of a drug is 100 mg and no child-specific dosing information is available, what would the weight-adjusted dose be for a child who weighs 40 kg?

$$child\,dose = 100\,mg \times \frac{40\,kg}{70\,kg} = 57\,mg$$

Dosing Based on Body Surface Area

Dosing based on body surface area requires an estimation of the patient's body surface area (BSA) expressed in square meters (m^2). That parameter might be estimated from a nomogram using height and weight or, for adults, by using an equation such as the Mosteller formula:

$$BSA = \sqrt{\frac{ht\,(cm) \times wt\,(kg)}{3600}}$$

Example: What is the computed BSA for an adult who weighs 194 lb and is 5 ft 10 in tall?

$$height = 70\,in \times 2.54\,cm/in = 178\,cm$$

$$weight = 194\,lb/2.2\,lb/kg = 88\,kg$$

$$BSA = \sqrt{\frac{178 \times 88}{3600}} = 2.09\,m^2$$

The average adult BSA is 1.73 m^2. That value can be used to obtain an estimated child's dose, given the usual dose for an adult and the child's calculated BSA.

Example: If the adult dose of a drug is 50 mg, what would be the BSA-adjusted dose for a child with an estimated BSA of 0.55 m²?

$$\text{child dose} = 50 \, \text{mg} \times \frac{0.55 \, \text{m}^2}{1.73 \, \text{m}^2} = 16 \, \text{mg}$$

Dosing Based on Creatinine Clearance

For many drugs, the rate of elimination depends on kidney function. As kidney function declines there is a decrease in drug clearance. Creatinine clearance (CrCl) estimates kidney function as a measure of the volume of blood plasma that is cleared of creatinine by kidney filtration per minute, and it is expressed in mL/min. CrCl can be calculated using the Cockcroft–Gault equation as a function of patient sex, age, weight, and serum creatinine for adults and by the Schwartz equation for children.

Cockcroft–Gault equation

For males:

$$\text{CrCl (mL/min)} = \frac{(140 - \text{age [years]}) \times \text{body weight (kg)}}{72 \times \text{serum creatinine (mg/dL)}}$$

For females:

$$\text{CrCl} = 0.85 \times \text{CrCl for males}$$

Example: Using the Cockcroft–Gault equation, calculate the CrCl rate for a 76-year-old female weighing 65 kg and having a serum creatinine of 0.52 mg/dL.

$$\text{CrCl(mL/min)} = \frac{0.85 \times (140 - 76 \text{ years}) \times 65 \text{ kg}}{72 \times 0.52 \text{ mg/dL}} = 94 \text{ mL/min}$$

Bedside Schwartz equation for estimating GFR in children:

$$\text{eGFR} = 0.413 \times \left[\frac{\text{height (cm)}}{\text{serum creatinine (mg/dL)}} \right]$$

The maintenance dose for some drugs is based on IBW and CrCl. See Chapter 7 for more detailed information.

3-9   Use of Batch Preparation Formulas

The relative amounts of ingredients in a pharmaceutical product are specified in a formula. A pharmacist may be required to reduce or enlarge the formula to prepare a lesser or greater amount of product. A formula might specify either the actual amount (weight or volume) of each ingredient for a specified total amount of product or the relative amount (part) of each ingredient. In the latter case, the ingredients must all be of the same measure (e.g., weight in grams).

Example: From the following lotion formula, calculate the quantity of triethanolamine required to make 200 mL of lotion.

Triethanolamine   10 mL
Oleic acid   25 mL
Benzyl benzoate   250 mL
Water to make   1000 mL

$$\frac{x}{10 \text{ mL}} = \frac{200 \text{ mL}}{1000 \text{ mL}}$$

$$x = \frac{200 \text{ mL} \times 10 \text{ mL}}{1000 \text{ mL}} = 2 \text{ mL}$$

Example: From the following formula, calculate the quantity of chlorpheniramine maleate required to make 400 g of product.

Chlorpheniramine maleate   10 parts
Phenindamine   20 parts
Phenylpropanolamine HCl   50 parts

Note that the formula will give a total of 80 parts, which will correspond to the desired quantity of 400 g. Then,

$$\frac{x}{400 \text{ g}} = \frac{10 \text{ parts}}{80 \text{ parts}}$$

$$x = 400 \text{ g} \times \frac{10 \text{ parts}}{80 \text{ parts}} = 50 \text{ g}$$

3-10 Conventions in Expression of Concentration

Drug concentrations are expressed in a variety of units. One must be prepared to calculate drug concentration units directly from their definitions and to interconvert among them.

Percentage Strength

Percentage specifies the number of parts per 100 parts. In pharmacy, *percentage strength* can be expressed three ways:

- Percent weight-in-volume = % (w/v) = g/100 mL of product (e.g., 0.9% normal saline)
- Percent weight-in-weight = % (w/w) = g/100 g of product (e.g., 1% hydrocortisone ointment)
- Percent volume-in-volume = % (v/v) = mL/100 mL of product (e.g., 70% isopropyl alcohol)

Example: What is the percentage strength % (w/v) for a preparation containing 250 mg of drug in 50 mL of solution? Note that % (w/v) is defined as g/100 mL. Thus,

$$250 \text{ mg} = 0.25 \text{ g}$$

$$\frac{0.25 \text{ g}}{50 \text{ mL}} = \frac{x}{100 \text{ mL}}$$

$$x = 100 \text{ mL} \times \frac{0.25 \text{ g}}{50 \text{ mL}} = 0.5 \text{ g}/100 \text{ mL} = 0.5\%$$

Parts (Ratio Strength)

Concentrations may be expressed in "parts" or *ratio strength* when the active ingredient is highly diluted. Assumptions concerning (w/w), (v/v), and (w/v) ratios are identical to those for percentages.

Example: Convert the ratio strength 1:2500 to percentage strength.

$$\frac{1 \text{ part}}{2500 \text{ parts}} = \frac{x}{100\%}$$

$$x\% = \frac{100 \text{ parts}}{2500 \text{ parts}} = 0.04\% \text{ (w/v)}$$

Millimoles

A 1 molar solution contains the molecular weight (mw) of the substance in g/L of solution. The *molarity* expresses the number of moles per liter. The *millimolarity* (mmol/L) is 1000 times the molarity of a solution or the molecular weight of a substance in mg/L of solution.

Example: What is the millimolar concentration of a solution consisting of 0.9 g of sodium chloride (NaCl, mw = 58.5) in 100 mL of water? The quantity of 0.9 g/100 mL corresponds to 9 g/1000 mL or 9000 mg/L.

$$\text{millimolarity} = \frac{9000 \text{ mg}}{58.5 \text{ mg/mmol}} = 154 \text{ mmol}$$

Milliequivalents

A milliequivalent (mEq) is a measure of the total number of ionic charges in a solution. The equivalent weight of an ion is the molecular weight in grams of the ion divided by the valence. Thus, the equivalent weight of a sodium ion (Na^+, mw = 23, valence = 1) is 23 g, and for calcium (Ca^{2+}, mw = 40, valence = 2), it is 20 g. A milliequivalent is the molecular weight of an ion in milligrams. For a molecule, the equivalent weight is obtained by dividing the molecular weight by the total valence of the positive or negative ion. For example, the milliequivalent weight of magnesium chloride ($MgCl_2$, mw = 95.3 mg, valence = 2) is 47.7 mg.

Example: What is the concentration, in milliequivalents per liter, of a solution containing 14.9 g of potassium chloride (KCl, mw = 74.5, valence = 1) in 1 liter? Accordingly,

$$\text{milliequivalent weight KCl} = 74.5 \text{ mg}$$

$$14.9 \text{ g KCl} = 14{,}900 \text{ mg}$$

$$\frac{14{,}900 \text{ mg}}{74.5 \text{ mg/mEq}} = 200 \text{ mEq}$$

Example: What weight in grams of magnesium sulfate ($MgSO_4$, mw = 120, valence = 2) is required to prepare 1 liter of a solution that is 25 mEq/L? The milliequivalent weight of $MgSO_4$ is 120/2 = 60 mg. Accordingly, 60 mg corresponds to 1 mEq of $MgSO_4$. Then,

$$\frac{x}{60\,mg} = \frac{25\,mEq}{1\,mEq}$$

$$x = 60\,mg \times \frac{25\,mEq}{1\,mEq} = 1500\,mg = 1.5\,g$$

Example: How many milliequivalents of calcium chloride ($CaCl_2$) are contained in 100 mL of a 5% (w/v) solution (mw = 111, valence = 2, 1 mEq = 55.5 mg)? The solution contains 5 g/100 mL $CaCl_2$, or 5000 mg/100 mL.

$$\frac{5000\,mg}{55.5\,mg/mEq} = 90\,mEq$$

Milliosmoles

Osmotic concentration is a measure of the total number of particles in solution and is expressed in milliosmoles (mOsm). The number of milliosmoles is based on the total number of cations and the total number of anions. The *milliosmolarity* of a solution is the number of milliosmoles per liter of solution (mOsm/L), where

$$mOsm/L = mmol/L \times number\ of\ species$$

$$number\ of\ species = number\ of\ ionic\ species\ upon\ complete\ dissociation$$

$$dextrose = 1\ specie$$

$$NaCl = 2\ species$$

$$CaCl_2 = 3\ species$$

The total osmolarity of a solution is the sum of the osmolarity of all of the solute components of the solution. When calculating osmolarity, assume that salts (e.g., NaCl) dissociate completely. Note the distinction between the terms *milliosmolarity* (mOsm/L of solution) and *milliosmolality* (mOsm/kg of solution). To convert mEq/L to mOsm/L, multiply mEq/L by the number of species.

Example: What is the concentration, in mOsm/L, of a 1 L solution that contains 5% dextrose + 0.45% NaCl + 20 mEq/L of KCl (dextrose mw = 180, NaCl mw = 58.5, KCl mw = 74.5)?

$$5\%\ dextrose = 5\,g/100\,mL = 50\,g/1000\,mL = 50,000\,mg/1000\,mL$$

$$\frac{50,000\,mg}{180\,mg/mmoL} \times 1\,specie = 278\,mOsm/L$$

$$0.45\%\ NaCL = 0.45\,g/100\,mL = 4.5\,g/1000\,mL = 4500\,mg/1000\,mL$$

$$\frac{4500\,mg}{58.5\,mg/mmoL} \times 2\,species = 154\,mOsm/L$$

$$20\,mEq/L\ KCl \times 2\,species = 40\,mOsm/L$$

$$278\,mOsm + 154\,mOsm + 40\,mOsm = 472\,mOsm$$

Units of Potency

The concentrations for some drugs (e.g., antibiotics and vitamins) are expressed as "units" of activity per micrograms or milligram (i.e., units/mcg or units/mg) as determined by a standardized bioassay.

Example: Each gram of a preparation of Cortisporin cream contains polymyxin B 10,000 units (polymyxin B 6000 units/mg). How many milligrams of polymyxin B are contained in 7.5 g cream?

$$10,000 \text{ units/g} \times 7.5 \text{ g} = 75,000 \text{ units}$$

$$\frac{75,000 \text{ units}}{6000 \text{ units/mg}} = 12.5 \text{ mg}$$

Parts per Million and Parts per Billion

Very low concentrations often are expressed in terms of parts per million (ppm) or parts per billion (ppb) (i.e., the number of parts of ingredient per million or billion parts of mixture or solution). Thus, ppm and ppb are special cases of ratio strength concentrations.

Example: Express 1:25,000 as parts per million.

$$\frac{1}{25,000} = \frac{x}{1,000,000}$$

$$x = 40 \text{ ppm}$$

Example: Express 100 ppm as a ratio strength, percentage strength, and mg/mL.

$$\frac{100 \text{ parts}}{1,000,000 \text{ parts}} = 1:10,000 = \frac{0.01 \text{g}}{100 \text{ mL}} = 0.01\% = \frac{10 \text{ mg}}{100 \text{ mL}} = 0.1 \text{mg/mL}$$

3-11   Dilutions and Concentrations

Simple Dilutions

In simple dilutions, a desired drug concentration is obtained by adding more solvent (diluent) to an existing solution or mixture. Mathematically, the key feature of this process, the amount of drug present, remains unchanged. The amount of drug in any solution is proportional to the concentration times the quantity of the solution. Thus, taking the initial concentration as C_1, the initial quantity of solution as Q_1, the final concentration as C_2, and the final quantity of solution as Q_2, one has the relationship: $C_1 \times Q_1 = C_2 \times Q_2$. When provided with values for any three of those variables, one can calculate the fourth variable. (Because the equation can be rearranged to $C_1/C_2 = Q_2/Q_1$, it sometimes is referred to as an inverse proportionality.)

Example: How much water should be added to 250 mL of a solution of 0.2% (w/v) benzalkonium chloride to make a 0.05% (w/v) solution?

$$C_1 = 0.2\% \text{ (w/v)}$$

$$Q_1 = 250 \text{ mL}$$

$$C_2 = 0.05\% \text{ (w/v)}$$

$$Q_2 = x$$

$$C_1 \times Q_1 = C_2 \times Q_2$$

$$0.2\% \times 250 \text{ mL} = 0.05\% \times x$$

$$x = 1000 \text{ mL}$$

$$1000 \text{ mL} - 250 \text{ mL} = 750 \text{ mL}$$

750 mL of water to be added

Simple Concentrations

In simple concentrations, a desired drug concentration is obtained by adding pure drug to an existing solution or mixture; therefore, the absolute amount of base or diluent remains unchanged. In contrast to simple dilution, the amount of base or diluent in any solution or mixture is proportional to the concentration times the quantity of the solution or mixture. Thus, taking the initial base concentration as C_1, the initial quantity of mixture as Q_1, the final base concentration as C_2, and the final quantity of mixture as Q_2, one has the relationship: $C_1 \times Q_1 = C_2 \times Q_2$. When provided with values for any three of those variables, one can calculate the fourth variable.

Example: How many grams of zinc oxide should be added to 3200 g of 5% (w/w) zinc oxide ointment to prepare an ointment containing 20% (w/w) zinc oxide?

$C_1 = 95\%$ (Concentration of the initial base)

$Q_1 = 3200$ g

$C_2 = 80\%$ (Concentration of final base)

$Q_2 = x$

$C_1 \times Q_1 = C_2 \times Q_2$

$95\% \times 3200$ g $= 80\% \times x$

$x = 3800$ g

3800 g $- 3200$ g $= 600$ g

600 g of zinc oxide is added

Alligation Alternate Method

Sometimes a drug concentration is required that is in between the concentrations of two (or more) stock solutions (or available drug products). In that case, the alligation alternate method may be used to quickly obtain the relative parts of each of the stock solutions needed to yield the desired concentration. If stock solutions of concentrations A% and B% (A% > B%) are to be used to make a solution of concentration C%, one sets up the following diagram to obtain the relative parts of solutions A and B.

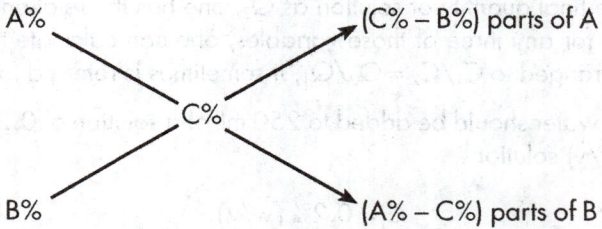

Example: In what proportion should 20% (w/v) dextrose be mixed with 5% (w/v) dextrose to obtain 15% (w/v) dextrose? How much of each is required to make 75 mL of 15% (w/v) solution?

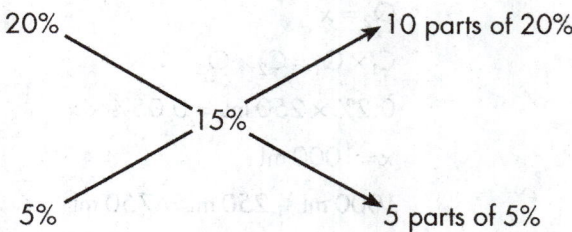

Thus, combine the stock solutions in the ratio of 10 parts of 20% (w/v) dextrose and 5 parts of 5% (w/v) dextrose (total of 15 parts). Accordingly, to make 75 mL of 15% solution (75 mL/15 parts = 5 mL/part), mix 50 mL (10 parts × 5 mL/part) of 20% solution with 25 mL (5 parts × 5 mL/part) of 5% solution.

Alligation Medial Method

Sometimes one may need to know the final concentration of a solution obtained by mixing specified volumes of two or more stock solutions. In that case, the alligation medial method may be used.

Example: What is the concentration of a solution prepared by combining 100 mL of a 10% solution, 200 mL of a 20% solution, and 300 mL of a 30% solution? Proceed as follows:

$$0.1 \times 100 \text{ mL} = 10 \text{ mL}$$
$$0.2 \times 200 \text{ mL} = 40 \text{ mL}$$
$$\underline{0.3 \times 300 \text{ mL} = 90 \text{ mL}}$$
$$600 \text{ mL} \quad 140 \text{ mL}$$
$$140 \text{ mL}/600 \text{ mL} \times 100 = 23.3\%$$

3-12 Isotonic Solutions

The preparation of many solutions requires attention to tonicity, a property based on the osmotic pressure that different concentrations of solutes exert as the solvent passes through a semipermeable membrane from a dilute solution to a more concentrated solution. Here, the term *solute* corresponds to cations, anions, and neutral undissociated molecules. A solution that has the same osmotic pressure as bodily fluids (blood or tears) is said to be *isotonic* (and isosmotic). As a point of reference, 0.9% (w/v) sodium chloride is isotonic.

Sodium Chloride Equivalents or E value

When preparing isotonic drug solutions, one must consider the tonicity contribution of the drug. That is accomplished by using the *sodium chloride equivalent* (E value) for the drug, which is defined as the number of grams of sodium chloride that would produce the same tonicity effect as 1 gram of the drug.

Using the total volume of isotonic solution to be prepared, first calculate the hypothetical weight, x, of sodium chloride (alone) that would be required to make that volume of water isotonic (0.9%). Next, using the weight of drug to be incorporated in the solution and its sodium chloride equivalent, calculate the weight of sodium chloride, y, that would correspond to the weight of the drug. Then, calculate the weight of sodium chloride, z, to be added to the preparation as: $z = x - y$.

Example: What weight of sodium chloride would be required to prepare 50 mL of an isotonic solution containing 1000 mg of pilocarpine nitrate (E = 0.23)?

Because isotonic saline requires 0.9 g/100 mL, 50 mL of isotonic saline will require 0.45 g (x). The 1000 mg of pilocarpine nitrate will correspond to 1 g × 0.23 = 0.23 g sodium chloride (y). Thus, the weight of sodium chloride (z) needed to make an isotonic solution is

$$0.45 \text{ g} - 0.23 \text{ g} = 0.22 \text{ g}$$

Example: Fluorescein sodium (mw = 376, E = 0.22) is to be provided as 500 mg in 60 mL of solution made isotonic with sodium chloride. What is the required weight of sodium chloride?

Because isotonic saline requires 0.9 g/100 mL, 60 mL of isotonic saline will require 0.54 g (*x*). The 500 mg of fluorescein sodium will correspond to 0.5 g × 0.22 = 0.11 g of sodium chloride (*y*). Thus, the weight of sodium chloride (*z*) needed to make an isotonic solution is

$$0.54\,g - 0.11\,g = 0.43\,g$$

3-13   Intravenous Infusion Flow Rates

A physician may specify the rate of flow of IV fluids in drops per minute, amount of drug per hour, or the duration of time of administration of the total volume of the infusion. Therefore, to program an infusion pump to give the medication at the correct rate, one may need to calculate the infusion rate in per minute or per hour increments.

Example: If 250 mg of a drug is in a 500 mL D$_5$W bag, what should the flow rate be, in mL/h, to deliver 50 mg of drug per hour? The amount per hour is divided by the drug concentration to calculate the infusion rate.

$$\frac{250\,mg}{500\,mL} = 0.5\,mg/mL$$

$$\frac{50\,mg/h}{0.5\,mg/mL} = 100\,mL/h$$

Example: If an infusion flow rate is 100 mL/h and the infusion set delivers 15 drops/mL, what is the rate of flow in drops per minute?

$$15\,drops/mL \times 100\,mL/h = 1500\,drops/h$$

$$\frac{1500\,drops/h}{60\,min} = 25\,drops/min$$

Example: If 500 mL of an infusion is to be delivered at a flow rate of 1.25 mL/min, how long will it take to deliver the 500 mL in hours?

$$\text{Total time of delivery} = \frac{500\,mL}{1.25\,mL/min} = 400\,min$$

$$= 6.7\,h$$

3-14   Nutrition Calculations

Body Mass Index

A method for assessing weight status is to determine the body mass index (BMI). BMI is calculated by dividing the body weight in kg by the height in m^2.

$$BMI = \text{weight (kg)} \div \text{height}^2\,(m)$$

Weight status is an important patient assessment parameter. Weight status, as reflected by BMI, is assessed in adults by the following guidelines:

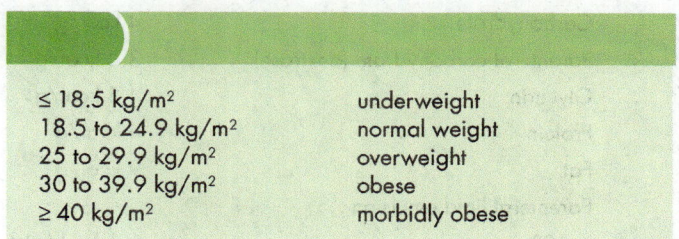

≤ 18.5 kg/m²	underweight
18.5 to 24.9 kg/m²	normal weight
25 to 29.9 kg/m²	overweight
30 to 39.9 kg/m²	obese
≥ 40 kg/m²	morbidly obese

Example: What is the weight status of an individual who is 6 ft tall and weighs 210 pounds.

$$\text{height(m)} = 6\,\text{ft} = 72\,\text{in} = 72\,\text{in} \times 2.54\,\text{cm/in} = 183\,\text{cm} = 1.83\,\text{m}$$

$$\text{weight(kg)} = 220\,\text{lb} \div 2.2\,\text{lb/kg} = 100\,\text{kg}$$

$$\text{BMI} = 100\,\text{kg}/1.83^2\,\text{m} = 29.9\,\text{kg/m}^2, \text{therefore overweight}$$

Nutritional Requirements

Daily fluid requirements for adults are 30 to 35 mL/kg or 1500 mL/m². The estimated daily fluid requirements for infants and children are provided in Table 3-3. Caloric estimate is 1 kilocalorie (kcal) for each mL of fluid required. These requirements are only estimates and the actual needs must be determined on the basis of an assessment of the patient. The recommended dietary intake of carbohydrates is 45% to 65% of total calories, fat is 20% to 35% of total calories, and protein is 10% to 35% of total calories. Adult protein needs range from 0.8 g/kg for a stable patient to 2.5 g/kg for patients with a critical illness or major burn. Pediatric protein needs range from 1 g/kg to 3 g/kg, are age dependent, and increase in conditions such as prematurity and critical illness. Table 3-4 provides the caloric content of the nutrients.

Example: What are the daily fluid and calorie needs for a 32-kg child?

$$\text{Fluids(mL/day)} = 1500\,\text{mL} + \left[20\,\text{mL/kg} \times (32\,\text{kg} - 20\,\text{kg})\right] = 1740\,\text{mL}$$

$$\text{Calories(kcal/day)} = 1740\,\text{mL} \times 1\,\text{kcal/mL} = 1740\,\text{kcal}$$

Example: A total nutrient admixture (TNA) order for 2400 mL contains 20% dextrose, 3% amino acids, and 3% lipid emulsion. How many calories does the TNA provide? (*Note:* the caloric density of lipid emulsion in a TNA is 10 kcal/g fat.)

TABLE 3-3. Maintenance Fluid and Caloric Requirements

Weight	Daily fluid and caloric requirement[a]
0 to 10 kg	100 mL/kg
10 to 20 kg	1000 mL + 50 mL/kg
> 20 kg	1500 mL + 20 mL/kg
Adult > 70 kg	2500 mL

a. Estimated caloric requirement is 1 kcal per mL of fluid requirement.

TABLE 3-4. Caloric Content of Nutrients

Nutrient	Calories
Carbohydrate	4 kcal/g
Parenteral carbohydrate (dextrose)	3.4 kcal/g
Glycerin	4.3 kcal/g
Protein	4 kcal/g
Fat	9 kcal/g
Parenteral lipid emulsion	
10%	1.1 kcal/mL
20%	2 kcal/mL
30%	3 kcal/mL

Dextrose calories = 2400 mL × 20 g/100 mL × 3.4 kcal/g = 1632 kcal

Protein calories = 2400 mL × 3 g/100 mL × 4 kcal/g = 288 kcal

Fat calories = 2400 mL × 3 g/100 mL × 10 kcal/g = 720 kcal

Total calories = 1632 kcal + 288 kcal + 720 kcal = 2640 kcal

NAPLEX Competency Statements

The questions in this chapter cover the following 2021 NAPLEX Competency Statements: **AREA 4:** 4.1; 4.2; 4.3; 4.4; 4.5; 4.6; 4.7.

 **3-15**   **Questions**

1. If 100 capsules contain 340 mg of active ingredient, what is the weight of active ingredient in 75 capsules?

A. 453 mg
B. 340 mg
C. 255 mg
D. 128 mg
E. 75 mg

2. What is the weight of 500 mL of a liquid with a specific gravity of 1.13?

A. 442 mg
B. 565 g
C. 442 g
D. 885 mg
E. 221 g

3. A pharmacist weighs out 325 mg of a substance on her class A prescription balance. Reweighing on a more sensitive analytical balance, she finds the weight is 312 mg. What is the percentage of error in the original weighing?

A. 4%
B. 5%
C. 6%
D. 10%
E. 12%

4. What is the minimum weighable quantity for a maximum of 5% error using a balance with a sensitivity requirement of 6 mg?

A. 80 mg
B. 100 mg
C. 120 mg
D. 150 mg
E. 240 mg

5. A patient weighing 175 lb is to receive an intramuscular dose of procainamide HCl of 50 mg/kg given in divided doses every 3 hours. How many milliliters from a 500 mg/mL vial should each injection contain?

A. 3.98 mL
B. 0.49 mL
C. 8.23 mL
D. 1.87 mL
E. 0.99 mL

6. What is the IBW of a female patient whose height is 5 ft 8 in?

A. 68 kg
B. 64 kg
C. 150 lb
D. 121 lb
E. 53 kg

7. What is the approximate BSA of an adult patient who weighs 154 lb and is 6 ft tall?

A. 1.73 m²
B. 3.15 m²
C. 1.89 m²
D. 0.70 m²
E. 2.67 m²

8. If the adult dose of a drug is 125 mg, what is the dose for a child whose BSA is estimated to be 0.68 m²?

A. 485 mg
B. 318 mg
C. 85 mg
D. 49 mg
E. 33 mg

9. What is the creatinine clearance for a 65-year-old female who weighs 50 kg and has a serum creatinine level of 1.3 mg/dL?

A. 34 mL/min
B. 40 mL/min
C. 26 mL/min
D. 82 mL/min
E. 100 mL/min

10. Using the formula that follows, determine how much zinc oxide is required to make 800 g of mixture:

Zinc oxide	150 g
Starch	250 g
Petrolatum	550 g
Coal tar	50 g

A. 200 g
B. 180 g
C. 420 g
D. 120 g
E. 40 g

11. Using the formula that follows, determine the weight of kaolin that would be required to produce 500 g of mixture:

Kaolin	12 parts
Magnesium oxide	3 parts
Bismuth subcarbonate	5 parts

A. 83 g
B. 300 g
C. 208 g
D. 333 g
E. 250 g

12. What weight of hexachlorophene is used in compounding 20 g of an ointment containing hexachlorophene at a concentration of 1:400?

A. 25 mcg
B. 50 mcg
C. 50 mg
D. 80 mg
E. 5 g

13. What weight of magnesium chloride ($MgCl_2$, mw = 95.3) is required to prepare 200 mL of a solution that is 5 millimolar?

A. 191 mg
B. 95.3 mg
C. 19.1 mg
D. 0.5 mg
E. 910 mcg

14. What is the milliosmolarity of normal saline (NaCl, formula weight = 58.5)?

A. 100 mOsm/L
B. 154 mOsm/L
C. 254 mOsm/L
D. 287 mOsm/L
E. 308 mOsm/L

15. How much water for injection is added to 250 mL of 20% dextrose to obtain 15% dextrose?

A. 333 mL
B. 83 mL
C. 250 mL
D. 166 mL
E. 58 mL

16. What volume of a 5% dextrose solution when added to a 20% dextrose solution would prepare 300 mL of a 15% dextrose solution?

A. 150 mL
B. 200 mL
C. 100 mL
D. 50 mL
E. 250 mL

17. What is the final concentration obtained by mixing 200 mL of 20% dextrose with 100 mL of 5% dextrose?

A. 10%
B. 15%
C. 7.5%
D. 12.5%
E. 17.5%

18. What weight of sodium chloride should be used in compounding the following prescription for ephedrine sulfate (mw = 429, E = 0.23)?

Ephedrine sulfate	0.25 g
Sodium chloride	qs
Purified water ad	30 mL
Make isotonic solution	

A. 1.22 g
B. 784 mcg
C. 212 mg
D. 527 mcg
E. 429 mg

19. A patient is to receive an infusion of 2 g of lidocaine in 500 mL D_5W at a rate of 2 mg/min. What is the flow rate in milliliters per hour?

A. 2 mL/h
B. 6.5 mL/h
C. 15 mL/h
D. 30 mL/h
E. 150 mL/h

20. How much boric acid is needed to prepare an isotonic solution of the following prescription?

Phenacaine HCl	1%	E value for phenacaine HCl is 0.2
Chlorobutanol	0.5%	E value for chlorobutanol is 0.24
Boric acid	qs	E value for boric acid is 0.52
Purified water ad	60 mL	

A. 0.55 g
B. 0.67 g
C. 0.75 g
D. 1.2 g
E. 2.2 g

21. How many milliequivalents of Na^+ are contained in a 30 mL dose of the following solution?

Disodium hydrogen phosphate	18 g	Na_2HPO_4 $7H_2O$ (mw = 268)
Sodium biphosphate	48 g	NaH_2PO_4 $4H_2O$ (mw =138)
Purified water ad	100 mL	

A. 144.63 mEq
B. 104.34 mEq
C. 40.29 mEq
D. 100 mEq
E. 52 mEq

22. What is the concentration (g/mL) of a solution containing 4 mEq of $CaCl_2$ $2H_2O$ per milliliter (mw = 147)?

A. 0.345 g/mL
B. 0.986 g/mL
C. 0.389 g/mL
D. 0.294 g/mL
E. 0.545 g/mL

23. An IV infusion for a patient weighing 132 lb calls for 7.5 mg metronidazole [Flagyl] per kilogram of body weight added to 1000 mL of 5% dextrose injection solution. How much drug is needed?

A. 250 mg
B. 350 mg
C. 150 mg
D. 450 mg
E. 900 mg

24. What is the total number of milliliters the patient receives per day for a 5% dextrose injection IV solution running at 52 mL/h?

A. 1350 mL
B. 1248 mL
C. 256 mL
D. 1000 mL
E. 1500 mL

25. What is the infusion rate in drops per minute (1 mL = 20 drops) for a 5% dextrose injection solution running at 52 mL/h?

A. 25 drops/min
B. 22 drops/min
C. 17 drops/min
D. 30 drops/min
E. 15 drops/min

26. If 50 mg of drug X is mixed with enough ointment base to obtain 20 grams of mixture, what is the concentration of drug X in ointment (expressed as a ratio)?

A. 1:300
B. 1:400
C. 1:200
D. 1:600
E. 1:100

27. When 23 mL of water for injection are added to drug-lyophilized powder, the resulting concentration is 200,000 units/mL. What is the volume of the dry powder if the amount of drug in the vial is 5,000,000 units?

A. 2 mL
B. 4 mL
C. 1 mL
D. 5 mL
E. 9 mL

28. If 20 grams of salicylic acid are mixed with enough hydrophilic petrolatum to obtain a concentration of 5%, how much ointment was used to prepare the prescription?

A. 400 g
B. 380 g
C. 250 g
D. 480 g
E. 280 g

29. A total nutrient admixture contains the following amounts: 20% dextrose, 3.5% amino acids, 3% lipid emulsion, 50 mEq/L sodium chloride, 25 mEq/L potassium chloride, and 10 mL multivitamin injection in a total volume of 2400 mL that will run at 100 mL/h. How many total calories will the patient receive on a daily basis?

A. 1632 kcal
B. 1968 kcal
C. 2352 kcal
D. 2400 kcal
E. 2688 kcal

30. What is the BMI of a person who is 5 ft 10 in and weighs 175 lb?

A. 30.0
B. 55.2
C. 25.1
D. 23.0
E. 18.5

 **3-16   Answers**

1. C.

$$x \text{ mg}:340 \text{ mg} = 75 \text{ cap}:100 \text{ cap}$$

$$x = 340 \text{ mg} \times 75 \text{ cap}/100 \text{ cap} = 255 \text{ mg}$$

2. B. A specific gravity of 1.13 corresponds to a density of 1.13 g/mL.

density = weight/volume; thus, weight

$$= \text{density} \times \text{volume} = 1.13 \text{ g/mL}$$

$$\times 500 \text{ mL} = 565 \text{ g}$$

3. A.

$$\% \text{ error} = \frac{(\text{error} \times 100\%)}{\text{quantity desired}}$$

$$= (325 - 312) \times \frac{100}{325} = 4\%$$

4. C.

$$\text{minimum weighable quantity} = \frac{SR \times 100\%}{5\%}$$

$$= 6 \text{ mg} \times \frac{100\%}{5\%}$$

$$= 120 \text{ mg}$$

5. E.

$$\text{daily dosage} = 50 \text{ mg/kg} \times \frac{175 \text{ lb}}{2.2 \text{ lb/kg}}$$

$$= 3977 \text{ mg}$$

$$\text{single IM injection} = (3977/8) \text{mg} \times \frac{1}{500 \text{ mg/mL}}$$

$$= 0.99 \text{ mL}$$

6. B.

$$\text{IBW} = 45.5 + (2.3 \times 8) = 64 \text{ kg}$$

7. C.

$$\text{weight} = \frac{154 \text{ lb}}{2.2 \text{ lb/kg}} = 70 \text{ kg}$$

$$\text{height} = 6 \text{ ft} \times 12 \text{ in/ft} \times 2.54 \text{ cm/in} = 183 \text{ cm}$$

$$\text{BSA} = \text{square root} \left[70 \times \frac{183}{3600} \right]$$

$$= \text{square root} [3.56] = 1.89 \text{ m}^2$$

8. D.

$$\text{child dose} = \text{adult dose} \times \frac{\text{child BSA}}{1.73} = 125 \text{ mg}$$

$$\times \frac{0.68 \text{ m}^2}{1.73 \text{ m}^2} = 49 \text{ mg}$$

9. A.

$$\text{CrCl} = 0.85 \times (140 - 65) \times \frac{50}{(72 \times 1.3)}$$

$$= 34 \text{ mL/min}$$

10. D. Note that the formula produces a total of 1000 g of the mixture. By proportions:

$$x \text{ g ZnO} : 150 \text{ g ZnO} = 800 \text{ g mix} : 1000 \text{ g}$$

$$x = 150 \text{ g} \times \frac{800 \text{ g}}{1000 \text{ g}} = 120 \text{ g}$$

11. B. Note that the formula produces a total of 20 parts of the mixture. By proportions:

$$x \text{ g kaolin} : 500 \text{ g mix}$$
$$= 12 \text{ parts kaolin} : 20 \text{ parts mix}$$

$$x = 500 \text{ g} \times \frac{12 \text{ parts}}{20 \text{ parts}} = 300 \text{ g}$$

12. C. By proportions:

$$x \text{ g hexachlorophene} : 20 \text{ g ung} = 1 \text{ part}$$

$$\text{hexachlorophene} : 400 \text{ parts ung}$$

$$x = 20 \text{ g} \times \frac{1 \text{ part}}{400 \text{ parts}} = 0.05 \text{ g} = 50 \text{ mg}$$

13. B. A 1 millimolar solution will contain 95.3 mg in 1000 mL. A 5 millimolar solution will contain 95.3 mg × 5 = 477 mg in 1000 mL. Thus, 200 mL of a 5 millimolar solution will contain 477 mg/5 = 95.3 mg in 200 mL.

14. E. Normal saline is 0.9% (w/v), or 0.9 g/100 mL = 9 g/1000 mL.

$$\text{milliosmolarity} = \left(\frac{9 \text{ g}}{58.5} \right) \times 2 \times 1000$$

$$= 308 \text{ mOsm/L}$$

15. B.

$$C_1 = 20\%, Q_1 = 250 \text{ mL}$$

$$C_2 = 15\%, Q_2 = x$$

$$C_1 \times Q_1 = C_2 \times Q_2$$

$$Q_2 = C_1 \times \frac{Q_1}{C_2} = 20\% \times \frac{250 \text{ mL}}{15\%}$$

$$= 333 \text{ mL}$$

added water = 333 mL – 250 mL = 83 mL

16. C.

20% (concentration of stock A)   15 – 5 = 10 = parts of A

15% (desired concentration)

5% (concentration of stock B)   20 – 15 = 5 = parts of B

Relative volumes are 10:5, or 2:1. Thus, 200 mL of a 20% dextrose solution (A) will require 100 mL of a 5% dextrose solution (B) to produce 300 mL of a 15% dextrose solution.

17. B.

$$20\% \times 200 \text{ mL} = 4000\% \text{ mL}$$

$$5\% \times 100 \text{ mL} = 500\% \text{ mL}$$

$$300 \text{ mL} = 4500\% \text{ mL}$$

$$\text{Mixture concentration} = \frac{4500\% \text{ mL}}{300 \text{ mL}} = 15\%$$

18. C.

900 mg of sodium chloride in 100 mL is isotonic:

$$x : 900 \text{ mg} = 30 \text{ mL} : 100 \text{ mL}$$

$$x = 900 \times \frac{30}{100} = 270 \text{ mg},$$

270 mg of sodium chloride would make 30 mL isotonic. But 1 g of ephedrine sulfate is equivalent to 0.23 g of sodium; thus,

$$y = 0.25 \text{ g} \times 0.23 = 0.058 \text{ g}$$

$$= 58 \text{ mg of sodium chloride}$$

Accordingly, the amount of sodium chloride to add $(z = x - y)$ is (270 mg – 58 mg) = 212 mg.

19. D. The bag contains 2000 mg in 500 mL, or 4 mg/mL. Therefore, a rate of 2 mg/min corresponds to 0.5 mL/min, which corresponds to 30 mL/h.

20. B. The 1% phenacaine HCl equals 0.6 g, and the 0.5% chlorobutanol equals 0.3 g. Using the E value of phenacaine HCl, we can write the ratio as follows:

$$\frac{0.6 \text{ g drug}}{1 \text{ g drug}} = \frac{x \text{ g NaCl}}{0.2 \text{ g NaCl}}$$

$$x = \frac{(0.2 \times 0.6)}{1}$$

= 0.12 g NaCl (amount of sodium chloride that is equivalent to 0.6 g drug)

Using the E value of chlorobutanol, we can write the ratio as follows:

$$\frac{0.3 \text{ g}}{1 \text{ g}} = \frac{x \text{ g NaCl}}{0.24 \text{ g NaCl}}$$

$$x = \frac{(0.3 \times 0.24)}{1}$$

= 0.072 g NaCl (amount of sodium chloride that is equivalent to 0.3 g chlorobutanol)

The amount of sodium chloride needed to make 60 mL of solution isotonic is calculated as follows:

$$\frac{0.9 \text{ g NaCl}}{x \text{ g NaCl}} = \frac{100 \text{ mL}}{60 \text{ mL}}$$

$$x = \frac{(0.9 \times 60)}{100}$$

= 0.54 g NaCl (amount of sodium chloride needed to make 60 mL of water isotonic if no drug or preservative were present)

amount of sodium chloride needed

$$= 0.54 \text{ g} - (0.12 \text{ g} + 0.072 \text{ g})$$

$$= 0.348 \text{ g NaCl}$$

Using the E value for boric acid, we can write the ratio as follows:

$$\frac{1\,g}{x\,g} = \frac{0.52\,g\,NaCl}{0.348\,g\,NaCl}$$

$$x = \frac{(1\,g \times 0.348\,g)}{0.52\,g}$$

$$= 0.67\,g \text{ (boric acid needed to make the prescription isotonic)}$$

21. A.

1 mEq of disodium hydrogen phosphate

$$= \frac{268\,mg}{2} = 134\,mg$$

1 mEq of disodium biphosphate

$$= \frac{138\,mg}{1} = 138\,mg$$

We can write the ratio as follows:

$$\frac{1\,mEq}{x\,mEq} = \frac{134\,mg}{18,000\,mg}$$

$$x = \frac{(18,000 \times 1)}{134} = 134.33\,mEq \text{ disodium hydrogen phosphate}$$

We can also write the ratio as follows:

$$\frac{1\,mEq}{x} = \frac{138\,mg}{48,000\,mg}$$

$$x = \frac{(1 \times 48,000)}{138} = 347.83\,mEq \text{ sodium biphosphate}$$

To adjust for volumes, we can write the ratios as follows:

$$\frac{134.33\,mEq}{x_1\,mEq} = \frac{100\,mL}{30\,mL} \text{ and}$$

$$\frac{347.83\,mEq}{x_2\,mEq} = \frac{100\,mL}{30\,mL}$$

Thus, $x_1 = 40.29$ mEq disodium hydrogen phosphate, and $x_2 = 104.34$ Eq sodium biphosphate. The total Na^+ mEq = 104.34 + 40.29 = 144.63 mEq.

22. D.

$$1\,mEq = \frac{147}{2} = 73.5\,mg$$

$$4\,mEq = 4 \times 73.5\,mg = 294\,mg/mL$$

$$= 0.294\,g/mL$$

23. D.

$$7.5\,mg/kg \times 60\,kg = 450\,mg$$

24. B.

$$52\,mL/h \times 1\,h \times 24 = 1248\,mL$$

25. C.

$$\frac{(52 \times 20)}{60} = \frac{x}{1\,min} = 17\,drops/min$$

26. B.

$$\frac{0.05\,g}{20\,g} = \frac{1}{x}, \text{ so } x = 400$$

27. A.

$$\frac{200,000\,units/mL}{1\,mL} = \frac{5,000,000}{x},$$

so $x = 25$ mL, and the volume of powder is $25 - 23 = 2$ mL

28. B.

$$\frac{5}{100} = \frac{20}{x}, \text{ so } x = 400\,g,$$

and the amount of ointment is $400 - 20 = 380$ g

29. E.

Dextrose kcal = 2400 mL × 0.2 g/mL × 3.4 kcal/g = 1632 kcal
Protein kcal = 2400 × 0.035 g/mL × 4 kcal/g = 336 kcal
Fat kcal = 2400 × 0.03 g/mL × 10 kcal/g = 720 kcal
Total kcal = 1632 kcal + 336 kcal + 720 kcal = 2688 kcal

30. C.

BMI = weight (kg)/height^2 (m)

weight = 175 lb ÷ 2.2 lb/kg = 79.5 kg

height = 5 ft 10 in = 70 in   70 in × 2.54 cm/in = 177.8 cm = 1.78 m

BMI = $79.5/1.78^2 = 25.1$

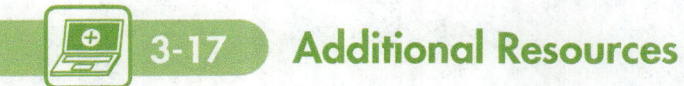

3-17   Additional Resources

Agarwal P. *Pharmaceutical Calculations*. Burlington, MA: Jones & Bartlett Learning; 2016.

Ansel HC, Stockton SJ. *Pharmaceutical Calculations*. 15th ed. Philadelphia: Wolters Kluwer and Lippincott Williams & Wilkins; 2017.

Holliday MA, Segar WE. The maintenance need for water in parenteral fluid therapy. *Pediatrics* 1957;19:823–832.

Mosteller RD: Simplified calculation of body-surface area. *N Engl J Med* 1987;317:1098.

O'Sullivan TA, Albrecht LS. *Understanding Pharmacy Calculations*. 2nd ed. Washington, DC: American Pharmacists Association; 2012.

Dosage Forms and Drug Delivery Systems

4

HASSAN ALMOAZEN

 4-1 KEY POINTS

- The drug delivery system deals with the pharmaceutical formulation of the drug and the dynamic interactions among the drug, its formulation matrix, its container, and the physiologic milieu of the patient. These dynamic interactions are the subject of pharmaceutics.
- The pharmaceutical dosage form contains the active drug ingredient in association with nondrug (usually inert) ingredients (excipients). Together they form the vehicle, or formulation matrix.
- Drug absorption depends on the fraction of the un-ionized form of the drug in gastrointestinal fluids and tissue surfaces plus the surface area available for absorption.
- Understand the relationship between the dissolution rate of a drug from its dosage form and drug solubility.
- Surfactants consist of hydrophilic and hydrophobic groups and can be used as emulsifying agents to reduce interfacial tensions and aid absorption.
- Water-soluble drugs are often formulated as sustained-release tablets to prolong drug release and control dissolution rates, whereas enteric-coated tablets are used to protect drugs from degradation in the stomach.
- Capsules are solid dosage forms with hard or soft gelatin shells that contain drugs and excipients.
- Aerosols are pressurized dosage forms designed to deliver drugs to pulmonary tissues with the aid of a liquefied or propelled gas.
- Transdermal patches deliver drugs through the skin into the bloodstream at a controlled rate.
- Macromolecular drug carriers, such as protein–polymer conjugates, and particulate delivery systems, such as microspheres and liposomes, are commonly used for delivery of drugs with low molecular weight, such as peptides and proteins, to different disease targets.
- Targeted or site-specific drug delivery systems deliver drugs to a tissue target or receptor site. These systems provide maximum therapeutic activity by preventing degradation during transit to the target site while avoiding delivery to nontarget sites.
- Several medications with high abuse potential have been formulated with abuse-deterrent properties.

 4-2 STUDY GUIDE CHECKLIST

The following topics may guide your study of this subject area:

- ☐ The relationship between the pH and the dissociation constant (pK_a) for a weak acid or a weak base drug and the way this relationship affects drug absorption.
- ☐ The relationship between solubility and dissolution rate for any drug and the major factors that affect both.
- ☐ Surfactants and micelles.
- ☐ Hydrophilic–lipophilic balance and the way it influences the formation of emulsions.
- ☐ Dispersed systems and different colloidal systems.
- ☐ Excipients and their functions in different dosage forms.

4-3   Introduction

Basic *pharmaceutics* includes the physicochemical properties of a drug—such as solubility and dissolution rate, hydrophilicity and hydrophobicity as characterized by oil-to-water partition coefficient ($K_{o/w}$), dissociation constant (pK_a), viscosity, and solid-state chemistry (amorphous and crystalline forms). A pharmaceutical *dosage form* is the delivery system that is administered to the patient so that an effective and safe dose of the drug is delivered. Typical examples of dosage forms are tablets, capsules, suppositories, parenterals, oral and nasal solutions, oral suspensions, metered dose inhalers, and transdermal patches. Achieving an optimal dose–response curve requires delivery of the drug to its site of action at a rate and a concentration that minimize its side effects and maximize its therapeutic effects. The development of safe and effective pharmaceutical dosage forms and delivery systems requires a thorough understanding of the basic pharmaceutics concepts that enable the drug to be formulated into a pharmaceutical dosage form. The successful design of a delivery system depends on the factors list in Box 4-1.

The pH Partition Theory and Dissociation Constant pK_a

The *pH partition theory* states that drugs are absorbed from the biological membranes by passive diffusion depending on the fraction of the un-ionized form of the drug at the pH of the fluids close to that of the biological membrane. The degree of ionization of the drug depends on both the pK_a and the pH of the drug solution. The gastrointestinal (GI) tract acts as a lipophilic barrier, and, thus, ionized drugs are more hydrophilic than un-ionized ones and have minimal membrane transport. The solution pH affects the overall partition coefficient of an ionizable substance. The pK_a of a molecule is the pH at which a 50:50 mixture of acid and conjugated base coexists in equilibrium. For an acidic drug, the acid form predominates at a pH lower than the pK_a, and the conjugated base form dominates at a pH higher than the pK_a. For a basic drug, the base form (un-ionized) dominates at pH values higher than the pK_a, and the conjugated acidic form (ionized) dominates at pH values below the pK_a. The extent of ionization of a drug molecule is given by the following Henderson–Hasselbalch equations, which describe a relationship between ionized and un-ionized species of a weak acid or base:

<table>
<tr><td>Weakly acidic drugs</td><td>Weakly basic drugs</td></tr>
<tr><td>$$pH = pK_a + \log\frac{[A^-]}{[HA]}$$</td><td>$$pH = pK_a + \log\frac{[B]}{[BH^+]}$$</td></tr>
</table>

where [HA] is the concentration of un-ionized acid, [A⁻] is the concentration of ionized acid, [B] is the concentration of un-ionized base, and [BH⁺] is the concentration of ionized base. Although pH partition theory is useful, it often does not hold true. For example, most weak acids are well absorbed from the small intestine, which is contrary to the prediction of the pH partition hypothesis. Similarly, quaternary ammonium compounds are ionized at all pH levels but are readily absorbed from the GI tract. These discrepancies arise because pH partition theory does not take into consideration the following factors, among others:

- Large epithelial surface areas of the small intestine compensate for ionization effects.
- Long residence time in the small intestine also compensates for ionization effects.

BOX 4-1. Factors of a Successful Delivery System

- Dose of the drug
- Route of administration
- Drug delivery system compatible with the drug's properties
- Rate and extent of drug release from the delivery system
- Bioavailability of the drug

- Charged drugs, such as quaternary ammonium compounds and tetracyclines, may interact with opposite-charged organic ions, resulting in a neutral species that is absorbable.
- Some drugs are absorbed by means of active transport.

Solubility

Drug solubility is the maximum amount of the drug that is soluble in unit volume of the solvent. For most drugs, the rate at which the solid drug dissolves in a solvent (dissolution) is often the rate-limiting step in the drug's bioavailability.

The following factors influence the dissolution rate:

- The conditions in the GI tract affect the dissolution rate. For example, the presence of foods that increase the viscosity of GI fluids decreases the movement of a drug and its dissolution rate.
- The degree of agitation experienced by each drug particle in the GI tract. Hence, an increase in gastric or intestinal motility may increase the dissolution rate of poorly soluble drugs.
- The dissolution rate of a weakly acidic drug in GI fluids is influenced by the drug solubility in the diffusion layer surrounding each dissolving drug particle. The pH of the diffusion layer significantly affects the solubility of a drug and its subsequent dissolution rate. The dissolution rate of a weakly acidic drug in GI fluid (pH 1 to 3) is relatively low because of its low solubility in the diffusion layer. If the pH in the diffusion layer could be increased, the solubility exhibited by the weakly acidic drug in this layer (and hence the dissolution rate of the drug in GI fluids) could be increased. The potassium or sodium salt form of the weakly acidic drug has a relatively high solubility at the elevated pH in the diffusion layer. Thus, the dissolution of the drug particles occurs at a faster rate. The reverse is true for weakly basic drugs; a reduction in pH of the diffusion layer would increase its solubility in the GI tract.
- Particle size and the surface area of the drug significantly influence the drug dissolution rate. An increase in the total effective surface area of the drug in contact with GI fluids causes an increase in its dissolution rate. The smaller the particle size is, the greater will be the effective surface area exhibited by a given mass of drug and the higher will be the dissolution rate. However, particle size reduction is not always helpful and may fail to increase the bioavailability of a drug. In the case of certain hydrophobic drugs, excessive particle size reduction tends to cause aggregation into larger particles. Preventing the formation of aggregates requires the dispersion of small drug particles in polyethylene glycol (PEG), polyvinylpyrrolidone (PVP), dextrose, or other agents. For example, a dispersion of griseofulvin in PEG 4000 enhances its dissolution rate and bioavailability. Certain drugs, such as penicillin G and erythromycin, are unstable in gastric fluids and do not dissolve readily. For such drugs, particle size reduction increases the rate of drug dissolution in gastric fluid but also increases the extent of drug degradation.
- Amorphous or noncrystalline forms of a drug may have faster dissolution rates than crystalline forms.
- Surface-active agents will increase dissolution rates by lowering interfacial tension, which allows better wetting and penetration by the solvent. Weakly acidic and basic drugs may be brought into solution by the solubilizing action of surfactants.

4-4 ▶ Surfactants and Micelles

Surface-active agents, or *surfactants,* are substances that adsorb to surfaces or interfaces to reduce surface or interfacial tension. They may be used as emulsifying agents, solubilizing agents, detergents, and wetting agents. Surfactants have two distinct regions in one chemical structure. One area is hydrophilic (water loving); another is hydrophobic (water repelling). The existence of two such moieties in a molecule is known as *amphipathy,* and the molecules are consequently referred to as *amphipathic molecules* or *amphiphiles.* Depending on the number and nature of the polar and nonpolar groups present, the amphiphile may be predominantly hydrophilic or lipophilic, or somewhere in between. For example, alkyl chain alcohols, amines, and acids are amphiphiles that change from being predominantly hydrophilic to lipophilic as the number of carbon atoms in the alkyl chain is increased. The hydrophobic portions are usually saturated or unsaturated hydrocarbon chains or, less commonly, heterocyclic or aromatic ring systems.

Surfactants are classified according to the nature of the hydrophilic or hydrophobic groups. In addition, some surfactants possess both positively and negatively charged groups and can exist as either anionic or cationic, depending on the pH of the solution.

At low concentrations in solutions, amphiphiles exist as monomers. As the concentration increases, aggregation occurs over a narrow concentration range. These aggregates, which may contain 50 or more monomers, are called *micelles*. Therefore, micelles are small spherical structures composed of both hydrophilic and hydrophobic regions. The polar head groups of the surfactant molecules are arranged in an outer shell while their hydrocarbon chains are oriented toward the center, forming a hydrophobic core. The concentration of monomers at which micelles are formed is called the *critical micellization concentration* (CMC). Surface tension decreases up to the CMC but remains constant above the CMC. The longer the hydrophobic chain or the lower the polarity of the polar group, the greater the tendency for monomers to escape from the water to form micelles and hence lower the CMC.

Hydrophilic–Lipophilic Balance Systems

A method of selecting emulsifying agents is based on the balance between the hydrophilic and lipophilic portions of the emulsifying agent, now widely known as the *hydrophilic–lipophilic balance (HLB) system*. The higher the HLB value of an emulsifying agent, the more hydrophilic is the agent. The emulsifying agents with lower HLB values are less polar and more lipophilic. The Spans (i.e., sorbitan esters) are lipophilic and have low HLB values (1.8 to 10); the Tweens (polyoxyethylene derivatives of the Spans) are hydrophilic and have high HLB values (10 to 16.7). Surfactants with the proper balance of hydrophilic and lipophilic affinities are effective emulsifying agents because they concentrate at the oil-in-water (o/w) interface. The type of emulsion produced depends primarily on the property of the emulsifying agent. The HLB of an emulsifier or a combination of emulsifiers determines whether an o/w or water-in-oil (w/o) emulsion results. In general, o/w emulsions are formed when the HLB of the emulsifier is within the range of about 9 to 12; w/o emulsions are formed when the range is about 3 to 6. The type of emulsion is a function of the relative solubility of the supernatant. An emulsifying agent with high HLB is preferentially soluble in water and results in the formation of an o/w emulsion. The reverse situation is true with surfactants of low HLB value, which tend to form w/o emulsions.

Micellar Solubilization

Micelles can be used to increase the solubility of materials that are normally insoluble or poorly soluble in the dispersion medium used. The interior of a micelle is composed of a hydrophobic core in which compounds that are poorly soluble in the dispersion medium can be dissolved. For example, surfactants are often used to increase the solubility of poorly soluble steroids. The factors affecting micellar solubilization are the nature of surfactants, the nature of solubilizates, and the temperature.

4-5   Dispersed Systems

Dispersed systems consist of particulate matter, known as the *dispersed phase*, distributed throughout a continuous or dispersion medium. The particulate matter, or dispersed phase, consists of particles that range from 1 nanometer (nm) to 0.5 micrometer (μm) (10^{-9} m to 5×10^{-7} m). Depending on the dispersed phase, dispersed systems are classified as follows:

- **True solutions:** Less than 1 nm, invisible under electron microscopy. Examples are oxygen molecules, ions, and glucose.
- **Colloidal dispersions:** From 1 nm to 0.5 µm, visible under electron microscopy. Examples are colloidal silver sols and natural and synthetic polymers.
- **Coarse dispersions:** Greater than 0.5 µm, visible under light microscopy. Examples are grains of sand, activated charcoal, emulsions, suspensions, and red blood cells.

4-6   Pharmaceutical Ingredients

Turning a drug into a pharmaceutical dosage form or a drug delivery system requires a compatible and desirable combination of the active drug(s) with excipients (ingredients that add liquid or solid mass to the medication, facilitate drug dissolution or bioavailability, optimize palatability, aid the manufacturing process, and promote product stability among other reasons specific to the product's intended characteristics). For example, in the preparation of tablets, the addition of diluents or fillers increases the bulk of the formulation. Binders are added to promote adhesion of the powdered drug to other ingredients. Lubricants assist the smooth tableting process. Disintegrants promote tablet breakup after administration. Coatings improve stability, control disintegration, or enhance appearance. In the preparation of pharmaceutical solutions, preservatives are added to prevent microbial growth, stabilizers are added to prevent drug decomposition, and colorants and flavorants are added to ensure product appeal. Thus, for each dosage form, the pharmaceutical ingredients establish the primary features of the product and control the physicochemical properties, drug-release profiles, and bioavailability of the product. Table 4-1 lists some typical pharmaceutical ingredients used in different dosage forms. Excipients are important factors in a drug's bioavailability (the extent of a drug absorbed into the body that is estimated by the ratio of the area under the curve of drug serum concentrations versus time for oral products compared to the area under the curve of serum concentrations versus time for the intravenous form of the drug; see Chapter 7 on pharmacokinetics).

4-7   Types of Commonly Used Dosage Forms

Solutions

Solutions are homogeneous mixtures of one or more solutes dispersed in a dissolving medium (solvent). Aqueous solutions containing a sugar or sugar substitute with or without added flavoring agents and drugs are classified as *syrups*. Sweetened hydroalcoholic (combinations of water and ethanol) solutions are termed *elixirs*. Hydroalcoholic solutions of aromatic materials are termed *spirits*. *Tinctures* are alcoholic or hydroalcoholic solutions of chemical or soluble constituents of vegetable drugs. Most tinctures are prepared by an extraction process. *Mouthwashes* are solutions used to cleanse the mouth or treat diseases of the oral membrane. *Antibacterial topical solutions* (e.g., benzalkonium chloride and strong iodine) will kill bacteria when applied to the skin or mucous membrane.

Solutions intended for oral administration usually contain flavorants and colorants to make the medication more attractive and palatable to the patient. They may contain stabilizers to maintain the physicochemical stability of the drug and preservatives to prevent the growth of microorganisms in the solution. A drug dissolved in an aqueous solution is in the solution; no dissolution step is necessary before systemic absorption occurs. Solutions that are prepared to be sterile, that are pyrogen free, and that are intended for parenteral administration are classified as *injectables*.

TABLE 4-1. Typical Pharmaceutical Ingredients

Ingredient type	Definition	Examples
Antifungal preservative	Used in liquid and semisolid formulations to prevent growth of fungi	Benzoic acid, butylparaben, ethylparaben, sodium benzoate, sodium propionate
Antimicrobial preservative	Used in liquid and semisolid formulations to prevent growth of microorganisms	Benzalkonium chloride, benzyl alcohol, cetylpyridinium chloride, phenyl ethyl alcohol
Antioxidant	Used to prevent oxidation	Ascorbic acid, ascorbyl palmitate, sodium ascorbate, sodium bisulfite, sodium metabisulfite
Binder	Used to cause adhesion of powder particles in tablet granulations	Acacia, alginic acid, ethylcellulose, povidone, starch
Diluent	Used as fillers to create desired bulk, flow properties, and compression characteristics in tablet and capsule preparations	Cellulose, kaolin, lactose, mannitol, sorbitol, starch
Disintegrant	Used to promote disruption of solid mass into small particles	Alginic acid, carboxymethylcellulose calcium, microcrystalline cellulose, sodium alginate, sodium starch glycolate,
Emulsifying agent	Used to promote and maintain dispersion of finely divided droplets of a liquid in a vehicle in which it is immiscible	Acacia, cetyl alcohol, glyceryl monostearate, sorbitan monostearate
Glidant	Used to improve flow properties of powder mixture	Colloidal silica, cornstarch, talc
Humectant	Used for prevention of dryness of ointments and creams	Glycerin, propylene glycol, sorbitol
Lubricant	Used to reduce friction during tablet compression and to facilitate ejection of tablets from the die cavity	Calcium stearate, magnesium stearate, mineral oil, stearic acid, zinc stearate
Plasticizer	Used to enhance coat spread over tablets, beads, and granules	Diethyl palmitate, glycerin
Surfactant	Used to reduce surface or interfacial tension	Polysorbate 80, sodium lauryl sulfate, sorbitan monopalmitate
Suspending agent	Used to reduce sedimentation rate of drug particles dispersed throughout a vehicle in which they are not soluble	Carbopol, hydroxymethylcellulose, hydroxypropyl cellulose, methylcellulose, tragacanth

Some drugs, particularly certain antibiotics, have insufficient stability in aqueous solution to withstand long shelf lives. These drugs are formulated as dry powder or granule dosage forms for reconstitution with purified water immediately before dispensing to the patient. The dry powder mixture contains all of the formulation components—that is, drug, flavorant, colorant, buffers, and others—except for the solvent. Examples of dry powder mixtures intended for reconstitution to make oral solutions include cloxacillin sodium, nafcillin sodium, oxacillin sodium, and penicillin V potassium.

Sucrose is the sugar most frequently used in syrups; in special circumstances, it may be replaced in whole or in part by other sugars (e.g., dextrose) or nonsugars (e.g., sorbitol, glycerin, and propylene glycol). Most syrups consist of between 60% and 80% sucrose. Sucrose not only provides sweetness and viscosity to the solution but also renders the solution inherently stable (unlike dilute sucrose solutions, which are unstable).

Compared with syrups, elixirs are usually less sweet and less viscous because they contain a lower proportion of sugar, and they are consequently less effective than syrups in masking the taste of drugs. In contrast to aqueous syrups, elixirs are better able to maintain both water-soluble and alcohol-soluble components in solution because of their hydroalcoholic properties. These stable characteristics often make elixirs preferable to syrups. All elixirs contain flavoring and coloring agents to enhance their palatability and appearance. Elixirs containing over 10% to 12% ethanol are usually self-preserving and do not require the addition of antimicrobial agents for preservation. Alcohols precipitate tragacanth, acacia, agar, and inorganic salts from aqueous solutions; therefore, such substances should either be absent from the aqueous phase or be present in such low concentrations as not to promote precipitation on standing. Some commonly used elixirs contain dexamethasone, pentobarbital, diphenhydramine, and digoxin.

Tablets

Types of tablets

Depending on the physicochemical properties of the drug, site and extent of drug absorption in the GI tract, stability to heat or moisture, biocompatibility with other ingredients, solubility, and dose, the following types of tablets are commonly formulated:

- *Swallowable tablets* are intended to be swallowed whole and then disintegrate and release their medicaments in the GI tract.
- *Effervescent tablets* are dissolved in water before administration. In addition to the drug substance, these tablets contain sodium bicarbonate and an organic acid such as tartaric acid. These additives react in the presence of water, liberating carbon dioxide, which acts as a disintegrator and produces effervescence.
- *Chewable tablets* are used when a faster rate of dissolution or buccal absorption is desired. Chewable tablets consist of a mild effervescent drug complex dispersed throughout a gum base. The drug is released from the dosage form by physical disruption associated with chewing, chemical disruption caused by the interaction with the fluids in the oral cavity, and the presence of effervescent material. For example, antacid tablets should be chewed to obtain quick relief of indigestion.
- *Buccal* and *sublingual tablets* dissolve slowly in the mouth, cheek pouch (buccal), or under the tongue (sublingual). Buccal or sublingual absorption is often desirable for drugs subject to extensive hepatic metabolism, often referred to as the *first-pass effect*. Examples are isoprenaline sulfate (a bronchodilator), nitroglycerin (a vasodilator, also known as glyceryl trinitrate), and testosterone tablets. These tablets do not contain a disintegrant and are compressed lightly to produce a fairly soft tablet.
- *Lozenges* are compressed tablets that do not contain a disintegrant. Some lozenges contain antiseptics (e.g., benzalkonium) or antibiotics for local effects in the mouth.
- *Controlled-release tablets* are used to improve patient compliance and to reduce side effects. Some water-soluble drugs are formulated as sustained-release tablets so that their release and dissolution are controlled over a long period. The combination of high- and low-viscosity grades of hydroxypropyl methylcellulose (HPMC) was used as the matrix base to prepare zileuton sustained-release tablets. A ternary polymeric matrix system composed of protein, HPMC, and highly water-soluble drugs such as **diltiazem** hydrochloride was developed by the direct compression method. Sustained-release tablets can also be prepared by formulating inert polymers such as polyvinyl chloride, polyvinyl acetate, and methyl methacrylate. These polymers protect the tablet from disintegration and reduce the dissolution rate of the drug inside the tablet. Examples of commonly used sustained-release drug delivery products are listed in Table 4-2.
- *Coated tablets* are used to prevent decomposition or to minimize the unpleasant taste of certain drugs. The different types of coatings include tablets that are film coated, sugar coated, gelatin coated (gel caps), or enteric coated. Enteric coatings are resistant to gastric juices but readily dissolve in the small intestine. These enteric coatings can protect drugs against decomposition in the acidic environment of the stomach. Commonly used polymers for enteric coating are acid-impermeable polymers such as cellulose acetate trimellitate, HPMC phthalate, polyvinyl acetate phthalate, cellulose acetate phthalate, and EUDRAGIT. Film-coated tablets are compressed tablets coated with a thin layer of a water-insoluble or water-soluble polymer such as methylcellulose phthalate,

TABLE 4-2. Examples of Sustained-Release Drug Delivery Products

Dosage forms	Active ingredients	Indications
Controlled-release tablets		
Abacavir (Ziagen)	Nucleoside reverse transcriptase inhibitor	HIV-1 infection
Sinemet	Carbidopa + levodopa	Parkinson's disease
Voltaren	**Diclofenac sodium**	Osteoarthritis and rheumatoid arthritis
Capsules		
Dexedrine Spansules	**Dextroamphetamine**	Narcolepsy
Adderall XL	**Amphetamine + dextroamphetamine**	Attention-deficit/hyperactivity disorder (ADHD)
Ritalin LA	**Methylphenidate hydrochloride**	ADHD
Videx EC	Didanosine	HIV-1 infection
Aerosols		
Ventolin HFA	**Albuterol sulfate**	Bronchodilator
Serevent	**Salmeterol**	Bronchodilator
Osmotic systems		
Ditropan XL	**Oxybutynin chloride**	Overreactive bladder
Covera-HS	Verapamil	Antihypertensive
Concerta	**Methylphenidate HCl**	ADHD
Inserts		
Lacrisert	Hydroxypropyl cellulose	Ophthalmic moisturizer
Atridox	Doxycycline	Periodontal disease
Transdermal patches		
Alora	**Estradiol**	Menopausal symptoms
CombiPatch	**Estradiol/norethindrone acetate**	Vasomotor symptoms associated with menopause
Androderm	Testosterone	Testosterone deficiency
Nicotine transdermal system	Nicotine	Smoking cessation
PEGylated protein		
PEGASYS	PEGylated interferon + ribavirin	Hepatitis B, hepatitis C
Liposomes		
Doxil	Doxorubicin HCl	Kaposi's sarcoma
DaunoXome	Daunorubicin	Kaposi's sarcoma
Poly(lactic-co-glycolic acid)/polylactic acid microspheres		
Lupron Depot	Luteinizing hormone-releasing hormone agonist	Prostate cancer, endometriosis
Zoladex Depot	Goserelin acetate	Prostate cancer, endometriosis
Nutropin Depot	Recombinant human growth hormone	Growth deficiencies

Boldface indicates one of top 100 drugs for 2020 by prescription volume.
HIV, human immunodeficiency virus.

ethylcellulose, povidone, or PEG. Abacavir is a capsule-shaped, film-coated tablet containing a nucleoside reverse transcriptase inhibitor, which is a potent antiviral agent for the treatment of HIV (human immunodeficiency virus) infection.

Tablet formulation

In addition to the drug, the following materials are added to make the powder system compatible with tablet formulation by the compression or granulation methods:

- *Diluents* or bulking agents are invariably added to very-low-dose drugs to bring overall tablet weight to at least 50 mg, which is the minimum desirable tablet weight. Commonly used diluents are lactose, starches, microcrystalline cellulose, dextrose, sucrose, mannitol, and sodium chloride. Dicalcium phosphate absorbs less moisture than lactose and is, therefore, used with hygroscopic drugs such as meperidine hydrochloride.

- *Adsorbents* are substances capable of holding quantities of fluids in an apparently dry state. Oil-soluble drugs or fluid extracts can be mixed with adsorbents and then granulated and compressed into tablets. Examples are fumed silica, microcrystalline cellulose, magnesium carbonate, kaolin, and bentonite.

- *Moistening agents* are liquids that are used for wet granulation. Examples include water, industrial methylated spirits, and isopropanol.

- *Binding agents (adhesives)* bind powders together in the wet granulation process. They also help bind granules together during compression. Examples include starches, gelatin, PVP, alginic acid derivatives, cellulose derivatives, glucose, and sucrose. Choice of binders affects the dissolution rate. For example, the tablet formulation of **furosemide** with PVP as the binder has a t_{50} (time required for 50% of the drug to be released during an in vitro dissolution study) of 3.65 minutes, but with starch mucilage as the binder, the t_{50} of the tablets was 117 minutes.

- *Glidants* are added to tablet formulations to improve the flow properties of the granulations. They act by reducing interparticle friction. Commonly used glidants are fumed (colloidal) silica, starch, and talc.

- *Lubricants* have a number of functions in tablet manufacture. They prevent adherence of the tablet material to the surfaces of the punch faces and dies, reduce interparticle friction, and facilitate the smooth ejection of the tablet from the die cavity. Many lubricants also enhance the flow properties of the granules. Commonly used lubricants are magnesium stearate, talc, stearic acid and its derivatives, PEG, paraffin, and sodium or magnesium lauryl sulfate. Among these lubricants, magnesium stearate is the most popular because it is effective as both a die and a punch lubricant. However, for many drugs (e.g., **aspirin**), magnesium stearate is chemically incompatible; therefore, talc or stearic acid is often used. Most lubricants, with the exception of talc, are used in concentrations below 1%.

- *Disintegrating agents* are added to tablets to promote breakup or disintegration after administration, which increases the effective surface area and promotes rapid release of the drug. Disintegrants act either by bursting open the tablet or by promoting the rapid ingress of water into the center of the tablet or capsule. Examples include starches, cationic exchange resins, cross-linked PVP, celluloses, modified starches, alginic acid and alginates, magnesium aluminum silicate, and cross-linked sodium carboxymethylcellulose. Among these agents, starch is the most popular disintegrant because it has a great affinity for water and swells when moistened, thus facilitating the rupture of the tablet matrix.

Disintegration, dissolution, and absorption

A solid drug product must disintegrate into small particles and release the drug before absorption can take place. Tablets that are intended for chewing or sustained release do not have to undergo disintegration.

The various excipients for tablet formulation affect the rates of disintegration, dissolution, and absorption. Systemic absorption of most products consists of a succession of processes such as the following:

- Disintegration of the drug product and subsequent release of the drug
- Dissolution of the drug in an aqueous environment
- Absorption across cell membranes into the systemic circulation

In the process of tablet disintegration, dissolution, and absorption, the rate at which the drug reaches the circulatory system is determined by the slowest step in the sequence. Disintegration of a tablet is usually more rapid than drug dissolution and absorption. For the drug that has poor aqueous solubility, the rate at which the drug dissolves (dissolution) is often the slowest step, and it, therefore, exerts a rate-limiting effect on drug bioavailability. In contrast, for the drug that has a high aqueous solubility, the dissolution rate is rapid, and the rate at which the drug crosses or permeates cell membranes is the slowest, or rate-limiting, step.

Capsules

Capsules are the dosage forms in which unit doses of powder, semisolid, or liquid drugs are enclosed in a hard or soft, water-soluble container or shell of gelatin. Coating of the capsule shell or drug particles within the capsule can affect bioavailability. There are two types of capsules: hard and soft gelatin capsules. Hard gelatin capsules are more versatile for controlled drug delivery.

Hard gelatin capsules

A hard gelatin capsule consists of two pieces, a cap and a body, that fit one inside the other. They are produced empty and are then filled in a separate operation. Hard gelatin capsules are usually filled with powders, granules, or pellets containing the drug. After ingestion, the gelatin shell softens, swells, and begins to dissolve in the GI tract. Encapsulated drugs are released rapidly and dispersed easily, leading to high bioavailability. Capsules are supplied in a variety of sizes, and high-speed filling machinery capable of filling approximately 1500 capsules per minute is available. The empty hard gelatin capsules are numbered from 000, the largest size, to 5, the smallest. The approximate filling capacity of capsules ranges from 6000 to 30 mg, depending on the types and bulk densities of powdered drug materials. Capsule forms of nonprescription drugs must have their edges sealed to comply with the federal Tamper Resistant Packaging Act.

Powder formulations for encapsulation into hard gelatin capsules require careful consideration of the filling process, such as lubricity, compactibility, and fluidity. Additives present in the capsule formulations, such as the amount and choice of fillers and lubricants, the inclusion of disintegrants and surfactants, and the degree of plug compaction, can influence drug release from the capsule.

Soft gelatin capsules

Soft gelatin capsules are prepared from plasticized gelatin by a rotary die process. They are formed, filled, and sealed in a single operation. Soft gelatin capsules may contain a nonaqueous solution, a powder, or a drug suspension, none of which solubilizes the gelatin shell. In contrast to hard gelatin capsules, soft gelatin capsules contain about 30% glycerol as a plasticizer in addition to gelatin and water. The moisture uptake of soft gelatin capsules plasticized with glycerol is considerably higher than that of hard gelatin capsules. Therefore, oxygen-sensitive drugs should not be inserted into soft gelatin capsules, nor should emulsions, because they are unstable and crack the shell of the capsule when water is lost in the manufacturing process. Extreme acidic and basic pH ingredients must also be avoided because a pH below 2.5 hydrolyzes gelatin, whereas a pH above 9.0 has a tanning effect on the gelatin. Insoluble drugs should be dispersed with an agent such as beeswax, paraffin, or ethylcellulose. Surfactants are also often added to promote wetting of the ingredients. Drugs and other ingredients that are commercially prepared in soft capsules include Declomycin, chloral hydrate, vitamin A, and vitamin E.

Emulsions

An *emulsion* is a thermodynamically unstable system that consists of at least two immiscible liquid phases—one of which is dispersed as globules (dispersed phase) and the other as a liquid phase (continuous phase)—that are stabilized by the presence of an emulsifying agent. Emulsified systems range from lotions of relatively low viscosity to ointments and creams, which are semisolid in nature.

Types of emulsions

One liquid phase in an emulsion is essentially polar (e.g., aqueous), whereas the other is relatively nonpolar (e.g., an oil).

- *Oil-in-water emulsion:* When the oil phase is dispersed as globules throughout an aqueous continuous phase, the system is referred to as an oil-in-water emulsion.
- *Water-in-oil emulsion:* When the oil phase serves as the continuous phase, the emulsion is termed a *water-in-oil emulsion.*
- *Multiple (w/o/w or o/w/o) emulsions:* These are emulsions whose dispersed phase contains droplets of another phase. Multiple emulsions are of interest as delayed-action drug delivery systems.
- *Microemulsions:* These consist of homogeneous transparent systems of low viscosity that contain a high percentage of both oil and water and high concentrations of emulsifier mixture. Microemulsions form spontaneously when the components are mixed in the appropriate ratios, and they are thermodynamically stable.

Externally applied emulsions may be o/w or w/o. The o/w emulsions use the following emulsifiers: sodium lauryl sulfate, triethanolamine stearate, sodium oleate, and glyceryl monostearate. The w/o emulsions are used mainly for external applications and may contain one or several of the following emulsifiers: calcium palmitate, sorbitan esters (Spans), cholesterol, and wool fats.

Types of instability in emulsions

The stability of an emulsion is characterized by the absence of coalescence of the internal phase; the absence of creaming; and the maintenance of elegance with respect to appearance, odor, color, and other physical properties. An emulsion becomes unstable because of creaming, breaking, coalescence, phase inversion, and some other factors.

Creaming and sedimentation

Creaming is the upward movement of dispersed droplets relative to the continuous phase, whereas *sedimentation,* the reverse process, is the downward movement of particles. Density differences in the two phases cause these processes, which can be reversed by shaking. Creaming is undesirable, however, because a creamed emulsion increases the likelihood of coalescence owing to the proximity of the globules in the cream. Factors that influence the rate of creaming are similar to those involved in the sedimentation rate of suspension particles and are indicated by Stokes's law. The rate of creaming is decreased by the following:

- A reduction in the globule size
- A decrease in the density difference between the two phases
- An increase in the viscosity of the continuous phase

This decrease may be achieved by homogenizing the emulsion to reduce the globule size and increasing the viscosity of the continuous phase with the use of thickening agents such as tragacanth or methylcellulose.

Breaking, coalescence, and aggregation

Creaming is a reversible process, whereas breaking is irreversible. When *breaking* occurs, simple mixing fails to resuspend the globules in a stable emulsified form. Because the film surrounding the particles has been destroyed, the oil tends to coalesce. *Coalescence* is the process by which emulsified particles merge with each other to form large particles. The major factor preventing coalescence is the mechanical strength of the interfacial barrier. Formation of a thick interfacial film is essential for minimal coalescence. In *aggregation,* the dispersed droplets come together but do not fuse. Aggregation is to some extent reversible.

Phase inversion

An emulsion inverts when it changes from an o/w to a w/o emulsion or vice versa. Inversion can be caused by adding an electrolyte or by changing the phase-to-volume ratio. For example, an o/w emulsion stabilized with sodium stearate can be inverted to a w/o emulsion by adding calcium chloride to form calcium stearate.

Microbial growth

Growth of microorganisms in an emulsion can cause physical separation of the phases. Because bacteria can degrade nonionic and anionic emulsifying agents, preservatives must be added to the product in adequate concentrations to prevent bacterial growth.

Suspensions

Suspensions are dispersions of finely divided solid particles of a drug in a liquid medium in which the drug is not readily soluble. Suspending agents are often hydrophilic colloids (e.g., cellulose derivatives, acacia, or xanthan gum) added to suspensions to increase viscosity, inhibit agglomeration, and decrease sedimentation. Highly viscous suspensions may prolong gastric emptying time, slow drug dissolution, and decrease the absorption rate. A suspension that is thixotropic as well as pseudoplastic should prove useful because it forms a gel on standing and becomes fluid when disturbed.

Desired characteristics of suspensions are as follows:

- Suspended material should settle slowly and should readily disperse on gentle shaking of the container.
- Particle size of the suspension should remain fairly constant.
- The suspension should pour readily and evenly from its container.

Ointments, Creams, and Gels

Ointments, creams, and gels are semisolid preparations intended for topical applications. These semisolid formulations are designed for local or systemic drug absorption.

Ointments are typically used as follows:

- Emollients to make the skin more pliable
- Protective barriers to prevent harmful substances from coming in contact with the skin
- Vehicles in which to incorporate medication

Ointment bases are classified into four general groups: (1) hydrocarbon bases, (2) absorption bases, (3) water-removable bases, and (4) water-soluble bases.

Hydrocarbon bases

Hydrocarbon (oleaginous) bases are anhydrous and insoluble in water. They cannot absorb or contain water and are not washable in water.

Petrolatum is a good base for oil-insoluble ingredients. It forms an occlusive film on the skin and absorbs less than 5% water under normal conditions. Wax can be incorporated to stiffen the base. Synthetic esters are used as constituents of oleaginous bases. These esters include glycerol monostearate, isopropyl myristate, isopropyl palmitate, butyl stearate, and butyl palmitate.

Absorption bases

Absorption bases are of two types: (1) those that permit the incorporation of aqueous solutions, resulting in the formation of w/o emulsions (e.g., hydrophilic petrolatum and anhydrous lanolin), and (2) those that are already w/o emulsions (emulsion bases) and, thus, permit the incorporation of small additional quantities of aqueous solutions (e.g., lanolin and cold cream). These bases are useful as emollients although they do not provide the degree of occlusion afforded by the oleaginous bases. Absorption bases are also not easily removed from the skin with water. An aqueous solution may first be incorporated into the absorption base, and then this mixture is added to the oleaginous base.

Water-removable bases

Emulsion, water-washable, or water-removable bases, commonly referred to as creams, represent the most commonly used type of ointment base. The majority of dermatologic drug products are formulated in an emulsion or cream base. Emulsion bases are washable and removed easily from skin or clothing. An emulsion base can be subdivided into three component parts: the oil phase, the emulsifier, and the aqueous phase. Drugs can be included in one of these phases or added to the formed emulsion. The oil phase, also known as the *internal phase,* is typically made up of petrolatum or liquid petrolatum together with cetyl or stearyl alcohol. Types of emulsion bases are as follows:

- *Hydrophilic ointment* is an o/w emulsion that uses sodium lauryl sulfate as an emulsifying agent. It is readily miscible with water and is removed from the skin easily. The aqueous phase of an emulsion base contains the preservatives that are included to control microbial growth. The preservatives in the emulsion include methylparaben, propylparaben, benzyl alcohol, sorbic acid, or quaternary ammonium compounds. The aqueous phase also contains the water-soluble components of the emulsion system, together with any additional stabilizers, antioxidants, and buffers that may be necessary for stability and pH control.
- *Cold cream* is a semisolid white w/o emulsion prepared with cetyl ester wax, white wax, mineral oil, sodium borate, and purified water. Sodium borate combines with free fatty acids present in the waxes to form sodium soaps that act as the emulsifiers. Cold cream is used as an emollient and ointment base. Eucerin cream is a w/o emulsion of petrolatum, mineral oil, mineral wax, wool wax, alcohol, and bronopol. It is frequently prescribed as a vehicle for delivery of lactic acid and glycerin to treat dry skin.
- *Lanolin* is a w/o emulsion that contains approximately 25% water and acts as an emollient and occlusive film on the skin, effectively preventing epidermal water loss.
- *Vanishing cream* is an o/w emulsion that contains a large percentage of water as well as a humectant (e.g., glycerin or propylene glycol) that retards surface evaporation. An excess of stearic acid in the formula helps to form a thin film when the water evaporates.

Water-soluble bases

Water-soluble bases may be anhydrous or may contain some water. They are washable in water and absorb water to the point of solubility. PEG ointment is a blend of water-soluble PEG that forms a semi-solid base. This base can solubilize water-soluble drugs and some water-insoluble drugs. It is compatible with a wide variety of drugs. It contains 40% PEG 4000 and 60% PEG 400. Another water-soluble base is the ointment prepared with propylene glycol and ethanol, which form a clear gel when mixed with 2% hydroxypropyl cellulose. This base is a commonly used dermatologic vehicle.

Incorporation of drugs into an ointment

Drugs may be incorporated into an ointment base by levigation and fusion. Normally, drug substances are in fine-powdered forms before being dispersed in the vehicle. Levigation of powders into a small portion of base is facilitated by the use of a melted base or a small quantity of compatible levigation aid, such as mineral oil or glycerin. Water-soluble salts are incorporated by dissolving them in a small volume of water and incorporating the aqueous solution into a compatible base. Fusion is used when the base contains solids that have higher melting points (e.g., waxes, cetyl alcohol, or glyceryl monostearate).

Suppositories

A *suppository* is a solid dosage form intended for insertion into body orifices (e.g., rectum, vagina, or urethra). Once inserted, the suppository base melts, softens, or dissolves at body temperature, distributing its medications to the tissues of the region. Suppositories are used for local or systemic effects. Rectal suppositories intended for local action are often used to relieve the pain, irritation, itching, and inflammation associated with hemorrhoids. Vaginal suppositories intended for local effects are used mainly as contraceptives, antiseptics in feminine hygiene, and methods to combat invading pathogens.

The suppository base has a marked influence on the release of active constituents. Two main classes of suppository bases are in use: the glyceride-type fatty bases and the water-soluble ones. The main water-soluble and water-miscible suppository bases are glycerinated gelatin and PEGs. PEG suppositories do not melt at body temperature but rather dissolve slowly in the body's fluids. Examples of rectal suppositories include **acetaminophen** and promethazine.

Inserts, Implants, and Devices

Inserts, implants, and devices are used to control drug delivery for localized or systemic drug effects. In these systems, drugs are embedded into biodegradable or nonbiodegradable materials to allow slow release of the drug. The inserts, implants, and devices are inserted into a variety of cavities (e.g., vagina, buccal cavity, cul de sac of the eye) or subcutaneous tissue.

Transdermal Drug Delivery Systems

Transdermal drug delivery systems (often called *transdermal patches*) deliver drugs directly through the skin and into the bloodstream. Percutaneous absorption of a drug generally results from direct penetration of the drug through the stratum corneum. Once through the stratum corneum, drug molecules may pass through the deeper epidermal tissues and into the dermis. When the drug reaches the vascularized dermal area, it becomes available for absorption into the general circulation. Among the factors influencing percutaneous absorption are the physicochemical properties of the drug, including its molecular weight, solubility, and partition coefficient; the nature of the vehicle; and the condition of the skin. Chemical permeation enhancers or iontophoresis are often used to enhance the percutaneous absorption of a drug.

In general, patches are composed of three key components: a protective seal that forms the external surface and protects it from damage, a compartment that holds the medication itself and has an adhesive backing to hold the entire patch on the skin surface, and a release liner that protects the adhesive layer during storage and is removed just before application. Examples of transdermal patches include those with **estradiol** (Estraderm, Alora), nicotine (NicoDerm CQ), and testosterone (Testoderm, Androderm). Controlled release of scopolamine through the skin (Transderm Scōp) relies on rate-limiting polymeric membranes.

Aerosol Products

Aerosols are pressurized dosage forms designed to deliver drugs with the aid of a liquefied or propelled gas (propellant). Aerosol products consist of a pressurizable container, a valve that allows the pressurized product to be expelled from the container when the actuator is pressed, and a dip tube that conveys the formulation from the bottom of the container to the valve assembly. Inhalation devices broadly fall into three categories: pressurized metered dose inhalers (MDIs), nebulizers, and dry powder inhalers. The most commonly used inhalers on the market are MDIs. They contain an active ingredient as a solution or as a suspension of fine particles in a liquefied propellant held under high pressure. MDIs use special metering valves to regulate the amount of formulation dispensed with each dose. Nebulizers do not require propellants and can generate large quantities of small droplets capable of penetrating into the lung. Sustained release of drugs, such as bronchodilators and corticosteroids for the treatment of asthma and chronic obstructive pulmonary diseases, involves encapsulation of the drugs in slowly degrading particles that can be inhaled. For accumulation in the alveolar zone of the lungs, which has a very large surface area, inhaled liquid or dry powder aerosols should have particle sizes in the range of 1 to 5 μm. Inhaled drugs play a prominent role in the treatment of asthma because this route has significant advantages over oral or parenteral administration. Azmacort (triamcinolone acetonide), Ventolin HFA (**albuterol sulfate**), and Serevent Diskus (**salmeterol**) are examples of commercially available aerosols for the treatment of asthma.

4-8 ▶ Targeted Drug Delivery Systems

Targeted drug delivery systems are drug carrier systems that deliver the drug to the target or receptor site in a manner that provides maximum therapeutic activity, prevents degradation or inactivation during transit to the target sites, and protects the body from adverse reactions because of inappropriate disposition. Design of an effective delivery system requires a thorough understanding of the drug, the disease, and the target site (Figure 4-1). Examples include macromolecular drug carriers (protein drug carriers); particulate drug delivery systems (e.g., microspheres, nanospheres, and liposomes); monoclonal antibodies; and cells. Plasma clearance kinetics, tissue distribution, metabolism, and cellular interactions of a drug can be controlled by the use of a site-specific delivery system. Targeting of drugs to specific sites in the body can be achieved by linking particulate systems or macromolecular carriers to monoclonal antibodies or to cell-specific ligands (e.g., asialofetuin, glycoproteins, or immunoglobulins) or by altering the surface characteristics so that they are not recognized by the reticuloendothelial system.

Particulate Drug Delivery Systems

Many particulate carriers have been designed for drug delivery and targeting. They include liposomes, micelles (see discussion of micelles earlier in the chapter), microspheres, and nanoparticles.

Liposomes

Liposomes are microscopic phospholipid vesicles composed of uni- or multilamellar lipid bilayers surrounding compartments. Multilamellar vesicles have diameters in the range of 1.0 to 5.0 μm. Sonication of multilamellar vesicles results in the production of small unilamellar vesicles with diameters in the range of

FIGURE 4-1. Essential Components of Drug Delivery

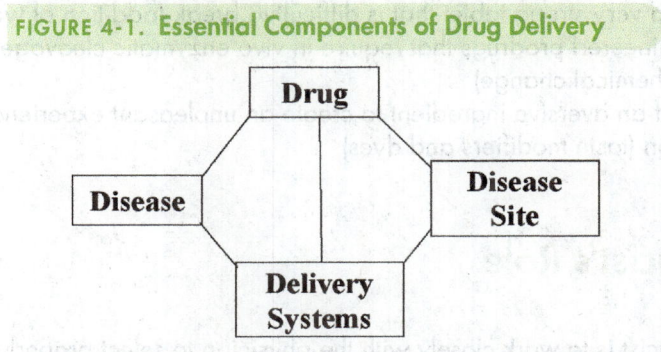

0.02 to 0.08 μm. The bilayer-forming lipid is the essential part of the lamellar structure, while the other compounds are added to impart certain characteristics to the vesicles. Water-soluble drugs can be entrapped in liposomes by intercalation in the aqueous bilayers, whereas lipid-soluble drugs can be entrapped within the hydrocarbon interiors of the lipid bilayers. Liposomes can encapsulate low-molecular-weight drugs, proteins, peptides, oligonucleotides, and genes. The antifungal agent amphotericin B is formulated in liposomes in the intravenous product AmBisome. Because conventional liposomes can be recognized by the immune system as foreign bodies, stealth liposomes evade recognition by the immune system on account of their unique PEG coating. Doxil is a stealth liposome formulation of doxorubicin that is used for the treatment of AIDS-related Kaposi's sarcoma.

Microparticles and nanoparticles

Microencapsulation is a technique that involves the encapsulation of small particles or the solution of drugs in a polymer film or coat. Different methods of microencapsulation result in either microcapsules or microspheres. For example, interfacial polymerization of a monomer usually produces microcapsules, whereas solvent evaporation may result in microspheres or microcapsules, depending on the amount of drug loading. A *microcapsule* is a reservoir-type system in which the drug is located centrally within the particle, whereas a *microsphere* is a matrix-type system in which the drug is dispersed throughout the particle. Microcapsules usually release their drug at a constant rate (*zero-order release*), whereas microspheres typically give a first-order release of drugs. Low-molecular-weight drugs, proteins, oligonucleotides, and genes can be encapsulated into microparticles to provide their sustained release at disease sites.

The hydrophilic substance, which acts as a coating material, may be selected from a variety of natural and synthetic polymers, including shellacs, waxes, gelatin, starches, cellulose acetate phthalate, and ethylcellulose among others. Following dissolution of the coating materials, the drug inside the microcapsule is available for dissolution and absorption.

Biodegradable polylactide and its copolymers with glycolide—poly(lactic-co-glycolic acid), or PLGA—are commonly used for preparation of microparticles from which the drug can be released slowly over a period of a month or so. Microspheres can be used in a wide variety of dosage forms, including tablets, capsules, and suspensions. Lupron Depot is a preparation of PLGA microspheres for sustained release of leuprolide, a small peptide analog of gonadotropin-releasing hormone.

Abuse-Deterrent Oral Dosage Forms

Abuse-deterrent formulations are designed to discourage and prevent attempts by the user to extract the active ingredient to enhance the euphorigenic effect by improvised methods of administration (e.g., injecting, chewing, snorting, or smoking). Several technologies are used in the pharmaceutical industry to design deterrent dosage forms (Table 4-3). These include the following:

- Incorporation of an excipient that gels when mixed with water, alcohol, or other solvents (viscosity modifiers)
- Incorporation of a physical barrier that resists crushing, dissolving, melting, or chemical extraction (insoluble plastic coating or incorporating of waxy materials)
- Formulation of a very strong tablet that is difficult to break (addition of waxy excipients)
- Chemically engineered prodrugs that require in vivo enzymatic cleavage to produce a pharmacological effect (chemical change)
- Incorporation of an aversive ingredient to create an unpleasant experience and thereby deter further extraction (taste modifiers and dyes)

4-9   Pharmacist's Role

The role of a pharmacist is to work closely with the physician to select properly the suitable dosage form for the patient. The dosage form should meet the clinical needs and age of the patient. For example, if

TABLE 4-3. Some Abuse-Deterrent Dosage Forms Currently on the Market

Drug(s)	Brand name	Dosage form	Abuse-deterrent mechanism
Buprenorphine + naloxone	**Suboxone**	Sublingual film	Naloxone is the deterrent component.
Hydrocodone bitartrate	Hysingla ER	Extended-release tablet	Tablet is difficult to crush or break and forms a thick gel when dissolved in water.
	Zohydro ER	Extended-release capsule	Capsule is a mixture of indistinguishable active immediate-release and active extended-release hydrocodone beads and inactive beads with no drug. Beads form a gel when crushed.
Hydromorphone HCl	Exalgo	Extended-release tablet	Tablet is crush and extraction resistant and uses push–pull osmotic delivery system.
Oxycodone HCl	**Oxaydo**	Immediate-release tablet	Tablet uses active and inactive ingredients that gel or cause nasal irritation.
	OxyContin	Controlled-release tablet	Tablet forms a gel that is difficult to inject or snort.

Boldface indicates one of top 100 drugs for 2020 by prescription volume.

a pediatric patient cannot swallow a tablet, the pharmacist should notify the physician that a liquid formulation is commercially available, instead of crushing regular tablets and mixing with juice or food for the patient. If the patient cannot take 3 or 4 tablets per day and a sustained release tablet is available, the pharmacist should inform the patient about the availability of sustained release tablets. If a patient is vomiting, a suppository dosage form is more convenient to take than an oral tablet. The pharmacist is the only health care provider who has an extensive knowledge of the composition and function of any dosage form and understands the advantages and disadvantages of the dosage forms available on the market.

NAPLEX Competency Statements

The questions in this chapter cover the following 2021 NAPLEX Competency Statements: **AREA 2:** 2.1 **AREA 3:** 3.5 **AREA 4:** 4.2; 4.5; 4.6.

 4-10 **Questions**

1. If the pK$_a$ of a weak acid drug is 2.5, at which pH will this drug become most ionized?

   A. pH 5
   B. pH 2.5
   C. pH 1.5
   D. pH 1
   E. pH 2

2. Which equation is used to calculate the pH of a buffer system?

   A. Henderson–Hasselbalch
   B. Noyes–Whitney
   C. Michaelis–Menten
   D. Yong's module
   E. Stokes–Einstein equation

3. If the pK$_a$ of a drug is 5, at which of the following pH values do the ionic and nonionic forms of the drug exist in equal ratio?

A. pH 1
B. pH 5
C. pH 7
D. pH 9
E. pH 3

4. What is bioavailability?

A. It is the measurement of the rate and extent of active drug that reaches the systemic circulation.
B. It is the relationship between the physical and chemical properties of a drug and its systemic absorption.
C. It is the movement of the drug into body tissues over time.
D. It is the dissolution of the drug in the GI tract.
E. It is the relationship between ionized drug and nonionized drug

5. What condition usually increases the rate of drug dissolution for a tablet? (Mark all that apply.)

A. Increase in the particle size of the drug
B. Decrease in the surface area of the drug
C. Use of the ionized, or salt, form of the drug
D. Use of the free acid or free base form of the drug
E. Use of coating on the tablet

6. If the pK$_a$ of a weak base drug is 8.3, at which of the following pH values does this drug become more ionized?

A. pH 4
B. pH 9
C. pH 10
D. pH 13
E. pH 8.3

7. Which of the following dosage forms may use surface-active agents in their formulations? (Mark all that apply.)

A. Emulsions
B. Suspensions
C. Colloidal dosage forms
D. Creams
E. Aerosols

8. Which of the following is true for tablet formulations? Select all that apply.

A. A disintegrating agent promotes granule flow.
B. Lubricants prevent adherence of granules to the punch faces of the tableting machine.
C. Glidants promote flow of the granules.
D. Binding agents are used for adhesion of powder into granules.
E. A disintegrating agent promotes disintegration of tablet into granules

9. Which of the following drug formulations leads to the most rapid absorption rate?

A. Controlled-release product
B. Hard gelatin capsule
C. Compressed tablet
D. Solution
E. Suppositories

10. What factor(s) affect drug dissolution rate? Select all that apply.

A. Crystalline or amorphous form of the drug
B. Decreased particle size of drug
C. Forming drug salts
D. Presence of surfactants in dosage form
E. Volume of aqueous media or fluids in GI tract

11. Which of the following properties of large molecules will be enhanced by adding PEG groups?

A. Absorption through the intestine
B. Solubility
C. Oxidation
D. Degradation
E. Evaporation

12. Which of the following statements is false?

A. The Henderson–Hasselbalch equation describes the effect of physical parameters on the stability of pharmaceutical suspensions.
B. The passive diffusion rate of hydrophobic drugs across biological membranes is higher than that of hydrophilic compounds.
C. When the dispersed phase in an emulsion formulation is lighter than the dispersion medium, creaming can occur.
D. Targeted drug delivery systems deliver the drug to the target or receptor site in a manner that provides maximum therapeutic activity.
E. Salts increase the solubility of drugs.

13. Which of the following is an emulsifying agent? (Mark all that apply.)

A. Sorbitan monooleate (Span 80)
B. Polyoxyethylene sorbitan monooleate (Tween 80)
C. Sodium lauryl sulfate
D. Gum acacia
E. Sucrose

14. Which of the following statements is false?

A. The partition coefficient is the ratio of drug solubility in n-octanol to that in water.
B. Absorption of a weak electrolyte drug does not depend on the extent to which the drug exists in its un-ionized form at the absorption site.
C. The drug dissolution rate of a drug can be influenced by pH
D. Amorphous forms of drugs have faster dissolution rates than do crystalline forms.
E. Crystalline form of the drug is less soluble than amorphous form of the drug

15. Which of the following agents may be used in the enteric coating of tablets? (Mark all that apply.)

A. Hydroxypropyl methylcellulose
B. Carboxymethylcellulose
C. Cellulose acetate phthalate
D. Acacia
E. Sucrose

16. Which statement is true about cold cream? Select all that apply.

A. Cold cream is water soluble base
B. Cold cream has sodium borate
C. Cold cream is w/o emulsion
D. Cold cream has cetyl ester wax
E. Cold cream has PEG

17. Which of the followings is/are incompatible with abuse-deterrent oral dosage form?

A. The use of fast dissolving tablets
B. The use of fast dissolving films
C. The use of waxy excipients
D. Difficult to break tablet
E. Immediate release tablet

18. What is the normal delivery route for targeted drug delivery?

A. Ophthalmic
B. Oral
C. Parenteral
D. Transdermal
E. Sublingual

19. Which of the followings is/are **not** characteristic(s) of microcapsule?

A. A *microcapsule* is a reservoir-type system in which the drug is located centrally within the particle
B. A *microcapsule* is a matrix-type system in which the drug is dispersed throughout the particle
C. A *microcapsule* usually releases the drug at a constant rate (*zero-order release*)
D. A *microcapsule* typically gives a first-order release of drugs
E. A protein drug can be incorporated in microcapsule

20. Which statement is true?

A. A tablet and transdermal drug delivery for the same drug are equivalent in dose
B. A tablet and parenteral drug delivery for the same drug are equivalent in dose
C. A tablet and an ointment for the same drug are equivalent in dose
D. An immediate release tablet and a sustained release tablet for the same drug are equivalent in dose
E. A brand name tablet and a generic tablet for the same drug can be equivalent in dose

 4-11   **Answers**

1. A. The answer is pH 5. For a weak acid, a higher pH increases ionization.

2. A. The Henderson–Hasselbalch equation for a weak acid and its salt is represented as pH = pK$_a$ + log [salt]/[acid], where pK$_a$ is the negative log of the dissolution constant of a weak acid, because [salt]/[acid] is the ratio of the molar concentration of salt and acid used to prepare a buffer.

3. B. The answer is pH 5. When pH equals pK_a, the ratio of ionized to un-ionized become the same.

4. A. Bioavailability is the measurement of the rate and extent of systemic circulation of an active drug.

5. C. The ionized, or salt, form of a drug is generally more water soluble and, therefore, dissolves more rapidly than the nonionized (free acid or free base) form of the drug. The dissolution rate is directly proportional to the surface area and inversely proportional to the particle size. Therefore, an increase in the particle size or a decrease in the surface area slows the dissolution rate.

6. A. The answer is pH 4. For a weak base, a lower pH value increases ionization of the molecule.

7. A, B, C. Surface-active agents facilitate emulsion formation by lowering the interfacial tension between the oil and water phases. Adsorption of surfactants on insoluble particles enables these particles to be dispersed in the form of a suspension.

8. B, C, D, E, disintegrating agents are added to the tablets to promote breakup of the tablet when placed in an aqueous environment. Lubricants are required to prevent adherence of the granules to the punch faces and dies. Glidants are added to tablet formulations to improve the flow properties of the granulations. Binding agents are added to bind powders together in the granulation process.

9. D. For a drug in solution, no dissolution is required before absorption. Consequently, compared with other drug formulations, a drug in aqueous solution has the highest bioavailability rate and is often used as the reference preparation for other formulations.

10. A, B, C, D, E All these factors affect drug dissolution rate.

11. B. PEG group increases the solubility of the molecule.

12. A. The Henderson–Hasselbalch equation describes the relationship between ionized and nonionized species of a weak electrolyte.

13. A, B, C, D. Sorbitan monooleate (Span 80), polyoxyethylene sorbitan monooleate (Tween 80), sodium lauryl sulfate, and gum acacia are surfactants used as emulsifiers.

14. B. According to pH partition theory, absorption of a weak electrolyte drug depends on the extent to which the drug exists in its un-ionized form at the absorption site. However, pH partition theory often does not hold true because most weakly acidic drugs are well absorbed from the small intestine, possibly because of the large epithelial surface areas of the organ.

15. C. An enteric-coated tablet has a coating that remains intact in the stomach but dissolves in the intestine when the pH exceeds 6. Enteric-coating materials include cellulose acetate phthalate, polyvinyl acetate phthalate, and hydroxypropyl methylcellulose phthalate.

16. B, C, D, are correct. Cold cream doesn't have PEG and is not soluble in water.

17. A, B, E are correct. We don't want the patient to be able remove the drug from the dosage form easily.

18. C is the correct answer. Targeted delivery will be destroyed by the other delivery routes.

19. B and **D** are correct answers. They are characteristics of microspheres.

20. E is correct. A brand name drug and a generic drug can have the same dose and should be bioequivalent.

4-12   Additional Resources

Adejare A, ed. *Remington: The Science and Practice of Pharmacy.* 22nd ed. Cambridge, MA: Elsevier; 2021.

Allen LV Jr, ed. *Ansel's Pharmaceutical Dosage Forms and Drug Delivery Systems.* 11th ed. Philadelphia, PA: Wolters Kluwer; 2018.

Sinko PJ. *Martin's Physical Pharmacy and Pharmaceutical Sciences.* 7th ed. Philadelphia, PA: Wolters Kluwer; 2017.

U.S. Food and Drug Administration. FDA facts: Abuse-deterrent opioid medications. Updated January 17, 2017. https://www.fda.gov/media/134150/download.

Compounding

JAMES W. TORR

5-1 KEY POINTS

- Pharmacists are the only health care professionals with the knowledge, training, and skills to compound medications.
- Compounded drug preparations are regulated differently than manufactured drug products.
- Traditional pharmacy compounding is regulated by state boards of pharmacy.
- Each extemporaneously compounded medication is prepared for a specific patient and involves a three-party relationship between the pharmacist, patient, and prescriber.
- The United States Pharmacopeia (USP) is a nongovernmental organization that develops standards for pharmaceuticals.
- A thorough knowledge of and proficiency in pharmacy math is essential for compounding.
- Beyond-use dates are assigned to compounded preparations when they are compounded.
- All weighing and measuring must be accurate; errors of 5% or more are to be avoided.
- Particle size reduction and geometric dilution are essential compounding methods to ensure uniform preparations.
- Care must be taken to minimize loss of ingredients (i.e., product loss) during compounding processes.

5-2 STUDY GUIDE CHECKLIST

The following topics may guide your study of this subject area:

- [ ] Compare and contrast the characteristics of a compounded preparation and a manufactured product.
- [ ] Apply regulatory and professional guidelines pertaining to pharmacy compounding.
- [ ] Describe equipment and supplies used for compounding nonsterile dosage forms.
- [ ] Recognize the chemical grades of components, specifically those preferred for use in pharmacy compounding.
- [ ] Understand methods of achieving accuracy in weighing and measuring ingredients.
- [ ] Apply calculations and procedures required for compounding various dosage forms.
- [ ] Describe the following terms and their application to compounding: geometric dilution, triturate (trituration), levigate (levigation), and eutectic mixture.
- [ ] Apply appropriate beyond-use dates to compounded preparations.
- [ ] Describe the physiochemical properties of pharmaceutical excipients.
- [ ] Demonstrate knowledge of compounding quality assurance, quality control, preparation testing, and necessary record-keeping requirements.

5-3   Introduction

Pharmacists compound medications to provide patients and prescribers additional options for medication therapy beyond commercially available products. Individualized, custom-prepared medications are needed because some therapeutic agents: (1) are not commercially available, (2) are not available in the dosage form or dose needed, and (3) may contain patient-averse components such as dyes, preservatives, fillers, flavors, fragrances, and binders. From time to time, commercially manufactured products may be unavailable for a variety of reasons. Several segments of the population, such as pediatric, geriatric, and veterinary patients, may not be sufficiently served by pharmaceutical manufacturers. Pharmacists, in collaboration with a prescriber, may improve the patient's quality of life by compounding medications to meet their unique drug therapy needs.

5-4   Philosophy of Compounding

- Compounding is extemporaneous for an individual patient.
- Compounding fulfills the need for unique dosage forms and sizes.
- The pharmacist collaborates as part of a three-party triad (Figure 5-1) with the prescriber and patient to satisfy drug therapy needs not met by commercially available products.
- The pharmacist follows up with the patient, the prescriber, or both to determine whether the compounded preparation needs further adjustment or refinement to be satisfactory.

5-5   Regulations and Guidelines for Compounding

Compounding is defined by the Drug Quality and Security Act (DQSA) of 2013, as "the combining, admixing, diluting, pooling, reconstituting, or otherwise altering of a drug or bulk drug substance to create a drug." The Food and Drug Administration (FDA) generally lacks authority over traditional pharmacy compounding. Pharmacy compounding is regulated by individual state boards of pharmacy. Because of this, compounding regulations will vary by state. As long as the compounding is performed in compliance with applicable state laws and certain provisions of the DQSA, the FDA typically does not get involved.

FIGURE 5-1. Triad Relationship of Pharmacy Compounding

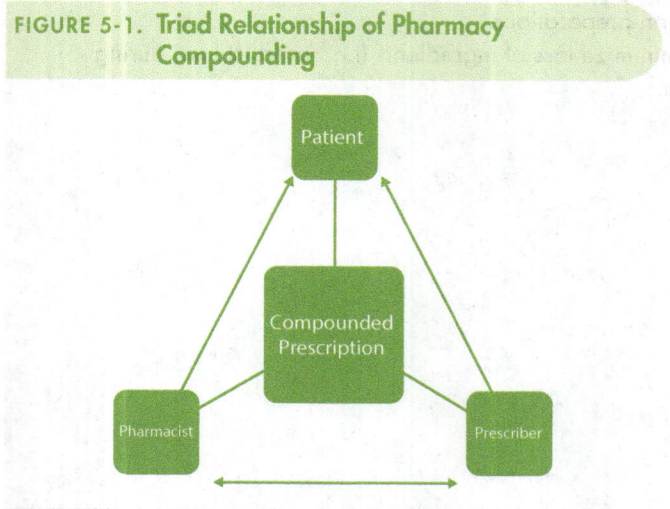

FIGURE 5-2. **Compounding vs Manufacturing**

Pharmacy Compounding (503A)	Manufacturing (503B)
• Patient specific	• Not patient specific
• Regulated by state boards of pharmacy	• Regulated by the FDA
• No clinical trials	• Clinical trials
• No NDA submission	• Submission of a New Drug Application (NDA)
• Good Compounding Practices (GCPs)	• Good Manufacturing Practices (GMPs)
• Beyond-Use Dates (BUDs)	• Expiration dates
• Exempt from FDA labeling requirements	• Follow FDA labeling requirements

The DQSA consists, in part, of Sections 503A and 503B. Section 503A addresses traditional pharmacy compounding where the three-party triad exists. It clarifies FDA involvement in compounding and recognizes that state boards of pharmacy are responsible for regulatory oversight. Section 503B addresses outsourcing facilities where sterile dosage forms are compounded in the absence of the traditional compounding three-party triad. Section 503B facilities may compound larger quantities of such dosage forms, register voluntarily with the FDA, must be compliant with Good Manufacturing Practices (GMPs), and are subject to inspection by the FDA.

The primary difference between a traditional compounding pharmacy (503A facility) and an outsourcing facility (503B), or compounding versus manufacturing, is the existence of the pharmacy triad relationship. This relationship is established via an individual prescription or medication order. Figure 5-2 illustrates some of the differences between pharmacy compounding and pharmaceutical manufacturing.

The FDA has the authority to update, modify, and withdraw its policies in regards to pharmacy compounding. In 2020 the FDA issued a guidance policy for the temporary compounding of certain alcohol-based and sanitizer products during the Coronavirus Disease 2019 (COVID-19) pandemic. During this public health emergency, manufacturers of alcohol-based hand sanitizer were not able to keep up with the demand for this product. Under this temporary guidance document, the FDA announced it did not intend to take action against pharmacies who compounded alcohol-based hand sanitizer for consumers and health care personnel, providing certain circumstances were met. This temporary policy allowed compounders to support a public health need without an individual prescription for each patient.

The United State Pharmacopeia (USP) is a nongovernmental organization that establishes quality standards for pharmaceuticals, including both manufactured products and compounded preparations. USP standards are not enforceable unless another regulatory agency defines their enforceability. General chapters numbered below 1000 are considered enforceable, whereas chapters numbered above 1000 are informational in nature. When preparing an official USP monograph, the preparation should meet the criteria described in such monographs. At the time this chapter was written, USP chapters related to pharmaceutical compounding were undergoing revisions. Individuals preparing for licensure examination should review the current and official compounding-related chapters of the USP.

5-6   Categories for Nonsterile Compounded Preparations

The USP <795>, Pharmaceutical Compounding—Nonsterile Preparations, describes three general categories of nonsterile compounded preparations. These categories are classified according to their complexity, desired site of action (local or systemic), and risk of harm to compounding personnel or patients. The categories are summarized in Table 5-1.

TABLE 5-1. Categories of Nonsterile Preparations

Category	Description/criteria
Simple	Preparations follow an official compendial monograph or peer-reviewed literature.
Moderate	Preparations require special procedures or calculations. Such preparations lack stability data.
Complex	Preparations require specialized processes, environment, or equipment to achieve desired outcomes (e.g., systemic effect, specialized drug delivery).

5-7   Pharmacy Requirements

Space

- An appropriate area is required; a dedicated area is recommended to reduce cross contamination. The area should provide limited traffic flow.
- Sufficient counter space for compounding and shelving for storage should be properly arranged and maintained, with components and equipment readily available.
- Appropriate lighting and temperature, humidity, and ventilation control are necessary.
- Separate areas are required for sterile and nonsterile compounding.
- A sink with potable and purified water should be readily available.
- Nonporous surfaces and materials should be used in the compounding area.

Equipment

- Appropriate equipment is required but varies based on the dosage form(s) being compounded.
- Compounding personnel must evaluate their equipment needs based on the type and volume of compounded medications they prepare. Table 5-2 lists examples of nonsterile compounding equipment.

TABLE 5-2. Examples of Nonsterile Compounding Equipment

Equipment category	Example(s)
Measuring (volumetric apparatus)	Graduated cylinders, pharmacy graduates, beakers, flasks, pipettes, and oral syringes
Weighing	Torsion balance (Class A) and electronic/analytical balance
Mixing	Mortars and pestles (Wedgewood, porcelain, and glass), spatulas (stainless steel and hard rubber), ointment slabs, stir bars (glass and polypropylene), rubber scrapers, and blenders
Processing	Casseroles, electronic mortar and pestles (EMPs), funnels, homogenizers, hot plates, magnetic stirrers, ointment mills, tablet pulverizers, pH analyzers, and thermometers
Specialty molds	Lollipops, rapid-dissolve tablets, tablet triturates, troches (lozenges), and suppositories
Personal protective equipment (PPE)	Gloves, face masks, hair covers, gowns, and goggles
Engineering controls	Compounding containment devices or powder containment enclosures
Packaging	Capsule-filling devices, tube-sealing equipment, and calibrated measuring and filling devices
Computer	Hardware and software for maintaining and processing labels, profiles, formulas, and required records

TABLE 5-3. Chemical Grades and Sources of Compounding Ingredients

USP/NF: United States Pharmacopeia/National Formulary (components meet official standards and are suitable for human use)

FCC: Food Chemicals Codex (food grade)

ACS: American Chemical Society (reagent grade)

AR: analytical reagent (high purity)

CP: chemically pure (uncertain quality)

Tech: technical (industrial quality)

Prefabricated/commercial dosage form (i.e., manufactured tablets or capsules of drugs)

Notes: (1) USP/NF or FCC components are preferred for compounding. Always obtain the certificate of analysis for every component used, and use components manufactured in an FDA-registered facility. (2) Excipients in prefabricated dosage forms must be considered (e.g., patient allergy to dyes).

Supplies

For the purpose of this chapter, supplies will be distinguished from equipment as perishable/disposable products. Supplies include items such as the following:

- Weigh boats, weighing paper (parchment and glassine), filter paper, ointment paper
- Containers of various types and sizes to properly package the dosage forms, such as prescription bottles, powder jars, capsule containers, ointment jars, ointment tubes, "ride-up" tubes, powder paper boxes, and suppository boxes

Components (Ingredients)

Components of compounded and other pharmaceutical dosage forms are either active pharmaceutical ingredients (APIs) or other added substances (excipients). Excipients aid in the preparation of the dosage form and contribute to the characteristics of the final dosage form. Table 5-3 lists various chemical grades of ingredients for use in compounding.

The number of available pharmaceutical excipients is vast and a complete discussion is beyond the scope of this chapter. Table 5-4 lists several excipients by their functional category. The function of a specific excipient may vary depending upon the dosage form prepared and the quantity of the excipient in the dosage form.

TABLE 5-4. Pharmaceutical Excipients

Antioxidant	Ascorbic acid
Humectant	Glycerin, propylene glycol, sorbitol
Levigating agent	Glycerin, mineral oil, propylene glycol
Preservative (antimicrobial)	Benzoic acid, parabens (e.g., methyl-, ethyl-, and propyl-parabens), sodium benzoate
Solvent	Alcohol, fixed oils, glycerin, mineral oil, propylene glycol, purified water
Stiffening agent	Cetyl alcohol, stearyl alcohol, white wax
Suspending agent	Bentonite, carbomer, cellulose derivatives (e.g., methylcellulose), tragacanth
Viscosity inducing agent	Bentonite, carbomer, cellulose derivatives (e.g., methylcellulose), poloxamer, tragacanth

Water and Alcohol

Unless otherwise indicated, USP <795> specifies that purified water should be used for nonsterile compounded preparations. Potable water should be used for washing hands and equipment. Alcohol USP (95% ethyl alcohol) is to be used for nonsterile compounded preparations when a specific alcohol is not identified in a compounding formulation.

Records and Record Keeping

Types of records include the following:

- A master formulation record must be in place for each preparation compounded, and it must be approved, signed, and dated by the pharmacist in charge.
- A compounding record of each compounded prescription must be made and maintained.
- A chronological record of each day's compounding activity should be made and kept for future reference and use.

Policies and Procedures

Types of policies and procedures include, among others, the following:

- Standard operating procedures (SOPs)
- Safety data sheets (SDS)—formerly Material Safety Data Sheets (MSDS)
- Certificates of analysis (COA)
- Quality assurance and control

Professional Considerations

- Is a commercial product in the desired dose and dosage form available?
- Is there an alternative product that will satisfy the patient's requirements?
- Can I perform the required pharmaceutical calculations?
- Can I accurately compound and package the preparation?

Quality Control Requirements

- Accurate calculations, weighing, and measuring
- Proper processing techniques
- Proper packaging
- Proper record keeping
- Proper labeling, including but not limited to beyond-use dates (BUDs)
- Proper documentation of quality assurance, quality control, and preparation testing

Beyond-Use Dates

- Pharmacists assign BUDs to compounded preparations to guide patients in the proper duration of use and storage of the preparation.
- BUDs are assigned from the date of preparation.
- The goal is to provide a BUD that will allow the patient enough time to fully use the amount of preparation dispensed but not enough time to allow the preparation to degrade, lose potency, or be stored for future use.
- In the absence of references on the stability of the specific dosage form compounded or sufficient experience with it, the section "General Guidelines for Assigning Beyond-Use Dates" in USP <795> is followed. BUDs are summarized in Table 5-5.

TABLE 5-5. Nonsterile Maximum Beyond-Use Dates[a]

Beyond-use date	14 days	30 days	6 months
Storage condition	Cold temperature (2°C to 8°C, 36°F to 46°F)	Room temperature (20°C to 25°C, 68°F to 77°F)	Room temperature (20°C to 25°C, 68°F to 77°F)
Preparation type	Oral preparations containing water	Liquid and semisolid topical, dermal, and mucosal preparations containing water	Preparations containing no water

a. The BUD cannot be greater than the expiration date of any component used to compound the preparation. Inclusion of an antimicrobial agent should be considered, if appropriate. Dispense in a container that reduces exposure to light and moisture.

5-8   General Compounding Process and Techniques

While the compounding procedure for different dosage forms and preparations may employ specific techniques, the general process can be broken down into a few distinct steps. These steps are illustrated in Figure 5-3.

Selected examples of specific compounding processes will be described in Section 5-9, Compounded Dosage Forms. Following the compounding of a nonsterile preparation, quality control should be performed prior to packaging and/or dispensing the prescription. Methods of quality control may include (1) visual inspection/appearance and (2) percent of error (i.e., weight or volume variance).

Weighing and Measuring

- Care should be taken during compounding to minimize the loss of ingredients and the preparation (i.e., product loss).
- The sensitivity of the pharmacy balance must be determined, and the minimum weighable quantity must be known for that particular balance.
- When weighing or measuring, the percentage of error should not exceed ±5% of the theoretical quantity or volume.

FIGURE 5-3. General Compounding Process*

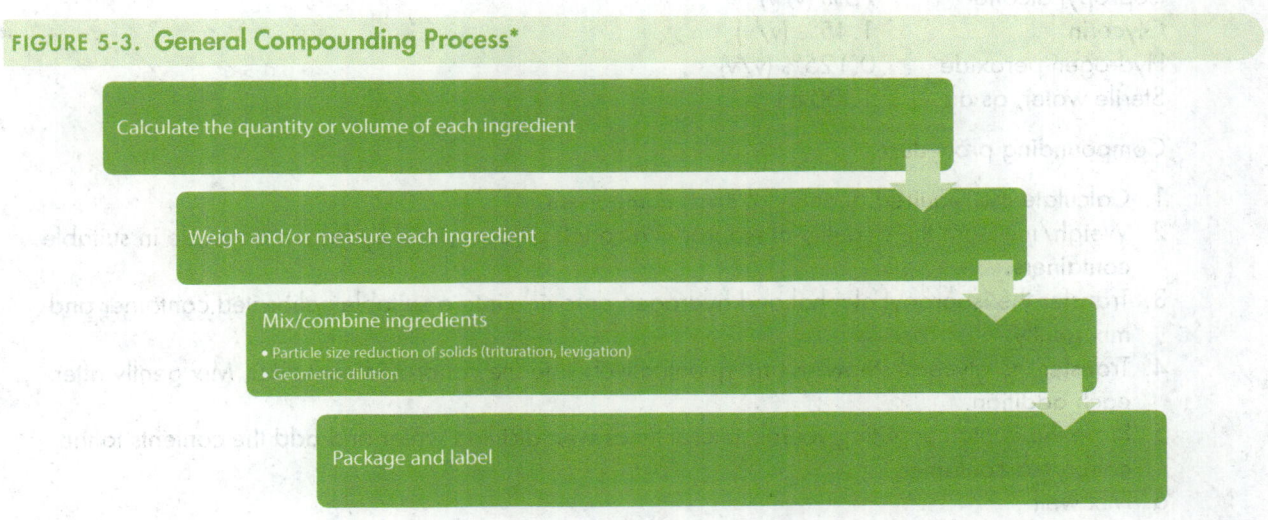

Calculate the quantity or volume of each ingredient

Weigh and/or measure each ingredient

Mix/combine ingredients
- Particle size reduction of solids (trituration, levigation)
- Geometric dilution

Package and label

*Note: This is a general overview of the compounding process. The mixing techniques utilized in the compounding process will vary based on the dosage form being compounded and the ingredients/components being utilized.

Mixing

- Geometric dilution is the preferred method for mixing components to achieve a uniform and homogenous preparation.
- Particle size reduction (comminution) is generally the first step when compounding with solid components to achieve uniform particle size.
- Comminution is achieved manually by trituration, levigation, or pulverization by intervention. It is achieved mechanically by grinders and various types of mills.
- Trituration is used to reduce the particle size of powders to make a greater surface area available (i.e., dry, solid components).
- Levigation is the process of mixing a powder with a liquid in which it is insoluble to reduce particle size and aid in incorporating the powder into a liquid or semisolid base (i.e., solid and liquid or semisolid components).
- Eutectic mixtures may be achieved by combining solid ingredients that liquefy when mixed together. Examples of eutectic chemicals include camphor, menthol, methyl salicylate, and thymol.

5-9 Compounded Dosage Forms

Solutions

- *Definition:* Solutions are chemically and physically homogenous liquid mixtures of two or more substances.
- *Types:* Examples include syrups, elixirs, aromatic waters, tinctures, and spirits. Solutions can be aqueous or nonaqueous.
- *Properties:* Examples include hypertonic, isotonic, hypotonic, osmolar, and osmolal.
- *Stability:* The stability of solutions may be enhanced by adjusting the pH, adding a preservative, and/or adding an antioxidant.
- *Rate of dissolution:* The rate of dissolution may be enhanced by stirring (agitation), heating, and reducing particle size.

An example of a solution is hand sanitizer.

Isopropyl alcohol	75% (v/v)
Glycerin	1.45% (v/v)
Hydrogen peroxide	0.125% (v/v)
Sterile water, qs ad	1000 mL

Compounding procedure:

1. Calculate the required quantity of each component.
2. Weigh/measure the quantity of isopropyl alcohol, glycerin, and hydrogen peroxide in suitable containers.
3. Transfer the isopropyl alcohol and hydrogen peroxide into a suitable calibrated container and mix gently.
4. Transfer the glycerol stepwise and quantitatively into the calibrated container. Mix gently after each addition.
5. Rinse the container with glycerol several times with distilled water and add the contents to the calibrated container.
6. Mix well.
7. Transfer the solution into suitable container(s).
8. Package and label the container(s).

Suspensions

- **Definition:** A suspension is a two-phased system containing a finely divided solid dispersed in a liquid vehicle.
- **Requirement:** The drug is uniformly dispersed throughout the vehicle.
- **Concentration:** Suspending agents are typically used in a concentration of 0.5% to 6%.
- **Viscosity:** The vehicle has enough viscosity to keep drug particles suspended separately.
- **Insolubility:** The active pharmaceutical ingredient is insoluble in the vehicle.
- **Tip:** Wet the insoluble powder with a vehicle-miscible liquid.
- **Stability:** Stability is enhanced by adding a preservative.
- **Advantage:** A suspension allows the preparation of a liquid form of an insoluble drug.

Categories of suspending agents and examples are as follows:

- **Natural hydrocolloids:** Acacia, alginic acid, gelatin, guar gum, sodium alginate, tragacanth, and xanthan gum
- **Semisynthetic hydrocolloids:** Ethylcellulose, methylcellulose, and sodium carboxymethyl cellulose
- **Synthetic hydrocolloids:** Carbomers (Carbopol), poloxamers (Pluronic), polyvinyl alcohol, and polyvinylpyrrolidone
- **Clays:** Bentonite and magnesium aluminum silicate (Veegum)

An example of an oral suspension follows:

Progesterone, micronized	1.2 g
Glycerin	3 mL
Methylcellulose 1% solution	30 mL
Flavored syrup, qs ad	60 mL

Compounding procedure:

1. Calculate the required quantity of each component.
2. Accurately weigh or measure each component.
3. In a glass mortar, wet the progesterone with the glycerin to form a thick paste.
4. Slowly add the methylcellulose solution while triturating.
5. When mixed thoroughly, pour the suspension into a graduate.
6. Add small amounts of syrup to the mortar, mix, and add to graduate until the desired volume is reached.
7. Package and label the container(s).

Emulsions

- **Definition:** An emulsion is a two-phase system of two immiscible liquids, one of which is dispersed throughout the other as small droplets.
- **Components:** An emulsion has an external, continuous phase or dispersion medium; an internal, discontinuous or dispersed phase; and an emulsifying agent.
- **Type:** Types are oil in water (o/w) and water in oil (w/o), depending on which is the internal or external phase.
- **Emulsifying agents:** Emulsifying agents can be natural gums (acacia, agar, chondrus, pectin, and tragacanth) or hydrophilic or lipophilic surfactants (the esters of sorbitan).
- **Lipophilic surfactants:** Commonly referred to as Spans.
- **Hydrophilic surfactants:** Commonly referred to as Tweens.
- **Hydrophilic–lipophilic balance:** A lower hydrophilic–lipophilic balance (HLB) value favors a w/o emulsion; a higher HLB value favors an o/w emulsion. Agents with an HLB value of 1 to 10 are considered to be lipophilic, while agents with an HLB value of > 10 are considered to be hydrophilic.

Emulsions with an HLB value of 3 to 8 are water in oil, while those emulsions with an HLB value of > 8 to 16 are oil in water.

- ■ *Other agents:* Other agents include bentonite, cholesterol, gelatin, lecithin, methylcellulose, soaps of fatty acids, sodium docusate, sodium lauryl sulfate, and triethanolamine.
- ■ *Solids:* Solid components should be dissolved before they are incorporated into the emulsion, or if a sizable quantity is added, a levigating or wetting agent may be needed.
- ■ *Flavors or fragrances:* Flavors or fragrances should generally be incorporated into the external phase.
- ■ *Preservatives:* Preservatives should be added in the aqueous phase but may also be added in the oily phase, if necessary.
- ■ *Stability:* Emulsions may separate over time via creaming, a reversible process, or cracking, which is irreversible.
- ■ *Continental method:* The continental or dry gum method of preparing an emulsion nucleus involves using the oil:water:dry gum emulsifier in a 4:2:1 ratio.
- ■ *Advantages:* An emulsion can be used to mask taste, improve palatability, increase absorption, and enhance bioavailability.

Capsules

- ■ *Definition:* This dosage form incorporates components into a shell called a *capsule*.
- ■ *Procedure:* Determine capsule size to fit total powder weight, triturate powders to reduce particle size, mix powders by geometric dilution, incorporate the diluent by geometric dilution if required, fill the capsules, and clean the outside of the filled capsules.
- ■ *Methods of filling:* Hand punch from powder on an ointment slab or use a capsule-filling machine.
- ■ *Sizing:* Capsules available, listed from largest to smallest, include 000, 00, 0, 1, 2, 3, 4, and 5. Determining the size of capsule to use for a particular dosage involves assessing the density or fluffiness of the powder, comparing it to known weights of various reference powders with published capsule-size capacities, and then filling and weighing the capsule. If the requested dosage does not fill a specific size of capsule, a filler should be added. Examples of filler for capsule preparation include, but are not limited to: (1) lactose, (2) citric acid, (3) cornstarch, (4) sodium bicarbonate, and (5) cellulose derivatives (e.g., methylcellulose and hydroxypropyl methylcellulose [HPMC]). The addition of a cellulose derivative provides a slower rate of release of the API.
- ■ *Advantages:* Capsules: (1) mask unpleasant taste of APIs and excipients, (2) allow incorporation of several components into one dosage form, (3) provide an accurate dosage size for liquids, semisolids, and powders, and (4) provide a dosage form that may be easier to swallow and is more acceptable to the patient. Capsules come in a variety of colors, which may aid in drug identification.

An example of an altered-release capsule formula follows:

Progesterone, micronized	25 mg
Hydroxypropyl methylcellulose (HPMC)	50%
Lactose, qs ad	per capsule size
M. ft. capsules	15 doses

Compounding procedure:

1. Calculate the required quantity of each ingredient.
2. Select the appropriate capsule size. *Note:* The quantity of lactose (filler) needed depends on the selected capsule size.
3. Accurately weigh each component.
4. If necessary, reduce particle size, and mix thoroughly by geometric dilution.

5. Fill capsules.
6. Weigh capsules (quality control).
7. Package and label the container(s).

Tablet Triturates

- **Definition:** A tablet triturate is a small tablet that is made in a mold and intended for sublingual administration. The molded tablet usually weighs about 60 to 200 mg.
- **Components:** Tablet triturates consist of an active pharmaceutical ingredient and a base, which may consist of lactose, sucrose, dextrose, and mannitol.
- **Formulation:** Molds that make 50 tablets are generally available in approximately 60-, 100-, and 200 mg tablet sizes. Formulations must be calculated to fit the size of the mold that will be used. If this capacity is not known, the capacity must be determined by filling the mold holes with the tablet triturate base and weighing the resulting tablets. On the basis of the size of the mold holes, mix the active pharmaceutical ingredient with the base, which often consists of four parts lactose and one part sucrose. Thoroughly triturate powders, mix by geometric dilution, and then moisten with a wetting solution containing four parts 95% ethyl alcohol and one part purified water until the powder mixture is adhesive. Press into mold uniformly.
- **Tip:** Tablets may be flavored by adding a flavor to the wetting solution. Color may be added by adding a small amount of powdered color to the powder mixture.
- **Advantages:** A tablet triturate rapidly dissolves under the tongue, is rapidly absorbed, avoids the first pass through the liver, and provides a rapid therapeutic response.

Troches, Lozenges, and Lollipops

- **Definition:** Troches, lozenges, and lollipops or suckers are solid dosage forms intended to be slowly dissolved in the mouth for local or systemic effects.
- **Formulation:** Troches, lozenges, and lollipops are composed of an active pharmaceutical ingredient and a base that may consist of (1) sugar and other carbohydrates that produce a hard preparation, (2) polyethylene glycols (PEGs) and other components that produce a softer preparation, or (3) a glycerin–gelatin combination that produces a chewable preparation.
  - Formulations must be calculated to fit the size of the mold that will be used. If this capacity is not known, the capacity must be determined by filling the mold cavities with the base and weighing the resulting troches, lozenges, or lollipops.
  - Flavors and colors are typically added just before the molds are filled.
- **Advantages:** Troches, lozenges, and lollipops are easy to administer, are convenient for patients who cannot swallow oral dosage forms, maintain a constant level of drug in the oral cavity and throat, and can have a pleasant taste.

Ointments, Creams, and Pastes

- **Definition:** Ointments, creams, and pastes are semisolid dosage forms for external application. Properties are typically characteristic of the base selected (e.g., white petrolatum, hydrophilic petrolatum, cold cream, hydrophilic ointment, polyethylene glycol ointment). These semisolid dosage forms protect the skin and mucous membranes, moisturize the skin, and provide a vehicle for various types of medications. Ointments and ointment bases may be classified by their water content or the extent of skin penetration. Characteristics of ointment bases, as defined by their water content are summarized in Figure 5-4.
- **Preparation:** Ointments are typically prepared by fusion or levigation. Powders should be comminuted to fine particles; some powders may be dissolved. If using the fusion method, use only enough heat to melt the component with the highest melting point. For the levigation method,

FIGURE 5-4. Characteristics of Ointment Bases

Oleaginous or Hydrocarbon Base	Absorption Base	Water-in-Oil (w/o) Emulsion Base	Oil-in-Water (o/w) Emulsion Base	Water-Soluble Base
• Occlusive • Greasy • Emollient • Not water washable • Not water absorbing • Insoluble in water	• Occlusive • Greasy • Emollient • Insoluble in water • Not water washable • Water absorbing	• Occlusive • Greasy • Emollient • Not water washable • Water absorbing • Insoluble in water	• Non-occlusive • Non-greasy • Water washable • Water absorbing • Insoluble in water	• Non-occlusive • Non-greasy • Water washable • Water absorbing • Water soluble

an ointment slab and metal spatula usually work well. Levigating agents should be carefully selected, considering both the component(s) to be incorporated and the base. Table 5-6 shows commonly used levigating agents grouped by type and matched with the appropriate group of ointment base classifications.

■ **Uses:** Ointments or creams are an effective dosage form for treating skin and mucous membranes. On occasion, an ointment or cream will move sufficient quantities of medication through the skin to produce a systemic effect. Some formulations provide effective protection for the skin and mucous membranes.

■ **Packaging:** Typically, ointments and creams are packaged in ointment jars. Ointment tubes may provide an ideal alternative package because it protects the preparation until it is squeezed out and used.

An example of an oleaginous ointment follows:

Salicylic acid	3%
Mineral oil	qs
White petrolatum, qs ad	30 g

TABLE 5-6. Levigating Agents by Type and Ointment Base Classification

Type of agent	Ointment base classification
Aqueous	
Glycerin	Oil-in-water emulsion
Propylene glycol	Water soluble
Polyethylene glycol 400	Water washable
Oily	
Mineral oil	Oleaginous or hydrocarbon
Castor oil	Absorption
Cottonseed oil	Water-in-oil emulsion

Note: Other agents may be useful for certain preparations, such as Tween 80 for incorporating coal tar. Castor oil is useful for incorporating ichthammol and Peru balsam.

Compounding procedure:

1. Calculate the required quantity of each component.
2. Accurately weigh each component.
3. Triturate the salicylic acid, if necessary, to reduce particle size.
4. Levigate with a small quantity of mineral oil.
5. By geometric dilution, incorporate the levigated salicylic acid into the white petrolatum.
6. Continue mixing (e.g., spatulation) until a uniform preparation is formed.
7. Package and label container(s).

Gels

- **Definition:** Gels are semisolid preparations consisting of particles suspended in a liquid that provides a rigid framework.
- **Components:** Gels generally consist of the following components: (1) an API, (2) a gelling agent (e.g., carbomers, cellulose derivatives, and poloxamers), (3) a wetting or levigating agent (e.g., propylene glycol and glycerin), (4) a suspending or dispersing agent (e.g., bentonite and silica gel), and (5) a penetration-enhancing agent (e.g., lecithin, dimethyl sulfoxide [DMSO]). Penetration-enhancers are specifically used when transdermal drug delivery is desired.
- **Formulation:** Use proper techniques for creating the gel to minimize the incorporation of air into the preparation, use small amounts of nonaqueous solvents, and, if possible, keep electrolyte components to a minimum. The adjustment of pH is necessary for carbomer gels. Aqueous solutions of poloxamer gels exhibit reverse thermal properties in relation to viscosity.
- **Advantages:** Gels are convenient, effective, and acceptable to patients. Gels have a variety of therapeutic applications. The gels avoid some problems that other dosage forms have, such as gastrointestinal irritation from oral dosages, pain from injections, and the undesirability of suppositories.

An example of transdermal gel using pluronic lecithin organogel (PLO) as the base follows:

Ketoprofen	5%
Propylene glycol	10%
Lecithin isopropyl palmitate liquid	20%
Poloxamer 407 20% aqueous solution, qs ad	100 mL

Compounding procedure:

1. Calculate the required quantity of each component.
2. Accurately weigh or measure each component.
3. In a glass mortar, triturate the ketoprofen with the propylene glycol to make a smooth paste.
4. Add the lecithin isopropyl palmitate liquid, and mix well.
5. Add sufficient poloxamer 407 20% gel to measure 100 mL.
6. Triturate until a high-quality gel is produced.
7. Package in a light-resistant container and label.

Note: The lecithin isopropyl palmitate liquid and the poloxamer 407 20% aqueous solution should be prepared before compounding the gel.

Suppositories

- **Definition:** Suppositories are solid dosage forms for insertion into the rectum, vagina, or urethra to provide localized or systemic therapy.
- **Sizes:** Rectal suppositories are approximately 2 g, vaginal suppositories are 3 to 5 g, and urethral suppositories are 2 g (female) or 4 g (male). Urethral suppositories were formerly called *bougies*.

- *Formulation:* Suppositories are usually made by fusion with either a fatty or a water-miscible base. They can also be hand molded or made by compression.
    - Suppositories are usually made in a metal or plastic mold. A plastic mold is called a shell.
    - The active pharmaceutical ingredient in powder form should be triturated (comminuted) to reduce particle size and should be levigated with a wetting agent before incorporation into the melted base.
    - The melted formulation should be poured continuously into the mold to prevent layering.
- *Calculations:* The capacity in grams of the suppository mold must be known to determine the quantity of base needed. If this capacity is not known, the capacity must be determined by filling the mold with the suppository base and weighing the resulting suppositories. The space in the suppository occupied by the active pharmaceutical ingredient(s) must be calculated using the density factor of each active ingredient. If the density factor is not known, it can be calculated by making a suppository containing a known amount of the active ingredient.
- *Advantages:* Suppositories deliver medication for local or systemic effects. The systemically absorbed medication avoids the first pass through the liver. They can be used when patients cannot take medication orally or by injection.

An example of a rectal suppository follows:

Progesterone, micronized	25 mg
PEG base	qs
M. ft. suppositories	12 doses

Formula for the suppository base follows:

PEG 300	50%
PEG 6000	50%

Compounding procedure:

1. Calibrate the mold for the base being used. On the basis of the weight of the suppositories made, calculate the required amount of each component.
2. Accurately weigh or measure each component.
3. Carefully heat the PEG 6000 until it melts.
4. Add the PEG 300, and mix well.
5. Very slowly add the micronized progesterone, and mix thoroughly.
6. Pour the mixture into the suppository mold.
7. Package and label in an appropriate container.

Note: When using the plastic molds, if the melted mixture is too hot it will melt the shell.

Powders

- *Definition:* Powders are fine particles that result from the comminution of dry substances. Particle sizes are usually determined by the size of sieve they will pass through and may be described as very coarse, coarse, moderately coarse, fine, and very fine.
- *Mixtures:* Mixtures of powders should have the same or similar size particles, and mixing should be accomplished by geometric dilution.
- *Preparation:* Comminution is the process of reducing particle size in powders. Powders are incorporated by geometric dilution.
- *Uses:* Powders taken by mouth may provide systemic effects, whereas powders applied topically provide localized effects. Powders that contain mucoadhesive components, when insufflated into body cavities, adhere to moist body surfaces.
- *Advantages:* Because they are dry, powders often have greater stability and may not react with components with which they are otherwise incompatible.

An example of a topical (dusting) powder:

Calamine
Zinc oxide, of each   8%
Red mercuric oxide   1%
Magnesium oxide, heavy, qs ad   60 g

Compounding procedure:

1. Calculate the required amount of each component.
2. Accurately weigh each component.
3. Thoroughly mix the powders by geometric dilution using a porcelain mortar.
4. To determine when the mixture is totally homogeneous, use the *spread test,* which is performed by using a spatula to spread a small amount of the mixed powders into a thin layer on a sheet of weighing paper.
5. Package and label in an appropriate container.

Powder Papers

- *Definition:* Powders or mixtures of powders are enfolded in papers containing one dose each and dispensed in an appropriate box or container.
- *Preparation:* Powder papers or charts contain finely subdivided (comminuted) powders, mixed by geometric dilution, with a dose of the appropriate size placed on a powder paper and properly folded. The appropriate size can be obtained by weighing.
- *Advantages:* For patients who have difficulty swallowing tablets or capsules and those who have indwelling nasogastric tubes, powder papers are a useful dosage form. Multiple medications can be combined and administered as one dose. The medication is in powder form and ready to be absorbed once it is in the gastrointestinal tract.

Sticks

- *Definition:* This topical dosage form is made in the shape of a rod, stick, or variation thereof and packaged in a container that allows it to be advanced upward as it is used.
- *Preparation:* Select a semisolid vehicle from a variety of polyethylene glycols, waxes, and oils that will produce the consistency desired. Triturate solid components, wet them with an appropriate wetting or levigating agent, and add them along with any liquid components to the melted vehicle. Mix thoroughly. Pour into an appropriate *ride-up* container.
- *Advantages:* Sticks are an effective, convenient method of applying a topical agent exactly in the location desired. They are very portable and can deliver a variety of agents, including those that are therapeutic, protective, and cosmetic.

5-10   Quality Assurance and Preparation Testing

The assurance of high quality influences every facet of compounding. Factors such as the compounding environment, facility design, fixtures, equipment, components, containers, personnel expertise and experience, policies, procedures, and documentation play important roles in achieving the highest quality possible in the compounding of individualized, customized preparations. Each preparation should be reviewed before dispensing to determine that the calculations, components, compounding process, and documentation are accurate and correct and that the preparation has the appropriate appearance. The typical goal is to have the contents of the preparation vary no more than plus or minus 5% of the labeled concentration. An indicator that a compounding pharmacy is committed to a high-quality practice is voluntary accreditation by the Pharmacy Compounding Accreditation Board (PCAB). As a national organization, PCAB carefully evaluates all aspects of a pharmacy's compounding operation. It ensures that policies and procedures are in place and operational for a high-quality practice. Accreditation by PCAB is currently the only benchmark available to attest to the quality of a compounding pharmacy and should be considered by pharmacies that provide compounding services.

5-11   Pharmacist's Role

As mentioned earlier in this chapter, pharmacists are the only health care professionals with the knowledge and skills to compound medications. Compounding is an essential component of pharmacy practice to help meet the unique drug therapy needs of patients. Compounding offers pharmacists the opportunity to play an essential role in customizing drug therapy for patient care through collaboration with the patient and prescriber.

NAPLEX Competency Statements

The questions in this chapter cover the following 2021 NAPLEX Competency Statements: **AREA 5:** 5.1; 5.3; 5.4.

 5-12   Questions

1. What type of water should be used when compounding a nonsterile preparation if a specific water article is not identified in the formula?

   A. Tap water
   B. Potable water
   C. Purified water
   D. Water for Injection
   E. Sterile Water for Injection

2. Which of the following excipients may be added to a capsule formulation to provide a slower rate of release from the capsules?

   A. Cornstarch
   B. Citric acid
   C. Lactose
   D. Hydroxypropyl methylcellulose
   E. Sodium bicarbonate

3. You are about to counsel a patient on a new compounded prescription for diltiazem 0.2% ointment, which is prepared in an oleaginous ointment base. Which of the following characteristics should the patient expect from this dosage form?

   A. Emollient
   B. Water absorbing
   C. Occlusive
   D. Water washable
   E. Greasy

4. Which of the following statements describes the best process when adding a water-miscible flavor to an oral o/w emulsion?

   A. Incorporate the flavor into the external phase of the emulsion.
   B. Incorporate the flavor into the internal phase of the emulsion.
   C. Incorporate the flavor into the dispersed phase of the emulsion.
   D. Incorporate the flavor into the discontinuous phase of the emulsion.
   E. Incorporate the flavor into either phase because it does not matter.

5. According to USP <795>, and in the absence of stability data, what would be the most appropriate beyond-use date (BUD) for the formulation below?

Tri-estrogen + progesterone capsules; for quantity 100

Estriol powder, USP	50 mg
Estrone powder, USP	6.25 mg
Estradiol powder, USP	6.25 mg
Progesterone powder, USP	10 g
Lactose powder, USP	qs

A. The BUD is not later than the time remaining until the earliest expiration date of any API or 6 months, whichever is earlier.
B. The BUD is not later than 14 days when stored at controlled room temperatures.
C. The BUD is not later than 30 days.
D. The BUD is not later than 14 days when stored at controlled cold temperatures (refrigerated).
E. No BUD is necessary

6. Which of the following statements represents a characteristic of a preparation in USP <795>'s moderate compounding category?

A. It requires manipulation of a commercial product by adding a component.
B. It has a USP compounding monograph.
C. It requires special calculations to determine component quantities per preparation of individualized units.
D. It has appeared in a peer-reviewed journal.
E. The preparation lacks stability data.

7. According to USP <795> and in the absence of stability data, what would be the most appropriate BUD for the formulation below?

Indomethacin 1% Topical Gel; for 100 mL

Indomethacin powder	1%
Carbomer 941 resin	2%
Purified water	10 %
Triethanolamine, qs	pH
Ethanol 95%, qs ad	100 mL

A. The BUD is not later than the time remaining until the earliest expiration date of any API or 6 months, whichever is earlier.
B. The BUD is not later than 14 days when stored at controlled room temperatures.
C. The BUD is not later than 30 days.
D. The BUD is not later than 14 days when stored at controlled cold temperatures (refrigerated).
E. No BUD is necessary

8. When compounding a capsule formula, it is determined that the desired weight of each capsule is 350 mg. What is the acceptable weight range for the finished capsules?

A. 300 to 400 mg
B. 315 to 385 mg
C. 297.5 to 402.5 mg
D. 325.5 to 374.5 mg
E. 332.5 to 367.5 mg

9. Which federal legislation amended the Food, Drug, and Cosmetic Act to make a distinction between 503A and 503B facilities?

A. Drug Quality and Security Act
B. Food and Drug Administration Modernization Act
C. Pharmacy Compounding Compliance Act
D. American Medicinal Drug Use Clarification Act
E. Orphan Drug Act

10. Which of the following characteristics are consistent with a compounded prescription?

A. Produced according to current GMPs
B. Subject to an approved NDA
C. Patient specific in conjunction with the prescriber
D. Exempt from FDA labeling requirements
E. Undergoes clinical trials prior to use

11. What chemical grade(s) are preferred for use when compounding a drug preparation?

A. ACS
B. FCC
C. AR
D. USP
E. NF

12. What is the primary function of lecithin in the Ketoprofen 10% PLO gel formula below?

Ketoprofen	10 g
Propylene glycol	10 mL
Lecithin isopropyl palmitate liquid	22 mL
Poloxamer 407 20% aqueous solution, qs ad	100 mL

A. Gelling agent
B. Penetration enhancer
C. Stiffening agent
D. Preservative
E. Antioxidant

13. What is the primary function of poloxamer in this Ketoprofen 10% PLO gel formula below?

Ketoprofen   10 g
Propylene glycol   10 mL
Lecithin isopropyl palmitate liquid   22 mL
Poloxamer 407 20% aqueous   100 mL
  solution, qs ad

A. Penetration enhancer
B. Antioxidant
C. Solvent
D. Humectant
E. Gelling agent

14. Which of the following organizations (entities) generally has regulatory jurisdiction over traditional pharmacy compounding?

A. Food and Drug Administration
B. United States Pharmacopeia
C. Pharmacy Compounding Accreditation Board
D. State board of pharmacy
E. American Pharmacists Association

15. Which of the following techniques is used to ensure even dispersion of ingredients in compounded preparations?

A. Comminution
B. Geometric dilution
C. Levigation
D. Trituration
E. Pulverization by intervention

16. What type of mortar and pestle should be used when comminuting dyes and/or potent ingredients?

A. Ceramic
B. Glass
C. Plastic
D. Wedgewood
E. Porcelain

17. Below is the formula for a compounded preparation. Review the procedural steps following the formula and place them in the correct order (sequence) from start to finish.

Perphenazine 0.5 mg/mL   for 100 mL
  Oral Liquid
Perphenazine powder, USP   0.05 g
Glycerin, USP   5 mL
Simple syrup, qs   100 mL

Unordered procedure	Ordered procedure
Mix the perphenazine powder with the glycerin to form a smooth paste.	
Package and label.	
Weigh and/or measure each ingredient accurately.	
Calculate the quantity of each ingredient for the total amount to be prepared.	
Add sufficient simple syrup geometrically to final volume with mixing after each addition.	

18. Which of the following characteristics are expected with water-in-oil emulsion bases?

A. Not water washable
B. Nonocclusive
C. Nongreasy
D. Insoluble in water
E. Emollient

19. Which of the following excipients would be expected to exert humectant effects on a compounded preparation?

A. Glycerin
B. Alcohol
C. Propylene glycol
D. Purified water
E. Sorbitol

20. What type of alcohol should be used when compounding a nonsterile preparation if a specific alcohol article is not identified in the formula?

A. Ethyl alcohol 100%
B. Ethyl alcohol 95%
C. Ethyl alcohol 70%
D. Isopropyl alcohol 99%
E. Isopropyl alcohol 70%

 **5-13**   **Answers**

1. **C.** USP <795> specifies that purified water is preferred and should be used when a water article is not specified when compounding a nonsterile preparation. Purified water is prepared by the processes of distillation, reverse osmosis, or ion exchange. These methods remove heavy metals and other contaminants from the water. Water for injection is used in sterile compounding, and tap and potable water meet the requirements for drinking water but not for compounding. Potable water is for hand washing when compounding.

2. **D.** Cellulose derivatives (e.g., hydroxypropyl methylcellulose, methylcellulose) may be added to a capsule formulation to provide a slower-release of drug.

3. **A, C, and E.** Characteristics of oleaginous ointment bases include: (1) emollient, (2) occlusive, (3) greasy, (4) not water washable, (5) not water absorbing, and (6) insoluble in water.

4. **A.** For the flavoring agent to be tasted, it must be in the external or continuous phase. In an o/w emulsion, the oil is the internal, dispersed, or discontinuous phase and water is the external or continuous phase.

5. **A.** USP <795> allows a maximum 6-month BUD for a nonaqueous preparation, if all conditions are met.

6. **C and E.** USP <795> states that nonsterile compounded preparations in the moderate category require special procedures or calculations and lack stability data. The compounding of troches is an example of a preparation in the moderate category. The cavities of a troche mold require calibration for each formula.

7. **C.** The maximum BUD would be 30 days because the preparation is a water containing liquid or semisolid intended for topical, dermal, or mucosal administration.

8. **E.** When compounding, weighing and measuring accuracy within ± 5% of theoretical (desired) weight is generally considered acceptable. In other words, weighing and measuring must be not less than 95% and not more than 105% of the theoretical (desired) quantity or volume. Therefore, the acceptable range is: 350 mg × 0.95 = 332.5 mg

and 350 mg × 1.05 = 367.5 mg. If a different level of acceptable error (e.g., 10%) were determined to be appropriate the correct answer would be different.

9. **A.** The Drug Quality and Security Act was enacted in November 2013 and distinguished between traditional compounding pharmacies (i.e., 503A) and outsourcing facilities (503B).

10. **C and E.** Characteristics of a compounded prescription differ from a manufactured product. Characteristics of compounded prescriptions include: (1) patient specific and triad relationship, (2) exemption from FDA labeling requirements, (3) regulated by a state board of pharmacy, (4) No NDA submission, and (5) incorporation of BUDs.

11. **B.** USP/NF or FCC grade components are preferred for compounding. Always obtain the certificate of analysis (COA) for every component used, and use components manufactured in FDA-registered facilities. Other component grades may be used if the COA is reviewed to determine that they are appropriate for use.

12. **B.** Excipients such as lecithin and DMSO are lipophilic and serve as penetration enhancers in topical preparations.

13. **E.** Examples of gelling agents include, but are not limited to, poloxamers, carbomers, and cellulose derivatives. Aqueous solutions of poloxamer exhibit reverse-thermal properties in relation to their viscosity.

14. **D.** The regulation of pharmacy compounding is generally regulated by individual state boards of pharmacy. This is true for pharmacies operating as traditional pharmacies (i.e., compounding is performed for specific patients, pursuant to a valid prescription). Pharmacies operating outside of this scope may be subject to FDA jurisdiction.

15. **B.** Geometric dilution is a mixing process used for even dispersion of ingredients and promotion of a homogenous preparation. Comminution is a method for particle size reduction. Trituration and levigation are methods of comminution.

16. **B.** A glass mortar and pestle is preferred for potent chemicals and dyes because it is nonporous. This reduces the risk for cross-contamination compared to ceramic (i.e., porcelain) and Wedgewood equipment.

17.

Unordered procedure	Ordered procedure
Mix the perphenazine powder with the glycerin to form a smooth paste.	Calculate the quantity of each ingredient for the total amount to be prepared.
Package and label.	Weigh and/or measure each ingredient accurately.
Weigh and/or measure each ingredient accurately.	Mix the perphenazine powder with the glycerin to form a smooth paste.
Calculate the quantity of each ingredient for the total amount to be prepared.	Add sufficient simple syrup geometrically to final volume with mixing after each addition.
Add sufficient simple syrup geometrically to final volume with mixing after each addition.	Package and label.

The general process for compounding always starts with calculating the quantity of ingredients, following by weighing and measuring. Different techniques for particle size reduction and mixing (e.g., geometric dilution) are then employed before packaging and labeling the preparation. Quality control methods are also integral before dispensing to a patient.

18. **A, D,** and **E.** Characteristics of w/o emulsion ointment bases include: (1) emollient, (2) occlusive, (3) greasy, (4) not water washable, (5) water absorbing, and (6) insoluble in water.

19. **A, C,** and **E.** Glycerin, propylene glycol, and sorbitol exhibit humectant properties that aid in moisture (i.e., water) retention.

20. **B.** Alcohol, USP (95% ethyl alcohol), is to be used for nonsterile compounded preparations when the formula does not specify the type or percentage of alcohol.

 **5-14** **Additional Resources**

The following references should be considered as additional resources for pharmacy compounding.

Allen LV Jr. *The Art, Science, and Technology of Pharmaceutical Compounding.* 6th ed. Washington, DC: American Pharmacists Association; 2021.

Adejare A, ed. *Remington: The Science and Practice of Pharmacy.* 23rd ed. Cambridge, MA: Elsevier; 2021.

Allen LV Jr. *Ansel's Pharmaceutical Dosage Forms and Drug Delivery Systems.* 11th ed. Philadelphia, PA: Wolters Kluwer; 2018.

Ansel HC, Stockton SJ. *Pharmaceutical Calculations.* 15th ed. Baltimore, MD: Lippincott Williams & Wilkins; 2017.

Shrewsbury R. *Applied Pharmaceutics in Contemporary Compounding.* 4th ed. Englewood, CO: Morton; 2020.

Elder DL. *A Practical Guide to Contemporary Pharmacy Practice and Compounding.* 4th ed. Philadelphia, PA: Wolters Kluwer; 2018.

Trissel LA, Ashworth LD, Ashworth J. *Trissel's Stability of Compounded Formulations.* 6th ed. Washington, DC: American Pharmacists Association; 2018.

United States Pharmacopeial Convention. *U.S. Pharmacopeia 42/National Formulary 37.* Rockville, MD: United States Pharmacopeial Convention; 2019.

Sterile Products

6

SUSAN H. MORGAN

6-1 KEY POINTS

- Sterile compounding requires the maintenance of sterility when using sterile manufactured products and the achievement of sterility when using nonsterile ingredients or devices.
- The air in an International Organization for Standardization (ISO) class 5 area has no more than 3520 particles 0.5 micron and larger per cubic meter of air. The laminar flow workbench provides an ISO class 5 area.
- The high-efficiency particulate air (HEPA) filter is 99.97% efficient at filtering out particles 0.3 micron in size.
- The critical site is any opening or pathway between the compounded sterile preparation or product (CSP) and the environment. The larger the critical site is and the longer it is exposed to the environment, the greater the risk of contamination of the preparation.
- Any pharmacist preparing CSPs must initially complete three successful hand hygiene, garbing, and gloving exercises with finger touch plates showing no growth after incubation.
- A sterilizing filter (0.2 micron) is required to filter sterilize a CSP. The integrity of the filter must be verified, usually by the bubble point test.
- The unidirectional airflow in a horizontal laminar flow workbench flows toward the operator. The operator must never put his or her hands between the HEPA filter and the critical site.
- The unidirectional airflow in a vertical laminar flow workbench flows down onto the work surface.
- A biological safety cabinet should always be used for preparing cytotoxic drugs. All biological safety cabinets have vertical laminar airflow.
- The hot air oven is used to remove pyrogens from items used in compounding and to sterilize compounded preparations that cannot be sterilized by steam.
- Moist-heat sterilization is a common way to sterilize equipment used in the compounding process. Only items that can be moistened by steam can be sterilized by autoclaving.
- The sterility test and the bacterial endotoxin test should be performed on all high-risk CSPs prepared in groups of more than 25 identical individual single-dose packages or in multidose vials intended for injection into the vascular or central nervous system.

6-2 STUDY GUIDE CHECKLIST

The following topics may guide your study of this subject area:

- ☐ Routes of administration and the unique characteristics of each.
- ☐ ISO classifications 5, 7, and 8.
- ☐ Primary engineering controls and how they work.
- ☐ Required specifications of the HEPA filter.
- ☐ Requirements of the buffer area and the anteroom.
- ☐ Gowning qualification requirements.
- ☐ Media fills.
- ☐ Microbial risk levels and associated beyond-use dates.
- ☐ *USP* Chapter <800> Hazardous Drugs—Handling in Healthcare Settings.
- ☐ The Drug Quality and Security Act of 2013:
  - ○ Section 503A: Pharmacy Compounding.
  - ○ Section 503B: Outsourcing Facilities.
- ☐ Sources of physical incompatibilities.
- ☐ Chemical degradation pathways.
- ☐ Quality control tests specific to sterile products.

6-3   Parenteral Products

Parenteral products are administered by injection and, therefore, bypass the gastrointestinal (GI) tract. Parenteral products must be sterile and free of pyrogens and particulate matter. Drugs that are destroyed or inactivated in the GI tract, or are poorly absorbed, can be given by a parenteral route. Parenteral routes of administration may also be used when the patient is uncooperative, unconscious, or unable to swallow. This route is also used when rapid drug absorption is essential, such as in emergency situations.

Parenteral Routes of Administration

Intravenous route

An intravenous (I.V.) medication is administered directly into the vein. The I.V. route gives a rapid effect with a predictable response. This route does not have as much volume restriction as other parenteral routes.

A *bolus* is an injection of solution into the vein over a short period of time. A bolus is used to administer a relatively small volume of solution and is often ordered as an "I.V. push."

An *infusion* refers to the introduction of larger volumes of solution given intravenously over a longer period of time. A continuous infusion is used to administer a large volume of solution at a constant rate. Intermittent infusions are used to administer a relatively small volume of solution over a specified amount of time at specific intervals.

Intramuscular route

An intramuscular (I.M.) medication is injected deep into a large muscle mass, such as the upper arm, thigh, or buttocks. The medication is absorbed from the muscle tissue, acting more quickly than when given by the oral route but not as quickly as when given by the I.V. route. Up to 2 mL may be administered intramuscularly as a solution or suspension given in the upper arm, and up to 5 mL may be given in the gluteal medial muscle of each buttock. A sustained-release action can be achieved with certain drugs that have low solubility because they are released from muscle tissue at a slow rate. I.M. injections are often painful, and reversing adverse effects from medications given by this route is very difficult.

Subcutaneous route

Subcutaneous injections of solution or suspension are given beneath the surface of the skin. Medications administered by this route are not absorbed as well as and have a slower onset of action than medications given by the I.V. or I.M. route. The volume of solution or suspension that can be injected subcutaneously is 2 mL or less.

Intradermal route

An intradermal (I.D.) injection is injected into the top layer of the skin and not as deep as a subcutaneous injection. Medications used for diagnostic purposes, such as a tuberculin test or an allergy test, are often administered by this route. The volume of solution that can be administered intradermally is limited to 0.1 mL. The onset of action and the rate of absorption of medication from this route are slow.

Intra-arterial route

An intra-arterial (I.A.) injection is injected directly into an artery. It delivers a high drug concentration to the target site with little dilution by the circulation.

Other routes

- **Intracardiac:** An injection is made directly into the heart.
- **Intra-articular:** An injection is made into a joint space.
- **Intrathecal:** An injection is made into the lumbar intraspinal fluid sacs. Appropriate preservative-free drugs should be used for intrathecal administration.

6-4 ▶ Definitions for Compounding of Sterile Preparations

- **Admixture:** Parenteral dosage forms that are combined for administration as a single entity.
- **Ante area:** An International Organization for Standardization (ISO) class 8 or better area where hand hygiene and garbing procedures, sanitizing of supplies, and other particulate-generating activities are performed. The area contains a line of demarcation separating the clean side from the dirty side.
- **Aseptic processing:** The separate sterilization of a product and its components, containers, and closures, which are then brought together and assembled in an aseptic environment. The primary objective of aseptic processing is to create a sterile preparation.
- **Aseptic technique:** Performance of a procedure or procedures under controlled conditions in a manner that will minimize the chance of contamination. Contaminants can be introduced from the environment, equipment and supplies, or personnel (see the section on ISO classification).
- **Buffer area:** The area where the primary engineering control is located.
- **Compounding aseptic containment isolator (CACI):** An isolator that protects workers from exposure to undesirable levels of airborne drugs while providing an aseptic environment during the compounding of sterile preparations.
- **Compounding aseptic isolator (CAI):** An isolator that maintains an aseptic compounding environment within the isolator throughout the compounding and material transfer process during the compounding of sterile preparations.
- **Critical site:** Any opening or surface that can provide a pathway between the sterile product and the environment.
- **Hypertonic:** A solution that contains a higher concentration of dissolved substances than the red blood cell, thereby causing the red blood cell to shrink.
- **Hypotonic:** A solution that contains a lower concentration of dissolved substances than the red blood cell, thereby causing the red blood cell to swell and possibly burst.
- **Isotonic:** A solution that has an osmotic pressure close to that of bodily fluids, thus minimizing patient discomfort and damage to red blood cells. Dextrose 5% in water and sodium chloride 0.9% solutions are approximately isotonic.
- **Primary engineering control (PEC):** A device or room that provides an ISO class 5 environment for the exposure of critical sites when producing compounded sterile preparations (CSPs). These devices include laminar airflow workbenches, biological safety cabinets (BSC), CAIs, and CACIs.
- **Sterilizing filter:** A filter that, when challenged with the microorganism *Brevundimonas diminuta* at a minimum concentration of 10^7 organisms per cm^2 of filter surface, will produce a sterile effluent. A sterilizing filter has a nominal pore size rating of 0.2 or 0.22 micron.
- **Tonicity:** Osmotic pressure exerted by a solution from the solutes or dissolved solids present.
- **Validation:** Establishment of documented evidence providing a high degree of assurance that a specific process will consistently produce a product meeting predetermined specifications and quality attributes.

ISO Classification

The ISO Classification of Particulate Matter in Room Air is the standard for clean rooms and associated environments. Limits are expressed in particles 0.5 micron and larger per cubic meter.

ISO class 5 area

The air in an ISO class 5 area has no more than 3520 particles 0.5 micron or larger per cubic meter of air. This class is the quality of air provided by the PEC and required for sterile product preparation.

ISO class 7 area

The air in an ISO class 7 area has a count of no more than 352,000 particles 0.5 micron or larger per cubic meter. This class is the quality of air usually required in the buffer area.

ISO class 8 area

The air in an ISO class 8 area has a count of no more than 3,520,000 particles 0.5 micron or larger per cubic meter. The ante area should have ISO class 8 air or better.

6-5   Sterile Product Preparation Area

The following are examples of PECs that provide the ISO class 5 area for compounding of CSPs.

Horizontal Laminar Flow Workbench

The horizontal laminar flow workbench (HLFW) is an ISO class 5 area. In order to achieve this, the HLFW works by drawing air in through a prefilter. The prefilter protects the HEPA filter from prematurely clogging. Prefilters should be checked regularly and changed as needed. A record of these checks and changes of the prefilter must be kept.

The plenum of the HLFW is the space between the prefilter and the HEPA filter The prefiltered air is pressurized in the plenum for consistent distribution of air to the high-efficiency particulate air (HEPA) filter (Figure 6-1).

FIGURE 6-1. Horizontal Laminar Flow Workbench

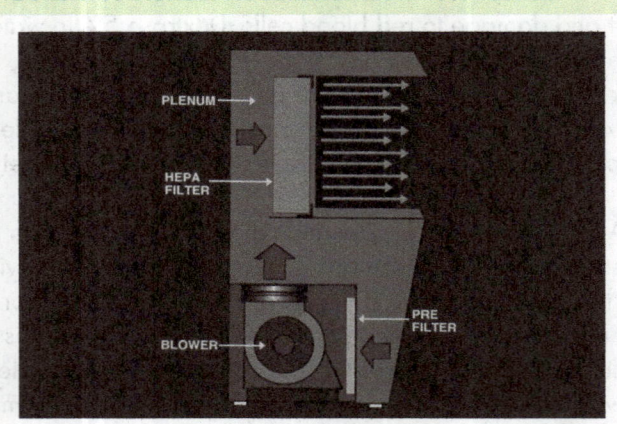

Laminar flow is the air in a confined space moving with uniform velocity along parallel lines. The term *unidirectional flow* has taken the place of laminar flow in more recent publications. Unidirectional flow is airflow moving in a single direction in a robust and uniform manner and at sufficient speed to sweep particles away from the critical processing area.

Vertical Laminar Flow Workbench

The vertical laminar flow workbench (VLFW) works like an HLFW in that the air is drawn in through the prefilter and is pressurized in the plenum for distribution over the HEPA filter. However, the air is blown down from the top of the workstation onto the work surface, not across it (Figure 6-2).

Working in vertical laminar flow requires different techniques than those used when working in horizontal laminar flow. In vertical laminar flow, an object or the hands of the operator must not be above an object in the hood. In horizontal laminar flow, an object or the hands of the operator must not be in back of another object. The hands of the operator must never come between the HEPA filter and the object.

A BSC, CAI, and CACI also use vertical unidirectional airflow to provide an ISO class 5 environment and are other examples of PECs.

HEPA Filter

The HEPA filter consists of a bank of filter media separated by corrugated pleats of aluminum. These pleats act as baffles to direct the air into laminar sheets. The HEPA filter is 99.97% efficient at removing particles 0.3 micron in size.

Certification of the HEPA filter

The velocity of air from the HEPA filter is checked with a velometer or hot wire anemometer. ISO 14644 recommends that the average air velocity should be greater than 0.2 m/second.

Integrity of the HEPA filter

The integrity of the HEPA filter is checked by introducing a high concentration of aerosolized Emery 3004 (a synthetic hydrocarbon) upstream of the filter on a continuous basis, while monitoring the penetration on the downstream side of the HEPA filter. The aerosol has an average particle size of 0.3 micron. An aerosol photometer is used to check for leaks by passing the wand slowly over the filter and the gasket.

FIGURE 6-2. Vertical Laminar Flow Workbench

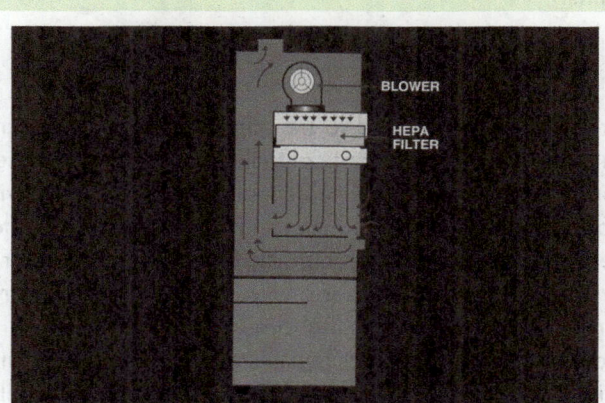

None of the surfaces shall yield greater than 0.01% of the upstream smoke concentration. Any value greater than 0.01% indicates that a serious leak is present and must be sealed. All repaired areas must be retested for compliance.

Buffer Area (Controlled Area)

The PEC provides an ISO class 5 workspace within the buffer area. The PEC must be located in a controlled environment, away from excess traffic, doors, air vents, or anything that could produce air currents greater than the velocity of the airflow from the HEPA filter because such air currents could introduce contaminants into the hood.

The buffer area shall be enclosed from other pharmacy operations. Floors, walls, ceiling, shelving, counters, and cabinets in the controlled area must be of nonshedding, smooth, and nonporous material to allow for easy cleaning and disinfecting. All surfaces shall be resistant to sanitizing agents. Cracks, crevices, and seams shall be avoided, as should ledges or other places that could collect dust. The floor of the buffer area shall be smooth and seamless with coved edges up the walls.

The walls of the buffer area can be sealed panels caulked with silicone or, if drywall is used, painted with epoxy paint, which is nonshedding. The corners of the ceiling and the walls shall be sealed to avoid cracks. A solid ceiling may be painted with epoxy paint, or nonshedding washable ceiling tiles that are caulked into place may be used.

Light fixtures shall be mounted flush with the ceiling and sealed. Anything that penetrates the ceiling or walls shall be sealed.

Air entering the room shall be fresh, HEPA filtered, and air conditioned. The room must be maintained at positive pressure (0.02 to 0.05 inch of water column) in relation to the adjoining rooms or corridors. At least 30 air changes per hour shall occur, with the PECs allowed to provide up to 15 of the 30 required air changes per hour.

Controlling the traffic in the buffer area is a critical factor in keeping the area clean. People entering the buffer area shall be properly scrubbed and gowned. Access to the buffer area shall be restricted to qualified personnel only. Only items required for compounding shall be brought into the buffer area. These items must be cleaned and sanitized before being taken into the buffer area and may be stored in the buffer area for a limited time. However, the number of items stored in the buffer area shall be kept to a minimum. All equipment used in the buffer area should remain in the room except during calibration or repair.

Because they can harbor many organisms, refrigerators and freezers should be located out of the buffer area. Computers and printers should be located outside of the buffer area because they generate many particles. However, if they are required to be in the buffer area, monitor the environment and evaluate their effect on the environment. Cardboard boxes shall not be stored in the buffer area. The items shall be removed from the boxes on the dirty side of the ante area and sanitized and transferred to the clean side of the ante area or to the buffer area for storage. Vials stored in laminated cardboard may be stored in the buffer area. Sinks or floor drains shall not be in the buffer area because potable water contains many organisms and endotoxins.

Preparation of Operators

An operator must be trained and evaluated to be capable of properly scrubbing and garbing before entering the buffer area. This requirement is critical to the maintenance of asepsis. People are the greatest source of contamination in a clean room. A seated or standing person without movement releases an average of 100,000 particles greater than 0.3 micron in diameter per minute. A person standing with full body movement releases an average of 2 million particles per minute greater than 0.3 micron in diameter, and if moving at a slow walk, he or she releases an average of 5 million particles per minute. Cleanroom garb is designed to help contain the particles that are being shed.

Before entering the ante area, an operator must remove all cosmetics and all hand, wrist, and other visible jewelry or piercings. Artificial nails or extenders are prohibited while working in the sterile compounding environment, and natural nails must be kept neat and trimmed. Garb is donned in an order proceeding from that considered dirtiest to that considered cleanest. Shoe covers, head and facial hair covers, and facemask or eye shields are donned before performing hand hygiene. Hands and forearms are then washed for 30 seconds with soap and water in the ante area, and hands and forearms are dried using a lint-free disposable towel or an electric hand dryer. While still in the ante area, an operator must don a nonshedding gown that zips or buttons up to the neck, falls below the knees, and has sleeves that fit snugly around the wrists.

After entering the buffer area, an operator must use a waterless, alcohol-based, surgical hand scrub with persistent activity to again cleanse the hands before putting on sterile gloves. Sterile contact agar plates must be used to sample the gloved fingertips of compounding personnel after garbing to assess garbing competency. For successful completion of this competency, no colony-forming units can be found on any of the agar plate samples. Three consecutive successful garbing and gloving exercises must be completed before sterile compounding is allowed. Routine application of sterile 70% isopropyl alcohol (IPA) must occur throughout the compounding process and whenever nonsterile surfaces are touched. After this initial evaluation, the entire process is repeated at least once a year for low- and medium-risk compounding and semiannually for high-risk compounding during any media-fill test procedure. The colony-forming unit action level for gloved hands will be based on the total number of colony-forming units on both gloves, not per hand.

Validation of the Operator

A *media fill* or *media transfer* is when a growth promotion media is used instead of the drug product, and all of the normal compounding manipulations are done. Ensuring that the process mimics the actual compounding process as closely as possible and represents worst-case conditions is critical. Usually, the medium used is soybean-casein digest, which is also known as trypticase soy broth (TSB). This medium will support the growth of organisms that are likely to be transmitted to CSPs from the compounding personnel and the environment. A media fill is used to check the quality of the compounding personnel's aseptic technique. It is also used to verify that the compounding process and the compounding environment are capable of producing sterile preparations.

Initially, before an operator can compound low- or medium-risk sterile injectable products, he or she must successfully complete one media fill using sterile fluid culture media such as 3% soybean-casein digest medium. Media fill units must be incubated at 20°C to 25°C for a minimum of 14 days or at 20°C to 25°C for a minimum of 7 days and then at 30°C to 35°C for a minimum of 7 days. A successful media fill is indicated by no growth in any of the media fill units. The media fill shall closely simulate the most challenging or stressful conditions encountered during the compounding of low- and medium-risk preparations. The compounding personnel shall perform a revalidation at a minimum of once a year by successfully completing one media fill. Validation for high-risk compounding focuses on ensuring that both the process and the compounding personnel are capable of producing a sterile preparation with all its purported quality attributes. Revalidation for high-risk compounding must be done on at least a semiannual basis. An example of a high-risk operation is the compounding of a sterile preparation from nonsterile drug powder. To mimic this operation, the compounder must use commercially available soybean-casein digest medium made up to a 3% concentration and perform normal processing steps, including filter sterilization. All media fills must occur in an ISO class 5 environment and must be completed without interruption.

6-6   Working in the Laminar Flow Workbench

Items not in a protective overwrap shall be wiped with a lint-free wipe soaked with sterile 70% IPA before being placed in the hood. Containers and packages must be inspected for cracks, tears, or particles as they are decontaminated and placed in the hood. Items in a protective overwrap, such as bags, must be taken from the overwrap at the edge of the hood (within the first 6 inches of the hood) and placed in the hood with the injection port facing the HEPA filter. The overwrap should not be placed in the hood, because doing so would introduce particles and organisms into the hood.

When working in the HLFW, an operator shall arrange supplies to the left or the right of the direct compounding area. The critical site must be in uninterrupted unidirectional airflow at all times. The compounder must be careful not to place an object or hand between the HEPA filter and the critical site because doing so would interrupt the airflow to the critical site and potentially cause particles to be washed from the hand or object onto the critical site.

All work performed in the HLFW must be done at least 6 inches inside the hood. The unidirectional airflow is blowing toward the operator, who acts as a barrier to the airflow, causing it to pass around the body and create backflow. This turbulence can cause room air to be carried into the front of the hood.

Items placed in the HLFW disturb the unidirectional airflow. The unidirectional airflow is disturbed downstream of the item for approximately 3 times the diameter of the object. If the item is placed next to the sidewall of the hood, the unidirectional airflow is disturbed downstream of the item for approximately 6 times the diameter of the object. The area downstream from the nonsterile object is no longer bathed in unidirectional airflow and may become contaminated with particles. For these reasons, ensuring that a direct path exists between the HEPA filter and the area where the manipulations will occur is very important.

With the VLFW, supplies in the hood should be placed so that the operator may work without placing a hand or object above the critical site. An operator can place many more items in the VLFW and still work without compromising the unidirectional airflow. The unidirectional airflow, which is coming down from the HEPA filter, strikes the work surface and changes direction to move horizontally across the work surface. Therefore, all work in the VLFW should be done at least 1 inch above the work surface. During the compounding of sterile preparations, all movements into and out of the hood must be minimized to decrease the risk of carrying contaminants into the direct compounding area.

6-7   Syringes, Needles, Ampuls, and Vials

Syringes

The basic parts of the syringe are the barrel, plunger, collar, rubber tip of the plunger, and tip of the syringe. Syringes are sterile and free of pyrogens. They are packaged either in paper or in a rigid plastic container. Syringe packages must be inspected to ensure that the wrap is intact. Syringes have either a Luer-Lok tip, in which the needle is screwed tightly onto the threaded tip, or a slip tip, in which the needle is held on by friction (Figure 6-3). Syringes are supplied with and without needles attached and

FIGURE 6-3. Types of Syringes

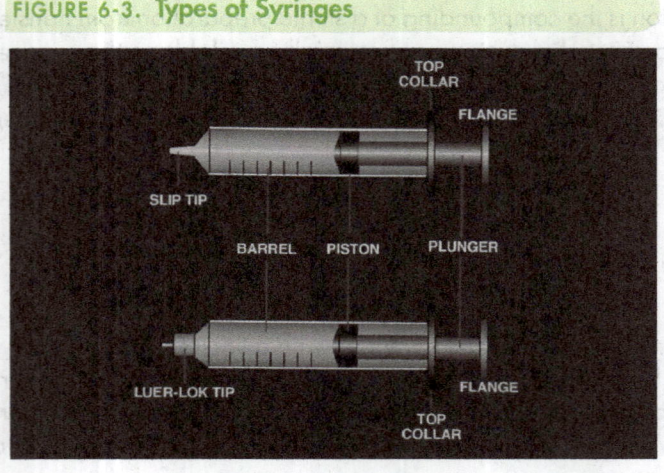

are available in a variety of sizes. When removing the syringe from its package, take care not to let the syringe tip touch any surface.

Calibration marks are on the barrel of the syringe. These marks are accurate to one-half the interval marked on the syringe. The critical sites on the syringe are the tip of the syringe and the ribs of the plunger. The ribs of the plunger go back inside the syringe on injection of the fluid from the syringe and could potentially contaminate the syringe.

Needles

The basic parts of a needle include the hub, needle shaft, bevel, bevel heel, and tip of the needle (Figure 6-4).

Needles are sterile and are wrapped either in plastic with a twist-off top or in paper. This wrap must be inspected for integrity before the needle is used. The gauge of the needle refers to its outer diameter. The larger the number, the smaller the bore of the needle. The smallest is 27 gauge, and the largest is 13 gauge. The length of the needle is measured in inches, and common lengths are 1 to 1.5 inches.

The critical sites on the needle are the hub of the needle, the entire needle shaft, and the tip of the needle.

Ampuls

Ampuls are single-dose containers. Before breaking the ampul, wipe the neck of the ampul with a sterile 70% IPA prep pad. Once ampuls are broken, they are an open-system container; air can pass freely in and out of the ampul. Any solution taken from an ampul must be filtered with a 5-micron filter needle or filter straw, because glass particles fall into the ampul when it is broken.

Vials

A vial is a molded glass or plastic container with a rubber closure secured in place with an aluminum seal. It may contain sterile solutions, dry-filled powders, or lyophilized drugs, or it may be an empty evacuated container. Vials may be single-dose or multiple-dose containers.

A single-dose container usually contains no preservative system to prevent the growth of microorganisms if they are accidentally introduced into the container. A single-dose vial punctured in an environment worse than ISO class 5 air must be used within 1 hour. A single-dose vial continuously exposed to ISO class 5 air may be used up to 6 hours after initial needle puncture. When the vial is first used, it should be labeled with the date, time, and initials of the person using the vial so the beyond-use date (BUD) can be determined. A multidose vial contains preservatives, and these vials can be entered more than once.

FIGURE 6-4. Basic Parts of a Needle

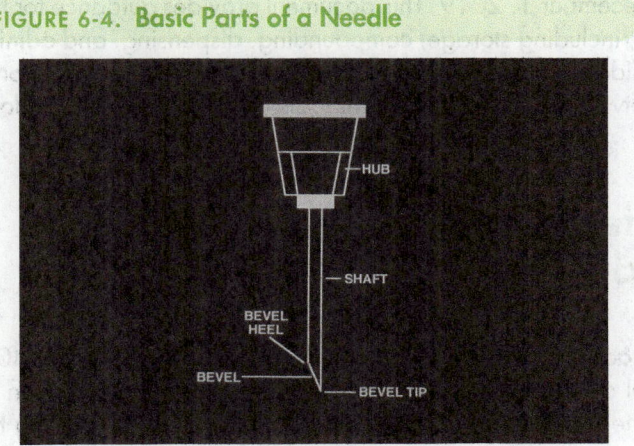

The pharmaceutical manufacturer has done studies to prove that the preservative system will remain effective and the closure will reseal after penetration by the needle. Therefore, the BUD for opened or entered multidose containers is 28 days, unless otherwise specified by the manufacturer.

6-8   Biological Safety Cabinets

A class II BSC should be used to prepare cytotoxic and other hazardous drugs. Four different types of class II BSCs exist. Types A1 and A2 exhaust 30% of HEPA-filtered air either into the room or to the outside through a canopy connection. Type A1 mixes the supply air in a common plenum and may have ducts and plenum under positive pressure. Type A2 has all contaminated ducts and plenum under negative pressure or surrounded by negative pressure. Type B1 exhausts 70% of total air through a dedicated exhaust duct and must be hard ducted. Type B2 exhausts 100% of total air to the outside without any recirculation and must be hard ducted also. With types B1 and B2, all the ducts and the plenum are under negative pressure and are surrounded by negative pressure.

Preparation of Hazardous Drugs

When working with hazardous drugs, personnel must wear appropriate protective equipment, including solid-front gowns, face masks, eye protection, hair and shoe covers, and double sterile chemotherapy-type gloves. Personnel must handle hazardous drugs with caution at all times, using appropriate chemotherapy gloves, not only during preparation but also during receiving, distribution, stocking, inventorying, and disposal.

Ensuring that positive pressure not be allowed to build up in the vial is imperative. On an annual basis, proper training on the use of closed-system transfer devices (CSTDs) or the negative pressure aseptic technique (if CSTDs are not available or do not fit the medication vial) to prevent the buildup of positive pressure within the vial must be done before preparing hazardous drugs. When a CSTD is used, it shall be used within the ISO class 5 environment of a BSC or CACI.

When compounding, personnel must use syringes and IV sets with Luer-Lok fittings if possible. Use a large enough syringe so that the plunger does not separate from the barrel of the syringe when filled with solution. Syringes should be filled with no more than 75% of their total volume. When possible, attach IV sets and prime them before adding the hazardous drug. Wipe the outside of the bag or bottle to remove any inadvertent contamination. The use of nonshedding, plastic-backed absorbent pads is also conducive to keeping the BSC as clean as possible.

The PEC shall be located in an ISO class 7 area physically separated from other preparation areas and maintained under negative pressure of not less than 0.01-inch water column to the surrounding area.

United States Pharmacopeia (USP) chapter <800>, Hazardous Drugs—Handling in Healthcare Settings, became effective December 1, 2019. This document provides guidance for handling hazardous drugs in all health care settings, including storage, compounding, dispensing, and administration. It incorporates previously developed guidance published by the National Institute for Occupational Safety and Health (NIOSH), the American Society of Health-System Pharmacists (ASHP), and the Oncology Nursing Society (ONS).

6-9   Overview of the Standard of Practice Related to Sterile Preparations

USP <797>, Pharmaceutical Compounding—Sterile Preparations in USP 40/NF (National Formulary) 35, became the official standard for sterile pharmaceutical compounding in June 2008. This chapter was revised and published on June 1, 2019, but received appeals regarding the BUD provisions. Therefore, the 2008 version of *USP* chapter <797> remains official until further notice, and the revised chapter is now with the Compounding Expert Committee to further explore the issues raised. USP <797> has three microbial risk levels of CSPs. The risk levels are determined on the basis of the potential for the introduction of microbial, chemical, or physical contamination into the product. The chapter covers topics such as validation of sterilization and of the aseptic process, environmental control and sampling, end-product testing, bacterial endotoxins, training, and a quality assurance program.

Low-Risk Compounding

Compounding is classified as *low risk* when all of the following conditions prevail:

- Commercially available sterile products, components, and devices are used in compounding within air quality of ISO class 5 or better.
- Compounding involves few aseptic manipulations, using not more than 3 commercially manufactured sterile products and not more than 2 entries into any 1 sterile container.
- Closed-system transfers are used. Withdrawal from an open ampul is classified as a closed system.
- In the absence of passage of a sterility test, the storage periods for the CSPs cannot exceed the following time periods before administration:
  - Storage for not more than 48 hours at a controlled room temperature of 20°C to 25°C
  - Storage for not more than 14 days at a cold temperature of 2°C to 8°C
  - Storage for not more than 45 days in a solid frozen state between −25°C and −10°C

Medium-Risk Compounding

Medium-risk CSPs are those compounded under low-risk conditions when one or more of the following conditions exist:

- Compounding involves pooling of additives for the administration to either multiple patients or one patient on multiple occasions.
- Compounding involves complex manipulations other than a single-volume transfer.
- The compounding process requires a long time period to complete dissolution or homogeneous mixing.
- In the absence of passage of a sterility test, the storage periods for the CSPs cannot exceed the following time periods before administration:
  - Exposure for not more than 30 hours at a controlled room temperature of 20°C to 25°C
  - Storage for not more than 9 days at a cold temperature of 2°C to 8°C
  - Storage for not more than 45 days in a solid frozen state between −25°C and −10°C

High-Risk Compounding

High-risk compounds are compounded under any of the following conditions and are either contaminated or at high risk to become contaminated with infectious microorganisms:

- A sterile preparation is compounded from nonsterile ingredients.
- Sterile ingredients or components are exposed to air quality inferior to ISO class 5 for more than 1 hour, including storage in environments inferior to ISO class 5 of opened or partially used packages of manufactured sterile products with no antimicrobial preservative system.
- Nonsterile water–containing preparations are exposed for more than 6 hours before being sterilized.
- No examination of labeling and documentation from suppliers or no direct determination that the chemical purity and content strength of ingredients meet their original or compendia specification occurs.
- Compounding personnel are improperly garbed and gloved.

■ In the absence of passage of a sterility test, the storage periods for the CSPs cannot exceed the following time periods before administration:
- Storage for not more than 24 hours at a controlled room temperature of 20°C to 25°C
- Storage for not more than 3 days at a cold temperature of 2°C to 8°C
- Storage for not more than 45 days in a solid frozen state between –25°C and –10°C

The Drug Quality and Security Act of 2013

The Drug Quality and Security Act (DQSA) of 2013 was passed by the U.S. Congress in an attempt to better define the difference between small pharmacy compounding and drug manufacturing. The DQSA applies to human drugs only. It does not apply to any veterinary products or to investigational drugs.

Title I of the DQSA, the Compounding Quality Act, addresses prescription drug compounding and divides pharmacy compounding into sections 503A and 503B.

Section 503A provides the requirements that must be met to allow exemption from the Food, Drug, and Cosmetic Act.

Section 503A requires that compounding must be performed by a licensed pharmacist in a licensed pharmacy, compounding must be performed in compliance with USP <795> and <797>, the compounded preparation must be packaged to promote safety and stability and labeled with the appropriate instructions to a patient, and the CSP can be made only upon receipt of a prescription for an individual patient. Some anticipatory compounding in limited quantities based on historical data is allowed.

Section 503B defines an outsourcing facility that mandates compliance with good manufacturing practices.

Title II of the DQSA, the Drug Supply Chain Security Act, establishes a track-and-trace system for monitoring the drug supply chain.

6-10   Sterilization Methods

Filtration

Filtration works by a combination of sieving, adsorption, and entrapment. Care must be taken to choose the correct filter to sterilize the preparation. Membrane filters generally are compatible with most pharmaceutical solutions, but interactions do occur—often because of sorption or leaching. *Sorption* is the binding of a drug or other formulation components to the filter, which can occur with peptide or protein formulations. Some filters have little or no affinity for peptides or proteins. *Leaching* is the extracting of components of the filter into the solution. Surfactants are often added to the filter to make it hydrophilic, and they may leach into the product. Large-molecular-weight peptides may be affected by filtration. Their passage through a filter with a small pore size may cause shear stress and alter the three-dimensional structure of the peptide. Solvents in the parenteral formulation may also affect filters. All filter manufacturers have compatibility data on their membrane type, and the data can be a source of information when choosing a membrane.

Filter choice

Choose the appropriate size and configuration of filtration device to accommodate the volume being filtered and to permit complete filtration without clogging of the membrane. A 25-mm syringe disk filter should filter no more than 100 mL of solution. If the solution being filtered has a heavy particulate load, a 5-micron filter should be used before the 0.2-micron filter to decrease the particulate load to the 0.2-micron filter. The filter membrane and housing must be physically and chemically compatible with the product to be filtered and capable of withstanding the temperature, pressures, and hydrostatic stress imposed on the system.

A pharmacy may rely on the certificate of quality provided by the vendor. Certification shall include microbial retention testing with *Brevundimonas diminuta* at a minimum concentration of 10^7 organisms per cm^2, as well as testing for membrane and housing integrity, nonpyrogenicity, and extractables.

Hydrophobic and hydrophilic filters

Hydrophilic membranes wet spontaneously with water. They are used for filtration of aqueous solutions and aqueous solutions containing water-miscible solvents. *Hydrophobic filters* do not wet spontaneously with water. They are used for filtering gases and solvents.

Filter integrity

A sterilizing filter assembly shall be tested for integrity after filtration has occurred. The *bubble point* is a simple, nondestructive check of the integrity of the filtration assembly, including the filter membrane. The basis for the test is that liquid is held in the capillary structure of the membrane by surface tension. The minimum pressure required to force the liquid out of the capillary space is a measure of the largest pores in the membrane.

A bubble point test is performed by wetting the filter with water, increasing the pressure of air upstream of the filter, and watching for air bubbles downstream to indicate passage of air through the filter capillaries. The typical water bubble point pressure of a sterilizing filter with a pore size rating of 0.2 micron is greater than 50 pounds per square inch gauge (psig). As pore size decreases, the bubble point increases. The bubble point given on the certificate of quality from the filter manufacturer is usually the water bubble point. Many drug formulations have a lower surface tension than water and will have a lower bubble point.

After the solution is filtered and before the integrity of the filter membrane is checked, the filter should be flushed with water to wash as much of the product off the membrane as possible. The integrity test may then be performed. Also, bubble points are often given for 70% IPA and water. Use the alcohol test for a hydrophobic filter.

Heat Sterilization

Moist-heat sterilization (autoclave)

Moist-heat sterilization is one of the most widely used methods of sterilization. Saturation of steam at high pressure is the foundation for the effectiveness of moist-heat sterilization. When steam makes contact with a cooler object, it condenses and loses latent heat to the object. The amount of energy released is approximately 524 kcal/g at 121°C. Most sterilization cycles are at 121°C at 15 psig for 20 to 60 minutes. Moist-heat sterilization is faster and does not require as high a temperature as dry-heat sterilization. Steam must make contact with the object to be sterilized. Oils cannot be sterilized by steam nor can an empty dry vial. Biological indicators of *Geobacillus stearothermophilus* and temperature-sensing devices shall be used to verify the effectiveness of the steam sterilization cycle.

Dry-heat sterilization

Dry-heat sterilization is usually done as a batch process in an oven designed for sterilization. It provides heated filtered air that is evenly distributed throughout the chamber by a blower. The oven is equipped with a system to control the temperature and exposure period. Dry-heat sterilization requires higher temperatures and longer exposure times than does moist-heat sterilization. Typical sterilization cycles are 120 to 180 minutes at 160°C or 90 to 120 minutes at 170°C. Biological indicators of *Bacillus subtilis* and temperature-sensing devices shall be used to verify the effectiveness of the dry-heat sterilization cycle.

Depyrogenation by dry heat

Dry heat also can be used for depyrogenation of glass and stainless steel equipment and of vials. The pyrogens are destroyed when the equipment is kept at 250°C for 30 minutes. The effectiveness of the dry-heat depyrogenation cycle shall be verified by using endotoxin challenge vials to determine whether the cycle is adequate to achieve a 3-log reduction in endotoxins.

Beyond-Use Date

Each CSP must have a label that specifies the correct names and amount of ingredients, total volume, storage requirements, route of administration, and BUD. The BUD is the date after which a compounded preparation is not to be used and is determined from the date the preparation is compounded. In the absence of passing the sterility test, the CSPs must comply with the microbial BUD. If the lot of CSPs has met the requirements of the sterility test, then the BUD may be based on chemical and physical stability. When assigning a BUD, compounding personnel should consult and apply drug-specific and general stability documentation and literature where available. They should consider the nature of the drug, its degradation mechanism, the container in which it is packaged, the expected storage conditions, and the intended duration of therapy.

6-11   Stability

Stability refers to physical, chemical, and microbial stability.

Instability usually refers to chemical reactions that are incessant and irreversible and result in distinctly different chemical entities. These new chemical entities can be therapeutically inactive and possibly exhibit greater toxicity.

Incompatibility usually refers to physicochemical phenomena such as concentration-dependent precipitation and acid–base reactions that occur when one drug is mixed with others to produce a product unsuitable for administration to the patient. An incompatibility could cause the patient not to receive the full therapeutic effect, or it could cause toxic decomposition products to form. A precipitated incompatibility may irritate the vein or cause occlusion of vessels.

There are three categories of incompatibilities: *therapeutic incompatibility, physical incompatibility,* and *chemical incompatibility.*

Therapeutic Incompatibility

Therapeutic incompatibility occurs when two or more drugs administered at the same time result in undesirable antagonistic or synergistic pharmacologic action.

Physical Incompatibility

Physical incompatibility is the combination of two or more drugs in a solution, resulting in a change in the appearance of the solution, a change in color, the formation of turbidity or a precipitate, or the evolution of a gas. Physical incompatibilities are related to solubility changes or container interactions rather than to molecular change to the drug entity itself.

Six major areas of concern about physical incompatibility

Compatibility or incompatibility of two or more drugs mixed in the same syringe

For example, preoperative medications—a combination of a narcotic, an analgesic, an antiemetic, and an anticholinergic—are mixed in the same syringe to save the patient from multiple intramuscular injections.

Compatibility of two or more drugs given through the same I.V. administration line

This concern is common in intensive care units, where patients are often on a number of I.V. medications and could be fluid restricted. For example, dopamine HCl 800 mg in 500 mL D_5W (5% dextrose in water) is prescribed. The nurse wants to push 2 amps of sodium bicarbonate through the I.V. line. The pH of dopamine is 3 to 4.5, and that of $NaHCO_3$ is approximately 8. If this push is done, a color change occurs because of decomposition of the product. The pH of the bicarbonate is too high for dopamine stability.

Compatibility of two or more drugs placed in the same bottle or bag of IV fluid

KCl, the most common additive, is a neutral salt composed of monovalent ions that are not likely to produce compatibility problems. Therefore, if a drug is compatible in a neutral salt, it is probably compatible in KCl.

Parenteral nutrition solutions can be especially difficult. The number of components, the long duration of contact time, and exposure to ambient temperature and light increase the potential for an adverse compatibility interaction to occur. The interaction of Ca and PO_4 to form $CaPO_4$, which appears as fine white particles that create a milky solution, is a problem.

Some ways to decrease the risk of injury are as follows:

- Calculate the solubility of the added calcium from the volume at the time when calcium is added. Flush the line in between the addition of any potentially incompatible components.
- Add the calcium before the lipid emulsion. Therefore, if a precipitate forms, the lipid will not obscure its presence.
- Periodically agitate the admixture, and check for precipitates. Train patients and caregivers to visually inspect for signs of precipitation and to stop the infusion if precipitation is noted.

The following factors enhance formation of precipitate of calcium and phosphate:

- High concentrations of calcium and phosphate
- Increases in solution pH
- Decreases in amino acid concentrations
- Increases in temperature
- Addition of calcium before phosphate
- Lengthy time delay or slow infusion rates
- Use of the chloride salt of calcium

Confirm that the calcium and phosphorus added together does not exceed 45 mEq/L.

Common practice is to use parenteral nutrition compounding software that predicts the likelihood of calcium phosphate precipitation and allows for adjustments in quantities of calcium and phosphorus before compounding.

Compatibility of the additive with the composition of the I.V. container

Nitroglycerin readily migrates into many plastics, especially polyvinylchloride (PVC). **Insulin** adsorbs to I.V. tubing, filters, and both glass and plastic containers.

Compatibility of the additive with the additional equipment used to prepare or administer the I.V. admixture

Cisplatin interacts with aluminum by forming a black precipitate when coming in contact with it.

Stability of the drug after admixture

Ampicillin sodium is stable for 72 hours when refrigerated and 24 hours at room temperature in normal saline. However, if it is added to D_5W, it is stable for only 4 hours when refrigerated and 2 hours at room temperature.

Other potential sources of physical incompatibilities

Concentration

A drug will remain in aqueous solution as long as its concentration is less than its saturation solubility.

Cosolvent system

Drugs that are poorly water soluble are often formulated using water-miscible cosolvents. Examples of water-miscible cosolvents include ethanol, propylene glycol, and polyethylene glycol. Dilution of drugs that are in a cosolvent system often causes precipitation of the drug. A good example is diazepam injection. Dilution of the drug results in precipitation in some concentrations, but sufficient dilution to a point below diazepam's saturation solubility results in a physically stable admixture.

pH

The greatest single factor in causing an incompatibility is a change in acid–base environment. Solubility of drugs that are weak acids or bases is a direct function of solution pH. The drug's dissociation constant and pH control the portion of drug in its ionized form and the solubility of the un-ionized form. A drug that is a weak acid may be formulated at a pH sufficient to yield the desired solubility. Sodium salts of barbiturates, phenytoin, and methotrexate are formulated at high pH values to achieve adequate solubility.

Sodium salts of weak acids precipitate as free acids when added to I.V. fluids having an acidic pH. If the pH of these drugs is lowered, the drug's solubility at the final pH may be exceeded, resulting in possible precipitation. Drugs that are salts of weak bases may precipitate in an alkaline solution.

Ionic interactions

Large organic anions and cations may also form precipitates, such as the precipitation that occurs when heparin (anionic) and aminoglycoside antibiotics (cationic) are mixed. These heparin salts of the cationic drug are relatively insoluble in water.

Sorption phenomena

With sorption phenomena, the intact drug is lost from the solution by adsorption to the surface or absorption into the matrix of container material, administration set, or filter.

Adsorption to the surface can result from interactions of functional groups within the drug's molecule to binding sites on the surfaces.

Absorption of lipid-soluble drugs into the matrix of plastic containers and administration sets, especially those made from PVC, does occur. The substantial amount of phthalate plasticizer used to make the PVC bag pliable and flexible allows the lipid-soluble drugs to diffuse from the solution into the plasticizer in the plastic matrix. Plastics such as polyethylene and polypropylene, which contain little or no phthalate plasticizer, do not readily absorb lipid-soluble drugs into the polymer core. Leaching of the phthalate plasticizer into the solution may also occur, especially if surface-active agents or a large amount of organic cosolvent is present in the formulation.

Chemical Incompatibility

Chemical incompatibilities are interactions resulting in molecular changes or rearrangements to different chemical entities. Most chemical interactions are not observable by the unaided eye.

Chemical degradation pathways

Hydrolysis is a common mode of chemical decomposition. Water attacks labile bonds in dissolved drug molecules. Functional groups labile to hydrolysis are carboxylic acid and phosphate esters, amides, lactams, and imines.

Oxidation is an electron loss that causes a positive increase in valence. Many drugs are in the reduced form, and oxygen creates stability problems. Steroids, epinephrine, and tricyclic compounds are sensitive to oxygen. For control of the stability problem, oxygen can be excluded, pH can be adjusted, and chelating agents or antioxidants can be added.

Reduction is when an electron is gained, causing a decrease in valence and the addition of halogen or hydrogen to the double bond. Beta-lactam antibiotics can produce reducing aldehydes on hydrolysis.

Photolysis is the catalysis by light of degradation reactions such as oxidation or hydrolysis. Examples of drugs that are light sensitive are amphotericin B, **furosemide**, and sodium nitroprusside. The reaction rate depends on the intensity and wavelength of light. Sodium nitroprusside in D_5W has a faint brownish cast, but exposure to light causes deterioration, which is evident by a change in color to blue caused by the reduction of the ferric ion to a ferrous ion.

Extreme pH can be a catalysis of drug degradation. Drug reaction rates are generally less at intermediate pH values than at high or low ranges. A buffer system is often used to ensure the maintenance of the proper pH.

Effects of temperature may be evident. Usually, but not always, an elevation in temperature may increase reaction rates.

An increase in drug concentration will usually increase the degradation rate exponentially. However, this rule does not always apply. Some drugs appear to have a lower rate of decomposition at a high concentration, such as the reduced hydrolysis of nafcillin in the presence of aminophylline. Greater buffer concentration at higher nafcillin concentrations protects the drug from aminophylline's high pH and slows the hydrolysis.

Expiration dates and removal of the IV bag overwrap are important. The overwrap protects against evaporation of the solution, desiccation of the container, drug oxidation, and photochemical inactivation of the drug. Substantial moisture loss may occur which would increase drug concentration. With ready-to-use dopamine or dobutamine injections, removal of the overwrap can allow oxygen to enter the container, thereby reducing drug stability. After removal of the overwrap, the expiration date should be changed at once.

6-12   Sterile Products Compounded from Nonsterile Drugs

When a sterile preparation is compounded from a nonsterile component, several concerns arise: how to sterilize the drug, how to sterilize the container and closure, and how to ensure that the drug and components are sterile. Every sterilization process must be verified, whether it is terminal sterilization of the CSP in the final container or aseptic processing of the CSP. Sterility testing must be done on all high-risk CSPs if they are prepared in groups of more than 25 single-dose packages or in multidose vials for administration to multiple patients. Such testing must also be done if before sterilization the preparations are exposed for more than 12 hours to temperatures of 2°C to 8°C or for more than 6 hours to temperatures above 8°C. If the high-risk CSPs are dispensed before the results of the sterility test are known, a method must be in place requiring daily observation of the test specimens and immediate recall of the CSP if there is evidence of microbial growth in the test sample.

Sterility Testing

There are two methods of sterility testing: *direct inoculation* and *membrane filtration*. The USP states that, when possible, membrane filtration should be performed and that two culture media are required: fluid thioglycollate medium (FTM) and TSB, which is also known as soybean-casein digest medium.

Media suitability test

Before beginning the test, one must confirm that the medium being used is sterile and will support the growth of microorganisms.

Sterility

Confirm the sterility of each sterilized batch of medium by (1) incubating a portion of the batch at the specified incubation temperature (TSB, 20°C to 25°C; FTM, 30°C to 35°C) for 14 days or (2) incubating uninoculated containers as negative controls during a sterility test procedure. When purchasing a new batch of sterile media from a vendor, incubate a portion for several days to ensure that it did not become contaminated during shipment.

Growth promotion test

Each lot of ready-prepared medium and each batch of dehydrated medium bearing the manufacturer's lot number must be tested for its growth-promoting qualities. Separately inoculate, in duplicate, containers of each medium with fewer than 100 viable microorganisms of each of the strains listed in the next paragraph. If visual evidence of growth appears in all inoculated media containers within 3 days of incubation in the case of bacteria and 5 days of incubation in the case of fungi, the test media is satisfactory. The test may be conducted simultaneously with testing of the media for sterility.

The organisms to be used for the growth promotion test of FTM are *Staphylococcus aureus* (*Bacillus subtilis* may be used instead), *Pseudomonas aeruginosa* (*Micrococcus luteus* may be used instead), and *Clostridium sporogenes* (*Bacteroides vulgatus* may be used instead). The test organisms for soybean-casein digest media are *Bacillus subtilis*, *Candida albicans*, and *Aspergillus brasiliensis* (formerly known as *Aspergillus niger*). Soybean-casein digest media are incubated at 20°C to 25°C, and FTM are incubated at 30°C to 35°C, both under aerobic conditions for a minimum of 14 days.

Validation test: Bacteriostasis and fungistasis test

The bacteriostasis and fungistasis test must be done on each product to determine if the product itself will inhibit the growth of microorganisms. This test needs to be done only once for each product tested. The organisms used are the same as those used for growth promotion. The test uses two sets of containers. One set is inoculated with the drug product and microorganisms, and the other set is inoculated with just the microorganisms. Both sets will be incubated at the appropriate temperature for no more than 5 days. The same amount of growth should be seen in both sets. If the drug is inhibiting the growth of the microorganisms, the conditions of the test must be modified so the drug will not inhibit growth. The modifications made will now become the method for performing the sterility test on the drug preparation.

Number of articles to test

The minimum number of articles to be tested in relation to the number of articles in the batch is as follows:

- For up to 100 articles, test 10% or 4 articles, whichever is greater.
- For more than 100 but not more than 500 articles, test 10 articles.

Interpretation of results

No growth

At days 3, 5, 7, 10, and 14, examine the media visually for growth. If no microbial growth is seen, the article complies with the test for sterility. Lack of growth of the media does not prove that all units in the lot are sterile.

Observed growth

When microbial growth is observed and confirmed microscopically, the article does not meet the requirements of the test for sterility. If there is no doubt that the microbial growth can be ascribed to faulty aseptic techniques or materials used in conducting the testing procedure, the test is invalid and must be repeated.

An investigation must occur, and the organism must be identified down to the species. All records must be reviewed, including all employee training procedures and records, aseptic gowning practices, equipment maintenance records, component sterilization data, and environmental monitoring data.

Visual inspection

Every unit compounded in the pharmacy should be subjected to a physical inspection against a white background and a black background. Any container whose contents show evidence of contamination with visible foreign material must be rejected.

Pyrogens

A pyrogen is a substance that produces fever. An endotoxin is a type of pyrogen.

Gram-negative bacteria produce more potent endotoxins than do gram-positive bacteria and fungi. The lipopolysaccharide (LPS) portion of the outer cell wall of gram-negative bacteria causes the pyrogenic response. The LPS can be sloughed off, and the bacteria do not have to be living for the LPS to be pyrogenic.

Some of the effects caused by pyrogens in the body are an increase in body temperature, chills, cutaneous vasoconstriction, decrease in respiration, increase in arterial blood pressure, nausea and malaise, and severe diarrhea.

The official endotoxin limits are 5 endotoxin units (EU)/kg per hour or 350 EU/total body per hour for drugs and biologicals. Drugs for intrathecal use have a much lower endotoxin limit of 0.2 EU/kg.

Water is the primary source of endotoxins because *Pseudomonas*, a gram-negative bacterium, grows readily in water. Other sources of endotoxins or pyrogens are raw material, equipment, processing, and human contamination. Endotoxins can be destroyed by dry heat; 3 to 5 hours at 200°C will depyrogenate glass vials and beakers. The endotoxin concentration can be reduced by rinsing with sterile water for injection. When a sterile preparation is compounded from a nonsterile product, any equipment that can withstand the heat of 200°C should be depyrogenated. An article that is depyrogenated is also sterile.

Pyrogen test (rabbit test)

The pyrogen test is designed to limit, to an acceptable level, the patient's risk of febrile reaction in the administration—by injection—of the product concerned. The test involves measuring the rise in temperature of rabbits following the IV injection of a test solution, and it is designed for products that can be tolerated by the test rabbit in a dose—not to exceed 10 mL/kg—injected intravenously within a period of no more than 10 minutes.

The rabbit test has several limitations. It is an in vivo method, it is an expensive and time-consuming test, and it is not a very sensitive test. Drugs that have pyretic side effects or that are antipyretics cannot be tested using the rabbit test. The test is not quantitative, and the pyrogenic response is dose dependent, not concentration dependent.

Bacterial endotoxin test (limulus amebocyte lysate test)

The bacterial endotoxin test (BET) provides a method for estimating the concentration of bacterial endotoxins that may be present in, or on the sample of, the article to which the test is applied using limulus amebocyte lysate (LAL) reagent. Because the blood cells of the horseshoe crab are sensitive to endotoxin and form a gel in its presence, LAL reagent is made from the lysate of amebocytes from the horseshoe crab.

There are two types of techniques for this test: the *gel-clot technique,* which is based on the formation of the gel, and the *photometric technique,* which is based on either the development of turbidity or the development of color in the test sample.

The routine gel-clot test requires 0.1 mL of test sample to be mixed with 0.1 mL of LAL reagent. This mixture is incubated for 1 hour at 37°C. A positive reaction is confirmed by the formation of a firm gel that remains intact when the tube is slowly inverted 180 degrees.

The BET is 5 to 50 times more sensitive, more simple and rapid, and less expensive than the pyrogen test. However, the clotting enzyme is heat sensitive, pH sensitive, and chemically related to trypsin. The test is dependable for detection of only pyrogens originating from gram-negative bacteria. Also, some drugs can inhibit the reaction, and other drugs can enhance the reaction.

The photometric technique requires the establishment of a standard regression curve. The test can be either an endpoint determination, in which the reading is made immediately at the end of the incubation period, or a kinetic test, in which the absorbance is measured throughout the reaction period.

All high-risk CSPs (except those for inhalation and ophthalmic use) that are prepared in groups of 25 or more individual single-dose units or in multidose vials for administration to multiple patients or that are exposed for more than 12 hours to temperatures of 2°C to 8°C and for more than 6 hours to temperatures above 8°C before sterilization must comply with the BET.

6-13 Pharmacist's Role

Since the advent of the Drug Quality and Security Act of 2013 and the pending revisions of several *USP* chapters, sterile compounding has become a focus of regulatory agencies, colleges of pharmacy, and compounding pharmacies. Pharmacists are in a perfect position to manage the processes related to sterile compounding and to ensure that these products are safe for their patients. Many of the roles that pharmacists have in sterile compounding require an in-depth knowledge of USP guidelines. With this foundation, pharmacists can prepare products to address specific needs of their patient population such as pediatric dosing and allergy concerns. Pharmacists are a resource for adaptive compounding if different routes of administration, compatibility requirements, dosing adjustment, or finding alternatives to drug supplies are required. Sterile compounding requires robust quality assurance programs and methods; pharmacists help with implementation, training, and monitoring for staff adherence. Environmental controls provide appropriate workplaces in which to compound products; pharmacists should ensure certifications are in order as well as providing remediation if issues are found. When pharmacists oversee sterility, ISO standards, and other topics covered in this chapter, the quality of the products prepared and the safety of the patients for whom they are caring can be ensured.

NAPLEX Competency Statements

The questions in this chapter cover the following 2021 NAPLEX Competency Statements: **AREA 5:** 5.1; 5.2; 5.3; 5.4; 5.5; 5.6.

6-14 Questions

1. Which of the following tests does *not* have to be completed on a high-risk CSP that will be administered by intravascular injection and is prepared in a lot size of 30 single-dose vials before release to a patient?

   A. Bacterial endotoxin test
   B. Visual inspection
   C. Sterility test
   D. Verification of the sterilizing filter integrity
   E. LAL test

2. Which of the following is correct concerning certification of a laminar flow workbench?

   A. The particles introduced into the plenum of the hood must be approximately 0.5 micron.
   B. Airflow from the HEPA filter must be 120 ft/min.
   C. A leak greater than 0.01% of the upstream smoke concentration through the filter is considered a serious leak.
   D. A total particle counter can be used to check the integrity of the HEPA filter.
   E. If a HEPA filter leaks, it cannot be patched; it must be replaced.

3. The bacterial endotoxin test is used to determine _____.

   A. the amount of pyrogens
   B. the level of pyrogens from gram-negative bacteria
   C. the fever-producing potential of bacterial endotoxins from gram-negative bacteria
   D. the level of bacterial endotoxin from gram-positive bacteria
   E. the amount of live bacteria present in the drug solution

4. Which of the following is correct concerning USP media transfers?

   A. An operator must successfully complete one media fill before compounding any CSPs.
   B. An operator who passes a written exam may compound sterile preparations until the chief pharmacist finds time to watch his or her aseptic technique.
   C. An operator who has successfully completed a media fill must requalify semiannually if he or she is preparing low-risk CSPs.
   D. When an operator successfully completes one media fill for high-risk compounding, he or she needs to revalidate quarterly by completing one media fill.
   E. Fluid thioglycollate media are used for media transfers.

5. For a transfer of product into the controlled area _____.

   A. bottles, bags, and syringes must be removed from brown cardboard boxes before being brought into the buffer area
   B. vials stored in laminated cardboard may not be brought into the controlled area
   C. stainless steel carts may be used to transfer items into the controlled area directly from the storage area
   D. large-volume parenteral bags of I.V. solution must be removed from their protective overwrap before being brought into the controlled area
   E. the refrigerator should be placed next to the laminar flow hood for easy access

6. Which of the following is correct concerning a vertical laminar flow hood?

   A. It is always a biological safety cabinet.
   B. In vertical laminar flow, the hands of the operator must not be behind an object.
   C. A vertical laminar flow hood has turbulent airflow within 1 inch of the work surface.
   D. A vertical laminar flow hood has the laminar airflow blowing at the operator.
   E. The operator works in a vertical flow hood and a horizontal flow hood in the same manner.

7. Certain factors may increase the risk of microbial contamination of a CSP. Which of the following would not be a risk factor?

   A. Very complex compounding steps
   B. Lengthy exposure of a critical site during compounding
   C. Use of appropriate aseptic technique
   D. Batch compounding without preservatives for multiple patients
   E. Preparation of a CSP from nonsterile powders

8. Which of the following is correct concerning the USP risk levels of CSPs?

   A. Preparations intended for administration over 3 days would be classified as low risk.
   B. A high-risk sterile preparation that has met the requirements of the sterility test can be stored for not more than 24 hours at a controlled room temperature.
   C. The storage time for a medium-risk preparation under refrigeration is for no more than 9 days.
   D. A CSP that will be administered to multiple patients or to a single patient multiple times is classified as a high-risk CSP.
   E. After meeting the requirements of the sterility test, a sterile preparation can be stored indefinitely.

9. Which of the following is correct?

A. For work done in a horizontal laminar flow workbench, arrange items in the hood so that your hand is never between the HEPA filter and an object.

B. For work done in a horizontal laminar flow workbench, vials that are not being used should be stacked up along the side of the hood to increase workspace in the hood.

C. Before each shift, 70% isopropyl alcohol is used to sterilize the laminar flow workbench.

D. An object placed in the horizontal laminar flow workbench disturbs the airflow downstream of the object equal to 2 times the diameter of the object.

E. Syringes and I.V. bags are placed in the hood in their protective overwrap.

10. Which of the following is correct concerning the necessity that operators in the buffer area be properly gowned?

A. Operators don gowns because they shed particles, and the nonshedding gowns keep them sterile.

B. Sterile gloves are used to avoid contamination of the CSP in case the operator accidentally touches a critical site during compounding of the preparation.

C. Frequent sanitization with sterile 70% isopropyl alcohol is essential to keep the operators' hands sterile during the compounding process.

D. Nonshedding garb and sterile gloves help contain the particles shed from the operators.

E. Operators must don gowns before working at the laminar flow workbench but not before entering the buffer area.

11. Which of the following is correct concerning placement of items and work performed in the laminar flow workstation?

A. Items in a horizontal flow hood should be placed in the center of the work area.

B. Items in a vertical laminar flow hood should be placed so that an operator's hand never goes over the top of a critical site while the operator is working in the hood.

C. An object placed in a horizontal laminar flow hood disturbs the airflow downstream of the object equal to 6 times the diameter of the object.

D. When working in a horizontal laminar flow workstation, an operator must perform all work at least 2 inches inside the hood.

E. Syringes and needles for immediate compounding work should be kept outside of vertical laminar flow hoods and inside of horizontal laminar flow hoods.

12. Which parts of the syringe are considered critical sites? (Mark all that apply.)

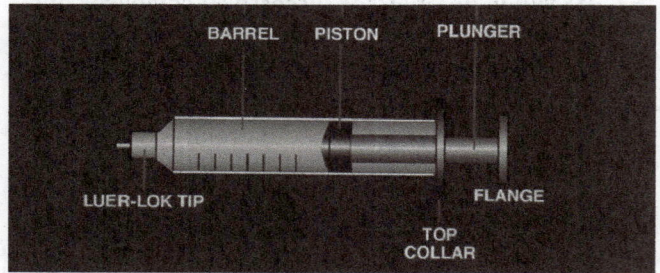

A. Plunger only
B. Collar only
C. Plunger and tip only
D. Collar and tip only
E. Plunger, collar, and tip

13. Which parts of the needle are considered critical sites? (Mark all that apply.)

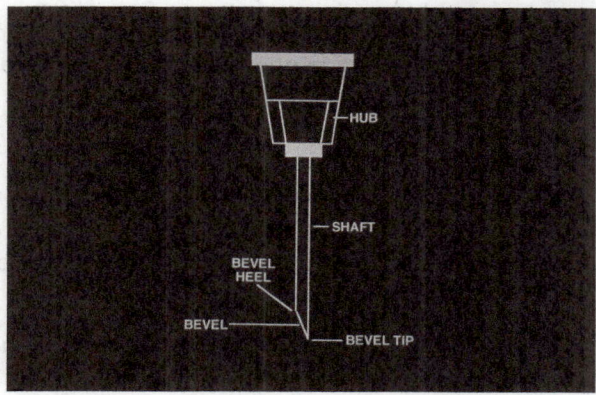

HUB

SHAFT

BEVEL HEEL

BEVEL

BEVEL TIP

A. The hub only
B. The needle shaft only
C. The hub and the bevel and bevel tip only
D. The needle shaft and the bevel and bevel tip only
E. The hub, the needle shaft, and the bevel and bevel tip

14. Which of the following statements is correct concerning ampuls?

A. Ampuls can be left in the hood and used for 2 days once opened.
B. Ampuls are single-dose containers and can be left in the hood and used for 7 days once opened.
C. Ampuls are single-dose containers and must have the neck wiped with a sterile alcohol pad before being broken.
D. Ampuls are multidose containers containing benzyl alcohol as preservative.
E. Ampuls should be broken outside the hood and then transported into the hood.

15. Which of the following statements is correct?

A. Filter integrity testing of the filter membrane is done to determine at what pressure the filter will break.
B. The manufacturer of the filter membrane determines the bubble point of the membrane; this value is always the same, no matter what solution has been filtered.
C. As the pore size of the filter membrane decreases, the pressure at which the air can be pushed from the largest pore increases.
D. The bubble point test is a destructive test.
E. Performing the bubble point test is not necessary if a certificate of quality from the filter manufacturer is provided.

16. Which of the following factors should be considered when choosing a sterilizing filter?

A. The temperature of the solution to be filtered
B. The compatibility of the membrane with the solution to be filtered
C. Whether the solution to be filtered is hydrophobic or hygrophobic
D. The compatibility of the filter housing with the filter membrane
E. The freezing point of the solution to be filtered

17. Which of the following statements is correct concerning the *USP* sterility test?

A. The validation test must be done on each CSP to determine if the article to be tested adversely affects the reliability of the test.
B. The growth promotion test does not require that the test organisms listed in the *USP* be used.
C. After inoculation, the media must be incubated for 14 days or fewer at the appropriate temperature.
D. No growth on the sterility test proves that the aseptically produced product is sterile.
E. Trypticase soy broth is incubated at 30°C to 35°C, and fluid thioglycollate is incubated at 20°C to 25°C.

18. Which of the following is correct?

A. Gram-negative bacteria must be alive to cause a pyrogenic response.

B. The lipopolysaccharide portion of the cell wall of gram-negative bacteria causes the pyrogenic response.

C. Endotoxin can be removed by a 0.2-micron filter.

D. Steam sterilization will depyrogenate an object just as well as the hot air oven.

E. An article that is depyrogenated is not necessarily sterile.

19. Which of the following statements is correct?

A. The rabbit test and the LAL test are the same test.

B. LAL reagent will determine the fever-producing potential of the pyrogens.

C. There are two types of techniques for the BET: the gel-clot technique and the photometric technique.

D. The CSP being tested has no effect on the test.

E. All CSPs may be tested using the rabbit test.

20. Which of the following statements is correct?

A. The rabbit test is the most sensitive because it can detect pyrogens from all sources.

B. The rabbit test is an in vitro test.

C. Some drugs may inhibit the formation of a gel in the BET.

D. No drug will enhance the formation of the gel in the BET.

E. The pyrogen test is a quantitative test.

21. The plenum in a laminar flow workbench is the area _____.

A. where the air is prefiltered

B. where air is pressurized for distribution over the HEPA filter

C. where compounding takes place

D. that serves no purpose

E. directly above the HEPA filter in a horizontal laminar flow hood

22. Calcium and phosphate can interact to form a precipitate in parenteral nutrition solutions. Of the following situations, which would not enhance calcium and phosphate precipitate formation?

A. High concentration of calcium and phosphate

B. Increase in solution pH

C. Decrease in temperature

D. Use of the chloride salt of calcium

E. A slow infusion rate

23. Which of the following is not a potential source of physical or chemical incompatibility?

A. Dilution of a drug in a cosolvent system into an aqueous system

B. Addition of a drug solution with a high pH into a solution with a low pH

C. Adsorption of a lipid-soluble drug into the matrix of a polypropylene container

D. A photosensitive drug such as sodium nitroprusside in 5% dextrose in water exposed to light

E. Leaching of phthalate plasticizer into the solution from a polyvinyl chloride container

 **6-15   Answers**

1. C. The bacterial endotoxin test (LAL test), visual inspection test, and bubble point test should all be completed before the CSP is dispensed. Because the sterility test takes 14 days, the preparation may be dispensed before the results are known. However, a system to recall the CSP must be in place if it does not meet the test's requirement.

2. C. Any leak greater than 0.01% of upstream smoke concentration is a serious leak. The smoke particles are 0.3 micron. The airflow from the HEPA filter should be 90 ft/min ± 20%. A total particle counter is used to classify the environment, not to certify the integrity of the HEPA filter. The HEPA filter can be patched.

3. B. The BET determines the level of bacterial endotoxin from gram-negative bacteria only. The BET cannot determine fever-producing potential of the endotoxins. The gram-negative bacteria do not have to be alive for the endotoxin to produce an effect.

4. A. The operator must successfully complete one media fill before compounding a sterile preparation. Once validated for low- or medium-risk compounding, the operator must revalidate annually. For high-risk compounding, the operator must revalidate semiannually. Passing only a written exam does not allow the operator to compound a CSP. Trypticase soy broth is the medium most often used in media fills.

5. **A.** Cardboard must be kept out of the buffer area. Vials stored in laminated cardboard may be stored in the buffer area. No items should be brought into the buffer area without being sanitized. Large-volume parenteral bags should be removed from their overwrap just before being used. The refrigerator should not be in the buffer room because it is a source of contamination.

6. **C.** There are several types of vertical laminar flow hoods of which the biological safety cabinet is one. The operator must never work over the top of items in the hood, and all work should be done at least 1 inch above the work surface.

7. **C.** Use of good aseptic technique is one way to ensure a good preparation.

8. **C.** A medium-risk CSP may not be stored for more than 9 days at cold temperature. USP <797> does not address administration at all; it applies only up to the time of administration. Once a CSP has met the requirement of the sterility test, the storage periods specified under the risk levels no longer apply. However, the BUD based on chemical stability always applies. A CSP that will be administered to multiple patients or to a single patient multiple times is a medium-risk CSP.

9. **A.** In an HLFW, never put your hand behind an object, and in a VLFW, never put your hand above an object. In an HLFW, a vial disturbs the laminar airflow equal to 3 times the diameter of the object. If the vial is next to the side wall, the airflow is disturbed equal to 6 times the diameter of the object. Syringes and I.V. bags should be taken from their overwrap at the edge of the hood.

10. **D.** Operators in the buffer area should wear clean, nonshedding gowns and gloves to help contain the particles that they shed. The sterile gloves are no longer sterile once they are out of the package. Proper aseptic technique must always be used.

11. **B.** Items in a vertical laminar flow hood should be placed so that an operator's hand never goes over the top of a critical site while the operator is working in the hood. Items should be placed in a horizontal flow hood to the right or left of the work

area. An object placed in a horizontal laminar flow hood disturbs the airflow downstream of the object equal to 3 times the diameter of the object. When working in a horizontal laminar flow workstation, an operator must perform all work at least 6 inches inside the hood.

12. **C.** The plunger and the tip of the syringe are critical sites of the syringe.

13. **E.** The hub, the needle shaft, and the bevel and bevel tip of the needle are all critical sites.

14. **C.** Once an ampul is opened, it must be used immediately.

15. **C.** The bubble point test is not a destructive test, and the value depends on the solution being filtered. When a CSP is filter sterilized, the bubble point test must be done before the preparation may be dispensed.

16. **B.** The compatibility of the membrane with the solution to be filtered should be considered. Other considerations include the volume of the solution to be filtered, whether the solution to be filtered is hydrophobic or hydrophilic, and the compatibility of the filter housing with the product to be filtered.

17. **A.** The validation (bacteriostasis and fungistasis test) must be completed one time for each CSP. The growth promotion organisms listed in the *USP* are used for the validation test and for the growth promotion test.

18. **B.** Endotoxin will pass through a 0.2-micron filter. Steam sterilization will not depyrogenate an article. Bacteria do not have to be alive to be pyrogenic.

19. **C.** The pyrogen test, also known as the rabbit test, determines the fever-producing potential of the pyrogens. The BET is also known as the LAL test. The drug product can inhibit or enhance the gel formation in the BET.

20. **C.** The pyrogen (rabbit) test is an in vivo test and is not as sensitive as the BET. It is not a quantitative test.

21. **B.** The plenum is the area behind the HEPA filter in an HLFW that allows air to be pressurized for even distribution over the filter.

22. **C.** An increase in temperature could enhance precipitate formation.

23. **C.** Absorption of a lipid-soluble drug into the matrix of polyvinylchloride containers does occur. Polypropylene and polyethylene contain little or no phthalate plasticizer.

6-16 Additional Resources

Akers MJ, Larrimore D, Guazzo D. *Parenteral Quality Control: Sterility, Pyrogen, Particulate and Package Integrity Testing.* 3rd ed. Boca Raton, FL: CRC Press; 2002.

American Society of Health-System Pharmacists. ASHP guidelines on compounding sterile preparations. *Am J Health-Syst Pharm.* 2014;71(2):145–166.

American Society of Health-System Pharmacists. ASHP guidelines on handling hazardous drugs. *Am J Health-Syst Pharm.* 2018; 75:1996–2031.

Trissel LA. *Handbook on Injectable Drugs.* 20th ed. Bethesda, MD: American Society of Health-System Pharmacists; 2018.

United States Pharmacopeial Convention. Bacterial endotoxin test. In: *United States Pharmacopeia 40/National Formulary 35.* Rockville, MD: United States Pharmacopeial Convention; 2017:163–169.

United States Pharmacopeial Convention. Hazardous drugs—handling in healthcare settings. In: *United States Pharmacopeia 40/National Formulary 35.* Rockville, MD: United States Pharmacopeial Convention; 2017:727–746.

United States Pharmacopeial Convention. Pharmaceutical compounding: sterile preparations. In: *United States Pharmacopeia 40/National Formulary 35.* Rockville, MD: United States Pharmacopeial Convention; 2017:683–727.

United States Pharmacopeial Convention. Pyrogen test. In: *United States Pharmacopeia 40/National Formulary 35.* Rockville, MD: United States Pharmacopeial Convention; 2017:234–236.

United States Pharmacopeial Convention. Sterility tests. In: *United States Pharmacopeia 40/National Formulary 35.* Rockville, MD: United States Pharmacopeial Convention; 2017:136–143.

Clinical Pharmacokinetics

7

S. CASEY LAIZURE

 7-1 KEY POINTS

- The steady-state drug concentration is determined by the clearance of the drug.
- Changes in the volume of distribution do not change the steady-state concentration.
- For a drug eliminated by first-order elimination the ratio of the dose to the steady-state drug concentration remains constant.
- Renal function can be quantitatively estimated from the serum creatinine and used to adjust the dose of renally eliminated drugs.
- Liver function tests measure liver damage not function and do not provide a quantitative estimate of liver drug metabolism.
- For high-extraction, hepatically eliminated drugs, there will be a large difference between the oral and intravenous dose due to the high first-pass metabolism when the drug is given orally.
- Absolute bioavailability is the difference in the AUC after oral dosing compared to intravenous dosing.
- The most commonly encountered pharmacokinetic drug interactions are due to changes in renal or hepatic drug elimination resulting in a change in the drug's clearance.

 7-2 STUDY GUIDE CHECKLIST

The following topics may guide your study of this subject area:

- ☐ Basic pharmacokinetic parameters including clearance, volume of distribution, and half-life.
- ☐ The half-life estimate from two plasma concentrations.
- ☐ Calculating how long it will take to drop from a higher to lower concentration using k.
- ☐ For a drug undergoing first-order elimination, calculating a new dose to achieve a target steady-state concentration from a measured steady-state drug concentration.
- ☐ The difference between first-order elimination and nonlinear elimination.
- ☐ The effect of controlled release ($k_a \ll k$) on drug disposition.
- ☐ Renal function estimate using the Cockcroft-Gault equation and understand the modification of diet in renal disease (MDRD) equation.
- ☐ Bioavailability estimate.
- ☐ The venous equilibrium model and how it applies to hepatic drug metabolism.
- ☐ Use of the venous equilibrium model to interpret hepatic drug interactions.

7-3   Introduction

Pharmacokinetics is the mathematical modeling of drug concentration-time used to understand drug disposition and make predictions on the relationship between drug dose and exposure. Understanding the numerous equations derived from models is an important part of clinical pharmacokinetics, but performing specific calculations based on pharmacokinetic equations is limited due to the lack of an adequate number of drug concentrations available from patients in clinical practice.

This review will focus on how we apply pharmacokinetics in the clinical setting to achieve therapeutic drug concentrations, interpret drug concentrations in patients, adjust doses, and assess drug interactions. It is expected that the reader has an understanding of basic pharmacokinetic equations.

Basic Pharmacokinetic Parameters

Volume of Distribution

The volume of distribution (V) is the theoretical volume based on the measured drug concentration in the plasma that would occur if the drug were allowed to completely distribute throughout the body without any drug elimination occurring. Knowing V, you can estimate the total amount of drug in the body from the measured drug plasma concentration. For example, if a 75-kg patient is taking digoxin, which has a V of 7.0 L/kg, and the digoxin plasma concentration is 0.5 ng/mL, then we estimate the total amount of digoxin in the body by:

$$Amt = Cp \times V$$

where Amt is amount of drug in the body, Cp is the measured drug plasma concentration, and V is the volume of distribution. For our patient the result is:

$$Amt = 0.5 \frac{\mu g}{L} \times \left(7.0 \frac{L}{kg} \times 75 \, kg \right) = 262.5 \, \mu g$$

Note the plasma concentration is changed from ng/mL to µg/L so that the units will properly cancel out giving the final answer in micrograms (g). When performing pharmacokinetic calculations always include units, which provides a check that your equation is correct and prevents incorrect answers due to a mismatch in the units.

Clinically we use the V to determine the amount of drug we need to give a patient in order to rapidly achieve a specific plasma concentration. In this case, Amt becomes what is most commonly referred to as the loading dose (LD), and can be estimated using the following equation:

$$LD = \frac{(C_t - C_{obs}) \times V}{F \times S}$$

where LD is a single dose to achieve the desired plasma concentration, C_t is the target plasma concentration we want to achieve, C_{obs} is the concentration of drug in the plasma before the loading dose (this will usually be 0), V is the volume of distribution, F is the bioavailability, and S the fraction of active drug in the salt form (this is usually 1). For most drugs the loading dose is based on the patient's body weight and will be in the units of mg/kg, which is derived from the V for the specific drug. Thus, it is not common to apply this equation directly in clinical practice although there are notable exceptions such as the dosing of theophylline in neonates for prevention of apnea. For example, if we are trying to achieve a theophylline plasma concentration of 8 µg/mL in an 18-day-old neonate who weighs 3.9 kg, we cannot use standard mg/kg dose estimates and must use the loading dose equation to estimate the proper loading dose as the V differs between adults and neonates:

$$LD = \frac{8\frac{mg}{L} \times \left(0.68\frac{L}{kg} \times 3.9\,kg\right)}{(1 \times 0.8)} = 26.5\,mg$$

where LD is the loading dose to achieve a plasma concentration of 8 μg/mL, 0.68 L/kg is V, 3.9 kg is the neonate's body weight, F = 1 (the dose is given intravenously) and S = 0.8 because the drug is given as aminophylline, which is 80% theophylline.

The range of volume of distribution for drugs is great from very small such as for **warfarin** at about 0.14 L/kg to extremely large such as for amiodarone with a V of about 66 L/kg. Drugs with small volumes tend to be more hydrophilic limiting their ability to cross lipophilic cell membranes, while drugs with large V's tend to be lipophilic compounds that can easily cross cell membranes and distribute to body tissues outside the plasma. Drugs with V's less than 0.5 L/kg such as **warfarin** and gentamicin have very limited distribution outside the plasma, drugs with V's around 0.8 to 1.0 L/kg usually distribute into total body water (vancomycin and theophylline), and drugs will large V's widely distribute into other body tissues such as fat (tetrahydrocannabinol) or muscle (digoxin). However, one cannot determine from V alone where a drug distributes as a large V by itself only indicates that the drug distributes outside the plasma compartment but not what tissue it goes into.

Clearance

The vast majority of drugs are eliminated by first-order elimination, which means a constant percentage of drug is eliminated per unit time. This means the actual elimination rate, amount per unit of time such as mg/h, changes with changes in the drug's plasma concentration. Where V is the parameter that relates the plasma concentration to the total amount of drug in the body, clearance (Cl) is the parameter that relates the actual drug elimination rate to the plasma concentration. For example, if the plasma concentration of a drug is 2.0 μg/mL and the Cl is 1.0 L/min, then we can determine the actual rate of drug elimination using the following equation:

$$ER = C_p \times Cl$$

where ER is the elimination rate, C_p is the plasma concentration, and Cl is the clearance. Thus, when the plasma concentration is 2.0 μg/mL, the rate of drug elimination is calculated as follows.

$$ER = 2.0\frac{mg}{L} \times 1.0\frac{L}{min} = 20\frac{mg}{min}$$

The Cl of a drug determines what the steady-state plasma concentration will be if a patient is chronically administered a consistent dose of the drug. Taking lidocaine as an example, we can predict the steady-state concentration that will be achieved if we administer a constant intravenous (I.V.) infusion at 4 mg/min in a patient with a lidocaine clearance of 1.0 L/min using the following equation:

$$C_{ss} = \frac{X_o}{Cl}$$

where C_{ss} is the steady-state plasma concentration that will occur, X_o is the drug dose in this case administered as a constant I.V. infusion, and Cl is the clearance. Thus, for our patient:

$$C_{ss} = \frac{4\,mg/min}{1.0\,L/min} = 4\frac{mg}{L}$$

and the steady-state plasma concentration achieved when we give a constant I.V. infusion at a rate of 4 mg/min will be 4 µg/mL. Steady state occurs when the amount of drug going into the body (X_o) is equivalent to the amount being eliminated from the body (ER). In this lidocaine example X_o is 4 mg/min, and the ER when the concentration reaches 4 µg/mL is 4.0 mg/min. Thus, clearance tells us at what plasma concentration the elimination rate will become equivalent to the dosing rate and steady state achieved. However, in clinical practice this C_{ss} equation is not useful as we do not know the patient's actual drug clearance. Also, the vast majority of drugs are given by chronic oral dosing not by constant I.V. infusion, and when plasma concentrations are measured it is most commonly going to be a trough concentration. Additionally, with oral dosing we would also have to account for bioavailability (F). Thus, this equation is not used in clinical practice. However, the equation can be rearranged to:

$$Cl = \frac{X_o}{C_{ss}}$$

This provides a clinically useful relationship between the dose and steady-state plasma concentration. As long as the Cl does not change the ratio of X_o to C_{ss} cannot change, which leads to the following equation commonly used to adjust dosing based on a measured drug plasma concentration:

$$\frac{D_{obs}}{C_{ss,obs}} = \frac{D_{new}}{C_{ss,target}}$$

where D_{obs} is the present dose the patient is receiving that resulted in the steady-state plasma concentration of $C_{ss,obs}$ and D_{new} is the new dose to achieve the new targeted steady-state plasma concentration $C_{ss,target}$. This relationship remains valid as long as the Cl and bioavailability have not changed. Thus, if a patient takes 300 mg of lithium 3 times per day and has a steady-state trough concentration of 0.55 mEq/L, then the dose required to achieve a lithium steady-state trough concentration of 0.8 mEq/L can be estimated as:

$$\frac{900 \text{ mg/d}}{0.55 \text{ mEq/L}} = \frac{D_{NEW}}{0.8 \text{ mEq/L}}$$

$$Dose_{new} = \frac{900 \frac{mg}{d} \times 0.8 \text{ mEq/L}}{0.55 \text{ mEq/L}} = 1309 \text{ mg/d}$$

which divided into 3 doses gives 436 mg leading to a recommendation of 450 mg of lithium 3 times per day to achieve a steady-state plasma trough concentration of 0.8 mEq/L.

The vast majority of drugs obey this first-order pharmacokinetics, which means that a plot of the natural log of the plasma concentration versus times results in a straight line, and that the clearance remains constant at usual therapeutic doses. However, there are hepatically eliminated drugs that are subject to nonlinear elimination when dosed in the normal therapeutic range, the most common example being the anticonvulsant drug phenytoin. When a drug is eliminated by enzymes in the liver, the velocity (v) of drug elimination by metabolism is described by the following equation:

$$v = \frac{V_{max} \times C}{K_m + C}$$

where V_{max} is the maximum rate of metabolism by hepatic enzymes possible, C is the plasma concentration of the drug, and K_m is the plasma concentration at the point of one-half of the V_{max}. The reason most drugs follow first-order (clearance remains constant) pharmacokinetics is because the K_m is much greater than the plasma concentration ($K_m \gg C$). As long is this remains true, then $K_m + C$ is approximately equal to K_m and the equation becomes:

$$v = \frac{V_{max} \times C}{K_m}$$

For this equation V_{max} over K_m is a constant that becomes the Cl in first-order pharmacokinetics. However, for phenytoin and a few other drugs and potentially for many hepatically eliminated drugs, if taken in overdoses, the plasma concentration approaches the K_m and the equation cannot be simplified. In this case the clearance of the drug becomes concentration dependent, which means the clearance decreases as the plasma concentration of the drug increases. Thus, if one doubles the dose of a first-order elimination drug, then the steady-state plasma concentration will double, and doubling the dose of a drug that undergoes nonlinear elimination will result in a greater than doubling of the steady-state plasma concentration. The converse is true also, if one decreases the dose of a drug with nonlinear elimination by half, the new steady-state plasma concentration will decrease by more than half. This unpredictability in the relationship between dose and steady-state plasma concentration makes dosing nonlinearly eliminated drugs more difficult.

Half-Life

The half-life ($t_{1/2}$) of a drug is the time it takes for the drug concentration (or the total amount of drug in the body) to decrease by 50%. First-order drug elimination is mathematically identical to radioactive decay with the $t_{1/2}$ being a parameter of an asymptotic decay function. It is commonly accepted that it takes 5 half-lives for a drug to be completely eliminated from the body once dosing is stopped, but technically there will still be 3.125% left after 5 half-lives (100%, 50%, 25%, 12.5%, 6.25%, 3.125%). The converse is also true; steady state is considered to be achieved after 5 half-lives, though actually the drug is still 3.125% from the steady-state concentration (0%, 50%, 75%, 87.5%, 93.75%, 96.875%). It is important to know these percent values so that one may apply them clinically. If a patient had a digoxin trough concentration determined after being dosed for 4 half-lives one would not want to ignore this concentration because it has not reached the 5 half-life threshold to be considered steady state. The concentration is 93.75% of the way there, which makes this concentration close to the steady-state concentration.

It is common to equate $t_{1/2}$ as the pharmacokinetic parameter determining how fast a drug is eliminated from the body. However, the $t_{1/2}$ of a drug is dependent on the V and the Cl of the drug as described by the following equation.

$$t_{1/2} = \frac{0.693 \times V}{Cl}$$

where V is the volume of distribution and Cl is the clearance of the drug. Thus, if the $t_{1/2}$ of a drug in a patient changes, it is due to a change in V, Cl, or both. However, the vast majority of the time when a patient's $t_{1/2}$ changes or when there are differences in half-lives between patients, it will be due to a change in the Cl or the variability in drug Cl between patients and not due to differences in the V. This is for the simple reason that large changes in V are unusual as opposed to large changes in Cl, which are quite common due to the variability and lability of renal and hepatic drug elimination. Variability in a drug's V between patients is significant, but Cl variability between patients is generally much greater.

Normally we think of the terminal elimination phase of a drug's disposition as defining the elimination rate constant, k, and thus, as shown below the half-life.

$$-m = k; \quad t_{1/2} = \frac{0.693}{k}$$

where m is the slope of line of the semilog plot of the terminal elimination phase and k is the first-order elimination rate constant. This equation presumes that for an orally administered drug, the absorption rate is rapid compared to the elimination rate ($k_a \gg k$). If this is true, then the drug is completely absorbed prior to the terminal elimination phase and the slope of the terminal elimination phase is determined by the elimination $t_{1/2}$ of the drug. However, if a drug is given in a controlled-release dosage form in which $k_a \gg k$, then the absorption rate becomes rate limiting and the semilog plot of the terminal elimination phase is determined by the absorption rate rather than the elimination rate, and the slope of the terminal elimination phase is dependent on k_a instead of k. This is referred to as the "flip-flop" in pharmacokinetics. This flip-flop affects the time to reach steady-state and the time to eliminate all drug from the body once dosing is stopped. For a controlled-release drug in which $k_a \gg k$, the time to reach steady state is 5 absorption rate half-lives ($t_{1/2, ABS}$), and the time to eliminate drug from the body is also 5 $t_{1/2, ABS}$.

A final consideration is the effect of nonlinear drug elimination on the $t_{1/2}$. As discussed previously, the clearance decreases as the drug plasma concentration increases and increases as the plasma concentration decreases. Thus, since the $t_{1/2}$ is inversely affected by the Cl, the $t_{1/2}$ is constantly changing as the drug plasma concentration changes for a drug exhibiting nonlinear elimination such as phenytoin. Though it is common that phenytoin is referred to as having a $t_{1/2}$ of about one day, technically $t_{1/2}$ is not a parameter of a drug that exhibits nonlinear elimination.

Drug Elimination

The two primary routes of drug elimination are by the kidneys (renal) and the liver (hepatic). The kidney removes drugs from the body, while the liver metabolizes drugs generally to a more water-soluble form that promotes renal elimination. Generally, we worry about the patient's renal function when dosed with a renally eliminated drug and the patient's liver function when dosed with a hepatically eliminated drug. However, hepatic elimination results in the formation of a metabolite, which may have therapeutic or toxic activity, that must be considered when a patient has renal disease. Morphine would be a typical example of a drug that is rapidly eliminated by hepatic metabolism (glucuronidation) with the removal of the glucuronides, morphine-3-glucuronide and morphine-6-glucuronide, by the kidneys. Though one might expect morphine dosing to be the same in patients with normal and poor renal function, this would be incorrect. The morphine-6-glucuronide retains opiate activity and will accumulate in patients with renal failure potentially leading to respiratory depression. Thus, even though morphine is rapidly metabolized by the liver, renal function must still be considered when dosing this drug.

Renal Drug Elimination

For drugs primarily eliminated by the kidneys, we can adjust the dose based on an assessment of their kidney function using the serum creatinine (SCr). The two most commonly used equations are the Cockcroft-Gault (CG) and the modified diet in renal disease (MDRD) equations. Both equations provide a quantitative estimate of a patient's renal function. The CC is the older equation, which was developed to estimate the creatinine clearance from the serum creatinine.

$$CrCl = \frac{(140 - Age)BW}{(72 \times SCr)}$$

where CrCl is the creatinine clearance in mL/min, Age is the patient's age in years, BW is the body weight in kilograms, and SCr is the serum creatinine in g/dL. If the patient is female, you must multiply your estimate by 0.85. The body weight should be the adjusted body weight as shown below.

$$ABW = IBW + 0.4(TBW - IBW)$$

where ABW is the adjusted body weight in kilograms, IBW is the ideal body weight, and TBW is the patient's actual total body weight. If a patient is overweight, using the IBW will underestimate their

CrCl and using their actual total body weight will overestimate the CrCl. The more overweight the patient is the greater the difference in the CrCl estimate that will occur using the different weights (IBW, ABW, TBW).

The MDRD equations uses the SCr just like the CC equation, but the equation was developed to estimate the relationship between the SCr and the glomerular filtration rate (GFR) rather than the CrCl.

$$GFR = 175 \times SCr^{-1.154} \times Age^{-0.203}$$

where GFR is the glomerular filtration rate in mL/min/1.73 m², SCr is the serum creatinine in g/dL, and Age is the patient's age in years. If the patient is female you must multiply the estimate by 0.742, and if the patient is African American you must multiply the estimate by 1.212. The resulting answer is in units of mL/min/1.73 m². In order to get the patients actual GFR in mL/min, you must multiply the estimate by the patient's body surface area divided by 1.73. Both equation estimates are affected by the patient's gender (male vs. female), and both are affected by weight (body surface area includes patient's weight). However, weight has a much bigger effect on the CC than the MDRD equation, and there is a bigger gap between these estimates as the patient weight increases. The MDRD equation also has a factor for ethnicity (African American) that is not included in the CC equation. Many dosing nomograms that adjust drug dose based on patient's estimated renal function still use the CC equation though arguments are being made to use the MDRD equation instead, and hospitals generally report the GFR estimated from the MDRD equation on patient laboratory results rather than a CC estimate. Be careful when using a GFR laboratory result as it is most likely the units will be mL/min/1.73 m², and you must convert to the patient's actual GFR using their body surface area for the purposes of adjusting drug doses.

Hepatic Drug Elimination

Unlike renal function, one cannot derive a quantitative estimate of liver function from a laboratory test. The group of tests often referred to as liver function tests, alanine transaminase (ALT), aspartate transaminase (AST), gamma-glutamyl transpeptidase (GTT), and alkaline phosphatase (Alk Phos) cannot be used to estimate drug elimination. These tests measure enzymes produced by cells in the liver that are released when the cells are damaged and release intracellular contents into the blood stream. Thus, the tests indicate damage to the liver, but they do not correlate quantitatively with the liver's metabolic capacity. All we can say is, therefore, that the elimination of a hepatically eliminated drug is most likely decreased, but we cannot say by how much, and there are no dosing nomograms for adjusting drug dose based on any hepatic laboratory parameter analogous to how we use the SCr in the dosing of renally eliminated drugs. Instead there are general statements such as start at a lower dose if patient has abnormal liver function tests or avoid the use of the drug in patients with severe hepatic disease.

The role of the liver in drug elimination is also unique because any drug consumed by oral dosing must pass through the liver before reaching the systemic circulation. All the drug that is absorbed from the gastrointestinal (GI) tract passes through the liver before reaching the systemic circulation and distributing to body tissues. The drug metabolism that occurs upon this first pass of the entire drug dose through the liver is referred to as first-pass metabolism. The model explaining hepatic drug metabolism, including first-pass metabolism after oral dosing, is called the venous equilibrium model (VEM). Understanding this model is necessary to properly interpret the pharmacokinetics of hepatically eliminated drugs and the effects of drug interactions and disease states on their disposition. This model has three parameters that determine hepatic drug clearance, the free fraction of drug in the plasma (f_{up}), the maximum clearance of the drug possible by hepatic metabolism referred to as the intrinsic clearance (Cl_{int}), and the liver blood flow (Q). Hepatically eliminated drugs are divided into three classes—low, intermediate, and high extraction—which are determined by the drug's extraction ratio.

$$ER = \frac{Cl_H}{Q}$$

where ER is the drug's extraction ratio, Cl_H is the hepatic clearance of the drug, and Q is the liver blood flow (approximately 1350 mL/min in humans). Low extraction drugs have an ER $\leq$ 0.3, high extraction drugs have an ER $\geq$ 0.7, and intermediate extraction drugs have an ER between 0.3 and 0.7. Thus, for **propranolol**, which has a hepatic clearance of about 1100 mL/min the ER is:

$$ER = \frac{1100 \text{ mL/min}}{1350 \text{ mL/min}} = 0.81$$

making it a high extraction drug. Drugs with high ERs are eliminated as fast as they are presented to the liver making their elimination flow dependent. Thus, their drug clearance is approximately equal to the liver blood flow.

$$Cl = Q$$

This is in contrast to low extraction drugs in which the clearance is dependent on f_{up} and Cl_{int}.

$$Cl = f_{up} \times Cl_{int}$$

and the Cl value is much less than the liver blood flow (Q). When a hepatically eliminated drug is given orally, it will undergo first-pass metabolism, which is described by the following equation.

$$F^* = 1 - ER$$

where F^* is the fraction of the absorbed drug dose that escapes first-pass metabolism. For high extraction drugs ER is $\geq$ 0.7 and a large proportion of the drug is metabolized before reaching the systemic circulation, which is in contrast to low extraction drugs that will have only a small portion of the drug dose metabolized before reaching the systemic circulation. Thus, for low extraction drugs, F^* is approximately equal to 1, and for high extraction drugs ($f_{up} \times Cl_{int} \gg Q$):

$$F^* = \frac{Q}{f_{up} \times Cl_{int}}$$

These equations based on the venous equilibrium model cannot be used quantitatively, but they are important in understanding what factors affect the steady-state plasma concentrations of hepatically eliminated drugs and the differences between low- and high-extraction drug disposition. The following equations show the factors that determine the free steady state (the pharmacologically active drug concentration) and the total steady-state (free concentration plus concentration bound to plasma proteins) drug concentrations.

Low-extraction drug (given intravenously or orally):

$$C_{ss,Total} = \frac{D}{f_{up} \times Cl_{int}}$$

$$C_{ss,Free} = f_{up} \times \frac{D}{f_{up} \times Cl_{int}} = \frac{D}{Cl_{int}}$$

In the case of a low-extraction drug, there is no first-pass metabolism (no F^*), and the Cl of the drug is equivalent to $f_{up} \times Cl_{int}$.

High-extraction drug (given intravenously)

$$C_{ss,Total} = \frac{D}{Q}$$

$$C_{ss,Free} = f_{up} \times \frac{D}{Q} = \frac{f_{up} \times D}{Q}$$

For a high-extraction drug, the Cl is equal to Q, and when the drug is given intravenously, hepatic first-pass metabolism is bypassed so there is no F*.

High-extraction drug (given orally)

$$C_{ss,Total} = \frac{F^* \times D}{Q} = \frac{\dfrac{Q}{f_{up} \times Cl_{int}} \times D}{Q} = \frac{D}{f_{up} \times Cl_{int}}$$

$$C_{ss,Free} = f_{up} \times \frac{F^* \times D}{Q} = \frac{f_{up} \times \dfrac{Q}{f_{up} \times Cl_{int}} \times D}{Q} = \frac{D}{Cl_{int}}$$

When a high-extraction drug is given orally, then the first-pass metabolism is significant. When we substitute in the equation for F* ($Q/f_{up} \times Cl_{int}$), the equations for the steady-state total and free concentrations simplify to the equations identical to a low-extraction drug. Using these equations, we can predict the effect of changes in f_{up}, Cl_{int}, and Q will have on the steady-state total and free concentrations, and whether this is likely to alter the therapeutic effect of the drug.

Bioavailability

The U.S. Food and Drug Administration defines *bioavailability* as "the rate and extent to which the active ingredient or active moiety is absorbed from a drug product and becomes available at the site of action." In practice, drug concentrations are rarely determined at the site of action (e.g., at a receptor site); therefore, bioavailability is more commonly defined as "the rate and extent that the active drug is absorbed from a dosage form and becomes available in the systemic circulation." The following factors affect bioavailability:

- Drug product formulation
- Properties of the drug (salt form, crystalline structure, formation of solvates, and solubility)
- Composition of the finished dosage form (presence or absence of excipients and special coatings)
- Manufacturing variables (tablet compression force, processing variables, particle size of drug or excipients, and environmental conditions)
- Rate and site of dissolution in the GI tract
- Physiologic determinants
- Contents of the GI tract (fluid volume and pH, diet, presence or absence of food, bacterial activity, and presence of other drugs)
- Rate of GI tract transit (influenced by disease, physical activity, drugs, emotional status of subject, and composition of the GI tract contents)
- Presystemic drug metabolism or degradation (influenced by local blood flow; condition of the GI tract membranes; and drug transport, metabolism, or degradation in the GI tract or during the first pass of the drug through the liver)

Absolute bioavailability

Absolute bioavailability is the fraction (or percentage) of a dose administered nonintravenously (or extravascularly) that is systemically available as compared to an intravenous [I.V.]) dose. If given orally, absolute *bioavailability* (F) is:

$$F = \frac{AUC_{PO}}{AUC_{IV}} \times \frac{D_{IV}}{D_{PO}}$$

where F is the fraction of the oral dose (PO) that is absorbed into the systemic circulation relative to an I.V. administration, AUC_{PO} and AUC_{IV} are the areas-under-the-curve for oral and intravenous administrations, respectively, and D_{IV} and D_{PO} are the doses administered intravenously and orally, respectively. When a drug is given intravenously the F is always considered to be 1.0.

Relative bioavailability

Relative bioavailability refers to a comparison of 2 or more dosage forms in terms of their relative rate and extent of absorption:

$$F = \frac{AUC_{test}}{AUC_{ref}} \times \frac{D_{ref}}{D_{test}}$$

Where F is the relative bioavailability of the test drug (test) to the reference drug (ref) in a dosage form other than intravenous. The equation is identical to the previous equation for absolute bioavailability with the exception that one is not comparing it to the drug administered intravenously. This is often done when one wants to compare two different oral formulations of the same drug against each other. Thus, if F is near 1, then the 2 dosage forms have the same bioavailability. This is not the same thing as bioequivalence, which includes assessing the rate as well as the extent of drug absorption.

Bioequivalence

Two dosage forms that do not differ significantly in their rate and extent of absorption are termed *bioequivalent*. In general, bioequivalence evaluations involve comparisons of dosage forms that are pharmaceutical equivalents or pharmaceutical alternatives. Pharmaceutical equivalents are drug products that contain identical amounts of the identical active drug ingredient (i.e., the same salt or ester of the same therapeutic moiety in identical dosage forms). Pharmaceutical alternatives are drug products that contain the identical therapeutic moiety, or its precursor, but not necessarily in the same amount or dosage form or as the same salt or ester.

Drug Interactions

Pharmacists are expected to be experts in drug interactions, and it is an area of therapeutics about which they are commonly asked questions by both patients and other health care providers. Databases on drug information provide an invaluable source for identifying drug interactions, but pharmacists should have an understanding of the underlying mechanisms and pharmacodynamics of drug interactions. Drug interactions can be divided into four major areas: (1) drug–drug interactions, (2) drug–disease interactions, (3) drug–food interactions, and (4) drug–polymorphism interactions.

Drug–drug interactions are either pharmacokinetic or pharmacodynamics. Pharmacokinetic interactions occur when a drug alters the disposition of another, such as **lovastatin** and ketoconazole.

Ketoconazole is a potent CYP3A4 inhibitor that decreases the metabolism of **lovastatin**, potentially increasing the risk of rhabdomyolysis. Inhibition of drug transporters is another type of pharmacokinetic interaction in which drug transport across a cell membrane is affected by another drug, such as digoxin and amiodarone. Amiodarone is a potent inhibitor to p-glycoprotein, an active transporter, that pumps substrates in the intestinal cell wall back into the lumen of the gut reducing absorption. Digoxin is a p-glycoprotein substrate-drug whose bioavailability is increased by amiodarone due to inhibition of this drug transporter. Drug–drug pharmacodynamics interactions occur when two drugs have overlapping pharmacological activity such as **alprazolam** and alcohol. Alcohol and **alprazolam** are both central nervous system depressants and when taken together synergistically interact increasing the risk of death by respiratory depression.

Drug–disease interactions are most commonly result from renal or hepatic disease, though there are other less common drug–disease interactions. Gentamicin is completely eliminated by the kidneys, and its elimination directly correlates with the patient's renal function. Hepatically eliminated drugs, such as phenytoin, have reduced elimination in patients with liver disease, increasing the risk of adverse effects.

Drug–food interactions are often due to some interaction that reduces absorption, such as tetracycline and milk. Milk has calcium in it, which combines with tetracycline to form an insoluble salt reducing the bioavailability and effectiveness of this antibiotic. The intestines contain drug-metabolizing enzymes, such as CYP3A4, which can be inhibited by grapefruit juice, resulting in an increase in bioavailability of a CYP3A4 substrate-drug such as **lovastatin**.

Drug–polymorphism interaction is an intense area of research. Like pharmacokinetic interactions, we can divide this class of drug interactions into pharmacokinetic or pharmacodynamic interactions. Pharmacokinetic interactions affect drug disposition, such as the interaction between codeine and CYP2D6 polymorphisms. Codeine is an opiate analgesic that is a prodrug requiring metabolism by CYP2D6 to morphine to exert its analgesic effect. CYP2D6-poor metabolizers will not convert codeine to morphine; the patient will not have a significant analgesic response when given codeine. The interaction between **warfarin** and VKORC1 G/A is a pharmacodynamics interaction in which carriers of the A allele are more sensitive to the anticoagulant effect of **warfarin** and, therefore, require lower doses.

Changes in Drug Clearance

Most clinically significant drug interactions result from a change in the clearance of a drug. For renally eliminated drugs, this is most commonly a decrease in clearance due to renal disease; but, for hepatically eliminated drugs, both decreases and increases in clearance are common. Decreases in hepatic metabolism can occur as a result of one drug inhibiting the metabolism of another, a genetic polymorphism associated with decreased enzyme activity, and loss of enzyme due to hepatic disease. Increases in clearance occur when one drug induces the metabolism of another by increasing the amount of the hepatic enzyme responsible for the drug's metabolism, or because of genetic polymorphisms resulting in gene duplication of the drug metabolizing enzyme.

Changes in hepatic clearance are most commonly either a decrease in hepatic drug clearance because of competitive enzyme inhibition or an increase in drug clearance because of enzyme induction. In competitive enzyme inhibition, one drug competes with another drug for the site of hepatic drug metabolism causing an increase in the K_m.

$$\downarrow v = \frac{V_{max} \times C}{\uparrow K_m + C}$$

The higher the concentration of the interacting drug, the greater the decrease in the elimination of the affected drug. Thus, the maximum reduction in drug clearance will occur when the interacting drug has reached steady-steady state, and the interaction will cease after the interacting drug dosing has been stopped for 5 half-lives. Enzyme induction does not cause any change in K_m, in the case of enzyme induction the V_{max} is increased.

$$\uparrow v = \frac{\uparrow V_{max} \times C}{K_m + C}$$

The higher the concentration of the interacting drug, the greater the enzyme induction and the larger the increase in the clearance of the affected drug, but because enzyme induction requires the production of more enzyme by the liver it will take 2 to 4 weeks after the interacting drug reaches steady state for the maximum effect to occur. Conversely, after the interacting drug is stopped, it will take 2 to 4 weeks for hepatic enzyme levels to return to baseline. Thus, the onset and offset of enzyme induction interactions are generally longer than the interactions due to competitive inhibition.

Changes in Volume of Distribution

When considering changes in the volume of distribution, we need to consider both the change relative to the total drug concentration and the pharmacologically active free drug concentration. The following equation defines the volume of distribution at steady state (V_{ss}).

$$V_{ss} = V_p + \frac{f_{up}}{f_{ut}} \times V_t$$

where V_p is the volume of the plasma, V_t is the volume of the tissues, f_{up} is the fraction unbound in the plasma, and f_{ut} is the fraction unbound in tissues. The V_p is small and usually does not contribute significantly to the total volume simplifying the equation to:

$$V_{ss} = \frac{f_{up}}{f_{ut}} \times V_t$$

However, the volume of distribution of the pharmacologically active drug is determined by the free drug concentration, which is the V_{ss} divided by the fraction unbound in the plasma.

$$V_{ss,u} = \frac{V_{ss}}{f_{up}} = \frac{\frac{f_{up}}{f_{ut}} \times V_t}{f_{up}} = \frac{V_t}{f_{ut}}$$

where $V_{ss,u}$ is the unbound volume of distribution at steady state, V_{ss} is the volume of distribution at steady state based on the total drug concentration, f_{up} is the fraction unbound in the plasma, and f_{ut} is the fraction unbound in the tissues. Thus, in a patient, V_t is generally a constant, and changes in the active drug concentration will only occur if the f_{ut} changes. There are no clinically documented changes in f_{ut}. Do not interpret this to mean that changes in f_{ut} do not occur as a result of drug interactions. The problem is that we have no way to measure f_{ut} unlike the f_{up}, which is simply the free drug concentration in the plasma divided by the total concentration in the plasma. Clinically, however, there are no drug interactions known that alter the unbound volume of distribution and require a change in the loading dose of a drug.

NAPLEX Competency Statements

The questions in this chapter cover the following 2021 NAPLEX Competency Statements:
AREA 1: 1.1 **AREA 3:** 3.4; 3.8; 3.9; 3.10 **AREA 4:** 4.1; 4.3; 4.9 **AREA 5:** 5.1.

7-4 Questions

1. A patient with decreased renal function (serum creatinine 2.4 g/dL) has been given a 600 mg dose of gentamicin at 09:30 on 5/10. Gentamicin plasma concentrations measured at 13:20 on 5/10 and 06:30 on 5/11 were 21.2 and 7.1 µg/mL, respectively. What is the half-life of gentamicin in this patient?

   A. 8.7 hours
   B. 14.3 hours
   C. 17.9 hours
   D. 10.8 hours
   E. 9.4 hours

2. The half-life of gentamicin in a patient is 4.6 hours. A plasma concentration drawn 2 hours after the 30-minute dosing infusion was started is 12.3 µg/mL. How long will it take for the gentamicin plasma concentration to fall from 12.3 to 1.0 g/mL?

   A. 8.6 hours
   B. 12.7 hours
   C. 16.6 hours
   D. 21.4 hours
   E. 19.4 hours

3. A drug given by constant I.V. infusion has a half-life of 18 hours. If the drug has been infusing for 48 hours, then what percent of the steady-state concentration have we reached?

   A. 38%
   B. 54%
   C. 85%
   D. 75%
   E. 93%

4. A patient has been taking 250 mg of valproic acid 4 times per day for 2 weeks ($t_{1/2}$ = 16 h) and a trough concentration drawn is 27 µg/mL. What dose would come closest to achieving a target steady-state trough concentration of 85 g/mL?

   A. 750 mg 2 times per day
   B. 750 mg 3 times per day
   C. 500 mg 3 times per day
   D. 500 mg 4 times per day
   E. 750 mg 4 times per day

5. A patient has come to the emergency room after overdosing on a medication. The plasma concentration is 38 µg/mL. The medication has k of 0.175 h⁻¹ and k_a of 0.052 h⁻¹. How long will it take for the plasma concentration to decrease to 5 µg/mL?

   A. 39 hours
   B. 53 hours
   C. 12 hours
   D. 19 hours
   E. 27 hours

6. Phenytoin has a volume of distribution of 0.7 L/kg. What I.V. loading dose (S = 0.92) would be required to achieve a target plasma concentration of 20 µg/mL in a patient weighing 212 pounds?

   A. 1500 mg
   B. 800 mg
   C. 900 mg
   D. 1800 mg
   E. 1350 mg

7. A pediatric patient receives immunosuppressive therapy with oral cyclosporine solution. His concentration-adjusted dosing regimen is 85 mg every 12 hours. Because of a recent change in his insurance coverage, he needs to be switched from the product he is currently using to a generic solution dosage form of cyclosporine that is covered by his insurance. The bioavailability of the dosage form he previously used is 43%; the bioavailability of the generic dosage form is 28%. What is the appropriate dosage regimen for the generic dosage form to maintain the same systemic exposure as obtained from the previously used dosage form?

   A. 25 mg every 12 hours
   B. 55 mg every 12 hours
   C. 184 mg every 12 hours
   D. 130 mg every 12 hours
   E. 95 mg every 12 hours

8. For a drug product in clinical drug development, an oral dosing regimen needs to be established for a phase III study that maintains an average steady-state concentration of 50 ng/mL. In single-dose studies, an oral dose of 80 mg resulted in an AUC of 962 ng/mL x h and an elimination half-life of 10.3 hours. What dosing regimen should be used?

A. 35 mg every 12 hours
B. 50 mg every 12 hours
C. 72 mg every 12 hours
D. 95 mg every 12 hours
E. 100 mg every 24 hours

9. Beth R. (58 kg, 63 years old) is suffering from symptomatic ventricular arrhythmia. She will be started on an oral multiple-dose regimen with the antiarrhythmic mexiletine. The population average values of mexiletine for clearance and volume of distribution are Cl = 0.5 L/h/kg and V = 6 L/kg. Although a therapeutic range of 0.5 to 2.0 mg/L has been described, avoiding large peak-to-trough fluctuations is recommended. The available oral dosage forms are 150-, 200-, and 250 mg capsules with an oral bioavailability of 0.9. Design an appropriate and practically reasonable oral-dosing regimen that keeps the plasma concentrations at an average concentration of approximately 1 mg/L, with a peak-to-trough fluctuation of ≤ 100% (between 0.75 and 1.5 mg/L).

A. 400 mg every 12 hours
B. 200 mg every 6 hours
C. 200 mg every 8 hours
D. 250 mg every 6 hours
E. 250 mg every 8 hours

10. The hospital laboratory results report an eGFR (estimated glomerular filtration rate) of 47 ml/min/1.73 m². The patient weighs 212 pounds and has a body surface are of 1.92 m². What is the estimated GFR you should use for adjusting a drug dose?

A. 47 ml/min
B. 42 ml/min
C. 63 ml/min
D. 52 ml/min
E. 38 ml/min

11. Dabigatran is a direct thrombin inhibitor used for stroke prevention in patients with nonvalvular atrial fibrillation and has a risk of bleeding complications if inappropriately dosed. A patient you have not previously evaluated is to be started on dabigatran, and you have the following information from today's labs: eGFR 24 mL/min/1.73 m² (reported by lab); BSA 2.30 m²; estimated CrCl by CG using adjusted body weight: 33 mL/min. What is the most appropriate recommendation for initial dosing of dabigatran in this patient?

Dabigatran (Pradaxa): Dosing for atrial fibrillation

- CrCl > 30 mL/min   150 mg orally twice daily
- CrCl 15 to 30   75 mg orally twice daily
- CrCl < 15   No recommendation provided

A. Start 75 mg twice daily and closely monitor for signs of bleeding.
B. Start 150 mg twice daily and closely monitor for signs of bleeding.
C. Confirm the patient's kidney function is stable before recommending a dosing regimen.
D. Inform the team this agent should not be used because of the patient's poor kidney function.
E. Start 75 mg once daily and closely monitor for sign of bleeding.

12. A new drug given to a subject orally (with normal CYP2D6 genotype) has a bioavailability of 12%. When the same subject is given a 10 mg I.V. dose the calculated AUC is 1260 ng/mL x h. The drug is completely metabolized by CYP2D6 to an inactive metabolite that is excreted in the urine. What can you conclude from this information?

A. This new drug must be a p-glycoprotein substrate.
B. This is a high-extraction drug that undergoes extensive first-pass metabolism.
C. This is a low extraction drug with poor oral absorption.
D. The subject taking this drug must be a CYP2D6 ultra-rapid metabolizer.
E. It is not possible to make any conclusions from this information without knowing the volume of distribution.

13. A patient has been taking oral phenytoin (F = 0.9) 300 mg/d for 7 years. During this time her kidney function has gradually declined from an eGFR of 85 mL/min to 32 mL/min and her albumin has declined from 4.5 to 2.4 g/dL. Phenytoin is highly bound to albumin, so in this patient phenytoin binding in the plasma will be lower than normal. How will her steady-state total and free phenytoin concentrations change with this decrease in protein binding?

A. The total and free concentrations will not change.

B. The total and free concentrations will decrease.

C. The total concentration will increase, and the free concentration will decrease.

D. The total concentration will decrease, and the free concentration will be unchanged.

E. It cannot be determined how the total and free concentrations will be affected by the change in protein binding.

14. Phenytoin is 90% bound to plasma proteins with a therapeutic range based on total drug concentration of 10 to 20 μg/mL. Thus, the therapeutic range based on the pharmacologically active drug concentration (the free concentration) is 1 to 2 g/mL (0.1 × 10 = 1; 0.1 × 20 = 2). If the plasma protein binding of phenytoin is reduced to 85%, then what is the therapeutic range based on the total phenytoin plasma concentration?

A. 10 to 20 μg/mL

B. 12.5 to 24.6 μg/mL

C. 6.7 to 13.3 μg/mL

D. 8 to 17 μg/mL

E. 13.3 to 25.7 g/mL

15. A patient weighing 85 kg is taking metoprolol 100 mg orally twice per day with good control of his blood pressure. Metoprolol is a CYP2D6 substrate with a volume of 4.2 L/kg, a clearance of 15 mL/min/kg, and a half-life of 3.2 h. He was recently started on paroxetine (a CYP2D6 inhibitor) 20 mg/d. What effect would you expect paroxetine to have on metoprolol?

A. Metoprolol free and total concentrations will not change.

B. Metoprolol free and total concentrations will increase.

C. Metoprolol free and total concentrations will decrease.

D. Metoprolol total concentration will decrease, and the free concentration will remain unchanged.

E. Metoprolol total concentration will increase, and the free concentration will remain unchanged.

16. A patient is taking digoxin 0.125 mg/day with a measured steady state of 1.7 ng/mL drawn 5 hours after his last digoxin dose. His heart rate is 81 beats per minute at this time. The desired steady-state concentration is 1.0 ng/mL. What is the most appropriate course of action?

A. Stop dosing and wait for the concentration to fall to 1 ng/mL and restart dosing at 0.125 mg every other day.

B. Decrease dose to 0.125 mg every other day now.

C. Check the patient's renal function.

D. Redraw the level later in the dosing interval.

E. Administer Digibind to bring the digoxin plasma concentration down into the therapeutic range.

17. As part of a patient medication reconciliation, you note that the patient is on warfarin and carbamazepine. Since carbamazepine induces the elimination of warfarin you should _____.

A. call the patient's physician with a warning that the anticoagulant effect of warfarin is going to decrease

B. find out how long he has been on this combination and recent INR values

C. stop the warfarin now and then call the physician

D. call the patient's physician and suggest using an anticonvulsant that does not induce warfarin's metabolism

E. recommend that the patient's warfarin dose be doubled to compensate for increased clearance of warfarin caused by carbamazepine-induced hepatic metabolism

18. Use the Cockcroft-Gault equation to calculate the creatinine clearance of a 67-year-old female weighing 187 pounds and 5 feet 4 inches tall with a serum creatinine of 2.8 g/dL.

A. 21 mL/min
B. 25 mL/min
C. 33 mL/min
D. 18 mL/min
E. 42 mL/min

19. A patient has been taking warfarin, a hepatically eliminated drug with a Cl of 3.5 mL/min, V of 10 L, and $t_{1/2}$ of 37 hours, and rifampin (a potent inducer of warfarin metabolism) for the past 6 months. His dose has been adjusted to keep his international normalized ratio (INR) between 2.0 and 2.5. His treatment with rifampin is being discontinued. What will happen to the steady-state free and total concentration of warfarin and his INR after stopping rifampin?

A. The total concentration will increase, and the free concentration will remain unchanged with no change in his INR.

B. The total concentration and the free concentration will increase causing an increase in his INR.

C. The total and free concentration will decrease causing a decrease in his INR.

D. The total concentration will remain unchanged and the free concentration will increase causing an increase in his INR.

E. The total and free concentration will be unchanged with no change in the INR.

20. It has been reported that myocardial infarction increases levels of alpha-1-acid glycoprotein, the major binding protein of lidocaine. What effect would you expect the increase in alpha-1-acid glycoprotein to have on lidocaine disposition (Cl = 1.0 L/min; V = 1.1 L/kg; $t_{1/2}$ = 2 hours, hepatic elimination?

A. $C_{ss,total}$ will increase and $C_{ss,free}$ will increase.

B. $C_{ss,total}$ and $C_{ss,free}$ will be unchanged.

C. $C_{ss,total}$ will increase and $C_{ss,free}$ will be unchanged.

D. $C_{ss,total}$ will be unchanged and $C_{ss,free}$ will increase.

E. $C_{ss,total}$ will be unchanged and $C_{ss,free}$ will decrease.

 **7-5** **Answers**

1. D. Estimation of k from two plasma concentrations is:

$$k = \frac{\ln\left(\frac{C1}{C2}\right)}{\Delta t}$$

C1 = 21.2 µg/mL
C2 = 7.1 µg/mL
Δt = time interval between C1 and C2

Time in this case is 24-hour clock time, which is what is used in all hospitals. We need to calculate the time interval from 5/10 13:20 to 5/11 06:30. Calculate the time interval from 13:20 to 24:00 and add 06:30.

Calculate time interval:

~~23:60~~
~~24:00~~
−13:20
10:40
+06:30
16:00 → 17:10 → 17:17 h

Calculate k:

$$k = \frac{\ln\left(\frac{21.2\ \mu g/mL}{7.1\ \mu g/mL}\right)}{17.17\ h} = 0.064\ h^{-1}$$

Calculate half-life

$$t_{1/2} = \frac{0.693}{0.064 \, h^{-1}} = 10.8 \, h$$

2. C. Calculate the time it takes (Δt) the plasma concentration to drop from 12.3 to 1.0 µg/mL.

$$\Delta t = \frac{\ln\left(\dfrac{C1}{C2}\right)}{k}$$

C1 = 12.3 µg/mL
C2 = 1.0 µg/mL
k = 0.693/4.6 h = 0.151 h⁻¹

$$\Delta t = \frac{\ln\left(\dfrac{12.3 \, \mu g/mL}{1.0 \, \mu g/mL}\right)}{0.151 \, h^{-1}} = 16.6 \, h$$

3. C. Since the half-life is 18 hours and the drug has been given for 48 hours, we know that the percent of steady-state concentration is between 75% (two half-lives = 36 hours) and 87.5% (three half-lives = 54 hours). To calculate the exact percent of steady state simply calculate k (k = 0.693/18 = 0.039) and use the following formula.

$$f_{ss} = 1 - e^{-k \times t}$$

where f_{ss} is the fraction of the steady-state concentration, k is the elimination rate constant, and t is the time since the start of the infusion. Thus,

$$f_{ss} = 1 - e^{-0.039 \times 48} = 0.846 \times 100 = 85\%$$

4. E. Use the ratio between the dose and steady-state trough concentration.

$$\frac{D_{obs}}{Css_{obs}} = \frac{D_{NEW}}{Css_{Target}}$$

$$\frac{1000 \, mg/day}{27 \, \mu g/ml} = \frac{D_{NEW}}{85 \, \mu g/ml}$$

$$D_{new} = \frac{3148 \, \dfrac{mg}{day}}{4}$$

$$= 787 \, mg \ 4 \text{ times per day}$$

$$\sim 750 \, mg \ 4 \text{ times per day}$$

5. A. This is the pharmacokinetic "flip-flop" with the $k_a \ll k$. Thus, we must use the k_a to calculate how long it will take the concentration to drop from 38 to 5 µg/mL rather than the k.

$$\Delta t = \frac{\ln\left(\dfrac{38 \, \mu g/mL}{5 \, \mu g/mL}\right)}{0.052 \, h^{-1}} = 39 \, h$$

6. A. Use the loading dose equation:

$$LD = \frac{(C_t - C_{obs}) \times V}{F \times S} = \frac{\left(20\dfrac{mg}{L} - 0\right) \times \left(0.7\dfrac{L}{kg} \times 96.4 \, kg\right)}{(1.0 \times 0.92)}$$

$$= 1467 \, mg \sim 1500 \, mg$$

7. D. First calculate how much cyclosporine he presently gets every 12 hours based on bioavailability of 43%. Then calculate the dose needed based on bioavailability of the new dosage form (28%)

$$85 \, mg \times 0.43 = 36.55 \, mg \text{ every 12 hours}$$

$$\frac{36.55 \, mg}{0.28} = 130.5 \, mg \sim 130 \, mg \text{ every 12 hours}$$

8. B. From the single-dose study we can calculate Cl/F. Using the oral clearance (Cl/F), calculate the dose that will achieve a mean steady-state concentration of 50 ng/mL when given every 12 hours, which is a reasonable time interval given the half-life of about 10 hours. For this calculation you are assuming the F remains constant between the single-dose study and your steady-state dosing estimate.

$$\frac{Cl}{F} = \frac{D}{AUC} = \frac{80 \, mg}{962 \dfrac{ng}{ml} \times h} = \frac{80,000 \, \mu g}{962 \dfrac{\mu g}{L} \times h} = 83.2 \, L/h$$

$$D = 50\frac{ng}{ml} \times 83.2\frac{L}{h} = 50\frac{\mu g}{L} \times 83.2\frac{L}{h}$$

$$= 4160\frac{\mu g}{h}$$

$$= 4.16\frac{mg}{h} \times 12 \, h \sim 50 \, mg \text{ every 12 hours}$$

9. E. The dose needed to achieve a mean steady state concentration of 1 mg/L is determined by the clearance in this patient, which is 29 L/h (0.5 L/h/kg × 58 kg). The dosing interval required that will keep the fluctuation between the peak and trough between 1.5 and 0.75 mg/L is determined by the k, which is equal to the Cl/V. Use k to determine how long it will take the concentration to drop from 1.5 to 0.75 mg/L. Calculate the dose based on the chosen time interval.

$$D/h = \frac{Css \times Cl}{F} = \frac{1\frac{mg}{L} \times 29\frac{L}{h}}{0.9} = 32.2 \text{ mg/h}$$

$$k = \frac{Cl}{V} = \frac{29\frac{L}{h}}{\left(6\frac{L}{kg} \times 58 \text{ kg}\right)} = 0.083 \text{ h}^{-1}$$

$$\Delta t = \frac{\ln\left(\frac{1.5 \text{ mg/L}}{0.75 \text{ mg/L}}\right)}{0.083 \text{ h}^{-1}} = 8.35 \text{ h}$$

$$D \text{ per } 8 \text{ h} = 32.2\frac{mg}{h} \times 8 \text{ h} = 257.6 \sim 250 \text{ mg every } 8 \text{ h}$$

10. **D.** The eGFR is in units of mL/min/1.73 m² and must be converted to mL/min by multiplying the eGFR by the patient's BSA divided by 1.73 m² before using it to adjust the dose of a renally eliminated drug in the patient.

$$GFR = eGFR \times \left(\frac{BSA_{Patient}}{1.73 \text{ m}^2}\right) = 47\frac{ml}{min} \times \left(\frac{1.92 \text{ m}^2}{1.73 \text{ m}^2}\right)$$
$$= 52 \text{ mL/min}$$

11. **C.** The correct answer to the question highlights the importance of knowing more about the patient than just the reported lab value and making assumptions that may not be accurate. In this case, the estimated renal function by the Cockcroft-Gault equation (33 mL/min) and the MDRD equation (31 mL/min) both result in a recommendation of 150 mg orally twice daily, but because you have no information on whether the patient's renal function is stable, it would be inappropriate to base a dose on this lab value. The serum creatinine has a long half-life, so, as renal function declines, it may continue to rise for several days in a patient who has an acute kidney injury. Thus, in this patient you don't know if the kidney function is still declining.

12. **C.** This is a hepatically eliminated drug, so the first step is to determine its extraction ratio.

$$ER = \frac{Cl_{Drug}}{Q} = \frac{\frac{D}{AUC}}{1350 \text{mL/min}} = \frac{\frac{10,000\,\mu g}{1260\,\mu g/L \times h}}{81 \text{ L/h}} = 0.098$$

Because this is a low-extraction drug (ER ≤ 0.3) there is no significant first-pass metabolism that could explain the low bioavailability of 12%. The drug could have reduced absorption if it is a substrate of p-glycoprotein, but there is no information given that would allow that conclusion. However, we do know that the bioavailability is due to poor absorption.

13. **D.** Phenytoin is a low-extraction, hepatically eliminated drug highly bound to albumin. A decline in protein binding results in an increase in the f_{up}. Thus, we can apply the venous equilibrium model equations to determine that the total steady-state concentration of phenytoin will decrease, and the free steady-state concentration will remain unchanged.

$$\downarrow C_{ss,Total} = \frac{D}{\uparrow f_{up} \times Cl_{int}}$$

$$\leftrightarrow C_{ss,Free} = \frac{D}{Cl_{int}}$$

14. **C.** To determine the total concentration that corresponds to a free concentration range of 1.0 to 2.0 simply divide the free concentration range by the f_{up}.

$$\text{Range} = \frac{1.0\,\mu g/mL}{0.15} \text{ to } \frac{2.0\,\mu g/mL}{0.15} = 6.7 \text{ to } 13.3\,\mu g/mL$$

Thus, as the protein binding decreases, the therapeutic range based on the total steady-state drug concentration decreases. Patients with kidney and liver disease have decreased albumin, which could lead to an inappropriate dosage increase resulting in toxicity if you apply a normal therapeutic range of 10 to 20 µg/mL as your target range.

15. **B.** Because metoprolol is a hepatically eliminated drug we need to determine its extraction ratio.

$$ER = \frac{Cl_{Drug}}{Q} = \frac{15\frac{ml}{min}}{1350 \text{ ml/min}} \times 85 \, kg = 0.94$$

Thus, this is a high-extraction drug being given orally. The inhibition of CYP2D6 by paroxetine would be a decrease in the Cl_{int}. Thus, applying the venous equilibrium model we would conclude that both the total and free steady-state concentrations would increase, possibly resulting in an unexpected decrease in blood pressure and heart rate.

$$\uparrow C_{ss,Total} = \frac{D}{f_{up} \times \downarrow Cl_{int}}$$

$$\uparrow C_{ss,Free} = \frac{D}{\downarrow Cl_{int}}$$

16. D. Digoxin has a significant distribution phase (two-compartment model), but the therapeutic range is based on digoxin trough concentrations. If you draw a level less than 8 hours after the dose, then the digoxin concentration will be falsely elevated. The patient's heart rate is 81, which also does not suggest the dose is too high. You should redraw an appropriate trough level in this case. The graph below shows the problem.

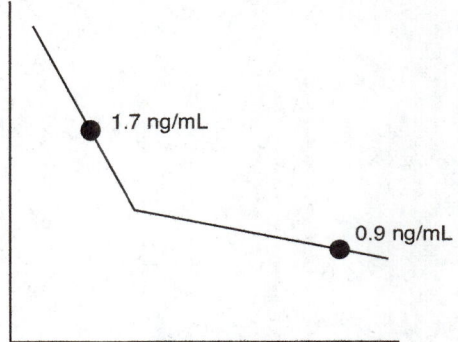

1.7 ng/mL

0.9 ng/mL

The level of 1.7 ng/mL is not a true trough level and may be significantly higher than the true trough level. To properly interpret drug level, you must know when the level was drawn in relation to the last dose.

17. B. There is a significant drug interaction between warfarin and carbamazepine with carbamazepine inducing the metabolism of warfarin leading to a decrease in warfarin's effect (decrease in INR) potentially increasing the risk of blood clot formation. However, if the patient were on carbamazepine before the initiation of warfarin therapy, then the warfarin dose would be stabilized under the condition of enzyme induction. In this case, it would not be appropriate to discontinue carbamazepine as it would lead to an increase in the warfarin level, which could lead to dangerous bleeding. You need more information to make an appropriate therapeutic decision.

18. A. The first step is to calculate the patient's ABW. Then use the ABW to calculate the CrCl.

$$ABW = IBW + 0.4(TBW - IBW)$$
$$= 54.7 \text{ kg} + 0.4(85 \text{ kg} - 54.7 \text{ kg}) = 66.8 \text{ kg}$$
$$CrCl = \frac{(140 - 67)66.8 \text{ kg}}{(72 \times 2.8 \text{ g/dl})} \times 0.85 = 20.6 \text{ mL/min}$$

19. B. Warfarin is a low-extraction hepatically eliminated drug. The dose was stabilized while the patient's hepatic enzymes were induced by rifampin. When rifampin is stopped the Cl_{int} will decrease.

$$\uparrow C_{ss,Total} = \frac{D}{f_{up} \times \downarrow Cl_{int}}$$

$$\uparrow C_{ss,Free} = \frac{D}{\downarrow Cl_{int}}$$

Remember that the maximal decrease in enzyme activity will take 2 to 4 weeks; therefore, you would expect the INR to increase over the next 2 to 4 weeks.

20. E. Lidocaine is a high-extraction hepatically eliminated drug given by I.V. infusion. The increase in alpha-1-acid glycoprotein will cause an increase in the protein binding resulting in a decrease in the f_{up}.

$$\leftrightarrow C_{ss,Total} = \frac{D}{Q}$$

$$\downarrow C_{ss,Free} = \frac{\downarrow f_{up} \times D}{Q}$$

Thus, the decrease in f_{up} would be expected to decrease the active free-drug concentration resulting in a decrease in the effects of the lidocaine infusion.

7-6 Additional Resources

Atkinson A, Daniels C, Dedrick R, et al. *Principles of Clinical Pharmacology.* San Diego, CA; Academic Press; 2001.

Ensom MH, Davis GA, Cropp CD, et al. Clinical pharmacokinetics in the 21st century: does the evidence support definitive outcomes? *Clin Pharmacokinet.* 1998;34(4):265–279.

Levy RH, Bauer LA. Basic pharmacokinetics. *Ther Drug Monit.* 1986;8(1):47–58.

Meibohm B, Derendorf H. Basic concepts of pharmacokinetic/pharmacodynamic (PK/PD) modelling. *Int J Clin Pharmacol Ther.* 1997;35:401–413.

Rolan PE. Plasma protein binding displacement interactions: why are they still regarded as clinically important? *Br J Clin Pharmacol.* 1994;37:125–128.

Rowland M, Tozer T. *Clinical Pharmacokinetics and Pharmacodynamics.* 4th ed. Media, PA: Williams & Wilkins; 2011.

Saitoh A, Jinbayashi H, Saitoh AK, et al. Parameter estimation and dosage adjustment in the treatment with vancomycin of methicillin-resistant *Staphylococcus aureus* ocular infections. *Ophthalmologica.* 1997;211(4):232–235.

Sawchuk RJ, Zaske DE, Cipolle RJ, et al. Kinetic model for gentamicin dosing with the use of individual patient parameters. *Clin Pharmacol Ther.* 1977;21:362–369.

Tod MM, Padoin C, Petitjean O. Individualising aminoglycoside dosage regimens after therapeutic drug monitoring: simple or complex pharmacokinetic methods? *Clin Pharmacokinet.* 2001;40:803–814.

Wilkinson GR, Shand DG. Commentary: a physiological approach to hepatic drug clearance. *Clin Pharmacol Ther.* 1975;18:377–390.

Biotechnology and Pharmacogenomics

8

HENRY M. DUNNENBERGER   GILLIAN C. BELL

8-1 KEY POINTS

- *Biotechnology*, as defined by the *Merriam-Webster Dictionary*, is "the manipulation (as through genetic engineering) of living organisms or their components to produce useful usually commercial products (as pest resistant crops, new bacterial strains, or novel pharmaceuticals)."
- The central dogma of molecular biology is that deoxyribonucleic acid (DNA) encodes ribonucleic acid (RNA), which, in turn, encodes protein.
- Recombinant DNA technology allows for the placement of a desired DNA fragment in proximity to other DNA fragments within a DNA molecule for a specific purpose.
- Cytokines secreted by cells orchestrate the immune response by activating immune cells such as lymphocytes, macrophages, monocytes, and neutrophils.
- Enzymes are proteins that catalyze a specific chemical reaction.
- Hormones are chemical substances transmitted by the bloodstream to cells distant from their physiologic source that impart specific cellular effects.
- Vaccines are antigenic preparations administered to stimulate the development of antibodies for the purpose of conferring active immunity against a particular pathogen or disease.
- Subsets of β-lymphocyte clones produce identical antibodies that recognize the same antigen. These identical antibodies are said to be monoclonal. Fusing β-lymphocytes with lymphocyte tumor cells produces a hybridoma that can be cultured in large quantities for the mass production of a given monoclonal antibody.
- Biotechnology has facilitated the development of novel drug delivery strategies, including liposomal technology, immunotoxins, and PEGylation.
- Pharmacogenomics is the scientific discipline of using genomewide approaches to understand the inherited basis of differences between individual responses to drugs.

8-2 STUDY GUIDE CHECKLIST

The following topics may guide your study of this subject area:

- [ ] Familiarize yourself with marketed biological products (Table 8-1).
- [ ] Gain a general sense of the types of biological products that are currently approved by the U.S. Food and Drug Administration.
- [ ] Study recombinant technology and the production of vaccines.
- [ ] Review the nomenclature of monoclonal antibodies.
- [ ] Familiarize yourself with concepts and terms related to pharmacogenomics.
- [ ] Review drugs with strong evidence between drug response and genetic variation (Tables 8-2 and 8-4).

8-3 ▶ Key Terms

- **Antibody (immunoglobulin):** A protein produced by β-lymphocytes in response to antigen molecules determined to be non-self. Antibodies recognize and bind to antigens, resulting in the antigens' inactivation or opsonization for phagocytosis or complement-mediated destruction. For example, a number of immunoglobulin G products have been developed for therapeutic use in various immune disorders.
- **Antigen:** A molecule that elicits an antibody-mediated immune response.
- **Clotting factor (blood factor):** Chemical blood constituents that interact to cause blood coagulation.
- **Cytokine:** An extracellular signaling protein that mediates communication between cells.
- **Gene:** A region of deoxyribonucleic acid (DNA) that encodes a specific ribonucleic acid (RNA) or protein responsible for a specific hereditary characteristic.
- **Gene therapy:** Therapeutic technologies that directly target human genes responsible for disease.
- **Genome:** The complete set of genetic information for a given organism.
- **Genomics:** The scientific discipline of mapping, sequencing, and analyzing genomes. It encompasses structural genomics, functional genomics, and pharmacogenomics.
- **Genotype:** An individual's collection of genes. Two alleles are inherited for a particular gene.
- **Hybridoma:** A cell line generated by the fusion of antibody-producing β-lymphocytes with lymphocyte tumor cells for the production of monoclonal antibodies.
- **Interferon:** A member of a group of cytokines that prevents viral replication and slows the growth and replication of cancer cells.
- **Interleukin:** A member of a group of cytokines involved in orchestration and regulation of the immune response.
- **Liposome:** A microscopic, sphere-like lipid droplet that functions as a therapeutic carrier.
- **Monoclonal antibody:** An antibody derived from a hybridoma cell line.
- **Pharmacogenomics:** The scientific discipline of using genomewide approaches to understand the inherited basis of differences between individuals in the response to drugs. *Pharmacogenetics* is a related term and field that traditionally considered such inherited differences on a gene-by-gene basis. These terms may be use interchangeably in clinical practice.
- **Phenotype:** Observable physical characteristic (such as enzyme activity).
- **Plasmid:** A small, circular, extrachromosomal DNA molecule capable of replication independent of that of the genome.
- **Polymerase chain reaction (PCR):** A molecular biologic technique for amplification of specific DNA molecules.
- **Polymorphism:** Variation within a gene.
- **Recombinant DNA (rDNA) technology:** The application of DNA molecules derived by joining two DNA molecules from different sources.
- **Restriction endonuclease:** An enzyme capable of cleaving a DNA molecule in a site-specific manner.
- **Ribozymes:** RNA molecules with intrinsic enzymatic activity.
- **Single nucleotide polymorphism (SNP):** Single base-pair substitution, a common type of DNA sequence variation.
- **Vaccine:** A preparation of antigenic material administered to stimulate the development of antibodies conferring active immunity against a particular pathogen or disease.

8-4 ▶ Overview

Biotechnology, defined by the *Merriam-Webster Dictionary* as "the manipulation (as through genetic engineering) of living organisms or their components to produce useful usually commercial products (as pest resistant crops, new bacterial strains, or novel pharmaceuticals)," has revolutionized the pharmaceutical industry by imparting the ability to mass produce safe and pure versions of chemicals produced naturally in the body. A multitude of disease states have been affected by therapeutic agents derived through biotechnology, including acquired immune deficiency syndrome (AIDS), anemia, cancer, congestive heart failure, cystic fibrosis, diabetes, growth hormone deficiency, hemophilia, hepatitis B and C, and multiple sclerosis. Additionally, our increased understanding of how to map an individual's response to a drug based on genetic makeup and the expanding field of pharmacogenomics shows great promise to revolutionize the way pharmacy and medicine are practiced. This chapter highlights key concepts relevant to the practicing pharmacist in the areas of biotechnology and pharmacogenomics.

Biological Products

Many U.S. Food and Drug Administration (FDA)–approved biological products are currently on the market, including blood factors, cytokines, enzymes, growth factors, hormones, interferons, monoclonal antibodies, and vaccines. A list of such biological products is provided in Table 8-1. Due to the nature of these products, a patient may experience hypersensitivity reactions or neutralizing reactions from these agents, thus, altering their therapeutic response. The risk of these types of reactions vary depending on the specific agent and should be considered when selecting the treatment of choice for a patient.

TABLE 8-1. Approved Biological Products[a]

Generic name	Brand name (manufacturer)	Indications
Blood factors		
Coagulation factor Xa (recombinant)	ANDEXXA (Portola Pharmaceuticals)	Reversal of anticoagulation from rivaroxaban or **apixaban**, as result of life-threatening or uncontrolled bleeding
Factor VII ⚠	NovoSeven, NovoSeven RT (Novo Nordisk)	Hemophilia
Factor VIII	Bioclate, Recombinate, Advate, Obizur (Baxter); Kogenate, Helixate, Kovaltry (Bayer); ReFacto (Genetics Institute); Xyntha (Wyeth); Nuwiq (Octapharma); Novoeight (Novo Nordisk); Adynovate (Baxalta); Afstyla (CSL Behring)	Hemophilia A
Factor IX	BeneFix (Genetics Institute); Alprolix (Biogen); Ixinity (Cangene); Rixubis (Baxter); Idelvion (CSL Behring)	Hemophilia B
Factor X	Coagadex (Bio Products)	Hereditary factor X deficiency
Factor XIII	Tretten (Novo Nordisk); Corifact (CSL Behring)	Congenital factor XIII deficiency
Cytokines		
Aldesleukin (IL-2) ⚠	Proleukin (Chiron)	Metastatic renal cell carcinoma and melanoma
Interferon alfa-2b ⚠	Intron-A (Schering)	Hairy cell leukemia; AIDS-related Kaposi's sarcoma; chronic hepatitis B and C; condylomata acuminata; malignant melanoma; follicular lymphoma; viral hepatitis B
Interferon beta-1b	Betaseron (Bayer); Extavia (Novartis)	Acute relapsing–remitting multiple sclerosis
Interferon beta-1a	Avonex (Biogen); Rebif (EMD Serono)	Acute relapsing–remitting multiple sclerosis
Interferon gamma-1b	Actimmune (InterMune)	Chronic granulomatous disease; osteoporosis
Oprelvekin (IL-11)	Neumega (Genetics Institute)	Thrombocytopenia from chemotherapy
Peginterferon alfa-2a ⚠	Pegasys (Roche)	Hepatitis C; active viral hepatitis B

(continued)

TABLE 8-1. Approved Biological Products^a *(Continued)*

Generic name	Brand name (manufacturer)	Indications
Peginterferon alfa-2b ⚠	PegIntron (Schering); Sylatron (Merck)	Hepatitis C; malignant melanoma
Peginterferon beta-1a	Plegridy (Biogen)	Relapsing forms of multiple sclerosis
Enzymes		
Alteplase	Activase (Genentech)	Acute myocardial infarction; pulmonary embolism; stroke; venous catheter occlusion
Bivalirudin	Angiomax (Medicines Co.)	Heparin-induced thrombocytopenia with thrombosis; coronary angioplasty (PTCA); unstable angina
Dornase alfa	Pulmozyme (Genentech)	Respiratory complication from cystic fibrosis
Eptifibatide	Integrilin (Millennium)	Acute coronary syndromes; percutaneous coronary intervention
Lepirudin	Refludan (Berlex)	Heparin-induced thrombocytopenia
Pancrelipase	Pancreaze (Ortho-McNeil-Janssen)	Exocrine pancreatic insufficiency; cystic fibrosis–associated pancreatic insufficiency
Pegloticase ⚠	Krystexxa (Savient)	Treatment of severe, treatment-refractory, chronic gout
Rasburicase ⚠	Elitek (Sanofi-Synthelabo)	Elevated plasma uric acid in pediatric malignancy
Reteplase	Retavase (Centocor/J&J)	Acute myocardial infarction
Sebelipase alfa	Kanuma (Alexion)	Lysosomal acid lipase deficiency
Tenecteplase	TNKase (Genentech)	Acute myocardial infarction
Tirofiban	Aggrastat (Merck)	Acute coronary syndromes
Growth factors		
Darbepoetin alfa ⚠	Aranesp (Amgen)	Anemia attributable to chemotherapy; anemia associated with end-stage renal disease and chronic renal insufficiency
Epoetin alfa ⚠	Epogen (Amgen); Procrit (Janssen Pharmaceuticals)	Anemia attributable to chronic renal disease; zidovudine-induced anemia; anemia attributable to chemotherapy; surgical procedure–associated transfusion
Filgrastim	Neupogen (Amgen)	Febrile neutropenia in nonmyeloid malignancies in patients undergoing myeloablative chemotherapy followed by marrow transplantation; febrile neutropenia in nonmyeloid malignancies following myelosuppressive chemotherapy; febrile neutropenia in patients with acute myeloid leukemia receiving chemotherapy; harvesting of peripheral blood stem cells; chronic neutropenia; radiation injury of bone marrow
Pegfilgrastim	Neulasta (Amgen)	Febrile neutropenia attributable to myelosuppressive chemotherapy; radiation injury of bone marrow
Sargramostim	Leukine (Berlex)	Acute myeloid leukemia–neutrophil recovery; allogeneic and autologous bone marrow transplant; autologous peripheral blood stem cell transplant; mobilization of hematopoietic progenitor cells into peripheral blood for collection by leukapheresis
Hormones		
Choriogonadotropin alfa	Ovidrel (Serono)	Fertility
Exenatide ⚠	Byetta (Amylin)	Diabetes mellitus type 2
Follitropin alfa	Gonal-F (Serono)	Ovulatory failure; male hypogonadotropic hypogonadism
Human growth hormone	Nutropin (Genentech)	Growth hormone deficiency in pediatric patients
	Genotropin (Pharmacia)	Growth hormone deficiency in adults

TABLE 8-1. Approved Biological Products[a] (Continued)

Generic name	Brand name (manufacturer)	Indications
Human insulin	Humulin, **Humalog** (Eli Lilly); Novolin, **NovoLog, Levemir** (Novo Nordisk); **Lantus** (Sanofi-Aventis)	Insulin-dependent diabetes mellitus
Ganirelix	Antagon (Organon)	Luteinizing hormone surge during fertility therapy
Glucagon	GlucaGen (Novo Nordisk)	Hypoglycemia; radiography of gastrointestinal tract
Liraglutide recombinant	Victoza (Novo Nordisk)	Diabetes mellitus type 2; obesity
Parathyroid hormone ⚠	Natpara (NPS Pharma)	Hypocalcemia in patients with hypoparathyroidism
Testosterone cypionate	Testosterone Cypionate Injection, USP (Sun Pharma)	Primary hypogonadism; hypogonadotropic hypogonadism
Testosterone undecanoate ⚠	Aveed (Endo Pharma)	Primary hypogonadism; hypogonadotropic hypogonadism
Thyrotropin	Thyrogen (Genzyme)	Thyroid cancer
Monoclonal antibodies		
Abciximab	ReoPro (Centocor)	Prevention of blood clots following percutaneous coronary intervention; unstable angina before percutaneous coronary intervention
Adalimumab ⚠	Humira (AbbVie)	Ankylosing spondylitis; acute rheumatoid arthritis; psoriatic arthritis; Crohn's disease; ulcerative colitis; hidradenitis suppurativa; plaque psoriasis; uveitis
Alemtuzumab ⚠	Campath (Berlex)	Chronic lymphocytic leukemia; acute relapsing-remitting multiple sclerosis
Basiliximab ⚠	Simulect (Novartis)	Acute organ transplant rejection
Bevacizumab	Avastin (Genentech)	Colorectal cancer; cervical cancer; glioblastoma multiforme of brain; metastatic renal cell carcinoma; nonsquamous non–small cell lung cancer; ovarian cancer
Blinatumomab ⚠	Blincyto (Amgen)	Acute lymphoblastic leukemia
Certolizumab pegol ⚠	Cimzia (UCB)	Ankylosing spondylitis; Crohn's disease; psoriatic arthritis; rheumatoid arthritis
Cetuximab ⚠	Erbitux (ImClone Systems)	Colorectal cancer; squamous cell carcinoma of the head and neck
Crizanlizumab	Adakveo (Novartis)	Vasoocclusive crises in adults and pediatric patients aged 16 years and older with sickle cell disease
Daclizumab	Zenapax (Roche); Zinbryta (Biogen)	Acute rejection of kidney transplant; relapsing forms of multiple sclerosis
Daratumumab	Darzalex (Janssen Biotech)	Multiple myeloma
Dinutuximab ⚠	Unituxin (United Therapeutics)	High-risk neuroblastoma in pediatric patients
Eculizumab ⚠	Soliris (Alexion)	Paroxysmal nocturnal hemoglobinuria; hemolytic uremic syndrome
Elotuzumab	Empliciti (Bristol-Myers Squibb)	Multiple myeloma
Golimumab ⚠	Simponi Aria (Janssen Biotech)	Rheumatoid arthritis; psoriatic arthritis; ankylosing spondylitis; ulcerative colitis
Ibritumomab (tiuxetan) ⚠	Zevalin (IDEC)	B-cell non-Hodgkin's lymphoma
Idarucizumab	Praxbind (Boehringer Ingelheim)	Anticoagulation reversal attributable to the effects of dabigatran
Infliximab	Remicade (Janssen Biotech)	Ankylosing spondylitis; Crohn's disease; psoriatic arthritis; rheumatoid arthritis; ulcerative colitis

(continued)

TABLE 8-1. Approved Biological Products[a] *(Continued)*

Generic name	Brand name (manufacturer)	Indications
Ixekizumab	Taltz (Eli Lilly)	Plaque psoriasis
Mepolizumab	Nucala (GlaxoSmithKline)	Asthma
Necitumumab	Portrazza (Eli Lilly)	Metastatic squamous non–small cell lung cancer
Nivolumab	Opdivo (Bristol-Myers Squibb)	Melanoma; non–small cell lung cancer; small cell lung cancer; renal cell carcinoma
Omalizumab ⚠	Xolair (Genentech)	Asthma; idiopathic urticaria
Panitumumab ⚠	Vectibix (Amgen)	Metastatic colorectal cancer
Pembrolizumab	Keytruda (Merck)	Metastatic or unresectable melanoma
Ranibizumab	Lucentis (Genentech)	Diabetic macular edema; exudative age-related macular degeneration; macular retinal edema
Reslizumab ⚠	Cinqair (Teva)	Asthma
Rituximab ⚠	Rituxan (IDEC/Genentech)	Chronic lymphoid leukemia; microscopic polyarteritis nodosa; non-Hodgkin's lymphoma; rheumatoid arthritis; Wegener's granulomatosis
Secukinumab	Cosentyx (Novartis)	Plaque psoriasis; psoriatic arthritis; ankylosing spondylitis
Trastuzumab ⚠	Herceptin (Genentech/PDL)	Metastatic breast cancer (Her 2 overexpression); metastatic gastric cancer (Her 2 overexpression); malignant neoplasm of cardioesophageal junction of stomach (Her 2 overexpression)
Others		
Abatacept	Orencia (Bristol-Meyers Squibb)	Rheumatoid arthritis
Albiglutide ⚠	Tanzeum (GlaxoSmithKline)	Diabetes mellitus type 2
Anakinra	Kineret (Amgen)	Chronic infantile neurological, cutaneous, and articular syndrome; rheumatoid arthritis
BCNU polymer	Gliadel (Guilford)	Recurrent glioblastoma multiforme; Hodgkin's disease; malignant intracranial tumor; malignant glioma; malignant glioma of the brain; multiple myeloma; non-Hodgkin's lymphoma
Daunorubicin-liposomal ⚠	DaunoXome (Gilead)	Kaposi's sarcoma
Doxorubicin-liposomal ⚠	DOXIL (Alza)	Kaposi's sarcoma; ovarian cancer
Dulaglutide ⚠	Trulicity (Eli Lilly)	Diabetes mellitus type 2
Etanercept ⚠	Enbrel (Amgen)	Ankylosing spondylitis; rheumatoid arthritis; psoriatic arthritis; chronic plaque psoriasis
Fomivirsen	Vitravene (Isis)	Cytomegalovirus retinitis
Glatiramer	Copaxone (Teva)	Relapsing multiple sclerosis
Lipid-based amphotericin B	Abelcet (Elan); Amphotec (Sequus); AmBisome (Fujisawa/Gilead)	Aspergillosis; cryptococcal meningitis in HIV; systemic fungal infections
Nesiritide	Natrecor (Scios/Innovex)	Congestive heart failure
Onasemnogene abeparvovec	Zolgensma (AveXis)	Spinal muscular atrophy in pediatric patients under 2 years old with bi-allelic mutations in the survival motor neuron 1 gene

Boldface indicates one of top 100 drugs for 2020 by prescription volume.
AIDS, acquired immune deficiency syndrome; BCNU, bis-chlorethylnitrosourea; HIV, human immunodeficiency virus; IL, interleukin; PTCA, percutaneous transluminal coronary angioplasty.
a. This table is not a comprehensive list of approved products.

FDA BOXED WARNINGS

Factor VII

Serious arterial and venous thrombotic events following administration of Factor VIIa (recombinant) have been reported.

Aldesleukin (IL-2)

Use aldesleukin with extreme caution in patients who have a history of cardiac or pulmonary disease. Withhold aldesleukin administration in patients developing moderate-to-severe lethargy or somnolence. Aldesleukin treatment is associated with an increased risk of disseminated infection, including sepsis and bacterial endocarditis. Aldesleukin administration has been associated with capillary leak syndrome. Administer aldesleukin in a hospital setting under the supervision of a qualified physician experienced in the use of anticancer agents.

Interferon alfa-2b

Alpha interferons, including interferon alfa-2b, cause or aggravate fatal or life-threatening neuropsychiatric, autoimmune, ischemic, and infectious disorders.

Peginterferon alfa-2a

Peginterferon alfa-2a may cause or aggravate fatal or life-threatening neuropsychiatric, autoimmune, ischemic, and infectious disorders.

Peginterferon alfa-2b

Alpha interferons, including peginterferon alfa-2b, cause or aggravate fatal or life-threatening neuropsychiatric, autoimmune, ischemic, and infectious disorders.

Pegloticase

Anaphylaxis and infusion reactions have been reported to occur during and after administration of pegloticase. Screen patients at risk for G6PD deficiency prior to starting pegloticase.

Rasburicase

Rasburicase may cause serious and fatal hypersensitivity reactions, including anaphylaxis. Do not administer rasburicase to patients with glucose-6-phosphate dehydrogenase (G6PD) deficiency. Rasburicase can result in methemoglobinemia. Rasburicase may interfere with uric acid measurements.

Darbepoetin alfa

Erythropoiesis-stimulating agents (ESAs) increase the risk of death, myocardial infarction (MI), stroke, venous thromboembolism, and thrombosis of vascular access. Use the lowest effective dose.

Epoetin alfa

Erythropoiesis-stimulating agents (ESAs) increase the risk of death, myocardial infarction (MI), stroke, venous thromboembolism, and thrombosis of vascular access. Use the lowest effective dose.

Exenatide

Exenatide extended release (ER) causes an increased incidence in thyroid C-cell tumors in animal studies.

Parathyroid hormone

In male and female rats, parathyroid hormone caused an increase in the incidence of osteosarcoma. Natpara has a REMS Program.

Testosterone undecanoate

Testosterone undecanoate and testosterone enanthate can cause blood pressure (BP) increases that can increase the risk of major adverse cardiovascular events. Virilization has been reported in children who were secondarily exposed to topical testosterone gel and solution. Because of the risks of serious POME reactions and anaphylaxis, testosterone undecanoate is available only through a restricted program under a risk evaluation and mitigation strategy (REMS) called the Aveed REMS Program.

Adalimumab

Patients treated with adalimumab are at an increased risk of developing serious infections, especially if these patients are also taking immunosuppressants. These infections include tuberculosis, invasive fungal infections, and opportunistic bacterial, viral, and other infections.

Patients treated with adalimumab have also developed certain malignancies, including lymphoma.

(continued)

FDA BOXED WARNINGS (Continued)

Alemtuzumab

Serious, including fatal, pancytopenia/marrow hypoplasia, autoimmune idiopathic thrombocytopenia, and autoimmune hemolytic anemia can occur in patients receiving alemtuzumab. Alemtuzumab causes serious and life-threatening infusion reactions. Alemtuzumab may cause an increased risk of stroke, serious, including fatal, bacterial, viral, fungal, and protozoan infections, and malignancies, including thyroid cancer, melanoma, and lymphoproliferative disorders. Lemtrada has a REMS program.

Basiliximab

Only physicians experienced in immunosuppression therapy and management of organ transplantation patients should prescribe basiliximab.

Blinatumomab

Cytokine release syndrome (CRS) and neurological toxicities, which may be life-threatening or fatal, occurred in patients receiving blinatumomab.

Certolizumab pegol

Patients treated with certolizumab are at an increased risk of developing serious infections, especially if these patients are also taking immunosuppressants. These infections include tuberculosis, invasive fungal infections, and opportunistic bacterial, viral, and other infections. Patients treated with certolizumab have also developed certain malignancies, including lymphoma.

Cetuximab

Cetuximab may cause serious and fatal infusion reactions. Cardiopulmonary arrest or sudden death occurred in patients with squamous cell carcinoma of the head and neck receiving cetuximab.

Dinutuximab

Neurotoxicities and serious and potentially life-threatening infusion reactions can occur in patients treated with dinutuximab.

Eculizumab

Life-threatening and fatal meningococcal infections have occurred in patients treated with eculizumab. Eculizumab is available only through a restricted program under a Risk Evaluation and Mitigation Strategy (REMS).

Golimumab

Patients treated with golimumab are at an increased risk of developing serious infections, especially if these patients are also taking immunosuppressants. These infections include tuberculosis, invasive fungal infections, and opportunistic bacterial, viral, and other infections. Patients treated with golimumab have also developed certain malignancies, including lymphoma.

Ibritumomab (tiuxetan)

Severe and prolonged cytopenias, severe cutaneous and mucocutaneous reactions, and death can occur with the ibritumomab tiuxetan therapeutic regimen. The dose of Y-90 ibritumomab tiuxetan should not exceed 32 mCi (1184 MBq).

Omalizumab

Anaphylaxis, presenting as bronchospasm, hypotension, syncope, urticaria, and/or angioedema of the throat or tongue, has been reported to occur after administration of omalizumab.

Panitumumab

Patients who received panitumumab are likely to have dermatologic toxicity and these can be severe.

Reslizumab

Anaphylaxis has been observed with reslizumab infusion.

Rituximab

Serious infusion-related reactions, progressive multifocal leukoencephalopathy, severe, including fatal, mucocutaneous reactions, and hepatitis B virus (HBV) reactivation can occur in patients treated with rituximab products.

Trastuzumab

Trastuzumab product administration can result in subclinical and clinical cardiac failure. Trastuzumab product administration can result in serious and fatal infusion reactions and pulmonary toxicity. Exposure to trastuzumab products during pregnancy can result in oligohydramnios and oligohydramnios sequence manifesting as pulmonary hypoplasia, skeletal abnormalities, and neonatal death.

FDA BOXED WARNINGS (Continued)

Albiglutide
Albiglutide is contraindicated in patients with a personal or family history of medullary thyroid carcinoma or in patients with multiple endocrine neoplasia type 2 (MEN2).

Daunorubicin-liposomal
Patients receiving liposomal daunorubicin can experience infusion reactions, hepatic impairment, bone marrow suppression, and myocardial toxicity. Administer liposomal daunorubicin only under the supervision of a physician who is experienced in the use of cancer chemotherapeutic agents.

Doxorubicin-liposomal
Doxorubicin (liposomal) can cause myocardial damage, including acute left ventricular failure. Serious, life-threatening, and fatal infusion-related reactions can occur with doxorubicin (liposomal).

Dulaglutide
Dulaglutide is contraindicated in patients with a personal or family history of medullary thyroid carcinoma and in patients with multiple endocrine neoplasia syndrome type 2 (MEN 2).

Etanercept
Patients treated with etanercept are at an increased risk of developing serious infections, especially if these patients are also taking immunosuppressants. These infections include tuberculosis, invasive fungal infections, and opportunistic bacterial, viral, and other infections.
Patients treated with etanercept have also developed certain malignancies, including lymphoma.

Gene Expression and Protein Synthesis

Proteins are the major macromolecular component of the cell and are responsible for conducting most of a cell's biological activity. Proteins consist of a linear polymer of amino acids linked together in a specific sequence. This specific sequence is responsible for a protein's structure and function. The initial code for the synthesis of a given protein is stored in a gene on a sequence of DNA that is part of a chromosome within the nucleus of a cell.

The central dogma of molecular biology is that DNA encodes RNA, which, in turn, encodes protein. A given amino acid within a protein is encoded by a triplet of nucleic acid base pairs within the gene encoding the protein. This triplet is called a *codon*. There are 64 codons encoding 20 different amino acids as dictated by the genetic code.

An overview of transcription, translation, and post-translational modification is shown in Figure 8-1.

Recombinant DNA Technology

Recombinant DNA technology uses several molecular biological tools to insert a desired DNA fragment with a specific purpose within a DNA molecule. Genes encoding a desired protein of interest can be easily excised through use of enzymes called *restriction endonucleases,* which allows for the cleavage of DNA in a plasmid or genome at very specific locations. The gene is then ligated into a vector, such as a plasmid, for gene cloning or for control of the expression of the encoded protein.

An expression vector is a plasmid designed to allow inducible expression of the inserted gene within a host cell (such as the bacterium *Escherichia coli*). This mechanism permits production of large quantities of the desired protein. The protein must then be isolated and purified for further use. Such techniques, used on an industrial scale, mass produce therapeutically useful biological products such as cytokines, enzymes, hormones, blood factors, and vaccines (Figure 8-2).

Cytokines (i.e., molecules secreted by cells) orchestrate the immune response and activate immune cells such as lymphocytes, monocytes, macrophages, and neutrophils. Therapeutically useful recombinant cytokines include interferons, interleukins, and colony-stimulating factors. Examples of these include interferon

FIGURE 8-1. Gene Expression: The Synthesis of Proteins

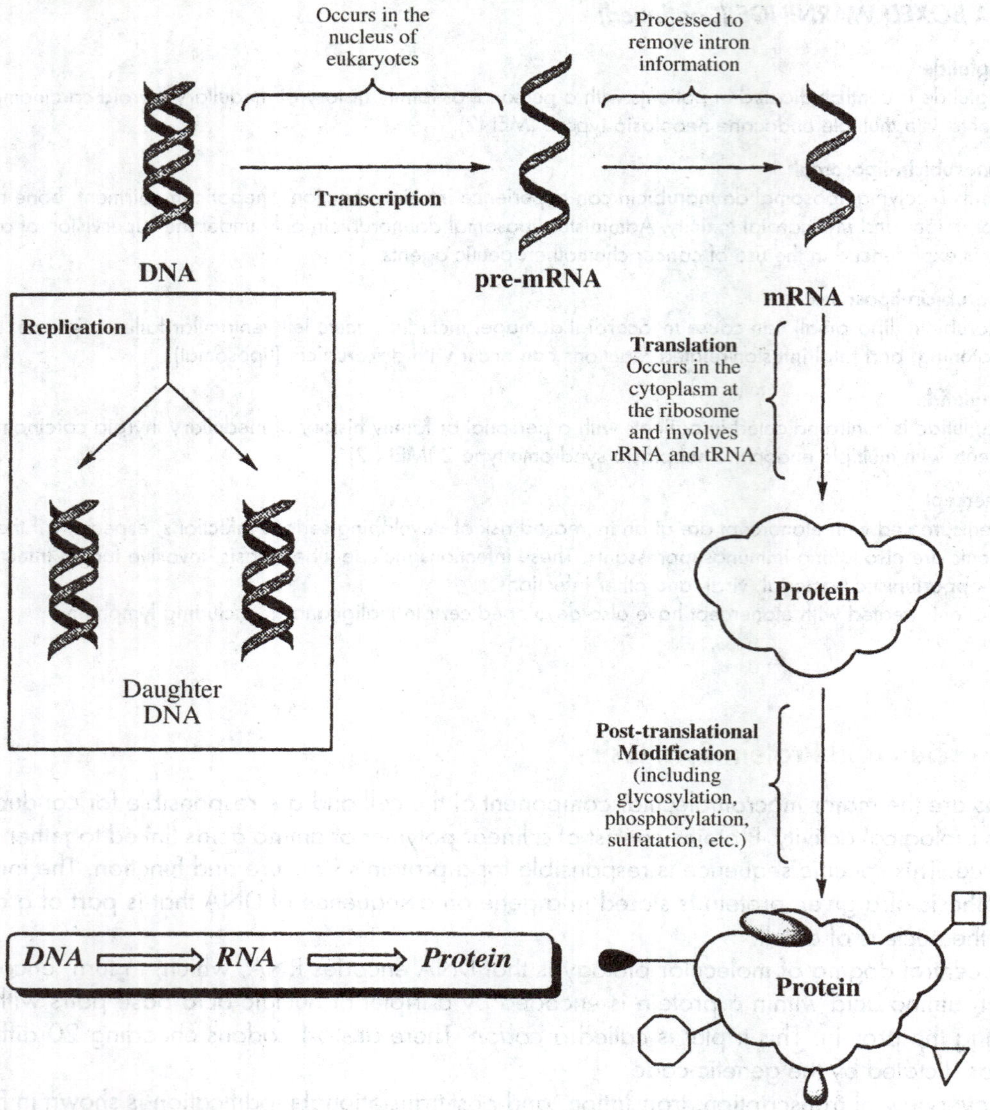

Reproduced from Sindelar, 2002.
mRNA, messenger ribonucleic acid; rRNA, ribosomal ribonucleic acid; tRNA, transfer ribonucleic acid.

beta-1b (Betaseron), which is used to treat acute relapsing–remitting multiple sclerosis, and oprelvekin (Neumega), which treats thrombocytopenia caused by chemotherapy.

An enzyme is a protein that catalyzes a specific chemical reaction. Numerous different enzymes with therapeutic use have been produced using rDNA technology. Alteplase (Activase), for example, treats acute myocardial infarction, pulmonary embolism, and stroke. Dornase alfa (Pulmozyme) treats respiratory complications that develop in cystic fibrosis. Eptifibatide (Integrilin) is used to treat acute coronary syndromes.

Hormones, chemical substances transmitted through the bloodstream, are designed to impart specific cellular effects to cells distant from their physiologic source. Since the introduction and success of recombinant **human insulin** in 1982, many other recombinant hormones have been developed, such as human growth hormone, which treats growth hormone deficiency in pediatric patients, and follitropin alfa (Gonal-F), which is used to remedy ovulatory failure.

FIGURE 8-2. Summary of Typical rDNA Production of a Protein from Either Genomic DNA or cDNA

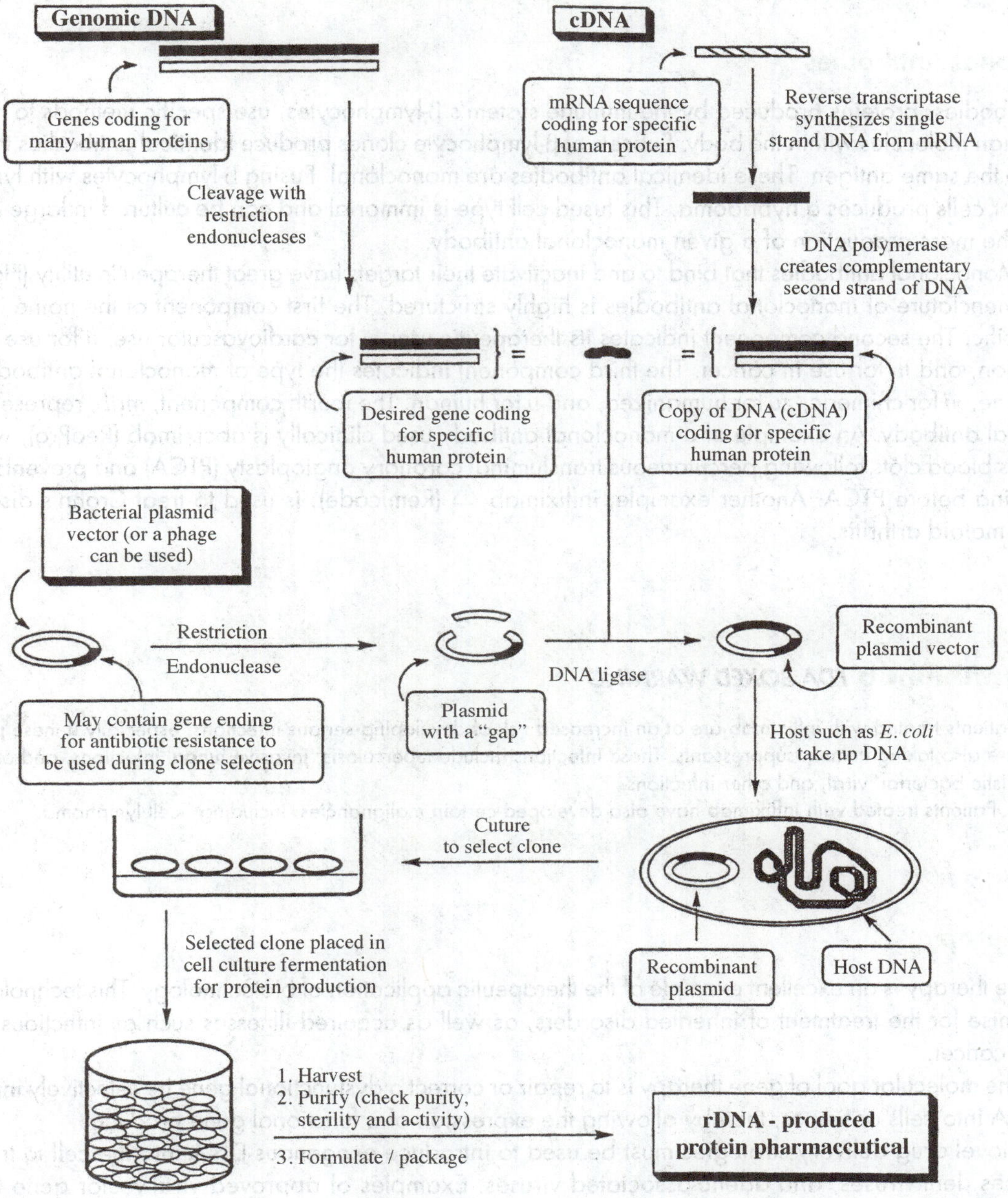

Reprinted with permission from Sindelar, 2002.
cDNA, complementary DNA; mRNA, messenger ribonucleic acid.

Clotting or blood factors are chemical blood constituents that interact to cause blood coagulation. Patients suffering from hemophilia A (caused by factor VIII deficiency) or hemophilia B (caused by factor IX deficiency) have benefited greatly from rDNA technology. Factors VII, VIII, and IX are available in recombinant forms for clinical use.

Vaccines, preparations of antigenic material administered to stimulate the development of antibodies, confer active immunity against a particular pathogen or disease. Vaccine development has also benefited from advances in rDNA technology. Traditional vaccine production used killed or nonvirulent organisms, microbial toxins, or actual microbial components to elicit long-term immune protection. Safer and more specific vaccine antigens have been devised as recombinant proteins. This technology has led to the very successful recombinant hepatitis B vaccine.

Monoclonal Antibodies

Antibodies, proteins produced by the immune system's β-lymphocytes, use specific methods to recognize foreign molecules within the body. Subsets of β-lymphocyte clones produce identical antibodies that recognize the same antigen. These identical antibodies are monoclonal. Fusing β-lymphocytes with lymphocyte tumor cells produces a hybridoma. This fused cell type is immortal and can be cultured in large quantities for the mass production of a given monoclonal antibody.

Monoclonal antibodies that bind to and inactivate their targets have great therapeutic utility (Figure 8-3). Nomenclature of monoclonal antibodies is highly structured. The first component of the name is product specific. The second component indicates its therapeutic use: *ci* for cardiovascular use, *li* for use in inflammation, and *tu* for use in cancer. The third component indicates the type of monoclonal antibody: *mo* for murine, *xi* for chimeric, *zu* for humanized, and *u* for human. The fourth component, *mab*, represents monoclonal antibody. An example of a monoclonal antibody used clinically is abciximab (ReoPro), which prevents blood clots following percutaneous transluminal coronary angioplasty (PTCA) and prevents unstable angina before PTCA. Another example, infliximab (Remicade), is used to treat Crohn's disease and rheumatoid arthritis.

> ⚠️ **Infliximab** *FDA BOXED WARNING*
>
> Patients treated with infliximab are at an increased risk of developing serious infections, especially if these patients are also taking immunosuppressants. These infections include tuberculosis, invasive fungal infections, and opportunistic bacterial, viral, and other infections.
>
> Patients treated with infliximab have also developed certain malignancies, including T-cell lymphoma.

Gene Therapy

Gene therapy is an excellent example of the therapeutic application of biotechnology. This technology holds promise for the treatment of inherited disorders, as well as acquired illnesses such as infectious diseases and cancer.

The molecular goal of gene therapy is to repair or correct a dysfunctional gene by selectively introducing rDNA into cells or tissues, thereby allowing the expression of a functional gene product.

Novel drug delivery strategies must be used to introduce exogenous DNA into the cell to treat retroviruses, lentiviruses, and adeno-associated viruses. Examples of approved viral-vector gene therapies are voretigene neparvovec (Luxturna) for Leber's congenital amaurosis, an inherited form of vision loss, and onasemnogene abeparvovec (Zolgensma) for pediatric patients less than 2 years of age with spinal muscular atrophy. These strategies also have applications for nonviral delivery systems (e.g., liposomes or uncomplexed plasmid DNA).

Alternative approaches using ribozymes (e.g., RNA repair) may also prove effective. The enzymatic activity of these RNA molecules can be used to repair defective messenger RNA (mRNA).

Chimeric RNA and DNA oligonucleotides make use of the cell's DNA mismatch repair apparatus to correct mutations at the genomic level. Antisense oligonucleotides for gene inactivation have proved clinically useful. Fomivirsen (Vitravene) targets the mRNA of human cytomegalovirus (CMV) and is indicated for the treatment of human CMV retinitis in patients with AIDS. Golodirsen (Vyondys 53) is an antisense oligonucleotide indicated for the treatment of Duchenne muscular dystrophy in patients who have a confirmed mutation of the *DMD* gene that is amenable to exon 53 skipping.

FIGURE 8-3. Production of Monoclonal Antibodies

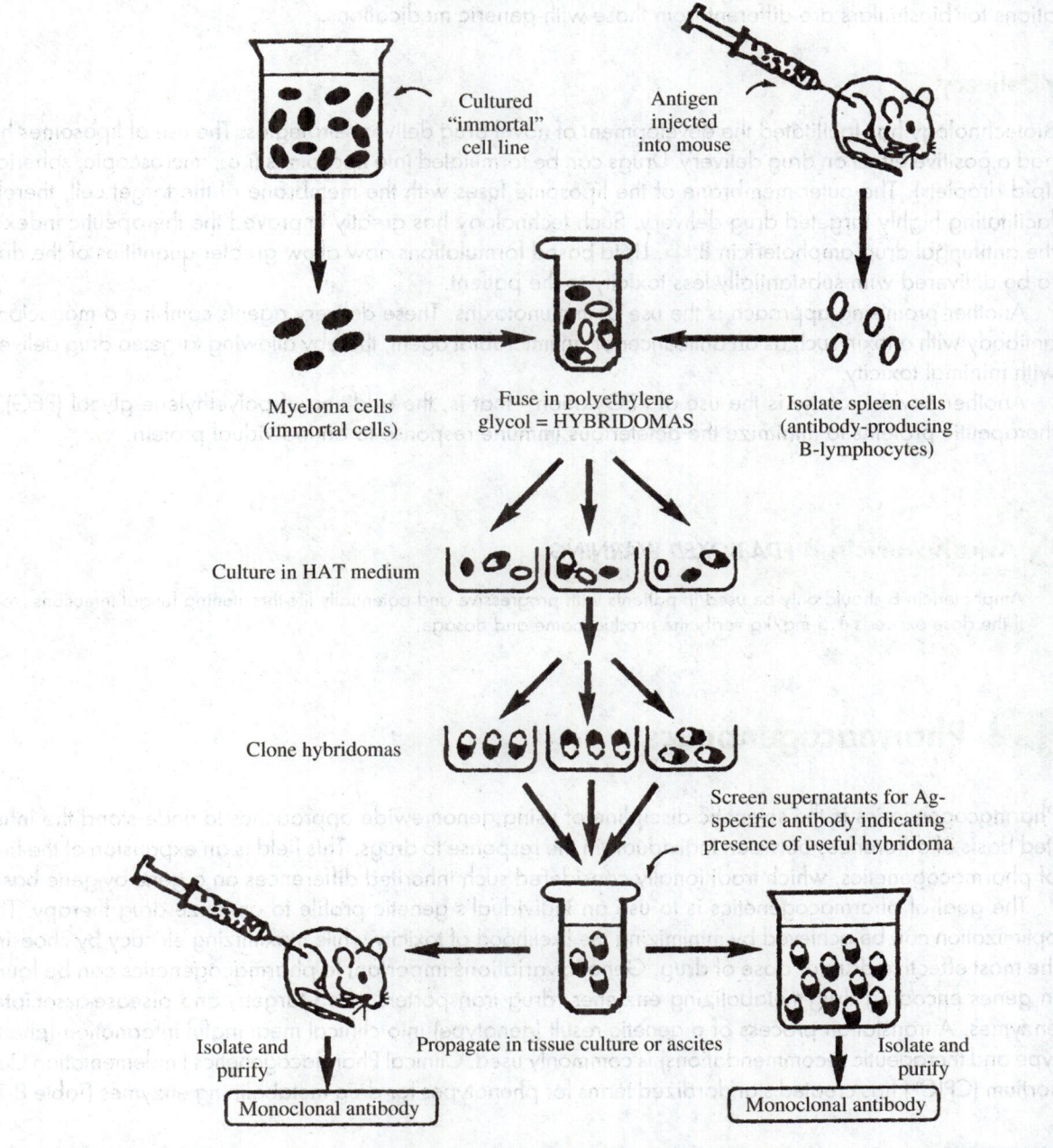

Cultured "immortal" cell line

Antigen injected into mouse

Myeloma cells (immortal cells)

Fuse in polyethylene glycol = HYBRIDOMAS

Isolate spleen cells (antibody-producing B-lymphocytes)

Culture in HAT medium

Clone hybridomas

Screen supernatants for Ag-specific antibody indicating presence of useful hybridoma

Isolate and purify

Propagate in tissue culture or ascites

Isolate and purify

Monoclonal antibody

Monoclonal antibody

Reproduced from Sindelar, 2002.

HAT, hypoxanthine-aminopterin-thymidine.

Biosimilar

The FDA defines a biosimilar as a biological product that is highly similar to a licensed reference biological product notwithstanding minor differences in clinically inactive components and that there are no clinically meaningful differences between the biological product and the reference product in terms of safety, purity, and potency. Biosimilars are not the same as generic medicines because of the complexities of the molecules derived from a living cell or organism. Therefore, the approval process and interchangeability considerations for biosimilars are different from those with generic medications.

Drug Delivery

Biotechnology has facilitated the development of novel drug delivery strategies. The use of liposomes has had a positive effect on drug delivery. Drugs can be formulated into liposomes (i.e., microscopic, spherical lipid droplets). The outer membrane of the liposome fuses with the membrane of the target cell, thereby facilitating highly targeted drug delivery. Such technology has greatly improved the therapeutic index of the antifungal drug amphotericin B . Lipid-based formulations now allow greater quantities of the drug to be delivered with substantially less toxicity to the patient.

Another promising approach is the use of immunotoxins. These delivery agents combine a monoclonal antibody with a toxin such as an anticancer or antimicrobial agent, thereby allowing targeted drug delivery with minimal toxicity.

Another novel strategy is the use of PEGylation—that is, the addition of polyethylene glycol (PEG) to therapeutic proteins to minimize the deleterious immune response to an individual protein.

> ⚠ **Amphotericin B** *FDA BOXED WARNING*
>
> Amphotericin B should only be used in patients with progressive and potentially life-threatening fungal infections. If the dose exceeds 1.5 mg/kg verify the product name and dosage.

8-5   Pharmacogenomics

Pharmacogenomics is the scientific discipline of using genomewide approaches to understand the inherited basis of differences between individuals in the response to drugs. This field is an expansion of the field of pharmacogenetics, which traditionally considered such inherited differences on a gene-by-gene basis.

The goal of pharmacogenetics is to use an individual's genetic profile to optimize drug therapy. This optimization can be achieved by minimizing the likelihood of toxicity while maximizing efficacy by choosing the most effective drug or dose of drug. Genetic variations important to pharmacogenetics can be found in genes encoding drug-metabolizing enzymes, drug transporters, drug targets, and disease-associated enzymes. A translation process of a genetic result (genotype) into clinical meaningful information (phenotype and therapeutic recommendations) is commonly used. Clinical Pharmacogenetics Implementation Consortium (CPIC®) has created standardized terms for phenotypes for drug metabolizing enzymes (Table 8-2).

Polymorphisms in Genes Involving Drug Metabolism

Genetic variants in genes encoding drug-metabolizing enzymes play a major role in determining drug concentrations that can influence drug efficacy and toxicity. Enzyme pharmacogenetics has been studied in great detail for many phase I enzymes, including cytochrome P450 isoenzymes, esterases, and dehydrogenases, as well as conjugating phase II enzymes. A few examples are discussed in this section and several polymorphic genes are included in Table 8-3.

TABLE 8-2. Effect of Phenotype on Metabolism of Medications

Metabolizer	Activity	Effect
Ultrarapid (UM) and rapid metabolizer (RM)	Higher-than-normal enzymatic activity	• Increased metabolism of active drugs that are inactivated by enzyme • Generation of active drug metabolites to a greater extent
Normal metabolizer (NM)	Full function enzymatic activity	• Expected metabolism of drugs inactivated by enzyme • Expected generation of active drug metabolites
Intermediate metabolizer (IM)	Decreased enzymatic activity (between normal and poor)	• Decreased metabolism of active drugs that are inactivated by enzyme compared to normal metabolizers • Generation of active drug metabolites to a lesser extent than normal metabolizers
Poor metabolizer (PM)	Little to no enzymatic activity	• Greatly decreased metabolism of active drugs that are inactivated by enzyme compared to normal metabolizers • Generation of active drug metabolites to much less extent than normal metabolizers

TABLE 8-3. Examples of Polymorphic Drug-Metabolizing Enzymes Affecting Drug Response[a]

Gene	Medication	Therapeutic implication
CYP2C19	**Clopidogrel**	Reduced platelet inhibition and increased risk for adverse cardiovascular events in IMs and PMs
	Voriconazole	Decreased likelihood of achieving therapeutic concentrations in UMs with standard dosing
	SSRIs (**citalopram, escitalopram**)	Possible decreased efficacy in UMs and increased adverse effects in PMs
	Tricyclic antidepressants	Possible decreased efficacy in UMs and increased adverse effects in PMs
	Proton pump inhibitors (**Omeprazole**, lansoprazole, dexlansoprazole)	Increased doses in UM and RMs for *Helicobacter pylori* treatment (with other medications) and decreased initial doses for chronic treatment in PMs
CYP2C9	Phenytoin	Increased risk for adverse effects in IMs and PMs
	Warfarin	Decreased metabolism in IMs and PMs; lower initial dosing may be warranted in those with concomitant variations in VKORC1 and CYP4F2
	Siponimod	Test patients for CYP2C9 variants to determine dosage Contraindicated in *3/*3 genotype
	NSAIDs	Increased risk for adverse effects in PMs
CYP2D6	Opioid analgesics (codeine, **tramadol**)	Possible lack of efficacy because of decreased formation of more active metabolites in PMs; possible risk of adverse effects in UMs
	Ondansetron, tropisetron	Decreased likelihood of achieving therapeutic concentrations in UMs with standard dosing
	SSRIs (**paroxetine**, fluvoxamine ⚠)	Possible decreased efficacy in UMs and increased adverse effects in PMs

(continued)

TABLE 8-3. Examples of Polymorphic Drug-Metabolizing Enzymes Affecting Drug Response[a] *(Continued)*

Gene	Medication	Therapeutic implication
	Tricyclic antidepressants	Possible decreased efficacy in UMs and increased adverse effects in PMs
	Eliglustat	Approved for adult patients with Gaucher disease type 1 who are CYP2D6 NMs, IMs, or PMs as detected by an FDA-cleared test
	Tetrabenazine ⚠	Doses above 50 mg/day should be genotyped for CYP2D6
		CYP2D6 poor metabolizer genotypes should be treated with lower doses
	Pimozide	CYP2D6 genotyping should be performed at doses above 0.05 mg/kg/day in children or above 4 mg/day in adults; should not exceed those doses, and doses should not be increased earlier than 14 days
	Antipsychotics (aripiprazole ⚠, risperidone ⚠, brexpiprazole ⚠)	Increased risk of adverse effects in PMs with standard dosing
	Atomoxetine ⚠	Increased risk of adverse effects in PMs with standard dosing
DPYD	Capecitabine ⚠, fluorouracil, tegafur	Reduced or absent DPYD activity can result in severe toxicity (neutropenia, nausea, vomiting, severe diarrhea, stomatitis, mucositis, hand–foot syndrome)
TPMT	Thiopurines (azathioprine, mercaptopurine, thioguanine)	Increased concentrations of active metabolites and risk of myelosuppression in IMs and PMs; risk of life-threatening myelosuppression in PMs with standard dosing
UGT1A1	Atazanavir	High likelihood of bilirubin-related discontinuation in PMs
	Irinotecan	Increased risk of neutropenia in PMs
	Belinostat	Reduce starting dose to 750 mg/m^2 in PMs

PharmGKB (https://www.pharmgkb.org); Clinical Pharmacogenetics Implementation Consortium (https://cpicpgx.org. Table of Pharmacogenetic Associations (https://www.fda.gov/medical-devices/precision-medicine/table-pharmacogenetic-associations).
Boldface indicates one of top 100 drugs for 2020 by prescription volume.
IM, intermediate metabolizer; NM, normal metabolizer; NSAID, nonsteroidal anti-inflammatory drug; PM, poor metabolizer; SSRI, selective serotonin reuptake inhibitor; UM, ultrarapid metabolizer.
a. This table is not a comprehensive list of approved products.

 FDA BOXED WARNINGS

Fluvoxamine
Patients aged 24 years and younger who take **paroxetine** or fluvoxamine are at increased risk of suicidal thoughts and behaviors.

Tetrabenazine
Tetrabenazine can increase the risk of depression and suicidal thoughts and behavior (suicidality) in patients with Huntington disease.

Aripiprazole
Elderly patients with dementia-related psychosis treated with aripiprazole are at an increased risk of death. Patients aged 24 years and younger who take aripiprazole are at increased risk of suicidal thoughts and behaviors.

Risperidone
Elderly patients with dementia-related psychosis treated with risperidone are at an increased risk of death.

Brexpiprazole
Elderly patients with dementia-related psychosis treated with brexpiprazole are at an increased risk of death. Patients aged 24 years and younger who take brexpiprazole are at increased risk of suicidal thoughts and behaviors.

FDA BOXED WARNINGS (Continued)

Atomoxetine
Atomoxetine increased the risk of suicidal ideation in short-term studies in children or adolescents with attention deficit hyperactivity disorder (ADHD).

Capecitabine
Patients receiving concomitant capecitabine and oral coumarin-derivative anticoagulant therapy should have their anticoagulant response (INR or PT) monitored frequently in order to adjust the anticoagulant dose accordingly.

Polymorphic Phase I Enzymes

CYP2D6 has the largest number of variations of all the CYP enzymes with more than 100 known alleles, and as much as 25% of all medications are metabolized by CYP2D6. Poor metabolizers possess two or more nonfunctional alleles, while ultrarapid metabolizers possess multiple copies of functional alleles. CYP2D6 poor metabolizers are at an increased risk of toxicity during therapy with many antidepressant and antipsychotic drugs because of the decreased metabolism of active metabolites. Conversely, CYP2D6 poor metabolizers are at risk of analgesic response to codeine ⚠ and **tramadol** ⚠ therapy.

 Codeine *FDA BOXED WARNING*

Codeine has a REMS program to ensure that the benefits of opioid analgesics outweigh the risks of addiction, abuse, and misuse. Prolonged use of codeine during pregnancy can result in neonatal opioid withdrawal syndrome. Serious, life-threatening, or fatal respiratory depression may occur with use of codeine. Concomitant use of opioids with benzodiazepines or other CNS depressants, including alcohol, may result in profound sedation, respiratory depression, coma, and death. Use of cytochrome P450 3A4 inducers, 3A4 inhibitors, or 2D6 inhibitors with codeine requires careful consideration of the effects on the parent drug, codeine, and the active metabolite morphine. CYP2D6 ultra-rapid metabolism and other risk factors for life-threatening respiratory depression may occur in children who receive codeine.

 Tramadol *FDA BOXED WARNING*

Tramadol has a REMS program to ensure that the benefits of opioid analgesics outweigh the risks of addiction, abuse, and misuse. Prolonged use of **tramadol** during pregnancy can result in neonatal opioid withdrawal syndrome. Serious, life-threatening, or fatal respiratory depression may occur with use of **tramadol**. Concomitant use of opioids with benzodiazepines or other CNS depressants, including alcohol, may result in profound sedation, respiratory depression, coma, and death. Use of cytochrome P450 3A4 inducers, 3A4 inhibitors, or 2D6 inhibitors with **tramadol** requires careful consideration of the effects on the parent drug, **tramadol**, and the active metabolites. CYP2D6 ultra-rapid metabolism and other risk factors for life-threatening respiratory depression may occur in children who receive **tramadol**.

CYP2C19 is responsible for inactivating proton pump inhibitors such as **omeprazole**. Polymorphisms resulting in poor metabolism of proton pump inhibitors by CYP2C19 can cause increased drug concentrations and, consequently, increased gastric pH, thus leading to not only increased symptom control but also an increased risk of side effects with chronic therapy. CYP2C19 is responsible for the bioactivation of clopidogrel ⚠ to the active thiol metabolite in a two-step process. Poor metabolizers of CYP2C19 can have reduced platelet inhibition and can be at an increased risk for adverse cardiovascular events. CYP2C19 ultrarapid metabolizers may have decreased efficacy with the selective serotonin reuptake inhibitors (SSRIs) **citalopram** and **escitalopram** , tertiary amine tricyclic antidepressants, and voriconazole because of increased metabolism of active metabolites.

CYP2C9 is responsible for the metabolism of the S-enantiomer of **warfarin** . As much as 10% of the population may have a homozygous variant phenotype resulting in low CYP2C9 activity. Low activity results in decreased **warfarin** clearance and subsequent increased risk of bleeding. Phenytoin and nonsteroidal anti-inflammatory drugs are also major substrates of *CYP2C9*; variations resulting in decreased metabolism can result in patients at risk for adverse effects with these drugs.

Clopidogrel *FDA BOXED WARNING*

Diminished antiplatelet effect may occur in patients with 2 loss-of-function alleles of the CYP2C19 gene.

Citalopram *FDA BOXED WARNING*

Patients aged 24 years and younger who take **citalopram** are at increased risk of suicidal thoughts and behaviors.

Escitalopram *FDA BOXED WARNING*

Patients aged 24 years and younger who take **escitalopram** are at increased risk of suicidal thoughts and behaviors.

Warfarin *FDA BOXED WARNING*

Warfarin can cause major or fatal bleeding.

Phenytoin *FDA BOXED WARNING*

Rapid infusions of phenytoin are associated with the risk of severe hypotension and cardiac arrhythmias.

Polymorphic Phase II Enzymes

N-acetyl transferase (NAT) is responsible for the acetylation of arylamine carcinogens and heterocyclic amines. Individuals with slow acetylation activity may experience toxicity, such as hydralazine- and procainamide-induced lupus-like syndrome and sulfonamide hypersensitivity.

Procainamide *FDA BOXED WARNING*

The prolonged administration of procainamide often leads to the development of a positive antinuclear antibody (ANA) test. Agranulocytosis, bone marrow depression, neutropenia, hypoplastic anemia, and thrombocytopenia in patients receiving procainamide. Due to the proarrhythmic properties of procainamide, it should be reserved for patients with life-threatening ventricular arrhythmias.

UDP-glucuronosyltransferase 1 family, peptide A1 (UGT1A1) isoenzyme is a member of the UGT1A1 superfamily of phase II drug-metabolizing enzymes. It is responsible for the catalysis of the glucuronidation reaction of xenobiotics. In colon cancer, irinotecan ⚠ is a common treatment option for metastatic disease as well as other types of solid tumors. Patients who have a protein-deactivating polymorphism in *UGT1A1* can experience severe toxicities, including myelosuppression and diarrhea.

Thiopurine methyltransferase, a protein encoded by the *TPMT* gene, is responsible for the inactivation of thiopurines (i.e., mercaptopurine, thioguanine, azathioprine ⚠). Polymorphisms in *TPMT* causing a loss of protein function can result in the accumulation of high levels of the cytotoxic thioguanine nucleotide (TGN) metabolites with standard dosing of thiopurines. Patients with loss of function *TPMT* polymorphism are at considerable risk for severe adverse effects, such as life-threatening myelosuppression, unless doses are drastically reduced.

 Irinotecan *FDA BOXED WARNING*

Patients receiving irinotecan may experience diarrhea and bone marrow suppression.

 Azathioprine *FDA BOXED WARNING*

Patients treated with azathioprine have also developed certain malignancies, including lymphoma.

Polymorphisms in Genes Encoding Drug Transporters

Genetic variations in drug transporters can affect the distribution of drugs, which can alter the concentration at the site of action. A few selected examples are discussed in this section. P-glycoprotein is a well-characterized member of the ATP (adenosine triphosphate)-binding cassette (ABC) transporter family. It is encoded by the *ABCB1* gene (also known as the *MDR1* gene), which is known to be highly polymorphic. Numerous studies have demonstrated associations between genetic variations in *ABCB1* and the efficacy or toxicity of medications, including digoxin, **simvastatin**, **ondansetron**, and methotrexate ⚠.

The solute carrier organic anion transporter family member 1B1 (*SLCO1B1*) gene encodes a membrane-bound organic anion transporter protein (OATP1B1) involved in active transport of endogenous and exogenous substances. It is responsible for the uptake of 3-hydroxy-3-methylglutaryl coenzyme A (HMG-CoA) reductase inhibitors (statins) into the liver. Variations in the *SLCO1B1* gene, resulting in decreased activity of the OATP1B1 transporter, have been associated with increased systemic exposure of **simvastatin** and increased risk of myopathy.

Methotrexate *FDA BOXED WARNING*

Serious adverse reactions, including death, have been reported with methotrexate. Other adverse reactions include bone marrow suppression, serious infections, renal toxicity and increased toxicity with renal impairment, GI toxicity, hepatic toxicity, pulmonary toxicity, hypersensitivity, and dermatologic reactions. Methotrexate can cause embryo-fetal toxicity, including fetal death and/or congenital anomalies. Methotrexate given concomitantly with radiotherapy may increase the risk of soft tissue necrosis and osteonecrosis. For intrathecal and high-dose therapy, use preservative-free formulation of methotrexate formulations and diluents for intrathecal and high-dose therapy. Methotrexate injection should be used only by health care providers whose knowledge and experience include the use of antimetabolite therapy.

Polymorphisms in Genes Encoding Drug Targets

Genetic variations in drug targets can alter response and affect efficacy.

The μ-opioid receptor gene (*OPRM1*) encodes the μ-opioid receptor, which is the primary binding site for endogenous opioid peptides and opioid analgesics. Numerous studies have examined the relationship of variations of *OPRM1* to opioid dose requirements and pain scores. Several studies reported higher consumption of intravenous opioids (morphine ⚠, fentanyl ⚠) postoperatively in patients with one or two copies of the variant allele, but other studies have reported no difference.

The *VKORC1* gene encodes vitamin K epoxide reductase complex subunit 1, the **warfarin** target enzyme, which is important for the carboxylation of vitamin K–dependent clotting factors. Polymorphisms in *VKORC1* have been found to account for about 30% of the variation in the required dose. Initial dosing recommendations based on *VKORC1* variations, in addition to *CYP2C9, CYP4F2*, and rs12777823, which is involved in the metabolism of **warfarin**, can be found in the FDA drug labeling. A more comprehensive dosing algorithm is also available at http://www.warfarindosing.org.

 Morphine *FDA BOXED WARNING*

Serious, life-threatening, or fatal respiratory depression has occurred with use of morphine especially with concomitant use of benzodiazepines or other CNS depressants. Prolonged use of morphine during pregnancy can result in neonatal opioid withdrawal syndrome. Ensure accuracy when prescribing, dispensing, and administering morphine oral solution. To ensure that the benefits of opioid analgesics outweigh the risks of addiction, abuse, and misuse, the FDA has required a REMS for morphine. Because of the risk of severe adverse effects when the epidural or intrathecal route of administration is employed, patients must be observed in a fully equipped and staffed environment for at least 24 hours after the initial dose.

 Fentanyl *FDA BOXED WARNING*

Serious, life-threatening, or fatal respiratory depression has occurred with use of fentanyl especially with concomitant use of CYP3A4 inhibitors, benzodiazepines, or other CNS depressants. Prolonged use of fentanyl during pregnancy can result in neonatal opioid withdrawal syndrome. Exposure of the fentanyl application site and surrounding area to direct external heat sources may increase fentanyl absorption and has resulted in fatal overdose of fentanyl. To ensure that the benefits of opioid analgesics outweigh the risks of addiction, abuse, and misuse, the FDA has required a REMS for fentanyl. Transdermal iontophoretic system (Ionsys) is for use only in patients in the hospital. Substantial differences exist in the pharmacokinetic profile of fentanyl buccal, intranasal, lozenge, and sublingual compared with other fentanyl products that result in clinically important differences in the extent of absorption of fentanyl that could result in fatal overdose.

Genes with Disease-Associated Polymorphisms

Genes that affect the disease itself or the risk of adverse effects when drugs are given are considered disease-associated genes. Polymorphisms occurring in disease-associated genes can influence the drug-associated efficacy and toxicity.

Variations in the coagulation factors prothrombin and factor V Leiden are associated with a higher risk of developing a deep vein thrombosis (DVT) and pulmonary embolism (PE). The use of estrogen-containing oral contraceptives is also associated with an increased risk of these thromboembolic disorders, and when they are used by individuals with these variations, the risk increases further. Long QT syndrome can be an inherited condition, which increases a patient's risk of arrhythmias and sudden death. Some variants in *KCNH2*, *KCNQ1*, and *SCN5A* are known to cause this condition. When drugs known to lengthen the QT interval are given to patients with variants in these genes the risk of arrhythmias and death is increased. In some cases, variants in genes may determine if a medication is likely to have a therapeutic effect on a patient. For example, poly (ADP-ribose) polymerase (PARP) inhibitors like olaparib (Lynparza) are indicated for the treatment of specific cancers in patients with certain *BRCA* variants. These same variants in *BRCA* also increase a patient's risk of developing certain types of cancers.

Genes with Hypersensitivity Reaction-Associated Polymorphisms

Genetic variants in genes encoding human leukocyte antigen mediate a patient's risk of developing hypersensitivity reaction like Stevens-Johnson Syndrome (SJS) while receiving specific drugs. Abacavir ⚠ is an antiviral used in the treatment of HIV/AIDS (human immunodeficiency virus/acquired immune deficiency syndrome) that can lead to life-threatening toxicities that have been associated with genetic variations. Studies suggest that patients who are treated with abacavir and have a specific human leukocyte antigen allele (*HLA-B*5701*) are at risk for developing abacavir hypersensitivity syndrome. The *HLA-B*5701* genetic test has been shown to reduce the incidence of this adverse outcome and provide more optimal treatment for patients affected by HIV/AIDS. Other examples of well-known drug/gene pairs are **allopurinol**/*HLA-B*58:01* and severe cutaneous adverse reactions and carbamazepine ⚠/*HLA-B*15:02* and *HLA-A*31:03* and Stevens-Johnson syndrome (SJS).

 Abacavir *FDA BOXED WARNING*

Patients who carry the HLA-B*5701 allele are at a higher risk of a hypersensitivity reaction to abacavir.

 Carbamazepine *FDA BOXED WARNING*

Patients who carry the HLA-B*5801 allele are at a higher risk of a hypersensitivity reaction to carbamazepine. Aplastic anemia and agranulocytosis have been reported in association with the use of carbamazepine.

Using Pharmacogenomics in Clinical Care

There are more than 140 medications with pharmacogenetic information in the FDA drug labeling. Although a large number of these are genetic biomarkers for targeted therapy in oncology, there are many other drugs with pharmacogenetic information associated with metabolism and hypersensitivity. This information can be found in various sections, including boxed warnings for several drugs. Abacavir and carbamazepine have boxed warnings recommending testing to help prevent hypersensitivity reactions. The boxed warning for codeine reports that respiratory depression and death have occurred in children who received

TABLE 8-4. Boxed Warnings per FDA Labeling Related to Pharmacogenomics Interactions

Gene or gene product	Medication	Drug effect associated with polymorphism
HLA-B*5701	Abacavir	Patients positive for HLA-B*5701 have a higher adverse reaction risk (hypersensitivity reactions). Do not use abacavir in patients positive for HLA-B*5701.
HLA-B*1502	Carbamazepine	Patients positive for HLA-B*1502 may be at increased risk of severe skin reactions with other drugs that are associated with a risk of Stevens Johnson syndrome/toxic epidermal necrolysis (SJS/TEN) Screening of patients with ancestry in genetically at-risk populations (patients of Asian descent) for the presence of the HLA-B*1502 allele should be carried out before treatment because of a high risk of serious and sometimes fatal dermatologic reactions.
CYP2C19	**Clopidogrel**	Results in lower systemic active metabolite concentrations in IMs and PMs, lower antiplatelet response, and may result in higher cardiovascular risk. Consider use of another platelet P2Y$_{12}$ inhibitor.
CYP2D6	Codeine and **tramadol**	Life-threatening respiratory depression and death have occurred in children who received codeine or tramadol; most cases with codeine followed tonsillectomy and/or adenoidectomy and many of the children had evidence of being an UM of codeine because of a CYP2D6 polymorphism. Codeine and tramadol are contraindicated in children younger than 12 years of age and in children younger than 18 years of age following tonsillectomy and/or adenoidectomy.

Table of Pharmacogenetic Associations (https://www.fda.gov/medical-devices/precision-medicine/table-pharmacogenetic-associations).
Boldface indicates one of top 100 drugs for 2020 by prescription volume.
IM, intermediate metabolizer; PM, poor metabolizer; UM, ultrarapid metabolizer.

codeine following tonsillectomy or adenoidectomy and had evidence of being ultrarapid metabolizers of codeine. Labeling for the antiplatelet drug clopidogrel warns that patients who are poor metabolizers of CYP2C19 may experience diminished effectiveness of clopidogrel compared with patients with normal function and that a different drug for these patients should be considered. Drugs with boxed warning related to pharmacogenomics are in Table 8-4. Several drugs have labeling that requires testing before administration. Additional drugs with pharmacogenetic information in FDA labeling can be found in the FDA table of pharmacogenomics biomarkers in drug labeling (https://www.fda.gov/medical-devices/precision-medicine/table-pharmacogenetic-associations).

Guidelines are now available to help clinicians translate pharmacogenetic results into actionable therapeutic recommendations. The Clinical Pharmacogenetics Implementation Consortium is an international group of more than 200 experts in the field of pharmacogenetics and laboratory medicine who help create peer-reviewed, evidence-based, detailed gene–drug clinical practice guidelines on how to use pharmacogenetic information to optimize prescribing. These guidelines use the genotype to phenotype to therapeutic recommendation model and can be found at https://cpicpgx.org. Additionally, the Pharmacogenetics Knowledge Base (PharmGKB) is a Web-based, comprehensive resource of curated knowledge about genetic variation affecting drug response (https://www.pharmgkb.org).

NAPLEX Competency Statements

The questions in this chapter cover the following 2021 NAPLEX Competency Statements: **AREA 1:** 1.1 **AREA 2:** 2.1; 2.2 **AREA 3:** 3.2; 3.3; 3.4; 3.5; 3.6; 3.7; 3.8; 3.10; 3.11 **AREA 5:** 5.1.

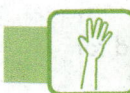 **8-6**   ## Questions

1. The process whereby the ribosome in the cytoplasm reads mRNA codons and matches them with the appropriate tRNA (which, in turn, carries amino acids responsible for protein synthesis) is referred to as _____.

   A. transcription
   B. translation
   C. transformation
   D. transfection
   E. transduction

2. Which of the following is an example of an rDNA-generated cytokine used for the management of acute relapsing–remitting multiple sclerosis?

   A. Interferon beta-1b (Betaseron)
   B. Aldesleukin (IL-2) (Proleukin)
   C. Eptifibatide (Integrilin)
   D. Bivalirudin (Angiomax)
   E. Abciximab (ReoPro)

3. Alteplase (Activase) is an rDNA protein of which of the following types?

   A. Hormone
   B. Enzyme
   C. Clotting factor
   D. Chemokine
   E. Cytokine

4. Which of the following biological agents is indicated for treatment of ovulatory failure?

   A. Ganirelix (Antagon)
   B. Glucagon (GlucaGen)
   C. Follitropin alfa (Gonal-F)
   D. Eptifibatide (Integrilin)
   E. Thyrotropin (Thyrogen)

5. Recombinant DNA technology has led to the development of vaccines for which of the following diseases _____.

   A. Hepatitis B
   B. Hepatitis A
   C. *Haemophilus influenzae* type B infection
   D. Malaria
   E. AIDS

6. As dictated by the nomenclature for monoclonal antibodies, which of the following is a chimeric monoclonal antibody therapeutically used for inflammatory disease?

   A. Abciximab
   B. Infliximab
   C. Palivizumab
   D. Rituximab
   E. Trastuzumab

7. Which of the following is best described as the repair or correction of a dysfunctional gene by selectively introducing rDNA into cells or tissues (ultimately leading to the expression of a functional gene product)?

   A. Monoclonal antibody therapy
   B. Gene therapy
   C. Antiviral therapy
   D. Cell therapy
   E. rDNA therapy

8. Fomivirsen (Vitravene) is an example of which of the following biological products?

   A. A liposomal formulation
   B. An antisense oligonucleotide
   C. An siRNA molecule
   D. An rDNA-produced protein
   E. A monoclonal antibody

9. The use of liposomal technology has favorably affected the therapeutic index of which of the following drugs?

   A. Cyclosporine
   B. Itraconazole
   C. Amphotericin B
   D. Cisplatin
   E. Propofol

10. Which of the following is best described as the scientific discipline of using genomewide approaches to understand the inherited basis of differences between individuals in their response to drugs?

    A. Pharmacogenomics
    B. Functional genomics
    C. Comparative genomics
    D. Pharmacodynamics
    E. Molecular genetics

11. An SNP always results in a change in which of the following?

A. The nucleotide sequence in the genome
B. The nucleotide sequence of a codon
C. The encoded amino acid of the codon
D. The encoded amino acid of the codon, with no change in function of the encoded protein
E. The encoded amino acid of the codon, with a clinically relevant change in the function of the encoded protein

12. Which of the following is best described as "the manipulation (as through genetic engineering) of living organisms or their components to produce useful usually commercial products (as pest-resistant crops, new bacterial strains, or novel pharmaceuticals)"?

A. Biology
B. Biotechnology
C. Biotherapy
D. Bioinformatics
E. Nanotechnology

13. Which of the following best outlines the central dogma of molecular biology?

A. mRNA→DNA→Protein
B. DNA→mRNA→Protein
C. Protein→RNA→DNA
D. DNA→Protein→mRNA
E. Protein→DNA→mRNA

14. Which of the following biotechnology agents is indicated for treating anemia caused by chronic renal disease?

A. Epoetin alfa
B. Bivalirudin
C. Filgrastim
D. Alemtuzumab
E. Sargramostim

15. Which of the following products is indicated for prevention of blood clots post-PTCA?

A. Abciximab
B. Basiliximab
C. Infliximab
D. Trastuzumab
E. Rasburicase

16. Which of the following products is indicated for respiratory complications in cystic fibrosis?

A. Dornase alfa
B. Pegloticase
C. Pancrelipase
D. Alteplase
E. Dulaglutide

17. Which of the following products is an example of a hormone?

A. Sargramostim
B. Tirofiban
C. Cetuximab
D. Oprelvekin
E. Exenatide

18. Which of the following genetic variations is important to the risk of hypersensitivity reactions after abacavir therapy?

A. *MGMT*
B. *HLA-B*5701*
C. *CYP2C19*
D. *TPMT*
E. *HLA-B*1502*

19. Thiopurine methyltransferase is important to the deactivation of which of the following drugs?

A. Azathioprine
B. Methotrexate
C. Warfarin
D. Irinotecan
E. Codeine

20. Which of the following genes is important to the risk of gastrointestinal toxicity after irinotecan therapy?

A. *PACSIN2*
B. *TPMT*
C. *UGT1A1*
D. *EGFR*
E. *DPYD*

 **8-7**   **Answers**

1. **B.** *Transcription* is the process by which RNA polymerase copies a strand of DNA into complementary RNA. *Transformation* refers to the alteration of the

heritable properties of a eukaryotic cell. *Transfection* is the introduction of foreign DNA into a eukaryotic cell. *Transduction* can refer to the transfer of DNA from one bacterium to another through a bacteriophage.

2. **A.** Aldesleukin (IL-2) (Proleukin) is a recombinant cytokine indicated for the treatment of metastatic renal cell carcinoma and melanoma. Eptifibatide (Integrilin) is a recombinant enzyme indicated for treatment of acute coronary syndromes. Bivalirudin (Angiomax) is an enzyme indicated for use in coronary angioplasty and unstable angina. Abciximab (ReoPro) is a monoclonal antibody indicated for prevention of blood clots post-PTCA and unstable angina before PTCA.

3. **B.** Alteplase (Activase) is an rDNA protein of the enzyme type.

4. **C.** Ganirelix (Antagon) is a recombinant hormone indicated for the treatment of luteinizing hormone surge during fertility therapy. Glucagon (GlucaGen) is a recombinant hormone indicated for treatment of hypoglycemia. Eptifibatide (Integrilin) is a recombinant enzyme indicated for the treatment of acute coronary syndromes. Thyrotropin (Thyrogen) is a recombinant hormone indicated for the treatment of thyroid cancer.

5. **A.** Although promising, this technology has not yet yielded vaccines for hepatitis A, malaria, AIDS, or infections caused by *Haemophilus influenzae* type B.

6. **B.** Nomenclature of monoclonal antibodies is highly structured. The first component of the name is product specific; the second component indicates its therapeutic use (*ci* for cardiovascular use, *li* for use in inflammation, *tu* for use in cancer); the third component indicates the type of monoclonal antibody (*mo* for murine, *xi* for chimeric, *zu* for humanized); and the fourth component (*mab*) represents monoclonal antibody.

7. **B.** The repair or correction of a dysfunctional gene by selectively introducing recombinant DNA into cells or tissues, ultimately leading to the expression of a functional gene product, is called *gene therapy*.

8. **B.** Fomivirsen (Vitravene) is the first product based on this technology to come to market.

9. **C.** Formulation of this antifungal agent as a liposomal preparation (AmBisome) has significantly reduced the nephrotoxicity and other adverse effects associated with this drug.

10. **A.** The scientific discipline of using genomewide approaches to understand the inherited basis of differences between individuals in their response to drugs best describes pharmacogenomics.

11. **A.** An SNP may occur outside of an open reading frame (coding region), it may induce a mutation where no change in encoded amino acid occurs, and it may or may not cause a functional change in an encoded protein.

12. **B.** This definition by the *Merriam-Webster Dictionary* best describes *biotechnology*.

13. **B.** DNA is transcribed into mRNA, which is translated ultimately to protein.

14. **A.** Bivalirudin is indicated for use in coronary angioplasty and unstable angina. Filgrastim is indicated for treatment of neutropenia. Alemtuzumab is indicated for treatment of chronic lymphocytic leukemia. Sargramostim is indicated for myeloid reconstitution after bone marrow transplant, after bone marrow transplant failure, as an adjunct to chemotherapy in acute myelogenous leukemia, and in peripheral blood progenitor cell transplant.

15. **A.** Basiliximab is indicated for management of acute organ transplant rejection. Infliximab is indicated for the treatment of Crohn's disease and rheumatoid arthritis. Trastuzumab is indicated for the management of metastatic breast cancer. Rasburicase is indicated for elevated uric acid levels.

16. **A.** Dornase alfa is indicated for respiratory complications in cystic fibrosis. Pegloticase is indicated for treatment of gout. Pancrelipase is indicated for pancreatic insufficiency in cystic fibrosis. Alteplase is indicated for acute myocardial infarction, pulmonary embolism, or stroke. Dulaglutide is indicated for diabetes mellitus type 2.

17. **E.** Exenatide is an example of a hormone. Sargramostim is considered a growth factor. Tirofiban is an enzyme. Cetuximab is a monoclonal antibody. Oprelvekin is a cytokine.

18. **B.** *HLA-B*5701* is a genetic variant that is associated with the risk for hypersensitivity reactions after abacavir therapy.

19. **A.** Thiopurine methyltransferase (TPMT) is responsible for the deactivation of thiopurine drugs (azathioprine, mercaptopurine, thioguanine).

20. **C.** *UGT1A1* variants are associated with the risk for gastrointestinal toxicity after irinotecan therapy.

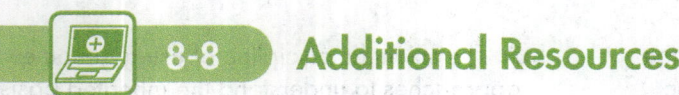

8-8   Additional Resources

Center for Biologics Evaluation and Research. U.S. Food and Drug Administration website. Available at: https://www.fda.gov/vaccines-blood-biologics.

Center for Drug Evaluation and Research. U.S. Food and Drug Administration website. Available at: https://www.fda.gov/drugs.

Clinical Pharmacogenetics Implementation Consortium (CPIC®) website. Available at: https://cpicpgx.org/.

Glick BR, Pasternak JJ, eds. *Molecular Biotechnology: Principles and Applications of Recombinant DNA*. 5th ed. Washington, DC: ASM Press; 2017.

Hollinger P, Hoogenboom H. Antibodies come back from the brink. *Nature Biotech*. 1998;16:1015–1016.

Relling MV, Evans WE. Pharmacogenomics in the Clinic. *Nature*. 2015 Oct 15;526(7573):343–350.

Sindelar RD. Pharmaceutical biotechnology. In: Williams DA, Lemke TL, eds. *Foye's Principles of Medicinal Chemistry*. 5th ed. Philadelphia, PA: Lippincott Williams & Wilkins; 2002:982–1015.

U.S. Food and Drug Administration. Table of Pharmacogenetic Associations. Available at: https://www.fda.gov/medical-devices/precision-medicine/table-pharmacogenetic-associations.

Vaughan TJ, Osbourn JK, Tempest PR. Human antibodies by design. *Nature Biotech*. 1998;16:535–539.

Weinshilboum R. Inheritance and drug response. *N Engl J Med*. 2003;348:529–537.

Biostatistics

9

JUNLING WANG

9-1 KEY POINTS

- In statistics, *data* are numbers that researchers can use to draw conclusions.
- When a characteristic can possess different values among the study subjects, this characteristic is a *variable*.
- When a variable's value is obtained by measuring, this variable is called a *quantitative variable*.
- When a variable's value is based on the nature of the attribute it measures and a counting process, the variable is called a *qualitative variable*.
- A *population* includes all study subjects that a researcher's research question concerns.
- A *sample* is a collection of study subjects that are not the entire population.
- Four statistical measures are usually used in a frequency distribution: frequency, cumulative frequency, relative frequency, and cumulative relative frequency.
- Commonly used measures for the central tendency are the mean, the median, and the mode.
- Commonly used measures for data dispersion are the range, the variance, and the standard deviation.
- A screening test can be evaluated from four aspects: sensitivity, specificity, predictive value positive, and predictive value negative.
- For each population parameter, we can compute two estimates: a point estimate and an interval estimate.
- The *null hypothesis* is the hypothesis to be tested for rejection or nonrejection. It is presumed to be true in the study population. The *alternative hypothesis* is usually consistent with the research hypothesis.
- Regression analysis evaluates the nature of the relationship between two variables and can predict the value of one variable based on the value of another variable. Correlation analysis assesses the strength of the relationships between two variables.
- We usually use the coefficient of determination to evaluate the simple linear regression. The value of the coefficient of determination ranges from 0 to 1.
- We usually use r to represent the sample correlation coefficient and ρ to represent the population correlation coefficient. The value of the correlation coefficient varies from −1 to 1.
- The chi-square test is frequently used when we handle frequency or count data and a categorical variable.
- We can use the nonparametric tests to analyze data that are rankings or classifications.

Editor's Note: Much of the material in the chapter is a summary of work done by Wayne W. Daniel (Daniel WW. *A Foundation for Analysis in the Health Sciences.* 8th ed. Hoboken, NJ: Wiley; 2005).

9-2 STUDY GUIDE CHECKLIST

The following topics may guide your study of this subject area:

- ☐ Basic concepts: variable, types of variables, population, sample, and simple random sample.
- ☐ Descriptive statistics: grouped data, measures of central tendency, and measures of dispersion.
- ☐ Evaluation of screening tests: sensitivity, specificity, predictive value positive, and predictive value negative.
- ☐ Concepts related to confidence interval: point estimate, interval estimate, reliability coefficient, precision, and margin of error.
- ☐ Basic concepts related to hypothesis testing: research hypothesis, statistical hypothesis, null hypothesis, alternative hypothesis, test statistic, rejection region and nonrejection region, significance level, type I and type II errors, P value, and one-sided and two-sided tests.
- ☐ Regression and correlation: independent and dependent variables, method of least squares, evaluation of the regression equation, correlation model.
- ☐ Chi-square tests: observed and expected frequencies.
- ☐ Nonparametric tests: advantages, disadvantages, and sign test.
- ☐ Limitations of statistical analysis.

9-3   Some Concepts

Some basic concepts are frequently used in statistics. Having a clear understanding of these concepts is crucial.

- *Data:* Data are numbers that researchers can use to draw conclusions. One can acquire data from two ways: measuring and counting. By measuring, we can get data such as height, weight, and blood pressure. We can also get data by counting, such as the number of prescriptions filled in a pharmacy or the number of hospitalizations in a hospital in a year. An individual number is a datum, and a collection of the numbers are data.
- *Statistics: Statistics* can be defined as a discipline dealing with two tasks: (1) acquiring and analyzing data and (2) drawing conclusions about study subjects based on the limited amount of data available rather than the entire study population.
- *Sources of data:* Statisticians can acquire data from a variety of sources:
  - *Routine records:* One convenient way for researchers to get data is from records kept by organizations of their daily operations. For example, pharmacy claims held by a pharmacy chain can facilitate research on the costs of medications for a given disease.
  - *Surveys:* Study subjects can answer questions in a survey to provide data for researchers if routine records are not available or sufficient. For instance, one can survey patients with a rare disease on the share of the prescription drug costs among their total health care costs.
  - *Experiments:* Some research questions call for an experiment such as a clinical trial because neither routine records or a patient survey is sufficient or available. For instance, a pharmacist may wish to determine whether pharmacy-based medication therapy management services can improve patient compliance with diabetes medications.
  - *External sources:* A researcher may need to search for external sources for the answers to a research question. These external sources may include data banks, practice guidelines, and academic journal articles.
- *Variable:* When a characteristic can possess different values among the study subjects, this characteristic is a *variable*. Some examples of variables include ages of patients vaccinated in a community pharmacy and the heights of patients in a clinic.
  - *Quantitative variable:* When a variable's value is determined by measuring (e.g., height, blood pressure, age), this variable is called a *quantitative variable*.
  - *Qualitative variable:* When a variable's value is based on the nature of the patient characteristic and a counting process, the variable is called a *qualitative variable*. An example of a qualitative variable is race, which can be White, Black, or other. A pharmacist may be interested in counting the number of female and male patients who visit the pharmacy. These counts are also called *frequencies*.
  - *Random variable:* When the value of a variable is determined randomly, and one cannot predict the value of the variable, the variable is called a random variable. One example of a random variable is adult height, which cannot be precisely predicted at birth. Another example of a random variable is the blood pressure; we cannot predict the exact value of someone's blood pressure unless we measure it.
  - *Discrete random variable:* To determine whether a variable is a *discrete random variable*, one just needs to find out whether there are gaps in the values of the variable. If there are gaps in between any two values, the variable is a discrete random variable. One example of a discrete random variable is the number of prescriptions filled in a chain pharmacy annually. The value of the number of prescriptions is always a whole number.
  - *Continuous random variable:* There are gaps between any two values of a *continuous random variable*. For instance, two individuals' annual health care expenses may be very close. Still, in theory, somebody else's health care expenses may be between the quantity of health care

costs for these two individuals. It is noteworthy though that some variables are continuous but are conventionally recorded as whole numbers. Health care cost, for example, is a continuous variable, but is frequently rounded to whole dollars.

- **Population:** A *population* in statistics includes all study subjects that a researcher's research question concerns. A population of values contains all values for a variable that the study population can take on. Based on the possible number of values in a population, a population can be further classified. If the number of possible values is limitless, we have an infinite population. If the number of possible values is fixed, we have a finite population.

- **Sample:** A *sample* is a collection of study subjects that are not the entire population. Suppose one's population comprises all patients who filled prescriptions through a pharmacy chain in a given month. If one only observes patients in a few pharmacies of the pharmacy chain, the collection of the patients is considered a sample.

- **Simple random sample:** A *simple random sample* is generated when the process is such that each individual has the same chance of being included. The method of making a simple random sample is termed *simple random sampling*.

9-4 Descriptive Statistics

To analyze data in statistics, one needs first to carry out descriptive analysis to "describe the data." Various descriptive analysis techniques are available, and they need to be selected carefully to serve our purposes.

Grouped Data

Grouping data into class intervals is a useful method to organize data. Class intervals need to be contiguous but nonoverlapping, and each datum needs to be grouped into one interval and not more than one interval. One can determine the number of intervals based on our preference. Generally, we do not want to use less than 6 or more than 15 class intervals, because otherwise, we run the risk of over- or under-summarizing the data. Grouping data involves producing a frequency distribution. Four measures are usually used in a frequency distribution: frequency, cumulative frequency, relative frequency, and cumulative relative frequency. *Frequency* is determined by counting the number of values in a class interval. *Cumulative frequency* is produced by totaling the number of values in a specific interval and its preceding intervals. *Relative frequency* is the percentage of values in a class interval among all values of the data. *Cumulative relative frequency* is produced by totaling the percentages of values in a class interval and its preceding intervals. Table 9-1 shows an example of a frequency distribution.

TABLE 9-1. A Frequency Distribution of the Ages of 100 Individuals

Class intervals (years)	Frequency	Cumulative frequency	Relative frequency	Cumulative relative frequency
10 to 19	10	10	0.1429	0.1429
20 to 29	15	25	0.2143	0.3571
30 to 39	15	40	0.2143	0.5714
40 to 49	10	50	0.1429	0.7143
50 to 59	15	65	0.2143	0.9286
60 to 69	5	70	0.0714	1.0000
Total	70		1.0000	

Measures of Central Tendency

To describe the central tendency for the data, we commonly use the mean, the median, and the mode. The *mean* is also called average, which can be produced by dividing the sum of the values taken on by a variable by the number of observations for the variable. The *median* is defined as a value such that there are an equal number of values greater than (or equal to) and lower than (or equal to) the value. The median can be determined by first ordering all values in the data. The median value is equal to the middle value when one has an odd number of observations. When one has an even number of observations, the median is equal to the average of the 2 middle observations. Mode refers to the most frequently occurring observation for a variable. If multiple values are occurring with equally high frequency, these values are all mode. In this case, there is more than 1 mode for the variable. If all observations possess different values for a variable, there is no mode.

Measures of Dispersion

Dispersion measures how the values are dispersed for a variable.

- **The range:** The range is computed as the difference between the largest value and the smallest value. Using the range is the simplest way to measure the dispersion of a variable.
- **Variance:** The variance describes how the values of the variable are scattered in relation to the mean of the variable. To estimate the variance, we first square the sum of the difference between each observation and the mean of the variable and then divide the result by the number of study subjects minus 1.
- **Standard deviation:** Standard deviation is calculated as the squared root of the variance. One advantage of the standard deviation compared to variance is that the unit of the variance is the squared unit of the variable. In contrast, the unit of the standard deviation is the original unit of the variable.
- **The coefficient of variation:** The coefficient of variation is calculated as the standard deviation divided by the mean. This measure is used when using other dispersion measures may produce erroneous conclusions. For example, one may be interested in comparing the dispersion of two variables measured in different units, such as serum cholesterol level and body weight. The former may be measured in milligrams per 100 milliliters, and the latter may be measured in pounds. Directly comparing them may produce erroneous findings. Because of the way the coefficient of variation is calculated and the units of the standard deviation and the mean cancel out, the coefficient of variation is unit free.

9-5   Evaluation of Screening Tests

A pharmacist needs to evaluate screening tests and diagnostics in clinical practice. Given a test result or the presence of specific symptoms, a pharmacist needs to determine whether the patient has or does not have the medical condition of interest. Both false positive and false negatives can result because screening tests and diagnostics are not perfect. A false positive occurs when a person has the disease but, for some reason, presents with a negative test result. A false negative happens when a person does not have the condition but presents with positive test results. To comprehensively evaluate a test, four measures are usually used at the same time: sensitivity, specificity, predictive value positive, and predictive value negative:

- *Sensitivity:* The sensitivity of a test is equal to the probability of a positive test among individuals with the medical condition. Using the system of symbols in Table 9-2, we can calculate the sensitivity of a test as follows:

$$x/(x + v)$$

TABLE 9-2. Individuals Cross-Classified Based on Disease and Test Results

Disease	Test results	
	Positive	Negative
Yes	x	v
No	y	w

Adapted from Daniel 2005.

- **Specificity:** The specificity is equal to the probability of a negative test among individuals without the medical condition. Using the system of symbols in Table 9-2, we can calculate the specificity of a test as follows:

$$w/(y + w)$$

- **Predictive value positive:** The predictive value positive is equal to the probability of a person having the medical condition among individuals with positive tests. Using the symbols in Table 9-2, we can calculate the predictive value positive as follows:

$$x/(x + y)$$

- **Predictive value negative:** The predictive value negative is equal to the probability of an individual not having the medical condition among individuals with negative test results. Using the symbols in Table 9-2, one can compute this probability as follows:

$$w/(v + w)$$

9-6   Estimation

In statistics concerning medical science, many populations have a fixed number of people. Studying every member of the population, however, is still generally impossible. Therefore, population parameters, such as population mean and population proportion, are usually estimated based on a sample. A researcher can generate two types of estimates for each parameter. A *point estimate* is produced when a single value is calculated to represent the population parameter of interest. For example, the sample mean is a point estimate of the population mean. An *interval estimate* comprises 2 values defining the range of the population parameter. Such an interval estimate is called a *confidence interval* because, with a certain level of confidence, one is certain that the interval contains the real value of the population parameter. The general formula for calculating a confidence interval is

point estimate ± (reliability coefficient) × (standard error)

In this formula, the point estimate of the parameter of interest is the center of the confidence interval. The reliability coefficient is a value that can be obtained based on the type of distribution concerning the sample. The standard error measures the dispersion of the estimates concerning the parameter. The product of the reliability coefficient and the standard error is also termed precision or margin of error.

We will illustrate as follows the construction of the confidence intervals for the population mean and population proportion. The method of the calculation for the confidence interval is not the focus of our illustration but rather its interpretation. Confidence intervals for other population parameters can be estimated similarly.

Confidence Interval for Population Mean

The first step for constructing a confidence interval is to estimate the sample mean, which is the center of the interval. The reliability coefficient can be determined on the basis of the standard normal distribution if the sample size is large. A good rule of thumb for determining a large sample is when the sample size is greater than 30, which holds in most cases. The reliability coefficients for 90%, 95%, and 99% confidence intervals are 1.645, 1.96, and 2.58, respectively.

For example, in a study of patients' punctuality for picking up their prescriptions, 35 patients were, on average, 17.2 minutes late for the scheduled pickup time with a standard deviation of 8 minutes. The 90% confidence interval for the population mean can be calculated as [15, 19.4]. The following is the interpretation of this confidence interval: one can be 90% confident that this interval [15, 19.4] contains the real value of the population mean.

Confidence Interval for Population Proportion

To produce an estimate on the population proportion, we will first need to calculate the sample proportion based on a sample that is drawn from the population. Then we can estimate the confidence interval for the population proportion following the same steps as for constructing the confidence interval for the population mean.

9-7   Hypothesis Testing

Hypothesis testing serves a similar function in statistics as estimation above, and both of them help us to draw conclusions about the population based on the data in a sample. They are closely related, although their techniques may appear different.

Basic Concepts

Null hypothesis and alternative hypothesis

We have two types of hypotheses when conducting research: a research hypothesis and a statistical hypothesis. The former is our theory or belief concerning a research idea that we are attempting to test rigorously. To test the research hypothesis though, we need to convert the research hypothesis into a statistical hypothesis. A statistical hypothesis is our theory of belief about a study topic that can be tested with statistical tests. A statistical hypothesis includes two statements, and they are conventionally named the null and the alternative hypotheses.

The null hypothesis is a proposition to be tested for rejection or nonrejection. It is usually termed H_0. The null hypothesis always contains an indication of equality (=, ≥, or ≤). The *alternative hypothesis* is a statement that may be true if the null hypothesis is rejected in the process of hypothesis testing. It perfectly complements the null hypothesis. Conventionally, the alternative hypothesis is called H_A. Usually, the alternative hypothesis is consistent with the research hypothesis, and the null hypothesis is the opposite of the research hypothesis.

One common mistake related to hypothesis testing is worth mentioning here. When a null hypothesis is not rejected in hypothesis testing, proof of the null hypothesis is not suggested. Based on hypothesis testing, we can only determine whether our data support the null hypothesis or do not support the null hypothesis.

Test statistic

A decision rule is used in hypothesis testing, and that rule is called test statistic. We first calculate the test statistic based on the data from the study sample and then decide whether or not to reject the null hypothesis. The values of the test statistic usually follow a specific distribution, and this distribution can be divided into 2 regions for the purpose of hypothesis testing: the rejection region and the nonrejection region. If the value of the test statistic falls in the rejection region, we will reject the null hypothesis. Otherwise, we do not reject the null hypothesis. This is because the values of the test statistic in the nonrejection region have a higher likelihood of occurring than the values in the rejection region for the purpose of hypothesis testing.

Significance level

The rejection and nonrejection regions are separated by a critical value in hypothesis testing. The level of significance, typically designated as α, determines the critical value of the test. Due to the importance of the level of significance in hypothesis testing, people also call hypothesis testing *significance testing*. Further, if the value of the test statistic is found to be within the rejection region, we often state that the statistical test is significant.

Type I and type II errors

We may possibly commit errors when performing hypothesis testing because the conclusion is related to a level of significance. Two types of errors can result from a hypothesis testing (Table 9-3) depending on the relationship between the status of the null hypothesis and our statistical conclusion. If we reject a true null hypothesis, our error is termed a *type I error*. If we do not reject a false null hypothesis, our error is termed *type II error*. The probability of a type I error is thus equal to the level of significance, which is α. The likelihood of a type II error is conventionally designated as β. Another important concept related to type II error is *power,* which is the probability of not committing a type II error.

We have control over the probability of type I error in hypothesis testing because this probability is equal to the level of significance. By selecting a low level of significance, we can lower the likelihood of type I error. The most widely used significance levels are 0.01, 0.05, and 0.1. We enjoy less control over type II error except that we know the probability of a type II error is usually higher than the likelihood of a type I error. As a matter of fact, in statistics, we do not typically know the exact status of the null hypothesis, so we cannot accurately determine the likelihood of a type II error. Therefore, we take more comfort when a null hypothesis is rejected, and we know we have a low probability of committing a type I error.

The *p* value

The *p* value is one of the essential values in hypothesis testing, and it is compared to the level of significance. When the *P* value is lower than the level of significance, or α, we conclude that the statistical test is significant.

One-sided and two-sided tests

In hypothesis testing, we also need to determine whether we want to use a two-sided or one-sided test. In a two-sided test, we will reject the null hypothesis both when the value of the test statistics is sufficiently large and adequately small. In a one-sided test, we will only reject the null hypothesis if the test statistic is sufficiently large or small, depending on the direction of the alternative hypothesis.

TABLE 9-3. Type I and Type II Errors

Null hypothesis	Statistical decision	
	Do not reject H_0	Reject H_0
True	Correct	Type I error
False	Type II error	Correct

Adapted from Daniel 2005.

9-8 Simple Linear Regression and Correlation Analyses

In medical sciences, we often need to conduct regression and correlation analysis when we need to examine the relationship between 2 numerical variables. Regression and correlation serve different purposes. We need to perform regression analysis when we are interested in the nature of the relationship and aim to predict and estimate the value of 1 variable based on the value of the other variable. We will conduct a correlation analysis if we need to determine the strength of the relationship. A variety of regression and correlation analyses are frequently used, but the most basic among them is the simple linear regression and correlation.

The Simple Linear Regression Model

Independent variable and dependent variable

The simple linear regression model addresses the relationship between 2 variables, and these 2 variables are usually called the independent variable, designated as *X*, and the dependent variable, *Y*. The value of *X* is fixed, and the researcher can control this variable by preselecting its values. For each preselected *X* value, there is at least one corresponding *Y* value. The purpose of the simple linear regression is to estimate the linear relationship between the independent variable and the dependent variable. The first step for the process is to visualize the relationship between the 2 variables by plotting a scatter diagram of the relationship between the 2 variables based on the data from the study sample. This is accomplished by assigning the values of the 2 variables to the horizontal axis and vertical axis, respectively. Usually, the value of the independent variable is assigned to the horizontal axis, and the value of the dependent variable is assigned to the vertical axis. By visualizing the relationship between the 2 variables, we can determine whether a linear relationship is a reasonable quantitative approximation for these 2 variables.

An example of such a diagram is the relationship between age and the forced expiratory volume (liters) among a group of children between 10 and 16 years of age (Figure 9-1). This diagram clearly shows that the older the children are, the higher the forced expiratory volume. In other words, a linear relationship may exist between the 2 variables.

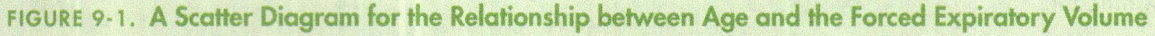

FIGURE 9-1. A Scatter Diagram for the Relationship between Age and the Forced Expiratory Volume

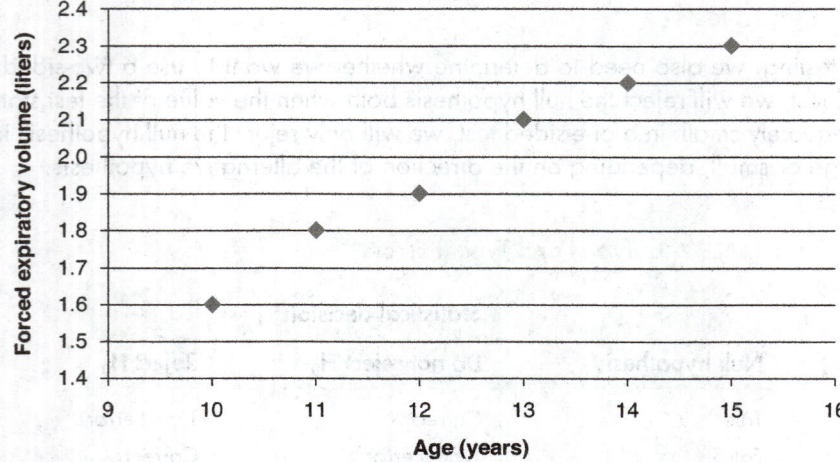

Estimation of the linear line

After we have determined that a linear relationship may be a reasonable depiction of the variables' relationship, there are multiple ways of estimating the linear line for the relationship. A most-widely used method is the *method of least squares*, and the line produced using this method is the *least squares line*.

The line produced by the simple linear regression analysis is of the following general format:

$$\hat{y} = a + bx$$

where *a* is the intercept of the line, and *b* is the slope of the line. Note that these are estimates of the intercept and the slope based on the study sample. The intercept and the slope of the line for the study population are typically designated as α and β, respectively. The estimated least squares line for the linear relationship depicted in Figure 9-1 is given by

$$\hat{y} = 0.23 + 0.14x$$

The intercept of the line has a positive sign, which suggests that the line meets the vertical axis where the dependent variable is positive. The slope of the line has a value of 0.14, which indicates that when *x* increases by 1 unit, *y* increases by 0.14 unit. The circumflex symbol above the *y* means that the values for the variable *y* are estimated based on this linear line. The exact values of the variable may be different from these estimates.

Evaluation of the regression equation

After we estimate a linear line, we must evaluate whether the linear line represents an adequate description of the variables' relationship. For this purpose, we usually use the coefficient of determination, designated as "R^2", which quantitatively measures how dispersed the data points distribute around the linear line. The possible values of the coefficient of determination are between 0 and 1. The higher this measure, the closer the data points distribute around the line. When this measure is equal to 0, the linear line is useless for explaining the relationship between the 2 variables. When this measure is equal to 1, all data points are on the linear line, and the linear line is a perfect representation of the relationship between the 2 variables. If the relationship between the 2 variables is approximately linear based on the scatter diagram, our estimate of the R^2 should be reasonably different from 0. Further, we rarely obtain a linear line with R^2 equal to 1 in our research because an exact linear relationship rarely occurs in the real world. The coefficient of determination for the preceding example in Figure 9-1 is 0.98.

Use of the regression equation

After obtaining a linear line, we can now predict and estimate the value of the dependent variable based on the value of the independent variable. For example, if $X = 11$ for the above line,

$$\hat{y} = 0.23 + 0.14(11) = 1.77$$

The Simple Linear Correlation Model

In a regression model, the roles of the independent variable and the dependent variable are different. However, in the framework of correlation analysis, the 2 variables have equal footing. The two variables in a simple linear correlation analysis do not serve different roles, although they are still designated as *X* and *Y* for ease of expression. In the regression analysis framework, we preselect the values of the independent variable, but in correlation analysis, we just measure the strength of the relationship between the 2 variables.

In the framework of a correlation analysis, we use the correlation coefficient to determine the relationship between the 2 variables. The correlation coefficient we calculate for the sample is designated r, and the population correlation coefficient is designated as ρ. The range of the correlation coefficient is between -1 and 1.

There are a few exceptional circumstances concerning the correlation coefficient. When $\rho = 1$, we consider the relationship between the 2 variables a perfect direct linear correlation. When $\rho = -1$, the 2 variables have a perfect inverse linear correlation. When $\rho = 0$, the 2 variables are not considered linearly correlated.

Some Caveats

As powerful as simple linear regression and correlation can be, they can only produce useless and even misleading information if they are not used properly. We need, therefore, to be mindful of some caveats when performing such analyses. First, when conducting simple linear regression and correlation, the variables must be measured on the same observation. Thus, analyzing the association between the age of a group of people and the disease status of another group of people typically would not produce credible information.

Second, when a strong linear relationship is discovered between the 2 variables, we should not take that as suggesting a causal effect of 1 variable on the other. Their actual relationship may turn out to be causal, but their relationship may not be causal, but rather, they may both be affected by a third factor directly or indirectly. Third, we must guard against extrapolation outside the range of the independent variables in the sample. This is because the relationship between the 2 variables may only be valid within the range of the independent variables in the sample. Outside this range, their actual relationship may even be nonlinear.

9-9   Chi-Square Tests

When we handle count data or frequency data and a categorical variable, we usually turn to the chi-square test. This test is rather simple to conduct, but it is widely used. We may have data on the number of pharmacy patients with different types of insurance at a pharmacy: private insurance, Medicaid, Medicare, and others. These are count data. We may be interested in comparing the insurance status between the patients at this pharmacy and those at another pharmacy. We may be interested in comparing rates of compliance with diabetes medications between females and males. The chi-square test is suitable for these scenarios because the variables are categorical.

To conduct a chi-square test, we need first to obtain 2 sets of frequencies: observed frequencies and expected frequencies. The *observed frequencies* are the number of study subjects who belong to various categories for the variable of interest (e.g., health insurance status). For example, among 100 pharmacy patients, 30 might be privately insured, 40 might have Medicare, 20 might have Medicaid, and 10 might not have any insurance. The *expected frequencies* are the number of study subjects that belong to each category of a variable if the null hypothesis is true. Again for our example, if the null hypothesis is that individuals are equally likely to fall in any 1 of the 4 insurance categories, 25 individuals are expected to have each of the 4 types of insurance.

The decision rule for a chi-square test is X^2, which measures whether the observed frequencies and the expected frequencies have high degrees of agreement. When their agreement is weak, the quantity of X^2 is high. We will reject the null hypothesis. The critical value for X^2 is determined based on a chi-square distribution.

The chi-square test also has its limitations. When the expected frequencies are too small, we will not be able to use the chi-square test to draw valid conclusions. Some statisticians believe that we should not use a chi-square test when any expected frequency in the data is lower than or equal to 5 or 10. Under those circumstances, we may choose an alternative analysis, such as Fisher's exact test.

9-10   Nonparametric Tests

Most of the statistical tests that we use are parametric statistics except that the chi-square test is not a parametric test. Two points differentiate parametric tests from nonparametric tests. First, when conducting a parametric analysis, population parameters are what we are interested in estimating or testing the hypothesis about. Nonparametric tests typically do not involve population parameters. Second, when conducting a parametric analysis, we usually must know the type of the population distribution, while this is generally untrue when performing a nonparametric test.

Nonparametric tests offer advantages over parametric tests when applied appropriately. First, when data are merely rankings or classifications, we may use nonparametric tests. In this situation, the measurement level may not be strong enough for parametric tests. Second, when the sample size is relatively small, applying nonparametric tests can be quick and easy.

Nonparametric tests do have limitations. Nonparametric tests are usually reserved for data that cannot be analyzed with parametric data. This is because in other situations applying nonparametric tests can lead to a waste of information. Further, carrying out nonparametric tests when the sample size is large can be time consuming.

One type of nonparametric test is the sign test, and it tests a hypothesis concerning the median of the distribution. The sign test is applicable as long as the variable of interest is continuous. To calculate the test statistic, we need plus and minus signs generated based on the study sample.

For example, the appearance scores among a group of study subjects are 4, 5, 8, 8, 9, 6, 10, 7, 6, and 6. Let us try to determine whether the median appearance score for this sample is 5. We first drop the appearance scores equal to 5 from further consideration. We then count the number of pluses as the number of appearance scores greater than 5 and number of minuses as the number of scores less than 5. We now have 8 pluses and 1 minus.

For this example, the null hypothesis is that the median for the scores is 5. If the null hypothesis is true, the numbers of plus and minus signs should be equal or relatively close. The probability of seeing a certain amount of plus and minus signs can be computed based on a binomial distribution. That precise probability turns out to be 0.039 for this example. Therefore, at the significance level of 0.05, we reject the null hypothesis and conclude that the median of the appearance scores in this sample may not be 5.

9-11   Limitations of Statistical Analysis

Statistics is a powerful tool for researchers in the health sciences. When applied correctly, statistics can effectively assist us in making decisions. However, statistical conclusions regarding an intervention or a program are not absolute and definitive and should be treated as only one source of information to facilitate decision making. Decision makers need to refer to other aspects of the intervention or program, such as safety, equity, accessibility. We also need to take into consideration the implications of statistical significance and the difference between statistical significance and clinical relevance. Statistical significance is more objective than clinical relevance because the latter may also reflect the perspective of a health care provider, a caregiver, and a patient. For instance, in a clinical experiment, a specific type of intervention may lead to a statistically significant reduction in blood pressure. However, if patients, doctors, and caregivers do not perceive patients as having improved, convincing the decision makers that implementing the program makes clinical sense would be hard.

9-12   Pharmacist's Role

Pharmacists play an important role related to statistics. A student pharmacist acquires knowledge from the literature in the process of training to become a pharmacist. After becoming a pharmacist, she/he is expected to be a life-long learner and is required to keep abreast of the development of the pharmacy and medical literature. Understanding statistics is essential for critically evaluating research for both student pharmacists and practicing pharmacists. Some pharmacists may even have the responsibility to teach statistics to the next generation of pharmacists and possibly to other health care providers. Using statistics is also inevitable when pharmacists carry out scholarship activities to advance pharmacy and medical literature.

NAPLEX Competency Statements

The questions in this chapter cover the following 2021 NAPLEX Competency Statements: **AREA 1:** 1.1; 1.7 **AREA 3:** 3.11 **AREA 4:** 4.8.

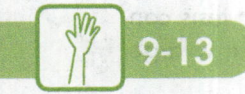 **9-13   Questions**

1. Which of the following statements about statistics is true?

   A. Data used in statistics have to include all individuals in a population.
   B. If an investigator has a research question, she or he has to collect original data.
   C. Statistical conclusions are drawn based on the data from the whole population.
   D. We do not need to study the entire population to draw conclusions about the study population.
   E. Data used in statistics are always from a survey.

2. Which of the following statements is *not* true for variables?

   A. A continuous random variable has gaps between its values.
   B. Height is a quantitative variable.
   C. Blood pressure can be a random variable.
   D. Weight is a continuous variable.
   E. A variable is not always random.

3. Which of the following is *not* true about frequency distribution?

   A. An observation in a sample may belong to more than one interval.
   B. Frequency as a statistical measure can be included in a frequency distribution.
   C. Relative frequency as a statistical measure can be included in a frequency distribution.
   D. Cumulative relative frequency as a statistical measure can be included in a frequency distribution.
   E. Cumulative frequency as a statistical measure can be included in a frequency distribution.

4. Which of the following is *not* true about central tendency?

   A. A set of values may not have a mode.
   B. When we have an odd number of values, the middle value is equal to the median after the data are ordered.
   C. Mean and median are equal.
   D. A set of values may have multiple modes.
   E. The mean, the median, and the mode are all measures of the central tendency.

5. Which of the following are measures of central tendency? (Mark all that apply.)

   A. Median
   B. Mean
   C. Range
   D. Coefficient of variation
   E. Standard deviation

6. Which of the following measures is unit free?

A. Range
B. Variance
C. Standard deviation
D. Coefficient of variation
E. Mean

Use the data from this table for Questions 7 to 10.

The following table shows 100 individuals cross-classified according to disease status and test results.

Test results	Disease		Total
	Present	Absent	
Positive	30	40	70
Negative	20	10	30
Total	50	50	100

7. What is the sensitivity for the test?

A. 30/50
B. 10/50
C. 30/70
D. 10/30
E. 30/100

8. What is the specificity of the test?

A. 30/50
B. 10/50
C. 30/70
D. 10/30
E. 30/100

9. What is the predictive value positive for the test?

A. 30/50
B. 10/50
C. 30/70
D. 10/30
E. 30/100

10. What is the predictive value negative for the test?

A. 10/30
B. 10/50
C. 30/50
D. 30/70
E. 30/100

11. Which of the following statements is true?

A. For a population parameter, we cannot generate both a point estimate and an interval estimate.
B. Precision refers to the lower limit of a confidence interval.
C. The reliability coefficient measures the dispersion of the estimates.
D. The reliability coefficient for the confidence interval can be determined on the basis of the standard normal distribution only when certain conditions are met.
E. A confidence interval cannot be calculated for the population parameters besides population mean and population proportion.

12. Which of the following statements is *not* true about statistical hypotheses?

A. The null hypothesis is a proposition presumed to be true.
B. The alternative hypothesis is usually consistent with the research hypothesis.
C. With a statistical test, we can prove or reject a null hypothesis.
D. A statistical analysis has to have a null hypothesis.
E. A statistical test does not need both null and alternative hypotheses.

13. Which of the following statements is true?

A. If the test statistic is included in the nonrejection region, the test is significant.
B. A typical level of significance is 0.95.
C. Researchers prefer higher levels of significance.
D. A typical level of significance is 0.05.
E. A typical level of significance is 0.90.

14. Which of the following statements is *not* true for type I and type II errors?

A. A statistical test always has either a type I or a type II error.
B. A type I error cannot occur at the same time as a type II error.
C. We can exercise less control over the likelihood of committing a type II error than a type I error.
D. We commit a type I error when we do not reject a false null hypothesis.
E. The probability of type I error is low when the level of significance is low.

15. Which of the following statements is *not* true?

A. We cannot estimate a linear regression line for any two variables.

B. A negative slope of a simple linear regression indicates the higher the independent variable, the lower the dependent variable.

C. A positive intercept means that the regression line meets the vertical line where the dependent variable is positive.

D. We have more control over the values of the dependent variable than the independent variable.

E. Regression and correlation are applicable when we are interested in analyzing the relationship between two numerical variables.

16. Which of the following statements is *not* true?

A. The coefficient of determination ranges from 0 to 1.

B. The correlation coefficient ranges from 0 to 1.

C. When $\rho = 1$, we consider the relationship between the 2 variables a perfect direct linear correlation.

D. When $\rho = -1$, the 2 variables have a perfect inverse linear correlation.

E. We can use the coefficient of determination to evaluate a linear regression line.

17. Which of the following statements is true?

A. Regression analysis can determine whether 2 variables have a causal relationship.

B. Correlation analysis can determine whether 2 variables have a causal relationship.

C. When the 2 variables have a linear relationship, we cannot always extrapolate this relationship to beyond the range of the independent variable in the sample.

D. A linear correlation model can be used to estimate the value of the dependent variable for the value of the independent variable.

E. If $\rho = -1$, X and Y have a perfect direct linear correlation.

18. Which of the following statements is true?

A. The two variables in correlation analysis do not have equal footing.

B. We can preselect values for both variables for simple linear correlation analysis.

C. We can preselect the values of the dependent variable in the framework of a simple linear regression analysis.

D. We have some control over the independent variable in the context of a simple linear regression analysis.

E. If $\rho = 0$, the 2 variables are linearly correlated.

19. Which of the following statements is *not* true about the chi-square test?

A. The chi-square test is a nonparametric test.

B. The test statistic of a chi-square test is determined based on a chi-square distribution.

C. We can always use the chi-square test for the analysis of categorical variables.

D. The rejection and nonrejection regions of the chi-square test are separated based on the chi-square distribution.

E. The chi-square test may be applicable when the variables are categorical.

20. Which of the following statements is true?

A. Nonparametric tests are always preferred over parametric tests.

B. When the sample size is large, applying a nonparametric test is easier than a parametric analysis.

C. We always need to know the type of population distribution to use a nonparametric test.

D. We need first to figure out the numbers of positive and negative signs in the data for the sign test.

E. Nonparametric tests are not applicable when the data are merely rankings or classifications.

9-14   Answers

1. **D.** We can draw conclusions about the population based on a sample.

2. **A.** A continuous variable does not have gaps between its values.

3. **A.** In a frequency distribution, each value can only be classified in one interval.

4. **C.** Mean and median are not always equal.

5. **A and B.** Median and mean are measures of central tendency. All other measures are measures of dispersion.

6. **D.** Because of the way the coefficient of variation is calculated and the units of the standard deviation and the mean cancel out, the coefficient of variation if unit free.

7. **A.** The sensitivity of a test is equal to the probability of a positive test among individuals with the medical condition.

8. **B.** The specificity is equal to the probability of a negative test among individuals without the medical condition.

9. **C.** The predictive value positive is equal to the likelihood of a person having the medical condition among individuals with positive test results.

10. **A.** The predictive value negative is equal to the probability of an individual not having the medical condition among individuals with negative test results.

11. **D.** When the sample size is greater than 30, reliability coefficients can be determined based on the standard normal distribution.

12. **C.** When we do not reject the null hypothesis, we have not proved the null hypothesis to be true.

13. **D.** Typical values of the level of significance are 0.01, 0.05, and 0.1.

14. **D.** We commit a type II error when we do not reject a false null hypothesis.

15. **D.** The independent variable has fixed values preselected by us for the simple linear regression. We have more control over the values of the independent variables than the dependent variable.

16. **B.** The value of the correlation coefficient ranges from −1 to 1.

17. **C.** Outside the range of the independent variable in the sample, the relationship between the dependent and independent variables is unknown.

18. **D.** The independent variable has fixed values preselected by us for the simple linear regression. We have control over the independent variable in the context of a simple linear regression analysis.

19. **C.** When an expected frequency is too small, we cannot use the chi-square test.

20. **D.** We need first to figure out the numbers of positive and negative signs based on the data for the sign test. We then will use these numbers to determine the significance of the test.

9-15   Additional Resource

Daniel WW. *A Foundation for Analysis in the Health Sciences*. 8th ed. Hoboken, NJ: Wiley; 2005.

Clinical Trial Design

10

BRADLEY A. BOUCHER

10-1 KEY POINTS

- Observational research may be prospective or retrospective.
- Experimental research is usually prospective.
- Experimental designs should seek to minimize bias, confounding variables, and random error.
- Cohort studies may be prospective or retrospective.
- Retrospective studies are ideally able to identify an association between variables.
- Well-designed randomized controlled trials (RCTs) can establish a cause-and-effect relationship between variables.
- Evidence-based medicine requires the critical appraisal of medical literature and the adoption of scientifically rigorous, relevant information into clinical practice.

10-2 STUDY GUIDE CHECKLIST

The following topics may guide your study of this subject area:

- ☐ Differences between observational and experimental studies.
- ☐ Similarities and differences between major experimental trial design types.
- ☐ Differences between parallel and crossover RCTs.
- ☐ Key aspects of RCTs to consider in reviewing published studies.
- ☐ Major blinding categories used in RCTs.
- ☐ Difference between *per protocol* and *intention-to-treat* data analysis techniques.
- ☐ Four major steps for critically appraising medical literature.
- ☐ Practical methods to assist practitioners in staying current with medical literature.
- ☐ Definition of evidence-based medicine.
- ☐ Major steps in practicing evidence-based pharmacy.

10-3 Introduction

Clinical research refers to studies conducted in humans seeking to answer a question regarding health care. It includes studies evaluating medical disease prevention, diagnosis, and treatment. Data derived from well-planned and well-executed clinical research studies are extremely important in advancing patient care. Although the basic principles of clinical research design techniques and processes are not particularly difficult to comprehend, actually conducting studies is a complex enough process that entire textbooks are devoted to trial design as well as to data processing and interpretation. Many health care practitioners lack the time and expertise to design and execute studies themselves without additional training, and practitioners may even be inadequately prepared to interpret published clinical data. Regardless, understanding the basics of clinical research design is essential for all practitioners to practice evidence-based medicine. Critical appraisal of medical literature and judicious use of new knowledge will aid clinicians in providing the best possible care to the patients they serve.

This chapter introduces the reader to the basic concepts of clinical research; clinical trial design, including the major types of clinical trials; and many of the key aspects of randomized controlled trials (RCTs). The chapter also addresses the basic principles for evaluating the primary literature and the techniques for reviewing such data and implementing useful findings in clinical practice.

10-4 Fundamentals of Research Design and Methodology

There are 2 basic types of clinical research: observational research and experimental research (Table 10-1). A brief description of each type follows:

- **Observational research:** In this type of research, the investigator observes what is occurring without intervening. Typically, descriptive statistics are used to summarize the study results. This method includes measures of central tendency (e.g., arithmetic mean, median, mode) and measures of variability (e.g., range, standard deviation, variance). Observational research may be retrospective or prospective. Retrospective studies involve looking back from the present, whereas prospective studies begin at the present time and observe study variables of interest from the present forward. One specific type of observational research that is very important within medicine is the case

TABLE 10-1. Summary of Major Clinical Study Designs

Type	Retrospective (R) vs. prospective (P)?	Prove causal relationship?*	Randomization possible?	Control group?
Descriptive/observational				
Case reports	R	No	No	No
Questionnaires/surveys	P	No	No	No
Case series	R or P	No	No	No
Cohort study	R or P	No	No	Yes
Case-control study	R	No	No	Yes
Randomized clinical trial				
Parallel	P	Yes	Yes	Yes
Crossover	P	Yes	Yes	Yes

* Causality based on inferential statistics.

report. A case report retrospectively describes a specific clinical case or a limited number of cases. Case reports cannot establish a causal relationship but may often be the first evidence of a previously unknown or unrecognized relationship. Another type of observational study is the questionnaire/survey. Other major observational clinical research designs are outlined below:

- *Case series:* This type of study is similar to a case report although it reports on a group of patients with similar clinical presentations or exposure to a particular treatment or condition compared with a single case or limited number of cases. A case series may be either retrospective or prospective. The lack of a control group and randomization limits the determination of a causal relationship and rigorous statistical analysis, respectively.
- *Cohort study:* A cohort study selects participants on the basis of one or more specific characteristics and compares them over time to either a different set of patients or the rest of the general population that serves as the control group. In either case, the study group of interest is exposed to the test treatment or condition at the beginning of the evaluation period, whereas the other group is not exposed. Cohort studies are essentially the same as RCTs (discussed below) except for the absence of randomization. A cohort study can be conducted prospectively, in which case participants are selected on the basis of the study characteristics of interest and then observed following exposure until the conclusion of the study. Cohort studies can also identify participants retrospectively, in which case participant records are used to identify and prospectively evaluate individuals with the selected characteristics thereafter. Yet another design is to study prospectively one group of patients possessing the study characteristics and having been exposed to the test treatment and to compare that group to a historical participant group evaluated retrospectively. A well-designed cohort study can provide convincing evidence of an association between study variables. However, the inability to randomize patients to one group or another is a major source of bias inherent in conducting cohort studies because the participant groups may not be comparable. *Bias* denotes systematic error within clinical investigations. Bias is distinct from *confounding variables.* The latter term is used to describe variables that are not systematically introduced into the study but that may affect the outcome of interest in clinical studies. Generally speaking, confounding variables cannot be controlled in clinical studies completely (e.g., use of concurrent medications during the course of a study).
- *Case-control study:* Case-control studies are similar to cohort studies in that one group of participants has a disease and is compared to a control group that does not have the disease. However, a best attempt is made to find patients within the control group who match the participants with the disease or condition on the basis of a predefined set of characteristics such as age or sex. Another difference is that case-control studies are always retrospective.
- *Experimental research:* In this type of research, a specific intervention or exposure to a condition is evaluated in a study group and typically compared with a control group. Experimental research is usually prospective in nature, but it may use historical controls or controls from medical literature for the comparator group. Familiarity with the terminology of experimental clinical study designs is useful from several vantage points. One aspect is the ability to efficiently plan and conduct clinical research on the basis of accepted methodologies by motivated investigators. Perhaps more important for most clinicians is the ability to interpret medical literature as previously noted. Upon identification of the methodology used within a published study, the clinician should be able to readily conceptualize how a study was conducted. The following list outlines each major experimental clinical study design:
  - *Randomized controlled trial (RCT):* In this type of trial, study participants are prospectively assigned randomly to one or more treatment or control groups upon meeting the inclusion criteria for the study. A well-designed and well-executed RCT provides evidence of a causal relationship between the intervention being investigated and the primary study outcome. The 2 most common design subtypes of RCTs are known as parallel and crossover.
    - *Parallel RCT:* In this study design, participants are randomized to one of the treatment or control arms of the study. Control groups may receive standard treatments, no treatment,

usual care, or placebos. *Placebos* are inactive substances that are often used in clinical drug studies. Typically, study participants receive the assigned treatment or control for the entire trial in a parallel RCT (Figure 10-1). Outcome responses for each treatment or control group are then compared at the conclusion of the study *between* patients assigned to each study group. Conditions being evaluated can be acute or chronic, which is one of the reasons that parallel RCTs are the most common prospective RCT design.

- *Crossover RCT:* In this design, the study participants receive one or more of the treatments or controls for a predefined period during the course of the study. Participants are then switched or "crossed over" to one or more of the other treatment or control arms (Figure 10-2). In this instance, outcome responses are compared *within* the same participants, resulting typically in less variability. Although crossover RCTs are efficient for evaluating causal effects of one treatment over another treatment within the same participant, a major limitation is that only stable, chronic, or episodic conditions can be studied. Examples of such conditions include glaucoma, epilepsy, and migraines. Even with chronic or episodic conditions, however, a return to the same baseline state is needed to use a crossover design. This return frequently requires a period of no treatment or usual treatment between study periods to avoid a carryover or residual effect as one treatment ends and the next one begins. This time period is referred to as a "washout" period.

Key Aspects of Randomized Controlled Trials

RCTs have a high weighting in the ranks of medical literature. Figure 10-3 is a diagram illustrating general considerations regarding scientific rigor of particular study designs. Understanding the basics of RCT design will aid in interpreting the results and applying new literature to study practice. This section reviews key considerations of RCT design. Many of the principles covered here may also be applied to other types of trials.

FIGURE 10-1. Example of Parallel Design

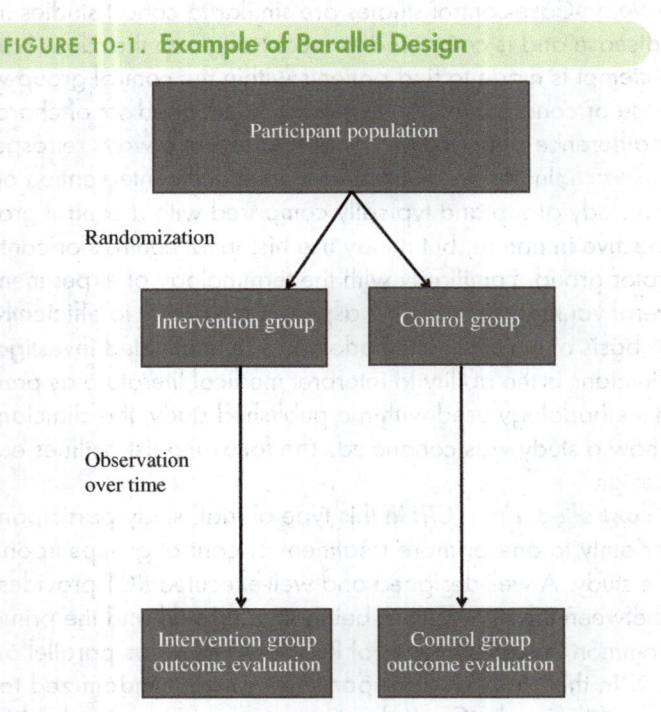

FIGURE 10-2. Example of Crossover Design

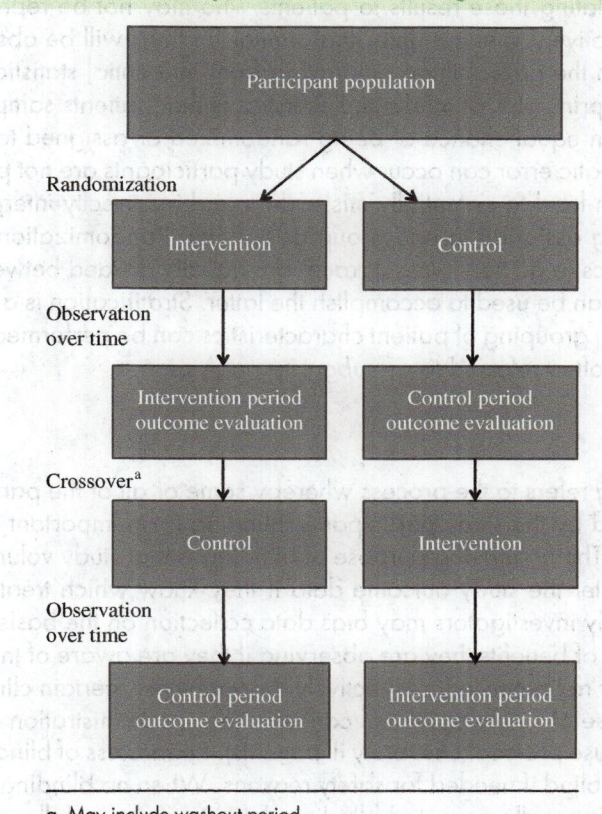

a. May include washout period.

Sampling and randomization

Sampling of a population is necessary in RCTs because enrolling every patient within a population with a particular disease state or condition in the study is not feasible. Key aspects of sampling are as follows:

- Study participants must be representative of the population to which the results of the study are to be applied.
- Patients enrolled in the study must meet all of the predetermined study inclusion criteria, and conversely, they must not have any of the characteristics listed as exclusion criteria.

FIGURE 10-3. Hierarchy of Literature Evidence

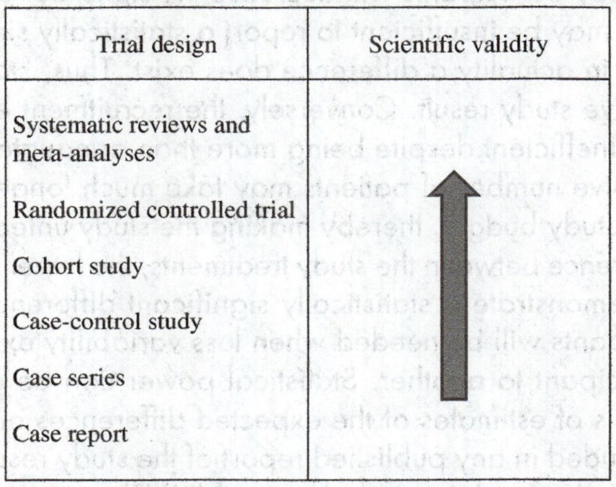

Trial design	Scientific validity
Systematic reviews and meta-analyses	
Randomized controlled trial	
Cohort study	
Case-control study	
Case series	
Case report	

Clinicians should consider the aforementioned inclusion and exclusion criteria when applying the study results to avoid extrapolating those results to patients who may not be representative of the population being evaluated. Alternatively, one can infer that similar findings will be observed in other patients who meet such criteria within the probabilities emanating from inferential statistics used to analyze the study data. One of the basic principles of inferential statistics is that patients sampled from a particular population of interest have an equal chance of being randomized or assigned to one of the study groups or another. As such, systematic error can occur when study participants are not properly randomized into the study groups, which can lead to potentially misleading and incorrectly interpreted study results because of bias in patients being assigned to one group or another. Randomization does not ensure that study participant characteristics (e.g., sex, weight, race) are equally divided between study groups. A process known as *stratification* can be used to accomplish the latter. Stratification is a grouping that occurs before randomization, although grouping of patient characteristics can be performed retrospectively. In this latter instance, the process is often referred to as *subgroup analysis*.

Blinding

In clinical trials, *blinding* refers to the process whereby some or all of the participants are unaware of the treatment being received by the study participants. Blinding is an important strategy for decreasing bias within any clinical trial. The underlying purpose of blinding is that study volunteers or patients may knowingly or unknowingly alter the study outcome data if they know which treatment or treatments they are receiving. Similarly, study investigators may bias data collection on the basis of the perceived benefits of the treatment or the lack of benefits they are observing if they are aware of the treatment the volunteers or patients are receiving or not receiving, respectively. Nevertheless, certain clinical studies may not be suitable for blinding because of safety or ethical concerns (e.g., administration of investigational treatments through compassionate-use protocols, severely ill patients). Regardless of blinding type, the processes must be in place to break the blind if needed for safety reasons. When no blinding is used, studies are referred to as *open-label* trials. Generally accepted blinding definitions are as follows:

- **Single blind:** Patients are unaware of which treatment they are receiving.
- **Double blind:** Neither the study patients nor the investigators are aware of the treatments. This method is the traditional gold standard within clinical research focused on treatment efficacy because this design has the greatest potential for minimizing bias from the study participants and investigators.
- **Triple blind (full blind):** Subjects, investigators as well as all personnel who organize and analyze the study data are blinded.

Sample size

Selection of sample size is an extremely important issue in designing randomized controlled trials. Inadequate numbers of study participants will decrease the statistical power of any clinical trial. In this instance, patient numbers may be insufficient to report a statistically significant difference between the study treatments although in actuality a difference does exist. Thus, *statistical power* is the probability of avoiding a false-negative study result. Conversely, the recruitment of an excessive number of study participants may be very inefficient despite being more than adequately powered statistically. Specifically, recruiting an excessive number of patients may take much longer than is necessary, and it may substantially increase the study budget, thereby making the study unfeasible to conduct. Generally, the greater the expected difference between the study treatments, the fewer the number of study participants who will be needed to demonstrate a statistically significant difference between the groups. Furthermore, fewer study participants will be needed when less variability exists in the study outcomes being measured from one participant to another. Statistical power can be calculated by investigators and biostatisticians on the basis of estimates of the expected differences and variability between the study groups and should be included in any published report of the study results. A related parameter related to sample size is known as the number needed to treat (NNT) to receive a benefit or to prevent a bad outcome for a particular treatment. It is the reciprocal of the absolute risk reduction (ARR) and can be calculated by dividing 100 by the ARR percentage. The ARR is the difference in outcome percentage between the treatment and control group. For example, if patients receive a treatment that reduces the risk of a heart attack from 3% to 1%, the ARR is 3% − 1% = 2%. The NNT to prevent one heart attack would be 100/2 = 50. The value of NNT provides a context for evaluating risk versus benefit of those receiving a given treatment. Yet another valuable parameter is known as the relative risk reduction (RRR). It is calculated by dividing the ARR by the incidence of the event in the control group. In the example above, this the RRR is 3% − 1%/3% = 66.6%

Controls

In the context of RCTs, controls are the comparator to the treatment of interest. In a crossover study design, patients serve as their own control. As previously noted, control groups may receive standard treatments, no treatment, usual care, or a placebo in both RCT crossover and parallel designs. Ideally, the placebo should have dosage form properties (e.g., color, shape, taste) that are identical to the active treatment dosage forms to avoid compromising study blinding. The potential for a "placebo effect" should always be considered. This occurs when the placebo has an effect on the study outcome despite receipt of an inactive substance. Use of placebos may not be suitable for all RCTs because of ethical considerations. In those instances, an active or usual treatment would be used as the control.

Follow-up

Any RCT must follow the study participants over a sufficient period of time to demonstrate adequate safety or efficacy data or both. The length of follow-up is determined by the following:

- The period of time intended for patients to receive the study intervention
- Long-term safety concerns
- The study objectives and outcome measures (e.g., pain scale, overall survival)

During the treatment and follow-up study periods, not all participants may remain in the study. More specifically, participants may drop out of the trial for a number of reasons, and investigators must plan how to handle the partial data in addition to the study sample size determination as previously noted. The 2 major analysis approaches are as follows:

- *Intention to treat:* This method includes all patients as a member of their respective study group, regardless of completion of the protocol since they began the study and were randomized. Data up to the point of withdrawal are used in the analysis.
- *Per protocol:* This method excludes data from participants with significant deviations from the protocol.

Importantly, the 2 analytical techniques are not mutually exclusive. Often investigators will report results from both techniques that allow the reader of the report to compare potential differences directly.

10-5 Pharmacist's Role

Evaluation for Medical Literature

Critical appraisal is an objective, systematic review of medical literature. Such a review is important in the context of caring for patients in a practice care sitting as well as at an institutional level. This could include analyses related to Pharmacy and Therapeutics Committee deliberations, formulary management, etc. The critical appraisal of original research articles can be time consuming; however, the skills required are not difficult to develop and are highly important to pharmacy practitioners.

Critical appraisal of the literature can be broken down into four steps:

- Search the literature for relevant evidence.
- Determine the applicability of the study.
- Evaluate basic study design.
- Critically evaluate the validity of the study results.

The following series of questions will aid in evaluating the design of a clinical trial and the validity of the results:

- Did the trial address a focused research question in terms of the following?
  - Population studied
  - Intervention given
  - Outcomes considered
- Did the authors use the correct type of study design?
- Was the assignment of participants randomized?
- Were all of the participants who entered the trial appropriately accounted for as well as those not enrolled in the study?
- Were participants and study personnel blinded? If not, were appropriate efforts made to blind the study treatments or was there appropriate justification for not blinding?
- Did the groups have similar baseline characteristics at the start of the study?
- Aside from the experimental interventions, were the groups treated equally?
- How large was the treatment effect?
- How precise was the estimate of the treatment effect?
- Can the study results be applied to the local population?
- Were all clinically important outcomes considered?
- Are the benefits worth the harm and costs?

Practicing Evidence-Based Medicine

Evidence-based medicine is the process of finding, appraising, and using contemporaneous research findings systematically. This process then serves as the basis for clinical decisions.

Steps to the Interdisciplinary Practices of Medicine and Pharmacy

The following steps can be applied broadly to the interdisciplinary practice of medicine, including the practice of pharmacy:

- Formulate a clear clinical question from a patient's problem.
- Search the literature for relevant clinical articles.
- Evaluate and critically appraise the evidence for validity usefulness.
- Implement useful findings in clinical practice.

Applying current evidence to clinical practice necessitates critical appraisal of the literature. Incorporating the following into routine practice will aid the reader of medical literature in reaching sound clinical decisions:

- Regularly review and keep up to date with relevant medical literature.
- Familiarize yourself with clinical practice guidelines that apply to your area of practice.
- Critically appraise literature to determine validity of study results and applicability to practice.

10-6   Glossary of Key Clinical Research Terms

Term	Definition
Bias	Systematic error within clinical investigations
Confounding variables	Variables that are not systematically introduced into the study but that may affect the outcome of interest in clinical studies
Randomization	Patients sampled from a particular population of interest have an equal chance of being randomized or assigned to one of the study groups or another
Stratification	Grouping that occurs before randomization based of specific patient characteristics
Blinding	Process whereby some or all of the participants are unaware of the treatment being received by the study participants. Three types: single blind, double blind, triple blind
Open label	No blinding of participants
Statistical power	Probability of avoiding a false-negative study result; largely a function of sample size and variability of differences between study groups
Controls	Comparator group to the treatment group in randomized clinical trials; controls may receive standard treatments, no treatment, usual care, or a placebo
Placebos	Inactive substances often used in clinical drug studies
Intention-to-treat analysis	Analysis that includes all patients as a member of their respective study group regardless of completion of the protocol since they began the study and were randomized
Per-protocol analysis	Analysis that excludes data from participants with significant deviations from the protocol

NAPLEX Competency Statements

The questions in this chapter cover the following 2021 NAPLEX Competency Statements: **AREA 1:** 1.7 **AREA 3:** 3.11.

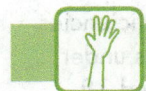 ## 10-7   Questions

1. Which of the following clinical study design characteristics is consistent with a case report?

    A. Observational
    B. Prospective
    C. Randomized
    D. Controlled
    E. Parallel

A study is conducted to determine the safety and efficacy of acetaminophen extended release (ER), 1300 mg orally 3 times daily compared to placebo relieving signs and symptoms of hip or knee osteoarthritis. The 542 patients, aged 60 years of age or older, were randomized to receive 1 of the 2 treatments. Mean pain score changes from baseline were lower for patients in the ER acetaminophen group compared to the placebo group ($P = 0.054$).

2. What is the study design used for this clinical trial?

    A. Case series
    B. Case-control study
    C. Parallel randomized control trial
    D. Crossover randomized control trial
    E. Cohort study

3. Which of the following is a true statement based on the study results in the study above?

A. ER acetaminophen is likely beneficial in patients with rheumatoid arthritis.
B. ER acetaminophen is not superior to placebo at a probability of less than 0.05.
C. Use of a placebo is not an ethical treatment in this study.
D. ER acetaminophen is ineffective in patients with osteoarthritis of the shoulder.
E. ER acetaminophen is likely superior to placebo in patients aged 20 to 50 with hip or knee osteoarthritis.

4. Which of the following statements is *true* regarding observational research design characteristics?

A. Participants are blinded.
B. They can be retrospective or prospective.
C. Randomization of participants is preferred.
D. They establish a causal relationship between variables of interest.
E. Results generally have limited clinical utility.

5. Which of the following research design types are considered experimental research? (Mark all that apply.)

A. Cohort study
B. Questionnaires/surveys
C. Case-control study
D. Randomized controlled trial
E. Retrospective epidemiologic study

6. Which of the following clinical trial designs evaluates intrasubject effects between 2 or more study treatments?

A. Crossover
B. Parallel
C. Case control
D. Case series
E. Cohort

7. Which of the following disease states are suitable for a crossover study design? (Mark all that apply.)

A. Glaucoma
B. Pneumonia
C. Migraine headaches
D. Epilepsy
E. Hypertension

8. Blinding of subjects is an important process within controlled trials to minimize which of the following?

A. Confounding variables
B. Systematic error
C. Bias
D. Variability
E. Sample size

Serum vitamin D concentrations were determined for 1200 non-Hispanic Whites and 1200 non-Hispanic Blacks aged 18 years and older from 2000 to 2006. Concentrations were linked to the average monthly solar ultraviolet light index. Of the non-Hispanic Blacks, 65% were deficient in vitamin D compared to 14.0% of non-Hispanic Whites in the month of January of the study year ($P < .001$).

9. What is the study design used for this clinical trial?

A. Cohort
B. Case control
C. Parallel randomized control
D. Crossover randomized control
E. Case series

10. Which of the following is a true statement based on the study results above?

A. Similar vitamin D deficiencies would be likely in Hispanic adults in January.
B. Normalization of the vitamin D concentrations can be expected in July.
C. Sun exposure during the winter months appears to be higher in adult non-Hispanic Blacks compared with non-Hispanic Whites.
D. A decreased incidence of vitamin D deficiencies can be expected in non-Hispanic Blacks under the age of 18 compared with those aged 18 and above based on greater ultraviolet light exposure.
E. There is no relationship between vitamin D deficiency and race.

11. Randomization is a key process within controlled trials to ensure which of the following?

A. Validity of inferential statistics
B. Avoidance of placebo effect
C. Avoidance of carryover effect
D. Normal distribution of study outcome
E. Maximization of biostatistical power

12. Which group of individuals is unaware of the subject treatment in a double-blind study?

A. Subjects only
B. Subjects and investigators
C. Investigators and data analysis personnel
D. Data analysis personnel and subjects
E. Subjects, data analysis personnel, and investigators

13. Which of the following is *true* regarding sample size in randomized controlled trials?

A. Increased sample size reduces statistical power.
B. Increased sample size is needed for a crossover design versus a parallel design.
C. Decreased sample size is needed when the expected difference in outcome between groups is large.
D. Decreased sample size is needed where large variability exists in the study outcome being measured.
E. Sample size is not a factor affecting statistical power.

14. Which of the following groups can serve as a control in a RCT? (Mark all that apply.)

A. Standard treatment
B. Placebo
C. No treatment
D. Historical
E. Usual care

15. Which of the following are acceptable techniques for managing data from those patients who withdraw from a study before completing the study protocol? (Mark all that apply.)

A. Analyzing the data using an intention-to-treat method
B. Analyzing the data using a per-protocol method with categorization of withdrawal subject characteristics including reason for withdrawal
C. Analyzing the data using both intention-to-treat and per-protocol methods
D. Analyzing the data in a blinded manner
E. Analyzing the data from those subjects completing the protocol following purging of withdrawal subject information from the study database

16. Which of the following are general steps in the critical appraisal of the literature relative to a published study? (Mark all that apply.)

A. Evaluating the validity of the study results
B. Searching for other studies published by the authors
C. Study funding source identification
D. Determining applicability of the study
E. Evaluating the basic study design

17. Which of the following questions aid in evaluating a published clinical trial? (Mark all that apply.)

A. Were all confounding variables avoided in the study?
B. Did the study groups have similar baseline characteristics?
C. How large was the treatment effect?
D. Are the benefits worth the harm and costs?
E. Was the study ethical?

18. Which of the following are essential vehicles for practitioners in keeping up to date with new literature? (Mark all that apply.)

A. Review articles
B. Clinical practice guidelines
C. Google Internet searches
D. Attendance at continuing education courses
E. Case reports

19. Which of the following are potential confounding variables? (Mark all that apply.)

A. Subject age differences
B. Concurrent medications
C. Medical complications that occur during study period
D. Study dropouts
E. Exclusion of patients with severe forms of the disease being studied

20. Which of the following are used to calculate a sample size? (Mark all that apply.)

A. Desired statistical power
B. Estimated effect size
C. Probability of the results affecting clinical practice
D. Variability and experimental error
E. Estimated time to complete the investigation

21. In a randomized controlled trial that follows a parallel design, which of the following is *true*?

A. Patients serve as their own control.
B. All patients end up receiving all of the interventions in random different orders, depending on group assignment.
C. Only patients who complete the entire protocol are included in the final analysis.
D. Patients are assigned to groups that receive a particular treatment over time; the only planned difference in the groups is the intervention.
E. Designs are limited to 2 study treatment arms.

22. The intention-to-treat analysis includes data from which patients?

A. All patients regardless of whether or not they completed the protocol
B. Only patients who complete a specified protocol
C. Only patients who complete the protocol with favorable outcomes
D. Only patients who complete the protocol with unfavorable outcomes
E. Only patients who complete entire trial and follow-up period

23. The major steps to the practice of evidence-based medicine include which of the following? (Mark all that apply.)

A. Formulate a clear clinical question from a patient's problem.
B. Search the literature for relevant clinical articles.
C. Use anecdotal evidence to guide practice for colleagues within an institution.
D. Evaluate and critically appraise the evidence for validity usefulness.
E. Implement useful findings in clinical practice.

A well-controlled, randomized clinical trial found that acute coronary syndrome patients receiving ticagrelor versus prasugrel had reduced primary outcomes of death, nonfatal myocardial infarction, or stroke from 10% to 6%, respectively, at 1 year.

24. What is the relative risk reduction for patients receiving prasugrel compared with ticagrelor?

A. 4%
B. 20%
C. 40%
D. 80%
E. 100%

25. What is the number of patients that need to receive prasugrel versus ticagrelor to prevent death, myocardial infarction, or stroke based on these study results?

A. 5
B. 10
C. 25
D. 50
E. 100

 **10-8   Answers**

1. A. Case reports are always observational. Prospective designs, randomization, and controls are all study design characteristics commonly used with randomized controlled trials and are not associated with case reports. Case reports do not employ a parallel or crossover designs. Therefore, Answers B, C, D, and E are incorrect.

2. C. The study described is a randomized parallel study of acetaminophen ER formulation compared to placebo in a group of patients with osteoarthritis. Patients did not crossover in this study to the other active treatment or placebo; therefore, answer D is incorrect. Also, patients were randomized in this study, which is not performed in a case series, case control, or cohort study (A, B, and E, respectively).

3. B. While patients with osteoarthritis receiving the acetaminophen ER formulation had lower pain scores than patients receiving placebo, the difference did not meet statistical significance probability of less than 0.05. The study design and results do not allow extrapolation to patients with rheumatoid arthritis (A) or those patients with osteoarthritis of the shoulder (D) nor a younger population aged 20 to 50 (E) as all patients in the study were greater than or equal to 60 years of age. The study is ethical because acetaminophen may or may not have a beneficial effect; therefore, C is incorrect.

4. B. Observational studies can be retrospective or prospective. Observational studies are unblinded, lack randomization, and are unable to establish a causal relationship between variables of interest; therefore, A, C, and D are incorrect. Results, however, may have substantial clinical utility despite these limitations. As such, E is incorrect.

5. **D.** Experimental research designs include randomized controlled trials. Cohort studies, case-control studies, questionnaires/surveys, and retrospective epidemiologic studies use observational designs; therefore, A, B, C, and E are incorrect.

6. **A.** Intrasubject effects are analyzed in crossover study designs. Parallel, case series, case-control, and cohort designs analyze intersubject effects; therefore, B, C, D, and E are incorrect.

7. **A, C, D, E.** Crossover study designs can be used only for stable, chronic, or episodic conditions. Glaucoma, migraine headaches, epilepsy, and hypertension meet one or more of these criteria; however, pneumonia is an acute condition and does not meet any of the criteria for a crossover study and is, thus, incorrect

8. **C.** Blinding of subjects is an important process within clinical trials to minimize bias. It does not minimize confounding variables, systematic error, variability, or sample size. A, B, D, and E, therefore, are incorrect.

9. **A.** In this study, serum vitamin D concentrations were prospectively measured in individuals from 2 different ethnic groups, non-Hispanic Whites and non-Hispanic Blacks over time. The key variable was exposure to solar ultraviolet light. This fits the definition of a cohort study. Patients were not matched to a control group; therefore, B is incorrect. Furthermore, individuals received no treatments nor were randomized, which one typically sees in a parallel or crossover study deign rendering C and D incorrect. A case series would be merely descriptive and involve far fewer patient than this study, E is incorrect.

10. **C.** There was a statistically significant deficiency in serum vitamin D concentrations in non-Hispanic Blacks compared to non-Hispanic Whites. This difference was linked to ultraviolet light exposure during the winter month of January. No conclusions can be extrapolated to Hispanic individuals since they were not studied (A). Furthermore, there are insufficient data to know vitamin D concentrations in July (B) or age-related differences, that is, under the age of 18 or 18 years of age and older (D). E is incorrect because race does appear to have a significant effect on vitamin D concentrations, at least during January.

11. **A.** Randomization is a key process within clinical trials to ensure the validity of inferential statistics used in analyzing the study results. It does not avoid the placebo effect, the carryover effect, ensure a normal distribution of the study outcome, or maximize biostatistical power (B, C, D, and E, respectively).

12. **B.** Subjects and investigators are unaware of the subject treatment in a double-blind study. In a single-blind study, only the subjects are unaware of the subject treatment. A triple-blind study refers to the blinding of all persons who come in contact with the study procedures or data; therefore, A, C, D, and E are incorrect.

13. **C.** Decreased sample size is needed when the expected difference in outcome between groups is large. Increased sample size increases statistical power and is needed when there is large variability in the study outcome being measured. Decreased sample size is needed for a crossover study design because patients are serving as their own controls. Sample size is a major factor that impacts statistical power. As such, A, B, D, and E are incorrect.

14. **A, B, C, E.** Randomized controlled trials can use standard treatment, usual care, no treatment, and placebo as controls. Historical controls cannot be used in a randomized clinical trial (D).

15. **A, B, C, D.** Patients who withdraw from a study before completing the study protocol can be managed by analyzing data using an intention-to-treat method or both an intention-to-treat method and a per-protocol method or by categorizing patients according to reason for withdrawal using a per-protocol method. Analyzing data in a blinded manner is not only acceptable but a standard practice. Purging data from the study database upon withdrawal from the study and including only subjects completing the protocol is inappropriate (E).

16. **A, D, E.** General steps in the critical appraisal of the literature relative to a published study include evaluating the validity of the study results, determining applicability of the study, and evaluating the basic study design. Searching for other studies published by the authors is not generally a step in appraising the literature (B) nor focusing on the study funding source (C).

17. **B, C, D.** Asking if the groups have similar baseline characteristics, determining the extent of the treatment effect, and asking if the benefits of the treatment are worth the harm and costs are all aids in

evaluating a clinical trial. Determining if all confounding variables were avoided in a study is not an aid in evaluating a clinical trial (A). Determining if the study meets ethical standards is the duty of the Institutional Review Board before conducting the trial (E).

18. **A, B, D.** Important vehicles for practitioners relative to keeping up to date with new literature include review articles, clinical practice guidelines, and attendance at continuing education events. Google internet searches are problematic to staying current with the literature because of the high degree of source variability (C). Case reports are generally not an important method for keeping up to date with new literature (E).

19. **A, B, C, D.** Potential confounding variables include subject age differences, concurrent medications, medical complications that occur during the study period, and study dropouts. Exclusion of patients with severe forms of the disease being studied is not a confounding variable because it can be controlled (E).

20. **A, B, D.** The desired statistical power, estimated effect size, and variability and experimental error are all used to calculate a sample size. The probability of the results affecting clinical practice is not generally used in calculating sample size (C) and neither is the estimated time to complete the investigation (E).

21. **D.** In a randomized controlled trial that follows a parallel design, patients are assigned to groups that receive a particular treatment over time; the only planned difference in the groups is the intervention. Patients do not serve as their own control (A). In general, patients receive only 1 study treatment depending on group assignment (B) and all patients are accounted for in the final analysis, including patients who do not complete the study protocol (C). Study treatment arms can be 2 or greater in number; therefore, E is incorrect.

22. **A.** The intention-to-treat analysis includes data from all patients regardless of whether they completed the protocol or type of outcome; therefore, B, C, D, and E are incorrect.

23. **A, B, D, E.** Formulating a clear clinical question from a patient's problem, searching the literature for relevant clinical articles, evaluating and critically appraising the evidence for validity usefulness, and implementing useful findings in clinical practice are all steps in the practice of evidence-based medicine. Using colleague anecdotal experience is not a routine element of practicing evidence-based medicine (C).

24. **C.** The absolute risk reduction in this study is the difference in the outcome of death, myocardial infarction, or stroke in those patients receiving ticagrelor (10%) and prasugrel (6%), which is 4% (A). The relative risk reduction is 4%/10% = 40%. The other choices (B, D, E) are incorrect.

25. **C.** The number of patients to prevent the outcome of death, myocardial infarction, or stroke in those receiving prasugrel versus ticagrelor. This number is calculated by dividing 100 by the absolute risk reduction between the 2 treatments or 100/4 = 25. The other choices (A, B, D, E) are incorrect.

10-9   Additional Resources

Aparasu RR, Bentley JP. *Principles of Research Design and Drug Literature Evaluation*. New York, NY: McGraw Hill Education; 2020.

Dawson B, Trapp RG. *Basic and Clinical Biostatistics*. 5th ed. New York, NY: McGraw-Hill; 2020.

Friedman LM, Furberg CD, DeMets DL, Reboussin DM, Granger CB. *Fundamentals of Clinical Trials*. 5th ed. New York, NY: Springer; 2015.

Greenhalgh T. *How to Read a Paper: The Basics of Evidence-Based Medicine*. 5th ed. London: BMJ Books; 2014.

Guyatt GH, Sackett DL, Cook DJ. Users' guides to the medical literature. II. How to use an article about therapy or prevention. *JAMA*. 1994;271(1):59–63.

Rosenberg W, Donald A. Evidence-based medicine: an approach to clinical problem solving. *BMJ*. 1995;310(6987):1122–1126.

Spilker B. *Guide to Clinical Trials*. New York, NY: Lippincott Williams and Wilkins; 1991.

Stroke

A. SHAUN ROWE

 ## 11-1 KEY POINTS

- Stroke is broadly defined as the death of brain cells secondary to a lack of perfusion.
- The primary reasons for a stroke are ischemia and hemorrhage.
- Ischemic stroke can be the result of an embolism, atherosclerosis, or cryptogenic condition.
- Hemorrhagic stroke involves either a hemorrhage in the parenchyma of the brain (i.e., intraparenchymal hemorrhage) or a hemorrhage in the subarachnoid space.
- The onset of symptoms associated with both ischemic and hemorrhagic stroke can be sudden.
- The acronym FAST (Facial drooping, Arm weakness, Speech difficulty, and Time is of the essence) describes many of the primary symptoms associated with stroke.
- Compared to an ischemic stroke, headache and loss of consciousness are more common with hemorrhagic stroke.
- Treatment goals for stroke are prevention of further neurologic injury, prevention of secondary damage, and prevention of reoccurrence of stroke.
- During the acute phase, pharmacotherapy for ischemic stroke focuses on fibrinolysis and pharmacotherapy for hemorrhagic stroke focuses on blood pressure control.
- In the subacute and postacute phases, treatment of ischemic stroke and hemorrhagic stroke secondary prevention are through modification of risk factors.
- Rapid treatment of ischemic stroke with alteplase not only improves the chance of a good outcome after stroke but also increases the risk of hemorrhage.
- Careful evaluation of inclusion and exclusion criteria for alteplase should be undertaken for every patient.
- Secondary prevention involves lifestyle modifications, hypertension and hyper-lipidemia treatment, and comorbid disease state management. All pharmacists can play a key role in the optimization of secondary prevention treatments.

 ## 11-2 STUDY GUIDE CHECKLIST

The following topics may guide your study of this subject area:

- [ ] General symptoms associated with both ischemic and hemorrhagic stroke.
- [ ] General goals of therapy for stroke.
- [ ] Properties of medications used in the acute treatment of ischemic and hemorrhagic stroke.
- [ ] Properties of subacute and post-acute treatment of ischemic and hemorrhagic stroke.
- [ ] Potential adverse drug events associated with medications used during the treatment of stroke.
- [ ] Significant drug–drug interactions associated with medications used during the treatment of stroke.
- [ ] Patient counseling points for the medications used during the treatment of stroke.

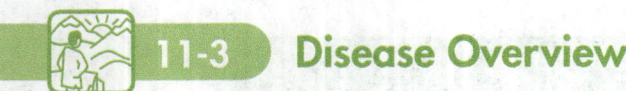

11-3   Disease Overview

Definition

Stroke generally can be defined as the death of brain cells secondary to a lack of perfusion. This lack of perfusion can be caused by a vessel blockage (ischemic stroke) or a vessel rupture (hemorrhagic stroke). Both types of stroke can be further subcategorized based on the etiology of the blockage and the location of the hemorrhage or ischemia.

In the United States, there are 130,000 deaths each year associated with stroke, and approximately 795,000 people experience a stroke each year. Though the incidence of stroke increases with age, the prevalence of stroke in younger people (20 to 64 years of age) is increasing. In 2013, 3,725,085 cases of hemorrhagic stroke and 7,258,216 cases of ischemic stroke occurred worldwide. This prevalence was almost double what was observed in 1990.

In addition, stroke has a significant effect on economic and disability outcomes. In the United States, the cost of care for patients who have experienced a stroke is estimated to be $34 billion yearly. This cost is approximately 1% of the U.S. yearly national health expenditures. Globally, stroke in young patients makes up approximately half of all disability-adjusted life years that are associated with stroke.

Classifications

Ischemic stroke accounts for 87% of strokes and can be secondary to an embolic event (e.g., cardioembolism, prothrombotic state), atherosclerosis, or cryptogenic condition. The remainder of strokes are hemorrhagic. Hemorrhagic strokes can be either intraparenchymal hemorrhages or subarachnoid in origin.

Clinical Presentation

In general, the clinical presentation of an ischemic stroke and the need for quick action can be summarized by the acronym FAST—Facial drooping, Arm weakness, Speech difficulty, and Time is of the essence (Table 11-1). Facial drooping can be minor (flattened nasolabial fold and asymmetry when smiling) to

TABLE 11-1. Clinical Symptoms Associated with Stroke

Type	Symptom
Facial	Partial to complete paralysis occurs on one side of the face that will be more prominent when the patient is smiling or raising his or her eyebrows.
Extremity weakness	Unilateral weakness may affect the arms, legs, or both. The weakness will vary from a mild drift to complete paralysis.
Uncoordinated movements	Limb ataxia may be present in the arms, legs, or both.
Difficulty speaking	Aphasia (inability to express or understand speech) and/or dysarthria (unclear articulation) may occur.
Sensory loss	Sensations may appear dull or different on one side of the body as compared to the other. The patient may not be able to feel touch at all.
Visual change	Partial to complete hemianopia (blindness over half the vision field) may occur.
Vertigo	Dizziness or a feeling of falling may occur. This is particularly true with strokes that affect the brain stem.
Pain	In general, ischemic strokes are not painful, but patients who experience a hemorrhagic stroke tend to report significant headache.

The FAST acronym (Facial drooping, Arm weakness, Slurred speech, Time is important) is suggested by the American Heart and American Stroke Associations as a quick public health reminder of the symptoms associated with stroke.

complete paralysis (unable to move the upper and lower face). Though arm weakness is mentioned in the acronym, both the arms and the legs can be involved. Generally, the observed weakness is unilateral and can vary from being unable to hold up the extremity against gravity to being unable to move it at all. In addition to weakness, patients experiencing a stroke can experience ataxia (uncoordinated movements) in their extremities. Patients can experience both aphasia (inability to speak fluently or comprehend speech) and dysarthria (unusually poor articulation).

In addition to these symptoms, patients who have experienced a hemorrhagic stroke may have additional symptoms. Generally, they have a severe headache. Patients may refer to this as the "worst headache of my life." Also, hemorrhagic stroke is more commonly associated with loss of consciousness and lower levels of consciousness on presentation. Though premorbid hypertension is associated with both ischemic and hemorrhagic stroke, patients who have experienced a hemorrhagic stroke may present for treatment with more severe hypertension.

Pathophysiology and Etiology

Because stroke is a form of vascular disease, many of the risk factors associated with cardiovascular disease also can be associated with stroke. An ischemic stroke is the result of an occlusion in an artery that supplies blood to the brain (Figure 11-1). Table 11-2 lists the modifiable and nonmodifiable risk factors associated with stroke.

Diagnostic Criteria

As previously mentioned, stroke is defined as the presence of cell death owing to lack of perfusion. This condition suggests the need for a tissue-based diagnosis of stroke; however, brain tissue rarely is obtained for such a diagnosis. Rather, the use of magnetic resonance imaging (MRI) is the gold

FIGURE 11-1. Common Cause of Ischemic Stroke: Blood Clot in the Cerebral Artery

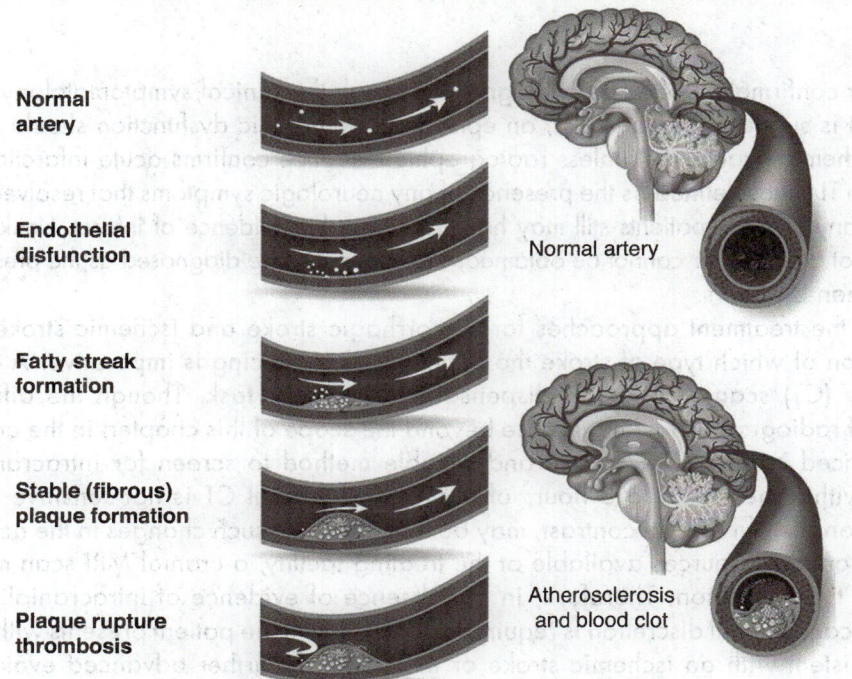

Normal artery

Endothelial disfunction

Normal artery

Fatty streak formation

Stable (fibrous) plaque formation

Atherosclerosis and blood clot

Plaque rupture thrombosis

TABLE 11-2. Risk Factors Associated with Stroke

Risk factor	Type
Modifiable	Hypertension
	Dyslipidemia
	Poor glucose control
	Obesity
	Physical inactivity
	Sleep apnea
	Cigarette smoking
	Excessive alcohol intake
	High-sodium diet
	Atrial fibrillation and other cardiac conditions requiring anticoagulation
	Sickle cell disease
	Migraine with aura
	Oral contraceptive use
	Drug abuse
	Hyperhomocysteinemia
	Acquired and hereditary hypercoagulable states
	Chronic inflammatory conditions
Nonmodifiable	Age
	Low birth weight
	Race and ethnicity (higher risk of stroke for African American and Hispanic/Latino ethnicity)
	Family history of stroke

standard for confirmation of a stroke diagnosis. Though the clinical symptomatology described earlier (Table 11-1) is suggestive of a stroke, an episode of neurologic dysfunction should be classified as a transient ischemic attack (TIA) unless radiographic evidence confirms acute infarction of brain tissue. Previously, a TIA was defined as the presence of any neurologic symptoms that resolved within 24 hours; however, many of those patients still may have radiographic evidence of infarct. Unlike a TIA, if clinical imaging is not available or cannot be obtained, stroke can also be diagnosed as the presence of symptoms for longer than 24 hours.

Because the treatment approaches for hemorrhagic stroke and ischemic stroke are distinct, the determination of which type of stroke the patient is experiencing is imperative. A cranial computed tomography (CT) scan or MRI is indispensable for such a task. Though the differences in these two types of radiographic techniques are beyond the scope of this chapter, in the acute stroke period an unenhanced cranial CT is a fast and reliable method to screen for intracranial hemorrhage. However, within the first 6 to 8 hours of a stroke, a cranial CT is not sensitive enough to detect ischemic changes. An MRI, in contrast, may be able to detect such changes in the acute stroke period. Depending on the resources available at the treating facility, a cranial MRI scan may be difficult to obtain in a timely fashion. Therefore, in the absence of evidence of intracranial hemorrhage in a cranial CT scan, clinical discretion is required to determine if the patient presents with symptomatology that is consistent with an ischemic stroke or that requires further advanced evaluation, such as a cranial MRI scan.

Treatment Principles and Goals

The goal of stroke treatment is the following:

- Prevention of further neurologic injury
- Prevention of secondary damage
- Prevention of reoccurrence of stroke

How these three goals are achieved depends on several variables—namely, the type of stroke the patient has experienced. The treatment approach for each stroke type is radically different in the acute period; however, in the subacute and postacute phases of treatment, many treatment similarities exist.

The acute phase of treatment focuses on the prevention of ongoing damage. In an ischemic stroke, treatment will focus on the lysis and removal of a potential thrombus that is causing ongoing damage. In a hemorrhagic stroke, the acute phase treatment will focus on management of blood pressure and surgical fixation of the bleeding source.

In the subacute and postacute treatment periods, the treatment focus for both hemorrhagic and ischemic stroke becomes similar. Because both hemorrhagic and ischemic stroke share similar risk factors, the focus shifts to secondary prevention techniques such as lifestyle modifications, blood pressure and cholesterol management, and comorbid disease state management.

11-4   Drug Therapy

Thrombolytic Agents

The mainstay of improved outcome poststroke (i.e., living independently with minimal to no deficit) is the rapid identification of stroke and treatment with alteplase, an intravenous (I.V.) fibrinolytic. Currently, no other thrombolytic (e.g., tenecteplase, reteplase, desmoteplase, urokinase) has labeling approved by the U.S. Food and Drug Administration (FDA) for the treatment of acute ischemic stroke and should not be recommended outside the setting of a clinical trial. Treatment with alteplase should be considered for all patients presenting within 4.5 hours of symptom onset. However, a thorough evaluation of the patient for potential contraindications (Table 11-3) to treatment should be completed before the initiation of therapy.

Activase (alteplase)

Mechanism of action

Alteplase, which is a tissue plasminogen activator (TPA), is a protease that rapidly converts plasminogen to plasmin in a thrombus. Thus, it effectively causes thrombolysis of a thrombus. However, it has limited conversion activity in the absence of bound fibrin.

Boxed warnings

- Alteplase has no boxed warning.

Dosing

For acute ischemic stroke, the alteplase dose is 0.9 mg/kg with a maximum dose of 90 mg. The dose is divided: 10% is administered as a bolus and the remainder as a 60-minute infusion. Table 11-3 lists the exclusion criteria for alteplase.

Patient instructions and counseling

- Do not take antiplatelet and anticoagulant agents within 24 hours of administration.
- Alteplase is Pregnancy Category C.
- Excretion in human milk is unknown.

TABLE 11-3. Criteria for Use of Alteplase in the Treatment of Ischemic Stroke

Patients with onset of symptoms in past 3 hours

Exclusion

Time-dependent factors:
- Head trauma—within past 3 months
- Arterial puncture at noncompressible site—within past 7 days
- Intracranial or intraspinal surgery—recent
- Heparin—within 48 hours
- Intracranial hemorrhage, neoplasm, arteriovenous malformation, or aneurysm—any history

Laboratory tests and imaging:
- Platelet count < 100,000/mm^3
- INR > 1.7 or PT > 15 seconds (If no recent use, administration should not be delayed pending laboratory test; however, treatment should be stopped if INR results are above exclusion criteria.)
- Blood glucose < 50 mg/dL
- CT scan significant for multilobar infarction

Physical examination:
- Symptoms of subarachnoid hemorrhage
- Blood pressure > 185/110 mmHg
- Active internal bleeding

Relative exclusion

Rapidly improving stroke symptoms

Pregnancy

Seizure at onset

Major surgery or trauma—within past 14 days

Gastrointestinal or urinary tract bleeding—within past 21 days

Myocardial infarction—within past 3 months

Additional criteria for patients with onset of symptoms between past 3 and 4.5 hours

Relative exclusion

Age greater than 80 years

NIHSS > 25

Ingestion of an oral anticoagulant regardless of INR

History of both diabetes and prior ischemic stroke

INR, international normalized ratio; PT, prothrombin time; NIHSS, National Institutes of Health Stroke Scale.

Adverse drug effects
- Bleeding
- Allergic reactions (anaphylaxis, angioedema, urticaria)

Drug–drug interactions
- No studies of specific drugs
- Anticoagulant: increased bleeding
- Antiplatelet: increased bleeding
- Angiotensin-converting enzyme inhibitors: increased risk of angioedema

Monitoring parameters

During the first 24 hours after administration, patient should be monitored to ensure blood pressure is maintained at less than 180/105 mmHg. In addition, neurological assessments for acute change should be conducted frequently during that time. A radiographic evaluation of the brain (i.e., CT or MRI) should be undertaken 24 hours after alteplase administration and before the initiation of antiplatelet or anti-coagulant medications.

Antihypertensive Agents

Antihypertensive therapy can play an important role in the acute treatment of both ischemic and hemorrhagic stroke. For ischemic stroke, blood pressure management becomes especially important if the patient has received alteplase. Maintaining the blood pressure below 180/105 mmHg decreases the risk of intracranial hemorrhage. Table 11-4 lists the recommended treatment algorithm for hypertensive patients for whom alteplase is being considered. In patients with hemorrhagic stroke, reduction of blood pressure is one of the primary means of reducing rebleeding and hematoma expansion. In addition, during the subacute and postacute treatment periods, reduction of blood pressure to normotensive levels is appropriate in both types of stroke. Because the treatment of hypertension is covered in Chapter 12, this portion of the chapter will focus on the intravenous agents used to treat the acute hypertension associated with stroke and agents specific to the treatment of subarachnoid hemorrhage. See Table 11-5 for dosages and properties of the most used acute I.V. antihypertensive agents.

Dihydropyridine calcium channel blockers

Mechanism of action

Dihydropyridine calcium channel blockers decrease the influx of calcium into cardiac and smooth muscle. Dihydropyridine calcium channel blockers are more selective for smooth muscle than cardiac muscle; therefore, the primary means of blood pressure reduction is through reduction in peripheral vascular resistance (i.e., arterial vasodilation).

Boxed warnings

Dihydropyridine calcium channel blockers has no boxed warning.

Patient counseling

- If the patient has heart failure or aortic stenosis, he or she should talk with a health care provider about changing to an alternate medication.
- Dihydropyridine calcium channel blockers are Pregnancy Category C.
- Excretion in human milk is minimal.

TABLE 11-4. Treatment of Excessive Hypertension When Considering Administration of Alteplase for Ischemic Stroke

Symptom	Treatment
Blood pressure > 185/110 mmHg and patient is otherwise a candidate for alteplase	Consider the use of bolus therapy over continuous infusion as first-line treatment: - Labetalol 10 to 20 mg - Nicardipine 5 mg/h, and titrate 2.5 mg/h every 5 to 15 minutes. - Hydralazine, enalaprilat, and others may be considered when appropriate.
Blood pressure > 180 to 230/105 to 120 mmHg	Consider the use of continuous infusion over bolus therapy as first-line treatment: - Labetalol 10 mg IV, and follow with infusion of 2 to 8 mg/min. - Nicardipine 5 mg/h, and titrate 2.5 mg/h every 5 to 15 minutes.
Unable to control blood pressure with above measure or diastolic blood pressure > 140 mmHg	- Consider sodium nitroprusside.

IV, intravenous.

TABLE 11-5. Commonly Used Intravenous Antihypertensive Agents

Drug	Class or mechanism of action	Route	Dose	Adverse drug reactions
Labetalol	β-blocker/α-blocker	IV push	10 to 20 mg over 1 to 2 minutes, and administer every 10 to 15 minutes.	Orthostatic hypotension
				Nausea
		IV infusion	2 mg/min to 8 mg/min	Dizziness
				Heart failure
				Bradycardia
Nicardipine	Dihydropyridine calcium channel blocker	IV infusion	Initial: 5 mg/h	Headache
			Titration: 2.5 mg/h every 5 to 15 minutes with a maximum dose of 15 mg/h	Hypotension
				Tachycardia
				Angina
				Nausea and vomiting
				Phlebitis
Clevidipine	Dihydropyridine calcium channel blocker	IV infusion	Initial: 1 to 2 mg/h	Headache
			Titration: double dose every 90 seconds to 3 minutes	Hypotension
				Tachycardia
				Angina
				Nausea and vomiting
				Hypertriglyceridemia
Hydralazine	Direct vasodilator	IV push	10 to 20 mg IV q2h prn	Angina
				Edema
				Nausea and vomiting
				Headache
Sodium nitroprusside	Venous and arterial vasodilation	IV infusion	Initial: 0.3 to 0.5 mcg/kg/min	Hypotension
			Titration: 0.5 mcg/kg every few minutes to desired effect	Phlebitis
				Dysrhythmias
			Maximum dose is 10 mcg/kg/min.	Cyanide poisoning
Enalaprilat	ACE inhibitor	IV push	0.625 to 1.25 mg IV q6h	Hyperkalemia
				Angioedema
				Acute kidney injury

ACE, angiotensin-converting enzyme; IV, intravenous.

Adverse drug effects

- Headache
- Hypotension
- Tachycardia
- Angina
- Nausea and vomiting
- Phlebitis

Drug–drug interactions

The 2 most used I.V. agents, clevidipine and nicardipine, have different metabolism pathways, and, therefore, different potential drug–drug interactions. Nicardipine is a substrate and inhibitor of the cytochrome

P450 (CYP450) 3A4 family of isoenzymes, and, therefore, substrates, inducers, and inhibitors of those isoenzymes can cause substantial changes in drug concentrations. Clevidipine does not have significant metabolic drug–drug interactions because it is not dependent on CYP isoenzymes for metabolism and undergoes hydrolysis by plasma and tissue esterase.

Monitoring parameters

Because the I.V. agents have rapid onset of action, careful and frequent monitoring of hemodynamics is required to avoid abrupt or excessive decreases in blood pressure. Because these agents, specifically nicardipine, can cause venous thrombosis, phlebitis, and local irritation, special attention should be paid to the infusion site. Health care providers should consider the need for infusion site changes every 12 hours to avoid such adverse events.

Nimotop and Nymalize (nimodipine)

Nimodipine ⚠ is the only medication labeled by the FDA to improve outcomes associated with subarachnoid hemorrhage. In general, therapy with nimodipine should begin within 96 hours of symptoms and continue for 21 days. The normal dose is 60 mg orally every 4 hours. However, patients who experience hypotension may choose to split the medication as 30 mg every 2 hours to decrease the risk of hypotension.

Mechanism of action

Though nimodipine is a dihydropyridine calcium channel blocker, its mechanism of action related to prevention of ischemic events after subarachnoid hemorrhage is not fully understood.

Patient instructions and counseling
- This medication may cause dizziness. Use caution when standing from a seated or lying position.
- Taking this medication for the full prescribed duration is important. Failure to do so will decrease the chance of having a good outcome.
- If administering nimodipine by a feeding tube, use the oral solution. Puncturing capsules with a needle to administer the liquid inside can lead to serious medication errors and needlestick injuries.
- Nimodipine is Pregnancy Category C.

Adverse drug effects
- Hypotension
- Diarrhea
- Headache
- Nausea

Drug–drug interactions

Because nimodipine is a CYP3A4 substrate, the use of strong inhibitors or inducers may lead to modified nimodipine concentrations. These changes may result in overexposure or underexposure to the medication.

⚠ **Nimodipine** *FDA BOXED WARNING*

Do not administer nimodipine intravenously or by other parenteral routes. Death and serious, life-threatening adverse events have occurred when the contents of nimodipine capsules have been injected parenterally.

Monitoring parameters

Because of the risk of hypotension, routine monitoring of blood pressure during administration of the medication is reasonable.

Labetalol

Mechanism of action

Labetalol is a nonselective, beta-adrenergic receptor antagonist and selective alpha-adrenergic (alpha-1) antagonist. Thus, it not only causes a decrease in cardiac workload but also reduces the systemic vascular resistance.

Boxed warnings

Labetalol has no boxed warning.

Patient instructions

- Avoid abrupt discontinuation, especially if the patient has heart disease, because it may result in angina or myocardial infarction.
- If the patient has heart failure, asthma, or slow heart rate, he or she should talk with a health care provider about changing to an alternate medication.

Adverse drug effects

- Orthostatic hypotension
- Nausea
- Dizziness
- Heart failure
- Bradycardia

Drug–drug interactions

Use of labetalol with other antihypertensive agents may increase the risk of hypotension and bradycardia.

Monitoring parameters

Blood pressure and heart rate should be monitored closely after administration. If use is to be prolonged, liver function tests should be periodically monitored.

Hydralazine

Mechanism of action

The mechanism of action associated with hydralazine is not fully understood; however, it decreases blood pressure through a direct relaxation of vascular smooth muscle. This leads to arterial vasodilation and decreased blood pressure.

Boxed warnings

Hydralazine has no boxed warning.

Patient counseling

- The drug may cause gastrointestinal discomfort such as diarrhea, nausea, and vomiting.
- The drug may cause nasal congestion.
- Report any symptoms of chest pain, palpitations, and shortness of breath to the health care provider.

Adverse drug effects

- Angina
- Edema

- Palpitations
- Tachycardia
- Diarrhea
- Nausea
- Vomiting
- Headache
- Agranulocytosis
- Systemic lupus erythematosus

Drug–drug interactions

Use of hydralazine with other antihypertensive agents may increase the risk of hypotension and bradycardia.

Monitoring parameters

Blood pressure and heart rate should be monitored frequently after administration. If prolonged use, monitoring of complete blood counts and antinuclear antibody titers should be conducted periodically.

Sodium nitroprusside

Mechanism of action

Through a reaction with oxyhemoglobin, sodium nitroprusside ⚠ produces methemoglobin, cyanide, and nitric oxide. The nitric oxide produces vasodilation through cyclic guanosine monophosphate (cGMP). This vasodilation occurs in both the veins and arteries; however, the effect is more pronounced in the veins. Thus, there is a significant reduction in preload with this medication.

Patient counseling

- This drug may cause increases or decreases in heart rate that the patient might feel. In addition, rash, nausea, and abdominal pain are not uncommon with this medication.

Adverse drug effects

- Hypotension
- Toxic epidermal necrolysis
- Metabolic acidosis
- Methemoglobinemia
- Cyanide poisoning

Drug–drug interactions

Sodium nitroprusside should not be used in patients who have taken sildenafil or other phosphodiesterase inhibitors as significant prolonged hypotension may occur.

Monitoring parameters

Blood pressure and heart rate should be monitored continuously while on sodium nitroprusside. If rate of medication exceeds 7 mg/kg/d, consider routine monitoring of plasma thiocyanate levels.

 Sodium nitroprusside *FDA BOXED WARNING*

Sodium nitroprusside may cause precipitous decreases in blood pressure and may lead to irreversible ischemic injuries or death. Continuous blood pressure monitoring is required. Sodium nitroprusside metabolism produces dose-related cyanide and may be lethal. Limit infusions at the maximum rate (10 mcg/kg/min) to the shortest duration possible as patient's ability to buffer cyanide will be exceeded in less than 1 hour at this rate.

Enalaprilat

Mechanism of action

Enalaprilat is an angiotensin converting enzyme (ACE) inhibitor that prevents the conversion of angiotensin I to angiotensin II; thus, leading to vasodilation and decreased aldosterone secretion.

Patient counseling

- This drug may cause nausea, vomiting, and headaches.
- If the patient thinks she is pregnant, she should stop taking this medication and discuss options for treatment of hypertension with a health care provider.
- This mediation may cause a dry cough. The patient should report this to the health care provider.

Adverse drug effects

- Hyperkalemia
- Nausea
- Headache
- Liver failure
- Angioedema

Drug–drug interactions

Use of any ACE inhibitor and aliskiren or sacubitril is contraindicated. Use of ACE inhibitors and mammalian target of rapamycin (mTOR) inhibitors or alteplase increases the risk of angioedema. Use of ACE inhibitors and angiotensin receptor blockers may increase the risk of hypotension. Use of an ACE inhibitor with a potassium sparing diuretic or **potassium** supplement may increase the risk of hyperkalemia.

Monitoring parameters

Blood pressure and heart rate should be monitored closely after administration. Monitor for signs and symptoms of angioedema. Monitor for signs of dry cough. Renal dysfunction can occur in patients soon after starting this medication; thus, monitoring of renal function indices is warranted for weeks after starting this medication.

> ⚠ **Enalaprilat** *FDA BOXED WARNING*
>
> When used in pregnancy during the second and third trimesters, ACE inhibitors can case injury and even death to the developing fetus. When pregnancy is detected, enalaprilat injection should be discontinued as soon as possible.

Antithrombotic Agents

Depending on the etiology of an ischemic stroke, antiplatelet agents or anticoagulant medications will be indicated to prevent a reoccurrence of stroke. In general, patients with atrial fibrillation who experience an embolic stroke will need anticoagulation, whereas patients without atrial fibrillation or other cardiac conditions requiring anticoagulation can be treated with antiplatelet agents. The use of an evaluating tool such as CHADS$_2$ (congestive heart failure, hypertension, age, diabetes, stroke [doubled]) or CHA$_2$DS$_2$-VASc (congestive heart failure, hypertension, age [2 points], diabetes, stroke/TIA/thromboembolism [2 points], vascular disease, sex) can help determine the risk of stroke in patients with atrial fibrillation and further define those patients for whom benefits outweigh the risks of treatment with anticoagulants versus antiplatelet therapy. These medications will not be started in the first 24 hours following thrombolytic administration, but they can be started in the first 24 hours if the patient is not a candidate for thrombolytic therapy. The chronic use of these medications will significantly reduce the chance of a second stroke.

Aspirin

Mechanism of action

Aspirin irreversibly inhibits cyclooxygenase, thereby preventing the conversion of arachidonic acid to thromboxane and platelet aggregation.

Boxed warnings

Aspirin has no boxed warning.

Patient instructions and counseling

- Discuss with a health care provider if experiencing dark tarry stools, coffee ground–like emesis, or other signs of excessive bleeding.
- Discuss with a health care provider any gastric discomfort because this may be sign of ulceration.
- Do not take with a nonsteroidal anti-inflammatory drug (NSAID).
- If the patient has asthma, he or she should consider talking with a health care provider about changing to an alternate medication.

Adverse drug effects

- Gastric ulcers
- Bleeding
- Bronchospasm

Drug–drug interactions

The use of **aspirin** with an NSAID may increase gastric adverse events and decrease the effectiveness of the antiplatelet properties of **aspirin**. The use of **aspirin** with anticoagulants such as **warfarin** or other antiplatelets such as clopidogrel may increase the risk of severe bleeding.

Monitoring parameters

In general, **aspirin** is a well-tolerated medication; however, monitoring for gastric ulceration and tolerability is important.

Aggrenox (aspirin and dipyridamole)

Mechanism of action

As previously discussed, **aspirin** irreversibly inhibits cyclooxygenase. The addition of dipyridamole, a phosphodiesterase and adenosine deaminase inhibitor, increases the antiplatelet effects.

Boxed warnings

Aspirin and dipyridamole have no boxed warnings.

Patient instructions and counseling

- Headaches are a common side effect of this medication. Contact a health care provider if they are intolerable.
- Medication should be taken whole; do not chew or crush. Capsules, however, may be opened so that the **aspirin** can be crushed and the delayed released beads suspended for feeding tube administration.
- Discuss with a health care provider if experiencing dark tarry stools, coffee ground–like emesis, or other signs of excessive bleeding.

- Discuss with a health care provider any gastric discomfort because this may be a sign of ulceration.
- Do not take with an NSAID.
- If the patient has asthma, he or she should consider talking with a health care provider about changing to an alternate medication.
- **Aspirin** and dipyridamole is Pregnancy Category D.

Adverse drug effects
- Headache
- Gastric ulcers
- Bleeding
- Bronchospasm

Drug–drug interactions

The use of **aspirin** and dipyridamole with an NSAID may increase gastric adverse events and decrease the effectiveness of the antiplatelet properties of **aspirin**. The use of **aspirin** and dipyridamole with anti-coagulants such as **warfarin** or other antiplatelets such as clopidogrel may increase the risk of severe bleeding.

Monitoring parameters

In addition to the gastric side effects of **aspirin**, the vasodilatory effects of dipyridamole commonly will cause headaches. Though many patients will be able to tolerate this side effect, it should be monitored and treated if intolerable to the patient.

Plavix (clopidogrel)

Mechanism of action

Clopidogrel ⚠ irreversibly binds the adenosine diphosphate receptor P2Y$_{12}$ on the platelet surface, thereby preventing platelet aggregation.

Patient instructions and counseling
- Discuss with a health care provider if experiencing dark tarry stools, coffee ground–like emesis, or other signs of excessive bleeding.
- Discuss with a health care provider any gastric discomfort because this may be a sign of ulceration.
- Do not take **clopidogrel** with an NSAID.
- **Clopidogrel** is Pregnancy Category B.

Adverse drug effects
- Bleeding
- Hepatitis
- Agranulocytosis
- Thrombotic thrombocytopenia purpura

 Clopidogrel *FDA BOXED WARNING*

Consider the use of another platelet inhibitor in patients identified as poor CYP2C19 metabolizers.

Drug–drug interactions

Because **clopidogrel** is a prodrug that requires conversion to its active form, there is a potential drug–drug interaction with agents that will inhibit CYP2C19. Agents such as **omeprazole** should be substituted with agents that have less effect on CYP2C19. In addition, the use of **clopidogrel** with other antiplatelet and anticoagulant medications will increase the risk of serious bleeding.

Monitoring parameters

Periodic testing of liver function tests is indicated. Consider CYP2C19 genotype testing to ensure the ability to convert **clopidogrel** to its active formulation.

Pletal (cilostazol)

Mechanism of action

Cilostazol ⚠ is a phosphodiesterase inhibitor. It blocks platelet inhibition through an increase in cyclic adenosine monophosphate (cAMP). In addition, as with other phosphodiesterase inhibitors, cilostazol can cause vasodilation.

Patient instructions and counseling

- Cilostazol is a Pregnancy Category C medication, and little information is known about the potential infant risk if used while lactating.
- This medication may cause changes in bowel habits (e.g., diarrhea). Any dark tarry stool should be reported to a health care provider because this may be a sign of bleeding.
- This medication should be taken on an empty stomach (i.e., 30 minutes before a meal or 2 hours after).
- The patient should not use this medication if he or she has heart failure of any severity. Phosphodiesterase inhibitors have been associated with decreased survival in patients with heart failure.

Adverse drug effects

- Peripheral edema
- Diarrhea
- Headache
- Palpitations
- Thrombocytopenia
- Leukopenia

Drug–drug interactions

Use caution with concomitant use of cilostazol and selective serotonin reuptake inhibitors (SSRIs) (e.g., **fluoxetine**, **paroxetine**) because the combination may increase the risk of bleeding. Because cilostazol is a substrate of CYP3A4, the concomitant use of strong inhibitors of CYP3A4 (e.g., clarithromycin, itraconazole, ketoconazole, protease inhibitors) may increase the drug concentrations of cilostazol and necessitate a dose reduction (i.e., 50 mg twice daily). The use of cilostazol is contraindicated in patients taking Adempas (riociguat). The combination may result in an increased risk of hypotension.

 Cilostazol *FDA BOXED WARNING*

Cilostazol is contraindicated in patients with congestive heart failure of any severity.

Monitoring parameters

Perform periodic monitoring of complete blood counts for thrombocytopenia and leukopenia.

Warfarin

Mechanism of action

Warfarin is an inhibitor of the vitamin K$_1$ epoxide reductase; therefore, at therapeutic concentrations, it prevents hepatic production of fully carboxylated vitamin K–dependent clotting factors (factors VII, IX, X, and II).

Patient instructions and counseling

- **Warfarin** is contraindicated in pregnancy unless there is a clear benefit of use as compared to the risk. In general, **warfarin** is probably safe to use while lactating.
- Because of the effect of vitamin K on **warfarin**, eat a diet with a consistent amount of vitamin K–containing foods (e.g., green leafy vegetables, broccoli, cabbage).
- Avoid the use of alcohol while taking this medication.
- Before starting a new prescription or over-the-counter medication, consult with the pharmacist about potential drug–drug interactions.
- Promptly report signs and symptoms of significant bleeding to a health care professional.
- Take the medication on a regular schedule.
- Regular monitoring is required. The patient should talk with the health care provider about how often he or she should have a blood test for monitoring drug.

Adverse drug effects

- Bleeding
- Potential for hypercoagulable state during initiation of medication

Drug–drug interactions

Warfarin is a substrate of many CYP enzymes. Primarily, it is metabolized through the CYP2C9 isoenzyme; however, CYP2C19, CYP2C18, CYP1A2, and CYP3A4 are also significantly involved with metabolism of **warfarin**. Thus, any inhibitors (e.g., amiodarone, statins, clarithromycin, systemic azole antifungals, fluoroquinolones, valproic acid, sulfamethoxazole) or inducers (e.g., carbamazepine, phenytoin, rifampin, ritonavir, modafinil) of these isoenzymes can significantly affect the narrow therapeutic range for **warfarin**. Increased INR monitoring should, therefore, occur with the initiation or discontinuation of interacting medications. In addition, antibiotics can disrupt the synthesis of vitamin K in the gastrointestinal tract by altering the normal flora that produce vitamin K.

Monitoring parameters

On initiation of therapy, daily monitoring of INR until in therapeutic range is indicated. The therapeutic range will depend on the indication for **warfarin**, but the most common INR target range is 2 to 3. Once the patient has a constantly stable INR in the therapeutic range, monitoring can be reduced gradually to every 3 months. In females of child-bearing age, a negative pregnancy test should be confirmed before the initiation of **warfarin**.

⚠ **Warfarin** *FDA BOXED WARNING*

Warfarin can cause major or fatal bleeding. Routine international normalized ratio (INR) monitoring should be performed on all patients.

Novel oral anticoagulants

Mechanism of action

The novel oral anticoagulants (NOACs) include both the oral direct thrombin inhibitor Pradaxa (dabigatran) and the oral factor Xa inhibitors Eliquis (**apixaban**), Savaysa (edoxaban), and Xarelto (rivaroxaban). In general, these medications disrupt the coagulation cascade through the reversible inhibition of either thrombin or factor Xa.

Patient instructions and counseling

- Promptly report any signs and symptoms of significant bleeding (e.g., dark tarry stools, blood in urine, incessant nosebleed).
- Avoid abrupt discontinuation of medication, and do not stop taking this medication without consulting a health care provider.
- A missed dose should be taken the same day.
- Take dose at the same time every day.
- **Apixaban** is Pregnancy Category B. All others are Pregnancy Category C.

Adverse drug effects

- Dabigatran: dyspepsia and gastritis
- Bleeding
- Potential allergic reactions

Drug–drug interactions

As with all anticoagulants, the use of other antithrombotic medications or agents with antithrombotic properties (e.g., NSAIDs) may increase the risk of bleeding. Use of NOACs with strong inhibitors of the P-glycoprotein transport system (e.g., itraconazole, quinidine, amiodarone) may increase drug concentrations, and concomitant use should occur only with caution.

Monitoring parameters

Unlike **warfarin**, NOACs do not require routine therapeutic monitoring. However, the periodic evaluation of laboratory tests for renal function changes is reasonable. Of note, Pradaxa (dabigatran) should be dispensed in its original bottle. Pradaxa should be used within 4 months of opening the manufacturer's bottle or blister package.

> ⚠ **Novel oral anticoagulants (NOACs)** *FDA BOXED WARNING*
>
> - Premature discontinuation of dabigatran, **apixaban**, rivaroxaban, and edoxaban increases the risk of thromboembolic events.
> - Spinal and epidural hematoma may occur when receiving neuraxial anesthesia or undergoing spinal procedures.
> - With edoxaban, there is reduced efficacy in nonvalvular atrial fibrillation patients with creatinine clearance greater than 95 mL/min.

11-5   Pharmacist's Role

The pharmacist's role in the management of patients with stroke occurs across the continuum of care. Pharmacists are involved from the initial care of patients who present to the emergency department with stroke-like symptoms all the way to care of patients in an outpatient setting. While in the hospital, pharmacists are involved with the initial screening and administration of thrombolysis for stroke patients, ensuring that patients receive the most appropriate medications given comorbidities that may complicate stroke treatment. In the outpatient setting, pharmacist education can help patients with medication adherence. In addition, pharmacists ensure that potential drug–drug and drug–disease state interactions do not complicate the care of the patient who has experienced a stroke.

NAPLEX Competency Statements

The questions in this chapter cover the following 2021 NAPLEX Competency Statements: **AREA 1:** 1.1; 1.2; 1.3; 1.4; 1.5; 1.6; 1.7 **AREA 2:** 2.1; 2.2 **AREA 3:** 3.1; 3.2; 3.3; 3.4; 3.5; 3.6; 3.7; 3.8; 3.9; 3.10; 3.11; 3.12 **AREA 5:** 5.5.

 **11-6** Questions

Use the following case study to answer Questions 1–3.

A 72-year-old man presents to the emergency department with complaints of right arm weakness and difficulty speaking. His wife reports that the symptoms started 1 hour ago. His past medical history is significant for hypertension, diabetes mellitus type 2, hypercholesterolemia, and atrial fibrillation. His medications include the following:

- Simvastatin 10 mg orally daily
- Warfarin 5 mg daily
- Lisinopril 10 mg daily
- Metformin 500 mg twice daily

The patient does not smoke or drink. His wife states that he had been holding his warfarin for the past 10 days for a dental procedure and that he had a stable INR of 2.2 to 2.6 for the past year. His current weight is 120 kg. His wife denies that he lost consciousness when the symptoms began. He has not had any recent procedures and denies any history of gastrointestinal and urinary bleeding.

1. The most likely cause of his arm weakness and difficulty speaking is _____.

A. an ischemic stroke
B. a hemorrhagic stroke
C. a seizure
D. a psychiatric condition
E. orthopedic injury

2. If the patient is diagnosed with an ischemic stroke, what other information must you have before administering alteplase?

A. Results of a cranial CT scan to rule out bleeding
B. Results of a cranial CT scan to confirm stroke
C. INR result
D. Confirmation of no seizure at onset of symptoms
E. MRI results to confirm stroke

3. What dose of alteplase should the patient receive if he is an appropriate candidate for fibrinolytic therapy?

A. 10.8 mg bolus over 1 minute with 97.2 mg over 60 minutes
B. 108 mg over 60 minutes
C. 9 mg bolus over 1 minute with 81 mg over 60 minutes
D. 90 mg bolus over 1 minute
E. 0.25 mg/kg bolus over 1 minute

4. In a patient who presents with an aneurysmal subarachnoid hemorrhage, which of the following medications has been shown to reduce the risk of delayed cerebral infarction?

A. Nicardipine
B. Verapamil
C. Nimodipine
D. Amlodipine
E. Hydralazine

5. When considering a patient for alteplase therapy, which medication is recommended as an initial treatment to achieve a blood pressure less than 185/110 mmHg?

A. Esmolol
B. Carvedilol
C. Metoprolol
D. Labetalol
E. Enalapril

6. A patient comes to your pharmacy with a prescription for Aggrenox. Which of the following is an appropriate counseling point?

A. Take on an empty stomach.
B. Do not open or crush a capsule.
C. Aggrenox may cause a headache.
D. Do not take with acetaminophen.
E. Do not take with anticoagulants.

7. Which of the following medications has a significant drug–drug interaction with warfarin?

A. Aspirin
B. Fluconazole
C. Acetaminophen
D. Atorvastatin
E. Water

8. Which of the following medications would be appropriate for the secondary prevention of stroke in a 75-year-old patient with hypertension and atrial fibrillation as a result of mitral stenosis (valvular damage)?

A. Aspirin
B. Pradaxa
C. Apixaban
D. Warfarin
E. Aggrenox

9. Which of the following would be the most appropriate counseling point for a patient prescribed Xarelto 20 mg orally daily?

A. Do not crush.
B. Take at the same time every day.
C. Take on an empty stomach.
D. If a dose is missed wait, until the next dose is due and take double the dose.
E. Do not take with aspirin.

10. Which of the following is a blood test used to monitor Eliquis?

A. aPTT
B. INR
C. PT
D. ACT
E. None of the above

11. Which of the following is a blood test used to monitor warfarin?

A. aPTT
B. INR
C. PT
D. anti-Xa level
E. None of the above

12. In a patient with a stroke secondary to atherosclerotic disease, who is not a candidate for fibrinolysis, how long should you wait from the time of symptom onset before starting an antiplatelet agent?

A. 12 hours
B. 24 hours
C. As soon as possible
D. Up to 2 weeks
E. 2 months

13. Which of the following is a modifiable risk factor for stroke?

A. Age
B. Obesity
C. Low birth weight
D. Family history of stroke
E. Family history of heart disease

14. Which medication has FDA approval for the treatment of ischemic stroke?

A. Streptokinase
B. Tenecteplase
C. Alteplase
D. Urokinase
E. Gentamicin

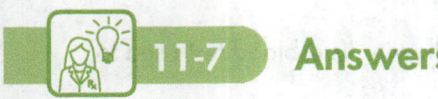

11-7   Answers

1. **A.** All the conditions should be considered in the differential diagnosis of this patient; however, based on his presenting symptoms, ischemic stroke is the most likely cause of his symptoms. Though the patient is taking warfarin, which increases his risk of intracerebral hemorrhage, he has not been taking the medication for the past 10 days. Seizure and psychiatric conditions can mimic a stroke, but the patient has no reported history of either condition.

2. **A.** A CT scan is not used to confirm stroke, but it is used to confirm there is no intracranial hemorrhage. Absence of intracranial hemorrhage must be confirmed before the administration of alteplase. Though the patient is taking warfarin, he has not taken the medication recently. Therefore, one would not need to delay alteplase administration to confirm his INR is less than 1.7. A seizure with stroke symptoms is only a relative contraindication.

3. **C.** Alteplase is given as 0.9 mg/kg of absolute body weight. Regardless of the patient's weight, the maximum dose is 90 mg. Ten percent of the dose is administered over 1 minute, and the remainder of the dose is administered over 60 minutes.

4. **C.** Nimodipine is the only FDA-approved medication for the prevention of delayed cerebral infarction in patients with aneurysmal subarachnoid hemorrhage.

5. **D.** Labetalol is a rapidly acting intravenous beta blocker with some alpha activity. It is recommended as a first-line treatment of excessive hypertension in a patient who would otherwise be a candidate for alteplase.

6. **C.** One of the most common side effects of Aggrenox (aspirin and dipyridamole) is headache. Aggrenox can be taken with or without food. The capsule can be opened with the aspirin inside crushed and extended release dipyridamole suspended for administration by a nasogastric tube or in apple sauce for patients with difficulty swallowing. There is no contraindication with taking it with acetaminophen.

7. **B.** Though aspirin can increase the risk of bleeding with warfarin, it has no significant drug–drug interaction if the combination of these medications is needed. Azole antifungals should be used with great caution in patients who are taking warfarin. There is no significant drug–drug interaction with acetaminophen or atorvastatin.

8. **D.** The patient has a $CHADS_2$ score of 4 placing him at high risk of recurrent stroke. He would benefit from the use of anticoagulation over antiplatelet therapy alone. NOACs are not indicated in those patients with valvular atrial fibrillation.

9. **B.** NOACs should be taken at approximately the same time every day. Dabigatran is the only NOAC that should not be crushed. Xarelto at doses above 10 mg should be taken with food. If a dose is missed, it should be taken as soon as possible in the same day. A dose should not be doubled if a missed dose is not remembered on the same day.

10. **D.** Though it is reasonable to monitor a chemistry panel to assess changes in renal function that may cause apixaban accumulation, there are no routine blood tests for apixaban.

11. **B.** In general, the INR is the standardized measure used to monitor warfarin. The INR is calculated based on a patient's PT, but the PT is not standardized and will vary in accordance with the method and lab test used. Thus, it is not a reliable measure used routinely to monitor warfarin.

12. **C.** If the patient does not receive fibrinolytic therapy, antiplatelet therapy should be started as soon as possible.

13. **B.** All the items listed are risk factors for stroke, but obesity is the only modifiable risk factor.

14. **C.** Alteplase is the only fibrinolytic with FDA approval for the treatment of ischemic stroke.

 **11-8   Additional Resources**

Baker WL, Marrs JC, Davis LE, et al. Key articles and guidelines in the primary prevention of ischemic stroke. *Pharmacotherapy.* 2013;33(6):e101–114.

Baker WL, Marrs JC, Davis LE, et al. Key articles and guidelines in the acute management and secondary prevention of ischemic stroke. *Pharmacotherapy.* 2013;33(6):e115–142.

Broderick JP, Jauch EC, Derdeyn CP. American Stroke Association Stroke Council update. *Stroke.* 2014;45:e5–7.

Centers for Disease Control and Prevention, National Center for Chronic Disease Prevention and Health Promotion, Division for Heart Disease and Stroke Prevention. Stroke facts. Available at: www.cdc.gov/stroke/facts.htm.

Connolly ES Jr, Rabinstein AA, Carhuapoma JR, et al. Guidelines for the management of aneurysmal subarachnoid hemorrhage: a guideline for healthcare professionals from the American Heart Association/American Stroke Association. *Stroke.* 2012;43(6):1711–1737.

Diringer MN, Bleck TP, Hemphill JC 3rd, et al. Critical care management of patients following aneurysmal subarachnoid hemorrhage: recommendations from the Neurocritical Care Society's Multidisciplinary Consensus Conference. *Neurocrit Care.* 2011;15(2):211–240.

Hemphill JC 3rd, Greenberg SM, Anderson CS, et al. Guidelines for the management of spontaneous intracerebral hemorrhage: a guideline for healthcare professionals from the American Heart Association/American Stroke Association. *Stroke.* 2015;46:2032–2060.

Kernan WN, Ovbiagele B, Black HR, et al. Guidelines for the prevention of stroke in patients with stroke and transient ischemic attack: a guideline for healthcare professionals from the American Heart Association/American Stroke Association. *Stroke.* 2014;45(7):2160–2236.

Meschia JF, Bushnell C, Boden-Albala B, et al. Guidelines for the primary prevention of stroke: a statement for healthcare professionals from the American Heart Association/American Stroke Association. *Stroke.* 2014;45(12):3754–3832.

Powers WJ, Rabinstein AA, Ackerson T, et al. Guidelines for the early management of patients with acute ischemic stroke: 2019 update to the 2018 guidelines for the early management of acute ischemic stroke: a guideline for healthcare professionals from the American Heart Association/American Stroke Association. *Stroke.* 2019;50:e344–e418.

Hypertension

BENJAMIN N. GROSS

12-1 KEY POINTS

- Blood pressure is categorized into 4 levels: normal, elevated, stage 1, or stage 2 hypertension. Elevated blood pressure is defined as a systolic blood pressure (SBP) 120 to 129 mmHg but with diastolic blood pressure (DBP) < 80 mmHg. Stage 1 hypertension is defined as a SBP between 130 and 139 mmHg or a DBP between 80 and 89 mmHg. Stage 2 hypertension is defined by SBP ≥ 140 mmHg or DBP ≥ 90 mmHg.
- Secondary causes of hypertension include renal parenchymal or renovascular disease, primary aldosteronism, obstructive sleep apnea, Cushing's syndrome, pheochromocytoma, hypothyroidism, hyperthyroidism, aortic coarctation, and drugs (steroids and estrogens, alcohol, cocaine, cyclosporine and tacrolimus, sympathomimetics, erythropoietin, licorice, monoamine oxidase inhibitors, tricyclic antidepressants, and nonsteroidal anti-inflammatory drugs).
- American College of Cardiology/American Heart Association (ACC/AHA) recommends similar treatment goals for all hypertensive populations.
- Thiazide diuretics, angiotensin converting enzyme inhibitors (ACEIs), angiotensin II receptor blockers (ARBs), or calcium channel blockers (CCBs) are considered the initial agent for treatment of hypertension for patients who are not Black.
- ACC/AHA considers thiazide diuretics and CCBs equivalent choices as initial therapy for hypertension in Black patients.
- ACC/AHA recommends ACEIs or ARBs alone or in combination with other drug classes in all patients with chronic kidney disease regardless of race and diabetes status.
- The classification and treatment of hypertensive urgencies and emergencies is determined by the presence or absence of acute target organ damage and not by blood pressure.
- All causes for inadequate response should be addressed before additional agents are added to a patient's antihypertensive regimen (i.e., pseudoresistance, nonadherence, volume overload, drug-related causes, associated conditions, and secondary causes of hypertension).

12-2 STUDY GUIDE CHECKLIST

The following topics may guide your study of this subject area:

- ☐ Proper BP measurement technique.
- ☐ Risk factors for hypertension.
- ☐ Secondary causes of hypertension with emphasis on drug-induced causes.
- ☐ General sense of lifestyle practices in management of hypertension with particular focus on the DASH (Dietary Approaches to Stop Hypertension) diet.
- ☐ Considerations for selection of antihypertensive drugs based on a patient's condition and prior drug experience.
- ☐ Actions of various categories of antihypertensive drugs.
- ☐ Trade names and available dosage forms, particularly of the "Top 100 Drugs."
- ☐ Frequency of dosing regimen.
- ☐ Major adverse drug reactions of antihypertensive drugs.
- ☐ Significant drug interactions of antihypertensive drugs.
- ☐ Any unique patient counseling points for specific antihypertensive drugs.
- ☐ Indications for drugs to treat hypertensive emergencies and urgencies.

12-3   Disease Overview

In the United States, 108 million (45%) adults are affected by hypertension. Onset most commonly occurs in the third to fifth decades of life, and the lifetime risk of hypertension is 90% for those surviving to age 80 years. Only 1 in 4 adults with high blood pressure have the condition under control. Half of adults with blood pressure ≥140/90 mmHg aren't prescribed or aren't taking medication despite the fact the individual should be taking medication for hypertension.

Classification

Blood pressure is categorized into 4 levels: normal, elevated, stage 1 or stage 2 hypertension (Table 12-1).

Clinical Presentation and Complications

Many individuals with uncontrolled hypertension are asymptomatic. Some individuals, however, may present with a number of cardiovascular effects including left ventricular hypertrophy, congestive heart failure (CHF), peripheral arterial disease, angina pectoris, myocardial infarction (MI), or sudden death. Individuals also may present with nephropathy, renal failure, transient ischemic attacks, stroke, retinal hemorrhage, retinopathy, or blindness.

Pathophysiology and Etiology

Cardiac output and peripheral resistance are important determinants of arterial pressure. Cardiac output is determined by stroke volume and heart rate. Stroke volume is determined by myocardial contractility. Peripheral resistance is determined by changes in small arteries and arterioles. The following factors are involved in regulation of both normal and elevated blood pressure.

Sympathetic nervous system activation

Central activation

Presynaptic alpha-2 stimulation is a negative feedback mechanism, leading to decreased norepinephrine release. Presynaptic beta stimulation leads to increased norepinephrine release.

Peripheral activation

Beta-1 stimulation leads to increased heart rate and contractility, causing increased cardiac output. Beta-2 stimulation leads to arterial vasodilation. Beta stimulation also causes increased renin release, resulting in increased angiotensin II production. Alpha-1 stimulation leads to arterial and venous vasoconstriction.

TABLE 12-1. Blood Pressure Categories

BP category	Systolic blood pressure		Diastolic blood pressure
Normal	≤120 mmHg	and	≤80 mmHg
Elevated	120 to 129 mmHg	and	<80 mmHg
Stage 1 hypertension	130 to 139 mmHg	or	80 to 89 mmHg
Stage 2 hypertension	≥140 mmHg	or	≥90 mmHg

Renin–angiotensin–aldosterone system

Decreased renal perfusion pressure causes increases in renin levels. Renin reacts with angiotensinogen to produce angiotensin I (AT-I). Angiotensin-converting enzyme (ACE) causes AT-I to become angiotensin II (AT-II). AT-II is a potent vasoconstrictor and stimulates aldosterone release, which increases sodium and fluid retention.

Water and sodium retention

Increased fluid volume causes increased cardiac output, which causes increased blood pressure (BP) acutely. Chronically, excess intracellular sodium causes vascular hypertrophy, which increases vascular resistance and response to vasoconstriction and, in turn, increases BP.

Etiology

Primary (essential) hypertension is found in 85% to 95% of all hypertension cases. The cause is unknown. Secondary hypertension is a result of other medical conditions, which could include any of the following: renal parenchymal or renovascular disease, primary aldosteronism, obstructive sleep apnea, Cushing's syndrome, pheochromocytoma, hypothyroidism, hyperthyroidism, or aortic coarctation. Medications may play a role in causing secondary (drug-induced) hypertension and making BP more difficult to control. Drug-induced hypertension has many causes (Box 12-1).

Diagnostic Criteria

Diagnosis and treatment begin with proper BP measurement, assessment, and follow-up planning (Table 12-2). The patient should avoid ingesting caffeine and smoking for 30 minutes before BP measurement and should be resting for 5 minutes before BP measurement. BP is measured as follows:

- Position arm (brachial artery) at heart level.
- Uncover arm; do not put cuff over clothes.
- Determine proper size cuff (Box 12-2).
- Position cuff 1 inch above antecubital crease.
- Ask patient about previous readings.
- Place stethoscope over brachial artery (medial to the center).
- Inflate cuff rapidly to approximately 30 mmHg above previous readings.
- Deflate cuff slowly.
- Remember to deflate cuff completely when done.

> **BOX 12-1. Causes of Drug-induced Hypertension**

- Steroids and estrogens (including oral contraceptives)
- Alcohol
- Cocaine
- Cyclosporine and tacrolimus
- Amphetamines
- Decongestants
- Caffeine
- Erythropoietin
- Licorice (in chewing tobacco)

- Monoamine oxidase inhibitors (MAOIs)
- Tricyclic antidepressants (TCAs)
- Serotonin norepinephrine reuptake inhibitors (SNRIs)
- Atypical antipsychotics
- Nonsteroidal anti-inflammatory drugs (NSAIDs)
- Angiogenesis inhibitors
- Tyrosine kinase inhibitors
- Herbal supplements: Ma Huang, St. John's Wort

TABLE 12-2. Recommendations for Follow-up Based on Initial BP Measurements for Adults

Initial BP (mmHg)[a]		
Systolic	Diastolic	Recommended follow-up
<120	<80	Reassess in 1 year.
120 to 129	>80	Reassess in 3 to 6 months.
130 to 139	80 to 89	Reassess in 1 month.
≥140	≥90	Reassess in 1 month.

a. If systolic and diastolic readings are different, follow recommendations for shorter time to follow-up (e.g., a person with a reading of 160/86 mmHg should be evaluated or referred to source of care within 1 month).

- Wait 1 to 2 minutes before repeating.
- Take pressure in both arms.
- If orthostatic hypotension is suspected, take BP while patient is sitting, standing, and supine.
- If 2 readings are taken at least 2 minutes apart, average the readings.
- If readings differ by >5 mmHg, take additional readings.

Treatment Principles and Goals

Table 12-3 outlines some important treatment principles involving secondary cause of hypertension which can impact response to treatment. Other treatment goals include reducing end-organ damage, minimizing or controlling other risk factors of CV disease, and maintaining BP (with minimal side effects) at or below the level appropriate for the patient's risk.

Monitoring and Evaluation

The initial evaluation of a patient with hypertension has the following goals: to identify known causes of high BP; to assess the presence or absence of target-organ damage and CV disease, the extent of disease, and the patient's response to therapies; and to identify other CV risk factors or concomitant disorders that may affect prognosis and guide therapy (Box 12-3).

The patient's history should be considered in the initial evaluation. History should include duration and levels of elevated BP; family history of hypertension, premature coronary heart disease (CHD), stroke, diabetes, dyslipidemia, or renal disease; history or symptoms of CHD, heart failure, cerebrovascular disease, pulmonary vascular disease, diabetes mellitus, renal disease, or dyslipidemia; and symptoms suggesting the cause of hypertension.

BOX 12-2. Blood Pressure Measurement Cuff Size Requirements

Upper arm circumference	Cuff size required
16 to 22 cm	Pediatric cuff
22 to 26 cm	Small adult cuff
27 to 34 cm	Adult cuff
35 to 44 cm	Large adult cuff
45 to 52 cm	Adult thigh

TABLE 12-3. Identifiable Causes, Diagnostic Tests, and Clinical Findings for Secondary Hypertension

Cause or diagnosis	Diagnostic test (clinical finding)
Chronic kidney disease	Estimated GFR (abdominal or flank mass for polycystic kidney disease)
Coarctation of the aorta	CT angiography (delayed or absent femoral pulse)
Cushing's syndrome and other glucocorticoid excess states, including chronic steroid therapy	History; dexamethasone suppression test (truncal obesity, moon facies, buffalo hump, abdominal striae, and hirsutism)
Drug-induced or drug-related condition	History, drug screening
Pheochromocytoma	24-hour urinary metanephrine and normetanephrine testing (headache, palpitations, and sweating)
Primary aldosteronism and other mineralocorticoid excess states	24-hour urinary aldosterone level or specific measurements of other mineralocorticoids (hypokalemia)
Renovascular hypertension	Doppler flow study; magnetic resonance angiography (abdominal bruit)
Sleep apnea	Sleep study with oxygen saturation (obesity, snoring, and fatigue during wake time)
Thyroid or parathyroid disease	Thyroid-stimulating hormone, serum parathyroid hormone (goiter, hypercalcemia)

CT, computed tomography; GFR, glomerular filtration rate.

BOX 12-3. Cardiovascular Risk Factors

Major Risk Factors

- Hypertension[a]
- Cigarette smoking
- Obesity[a] (body mass index ≥30 kg/m^2)
- Physical inactivity
- Dyslipidemia[a]
- Diabetes mellitus[a]
- Microalbuminuria or estimated GFR <60 mL/min
- Age (>55 years for men, >65 years for women)
- Family history of premature cardiovascular disease (men age <55 years, women age <65 years)

Target Organ Damage

Heart

- Left ventricular hypertrophy
- Angina or prior MI
- Prior coronary revascularization
- Heart failure

Brain

- Stroke or transient ischemic attack

Kidney

- Chronic kidney disease
- End-stage renal disease

Vascular System

- Peripheral arterial disease

Eyes

- Retinopathy

Adapted from JNC-7 Express, National Heart, Lung, and Blood Institute, 2003.
GFR, glomerular filtration rate.
a. Components of the metabolic syndrome.

BOX 12-4. General Guidelines to Improve Patient Adherence to Antihypertensive Therapy

- Be aware of signs of patient nonadherence to antihypertensive therapy.
- Establish the goal of therapy: to reduce blood pressure to nonhypertensive levels with minimal or no adverse effects.
- Educate patients about the disease, and involve them and their families in its treatment. Have them measure blood pressure at home.
- Maintain contact with patients; consider telecommunication.
- Keep patient's care inexpensive and simple.
- Encourage lifestyle modifications.
- Counsel patient to integrate pill taking into routine activities of daily living.

- Prescribe medications according to pharmacologic principles, favoring long-acting formulations.
- Be willing to stop unsuccessful therapy and try a different approach.
- Anticipate adverse effects. Adjust therapy to prevent, minimize, or ameliorate side effects.
- Continue to add effective and tolerated drugs, stepwise, in sufficient doses to achieve the goal of therapy.
- Encourage a positive attitude about achieving therapeutic goals.
- Consider using nurse case management.

Adapted from JNC-7 Express, National Heart, Lung, and Blood Institute, 2003.

Other items to consider in the patient's history include the following:

- Recent weight changes, physical activity levels, or smoking or other tobacco use
- Dietary assessment of intake of sodium, alcohol, saturated fat, and caffeine
- Complete medication history, including prescription, over-the-counter, and herbal or natural products that may increase BP or decrease effectiveness of antihypertensive agents
- Results and adverse effects of previous antihypertensive therapy
- Psychosocial and environmental factors that may influence hypertension control

Necessary routine laboratory tests include urinalysis; complete blood count (CBC); blood chemistries (sodium, potassium, creatinine, blood urea nitrogen [BUN], and glucose); creatinine clearance; fasting lipid profile: total cholesterol, triglycerides, high-density lipoprotein (HDL), and low-density lipoprotein (LDL); and electrocardiogram (ECG).

Follow-up evaluation

Follow-up evaluation includes any of the previous exams completed during the initial evaluation that are required to monitor both response to and possible adverse effects from prescribed antihypertensive therapies, in addition to the assessment of any new symptoms of target organ damage and the assessment of patient adherence to therapy (Box 12-4).

12-4   Nondrug Therapy

Lifestyle modifications are recommended to improve both BP and overall cardiovascular health (Table 12-4). Research has shown that the DASH (Dietary Approaches to Stop Hypertension) diet, which is rich in fruits, vegetables, and low-fat dairy foods and has reduced saturated and total fats, significantly lowers BP.

12-5   Drug Therapy

All patient factors (severity of BP elevation, presence of target organ damage, and presence of CV disease or other risk factors) must be considered when initiating therapy.

TABLE 12-4. Lifestyle Modifications to Manage Hypertension

Modification	Recommendation	Approximate SBP reduction (range)
Weight reduction	Maintain normal body weight (body mass index 18.5 to 24.9 kg/m²).	5 to 20 mmHg/ 10 kg weight loss
Adopt DASH eating plan	Consume a diet rich in fruits, vegetables, and low-fat dairy products with a reduced content of saturated and total fat.	8 to 14 mmHg
Dietary sodium reduction	Reduce dietary sodium intake to no more than 100 mmol per day (2.4 g sodium or 6 g sodium chloride).	2 to 8 mmHg
Physical activity	Engage in regular aerobic physical activity such as brisk walking (at least 30 minutes per day, most days of the week).	4 to 9 mmHg
Moderation of alcohol consumption	Limit consumption to no more than 2 drinks (1 oz or 30 mL ethanol; e.g., 24 oz beer, 10 oz wine, or 3 oz 80-proof whiskey) per day in most men and to no more than 1 drink per day in women and lighter-weight persons.	2 to 4 mmHg

Adapted from JNC-7 Express, National Heart, Lung, and Blood Institute, 2003.
DASH, Dietary Approaches to Stop Hypertension.

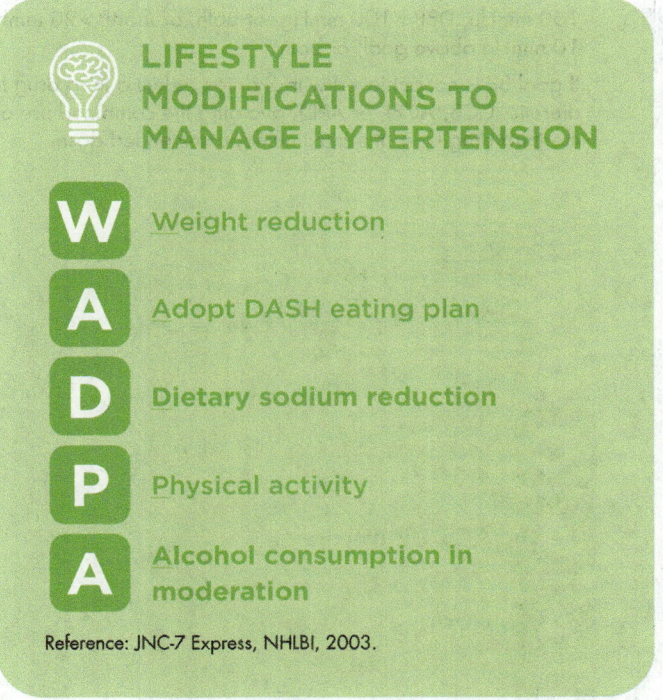

LIFESTYLE MODIFICATIONS TO MANAGE HYPERTENSION

W Weight reduction

A Adopt DASH eating plan

D Dietary sodium reduction

P Physical activity

A Alcohol consumption in moderation

Reference: JNC-7 Express, NHLBI, 2003.

Initial Therapy

Use of lifestyle modifications (Table 12-4) should continue to be stressed to patients after the decision to initiate drug therapy has been made to further decrease the risk of complications from cardiovascular disease. ACC/AHA recommends the use of thiazide diuretics, ACEIs, or ARBs or calcium channel blockers as initial therapy in non-Black patients, alone or in combination with other agents. ACC/AHA recommends CCBs and thiazide diuretics in Black patients, alone or in combination. ACC/AHA recommends ACEIs or ARBs alone or in combination with other drug types in chronic kidney disease (CKD) regardless of race or diabetes status.

TABLE 12-5. Strategies to Dose Antihypertensive Drugs

Strategy	Description	Details
A	Begin one drug, titrate to maximum dose, and then add a second drug.	If goal BP is not achieved with the initial drug, titrate the dose of the initial drug up to the maximum recommended dose to achieve goal BP.
		If goal BP is not achieved with the use of one drug despite titration to the maximum recommended dose, add a second drug from the list (thiazide-type diuretic, CCB, ACEI, or ARB) and titrate up to the maximum recommended dose of the second drug to achieve goal BP.
		If goal BP is not achieved with 2 drugs, select a third drug from the list (thiazide-type diuretic, CCB, ACEI, or ARB), avoiding the combined use of an ACEI and an ARB. Titrate the third drug up to the maximum recommended dose to achieve goal BP.
B	Begin one drug, and add a second drug before achieving maximum dose of the initial drug.	Begin one drug and add a second drug before achieving the maximum recommended dose of the initial drug, then titrate both drugs up to the maximum recommended doses of both to achieve goal BP.
		If goal BP is not achieved with 2 drugs, select a third drug from the list (thiazide-type diuretic, CCB, ACEI, or ARB), avoiding the combined use of an ACEI and an ARB. Titrate the third drug up to the maximum.
C	Begin with 2 drugs at the same time, either as 2 separate pills or as a single pill combination.	Initiate therapy with 2 drugs simultaneously, either as 2 separate drugs or as a single pill combination.
		Some committee members recommend beginning therapy with ≥2 drugs when SBP >160 mmHg, DBP >100 mmHg, or both, or if SBP >20 mmHg above goal, DBP >10 mmHg above goal, or both.
		If goal BP is not achieved with 2 drugs, select a third drug from the list (thiazide-type diuretic, CCB, ACEI, or ARB), avoiding the combined use of an ACEI and an ARB. Titrate the third drug up to the maximum recommended dose.

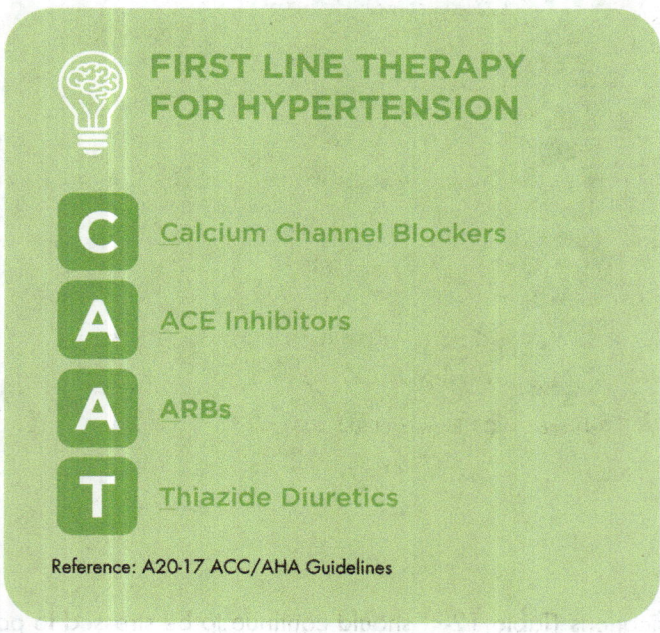

FIRST LINE THERAPY FOR HYPERTENSION

C Calcium Channel Blockers

A ACE Inhibitors

A ARBs

T Thiazide Diuretics

Reference: A20-17 ACC/AHA Guidelines

Guidelines recommend beginning with one drug, titrate to maximum dose, and then add a second drug from a second class (Table 12-5). For patients who are 20/10 mmHg greater than their goal BP, a 2-drug combination therapy should strongly be considered. All causes for an inadequate response should be addressed before additional agents are added to a patient's antihypertensive regimen (Box 12-5). Vasodilators, alpha-1-receptor antagonists, alpha-2-receptor agonists, and postganglionic adrenergic neuron blockers should be avoided as initial agents for hypertension.

BOX 12-5. Causes of Inadequate Responsiveness to Therapy

Pseudoresistance

- "White-coat hypertension" or office elevations
- Pseudohypertension in older patients
- Use of regular adult cuff on a very obese arm

Nonadherence to Therapy

Volume Overload

- Excess salt intake
- Progressive renal damage (nephrosclerosis)
- Fluid retention from reduction of blood pressure
- Inadequate diuretic therapy

Drug-Related Causes

- Doses too low
- Wrong type of diuretic
- Inappropriate combinations
- Rapid inactivation (e.g., hydralazine)
- Drug actions and interactions
- Steroids and estrogens (including oral contraceptives)
- Alcohol
- Cocaine
- Cyclosporine and tacrolimus
- Amphetamines
- Decongestants

- Caffeine
- Erythropoietin
- Licorice (in chewing tobacco)
- Monoamine oxidase inhibitors (MAOIs)
- Tricyclic antidepressants (TCAs)
- Serotonin norepinephrine reuptake inhibitors (SNRIs)
- Atypical antipsychotics
- Nonsteroidal anti-inflammatory drugs (NSAIDs)
- Angiogenesis inhibitors
- Tyrosine kinase inhibitors
- Herbal supplements: Ma Huang, St. John's Wort

Associated Conditions

- Smoking
- Increasing obesity
- Sleep apnea
- Insulin resistance or hyperinsulinemia
- Ethanol intake of more than 1 oz (30 mL) per day
- Anxiety-induced hyperventilation or panic attacks
- Chronic pain
- Intense vasoconstriction (arteritis)
- Organic brain syndrome (e.g., memory deficit)

Identifiable Causes of Hypertension

Adapted from JNC-7 Express, National Heart, Lung, and Blood Institute, 2003.

Diuretics

Thiazide and thiazide-like diuretics

See Table 12-6 for a list of thiazide and thiazide-like diuretics, their usual dosage range, and adverse effects associated with these medications.

Mechanism of action

Reduction of total fluid volume occurs through the inhibition of sodium reabsorption in the distal tubules, which causes increased excretion of sodium, water, potassium, and hydrogen. Direct arteriole dilation also occurs. The effectiveness of other antihypertensive agents is increased by preventing re-expansion of plasma volume. A significant decrease in efficacy occurs in patients with renal failure: serum creatinine >2 mg/dL or glomerular filtration rate (GFR) <30 mL/min with the exception of metolazone.

Diuretics also are available in combination with other medications (Table 12-7).

Patient instructions and counseling

- Take early in the day to avoid nocturia.
- Medication may increase sensitivity to sunlight. Consider using sunscreen with sun protection factor (SPF) >15.
- Medication may increase blood glucose in patients with diabetes.
- Medication can increase uric acid levels; use cautiously in patients with gout.
- Report problems with muscle cramps, which may indicate decreased potassium level.

TABLE 12-6. Thiazide Diuretics, Thiazide-Like Diuretics, Loop Diuretics, Potassium-Sparing Agents, and Aldosterone-Receptor Blockers

Drug	Trade name	Usual dosage range, total mg/d (frequency per day)	Adverse effects and comments[a]
Thiazide diuretics			
Chlorothiazide	Diuril	125 to 500 (1)	**Biochemical:** decreased potassium, sodium, and magnesium; increased uric acid and calcium
Chlorthalidone	Thalitone	12.5 to 25 (1)	**Rare:** blood dyscrasias, photosensitivity, pancreatitis, hyponatremia, and sulfonamide-type immune reactions
Hydrochlorothiazide	HydroDIURIL, **Microzide**	12.5 to 50 (1)	**Other:** impotence, fatigue, headache, rash, and vertigo
Thiazide-like diuretics			
Indapamide	Lozol	2.5 to 5 (1)	
Metolazone	Mykrox	2.5 to 10 (1)	
Metolazone	Zaroxolyn	2.5 to 5 (1)	(Decreased or no hypercholesterolemia compared to other thiazides; decreased microalbuminuria in diabetes)
Loop diuretics			
Bumetanide	Bumex	0.5 to 2 (2)	Ototoxicity at high doses
Furosemide	Lasix	20 to 80 (2)	(Short duration and no hypercalcemia)
Torsemide	Demadex	2.5 to 10 (1)	(Short duration and no hypercalcemia)
Potassium-sparing agents[b]			
Amiloride ⚠	Midamor	5 to 10 (1 to 2)	Hyperkalemia
Triamterene ⚠	Dyrenium	50 to 100 (1 to 2)	(No administration with history of kidney stones or hepatic disease)
Aldosterone-receptor blockers			
Eplerenone	Inspra	50 to 100 (1 to 2)	
Spironolactone	Aldactone	25 to 50 (1 to 2)	

Boldface indicates one of top 100 drugs for 2020 by prescription volume.
a. Adverse effects listed are for the class of drugs, except where noted for individual drugs (in parentheses).
b. See Table 12-7 for combination products.

⚠ **Furosemide** *FDA BOXED WARNING*

Furosemide is a potent diuretic which, if given in excessive amounts, can lead to a profound diuresis with water and electrolyte depletion. Therefore, careful medical supervision is required and dose and dosage interval must be adjusted to the individual patient's needs.

Amiloride *FDA BOXED WARNING*

Like other potassium-conserving agents, amiloride may cause hyperkalemia (serum potassium levels greater than 5.5 mEq per liter) which, if uncorrected, is potentially fatal. Hyperkalemia occurs commonly (about 10%) when amiloride is used without a kaliuretic diuretic. This incidence is greater in patients with renal impairment, diabetes mellitus (with or without recognized renal insufficiency), and in the elderly. When amiloride hydrochloride is used concomitantly with a thiazide diuretic in patients without these complications, the risk of hyperkalemia is reduced to about 1 to 2 percent. It is thus essential to monitor serum potassium levels carefully in any patient receiving amiloride, particularly when it is first introduced, at the time of diuretic dosage adjustments, and during any illness that could affect renal function.

 Triamterene *FDA BOXED WARNING*

May cause hyperkalemia, which if uncorrected, is potentially fatal. Hyperkalemia is more likely to occur in patients with renal impairment, diabetes mellitus (with or without recognized renal insufficiency), and in the elderly or severely ill. Monitor serum potassium levels carefully in any patient receiving triamterene.

TABLE 12-7. Combination Drugs for Hypertension

Fixed-dose combination (mg)[a]	Trade name
ACEIs and CCBs	
Amlodipine/benazepril hydrochloride (2.5/10, 5/10, 5/20, 10/20)	Lotrel
Trandolapril/verapamil (2/180, 1/240, 2/240, 4/240)	Tarka
Perindopril/**amlodipine** (3.5/2.5, 7/5, 14/10)	Prestalia
ACEIs and diuretics	
Benazepril/**hydrochlorothiazide** (5/6.25, 10/12.5, 20/12.5, 20/25)	Lotensin HCT
Captopril/**hydrochlorothiazide** (25/15, 25/25, 50/15, 50/25)	Capozide
Enalapril maleate/**hydrochlorothiazide** (5/12.5, 10/25)	Vaseretic
Lisinopril/hydrochlorothiazide (10/12.5, 20/12.5, 20/25)	Prinzide
Moexipril HCl/**hydrochlorothiazide** (7.5/12.5, 15/25)	Uniretic
Fosinopril HCl/**hydrochlorothiazide** (10/12.5, 20/12.5)	Monopril HCT
Quinapril HCl/**hydrochlorothiazide** (10/12.5, 20/12.5, 20/25)	Accuretic
ARBs and CCBs	
Amlodipine/valsartan (5/160, 5/320, 10/160, 10/320)	Exforge
Amlodipine/olmesartan (5/20, 5/40, 10/20, 10/40)	Azor
Amlodipine/telmisartan (5/40, 5/80, 10/40, 10/80)	Twynsta
ARBs and diuretics	
Candesartan cilexetil/**hydrochlorothiazide** (16/12.5, 32/12.5)	Atacand HCT
Olmesartan medoxomil/**hydrochlorothiazide** (20/12.5, 40/12.5, 40/25)	Benicar HCT
Eprosartan mesylate/**hydrochlorothiazide** (600/12.5, 600/25)	Teveten HCT
Irbesartan/**hydrochlorothiazide** (150/12.5, 300/12.5)	Avalide
Losartan potassium/**hydrochlorothiazide** (50/12.5, 100/25)	Hyzaar
Telmisartan/**hydrochlorothiazide** (40/12.5, 80/12.5, 80/25)	Micardis HCT
Valsartan/**hydrochlorothiazide** (80/12.5, 160/12.5)	Diovan HCT
Azilsartan medoxomil/chlorthalidone (40/12.5, 40/25)	Edarbyclor

(continued)

TABLE 12-7. Combination Drugs for Hypertension *(Continued)*

Fixed-dose combination (mg)[a]	Trade name
ARBs, CCBs, and diuretics	
Amlodipine/valsartan/hydrochlorothiazide (5/160/12.5, 5/160/25, 10/160/12.5, 10/160/25, 10/320/25)	Exforge HCT
Olmesartan/**amlodipine/hydrochlorothiazide** (20/5/12.5, 40/5/12.5, 40/5/25, 40/10/12.5, 40/10/25)	Tribenzor
Beta blockers and diuretics	
Atenolol/chlorthalidone (50/25, 100/25)	Tenoretic
Bisoprolol fumarate/**hydrochlorothiazide** (2.5/6.25, 5/6.25, 10/6.25)	Ziac
Propranolol HCl/hydrochlorothiazide (40/25, 80/25)	Inderide
Metoprolol tartrate/hydrochlorothiazide (50/25, 100/25)	Lopressor HCT
Nadolol/bendroflumethiazide (40/5, 80/5)	Corzide
Metoprolol succinate/hydrochlorothiazide (25/12.5, 50/12.5, 100/12.5)	Dutoprol
Beta blockers and ARBs	
Nebivolol HCl/**Valsartan** (5/80)	Byvalson
RI and diuretic	
Aliskiren/**hydrochlorothiazide** (150/12.5, 150/25, 300/12.5, 300/25)	Tekturna HCT
RI and CCB	
Aliskiren/**amlodipine** (150/5, 300/5, 150/10, 300/10)	Tekamlo
RI, CCB, and diuretic	
Aliskiren/**amlodipine/hydrochlorothiazide** (150/5/12.5, 300/5/12.5, 300/5/25, 300/10/12.5, 300/10/25)	Amturnide
Other combinations	
Amiloride HCl/**hydrochlorothiazide** (5/50)	Moduretic
Spironolactone/hydrochlorothiazide (25/25, 50/50)	Aldactazide
Triamterene/**hydrochlorothiazide** (37.5/25, 50/25, 75/50)	Dyazide, Maxzide

Adapted from JNC-7 Express, National Heart, Lung, and Blood Institute, 2003.
Boldface indicates one of top 100 drugs for 2020 by prescription volume.
RI, renin inhibitor.
a. Some drug combinations are available in multiple fixed doses. Each drug dose is reported in milligrams.

⚠️ **Amiloride HCl** *FDA BOXED WARNING*

May cause hyperkalemia, which is potentially fatal if uncorrected. The risk is higher in patients with renal impairment or diabetes mellitus. Monitor serum potassium levels carefully in any patient receiving therapy.

⚠️ **Spironolactone** *FDA BOXED WARNING*

This drug has been reported to be tumorigenic in rat chronic toxicity studies. Use this drug only as indicated. Fixed-dose **spironolactone/hydrochlorothiazide** is not indicated for the initial treatment of edema or hypertension.

Triamterene *FDA BOXED WARNING*

Abnormal elevation of serum potassium levels (greater than or equal to 5.5 mEq/L (5.5 mmol/L)) can occur with all potassium-sparing diuretic combinations, including **hydrochlorothiazide**/triamterene capsules. Hyperkalemia is more likely to occur in patients with renal impairment and diabetes (even without evidence of renal impairment), and in the elderly or severely ill. Since uncorrected hyperkalemia may be fatal, serum potassium levels must be monitored at frequent intervals, especially in patients first receiving **hydrochlorothiazide**/triamterene capsules, when dosages are changed or with any illness that may influence renal function.

Drug–drug and drug–disease interactions

- Steroids cause salt retention and antagonize thiazide action.
- NSAIDs blunt thiazide response.
- Class IA or III antiarrhythmics (that prolong the QT interval) may cause torsades de pointes with diuretic-induced hypokalemia.
- Probenecid and lithium block thiazide effects by interfering with thiazide excretion into the urine.
- Thiazides decrease lithium renal clearance and increase the risk of lithium toxicity.

Monitoring parameters

- BP
- Weight
- Serum electrolytes and uric acid
- BUN and creatinine
- Cholesterol levels

Loop diuretics

See Table 12-6 for a list of loop diuretics, their usual dosage range, and adverse effects associated with these medications.

Mechanism of action

Reduction of total fluid volume occurs through the inhibition of sodium and chloride reabsorption in the ascending loop of Henle, which causes increased excretion of water, sodium, chloride, magnesium, and calcium. Loop diuretics are more effective than thiazides in patients with renal failure: serum creatinine > 2 mg/dL or GFR <30 mL/min.

Patient instructions and counseling

- Take early in the day to avoid nocturia.
- Medication is less effective for hypertension and more effective reducing volume overload.
- Medication may increase sensitivity to sunlight. Consider using sunscreen with SPF >15.
- Medication can increase uric acid levels; use cautiously in patients with gout.
- Report problems with muscle cramps, which may indicate decreased potassium level.
- Rise slowly from a lying or sitting position.

Drug–drug and drug–disease interactions

- Aminoglycosides can precipitate ototoxicity when combined with loop diuretics.
- NSAIDs blunt diuretic response.
- Class IA or III antiarrhythmics (that prolong the QT interval) may cause torsades de pointes with diuretic-induced hypokalemia.

Monitoring parameters

- Weight
- Serum electrolytes
- BUN and creatinine
- Uric acid
- Hearing (in high doses)

Potassium-sparing diuretics

See Table 12-6 for a list of potassium-sparing diuretics, their usual dosage range, and adverse effects associated with these medications.

Mechanism of action

Potassium-sparing diuretics interfere with potassium and sodium exchange in the distal tubule, decrease calcium excretion, and increase magnesium loss.

Patient instructions and counseling

- Take early in the day to avoid nocturia.
- Medication is less effective than agents that lower BP.
- Take after meals.
- Avoid excessive ingestion of foods high in potassium and use of salt substitutes.
- Report problems with muscle cramps, which may indicate decreased potassium levels.
- Sexual dysfunction is possible.
- Avoid if creatinine clearance (CrCl) <30 mL/min.

Drug–drug and drug–disease interactions

- ACEIs may increase the risk of hyperkalemia.
- Indomethacin can cause a decrease in renal function when combined with triamterene.
- Cimetidine increases bioavailability and decreases clearance of triamterene.

Monitoring parameters

- Weight
- Serum electrolytes (especially potassium)
- BUN and creatinine

Adrenergic Inhibitors

Postganglionic adrenergic neuron blockers

Because this medication class is poorly tolerated, it is best avoided unless necessary to treat refractory hypertension that is unresponsive to all other agents. See Table 12-8 for the postganglionic adrenergic neuron blocker reserpine (Serpasil), its usual dosage range, and adverse effects associated with it.

TABLE 12-8. Postganglionic Adrenergic Neuron Blocker

Drug	Trade name	Usual dosage range, total mg/d (frequency per day)	Adverse effects and comments
Reserpine	Serpasil	0.05 to 0.25 (1)	Nasal congestion, sedation, depression, activation of peptic ulcer, dizziness, lethargy, memory impairment, sleep disturbances, and weight gain

Adapted from JNC-7 Express, National Heart, Lung, and Blood Institute, 2003.

Mechanism of action

Postganglionic adrenergic neuron blockers cause presynaptic inhibition of the release of the neurotransmitter from peripheral neurons by agonistic activity on the alpha-2 receptor and depletion of the neurotransmitter through competitive uptake into the neurosecretory vesicles.

Patient instructions and counseling

- Report symptoms of dizziness or hypotension.
- Do not take over-the-counter (OTC) cold products without first asking the health care provider or pharmacist.
- Rise slowly from a lying or sitting position.
- Report new fluid retention.
- Sexual dysfunction is possible.

Drug–drug and drug–disease interactions

- OTC sympathomimetics may potentiate an acute hypertensive effect.
- Tricyclic antidepressants and chlorpromazine antagonize the therapeutic effects of guanethidine.
- Pheochromocytoma is a contraindication to this class of medications.
- This medication class should be avoided in patients with CHF, angina, and cerebrovascular disease.

Monitoring parameters

- History of depression
- Sleep disturbances, drowsiness, and lethargy
- Symptoms of peptic ulcer

Centrally active alpha-2 agonists

This medication class (second-line agents) is best avoided unless necessary to treat refractory hypertension that is unresponsive to all other agents. See Table 12-9 for a list of centrally active alpha-2 agonists, their usual dosage range, and adverse effects associated with these medications.

Mechanism of action

These medications cause decreased sympathetic outflow to the cardiovascular system by agonistic activity on central alpha-2 receptors.

Patient instructions and counseling

- Report symptoms of dizziness or hypotension.
- Exercise sedation precautions.

TABLE 12-9. Centrally Active Alpha-2 Agonists

Drug	Trade name	Usual dosage range, total mg/d (frequency per day)	Adverse effects and comments[a]
Clonidine HCl[b]	Catapres	0.1 to 0.8 (2)	Sedation, dry mouth, bradycardia, withdrawal hypertension, orthostatic hypotension, depression, impotence, and sleep disturbances
Methyldopa	Aldomet	250 to 1000 (2)	(Hepatic and autoimmune disorders)

Adapted from JNC-7 Express, National Heart, Lung, and Blood Institute, 2003.
a. Adverse effects listed are for the class of drugs, except where noted for individual drugs (in parentheses).
b. Clonidine HCl is also available as a once-weekly transdermal patch.

- Fever and flu-like symptoms may represent hepatic dysfunction (methyldopa).
- Report new fluid retention.
- Sexual dysfunction is possible.

Drug–drug and drug–disease interactions

Use cautiously with other sedating medications.

Monitoring parameters

- CBC—positive Coombs test in 25% of those tested; <1% develop hemolytic anemia (methyldopa)
- Sleep disturbances, drowsiness, or dry mouth
- Symptoms of depression
- Impotence
- Pulse
- Rebound hypertension

Peripherally acting alpha-1 adrenergic blockers

This medication class (second-line agents) is best avoided unless necessary to treat refractory hypertension that is unresponsive to all other agents. See Table 12-10 for a list of peripherally acting alpha-1 adrenergic blockers, their usual dosage range, and adverse effects associated with these medications.

Mechanism of action

Peripheral alpha-1 postsynaptic receptors are blocked, which causes vasodilation of both arteries and veins (indirect vasodilators). These agents cause less reflex tachycardia than do direct vasodilators (hydralazine and minoxidil).

Patient instructions and counseling

- Take first dose of no more than 1 mg of any agent, and take at bedtime.
- Rise slowly from a lying or sitting position.
- Medication may cause dizziness.
- Priapism is possible.

Drug–drug and drug–disease interactions

- NSAIDs decrease antihypertensive effects of alpha-1 blockers.
- Increased antihypertensive effects occur with diuretics and beta blockers.

TABLE 12-10. Peripherally Acting Alpha-1 Adrenergic Blockers

Drug	Trade name	Usual dosage range, total mg/d (frequency per day)	Adverse effects and comments
Doxazosin mesylate	Cardura	1 to 16 (1)	Postural hypotension, syncopal episode with first dose, diarrhea, weight gain, peripheral edema, dry mouth, urinary urgency, constipation, priapism, nausea, dizziness, headache, palpitations, and sweating; no effects on glucose or cholesterol
Prazosin HCl	Minipress	2 to 20 (2 to 3)	
Terazosin HCl	Hytrin	1 to 20 (1 to 2)	

Reprinted with permission from JNC-VII, 2004.

Monitoring parameters

- BP and pulse
- Peripheral edema

Beta blockers

See Table 12-11 for a list of beta blockers, their usual dosage range, and adverse effects associated with these medications.

 Beta Blockers *FDA BOXED WARNING*

Abrupt withdrawal is not advised in patients with angina pectoris, coronary artery disease (CAD), or ischemic heart disease. Severe exacerbation of angina and the occurrence of MI and ventricular arrhythmias have been reported in angina patients following abrupt discontinuation. When discontinuation of these drugs is planned, patients should be observed carefully and advised to limit physical activity to a minimum. If the angina worsens or acute coronary insufficiency develops, promptly reinstituting **atenolol**, at least temporarily, is recommended. Because CAD is common and unrecognized, the prudent approach may be not to discontinue **atenolol**/nadolol/ **metoprolol** therapy abruptly in patients treated only for hypertension and in patients considered at risk of having occult atherosclerotic heart disease who are given **propranolol** for other reasons. Gradually reduce dosage over at least 1 to 2 weeks. If angina markedly worsens or acute coronary insufficiency develops on drug withdrawal, reinstate therapy, at least temporarily. Advise the patient against cessation or interruption of therapy without the advice of a physician.

Mechanism of action

These medications competitively block response to beta-adrenergic stimulation, which leads to the following: blocked secretion of renin, decreased cardiac output as a result of decreased cardiac contractility and decreased heart rate, and decreased central sympathetic output.

Patient instructions and counseling

- Report symptoms of dizziness or hypotension.
- Exercise sedation precautions (with lipid-soluble compounds).
- Abrupt withdrawal of the drug should be avoided. (See FDA boxed warning below.)
- Sexual dysfunction is possible.

Drug–drug and drug–disease interactions

- Use with caution in patients with diabetes because of the masking of hypoglycemic symptoms.
- Use with caution in patients with Raynaud's phenomenon or peripheral vascular disease.
- Beta blockers may decrease the effectiveness of sulfonylureas.
- Nondihydropyridines may increase the effect and toxicity of beta blockers.

Monitoring parameters

- ECG
- Rebound hypertension
- Cholesterol levels
- Pulse (apical and radial)
- Glucose levels

TABLE 12-11. Beta Blockers and Combination Alpha and Beta Blockers

Drug	Trade name	Lipid solubility/ primary (secondary) routes of elimination	Usual dosage range, total mg/d (frequency per day)	Adverse effects and comments[a]
Beta blockers				
Acebutolol[b,c]	Sectral	Low/H (R)	200 to 800 (1)	Bronchospasm, bradycardia, and heart failure; may mask insulin-induced hypoglycemia; *less serious:* impaired peripheral circulation, insomnia, fatigue, decreased exercise tolerance, and hypertriglyceridemia, except agents with intrinsic sympathomimetic activity
Atenolol[b] ⚠	Tenormin	Low/R (H)	25 to 100 (1)	
Betaxolol[b]	Kerlone	Low/H (R)	5 to 20 (1)	
Bisoprolol fumarate[b]	Zebeta	Low/R (H)	2.5 to 10 (1)	
Carteolol HCl[c]	Cartrol	Low/R	2.5 to 10 (1)	
Metoprolol tartrate[b] ⚠	Lopressor	Moderate/H (R)	50 to 100 (2)	
Metoprolol succinate[b] ⚠	Toprol-XL	Moderate/H (R)	50 to 100 (1)	
Nadolol ⚠	Corgard	Low/R	40 to 120 (1)	
Nebivolol[b]	Bystolic	High/H (R)	5 to 20 (1)	
Penbutolol sulfate[c]	Levatol	High/H (R)	10 to 20 (1)	
Pindolol[c]	Visken	Moderate/H (R)	10 to 60 (2)	
Propranolol HCl ⚠	Inderal	High/H	40 to 160 (2)	
Timolol maleate	Inderal LA	High/H	60 to 180 (1)	
	Blocadren	Low–moderate/H (R)	20 to 40 (2)	
Combined alpha and beta blockers				
Carvedilol	Coreg	Moderate/bile into feces	12.5 to 50 (2)	Postural hypotension, bronchospasm
Carvedilol	Coreg CR	Moderate/bile into feces	10 to 80 (1)	Postural hypotension, bronchospasm
Labetalol	Normodyne, Trandate	Moderate/R (H)	200 to 800 (2)	

Adapted from JNC-VII, 2004.
Boldface indicates one of top 100 drugs for 2020 by prescription volume.
H, hepatic; R, renal.
a. Adverse effects listed are for the class of drugs.
b. Cardioselective.
c. Intrinsic sympathomimetic activity.

 Atenolol *FDA BOXED WARNING*

Following abrupt cessation of certain beta-blocking agents, exacerbations of angina pectoris and, in some cases, myocardial infarction and ventricular arrhythmias have occurred. As with other beta blockers, when discontinuation of **atenolol** is planned, the patients should be carefully observed and advised to minimize physical activity. If the angina worsens or acute coronary insufficiency develops, promptly reinstitute **atenolol**, at least temporarily. Warn patients against interruption or discontinuation of therapy without advice of physician.

Metoprolol Tartrate *FDA BOXED WARNING*

Ischemic heart disease: Following abrupt cessation of therapy with certain beta-blocking agents, exacerbations of angina pectoris and, in some cases, myocardial infarction have occurred. When discontinuing chronically administered metoprolol succinate, particularly in patients with ischemic heart disease, the dosage should be gradually reduced over a period of 1 to 2 weeks and the patient should be carefully monitored. If angina markedly worsens or acute coronary insufficiency develops, metoprolol succinate administration should be reinstated promptly, at least temporarily, and other measures appropriate for the management of unstable angina should be taken. Warn patients against interruption or discontinuation of therapy without the physician's advice. Because coronary artery disease is common and may be unrecognized, it may be prudent not to discontinue metoprolol succinate therapy abruptly, even in patients treated only for hypertension.

 ## Metoprolol Succinate *FDA BOXED WARNING*

Ischemic heart disease: Following abrupt cessation of therapy with certain beta-blocking agents, exacerbations of angina pectoris and, in some cases, myocardial infarction have occurred. When discontinuing chronically administered metoprolol succinate, particularly in patients with ischemic heart disease, the dosage should be gradually reduced over a period of 1 to 2 weeks and the patient should be carefully monitored. If angina markedly worsens or acute coronary insufficiency develops, metoprolol succinate administration should be reinstated promptly, at least temporarily, and other measures appropriate for the management of unstable angina should be taken. Warn patients against interruption or discontinuation of therapy without the physician's advice. Because coronary artery disease is common and may be unrecognized, it may be prudent not to discontinue metoprolol succinate therapy abruptly, even in patients treated only for hypertension.

 ## Nadolol *FDA BOXED WARNING*

Following abrupt cessation of therapy with certain beta-blocking agents, exacerbations of angina pectoris and, in some cases, myocardial infarction have occurred. The dosage should be gradually reduced over a period of 1 to 2 weeks and the patient should be carefully monitored when discontinuing chronic therapy, particularly in patients with ischemic heart disease. If angina markedly worsens or acute coronary insufficiency develops, nadolol administration should be reinstated promptly, at least temporarily, and other measures appropriate for the management of unstable angina should be taken. Patients should be warned against interruption or discontinuation of therapy without the physician's advice.

 ## Propranolol HCl *FDA BOXED WARNING*

Following abrupt cessation of therapy with **propranolol**, exacerbations of angina pectoris and, in some cases, myocardial infarction have been reported. Even in the absence of overt angina pectoris, when discontinuing therapy, **propranolol** should not be withdrawn abruptly, and patients should be cautioned against interruption of therapy without the physician's advice.

Direct Vasodilators

This medication class (second-line agents) is best avoided unless necessary to treat refractory hypertension that is unresponsive to all other agents. These agents should *not* be used alone secondary to increases in plasma renin activity, cardiac output, and heart rate and, therefore, should be used only when beta blockers and diuretics are part of the antihypertensive regimen. See Table 12-12 for a list of direct vasodilators, their usual dosage range, and adverse effects associated with these medications.

Mechanism of action

These agents cause direct relaxation of peripheral arterial smooth muscle and thereby significantly decrease peripheral resistance.

Patient instructions and counseling

- Report symptoms of dizziness or hypotension.
- Hirsutism is possible (minoxidil).
- Report any new symptoms of fatigue, malaise, low-grade fever, and joint aches.
- Report rapid weight gain (>5 lb), unusual swelling, and pulse increases of >20 beats per minute above normal.
- Rise slowly from a lying or sitting position.

Drug–drug and drug–disease interactions

- Use with caution in patients with pulmonary hypertension.
- Use with caution in patients with significant renal failure or CHF.
- Use with caution in patients with coronary artery disease or a recent MI.

TABLE 12-12. Direct Vasodilators

Drug	Trade name	Usual dosage range, total mg/d (frequency per day)	Adverse effects and comments[a]
			Headaches, fluid retention, tachycardia, peripheral neuropathy, and postural hypotension
Hydralazine HCl	Apresoline	25 to 100 (2)	(Lupus syndrome)
Minoxidil	Loniten	2.5 to 80 (1 to 2)	(Hirsutism)

Adapted from JNC-7 Express, National Heart, Lung, and Blood Institute, 2003.
a. Adverse effects listed are for the class of drugs, except where noted for individual drugs (in parentheses).

⚠ Minoxidil *FDA BOXED WARNING*

Minoxidil can cause pericardial effusion, occasionally progressing to tamponade, and angina pectoris may be exacerbated. Minoxidil should be reserved for hypertensive patients who do not respond adequately to maximum therapeutic doses of a diuretic and two other antihypertensive agents. Minoxidil must be administered under close supervision, usually concomitantly with therapeutic doses of a beta-adrenergic blocking agent to prevent tachycardia and increased myocardial workload. It must also usually be given with a diuretic, frequently one acting in the ascending limb of the loop of Henle, to prevent serious fluid accumulation. Patients with malignant hypertension and those already receiving guanethidine should be hospitalized when minoxidil is first administered so that they can be monitored to avoid too rapid, or large orthostatic, decreases in blood pressure.

Monitoring parameters
- Weight (fluid status)
- BP and pulse
- CBC with antinuclear antibody test (hydralazine)

Calcium Antagonists

Low-renin hypertensive, Black, and elderly patients respond well to this class of medications. See Table 12-13 for a list of calcium antagonists, their usual dosage range, and adverse effects associated with these medications.

Mechanism of action

Calcium antagonists inhibit the influx of calcium ions through slow channels in vascular smooth muscle and cause relaxation of both coronary and peripheral arteries. These agents cause sinoatrial (SA) and atrioventricular (AV) nodal depression and a decrease in myocardial contractility (nondihydropyridines).

Patient instructions and counseling
- Report symptoms of dizziness or hypotension.
- Constipation is possible (verapamil).
- Report any new symptoms of shortness of breath, fatigue, or increased swelling of the extremities.
- Rise slowly from a lying or sitting position.

TABLE 12-13. Calcium Antagonists

Drug	Trade name	Usual dosage range, total mg/d (frequency per day)	Adverse effects and comments[a]
Nondihydropyridines			
Diltiazem HCl	Cardizem SR,	180 to 420 (1)	Conduction defects, worsening of systolic dysfunction, and gingival hyperplasia
	Cardizem CD, Dilacor XR, Tiazac	120 to 360 (1)	
Verapamil immediate-release	Calan, Isoptin	80 to 320 (2)	(Nausea and headache)
Verapamil long-acting	Calan SR, Isoptin SR	120 to 360 (1 to 2)	(Constipation)
Verapamil COER	Covera HS, Verelan PM	120 to 360 (1)	
Dihydropyridines			
Amlodipine besylate	**Norvasc**	2.5 to 10 (1)	Edema of the ankle, flushing, headache, and gingival hyperplasia
Felodipine	Plendil	2.5 to 20 (1)	
Isradipine	DynaCirc	2.5 to 10 (2)	
	DynaCirc CR	5 to 20 (1)	
Nicardipine HCl	Cardene SR	60 to 120 (1)	
Nifedipine	Procardia XL, Adalat CC	30 to 60 (1)	

Adapted from JNC-7 Express, National Heart, Lung, and Blood Institute, 2003.
Boldface indicates one of top 100 drugs for 2020 by prescription volume.
a. Adverse effects listed are for the class of drugs, except where noted for individual drugs (in parentheses).

Drug–drug and drug–disease interactions

- Use with caution in patients on beta blockers (nondihydropyridines), which may increase CHF and bradycardia. This combination also can cause conduction abnormalities to the AV node.
- Use with extreme caution in patients with conduction disturbances in the SA or AV node.
- Grapefruit juice may increase the levels of some dihydropyridines.

Monitoring parameters

- Peripheral edema
- BP and pulse
- Bowel habits

Angiotensin-Converting Enzyme Inhibitors and Angiotensin II Receptor Blockers

Ethnic differences exist in the response to these classes of medications. These agents are relatively ineffective as monotherapy in Black patients. However, the addition of diuretic therapy has been shown to sensitize Black patients to these agents to obtain similar responses as in non–Black patients. See Table 12-14 for a list of ACEIs and ARBs, their usual dosage range, and adverse effects associated with these medications.

TABLE 12-14. Angiotensin-Converting Enzyme Inhibitors and Angiotensin II Receptor Blockers

Drug	Trade name	Usual dose range, total mg/d (frequency per day)	Adverse effects and comments
ACEIs ⚠			
Benazepril HCl	Lotensin	10 to 40 (1 to 2)	**Common:** cough
Captopril	Capoten	25 to 100 (2 to 3)	**Rare:** angioedema, hyperkalemia, rash, loss of taste, and leucopenia
Enalapril maleate	Vasotec	2.5 to 40 (1 to 2)	**Other:** vertigo, headache, fatigue, first-dose hypotension, minor GI disturbances, acute renal insufficiency in patients with predisposing factors such as renal stenosis and coadministration with thiazide diuretics, and proteinuria (especially in patients with history of renal disease)
Fosinopril sodium	Monopril	10 to 40 (1 to 2)	
Lisinopril	**Prinivil, Zestril**	10 to 40 (1)	
Moexipril	Univasc	7.5 to 30 (1)	
Perindopril	Aceon	4 to 8 (1 to 2)	
Quinapril HCl	Accupril	10 to 40 (1 to 2)	
Ramipril	Altace	1.25 to 20 (1)	
Trandolapril	Mavik	1 to 4 (1)	
ARBs ⚠			
Azilsartan	Edarbi	40 to 80 (1)	Angioedema and hyperkalemia
Candesartan	Atacand	8 to 32 (1)	
Eprosartan	Teveten	400 to 800 (1 to 2)	
Irbesartan	Avapro	150 to 300 (1)	
Losartan	**Cozaar**	25 to 100 (1 to 2)	
Olmesartan	Benicar	20 (1)	
Telmisartan	Micardis	40 to 80 (1)	
Valsartan	**Diovan**	80 to 320 (1)	

Adapted from JNC-VII, 2004.
Boldface indicates one of top 100 drugs for 2020 by prescription volume.
GI, gastrointestinal.

ACEIs and ARBs *FDA BOXED WARNING*

- When pregnancy is detected, these drugs should be discontinued as soon as possible.
- Drugs that act directly on the renin-angiotensin system can cause injury and death to developing fetus.

Mechanism of action

ACEIs

ACEIs inhibit the conversion of angiotensin I to angiotensin II, a potent vasoconstrictor. These agents indirectly inhibit fluid volume increases by inhibiting angiotensin II–stimulated release of aldosterone.

ARBs

ARBs inhibit the binding of angiotensin II to the angiotensin II receptor, thereby inhibiting the vasoconstrictive properties of angiotensin II as well as its ability to stimulate the release of aldosterone. These agents currently are considered alternative therapy in patients not able to tolerate ACEIs because of cough.

Patient instructions and counseling

- Report symptoms of dizziness or hypotension.
- Symptoms of swelling of the lips, mouth, or face should be considered an emergency. Report immediately to a physician's office or an emergency department.
- Report new rashes (especially with captopril).
- Do not use salt substitutes containing potassium, and do not take OTC potassium supplements.
- Rise slowly from a lying or sitting position.

Drug–drug and drug–disease interactions

- NSAIDs will decrease the effectiveness of ACEIs and ARBs.
- Potassium-sparing diuretics, potassium supplements, and salt substitutes will increase the risk of hyperkalemia when used in combination with ACEIs and ARBs.
- ACEIs and ARBs should be avoided in patients with bilateral renal artery stenosis or stenosis in a single kidney.
- ACEIs and ARBs should be avoided in pregnant patients.

Monitoring parameters

- Serum electrolytes (especially creatinine and potassium)
- Symptoms of angioedema
- BP
- Symptoms of hypotension
- CBC (especially with captopril and enalapril) for neutropenia, which is more common in patients with preexisting renal impairment
- Cough (ACEIs)

Direct Renin Inhibitors ⚠

See Table 12-15 for the direct renin inhibitor aliskiren, its usual dosage range, and adverse effects associated with this medication.

Direct Renin Inhibitors *FDA BOXED WARNING*

When pregnancy is detected, these drugs should be discontinued as soon as possible. Drugs that act directly on the renin-angiotensin system can cause injury and death to a developing fetus.

TABLE 12-15. Direct Renin Inhibitor

Drug	Trade name	Usual dose range, total mg/d (frequency per day)	Adverse effects and comments
Aliskiren	Tekturna	150 to 300 mg (1)	**Common:** diarrhea **Rare:** elevated uric acid, gout, renal stone, angioedema, and rash **Other:** headache, nasopharyngitis, dizziness, fatigue, upper respiratory tract infection, back pain, and cough

Tekturna [package insert]. East Hanover, NJ: Novartis Pharmaceuticals; revised March 2012.

Mechanism of action

Direct renin inhibitors competitively inhibit human renin, which decreases plasma renin activity and inhibits the conversion of angiotensinogen to angiotensin I.

Patient instructions and counseling

- Establish a routine pattern for taking aliskiren with regard to meals. High-fat meals decrease absorption significantly.
- Store the medicine in a closed container at room temperature, away from heat, moisture, and direct light.
- Report symptoms of dizziness or hypotension.
- Symptoms of swelling of the lips, mouth, or face should be considered an emergency. Report immediately to a physician's office or an emergency department.

Drug–drug and drug–disease interactions

- Concomitant use of aliskiren with cyclosporine is not recommended.
- Potassium-sparing diuretics, potassium supplements, and salt substitutes will increase the risk of hyperkalemia when used in combination with aliskiren.
- Blood concentrations of **furosemide** are significantly reduced when given with aliskiren.
- Ketoconazole significantly increases aliskiren plasma levels.
- The combination of ACEIs or ARBs with aliskiren should be avoided.

Monitoring parameters

- Symptoms of angioedema
- BP
- Symptoms of hypotension
- Serum electrolytes (especially creatinine and potassium)

12-6   Hypertensive Urgencies and Emergencies

The classification of hypertensive urgencies and emergencies is determined by the presence or absence of acute target organ damage, not by BP; such presence or absence determines the appropriate treatment approach. The relative rise and rate of increase in BP is more important than the actual BP.

Hypertensive Urgencies

Hypertensive urgencies are accelerated, malignant, or perioperative elevations in BP in the absence of new or progressive target organ damage; therefore, immediate lowering of BP is not required.

Table 12-16 shows the agents used to treat hypertensive urgencies. No particular agent of choice exists; medications should be selected on the basis of patient characteristics. Oral therapy is preferred. However, onset of action should occur in 15 to 30 minutes, and peak effects should be seen in 2 to 3 hours. Check blood pressure every 15 to 30 minutes to ensure response. Use of immediate-release nifedipine is inappropriate to lower BP in patients with hypertensive urgencies.

Hypertensive Emergencies

Acute elevation of BP (>180 mmHg systolic or >120 mmHg diastolic) with the presence of acute or ongoing target organ damage constitutes a hypertensive emergency (Box 12-6). This situation requires immediate lowering of BP to prevent or minimize target organ damage.

TABLE 12-16. Agents Used to Treat Hypertensive Urgencies

Drug	Dose	Onset	Duration	Adverse effects
Captopril	25 mg, repeat in 1 to 2 hours as needed	5 to 15 min	4 to 6 h	Hypotension, acute renal failure, and angioedema
Clonidine	0.1 to 0.2 mg, repeat in 1 to 2 hours as needed (up to 0.6 mg)	5 to 15 min	6 to 12 h	Hypotension, drowsiness, sedation, and dry mouth
Labetalol	100 to 400 mg, repeat in 2 to 3 hours as needed	15 to 30 min	4 to 6 h	Hypotension, heart block, and bronchoconstriction

Boldface indicates one of top 100 drugs for 2020 by prescription volume.

BOX 12-6. Clinical Findings of Target Organ Damage

Target Organ Damage

- Hypertensive encephalopathy
- Intracranial hemorrhage
- Unstable angina
- Acute myocardial infarction
- Acute left ventricular failure with pulmonary edema
- Dissecting aortic aneurysm
- Eclampsia

Clinical Findings

- *Funduscopic:* papilledema, hemorrhage, exudates
- *Neurologic:* somnolence, confusion, seizures, coma, visual deficits or blindness
- *Cardiac:* S_4 gallop, ischemic changes on ECG, chest x-ray consistent with pulmonary edema, chest pain
- *Renal:* oliguria, progressive azotemia, hematuria, proteinuria
- *Other:* dyspnea

Reprinted with permission from JNC-VII, 2004.

Table 12-17 shows details of parenteral drugs used for treatment of hypertensive emergencies. As an initial goal, reduce mean arterial pressure (MAP) by no more than 25% within minutes to hours. Reach BP of 160/100 mmHg within 2 to 6 hours. Measure BP every 5 to 10 minutes until goal MAP is reached and life-threatening target organ damage resolves. Maintain goal BP for 1 to 2 days, and further reduce BP toward normal over several weeks. Excessive falls in BP may precipitate renal, cerebral, or coronary ischemia. Intravenous agents are preferred because of the ability to titrate dosages on the basis of BP response; however, specific agents should be chosen on the basis of patient findings (Table 12-18).

TABLE 12-17. Parenteral Drugs for Treatment of Hypertensive Emergencies

Drug	Dose	Onset of action	Duration of action	Adverse effects[a]	Special indications
Vasodilators					
Sodium nitroprusside	0.25 to 10 mcg/kg/min I.V. infusion[b] (maximal dose for 10 min only)	Immediate	1 to 2 min	Nausea, vomiting, muscle twitching, sweating, and thiocyanate and cyanide intoxication	Most hypertensive emergencies; caution with high intracranial pressure or azotemia
Nicardipine hydrochloride	5 to 15 mg/h I.V.	5 to 10 min	1 to 4 h	Tachycardia, headache, flushing, and local phlebitis	Most hypertensive emergencies except acute heart failure; caution with coronary ischemia
Clevidipine	1 to 2 mg/h, doubling every 90 seconds until BP approaches target, then increasing by less than double every 5 to 10 min; maximum dose 32 mg/h; maximum duration 72 h	2 min	5 to 15 min	Headache, nausea, and vomiting	Most hypertensive emergencies except in patients with severe aortic stenosis
Fenoldopam mesylate	0.1 to 0.3 mcg/kg/min I.V. infusion	<5 min	30 min	Tachycardia, headache, nausea, and flushing	
Nitroglycerin	5 to 100 mcg/min I.V. infusion[b]	2 to 5 min	3 to 5 min	Headache, vomiting, methemoglobinemia, and tolerance with prolonged use	Coronary ischemia
Enalaprilat	1.25 to 5 mg every 6 h I.V.	15 to 30 min	6 h	Precipitous fall in pressure in high-renin states; response variable	Acute left ventricular failure; avoid in acute MI
Hydralazine hydrochloride	10 to 20 mg I.V.; 10 to 50 mg I.M.	10 to 20 min; 20 to 30 min	3 to 8 h	Tachycardia, flushing, headache, vomiting, and aggravation of angina	Eclampsia
Adrenergic inhibitors					
Labetalol hydrochloride	20 to 80 mg I.V. bolus every 10 min; 0.5 to 2 mg/min I.V. infusion	5 to 10 min	3 to 6 h	Vomiting, scalp tingling, burning in throat, dizziness, nausea, heart block, and orthostatic hypotension	Most hypertensive emergencies except acute heart failure

TABLE 12-17. Parenteral Drugs for Treatment of Hypertensive Emergencies (Continued)

Drug	Dose	Onset of action	Duration of action	Adverse effects[a]	Special indications
Esmolol hydrochloride	250 to 500 mcg/kg/min I.V. infusion for 1 min, then 50 to 100 mcg/kg/min for 4 min; may repeat sequence	1 to 2 min	10 to 20 min	Hypotension and nausea	Aortic dissection, perioperative
Phentolamine	5 to 15 mg I.V.	1 to 2 min	3 to 10 min	Tachycardia, flushing, and headache	Catecholamine excess

Reprinted with permission from JNC-VII, 2004.
I.M., intramuscular; I.V., intravenous; MI, myocardial infarction.
a. Hypotension may occur with all agents.
b. Requires special delivery system.

TABLE 12-18. Selected Agents for Specific Hypertensive Emergencies

Emergency	Recommended therapy	Comments
Encephalopathy	Labetalol, nicardipine, and nitroprusside	Avoid methyldopa (sedation), diazoxide (reduces cerebral blood flow), reserpine (sedation), and hydralazine (increases intracranial pressure).
Myocardial infarction or unstable angina	Nitroglycerin, labetalol, nicardipine, and esmolol	Reduce BP until pain is relieved, and use in conjunction with conventional therapy for myocardial infarction or angina.
Congestive heart failure	Nitroprusside, nitroglycerin, clevidipine	Avoid diazoxide and hydralazine (increase oxygen demand), dihydropyridines (may worsen angina), and nitroprusside (coronary steal). Avoid labetalol, esmolol, and other beta blockers (reduce cardiac output).
Subarachnoid hemorrhage, intracerebral hemorrhage, and stroke	Multiple agents	BP reduction is controversial because it may cause hypoperfusion; generally recommended for severe hypertension (systolic BP > 220 mmHg or diastolic BP > 120 mmHg). Lower BP 15% during first 24 hours.
Dissecting aortic aneurysm	Esmolol and labetalol	Avoid diazoxide and hydralazine (increase shear force).
Pheochromocytoma and cocaine overdose	Phentolamine, nicardipine, and clevidipine	Requires rapid lowering of BP.
Renal insufficiency	Clevidipine, fenoldopam, nicardipine	
Perioperative hypertension	Clevidipine, nicardipine, esmolol, and nitroglycerin	BP levels > 180/110 mmHg should be controlled before surgery. Contributing factors to postoperative hypertension may include pain and increased intravascular volume, which may require parenteral loop diuretics.
Eclampsia or preeclampsia	Hydralazine, labetalol, nicardipine	Requires rapid BP lowering.

12-7   Pharmacist's Role

The role of a pharmacist in the management of hypertension is well documented in ambulatory and community settings. This includes medication therapy management, collaborative drug therapy management, and telehealth. Pharmacists can provide counseling on how to take medications for BP, what types of medications to avoid using, and recommendations of agents to health care providers. Those pharmacists working under collaborative practice agreements (state specific) can initiate, monitor, and manage therapy for patients with hypertension.

NAPLEX Competency Statements

The questions in this chapter cover the following 2021 NAPLEX Competency Statements: **AREA 1:** 1.3; 1.4; 1.5; 1.6; 1.7 **AREA 2:** 2.1; 2.2 **AREA 3:** 3.2; 3.3; 3.6; 3.7; 3.9; 3.10; 3.11; 3.12.

12-8   Questions

1. According to the ACC/AHA guidelines, which of the following agents are suitable as initial therapy for the treatment of uncomplicated hypertension? (Mark all that apply.)

   A. Hydrochlorothiazide
   B. Chlorthalidone
   C. Atenolol
   D. Hydralazine
   E. Amlodipine

2. Hyperkalemia is a possible adverse effect of which of the following medications? (Mark all that apply.)

   A. Felodipine
   B. Doxazosin
   C. Captopril
   D. Amiloride
   E. Candesartan

3. A 48-year-old patient with hypertension presents with a new diagnosis of chronic kidney disease. Which of the following agents would be an appropriate choice as initial therapy for this patient?

   A. Clonidine
   B. Hydralazine
   C. Diltiazem
   D. Lisinopril
   E. Nisoldipine

4. A 62-year-old patient with a history of hypertension and gout presents to begin pharmacotherapy for hypertension. Which agent is the most appropriate choice as initial therapy?

   A. Chlorothiazide
   B. Torsemide
   C. Tenormin
   D. Chlorthalidone
   E. Losartan

5. Which of the following medications can cause bradycardia? (Mark all that apply.)

   A. Terazosin
   B. Verapamil
   C. Diltiazem
   D. Ziac
   E. Clonidine

6. A patient requires a cardioselective beta blocker in his outpatient medication regimen after recent discharge from the hospital following a new MI. You suggest he take _____.

   A. labetalol
   B. esmolol
   C. propranolol
   D. atenolol
   E. carvedilol

7. A patient presents to your ambulatory clinic with a BP of 210/125 mmHg. Past medical history is significant for type 2 diabetes, CHF, and renal insufficiency. Which of the following would be considered a hypertensive emergency?

A. Blood glucose levels >300 mg/dL, which increase the patient's risk for acute renal failure

B. Serum creatinine of 3 mg/dL

C. Nausea, vomiting, and diarrhea for 3 days

D. S$_4$ gallop and a chest x-ray consistent with pulmonary edema

E. Polyuria combined with polydipsia

8. What are the treatment goals for a patient with hypertensive emergency?

A. Systolic pressure should be reduced to 120 mmHg within the first hour of treatment to reduce the risk of further end-organ damage.

B. Diastolic pressure should be reduced to 80 mmHg within the first hour of treatment to reduce the risk of further end-organ damage.

C. Blood pressure should be reduced to 160/100 mmHg in the first 2 to 6 hours of therapy.

D. Mean arterial pressure should be reduced by at least 50% within the first minutes to hours of therapy.

E. Blood pressure should be reduced to no lower than 180/110 mmHg in the first hour, because excessive drops in blood pressure may precipitate coronary ischemia.

9. A patient presents to your ambulatory clinic with a blood pressure of 210/125 mmHg. Past medical history is significant for type 2 diabetes, CHF, and renal insufficiency. What would be the recommended treatment for the patient's hypertensive emergency?

A. Clonidine orally, 0.1 to 0.2 mg; repeat in 1 to 2 hours as needed (up to 0.6 mg)

B. Labetalol orally, 100 to 400 mg; repeat in 2 to 3 hours as needed

C. Nifedipine sublingually, 10 mg; repeat in 0.5 to 1 hour as needed (up to 60 mg)

D. Labetalol intravenously, 20 to 80 mg bolus, followed by 0.5 to 2 mg/min infusion

E. Enalaprilat intravenously, 1.25 to 5 mg every 6 hours

10. Which of the following antihypertensive agents can cause first-dose syncope, palpitations, peripheral edema, and priapism?

A. Hydralazine

B. Nitroprusside

C. Prazosin

D. Verapamil

E. Moexipril

11. Which of the following antihypertensive agents is most likely to cause lupus syndrome, postural hypotension, and peripheral neuropathy?

A. Atenolol

B. Hydralazine

C. Guanfacine

D. Mibefradil

E. Nitroprusside

12. Which of the following medications is associated with drug-induced hypertension? (Mark all that apply.)

A. Prednisone

B. Indomethacin

C. Rosiglitazone

D. Albuterol

E. Cyclosporine

13. What is the best recommendation for antihypertensive medication in a patient who has atrial fibrillation, coronary artery disease with angina, and hyperthyroidism?

A. Minoxidil

B. Betaxolol

C. Telmisartan

D. Nicardipine

E. Amiloride

14. What antihypertensive agent should *not* be used in a patient with essential hypertension and a history of depression with suicidal ideation?

A. Captopril

B. Prazosin

C. Metolazone

D. Reserpine

E. Amlodipine

15. Which of the following are secondary causes of hypertension? (Mark all that apply.)

A. Renovascular disease
B. Pheochromocytoma
C. Systemic lupus erythematosus
D. Primary aldosteronism
E. Stevens–Johnson syndrome

Use Patient Profile 12-1 to answer Questions 16-20.

16. Possible complications that the patient is at risk of developing secondary to uncontrolled hypertension include which of the following?

A. Hyperaldosteronism, urinary tract infection
B. MI, blindness
C. Blindness, hyperaldosteronism
D. Urinary tract infection, blindness
E. Chronic obstructive pulmonary disease, pneumonia

17. Education regarding lifestyle modification issues in this patient should include which of the following? (Mark all that apply.)

A. Limit alcohol intake to no more than 2 drinks per day.
B. Reduce daily intake of dietary magnesium, calcium, and sodium.
C. Increase aerobic physical activity, decrease weight, and limit dietary saturated fat and cholesterol.
D. Consume a diet consistent with the Atkins Diet.
E. Stop smoking.

PATIENT PROFILE 12-1

Date: 4/20/17
Height: 5'11"
Patient: male, age 70 years
Race: Black
Known diseases: Diabetes (15 years), hypertension (20 years), obstructive sleep apnea (5 years), osteoarthritis
OTC use: Aleve, Actron

Date of birth: 4/14/47
Weight: 248 lb
Allergies: No known drug allergies
Pharmacist notes and other patient information: + tobacco, 1.5 packs/day; coffee, 4 to 5 cups/day; alcohol, 2 drinks/week

Date	Rx No.	Drug and strength	Route	Quantity	Regimen	Refills	Pharmacist	Prescriber
1/15/17	001	Glipizide 5 mg	Oral	30	1 daily	5	BCE	NTE
1/15/17	002	Lisinopril 5 mg	Oral	30	1 daily	5	BCE	NTE
1/15/17	003	Hydrodiuril 12.5 mg	Oral	30	1 daily	5	BCE	NTE
1/20/17	004	Ibuprofen 800 mg	Oral	90	1 3 times daily	5	REM	FTD
2/11/17	001-RF	Glipizide 5 mg	Oral	30	1 daily	4	BCE	NTE
2/11/17	003-RF	Hydrodiuril 12.5 mg	Oral	30	1 daily	4	BCE	NPR
2/11/17	004-RF	Ibuprofen 800 mg	Oral	90	1 3 times daily	4	REM	FTD
3/13/17	001-RF	Glipizide 5 mg	Oral	30	1 daily	3	BCE	NTE
3/13/17	002-RF	Lisinopril 5 mg	Oral	30	1 daily	4	BCE	NTE
3/13/17	004-RF	Ibuprofen 800 mg	Oral	90	1 3 times daily	3	REM	FTD

18. Possible reasons that the patient's BP is uncontrolled include which of the following?

   A. Use of NSAIDs, which causes decreased effectiveness of ACEI therapy, and drug interaction between glipizide and lisinopril

   B. Use of NSAIDs, which causes decreased effectiveness of ACEI therapy, and possible problems with adherence to antihypertensive therapy

   C. Lack of BP response to ACEI therapy, which should not be used in combination with diuretics in Black patients, and possible problems with adherence to antihypertensive therapy

   D. Lack of blood pressure response to ACEI therapy, which should not be used in combination with diuretics in Black patients, and drug interaction between glipizide and lisinopril

   E. Patients with osteoarthritis, who tend to have hypertension that is difficult to control

19. The appropriate initial antihypertensive agent in this patient could be _____.

   A. benazepril
   B. terazosin
   C. minoxidil
   D. metoprolol
   E. clonidine

20. If the patient is not able to tolerate lisinopril because of adverse effects such as cough, an appropriate alternative agent would be _____.

   A. telmisartan
   B. labetalol
   C. guanabenz
   D. reserpine
   E. prazosin

 **12-9 Answers**

1. A, B, E. Appropriate choices for initial agents in the treatment of uncomplicated hypertension include diuretics, ACEIs, ARBs, and CCBs. Hydralazine is a direct vasodilator, which would never be considered a first-line agent in the treatment of hypertension. Atenolol is a beta blocker and is no longer considered first-line therapy according to ACC/AHA guidelines.

2. C, D, E. Hyperkalemia is a possible side effect with ACEIs, ARBs, and potassium-sparing diuretics. Doxazosin is a peripherally acting alpha-1 blocker, which does not cause hyperkalemia. Felodipine is a calcium channel antagonist and is not linked to causing hyperkalemia.

3. D. For patients who have hypertension and chronic kidney disease, ACC/AHA recommends the use of ACEIs, diuretics, ARBs, and dihydropyridine CCBs. The only listed ACEI is perindopril.

4. E. For patients who have hypertension and gout, ACC/AHA recommends against using diuretic therapy, which increases the risk of gouty attacks. The only medications listed that are not diuretics are atenolol (Tenormin), which is a beta blocker, and losartan, which is an angiotensin II receptor blocker. Beta blockers are not considered first line, so the appropriate choice is losartan.

5. B, C, D, E. Verapamil and diltiazem are nondihydropyridine calcium channel blockers, Ziac (bisoprolol and hydrochlorothiazide) is a beta blocker, and clonidine is a centrally acting alpha-2 agonist. They all have negative inotropic effects on the myocardium. Terazosin is a peripherally acting alpha-1 blocker, which does not cause bradycardia.

6. D. Labetalol, propranolol, and carvedilol are all nonselective beta blockers. Esmolol is a cardioselective agent available only in injectable form and, therefore, would not be for outpatient use. Atenolol is a cardio-selective beta blocker that is available as an oral tablet and, therefore, can be used for outpatient dosing.

7. D. The classification of hypertensive urgencies and emergencies is determined by the presence or absence of acute target organ damage and not by the actual blood pressure measurement. Presence of an S_4 gallop and a chest x-ray consistent with pulmonary edema suggest acute left ventricular failure with pulmonary edema, which represents defined target organ damage and, in turn, means the patient should be classified as a hypertensive emergency.

8. C. According to ACC/AHA guidelines, in patients with hypertensive emergencies, the initial goal is a drop in mean arterial pressure of no more than 25% within minutes to hours followed by a drop to 160/100 mmHg within 2 to 6 hours.

9. E. In a patient with CHF and hypertensive emergency, recommended treatments include nitroglycerin, nitroprusside, and enalaprilat (Table 12-17). Clonidine and labetalol (orally) are incorrect choices because the patient requires IV therapy. Nifedipine SL is not indicated for immediate reduction of blood pressure. Labetalol IV is not an appropriate choice in a patient with CHF because it could decrease cardiac output.

10. C. Possible side effects of peripherally acting alpha-1 blockers (prazosin) include first-dose syncope, palpitations, peripheral edema, and priapism (Table 12-10).

11. B. Possible side effects of direct vasodilators (hydralazine) include postural hypotension and peripheral neuropathy. However, lupus syndrome is unique to hydralazine and does not occur with minoxidil (Table 12-12).

12. A, B, E. All agents listed except rosiglitazone and albuterol are possible causes of drug-induced hypertension through multiple mechanisms (Box 12-3).

13. B. The diagnoses of atrial fibrillation, coronary artery disease with angina, and hyperthyroidism are all considered comorbid conditions with hypertension in which the use of beta blockers may have favorable effects.

14. D. Because of its possible increased risk of depression, reserpine should not be used for patients for whom the risk for depression or suicide already exists.

15. C, E. All listed diseases except systemic lupus erythematosus and Stevens–Johnson syndrome are possible causes of secondary hypertension through various mechanisms.

16. B. Uncontrolled hypertension causes multiple organ system problems, including cardiovascular (CHF, MI, and peripheral arterial disease); ophthalmologic (retinopathy and blindness); cerebrovascular (transient ischemic attack and cerebrovascular accident); and renovascular (nephropathy, renal failure, and dialysis) issues. This patient, therefore, is at risk for MI and blindness, not for hyperaldosteronism or urinary tract infections.

17. A, C, E. Lifestyle modifications to be considered in hypertensive patients include weight loss; limit of alcohol intake; increased aerobic activity; reduced sodium intake; maintenance of adequate dietary potassium, calcium, and magnesium intake; and smoking cessation.

18. B. Other responses are untrue or not applicable with diabetes.

19. A. In patients with hypertension and comorbid conditions of CKD and diabetes, the initial agent should be an ACEI.

20. A. In patients who cannot tolerate ACEI therapy secondary to the adverse effect of cough, angiotensin II receptor blockers are considered good alternative agents.

12-10   Additional Resources

JNC-7 Express (Joint National Committee on Prevention, Detection, Evaluation, and Treatment of High Blood Pressure [JNC-7] Express). May 2003. NIH: National Heart, Lung, and Blood Institute Web site. NIH Publication 03-5233. Available at: www.nhlbi.nih.gov/files/docs/guidelines/express.pdf.

JNC-VIII (The Eighth Report of the Joint National Committee on Prevention, Detection, Evaluation, and Treatment of High Blood Pressure). *JAMA.* 2014;311:507–520.

Whelton PK, Carey RM, Aronow, WS, et al. 2017 ACC/AHA/AAPA/ABC/ACPM/AGS/APhA/ASH/ASPC/NMA/PCNA Guideline for the Prevention, Detection, Evaluation, and Management of High Blood Pressure in Adults: Executive Summary: A Report of the American College of Cardiology/American Heart Association Task Force on Clinical Practice Guidelines. *J Am Coll Cardiol.* 2018;71(19):2199–2269.

Saseen JL, Maclaughlin EJ. Hypertension. In: DiPiro JT, Talbert RL, Yee GC, et al., eds. *Pharmacotherapy: A Pathophysiologic Approach.* 10th ed. New York, NY: McGraw-Hill; 2017:45–78.

Heart Failure

13

ROBERT B. PARKER

 13-1 KEY POINTS

- Heart failure is a clinical syndrome resulting from the heart's inability to pump sufficient blood to meet the body's needs. Heart failure can be caused by any disorder that affects cardiac systolic and/or diastolic function.
- Patients with an ejection fraction of ≤40% are classified as having heart failure with reduced ejection fraction (HFrEF) whereas those with an ejection fraction of ≥50% have heart failure with preserved ejection fraction (HFpEF).
- Compensatory mechanisms are activated to help maintain adequate cardiac output; activation of those systems is responsible for heart failure symptoms and disease progression. Medications that improve patient outcomes antagonize those compensatory mechanisms.
- Drugs that can precipitate or worsen heart failure should be avoided (e.g., nonsteroidal anti-inflammatory drugs [NSAIDs], verapamil, **diltiazem**, and others).
- All patients with stage C heart failure with reduced ejection fraction (HFrEF) should be routinely treated with guideline directed medical therapy (GDMT) that includes an angiotensin II receptor blocker–neprilysin inhibitor (preferred)/angiotensin-converting enzyme inhibitors (ACEIs)/angiotensin II receptor blockers (ARBs), evidence-based beta blocker (bisoprolol, extended-release **metoprolol succinate**, or **carvedilol**), aldosterone antagonist, and sodium-glucose-cotransporter-2 (SGLT2) inhibitor, to reduce morbidity and mortality.
- Diuretics are used to reduce fluid retention, thus minimizing symptoms.
- Digoxin does not improve survival in patients with heart failure but does provide symptomatic benefits. The goal plasma concentration is 0.5 to 1 ng/mL.
- Patients with acute decompensated heart failure (ADHF) often require hospitalization and aggressive therapy with intravenous diuretics, positive inotropic drugs, and vasodilators.

 13-2 STUDY GUIDE CHECKLIST

The following topics may guide your study of this subject area:

- ☐ Risk factors for developing heart failure, including drugs that can precipitate or worsen the disorder.
- ☐ Clinical presentation of heart failure.
- ☐ Drugs that improve survival by affecting the pathophysiology of heart failure.
- ☐ Selection of appropriate pharmacotherapy based on treatment guidelines and patient characteristics.
- ☐ Mechanisms of action of classes of drugs used to treat heart failure and appropriate monitoring parameters.
- ☐ Major adverse drug reactions to drugs used to treat heart failure.
- ☐ Significant drug interactions involving medications used to treat heart failure.
- ☐ Trade names and generic names of medications used to treat heart failure.
- ☐ Patient counseling points for drugs used to treat heart failure.

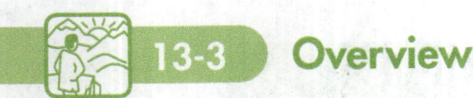

Overview

Heart failure is a clinical syndrome resulting from any disorder that affects the heart's structure and/or function and is confirmed by increased plasma natriuretic peptide concentrations and evidence of pulmonary or systemic congestion. Heart failure can result from abnormalities in systolic as well as diastolic function. Patients with heart failure symptoms and left ventricular ejection fraction (LVEF) ≤ 40% are classified as having heart failure with reduced ejection fraction (HFrEF), whereas those with LVEF ≥ 50% have heart failure with preserved ejection fraction (HFpEF). Approximately 50% of patients with heart failure have HFpEF. This distinction is important because decisions about the pharmacotherapy of heart failure are based on whether the patients has reduced or preserved ejection fraction.

More than 6 million people in the United States have heart failure; approximately 1 million new cases are diagnosed each year.

At the time of heart failure diagnosis, the 5-year mortality rate is approximately 50%.

Each year, more than 1 million hospital discharges for heart failure occur. The annual costs for treating heart failure exceed $37 billion.

Classification

The guidelines for heart failure evaluation and management from the American College of Cardiology (ACC) and the American Heart Association (AHA) classification scheme emphasize both the evolution and the progression of the disease. This scheme more objectively identifies patients within the course of the disease and links to treatments appropriate for each stage (Table 13-1).

TABLE 13-1. Stages of Heart Failure and Treatments

ACC/AHA heart failure stage	Examples	Goals of therapy	Usual therapy
A – High risk for developing HF but no symptoms or structural heart disease	Patients with HTN, coronary or other atherosclerotic vascular disease, diabetes, obesity	Risk factor identification and modification to prevent coronary artery or other vascular disease	ACEI or ARB for vascular disease, statins as indicated, treat HTN per current guidelines
B – Structural heart disease but no HF signs or symptoms (Pre-heart failure)	Patients with previous myocardial infarction, low EF, left ventricular hypertrophy	Prevent HF symptoms and further remodeling of the heart	ACEI, ARBs, beta blockers as indicated
C – Structural heart disease with current or prior HF symptoms	Patients with HF symptoms and either reduced EF (HFrEF) or preserved EF (HFpEF)	Minimize symptoms, reduce mortality, hospitalizations, HF progression, improve quality of life	HFrEF: ACEI/ARB/ARNI, beta blocker, aldosterone antagonist, SGLT2 inhibitor, diuretics for volume overload HFpEF: Diuretics for volume overload, guideline directed treatment of comorbidities (e.g., HTN, coronary artery disease, diabetes, atrial fibrillation)
D – Refractory HF requiring specialized interventions	Patients with marked symptoms at rest or requiring recurrent hospitalizations despite maximal medical therapy	Reduce symptoms and hospitalizations, improve quality of life, determine end of life goals	Chronic inotropes, mechanical circulatory support, palliative care and hospice

HF, heart failure; HTN, hypertension; EF, ejection fraction; HFrEF, heart failure with reduced ejection fraction; HFpEF, heart failure with preserved ejection fraction; ACEI, angiotensin-converting enzyme inhibitor; ARB, angiotensin II receptor blocker; ARNI, angiotensin receptor-neprilysin inhibitor; SGLT2, sodium-glucose cotransporter-2.

Acute Decompensated Heart Failure

Both the growing number of patients with heart failure and the progressive nature of the syndrome have led to substantial increases in hospitalizations for heart failure. *Acute decompensated heart failure* (ADHF) is defined as new or worsening signs or symptoms that are usually caused by (1) volume overload (pulmonary congestion, systemic congestion, or both), (2) hypoperfusion (hypotension, renal insufficiency, shock syndrome, or some combination), or (3) both volume overload and hypoperfusion. ADHF frequently requires hospitalization for acute treatment targeted at reducing volume overload and improving cardiac output.

Causes of ADHF include medication and dietary noncompliance, atrial fibrillation or other arrhythmias, myocardial ischemia, uncontrolled hypertension, pulmonary embolus, concurrent illnesses (e.g., pneumonia), recent addition of negative inotropic or cardiotoxic drugs, nonsteroidal anti-inflammatory drugs (NSAIDs), excessive alcohol or illicit drug use, and progression of heart failure.

Clinical Presentation

The primary manifestations of heart failure are (1) dyspnea and fatigue that may limit exercise tolerance and (2) fluid retention that may lead to pulmonary and peripheral edema. Some patients may have marked exercise intolerance but little evidence of fluid retention, whereas others may have prominent edema with few dyspnea or fatigue symptoms.

Other symptoms include paroxysmal nocturnal dyspnea, orthopnea, cough, weight gain, and nocturia. Other signs include ascites, jugular venous distension, hepatojugular reflux, hepatomegaly, tachypnea, bibasilar pulmonary rales, pulmonary and/or peripheral edema, pleural effusion, tachycardia, cool extremities, and S_3 gallop. Patients with ADHF experience similar symptoms, which may be more severe.

Pathophysiology

Heart failure can result from any disorder (see the next section on specific causes of heart failure) that impairs the heart's systolic function (i.e., pumping ability) or diastolic function (i.e., impaired cardiac relaxation). Many patients have manifestations of both abnormalities. In either case, the initiating event in heart failure is a decrease in cardiac output. The decrease in cardiac output leads to the activation of compensatory systems, including the renin-angiotensin and sympathetic nervous systems as well as other neurohormones that result in increased renal sodium and water retention, vasoconstriction, tachycardia, and other alterations in the function and structure of the heart.

Specific Causes of Heart Failure

Coronary artery disease is the cause of heart failure in about 65% of patients with HFrEF. Other causes include nonischemic cardiomyopathy (e.g., attributable to hypertension, thyroid disease, or valvular disease). Approximately 75% of patients with heart failure have antecedent hypertension. Other common risk factors for development of heart failure include diabetes and metabolic syndrome.

Approximately 50% of patients have HFpEF caused by impaired cardiac diastolic dysfunction. This type of heart failure is observed most often in elderly patients.

A number of drugs can precipitate or worsen heart failure: See Box 13-1.

Diagnostic Criteria

No single diagnostic test for heart failure exists; rather, the diagnosis is a clinical one based on history, signs and symptoms, and physical examination. A thorough history and physical examination are important for identifying cardiac and noncardiac disorders or behaviors (e.g., diet, adherence to medications) that may cause or hasten heart failure progression.

BOX 13-1. Drugs That Precipitate or Exacerbate Heart Failure

- Drugs with negative inotropic effects include antiarrhythmics (disopyramide, flecainide, propafenone, and others); beta blockers; calcium channel blockers (verapamil and **diltiazem**); and oral antifungals (itraconazole and terbinafine).

- Cardiotoxic drugs include the anthracyclines (doxorubicin, daunorubicin, epirubicin) cyclophosphamide, ethanol, amphetamines (cocaine and methamphetamine), trastuzumab, bevacizumab, mitoxantrone, ifosfamide, lapatinib, sunitinib, and imatinib.

- Drugs that cause sodium and water retention can precipitate or worsen heart failure and include NSAIDs (which can also attenuate the efficacy, and increase the toxicity, of diuretics and angiotensin-converting enzyme inhibitors [ACEIs]), glucocorticoids, rosiglitazone, and pioglitazone.

- Drugs with an uncertain mechanism for toxicity include infliximab, etanercept, dronedarone, and the dipeptidyl peptidase-4 (DPP-4) inhibitors (e.g., saxagliptin).

Boldface indicates one of top 100 drugs for 2020 by prescription volume.

The echocardiogram is one of the most useful diagnostic tests in patients with heart failure. It is used to determine the EF as well as the presence of other structural or functional abnormalities that could be causing heart failure. Most patients with newly diagnosed HFrEF undergo evaluation for the presence of coronary artery disease (CAD).

A rapid bedside assay for natriuretic peptides (B-type natriuretic peptide [BNP] or N-terminal pro B-type natriuretic peptide [NT-proBNP]) often is used in acute care settings (e.g., emergency departments) as an aid in the diagnosis of suspected heart failure. The assay is useful for differentiating between heart failure exacerbations and other causes of dyspnea, such as chronic obstructive pulmonary disease (COPD), asthma, or infection. Patients with dyspnea secondary to heart failure have elevated BNP or NT-proBNP concentrations.

Treatment Principles and Goals of Therapy

The goals of therapy include improving the patient's quality of life, minimizing symptoms, reducing hospitalizations for heart failure exacerbations, slowing progression of the disease, and improving survival.

The ACC/AHA guideline recommendations for treatment of stages A–D heart failure are available at https://www.ahajournals.org/doi/full/10.1161/cir.0b013e31829e8776 and https://www.ahajournals.org/doi/full/10.1161/CIR.0000000000000509. A 2021 update is available at https://www.jacc.org/doi/pdf/10.1016/j.jacc.2020.11.022. For stages A and B, therapy is targeted primarily toward preventing heart failure development; in stages C and D, however, the focus is targeted toward treatment of patients with symptomatic heart failure.

13-4 Drug Therapy of Heart Failure

This section on drug therapy focuses on the treatment of patients with stage C HFrEF. These patients should be routinely managed with a diuretic (if needed to control volume retention), an angiotensin receptor blocker–neprilysin inhibitor (ARNI, preferred) or ACEI or angiotensin II receptor blocker (ARB), a beta blocker, an aldosterone antagonist, and an SGLT2 inhibitor. Drug therapies that can be considered in selected patients include digoxin, hydralazine–isosorbide dinitrate, and ivabradine.

In contrast to patients with HFrEF, these same drug therapies have not been shown to improve important outcomes (e.g., mortality, hospitalizations) in patients with HFpEF with the exception of aldosterone antagonists, which may reduce hospitalizations. However, these same drugs often are used to treat HFpEF because these patients have many comorbidities (e.g., hypertension, diabetes, coronary artery disease) that require treatment using these agents.

Loop Diuretics

Only patients with signs or symptoms of volume overload need diuretic therapy. Most heart failure patients require use of the more potent loop diuretics (Table 13-2) instead of thiazide diuretics.

Mechanism of action

Loop diuretics inhibit the Na-K-Cl cotransporter 2 in the ascending limb of the loop of Henle resulting in increased renal excretion of sodium, chloride, potassium, magnesium, and water.

Patient instructions and counseling

- Patients should take their loop diuretic once a day in the morning or, if taking twice daily, in the morning and afternoon.
- Loop diuretics can cause frequent urination.
- Patients should weigh themselves daily (preferably in the morning, after urinating). Patients who gain more than 1 pound per day for several consecutive days or 3 to 5 pounds in 1 week should contact their health care provider.
- Patients should report muscle cramps, dizziness, excessive thirst, weakness, or confusion, as these may be signs of overdiuresis.
- Patients should avoid sun exposure or use sunscreen when taking loop diuretics.

Adverse drug effects

- Electrolyte depletion: hyponatremia, hypokalemia, hypomagnesemia
- Hypotension
- Renal insufficiency

Drug–drug and drug–disease interactions

- Food decreases the bioavailability of **furosemide** and bumetanide, so these agents should be taken on an empty stomach. Food does not affect torsemide absorption.
- Oral **furosemide** absorption is slowed significantly in patients with ADHF, resulting in decreased diuretic response. Therefore, these patients usually require intravenous (I.V.) **furosemide**.

Monitoring parameters

- Serum sodium, potassium, magnesium, creatinine, and blood urea nitrogen (BUN)
- Patient weight (a loss of 0.5 to 1 kg daily is desired until the patient achieves the desired dry weight)

TABLE 13-2. Loop Diuretics

Generic name	Trade name	Dosage form	Dosage range and frequency
Furosemide	**Lasix**	Tablet	20 to 160 mg daily or twice daily
Bumetanide	Bumex	Tablet	0.5 to 5 mg daily or twice daily
Torsemide	Demadex	Tablet	10 to 100 mg daily or twice daily

Boldface indicates one of top 100 drugs for 2020 by prescription volume.

- Urine output
- Blood pressure
- Jugular venous distension
- Improvement in heart failure symptoms (dyspnea and peripheral edema)

Angiotensin-Converting Enzyme Inhibitors ⚠

ACEIs are recommended for all patients with HFrEF and current or prior symptoms of heart failure, unless contraindicated (Table 13-3). ACEIs reduce symptoms, hospitalizations, and mortality, and they improve clinical status and quality of life.

Mechanism of action

ACEIs inhibit the angiotensin-converting enzyme, which is responsible for the conversion of angiotensin I to the potent vasoconstrictor angiotensin II, thus, decreasing plasma angiotensin II and aldosterone concentrations and reducing the adverse effects of those neurohormones. Inhibition of the angiotensin-converting enzyme also prevents the breakdown of the endogenous vasodilator bradykinin.

Patient instructions and counseling

- Patients who are pregnant or breast-feeding should not take ACEIs. If a patient becomes pregnant while taking an ACEI, she should contact her physician immediately.
- Salt substitutes containing potassium should be used cautiously.
- Patients should call their physician immediately if they experience swelling of the face, eyes, lips, tongue, arms, or legs or if they have difficulty breathing or swallowing.
- ACEIs may cause a cough.

Adverse drug effects

- Hypotension
- Dizziness
- Renal insufficiency
- Cough
- Angioedema
- Hyperkalemia

TABLE 13-3. Angiotensin-Converting Enzyme Inhibitors

Generic name	Trade name	Dosage form	Dosage range and frequency
Captopril	Capoten	Tablet	6.25 to 50 mg three times daily
Enalapril	Vasotec	Tablet	2.5 to 20 mg twice daily
Fosinopril	Monopril	Tablet	5 to 40 mg daily
Lisinopril	**Zestril, Prinivil**	Tablet	2.5 to 40 mg daily
Quinapril	Accupril	Tablet	5 to 20 mg twice daily
Ramipril	Altace	Capsule	1.25 to 10 mg daily
Perindopril	Aceon	Tablet	2 to 16 mg daily
Trandolapril	Mavik	Tablet	0.5 to 4 mg daily

Boldface indicates one of top 100 drugs for 2020 by prescription volume.

Angiotensin-Converting Enzyme Inhibitors (ACEIs) *FDA BOXED WARNING*

When used in pregnancy during the second and third trimesters, all ACE inhibitors can cause injury and even death to the developing fetus. When pregnancy is detected, these agents should be discontinued as soon as possible.

Drug–drug and drug–disease interactions
- NSAIDs increase the risk of renal insufficiency and attenuate the beneficial effects of ACEIs.
- Potassium supplements or potassium-sparing diuretics should be used with caution.
- Diuretics increase the risk of hypotension.
- Contraindicated in patients with bilateral renal artery stenosis.

Monitoring parameters
- Assess blood pressure, renal function, (BUN and creatinine), and potassium at baseline and 1 to 2 weeks after initiation or dose increase.
- Heart failure symptoms
- Dose (initiate therapy at low doses; if lower doses are tolerated well, follow with gradual increases)

Other
ACEIs are pregnancy category C during the first trimester and pregnancy category D during the second and third trimesters. ACEIs can cause fetal and neonatal morbidity and death when administered to pregnant women. ACEIs should be discontinued as soon as possible after pregnancy is determined.

Angiotensin II Receptor Blockers ⚠

Current guidelines recommend ARBs to reduce morbidity and mortality in patients with HFrEF intolerant to ACEIs because of cough or angioedema. Note that ARBs are just as likely as ACEIs to cause impaired renal function, hyperkalemia, or hypotension (Table 13-4).

Mechanism of action
- ARBs block the angiotensin I receptor and attenuate the effects of angiotensin II.
- Unlike ACEIs, ARBs do not affect the kinin system and, thus, are not associated with cough.
- ARBs reduce hospitalizations and improve survival.

TABLE 13-4. Angiotensin II Receptor Blockers

Generic name	Trade name	Dosage form	Dosage range and frequency
Candesartan	Atacand	Tablet	4 to 32 mg daily
Losartan	Cozaar	Tablet	25 to 150 mg daily
Valsartan	Diovan	Tablet	20 to 160 mg twice daily

Boldface indicates one of top 100 drugs for 2020 by prescription volume.

Patient instructions and counseling

- Patients who are pregnant or breast-feeding should not take ARBs. If a patient becomes pregnant while taking an ARB, she should contact her physician immediately.
- Salt substitutes containing potassium should be used cautiously.
- Dizziness or light-headedness may occur, especially in patients taking diuretics.

Adverse drug effects

- Hypotension
- Dizziness
- Renal insufficiency
- Hyperkalemia

Drug–drug and drug–disease interactions

- Potassium supplements or potassium-sparing diuretics should be used with caution.
- NSAIDs increase the risk of renal insufficiency.
- Diuretics increase the risk of hypotension.

Monitoring parameters

- Assess blood pressure, renal function, (BUN and creatinine), and potassium at baseline and 1 to 2 weeks after initiation or dose increase.
- Heart failure symptoms
- Dose (initiate therapy at low doses; if lower doses are tolerated well, follow with gradual increases)

Other

ARBs are pregnancy category D and can cause fetal and neonatal morbidity and death when administered to pregnant women. ARBs should be discontinued as soon as possible after pregnancy is determined.

Angiotensin II Receptor Blocker–Neprilysin Inhibitor ⚠

A combination product containing the ARB **valsartan** plus the neprilysin inhibitor sacubitril recently was approved for treatment of HFrEF to reduce the risk of cardiovascular death and heart failure hospitalization (Table 13-5). Recent guidelines state that sacubitril/**valsartan** is preferred over ACEIs or ARBs in patients

---

⚠ **Angiotensin II Receptor Blockers (ARBs)** *FDA BOXED WARNING*

When used in pregnancy, all ARBs can cause injury and even death to the developing fetus. When pregnancy is detected, these agents should be discontinued as soon as possible.

TABLE 13-5. Angiotensin II Receptor Blocker–Neprilysin Inhibitor

Generic name	Trade name	Dosage form	Dosage range and frequency
Sacubitril/**valsartan**	Entresto	Tablet	24/26 to 97/103 mg twice daily

Boldface indicates one of top 100 drugs for 2020 by prescription volume.

with HFrEF. Sacubitril/**valsartan** can be used as initial therapy in patients newly diagnosed with HFrEF or in patients tolerating an ACEI or ARB, replacement by sacubitril/**valsartan** can further reduce morbidity and mortality.

Mechanism of action
- **Valsartan** blocks the angiotensin I receptor and attenuates the effects of angiotensin II.
- Sacubitril inhibits neprilysin, an enzyme that breaks down numerous endogenous vasoactive substances, including natriuretic peptides, bradykinin, and others. As a result, the actions of these compounds are increased.
- Sacubitril/**valsartan** significantly reduces the risk of cardiovascular death or hospitalization for heart failure compared to enalapril.

Patient instructions and counseling
- Patients who are pregnant or breast-feeding should not take sacubitril/**valsartan**. If a patient becomes pregnant while taking sacubitril/**valsartan**, she should contact her physician immediately.
- Salt substitutes containing potassium should be used cautiously.
- Dizziness or light-headedness may occur, especially in patients taking diuretics.

Adverse drug effects
- Hypotension
- Dizziness
- Renal insufficiency
- Hyperkalemia
- Angioedema
- Cough

Drug–drug and drug–disease interactions
- Potassium supplements and potassium-sparing diuretics should be used with caution.
- Sacubitril/**valsartan** ⚠ is contraindicated for use with an ACE inhibitor. If switching from an ACE inhibitor to sacubitril/**valsartan**, discontinue the ACE inhibitor at least 36 hours before starting sacubitril/**valsartan**.
- NSAIDs increase the risk of renal insufficiency.
- Sacubitril/**valsartan** is contraindicated in patients with a history of ACE inhibitor–associated angioedema.

Monitoring parameters
- Assess blood pressure, renal function, (BUN and creatinine), and potassium at baseline and 1 to 2 weeks after initiation or dose increase
- Heart failure symptoms
- Dose (initiate therapy at low doses; if lower doses are tolerated well, follow with gradual increases)

⚠ **Sacubitril/valsartan (Entresto)** *FDA BOXED WARNING*

When used in pregnancy, this agent can cause injury and even death to the developing fetus. When pregnancy is detected, sacubitril/**valsartan** should be discontinued as soon as possible.

Other

Sacubitril/valsartan can cause fetal and neonatal morbidity and death when administered to pregnant women. It should be discontinued as soon as possible after pregnancy is determined.

Beta Blockers

Treatment with beta blockers reduces symptoms, improves clinical status, and decreases the risk of death and hospitalization. One of the 3 beta blockers shown to reduce mortality (bisoprolol, **carvedilol**, and extended-release **metoprolol succinate**) should be used in all stable patients with HFrEF and current or prior heart failure symptoms, unless contraindicated (Table 13-6).

Mechanism of action

- Blockade of beta receptors antagonizes increased sympathetic nervous system activity, which is one of the important mechanisms responsible for heart failure progression.
- Beta blockers should be used in combination with ACEIs, ARBs, or sacubitril/**valsartan**, diuretics, aldosterone antagonists, and SGLT2 inhibitors.

Patient instructions and counseling

- Beta blockers may cause fluid retention or worsening of heart failure upon initiation of therapy or after a dose increase. Patients should report body or leg swelling or increased shortness of breath. Patients should weigh themselves daily. Patients who gain more than 1 pound per day for several consecutive days or 3 to 5 pounds per week should contact their health care provider.
- Fatigue or weakness may occur early in treatment but usually will resolve spontaneously.
- Dizziness, light-headedness, or blurred vision, which may be caused by blood pressure that is too low or by bradycardia or heart block, should be reported.
- Patients should take **carvedilol** with food.
- Patients must not miss doses or abruptly stop taking these medications.

Adverse drug effects

The adverse effects that are most commonly observed in patients with heart failure receiving beta blockers are:

- Fluid retention and worsening heart failure
- Fatigue
- Bradycardia and heart block
- Hypotension
- Possible hypertension, tachycardia, or myocardial ischemia stemming from abrupt withdrawal

For other adverse effects, see Chapter 12 on hypertension and Chapter 15 on ischemic heart disease.

TABLE 13-6. Beta Blockers

Generic name	Trade name	Dosage form	Dosage range and frequency
Bisoprolol	Zebeta	Tablet	1.25 to 10 mg daily
Carvedilol	Coreg	Tablet	3.125 to 50 mg twice daily
Metoprolol succinate extended-release	Toprol-XL	Tablet	12.5 to 200 mg daily

Boldface indicates one of top 100 drugs for 2020 by prescription volume.

Drug–drug and drug–disease interactions

- Amiodarone can increase the risk of bradycardia, heart block, and hypotension.
- Quinidine, **fluoxetine**, **paroxetine**, and other inhibitors of cytochrome P4502D6 inhibit hepatic metabolism of **metoprolol** and **carvedilol** and may result in increased plasma concentrations and enhanced effects.
- Beta blockers may cause bronchoconstriction in patients with asthma or COPD.
- Beta blockers should not be used in patients with symptomatic bradycardia or heart block unless a pacemaker is present.
- Beta blockers may worsen blood glucose control in patients with diabetes and may mask the signs of hypoglycemia.

Monitoring parameters

- Blood pressure and heart rate
- Heart failure symptoms, especially signs/symptoms of volume overload
- Weight (daily)

Kinetics

- Bisoprolol is eliminated about 50% by the kidneys, so dosage adjustment may be required in patients with renal insufficiency.
- Both **metoprolol** and **carvedilol** are metabolized by the liver.

Other

- Patients should be stable (i.e., minimal evidence of fluid overload or volume retention) before beta blocker treatment is initiated.
- Treatment should be initiated with low doses and titrated slowly upward until the target dose is reached. Doses usually are increased no more frequently than every 2 weeks, with close monitoring of symptoms required during the titration period.
- Fluid accumulation during dose titration usually can be managed by adjusting diuretic doses.
- Staggering the schedule of other heart failure medications that lower blood pressure (e.g., ACEIs, diuretics) may help reduce the risk of hypotension.

Aldosterone Receptor Antagonists

Current guidelines recommend the addition of aldosterone antagonists (**spironolactone** or eplerenone) to reduce the risk of death and hospitalization in patients with New York Heart Association (NYHA) class II–IV HFrEF who can be monitored closely for renal function and serum potassium (Table 13-7). Aldosterone antagonists also are recommended for patients with acute myocardial infarction and an LVEF ≤ 40%, as well as heart failure symptoms or a history of diabetes.

TABLE 13-7. Aldosterone Receptor Antagonists

Generic name	Trade name	Dosage form	Dosage range and frequency
Spironolactone	Aldactone	Tablet	12.5 to 50 mg daily
Eplerenone	Inspra	Tablet	25 to 50 mg daily

Boldface indicates one of top 100 drugs for 2020 by prescription volume.

Mechanism of action

Aldosterone plays an important role in heart failure pathophysiology. In addition to increasing renal sodium and water retention and potassium loss, elevated plasma aldosterone is a key mediator of ventricular hypertrophy and remodeling, which drives the initiation and progression of heart failure. Antagonism of aldosterone receptors by **spironolactone** and eplerenone attenuates these harmful effects.

Patient instructions and counseling

- Salt substitutes containing potassium should be avoided.
- Patients should call their physician immediately if they experience muscle weakness or cramps; numbness or tingling in hands, feet, or lips; or slow or irregular heartbeat.
- **Spironolactone** may cause swollen or painful breasts in men.

Adverse drug effects

- Hyperkalemia
- Gynecomastia (only with **spironolactone**)
- Irregular menses

Drug–drug and drug–disease interactions

- ACEIs, ARBs, and NSAIDs increase the risk of hyperkalemia.
- Potassium supplements increase the risk of hyperkalemia. Supplements should not be used if serum potassium > 3.5 mEq/L.
- Elderly patients and patients with diabetes are at an increased risk of hyperkalemia.
- Erythromycin, clarithromycin, verapamil, ketoconazole, fluconazole, itraconazole, and other inhibitors of cytochrome P4503A4 inhibit hepatic metabolism of eplerenone and may result in increased plasma concentrations and enhanced effects.

Monitoring parameters

- Serum creatinine should be ≤2.5 mg/dL in men or ≤2 mg/dL in women (or estimated glomerular filtration rate > 30 mL/min for men and women) before therapy is initiated.
- Serum potassium should be ≤5 mEq/L before therapy is initiated. Potassium should be evaluated before and 2 to 3 days after therapy is started, again 1 week after therapy is started, and then at least monthly for the first 3 months of therapy, then every 3 months.

Sodium-Glucose Co-Transporter-2 (SGLT2) Inhibitors

Current guidelines recommend the addition of a SGLT2 inhibitor (dapagliflozin or empagliflozin) to reduce the risk of adverse outcomes (e.g., hospitalization or death) in patients with NYHA class II–IV HFrEF (LVEF ≤ 40%) with or without diabetes in conjunction with other recommended GDMT for HFrEF (Table 13-8).

TABLE 13-8. Sodium-Glucose Cotransporter-2 Inhibitors

Generic name	Trade name	Dosage form	Dosage range and frequency
Dapagliflozin	Farxiga	Tablet	10 mg daily
Empagliflozin	Jardiance	Tablet	10 mg daily

Mechanism of action

The sodium-glucose cotransporter-2 (SGLT2) inhibitors are agents to treat diabetes that reduce glucose reabsorption in the proximal tubule of the kidney resulting in diuresis and natriuresis. Beneficial improvements in myocardial energy metabolism, oxidative stress, and ventricular remodeling also likely play a role in improving outcomes. In patients with HFrEF, dapagliflozin and empagliflozin reduce the occurrence of adverse outcomes such as hospitalization or death in patients with and without type 2 diabetes. As a result, these two agents are recommended as first line therapy in current treatment guidelines.

Patient instructions and counseling

- In patients with diabetes, ketoacidosis can occur even if the blood sugar is less than 250 mg/dl. Patients should contact their health care provider immediately if they have nausea, vomiting, abdominal pain, fatigue, or shortness of breath.
- These medications should not be used in patients with type 1 diabetes.
- If you have diabetes and take other medications that can lower blood sugar, you could develop symptoms of low blood sugar such as headache, shaking or feeling jittery, irritability, weakness, drowsiness, sweating, confusion, dizziness, or hunger. The doses of your other medications for diabetes many need to be adjusted to reduce this risk.
- Dehydration resulting in low blood pressure can occur. Call your health care provider if you lose fluid from your body from vomiting or diarrhea.
- Call your health care provider if you experience signs or symptoms of a urinary tract infection such as burning when passing urine, a need to urinate frequently, pain in the lower abdomen, or blood in the urine. Other symptoms include fever, back pain, nausea, or vomiting.
- Genital yeast infections can occur, particularly in women and uncircumcised males. Women may have vaginal odor, white or yellowish vaginal discharge or itching. Men may have redness, itching, swelling of the penis or foul smelling discharge from the penis, or pain in the skin around the penis.
- Seek medical attention immediately if you have a fever or are feeling very weak, tired, or uncomfortable and you have pain, tenderness, swelling, or redness in the area between your anus and genitals.

Adverse drug effects

- Genital mycotic infections
- Urinary tract infections
- Necrotizing fasciitis of the perineum (Fournier's Gangrene)
- Hypoglycemia (usually in patients with type 2 diabetes taking other medications)
- Ketoacidosis in patients with diabetes regardless of blood glucose level
- Volume depletion and hypotension
- Increased serum creatinine

Drug–drug and drug–disease interactions

- The risk of hypoglycemia is increased in patients receiving sulfonylureas or insulin.
- Concomitant use of diuretics may increase the risk of volume depletion.

Monitoring parameters

- The eGFR should be ≥ 30 ml/min/1.73 m^2 in patients receiving dapagliflozin and ≥ 20 ml/min/1.73 m^2 for empagliflozin.
- Volume status

- Blood pressure
- Blood glucose
- Signs/symptoms of genital mycotic and urinary tract infections

Digoxin

Digoxin decreases hospitalizations and improves symptoms in patients with HFrEF but does not affect mortality.

Mechanism of action

- Digoxin inhibits the Na+-K+-ATPase pump, which results in an increase in intracellular calcium that, in turn, causes a positive inotropic effect.
- Digoxin increases parasympathetic activity and decreases sympathetic outflow from the central nervous system. These effects occur at low plasma concentrations, where little positive inotropic effect is seen.

Patient instructions and counseling

Patients should report any of the following to their health care provider:

- Dizziness, light-headedness, or fatigue
- Changes in vision (blurred or yellow vision)
- Irregular heartbeat
- Loss of appetite
- Nausea, vomiting, or diarrhea

Adverse drug effects

- Cardiovascular (cardiac arrhythmias, bradycardia, and heart block)
- Gastrointestinal (anorexia, abdominal pain, nausea, and vomiting)
- Neurological (visual disturbances, disorientation, confusion, and fatigue)

Toxicity typically is associated with serum digoxin concentrations >2 ng/mL but may occur at lower concentrations in elderly patients and in patients with hypokalemia or hypomagnesemia.

Drug–drug and drug–disease interactions

The following drugs increase serum digoxin concentrations:

- Quinidine, verapamil, dronedarone, and amiodarone (if these medications are added, the digoxin dose should be decreased by 50%)
- Propafenone
- Flecainide
- Macrolide antibiotics (erythromycin and clarithromycin)
- Itraconazole and ketoconazole
- **Spironolactone**
- Cyclosporine

Drugs that decrease serum digoxin concentrations include the following:

- Antacids
- Cholestyramine and colestipol

- Rifampin
- Metoclopramide

Diuretic-induced hypokalemia or hypomagnesemia increases the risk of digoxin toxicity.

Monitoring parameters

- The target serum digoxin concentration is 0.5 to 0.9 ng/mL. This can usually be achieved with a dose of 0.125 mg daily. Lower doses may be required in patients older than 70 and/or with reduced renal function or low lean body mass.
- No loading dose is needed in the treatment of heart failure.
- Blood samples to determine serum digoxin concentrations should be collected at least 6 hours, and preferably 12 hours or more, after the last dose.
- Heart rate
- Serum potassium and magnesium
- Renal function (serum BUN and creatinine)
- Heart failure symptoms

Ivabradine

Ivabradine (Corlanor) is approved for treatment of patients with HFrEF who are in sinus rhythm with a resting heart rate ≥ 70 bpm and who are on maximally tolerated beta blocker doses or have contraindications to beta blockers. Ivabradine reduces the risk of hospitalization for worsening heart failure.

Mechanism of action

Ivabradine blocks the I_f current in the sinus node, resulting in a reduction in heart rate.

Patient instructions and counseling

- Patients who are pregnant or breast-feeding should not take ivabradine. If a patient becomes pregnant while taking ivabradine, she should contact her physician immediately. Females who potentially could become pregnant while taking ivabradine should use effective contraception.
- The risk of an irregular heartbeat is increased. Patients experiencing palpitations, chest pain, or shortness of breath should contact their health care provider.
- Ivabradine increases the risk of a slow heart rate (bradycardia).
- Take with food.

Adverse drug effects

- Bradycardia
- Hypertension
- Atrial fibrillation
- Phosphenes (temporary brightness in the visual field)

Drug–drug and drug–disease interactions

- Ivabradine is contraindicated with strong CYP3A4 inhibitors (azole antifungals, macrolide antibiotics, HIV [human immunodeficiency virus] protease inhibitors).
- Moderate CYP3A4 inhibitors (**diltiazem**, verapamil, grapefruit juice) and inducers (St. John's wort, rifampin, barbiturates, phenytoin) should be avoided.
- The risk of bradycardia is increased in patients receiving β-blockers or other drugs that slow heart rate (e.g., digoxin, amiodarone).

Monitoring parameters

- The starting dose is 5 mg twice daily. The dose can be increased to 7.5 mg twice daily after 2 weeks to achieve a resting heart rate of 50 to 60 bpm.
- Heart rate and electrocardiogram
- Vision

Other

Ivabradine can cause fetal and neonatal morbidity and death when administered to pregnant women and should be discontinued as soon as possible after pregnancy is determined. Effective contraception should be used.

Hydralazine–Isosorbide Dinitrate

Guidelines recommend the use of hydralazine–isosorbide dinitrate to reduce morbidity and mortality in self-described Black patients with HFrEF and persistent symptoms despite treatment with sacubitril/**valsartan**/ACEI/ARB, beta blockers, aldosterone antagonists, and SGLT2 inhibitors. Hydralazine–isosorbide dinitrate also is an option in patients with HFrEF who experience drug intolerance, hypotension, or renal insufficiency with ACEI or ARB treatment. A fixed-dose combination product is available (BiDil). Adverse effects with the hydralazine–isosorbide dinitrate combination are common (primarily headache, dizziness, and gastrointestinal complaints), leading many patients to discontinue therapy.

13-5　Drug Therapy for Acute Decompensated Heart Failure

Patients with ADHF usually are admitted to the hospital for aggressive treatment with I.V. diuretics, vasodilators (Table 13-9), or positive inotropic drugs (Table 13-10). Treatment goals include improving symptoms, reducing volume overload, improving cardiac output, identifying and addressing precipitating factors, and optimizing chronic therapy before hospital discharge. Most cases of ADHF are the result of volume overload or hypoperfusion (low cardiac output), and treatment is directed at the underlying problem.

Volume Overload

- The goal is to reduce volume overload and minimize congestive symptoms.
- I.V. loop diuretics often are used. For patients who are unresponsive to loop diuretics, the addition of supplemental thiazide diuretics (e.g., metolazone) may be helpful.

TABLE 13-9. Vasodilators

Generic name	Trade name	Mechanism of action	Dose[a]	Adverse effects and comments
Nitroprusside	Nipride	Arterial and venous dilator	Initial dose is 0.1 to 0.25 mcg/kg/min, and titrate to response.	Hypotension, headache, tachycardia, cyanide and thiocyanate toxicity, myocardial ischemia
Nitroglycerin	Nitro-Bid, Nitrostat	Venous dilator but also an arterial dilator at higher doses	Initial dose is 5 to 10 mcg/min, and titrate to response.	Hypotension, headache, tachycardia, tolerance to hemodynamic effects

a. All are given by continuous I.V. infusion.

TABLE 13-10. Inotropes

Generic name	Trade name	Mechanism of action	Dose[a]	Adverse effects and comments
Dobutamine	Dobutrex	Beta-1- and beta-2-receptor agonist and weak alpha-1 agonist; increases cardiac output and vasodilates	2.5 to 20 mcg/kg/min	Increases heart rate, contractility, myocardial oxygen demand, myocardial ischemia, arrhythmias; not useful to increase blood pressure in hypotensive patients
Milrinone	Primacor	Inhibits phospho-diesterase III, resulting in positive inotropic and vasodilating effects	0.125 to 0.75 mcg/kg/min	Arrhythmias, hypotension, headache; alternative for patients not responding to dobutamine or dopamine; may be useful for patients receiving beta blockers because its positive inotropic effects are not mediated by beta receptors; dose adjustment needed in patients with renal insufficiency

a. All are given by continuous I.V. infusion.

- Inotropic therapy (dobutamine or milrinone) usually is not necessary, although it can be considered in patients who are not responding to I.V. loop diuretics or vasodilators. The addition of I.V. vasodilators (nitroglycerin, nitroprusside) also can reduce symptoms.

Volume Overload and Hypoperfusion

- Use inotropes to improve cardiac output first (i.e., before removing excess volume with I.V. loop diuretics).
- I.V. vasodilators also can be used to increase cardiac output.

Monitoring Parameters

- Daily weight
- Daily fluid intake and output
- Vital signs, at least daily
- Signs of heart failure, at least daily: edema, ascites, pulmonary rales, jugular venous pressure, hepatomegaly, and hepatojugular reflux
- Symptoms of heart failure, at least daily: orthopnea, paroxysmal nocturnal dyspnea, cough, dyspnea, fatigue, and light-headedness
- Electrolytes, at least daily: sodium, potassium, and magnesium
- Renal function, at least daily: BUN and serum creatinine

13-6 Nondrug Therapy

Nondrug therapies include the following:

- Ultrafiltration
- Intra-aortic balloon pump
- Left ventricular assist devices

- Cardiac resynchronization therapy
- Implantable cardioverter defibrillator
- Cardiac transplantation

13-7   Pharmacist's Role

Multidisciplinary team care of patients with HF involving physicians, pharmacists, nurses, and other health care professionals has been shown to reduce the risk of hospitalization and improve quality of life. Pharmacists play a key role in the team-based care of patients with HF. Studies show that patients receiving education from pharmacists are more likely to be adherent to medications and have fewer adverse drug reactions, medication errors, or hospitalizations. Pharmacists assist in the selection, initiation, dose titration, and follow-up monitoring needed to optimize guideline-directed medical therapy.

Pharmacists can:

- identify factors causing heart failure exacerbations including medication and dietary nonadherence and use of medications that worsen heart failure (e.g., NSAIDs).
- identify sources for medication nonadherence including costs, adverse effects, complexity of regimens, and physical or cognitive impairment and recommend approaches to address these problems.
- recommend appropriate dose adjustments in patients with impaired renal or hepatic function.
- screen for drug–drug interactions and recommend appropriate management.

Most patients with heart failure have numerous comorbidities (e.g., hypertension, diabetes, coronary artery disease, atrial fibrillation) requiring drug therapy so that the number of different medications patients receive is often large. Pharmacists can assist in optimizing the management of these disorders, assuring that optimal treatments are selected that will achieve goals of therapy but not worsen heart failure.

NAPLEX Competency Statements

The questions in this chapter cover the following 2021 NAPLEX Competency Statements: **AREA 1:** 1.1; 1.2; 1.3; 1.4; 1.5; 1.6; 1.7 **AREA 2:** 2.1; 2.2; 2.4 **AREA 3:** 3.1; 3.2; 3.3; 3.4; 3.5; 3.6; 3.7; 3.8; 3.9; 3.10; 3.11; 3.12 **AREA 5:** 5.5.

13-8  Questions

1. Which combinations represent optimal pharmacotherapy of patients with stage C HFrEF?

   A. Furosemide, clonidine, hydrochlorothiazide, and propranolol
   B. Furosemide, sacubitril/valsartan, spironolactone, dapagliflozin, and carvedilol
   C. Carvedilol, verapamil, amlodipine, and dobutamine
   D. Cardizem, hydrochlorothiazide, digoxin, and sotalol
   E. Dobutamine, amiodarone, furosemide, and nitroglycerin

2. Which mechanism most likely contributes to the benefits of beta blockers in the treatment of HFrEF?

   A. Stimulation of beta-2 receptors
   B. Increased heart rate and blood pressure
   C. Stimulation of beta-1 receptors
   D. Blockade of increased sympathetic nervous system activity
   E. Blockade of angiotensin II receptors

3. Appropriate monitoring parameters for enalapril therapy in the treatment of heart failure include, (Mark all that apply.)

   A. serum creatinine.
   B. blood pressure.
   C. thyroid stimulating hormone.
   D. serum potassium.
   E. hemoglobin A1C.

4. Patients taking eplerenone for heart failure should avoid taking _____.

   A. NSAIDs
   B. ACEIs
   C. beta blockers
   D. Demadex
   E. calcium supplements

5. Which are adverse effects of digoxin? (Mark all that apply.)

   A. Hepatotoxicity
   B. Anorexia
   C. Stroke
   D. Changes in color vision
   E. Bradycardia

6. Heart failure may be exacerbated by which medications? (Mark all that apply.)

   A. Naproxen
   B. Glipizide
   C. Diltiazem
   D. Crestor (rosuvastatin)
   E. Rosiglitazone

7. Cough is an adverse effect associated with which medication?

   A. Ramipril
   B. Valsartan
   C. Carvedilol
   D. Ivabradine
   E. Eplerenone

8. Which are adverse effects of Entresto? (Mark all that apply.)

   A. Bradycardia
   B. Hyperkalemia
   C. Angioedema
   D. Increased serum creatinine
   E. Hypertension

9. Which adverse effects of lisinopril can be avoided by switching to candesartan? (Mark all that apply.)

   A. Cough
   B. Renal insufficiency
   C. Hyperkalemia
   D. Hypotension
   E. Injury or death to developing fetus

10. Which medications increase digoxin serum concentrations? (Mark all that apply.)

    A. Biaxin (clarithromycin)
    B. Hydralazine
    C. Amiodarone
    D. Lipitor (atorvastatin)
    E. Warfarin

11. Which medications can cause bradycardia? (Mark all that apply.)

    A. Carvedilol
    B. Corlanor
    C. Ramipril
    D. Entresto
    E. Dobutamine

12. Which are contraindicated in patients with a history of lisinopril-induced angioedema? (Mark all that apply.)

    A. Captopril
    B. Torsemide
    C. Spironolactone
    D. Milrinone
    E. Entresto

13. Which statements are true about ivabradine use in patients with HFrEF? (Mark all that apply.)

    A. Indicated to reduce mortality
    B. Reduces the risk of HF hospitalizations
    C. Increases heart rate
    D. Indicated in patients receiving maximum tolerated beta-blocker doses with a heart rate > 70 bpm
    E. Increases the risk of hypokalemia in patients receiving Bumex.

14. Which best describes the use of furosemide in heart failure?

    A. Furosemide reduces mortality and slows heart failure progression.
    B. Hypokalemia is a common adverse effect.
    C. Response can be evaluated by monitoring hemoglobin A1C.
    D. Oral absorption is increased in patients with acute decompensated heart failure.
    E. Furosemide's bioavailability is not affected by food.

15. Which is an important consideration when using beta blockers for treating HFrEF?

A. They are effective only in patients who have had a myocardial infarction.
B. All beta blockers are equally effective for the treatment of HFrEF.
C. Therapy should be initiated at the target dose.
D. Patients with fluid overload are the optimal candidates for initiating therapy.
E. Therapy should be initiated at low doses and titrated upward slowly.

16. Which are adverse drug reactions with Jardiance? (Mark all that apply.)

A. Genital fungal infections
B. Tachycardia
C. Urinary tract infections
D. Hypertension
E. Hypoglycemia

17. Which is true regarding digoxin therapy in patients with HFrEF?

A. Digoxin reduces mortality.
B. Concomitant amiodarone therapy decreases digoxin plasma concentrations.
C. Digoxin is contraindicated in patients with HFrEF and atrial fibrillation.
D. The target digoxin plasma concentration is 0.5 to 0.9 ng/mL.
E. Concomitant glyburide therapy increases digoxin plasma concentrations.

18. Which beta blocker also blocks alpha-1 receptors and is effective for treating HFrEF?

A. Metoprolol
B. Carvedilol
C. Bisoprolol
D. Propranolol
E. Atenolol

19. Which are contraindicated in a patient with HFrEF receiving lisinopril?

A. Metoprolol succinate
B. Sacubitril/valsartan
C. Eplerenone
D. Bumex
E. Digoxin

20. Which is correct regarding the treatment of ADHF?

A. Nitroglycerin is the agent of choice in patients with ADHF and hypotension.
B. Milrinone is preferred over dobutamine in patients receiving concomitant beta-blocker therapy.
C. Absorption of oral loop diuretics is increased.
D. Dobutamine and milrinone improve survival.
E. Verapamil reduces volume overload and improves cardiac output.

Use Patient Profile 13-1 to answer Questions 21 and 22.

21. Which medications should be added to Mr. Johnson's regimen?

A. Spironolactone, and dapagliflozin
B. Valsartan and prazosin
C. Torsemide and amlodipine
D. Verapamil and amiodarone
E. Clonidine and hydrochlorothiazide

22. Mr. Johnson's serum potassium level of 2 mEq/L (normal 4 to 5 mEq/L) could _____.

A. increase the risk of Lanoxin (digoxin) toxicity
B. be treated by increasing the dose of Lasix (furosemide)
C. be considered a side effect of therapy with enteric-coated (EC) aspirin
D. be caused by an interaction between Crestor (rosuvastatin) and Lanoxin
E. increase the risk of bleeding from Plavix

PATIENT PROFILE 13-1

Patient Name: William Johnson   **Height:** 5'11"
Age: 64   **Weight:** 185 lb
Sex: Male   **Allergies:** NKA
Diagnosis: Myocardial infarction 2019
                   Hypertension
                   Heart failure
                   Hyperlipidemia

Laboratory and diagnostic tests

Echocardiogram in 12/19 showed LVEF 30%

Blood pressure on 4/1/20: 145/90 mmHg

Heart rate on 4/1/20: 88 bpm

Lipid profile on 4/1/20:

  Total cholesterol, 125 mg/dL

  LDL cholesterol, 55 mg/dL

  HDL cholesterol, 50 mg/dL

  Triglycerides, 100 mg/dL

  Serum potassium, 2 mEq/L

Medication record

Date	Rx #	Physician	Drug and strength	Quantity	Sig	Refills
4/1	1000	Smith	Lanoxin 0.125 mg	90	1 tab daily	2
4/1	1001	Smith	Lasix 40 mg	60	1 tab every morning	3
4/1	1002	Smith	KCl 20 mEq	90	1 tab every morning	1
4/1	1003	Smith	Crestor 40 mg	90	1 tab every night	3
4/1	1004	Smith	EC aspirin 81 mg	90	1 tab every morning	2
4/1	1005	Smith	Plavix 75 mg	90	1 tab every morning	3
4/1	1006	Smith	Entresto 47/103 mg	90	1 tab twice daily	3
4/1	1007	Smith	Carvedilol 25 mg	90	1 tab twice daily	3

Use Hospital Inpatient Profile 13-1 to answer Questions 23–25.

23. According to her profile, the recent worsening of Mrs. Smith's heart failure most likely is related to _____.

  A. Zestril (lisinopril)
  B. naproxen
  C. subtherapeutic serum digoxin concentration
  D. furosemide
  E. drug interaction between Zestril and furosemide

24. Toprol-XL is an agent that _____.

  A. is contraindicated in heart failure
  B. blocks beta-1, beta-2, and alpha-1 receptors
  C. blocks only beta-1 receptors
  D. should not be used in combination with Zestril
  E. increases the serum digoxin concentration

25. Which medications could improve this patient's symptoms and survival? (Select all that apply)

  A. Spironolactone
  B. Amlodipine
  C. Empagliflozin
  D. Dobutamine weekly infusion
  E. Warfarin

HOSPITAL INPATIENT PROFILE 13-1

Patient Name: Ellen Smith   **Height:** 5'4"

Age: 71   **Weight:** 150 lb

Sex: Female   **Allergies:** NKA

Diagnosis: Heart failure exacerbation with 20-lb weight gain over past 3–4 weeks

Hypertension

Osteoarthritis

Laboratory and diagnostic tests

Echocardiogram in 2/20 showed LVEF 25%

Blood pressure on 4/1/20: 130/85 mmHg

Heart rate on 4/1/20: 80 bpm

Serum digoxin concentration on 4/1/20: 0.8 ng/mL

Medication record

Date	Rx #	Physician	Drug and strength	Quantity	Sig	Refills
2/1	100	Jones	Lanoxin 0.125 mg	90	1 tab daily	2
3/1	101	Jones	Furosemide 80 mg	60	1 tab every morning	3
1/4	102	Jones	Zestril 20 mg	90	1 tab daily	1
1/4	103	Jones	Toprol-XL 50 mg	90	1 tab daily	3
3/1	104	Nelson	Naproxen 500 mg	90	1 tab twice daily with food	3

 13-9   Answers

1. **B.** Furosemide, sacubitril/valsartan, spironolactone (an aldosterone antagonist), dapagliflozin (SGLT2 inhibitor), and carvedilol (a beta blocker) in combination should be used routinely in patients with HFrEF to reduce mortality, improve symptoms, and slow heart failure progression as described in the 2021 ACC Consensus Decision Pathway for Optimization of Heart Failure Treatment.

2. **D.** Activation of the sympathetic nervous system plays an important role in the initiation and progression of heart failure. The benefits of beta blockers are thought to be due to the blockade of the sympathetic nervous system's increased activity.

3. **A, B, D.** Enalapril (and other ACEIs) can worsen renal function, lower blood pressure, and increase serum potassium. Thus, serum creatinine, blood pressure, and potassium should be monitored. ACEIs do not affect thyroid stimulating hormone or hemoglobin A1C.

4. **A.** Use of eplerenone is associated with renal potassium retention. Concomitant use of NSAIDs significantly increases the risk of hyperkalemia.

5. **B, D, E.** Anorexia, changes in color vision, and bradycardia are common symptoms of digoxin toxicity. Digoxin is not associated with hepatotoxicity or stroke.

6. **A, C, E.** Naproxen (an NSAID) can worsen heart failure by (1) increasing renal sodium and water retention and (2) attenuating the efficacy and enhancing the toxicity of ACEIs, ARBs, and diuretics. Diltiazem has negative inotropic effects and worsens heart failure in patients with HFrEF. Rosiglitazone is contraindicated in patients with heart failure as it increases fluid retention. Glipizide and Crestor do not affect heart failure.

7. **A.** Cough frequently is encountered as an adverse effect of ACEIs and is believed to be caused by bradykinin accumulation. The other agents do not cause cough.

8. **B, C, D.** Adverse effects of Entresto (sacubitril/valsartan) include hyperkalemia, angioedema,

and increased serum creatinine. It does not affect heart rate or increase blood pressure; it will decrease blood pressure.

9. **A.** The angiotensin receptor blocker candesartan is just as likely as lisinopril (or any other ACEI) to cause hypotension, hyperkalemia, renal insufficiency, and fetal injury. Candesartan (or other ARBs) are alternative agents for patients intolerant to ACEIs because of cough.

10. **A, C.** The macrolide antibiotic Biaxin (clarithromycin) and amiodarone are associated with 50% to 100% increases in serum digoxin concentrations. These agents do so by inhibiting the P-glycoprotein drug transporter. Hydralazine, Lipitor (atorvastatin), and warfarin do not affect digoxin pharmacokinetics.

11. **A, B.** Carvedilol is a beta blocker and is associated with a decreased heart rate (bradycardia). Corlanor (ivabradine) also can decrease heart rate. The other choices either increase (dobutamine) or do not affect (ramipril) heart rate.

12. **A, E.** Lisinopril is an ACEI, and angioedema is a known adverse effect of all agents in that drug class. Thus, captopril, which also is an ACEI, should not be used in this situation. Also, Entresto (sacubitril/valsartan) is contraindicated in patients with ACEI-associated angioedema because of the risk of a recurrent event. The other agents are not associated with angioedema.

13. **B, D.** Ivabradine is indicated in patients receiving maximum tolerated beta-blocker doses with a heart rate > 70 bpm to reduce the risk of heart failure hospitalizations. It does not affect mortality nor does it affect serum potassium concentrations.

14. **B.** Furosemide causes renal potassium loss and, thus, is associated with hypokalemia. It does not improve mortality or affect heart failure progression. Its oral absorption is slowed in patients with ADHF, and its bioavailability is reduced by food. Hemoglobin A1C is not useful for monitoring furosemide therapy.

15. **E.** When used to treat HFrEF, beta-blocker therapy should be started at low doses and gradually titrated upward until reaching the target dose that was shown in clinical trials to improve survival. Starting at the target dose or initiating treatment in patients with fluid overload increases the risk of worsening heart failure. Only carvedilol, bisoprolol,

and metoprolol succinate extended-release are the guideline-recommended agents as they are the only agents shown to be effective in HFrEF.

16. **A, C, E.** The SGLT2 inhibitors empagliflozin (Jardiance) and dapagliflozin (Farxiga) block the renal reabsorption of glucose resulting in increased glucosuria. Use of these agents is associated with increased risk of fungal infections of the genitals (highest risk in women and uncircumcised males), urinary tract infections, and hypoglycemia. Although the risk of hypoglycemia is generally low, the risk is increased in patients receiving insulin or insulin secretagogues). These agents do not cause tachycardia and can cause hypotension secondary to volume depletion, not hypertension.

17. **D.** The 2017 ACC–AHA Guidelines for the Management of Heart Failure suggest a target digoxin plasma concentration of 0.5–1 ng/mL. Digoxin does not improve survival in patients with heart failure—it only improves symptoms. Amiodarone increases digoxin plasma concentrations, and glyburide does not affect digoxin concentrations. Digoxin is useful in the management of patients with heart failure who also have atrial fibrillation.

18. **B.** Only carvedilol blocks alpha-1 receptors and has been shown to be effective in patients with HFrEF.

19. **B.** Sacubitril/valsartan (Entresto) is contraindicated for use with an ACEI because of increased risk of angioedema. The other agents can be used safely with an ACEI.

20. **B.** The positive inotropic effects of milrinone are not mediated through the beta-1 receptor; therefore, its effects are not diminished by concomitant beta-1 blocker therapy. Nitroglycerin is associated with an increased risk of hypotension. No inotropic agents are shown to improve survival. Absorption of oral loop diuretics is decreased in ADHF. Verapamil has negative inotropic effects and would worsen volume overload.

21. **A.** An aldosterone antagonist (spironolactone) and SGLT2 inhibitor (dapagliflozin) are indicated in this patient with HFrEF to improve survival and slow disease progression as described in the 2021 ACC Expert Decision Pathway for Optimization of Heart Failure Treatment.

22. **A.** Hypokalemia increases the risk of digoxin toxicity.

23. B. The addition of the NSAID naproxen approximately 3 to 4 weeks before admission likely is the cause of this episode of ADHF. Any NSAID can increase sodium and water retention and negate the effects of diuretics and ACEIs.

24. C. Toprol-XL (metoprolol succinate extended-release) is a cardioselective beta blocker. It blocks only the beta-1 receptor at usual therapeutic doses.

25. A and C. The addition of an aldosterone antagonist, either spironolactone or eplerenone, and a SGLT2 inhibitor (dapagliflzin or empagliflozin) are indicated to improve survival, reduce risk of hospitalization due to heart failure, and decrease symptoms in patients with HFrEF. Amlodipine would have no effect on these outcomes and weekly dobutamine infusions do not improve survival.

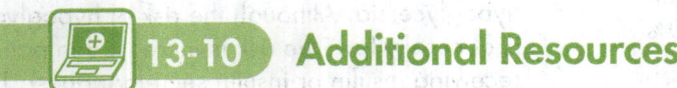 **13-10   Additional Resources**

Bozkurt B, Coats AJS, Tsutsui H, et al. Universal definition and classification of heart failure: a report of the Heart Failure Society of America, Heart Failure Association of the European Society of Cardiology, Japanese Heart Failure Society and Writing Committee of the Universal Definition of Heart Failure. *J Cardiac Fail* 2021;27:387–413.

Carlson MD, Eckman PM. Review of vasodilators in acute decompensated heart failure: the old and the new. *J Cardiac Fail.* 2013;19(7):478–493.

Ellison DH, Felker GM. Diuretic treatment in heart failure. *N Engl J Med.* 2017;377:1964–75.

Maddox TM, Januzzi JL, Allen LA, et al. 2021 update to the 2017 ACC expert decision pathway for optimization of heart failure treatment: answers to 10 pivotal issues about heart failure with reduced ejection fraction: a report of the American College of Cardiology Solution Set Oversight Committee. *J Am Coll Cardiol* 2021;77:772–810.

Page RL, O'Bryant CL, Cheng D, et al. Drugs that may cause or exacerbate heart failure: a scientific statement from the American Heart Association. *Circulation.* 2016;134:1–38.

Parker RB, Nappi JM, Cavallari LH. Chronic heart failure. In: DiPiro JT, Yee GC, Posey LM, et al., eds. *Pharmacotherapy: A Pathophysiologic Approach.* 11th ed. New York, NY. McGraw-Hill; 2019:79–115.

Reed BN, Rodgers JE. Acute decompensated heart failure. In: DiPiro JT, Yee GC, Posey LM, et al., eds. *Pharmacotherapy: A Pathophysiologic Approach.* 11th ed. New York, NY: McGraw-Hill; 2019:117–134.

Vardeny O, Miller R, Solomon SD. Combined neprilysin and renin-angiotensin system inhibition for the treatment of heart failure. *J Am Coll Cardiol HF.* 2014;2:663–670.

Yancy CW, Jessup M, Bozkurt B, et al. 2013 ACCF/AHA guideline for the management of heart failure: a report of the American College of Cardiology Foundation/American Heart Association Task Force on Practice Guidelines. *Circulation.* 2013;128:e240–e327.

Yancy CW, Jessup M, Bozkurt B, et al. 2017 ACC/AHA/HFSA focused update of the 2013 ACCF/AHA guideline for the management of heart failure: a report of the American College of Cardiology/American Heart Association Task Force on Clinical Practice Guidelines and the Heart Failure Society of America. *J Am Coll Cardiol.* 2017;70:776–803.

Cardiac Arrhythmias

ROBERT B. PARKER

14-1 KEY POINTS

- All antiarrhythmic drugs (AADs) are proarrhythmic.
- Cardiac arrhythmias range from benign to lethal.
- Antiarrhythmic drug therapy should be individualized to patient response while minimizing adverse effects.
- Many AADs are associated with significant drug interactions.
- Nonpharmacologic therapy is an important treatment modality, particularly to prevent life-threatening ventricular tachycardia and ventricular fibrillation and to maintain sinus rhythm in patients with atrial fibrillation.
- Treatment of atrial fibrillation always should include an assessment of antithrombotic therapy to reduce stroke risk.
- **Warfarin** or the direct-acting oral anticoagulants dabigatran, rivaroxaban, **apixaban**, and edoxaban are indicated to reduce the risk of stroke in patients with atrial fibrillation.

14-2 STUDY GUIDE CHECKLIST

The following topics may guide your study of this subject area:

- ☐ Risk factors for developing arrhythmias, especially atrial fibrillation.
- ☐ AADs are not proven to improve survival.
- ☐ Selection of appropriate pharmacotherapy for atrial fibrillation, including medications used for rate control, prevention of thromboembolism, and conversion to and maintenance of sinus rhythm, based on treatment guidelines and patient characteristics.
- ☐ Mechanisms of action of drug classes used to treat arrhythmias.
- ☐ Major adverse drug reactions of drugs used to treat arrhythmias.
- ☐ Significant drug interactions involving medications used to treat arrhythmias.
- ☐ Trade names and generic names of medications used to treat arrhythmias.
- ☐ Patient-counseling points for drugs used to treat arrhythmias.

14-3   Mechanisms of Arrhythmia

Normal Conduction System

The sinoatrial (SA) node, located in the right atrium, initiates an impulse that

- stimulates the left atrium and atrioventricular (AV) node, which
- stimulates the left and right bundle branches via the bundle of His, which then
- stimulates Purkinje fibers and causes ventricular contraction.

Cardiac arrhythmias arise secondary to abnormalities in impulse formation and/or conduction due to the following mechanisms (See Box 14-1 Mechanisms of Arrhythmias):

14-4   Clinical Manifestations

Symptoms

Both bradyarrhythmias and tachyarrhythmias can be associated with reduced cardiac output, producing symptoms that include dizziness, syncope, chest pain, fatigue, confusion, and exacerbation of heart failure. Patients with tachyarrhythmias also may report palpitations. With atrial fibrillation or flutter, patients may experience dizziness, palpitations, light-headedness, dyspnea, fatigue, and worsening heart failure, as well as symptoms of transient ischemic attack (TIA) or stroke. Ventricular arrhythmias can be asymptomatic or can cause loss of consciousness and death. Patients with ventricular tachycardia (VT) may be asymptomatic, but VT can result in hypotension, syncope, or death. Ventricular fibrillation produces no cardiac output and causes most cases of sudden cardiac death.

14-5   Diagnostic Criteria and Therapy According to Arrhythmia Classification

Arrhythmias are defined by the following:

- Anatomic location
  - Supraventricular arrhythmias arise from abnormalities in the SA node, the atrial tissue, the AV node, or the bundle of His.
  - Ventricular arrhythmias originate from below the bundle of His.

BOX 14-1. Mechanisms of Arrhythmias

- Automaticity (spontaneous impulse generation)
- Latent pacemaker (non-SA node pacemaker)
- Triggered automaticity (early or late after-depolarizations)
- Reentry
- Impulse conduction
- Automaticity and impulse conduction

- Ventricular rate
  - *Bradyarrhythmias:* Heart rate < 60 beats per minute (bpm).
  - *Tachyarrhythmias:* Heart rate > 100 bpm.

Bradyarrhythmias

Sinus bradycardia

Diagnostic criteria and characteristics

Heart rate is less than 60 bpm; otherwise, the electrocardiogram (ECG) is normal.

Clinical etiology

Causes include acute myocardial infarction (MI), hypothyroidism, drug-induced causes (beta blockers including ophthalmic agents, digoxin, calcium channel blockers [**diltiazem**, verapamil], **clonidine**, amiodarone, and cholinergic agents), and hyperkalemia.

Treatment goals

Restore normal sinus rhythm if the patient is clinically symptomatic.

Drug and nondrug therapy

For intermittent symptomatic episodes, administer atropine 0.5 to 1 mg intravenously, repeated up to maximum dose of 3 mg.

For persistent episodes, or if patient is unresponsive to atropine, place transvenous or transcutaneous pacemaker.

Atrioventricular block

Diagnostic criteria and characteristics

Criteria are as follows:

- *First-degree:* Prolonged PR interval > 0.20 seconds, 1:1 atrioventricular conduction
- *Second-degree Mobitz type I:* Gradual prolongation of PR interval followed by P wave without ventricular conduction
- *Second-degree Mobitz type II:* Constant PR interval with intermittent P wave without ventricular conduction; may have widened QRS complex
- *Third-degree:* Heart rate 30 to 60 bpm; no temporal relation between atrial and ventricular contraction; ventricular contraction initiated by AV junction or ventricular tissue

Clinical etiology

Causes include AV nodal disease, acute MI, myocarditis, increased vagal tone, drugs that slow AV nodal conduction (beta blockers, digoxin, calcium channel blockers [**diltiazem**, verapamil], **clonidine**, amiodarone, cholinergic agents), and hyperkalemia.

Treatment goals

Restore sinus rhythm if the patient is symptomatic.

Drug and nondrug therapy

Discontinue any drugs associated with slowing AV nodal conduction. If the cause is reversible, treat with a temporary pacemaker or intermittent atropine. If the condition is chronic, implant a permanent pacemaker.

Supraventricular Arrhythmias

Atrial fibrillation and atrial flutter (See Table 14-1)

Diagnostic criteria and characteristics

Criteria are as follows:

- *Atrial fibrillation:* No P waves; irregularly irregular QRS pattern
- *Atrial flutter:* Sawtooth P wave pattern; regular QRS pattern
- *Ventricular response:* Usually fast but also can be slow or normal

Clinical etiology

Causes and risk factors for developing atrial fibrillation and atrial flutter include valvular heart disease, heart failure, hypertension, ischemic heart disease, diabetes, obesity, obstructive sleep apnea, cardiac surgery, infection, alcohol abuse, hyperthyroidism, chronic obstructive pulmonary disease, pulmonary embolism, and idiopathic causes. Atrial fibrillation and flutter are the most commonly occurring arrhythmias, and risk increases with age.

Complications include stroke and heart failure exacerbation.

Specific treatment goals for atrial fibrillation

Figure 14-1 illustrates a treatment algorithm for atrial fibrillation.

Control the ventricular rate (See Figure 14-2)

Beta blockers (esmolol, **metoprolol**, **propranolol**, others) and calcium channel blockers (**diltiazem**, verapamil) are the most effective agents. Beta blockers are preferred in patients with compelling indications for use with a comorbid condition including previous MI or heart failure with reduced ejection fraction. Calcium channel blockers should not be used in patients with heart failure with reduced ejection fraction because of their negative inotropic effects.

Digoxin can be useful in patients with heart failure with reduced ejection fractions, especially when combined with a beta blocker; digoxin slows the ventricular rate but is more effective in reducing resting heart rate. It is not effective at controlling ventricular response associated with activity.

For rapid control of ventricular rate, intravenous (I.V.) beta blockers, calcium channel blockers, or digoxin should be used.

Digoxin, calcium channel blockers, and beta blockers do not restore sinus rhythm.

The target resting heart rate remains controversial, but current guidelines recommend a resting rate of <80 to 110 bpm.

TABLE 14-1. Classification of Atrial Fibrillation (as Defined by the 2014 AHA/ACC/HRS Atrial Fibrillation Treatment Guidelines)

Type of atrial fibrillation	Clinical features	Pattern
Paroxysmal	Terminates spontaneously or with intervention within 7 days of onset	± Recurrent
Persistent	Continuous AF sustained > 7 days	Recurrent
Longstanding Persistent	Continuous AF sustained > 12 months	Recurrent
Permanent	No further attempts to restore and/or maintain sinus rhythm will be pursued based on joint decision by patient and clinician	Established
Valvular AF	AF in the setting of moderate-to-severe mitral stenosis or the presence of a mechanical heart valve	N/A

FIGURE 14-1. A Treatment Algorithm for Atrial Fibrillation

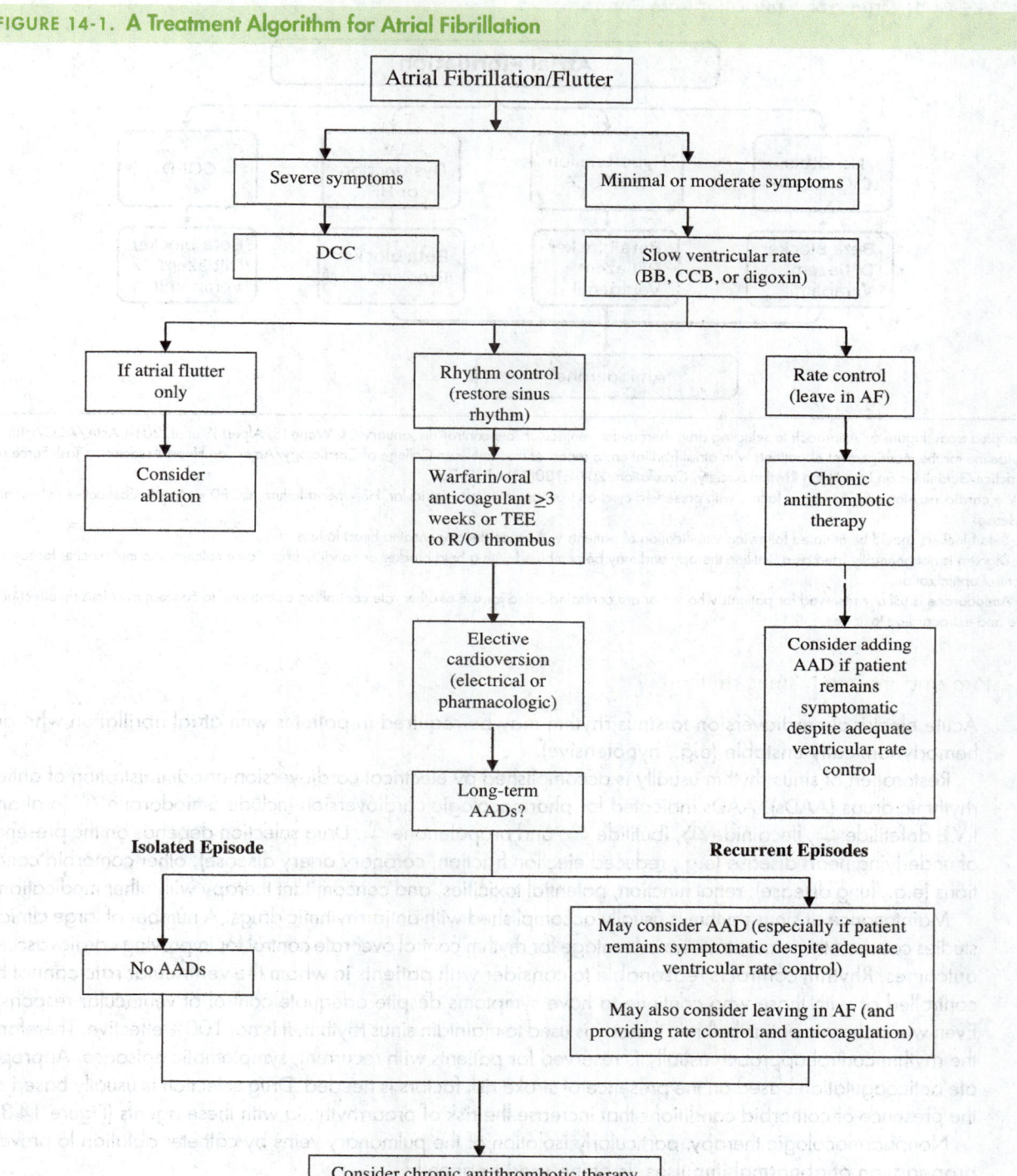

Reproduced with permission from Sanoski, Bauman, 2011.

AADs, antiarrhythmic drugs; AF, atrial fibrillation; BB, β-blocker; CCB, nondihydropyridine calcium channel blocker; DCC, direct-current cardioversion; R/O, rule out; TEE, transesophageal echocardiography.

a. Selection of the most appropriate antithrombotic therapy is based on the presence of risk factors for stroke, regardless of whether the rhythm or rate control approach is selected.

FIGURE 14-2. Drugs for Ventricular Rate Control

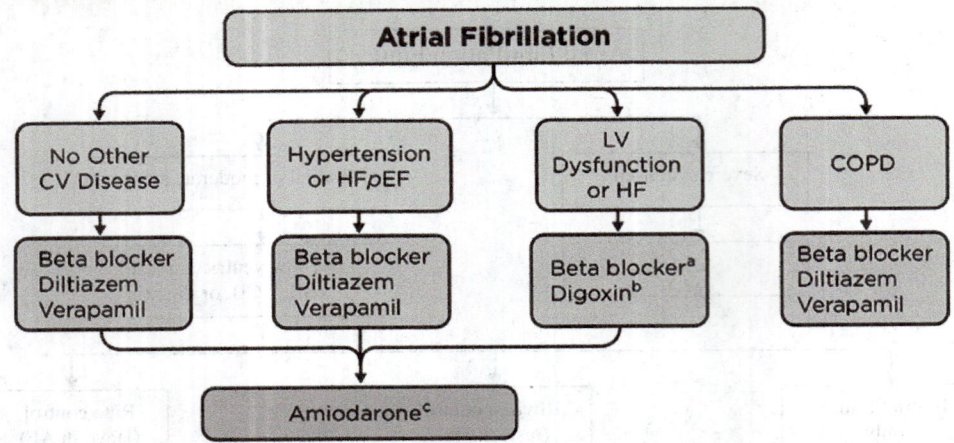

Adapted from: Figure 6 "Approach to selecting drug therapy for ventricular rate control" in January CT, Wann LS, Alpert JS et al. 2014 AHA/ACC/HRS guideline for the management of patients with atrial fibrillation: a report of the American College of Cardiology/American Heart Association Task Force on Practice Guidelines and the Heart Rhythm Society. *Circulation.* 2014;130(23):e199–267.

CV = cardiovascular, HFpEF = heart failure with preserved ejection fraction, LV = left ventricular, HF = heart failure, COPD = chronic obstructive pulmonary disease.

a. Beta blockers should be initiated following stabilization of patients with acute decompensated heart failure.

b. Digoxin is not generally used as a first-line therapy and may be combined with a beta blocker or nondihydropyridine calcium channel blocker for rate control optimization.

c. Amiodarone is usually reserved for patients who fail or are contraindicated for use of other rate controlling agents due to concern over its side effect profile and extracardiac toxicities.

Restore and maintain sinus rhythm

Acute electrical cardioversion to sinus rhythm may be required in patients with atrial fibrillation who are hemodynamically unstable (e.g., hypotensive).

Restoration of sinus rhythm usually is accomplished by electrical cardioversion or administration of antiarrhythmic drugs (AADs). AADs indicated for pharmacologic cardioversion include amiodarone ⚠ (oral and I.V.), dofetilide ⚠, flecainide ⚠, ibutilide ⚠, and propafenone ⚠. Drug selection depends on the presence of underlying heart disease (e.g., reduced ejection fraction, coronary artery disease), other comorbid conditions (e.g., lung disease), renal function, potential toxicities, and concomitant therapy with other medications.

Maintenance of sinus rhythm is usually accomplished with antiarrhythmic drugs. A number of large clinical studies consistently demonstrate no advantage for rhythm control over rate control for improving cardiovascular outcomes. Rhythm control is reasonable to consider with patients in whom the ventricular rate cannot be controlled or with those who continue to have symptoms despite adequate control of ventricular response. Even when chronic antiarrhythmic therapy is used to maintain sinus rhythm, it is not 100% effective. Therefore, the rhythm control approach usually is reserved for patients with recurrent, symptomatic episodes. Appropriate anticoagulation based on the presence of stroke risk factors is needed. Drug selection is usually based on the presence of comorbid conditions that increase the risk of proarrhythmia with these agents (Figure 14-3).

Nonpharmacologic therapy, particularly isolation of the pulmonary veins by catheter ablation to prevent propagation of abnormal impulses, is being used frequently.

Prevent thromboembolism

The following applies before use of pharmacologic or direct-current cardioversion. If atrial fibrillation is present for ≥48 hours or for an unknown duration, anticoagulate with **warfarin** (international normalized ratio [INR] 2 to 3), dabigatran, rivaroxaban, **apixaban**, or edoxaban for at least 3 weeks before cardioversion, and continue for at least 4 weeks after sinus rhythm has been restored. Long-term anticoagulation is based on the stroke risk as determined by the CHA$_2$DS$_2$-VASc score.

FDA BOXED WARNINGS

Amiodarone

May cause potentially fatal toxicities, including pulmonary toxicity, hepatotoxicity, liver injury and worsened arrhythmia. Intended for use only in patients with life-threatening arrhythmias when other treatments ineffective or not tolerated.

Dofetilide

To minimize the risk of induced arrhythmia, patients initiated or reinitiated on dofetilide should be placed for a minimum of 3 days in a facility that can provide calculations of creatinine clear-ance, continuous ECG monitoring, and cardiac resuscitation.

Flecainide

Increased mortality and nonfatal cardiac arrest in patients with non-life-threatening ventricular arrhythmias and structural heart disease; consider avoiding flecainide in these patients. Flecainide is not recommended for use in patients with chronic atrial fibrillation.

Ibutilide

Ibutilide fumarate can cause potentially fatal arrhythmias, particularly sustained polymorphic ventricular tachycardia, usually in association with QT prolongation (torsades de pointes), but sometimes without documented QT prolongation. These arrhythmias can be reversed if treated promptly. It is essential that ibutilide fumarate injection be administered in a setting of continuous ECG monitoring and by personnel trained in identification and treatment of acute ventricular arrhythmias, particularly polymorphic ventricular tachycardia. Patients with atrial fibrillation of more than 2 to 3 days' duration must be adequately anticoagulated, generally for at least 2 weeks. Patients with chronic atrial fibrillation have a strong tendency to revert after conversion to sinus rhythm and treatments to maintain sinus rhythm carry risks. Patients to be treated with ibutilide fumarate injection, therefore, should be carefully selected such that the expected benefits of maintaining sinus rhythm outweigh the immediate risks of ibutilide fumarate injection, and the risks of maintenance therapy, and are likely to offer an advantage compared with alternative management.

Propafenone

Given the lack of any evidence that these drugs improve survival, antiarrhythmic agents should generally be avoided in patients with non-life-threatening ventricular arrhythmias, even if the patients are experiencing unpleasant, but not life-threatening, symptoms or signs.

FIGURE 14-3. Selection of Antiarrhythmic Drugs to Maintain Sinus Rhythm

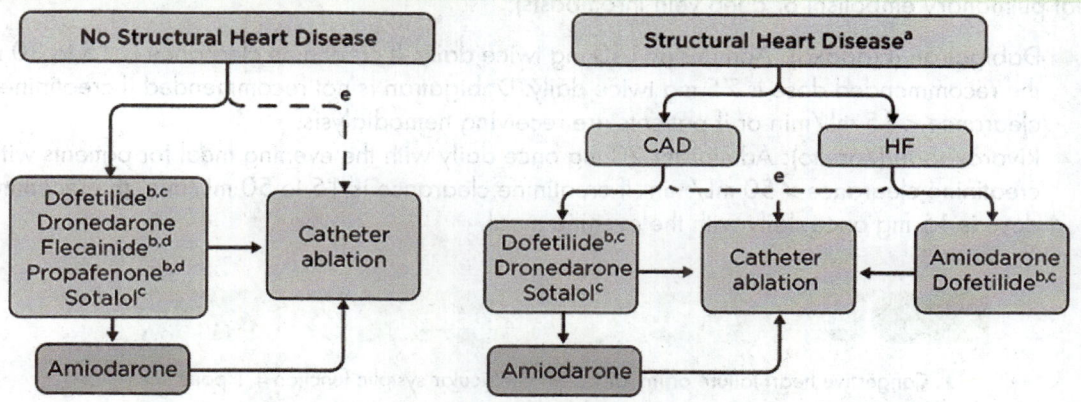

Adapted from Figure 7 "Strategies for rhythm control in patients with paroxysmal and persistent AF" in January CT, Wann LS, Alpert JS et al. 2014 AHA/ACC/HRS guidelines for the management of the patients with atrial fibrillation: a report of the American College of Cardiology/American Heart Association Task Force on Practice Guidelines and the Heart Rhythm Society. *Circulation.* 2014;130(23):e199–267.

CAD = coronary artery disease, HF = heart failure.

a. Structural heart disease is a broad term encompassing valvular heart disease, coronary heart disease, cardiomyopathies, congestive heart failure, left ventricular dysfunction, and significant left ventricular hypertrophy.

b. Agent not recommended for use in patients with severe left ventricular hypertrophy (wall thickness > 1.5 cm).

c. Agent should be used with caution in patients at risk for torsades de pointes (e.g., prolonged baseline QT/QTc interval, on concomitant meds that prolong QT/QTc interval, renal dysfunction).

d. Agent should be combined with an AV nodal blocking agent (e.g., beta blocker, nondihydropyridine calcium channel blocker).

e. Catheter ablation is only recommended as first-line therapy for patients with paroxysmal AF.

If atrial fibrillation is present for ≥48 hours or for an unknown duration and no anticoagulation therapy has been given in the preceding 3 weeks, transesophageal echocardiography (TEE) often is used to determine the presence of atrial thrombus. If no thrombus is seen, cardioversion can be attempted provided anticoagulation has been achieved before TEE and is continued for at least 4 weeks afterward. If atrial thrombus is seen on TEE, anticoagulation should be initiated and a repeat TEE should be performed before attempting later cardioversion.

Recommended chronic antithrombotic therapy

The choice of the optimal antithrombotic agent is based on the patient-specific risks of stroke and bleeding and should involve shared decision making with patients based on their values and preferences. Current guidelines now recommend the use of the CHA_2DS_2-VASc score to calculate stroke risk in patients with nonvalvular atrial fibrillation. Each stroke risk factor is assigned a point value, and the total number of points is associated with an annual risk of stroke. The CHA_2DS_2-VASc risk factors for stroke are as follows (See Box 14-2 CHA_2DS_2-VASc Stroke Risk Factors):

The following treatments are recommended according to a patient's CHA_2DS_2-VASc score:

- CHA_2DS_2-VASc score is 0 in men or 1 in women: omitting anticoagulant therapy is reasonable.
- CHA_2DS_2-VASc score is 1 in men or 2 in women: oral anticoagulation may be considered.
- CHA_2DS_2-VASc score ≥ 2 in men or ≥ 3 in women: oral anticoagulation is recommended.
- For patients with atrial fibrillation who have mechanical heart valves or moderate-to-severe mitral stenosis, **warfarin** therapy is recommended.

Oral anticoagulation

The use of oral anticoagulants significantly reduces the risk of stroke in patients with atrial fibrillation. Options include **warfarin** with the dose titrated to achieve an INR 2–3 or the direct-acting oral anticoagulants (DOACs) dabigatran, rivaroxaban, **apixaban**, or edoxaban. In DOAC-eligible patients, DOACs are recommended over **warfarin**. DOACs are either noninferior or, as shown in some clinical trials, superior to **warfarin** for prevention of stroke or systemic embolism and have a reduced risk of bleeding. Detailed information about these agents' mechanism of action, adverse effects, drug interactions, monitoring, and patient counseling can be found in Chapter 30, on thromboembolic disease. The recommended DOAC doses for treatment of atrial fibrillation are as follows (note that these doses may differ from those used to treat pulmonary embolism or deep vein thrombosis):

- Dabigatran (Pradaxa): Administer 150 mg twice daily. If creatinine clearance is 15 to 30 mL/min, the recommended dose is 75 mg twice daily. Dabigatran is not recommended if creatinine clearance < 15 mL/min or if patients are receiving hemodialysis.
- Rivaroxaban (Xarelto): Administer 20 mg once daily with the evening meal for patients with creatinine clearance > 50 mL/min. If creatinine clearance is 15 to 50 mL/min, the recommended dose is 15 mg once daily with the evening meal.

> **BOX 14-2. CHA_2DS_2-VASc Risk Factors for Stroke**
>
> - **C**ongestive heart failure or impaired left ventricular systolic function = 1 point
> - **H**ypertension = 1 point
> - **A**ge ≥ 75 years = 2 points
> - **D**iabetes = 1 point
> - **S**troke/TIA/thromboembolism = 2 points
> - **V**ascular disease (MI, peripheral artery disease, or aortic plaque) = 1 point
> - **A**ge 65 to 74 years = 1 point
> - **S**ex category (female) = 1 point

- **Apixaban** (Eliquis): The recommended dose is 5 mg twice daily. The dose should be reduced to 2.5 mg twice daily in patients with any two of the following characteristics: age ≥ 80 years, weight ≤ 60 kg, or serum creatinine ≥ 1.5 mg/dL.
- **Edoxaban** (Savaysa): The recommended dose is 60 mg once daily in patients with creatinine clearance > 50 mL/min and ≤ 95 mL/min. In patients with creatinine clearance of 15 to 50 mL/min, the dose should be reduced to 30 mg once daily. Edoxaban should not be used in patients with a creatinine clearance > 95 mL/min.
- DOACs should not be used in patients with atrial fibrillation and a mechanical heart valve.
- In patients receiving dialysis or with end-stage chronic kidney disease, dabigatran, rivaroxaban, and edoxaban are not recommended, but it is reasonable to use **warfarin** (INR 2–3) or **apixaban** for anticoagulation.

Paroxysmal supraventricular tachycardia

Diagnostic criteria and characteristics

Criteria for paroxysmal supraventricular tachycardia (PSVT) are as follows:

- Heart rate of 160 to 240 bpm that is abrupt in onset and termination with a normal QRS interval
- 1:1 AV conduction

Mechanism of arrhythmia

The mechanism of arrhythmia is reentry.

Clinical etiology

Causes include idiopathic causes, fever, and drug-induced causes (sympathomimetics, anticholinergics, beta agonists).

Treatment goals

- ***Acute:*** Terminate reentry circuit by prolonging refractoriness and slowing conduction. For hemodynamically unstable patients, synchronized cardioversion is the treatment of choice. In hemodynamically stable patients, vagal maneuvers (carotid massage and Valsalva maneuver [the most common], squatting, deep breathing, coughing, inducement of eyeball pressure, and diving reflex [less common]), and/or I.V. adenosine are the initial treatments. If these are not effective or not available, then I.V. **diltiazem** or verapamil can be used. I.V. beta blockers are also reasonable for acute treatment.
- ***Chronic:*** Prevent or minimize the number and severity of episodes. AADs no longer are the treatment of choice to prevent recurrences. Most patients undergo radiofrequency catheter ablation of the reentrant substrate, which is curative and is associated with a low complication rate.

Ventricular Arrhythmias

Major classifications and diagnostic criteria

- Premature ventricular contractions (PVCs)
  - PVCs are extra abnormal heartbeats that originate in the ventricles. They are termed *premature* because they occur before the normal heartbeat.
  - PVCs often are asymptomatic or cause only palpitations.
- Ventricular tachycardia
  - VT is defined as three or more consecutive PVCs at a rate exceeding 100 bpm and a wide QRS interval (> 0.12 seconds), usually with a regular pattern.
  - Nonsustained VT (NSVT) is defined as an episode that lasts less than 30 seconds.
  - Sustained VT is defined as an episode that lasts more than 30 seconds.
- Ventricular fibrillation
  - Ventricular fibrillation is defined as an absence of organized cardiac electrical or mechanical activity and no recognizable P waves, QRS complexes, or T waves on the ECG.
  - Ventricular fibrillation rapidly results in no effective cardiac output, blood pressure, or pulse.

Clinical etiology

Causes include acute MI, electrolyte disturbances, catecholamines, and drug-induced causes.

Treatment goals

- Treat acute symptoms and precipitating causes.
- Restore sinus rhythm.
- Prevent or minimize recurrences.

14-6   Drug and Nondrug Therapy

Premature Ventricular Contractions

Apparently healthy patients without underlying structural heart disease are not at increased risk for VT or sudden cardiac death; therefore, no drug therapy is necessary.

Patients with PVCs and underlying heart disease (e.g., previous MI, decreased ejection fraction) are at increased risk for more serious arrhythmias. However, AADs do not reduce this risk; in fact, their use is associated with increased risk of lethal arrhythmias. All such patients should receive medications proven to improve survival, including beta blockers, antiplatelet agents, statins, angiotensin-converting enzyme inhibitors (ACEIs) or angiotensin receptor blockers (ARBs), and aldosterone antagonists if appropriate. To reduce mortality in such patients with a left ventricular ejection fraction (LVEF) ≤ 30% to 40%, an implantable cardioverter defibrillator (ICD) is indicated.

Nonsustained Ventricular Tachycardia

For patients with heart disease and LVEF > 40%, maximize other cardiovascular medications with proven effects on survival (see previous paragraph).

Recent studies indicate that patients with heart disease and LVEF ≤ 30% to 40% are at increased risk for sudden cardiac death (usually from ventricular fibrillation). Use of an ICD improves survival in this group, but amiodarone does not affect survival. Even in the absence of PVCs or NSVT in this patient group, these patients are at increased risk for sudden cardiac death, and an ICD is indicated to improve survival. Unless contraindicated, these patients also should receive guideline-recommended medical therapy, which could include angiotensin receptor blocker/neprilysin inhibitor/ACEIs/ARBs, beta blockers, diuretics, aldosterone antagonists, and serum-glucose co-transporter-2 inhibitors.

Sustained Ventricular Tachycardia or Ventricular Fibrillation (Postresuscitation)

If the event occurs within 24 to 48 hours of MI or because of other reversible causes, no antiarrhythmic drug therapy is needed except beta blockers.

If the event is not secondary to MI or another reversible cause, ICD placement is recommended.

AADs (i.e., amiodarone or sotalol) may still be required to decrease the number of defibrillator discharges, increase patient comfort, and prolong ICD battery life.

Amiodarone can be considered if the patient refuses ICD placement.

Torsades de Pointes

This is a specific type of ventricular tachycardia with QRS complexes that appear to twist around the ECG baseline. It is associated with a prolonged QT interval.

Clinical etiology

Causes are as follows:

- Genetic abnormalities in cardiac potassium channels
- Acquired
  - Hypokalemia or hypomagnesemia
  - Myocardial ischemia or infarction
  - Subarachnoid hemorrhage
  - Hypothyroidism
  - Myocarditis or cardiomyopathy
  - Arsenic poisoning
  - Drug-induced causes (known association with torsades de pointes)
    - *Antiarrhythmics:* quinidine, procainamide, disopyramide, sotalol ⚠, ibutilide, dofetilide, amiodarone, dronedarone ⚠
    - *Antipsychotics:* chlorpromazine, haloperidol, mesoridazine, thioridazine, pimozide, **citalopram**, atypical antipsychotics (e.g., **quetiapine**, ziprasidone)
    - *Antidepressants:* **amitriptyline**, desipramine, doxepin, imipramine, nortriptyline
    - *Antibiotics:* erythromycin, clarithromycin, **azithromycin**, levofloxacin, moxifloxacin, pentamidine, trimethoprim-sulfamethoxazole, hydroxychloroquine
    - *Others:* methadone, droperidol, **ondansetron**

Treatment

- Stop the offending drug if possible.
- Administer direct-current cardioversion for hemodynamically unstable patients.
- Administer magnesium sulfate 2 g over 1 minute I.V.
- Use a pacemaker or isoproterenol infusion to increase heart rate.
- Correct hypokalemia or hypomagnesemia.

Drug therapy

See Tables 14-2, 14-3, and 14-4 for information about AADs. AADs terminate or minimize arrhythmias by:

- decreasing automaticity of abnormal pacemaker tissues,
- altering conduction characteristics of reentry,
- increasing refractory period, or
- eliminating premature impulses that trigger reentry.

 FDA BOXED WARNINGS

Sotalol

Sotalol can cause life threatening ventricular tachycardia associated with QT interval prolongation. To minimize the risk of drug-induced arrhythmia, initiate or reinitiate oral sotalol in a facility that can provide cardiac resuscitation and continuous electrocardiographic monitoring. Sotalol can cause life threatening ventricular tachycardia associated with QT interval prolongation. If the QT interval prolongs to 500 msec or greater, reduce the dose, lengthen the dosing interval, or discontinue the drug. Calculate creatinine clearance to determine appropriate dosing.

Dronedarone

Increased risk of death, stroke and heart failure in patients with decompensated heart failure or permanent atrial fibrillation. In patients with symptomatic heart failure and recent decompensation requiring hospitalization or NYHA Class IV heart failure, dronedarone hydrochloride doubles the risk of death. Dronedarone hydrochloride is contraindicated in patients with symptomatic heart failure with recent de-compensation requiring hospitalization or NYHA Class IV heart failure. In patients with permanent atrial fibrillation, dronedarone hydrochloride doubles the risk of death, stroke, and hospitalization for heart failure. Dronedarone hydrochloride is contraindicated in patients in atrial fibrillation (AF) who will not or cannot be cardioverted into normal sinus rhythm.

TABLE 14-2. Effects of Antiarrhythmic Drugs on Cardiac Electrophysiology

Drug class	Ion block	Conduction	Refractory period	Automaticity
Ia	Sodium and **potassium**	↓	↑	↓
Ib	Sodium	0/↓	↓	↓
Ic	Sodium	↓↓	↓	↓
II	Calcium (indirect effect)	↓	↑	↓
III[a]	**Potassium**	0	↑↑	0
IV	Calcium	↓	↑	↓

↓, decreases; ↑, increases.
a. Sotalol also possesses beta-blocking activity. Amiodarone also possesses sodium and calcium channel blockade.

TABLE 14-3. Class I and III Antiarrhythmic Drug Availability and Standard Dosing Regimens

Generic name	Trade name	Dosage forms	Loading dose	Maintenance dose
Class Ia				
Quinidine gluconate	Generic	324 mg tablets		328 to 648 mg 3 times daily
Quinidine sulfate	Generic	200, 300 mg tablets		200 to 400 mg 4 times daily
Procainamide	Generic	100, 500 mg/mL injection Oral procainamide not available	I.V.: 15 to 18 mg/kg at 20 to 50 mg/min	I.V.: 1 to 6 mg/min
Disopyramide	Norpace	100, 150 mg capsules		150 to 300 mg 4 times daily
	Norpace CR	100, 150 mg capsules		300 to 600 mg twice daily
Class Ib				
Lidocaine	Xylocaine	0.5, 1, 1.5, 2, 4, and 20% solutions	I.V.: 100 mg repeat up to 2 times	I.V.: 1 to 4 mg/min
Mexiletine	Mexitil	150, 200, 250 mg capsules		100 to 300 mg 3 times daily
Class Ic				
Flecainide	Tambocor	50, 100, 150, 200 mg tablets	200 to 300 mg for conversion of atrial fibrillation to sinus rhythm	50 to 200 mg twice daily
Propafenone	Rythmol, Rythmol-SR	150, 225, 300 mg tablets	450 to 600 mg for conversion of atrial fibrillation to sinus rhythm	150 to 300 mg 3 times daily
		225, 325, 425 mg capsules		225 to 425 mg twice daily
Class III				
Amiodarone	Cordarone, Pacerone, Nexterone (premixed I.V. injection)	100, 200, 300, 400 mg tablets premix: 150 mg/100 mL and 360 mg/200 mL	800 to 1600 mg/day in divided doses × 2 to 4 weeks for total of 10 g I.V. (VT/VF): 150 mg/10 min or 900 mg in 500 mL D5W at 1 mg/min × 6 h I.V. (cardiac arrest): 300 mg	orally: 100 to 400 mg daily I.V.: 0.5 mg/min

TABLE 14-3. Class I and III Antiarrhythmic Drug Availability and Standard Dosing Regimens *(Continued)*

Generic name	Trade name	Dosage forms	Loading dose	Maintenance dose
Sotalol	Betapace, Betapace AF	80, 120, 160, 240 mg tablets		80 to 160 mg q12 h
Ibutilide	Corvert	0.1 mg/mL (10 mL) injection	I.V.: 1 mg over 10 min; repeat × 1 if needed	Not applicable
Dofetilide	Tikosyn	125, 250, 500 mcg capsules		CrCl > 60 mL/min = 500 mcg twice daily; 40 to 60 mL/min = 250 mcg twice daily; 20 to 39 mL/min = 125 mcg twice daily; <20 mL/min = not recommended
Dronedarone	Multaq	400 mg tablets		400 mg twice daily
Miscellaneous				
Atropine		0.1, 0.3, 0.4, 0.5, 0.6, 0.8, 1 mg/mL injection	0.5 to 1 mg every 5 minutes up to 3 mg total	
Adenosine	Adenocard	3 mg/mL injection		Initial dose: 6 mg I.V. bolus; if necessary, can be followed by 12 mg every 2 minutes as I.V. bolus; flush I.V. line after each administration
Digoxin	Lanoxin	0.0625, 0.125, 0.1875, 0.25 mg tablets 50 mcg/mL elixir 100, 250 mcg/mL injection	I.V. and orally : 0.25 mg every 2 hours up to 1.5 mg	I.V. and orally : 0.125 to 0.375 mg daily

TABLE 14-4. Selected Antiarrhythmic Drug Interactions and Significant Adverse Effects

Drug	Effect of disease/drugs on antiarrhythmic drug concentrations	Effect of antiarrhythmic drug on other drug concentrations	Common or severe adverse effects
Lidocaine	*Elevated:* with decreased cardiac output		Central nervous system (CNS) toxicity: paresthesias, dizziness, muscle twitching, confusion, nausea and vomiting, slurred speech, seizures, sinus arrest
Mexiletine	*Reduced:* enzyme inducers *Elevated:* quinidine, amiodarone, ritonavir	*Elevated:* theophylline	GI distress; CNS: tremor, dizziness, confusion, vertigo, nystagmus, diplopia, tremor, ataxia; hypotension; sinus bradycardia; AV block
Flecainide	*Elevated:* CYP2D6 inhibitors (e.g., **fluoxetine**, **paroxetine**, tricyclics)	*Elevated:* digoxin	Proarrhythmia, prolonged PR interval and QRS complex, dizziness, blurred vision, headache, tremor, heart failure
Propafenone	*Reduced:* enzyme inducers *Elevated:* CYP2D6 inhibitors	*Elevated:* **warfarin**, digoxin, cyclosporine, theophylline	Metallic/bitter taste; CNS: dizziness, paresthesias, fatigue; GI distress; heart failure; liver injury; bradycardia; AV block; proarrhythmia

(continued)

TABLE 14-4. Selected Antiarrhythmic Drug Interactions and Significant Adverse Effects *(Continued)*

Drug	Effect of disease/drugs on antiarrhythmic drug concentrations	Effect of antiarrhythmic drug on other drug concentrations	Common or severe adverse effects
Amiodarone[a]	*Elevated:* Grapefruit juice	*Elevated:* inhibits most CYP450 enzymes and P-glycoprotein. **warfarin**, digoxin, phenytoin, cyclosporine, **lovastatin**, **simvastatin**, **atorvastatin**	I.V.: phlebitis; general: corneal microdeposits, photophobia, increased liver enzymes, photosensitivity, blue-gray skin discoloration, pulmonary fibrosis, hyper- and hypothyroidism, polyneuropathy
Sotalol	*Elevated:* Adjust dose for renal function		Beta-blocking effects: bradycardia, fatigue, dyspnea, bronchospasm, heart failure; QTc prolongation; torsades de pointes
Ibutilide			QTc prolongation, torsades de pointes
Dofetilide	*Elevated:* verapamil, cimetidine, ketoconazole, trimethoprim, megestrol, prochlorperazine, **hydrochlorothiazide**, adjust dose for renal function		QTc prolongation, torsades de pointes
Digoxin	*Elevated:* amiodarone, verapamil, **diltiazem**		
Dronedarone	*Elevated:* nefazodone, ritonavir, ketoconazole, itraconazole, voriconazole, telithromycin, clarithromycin, cyclosporine, grapefruit juice, verapamil, **diltiazem** *Reduced:* rifampin, phenobarbital, carbamazepine, phenytoin, St. John's wort	*Elevated:* Inhibits CYP3A4, CYP2D6, and P-glycoprotein; **simvastatin**, verapamil, **diltiazem**, nifedipine, sirolimus, tacrolimus, beta blockers, tricyclic antidepressants, selective serotonin reuptake inhibitors that are CYP2D6 substrates, digoxin, dabigatran	Contraindicated in patients with NYHA (New York Heart Association) class IV heart failure or NYHA class II-III heart failure with a recent decompensation requiring hospitalization or in patients with permanent atrial fibrillation, new or worsening heart failure, hepatocellular liver injury and acute liver failure, QTc prolongation, bradycardia, hypokalemia and hypomagnesemia when used with potassium-depleting diuretics; diarrhea, nausea, vomiting, abdominal pain, indigestion, weakness, fatigue, rash, itching

Boldface indicates one of top 100 drugs for 2020 by prescription volume.
a. See Table 14-5.

Patient counseling

Patients should be counseled to take medication as prescribed. If a dose is missed, the patient should take the dose as soon as it is remembered, unless it is close to the next scheduled dose. In that case, the patient should skip the missed dose and continue the regular regimen; doses should not be doubled.

Many drug interactions are possible. Patients should inform health care providers of medications prescribed before starting new medications, including over-the-counter medications (Table 14-4).

Periodic ECG and laboratory assessments may be required to minimize or prevent adverse effects.

Patients should be informed that complete remission of their arrhythmia is unlikely. However, symptomatic arrhythmias that have increased in frequency or severity should be reported to the physician immediately.

Patients with atrial fibrillation or flutter should be informed about the importance of antithrombotic therapy as well as the signs and symptoms of stroke. Patients with symptoms such as sudden onset of slurred speech, facial drooping, or muscle weakness should seek emergency care.

AADs that are administered as extended-release formulations should not be crushed, opened, or chewed. Advise patients to swallow the dose whole.

Drug-specific information

Amiodarone

Amiodarone is the least proarrhythmic of the class I and class III antiarrhythmic drugs.

The U.S. Food and Drug Administration now requires that a medication guide be distributed directly to each patient to whom amiodarone is dispensed.

Visual disturbances are rare but should be reported immediately to the physician.

Difficulty breathing, shortness of breath, wheezing, or persistent cough should be reported immediately to the physician.

If the patient experiences nausea or vomiting, passes brown or dark-colored urine, feels more tired than usual, or experiences stomach pain, or if the patient's skin or whites of the eyes turn yellow, the patient should report the symptoms to the physician immediately.

Cardiac symptoms such as pounding heart, skipping of a beat, or very rapid or slow heartbeats, as well as light-headedness or feeling faint, should be reported to the physician immediately.

Periodic laboratory tests to evaluate thyroid function, liver function, and pulmonary function, as well as diagnostic tests such as chest x-ray, ECG, and eye exams, may be necessary to assess and prevent adverse effects (Table 14-5).

Amiodarone may cause skin photosensitivity. Patients should be advised to wear protective clothing and sunscreen when exposed to sunlight or ultraviolet light.

Prolonged use may cause blue-gray skin discoloration.

Patients should tell their physicians and pharmacists about all other medications they are taking, including prescription and nonprescription medications, vitamins, and herbal supplements.

Frequent administration with grapefruit juice may increase oral absorption. Encourage patients to drink water with amiodarone or to separate grapefruit juice consumption by at least 2 hours.

Beta blockers (including sotalol)

Patients with asthma and chronic obstructive pulmonary disease should be advised that beta blockers may worsen their symptoms of airway disease. Advise patients to notify a physician immediately if this occurs.

TABLE 14-5. Suggested Monitoring Guidelines for Amiodarone

Test	Baseline		6 months	12 months
Electrocardiogram	•		•	•
Pulmonary function tests	•	Routine monitoring is controversial; may repeat tests if patient becomes symptomatic.		
Ophthalmologic examination	•	Periodic exam is recommended.	•	•
Chest x-ray	•	Repeat earlier if patient becomes symptomatic.	•	•
Thyroid function tests	•		•	•
Liver enzymes	•		•	•

Patients with diabetes should be advised that beta blockers may mask symptoms of hypoglycemia. Patients should avoid abrupt withdrawal of beta-blocker therapy. If withdrawal of beta-blocker therapy is desired, the patient should contact the physician for the dosage-tapering regimen, if necessary.

Digoxin

Refer to Chapter 13 on heart failure.

Dronedarone

Dronedarone is indicated to reduce the risk of cardiovascular hospitalization in patients with paroxysmal or persistent atrial fibrillation or atrial flutter who are in sinus rhythm or who will be cardioverted.

Dronedarone should not be used in patients with permanent atrial fibrillation (i.e., heart rhythm remains in atrial fibrillation and cannot be changed back to normal rhythm).

Dronedarone should not be used in patients with severe heart failure because it may increase the risk of death. If patients have been hospitalized for heart failure within the past month, they should not take dronedarone even if they feel better now.

Patients should be counseled to call their health care provider immediately if they experience signs and symptoms of worsening heart failure:

- Shortness of breath or wheezing at rest
- Wheezing, chest tightness, or coughing up of frothy sputum at rest, nighttime, or after minor exercise
- Trouble sleeping at night, or waking up at night with problems breathing
- Use of more pillows to prop themselves up at night to breathe easier
- Rapid weight gain of more than 5 pounds
- Increased swelling in feet or legs

Dronedarone can be hepatotoxic, including causing liver failure. Advise patients to report any symptoms of potential liver injury:

- Anorexia, nausea, or vomiting
- Fever or malaise
- Right upper quadrant abdominal pain or discomfort
- Jaundice, dark urine, or itching

Dronedarone can interact with many other medications. Patients should report to their health care provider and pharmacist all prescription and nonprescription medications, vitamins, or herbal supplements they are taking.

Dronedarone should be taken twice daily with food, once with the morning meal and once with the evening meal. If a dose is missed, the patient should wait and take the next dose at the regular time. The patient should not take 2 doses at the same time.

Do not drink grapefruit juice while taking dronedarone. Grapefruit juice can increase dronedarone plasma concentrations.

The most common adverse effects are diarrhea, nausea, vomiting, abdominal pain and indigestion, weakness, fatigue, rash, and itching.

A medication guide should be dispensed with dronedarone.

14-7   Pharmacist's Role

- Multidisciplinary team care of patients with arrhythmias, especially atrial fibrillation, involving physicians, pharmacists, nurses, and other health care professionals is key to ensure optimization of therapy.

- Pharmacists play a key role in the team-based care of patients with arrhythmias. Patients receiving education from pharmacists are more likely to be adherent to medications and have fewer adverse drug reactions, medication errors, or hospitalizations.
- Pharmacists assist in the selection, initiation, dose titration, and follow-up monitoring needed to optimize pharmacotherapy.
- Pharmacists can identify sources for medication nonadherence including costs, adverse effects, complexity of regimens, and physical or cognitive impairment and recommend approaches to address these problems.
- Recommend appropriate dosing and dose adjustments in patients with impaired renal or hepatic function. This is especially important with DOACs used to prevent stroke in patients with atrial fibrillation.
- Screen for drug–drug interactions and recommend appropriate management.

Most patients with arrhythmias have numerous comorbidities (e.g., hypertension, diabetes, coronary artery disease, heart failure) requiring drug therapy so that the number of different medications patients receive is often large. Pharmacists can assist in optimizing the management of these disorders, assuring that optimal treatments are selected that will achieve goals of therapy but not worsen heart failure.

NAPLEX Competency Statements

The questions in this chapter cover the following 2021 NAPLEX Competency Statements: **AREA 1:** 1.1; 1.2; 1.3; 1.4; 1.5; 1.6; 1.7 **AREA 2:** 2.1; 2.2; 2.3; 2.4 **AREA 3:** 3.1; 3.2; 3.3; 3.4; 3.5; 3.6; 3.7; 3.8; 3.9; 3.10; 3.11; 3.12 **AREA 5:** 5.5.

 **14-8** **Questions**

1. Which are adverse effects of oral amiodarone? (Mark all that apply.)

    A. Photosensitivity
    B. Pulmonary fibrosis
    C. Phlebitis
    D. Hyperkalemia
    E. Hypothyroidism

2. Which antiarrhythmic agents' mechanism of action is primarily the result of sodium ion transport blockade?

    A. Propafenone
    B. Ibutilide
    C. Sotalol
    D. Verapamil
    E. Diltiazem

3. Which medications can cause atrioventricular block? (Mark all that apply.)

    A. Diltiazem
    B. Amlodipine
    C. Sotalol
    D. Dofetilide
    E. Amiodarone

4. Which can be symptoms of atrial fibrillation? (Mark all that apply.)

    A. Dizziness
    B. Palpitations
    C. Angina
    D. Hypertension
    E. Sudden-onset slurred speech

5. Which are recommended for monitoring patients requiring chronic amiodarone therapy? (Mark all that apply.)

    A. Electrocardiogram
    B. Coagulation tests
    C. Thyroid function tests
    D. Liver function tests
    E. Chest x-ray

6. For the treatment of chronic atrial fibrillation, apixaban would be indicated in which patients? (Mark all that apply.)

A. A male with heart failure and diabetes
B. A female over 75 years old with hypertension
C. A 50-year-old male with no risk factors for thromboembolism
D. A 77-year-old female with diabetes and a previous MI
E. A 63-year-old male who has had a previous stroke

7. The anticoagulant effect of dabigatran is mediated by _____.

A. inhibiting synthesis of vitamin K–dependent clotting factors
B. blocking the platelet P2Y$_{12}$ receptor
C. inhibiting clotting factor Xa
D. direct thrombin inhibition
E. inhibiting the VKORC1 enzyme

8. Which medications are preferred for control of ventricular response in patients with atrial fibrillation and heart failure with reduced ejection fraction?

A. Metoprolol succinate
B. Verapamil
C. Diltiazem
D. Amlodipine
E. Dofetilide

9. Which medications are associated with torsades de pointes? (Mark all that apply.)

A. Erythromycin
B. Ampicillin
C. Atenolol
D. Methadone
E. Verapamil

10. Which are important determinants of the anti-coagulant response to warfarin? (Mark all that apply.)

A. CYP2C9 genotype
B. CYP2D6 genotype
C. VKORC1 genotype
D. Dietary vitamin C intake
E. Creatinine clearance

11. What is the recommended dosage regimen for dofetilide in a patient with a calculated creatinine clearance of 30 mL per minute?

A. Dofetilide therapy is not recommended.
B. 125 mcg orally twice daily
C. 125 mg orally twice daily
D. 500 mcg orally twice daily
E. 500 mg orally twice daily

12. A patient with atrial fibrillation receiving rivaroxaban should avoid _____.

A. calcium supplements
B. orange juice
C. Digoxin
D. Clarithromycin
E. Pravastatin

13. Which will increase dronedarone plasma concentrations and should be avoided in patients taking this medication?

A. Grapefruit juice
B. Ranitidine
C. Atenolol
D. Nitroglycerin
E. Warfarin

14. A 66-year-old male with a past medical history of heart failure with reduced ejection fraction and hypertension presents to the emergency room with a 1-week history of intermittent palpitations and dizziness. The ECG reveals atrial fibrillation with a ventricular rate of 130 bpm. The decision is made to attempt to restore normal sinus rhythm. Which of the following represents the best therapeutic approach to cardioverting the patient?

A. Perform TEE; if no thrombus is present, cardiovert; anticoagulation is not necessary.
B. Perform TEE; if no thrombus is present, cardio-vert; anticoagulate for at least 4 weeks postcardioversion.
C. Anticoagulate for 4 weeks before cardioversion; discontinue anticoagulation postcardioversion.
D. Anticoagulate for 2 weeks before cardioversion; continue anticoagulation for at least 4 weeks postcardioversion.
E. Direct-current cardiovert immediately.

15. Which would be the best agent to maintain sinus rhythm in a patient with atrial fibrillation and heart failure with reduced ejection fraction?

    A. Flecainide
    B. Amiodarone
    C. Digoxin
    D. Ibutilide
    E. Dronedarone

16. Which agent should be taken with the evening meal to enhance bioavailability?

    A. Rivaroxaban
    B. Dabigatran
    C. Warfarin
    D. Amiodarone
    E. Dofetilide

17. Which are indicated to reduce the risk of stroke in a patient with atrial fibrillation that has a CHA_2DS_2-VASc score of 4 and a creatinine clearance of 105 mL/min? (Mark all that apply.)

    A. Aspirin
    B. Edoxaban
    C. Apixaban
    D. Rivaroxaban
    E. Amiodarone

18. Which can be used to treat a patient with drug-induced torsades de pointes? (Mark all that apply.)

    A. Discontinuation of any drugs associated with prolonged QT interval
    B. Pacemaker to increase heart rate
    C. Adenosine
    D. Magnesium sulfate
    E. Ibutilide

19. Which antiarrhythmic agents require dosage adjustment in patients with impaired renal function? (Mark all that apply.)

    A. Digoxin
    B. Amiodarone
    C. Lidocaine
    D. Verapamil
    E. Propafenone

20. Which is *not* a characteristic of atrial fibrillation?

    A. No discernible P waves
    B. Ventricular rate of 100 to 130 bpm
    C. Regular QRS pattern
    D. Narrow QRS complex
    E. Chaotic atrial contractions

21. Which would be the best choice for ventricular rate control in atrial fibrillation secondary to hyperthyroidism?

    A. Adenosine
    B. Digoxin
    C. Apixaban
    D. Propranolol
    E. Atropine

22. A dose-limiting adverse effect of sotalol is _____.

    A. bradycardia
    B. polyneuropathy
    C. metallic taste
    D. agranulocytosis
    E. lupus-like syndrome

23. Which laboratory tests should be performed in a patient beginning dofetilide therapy? (Mark all that apply.)

    A. Serum albumin
    B. Serum potassium
    C. Creatinine clearance
    D. Hemoglobin A1C
    E. Electrocardiogram

24. Warfarin dosage reduction should be considered when administered with which drugs? (Mark all that apply.)

    A. Amiodarone
    B. Sotalol
    C. Trimethoprim-sulfamethoxazole
    D. Rifampin
    E. Lisinopril

25. The anticoagulant effect of apixaban is mediated by _____.

    A. inhibiting synthesis of vitamin K–dependent clotting factors
    B. blocking the platelet $P2Y_{12}$ receptor
    C. inhibiting clotting factor Xa
    D. direct thrombin inhibition
    E. inhibiting the VKORC1 enzyme

14-9   Answers

1. A, B, E. Photosensitivity is a common adverse effect of oral amiodarone. Patients should be counseled to limit sun exposure and use sunscreen. Pulmonary fibrosis usually is seen in patients receiving long-term amiodarone therapy (months to years). The amiodarone molecule contains iodine and can cause hypo- or hyperthyroidism. Phlebitis would be expected to occur only during I.V. amiodarone infusion, particularly through a peripheral I.V. line. Amiodarone does not affect serum potassium.

2. A. Propafenone blocks sodium entry into the cardiac cell, slowing depolarization. Ibutilide and sotalol primarily act by blocking potassium transport, whereas verapamil and diltiazem inhibit the calcium channel.

3. A, C, E. Drug-induced AV heart block is caused by agents that slow conduction through the AV node. Diltiazem (the nondihydropyridine calcium channel blocker), sotalol (which has beta-blocking properties), and amiodarone all slow AV node conduction. The dihydropyridine calcium channel blocker amlodipine does not usually affect AV conduction, nor does dofetilide.

4. A, B, C, E. Because of functional atrial contraction loss and rapid ventricular rate (producing palpitations), cardiac output may decrease, resulting in decreased perfusion of major organs, particularly the brain (dizziness, confusion, etc.) and heart (angina and heart failure exacerbation). Depending on the vascular tone, blood pressure may remain stable or may fall as a direct result of decreased cardiac output; however, hypertension would not be expected. Patients with atrial fibrillation are at increased risk of thrombosis, particularly stroke (sudden onset slurred speech), secondary to pooling of blood in the left atrium and subsequent thrombus formation.

5. A, C, D, E. All of these tests are used to monitor for amiodarone adverse effects. They all should be performed at baseline and periodically after treatment is started.

6. A, B, D, E. All of these patients have a $CHA_2DS_2\text{-}VASc$ score of 2 or greater, and oral anticoagulant therapy is indicated to reduce the risk of stroke. Patients younger than age 65 with no thromboembolic risk factors are at low risk of stroke; current guidelines do not recommend antithrombotic therapy for such patients.

7. D. Dabigatran is a direct thrombin inhibitor. It does not affect synthesis of the vitamin K–dependent clotting factors or platelet activity.

8. A. Metoprolol succinate would be the drug of first choice, because it helps slow the ventricular rate and improves survival as well as other important outcomes (e.g., reduces hospitalizations) in patients with heart failure with reduced ejection fraction. Both verapamil and diltiazem are negative inotropes and should not be used in patients with heart failure and low ejection fractions. Although it is a calcium channel blocker, amlodipine does not affect AV nodal conduction. Dofetilide is used for conversion to and maintenance of sinus rhythm, not rate control.

9. A, D. Erythromycin and methadone can prolong the QTc interval and increase the risk of torsades de pointes.

10. A, C. The *VKORC1* gene determines the activity of the vitamin K epoxide-reductase enzyme, which is the target for warfarin. The *S*-isomer of warfarin is the most potent and is metabolized primarily by hepatic CYP2C9. Loss-of-function mutations in the *CYP2C9* gene are associated with reduced warfarin dose requirements. Warfarin is not metabolized by hepatic CYP2D6, and its elimination is not affected by renal function. Dietary vitamin K intake, but not vitamin C, also affects warfarin dose requirements.

11. B. Dofetilide is eliminated renally and, therefore, must be adjusted according to creatinine clearance to decrease the significant risk of torsades de pointes. See Table 14-3.

12. D. Patients receiving rivaroxaban should avoid clarithromycin because it is a combined P-glycoprotein inhibitor and strong CYP3A4 inhibitor. Concomitant administration increases rivaroxaban plasma concentrations and increases bleeding risk.

13. A. Dronedarone is metabolized by CYP3A4, and grapefruit juice is a potent CYP3A4 inhibitor. Grapefruit juice should not be used by patients taking dronedarone. This combination results in significant increases in dronedarone plasma concentrations and the risk of adverse effects.

14. B. Because the patient appears to have been in atrial fibrillation for 1 week by history, the risk of thromboembolism during conversion to sinus rhythm is significant. Proper treatment would require at least 3 to 4 weeks of anticoagulation (warfarin INR 2–3 or a DOAC) before cardioversion, followed by at least 4 weeks of anticoagulation postcardioversion. Alternatively, a TEE can be used to rule out an atrial thrombus, allowing immediate cardioversion. Because the atria will require time to recover normal contractile activity, anticoagulation will be required for at least 4 weeks postconversion.

15. B. Because the patient has heart failure with reduced ejection fraction, the results of the Cardiac Arrhythmia Suppression Trial (CAST) indicate that class Ic agents should be avoided because of increased risk of death. Sotalol may worsen heart failure. Ibutilide is indicated for conversion only, not for maintenance of sinus rhythm. Dronedarone is contraindicated in patients with heart failure because of increased mortality risk.

16. A. Rivaroxaban should be taken with the evening meal to increase bioavailability. The pharmacokinetics of the other medications are not affected by food.

17. C, D. In a patient with a CHA_2DS_2-VASc score of 4, anticoagulation is indicated to reduce the risk of stroke. Aspirin would not be effective. Edoxaban should not be used in patients with creatinine clearance > 95 mL/min. Either apixaban or rivaroxaban would be effective in this patient. Amiodarone does not affect the risk of stroke.

18. A, B, D. Discontinuation of drugs that prolong the QT interval is essential in order to terminate torsades de pointes and prevent recurrences. Treatment should consist of I.V. magnesium sulfate and a pacemaker to increase heart rate and shorten the QT interval. Adenosine typically is used only to terminate PSVT. Ibutilide is a class 3 antiarrhythmic drug that is associated with torsades de pointes and should not be used to treat this arrhythmia.

19. A. Digoxin requires dosage adjustment in patients with impaired renal function.

20. C. Atrial fibrillation represents chaotic atrial activity resulting in no identifiable P wave. Because atrial fibrillation originates above the AV node, the QRS complex is narrow and the ventricular rate is typically greater than 100 bpm.

21. D. Beta blockers are the preferred rate-controlling agent for hyperthyroidism because they inhibit the adrenergic response and decrease thyroid hormone conversion (especially propranolol). Digoxin is not as effective in controlling the ventricular rate related to a hyperadrenergic state (hyperthyroidism).

22. A. Sotalol possesses significant beta-blocking activity; therefore, the patient may experience adverse effects similar to traditional beta blockers.

23. B, C, E. Serum potassium should be evaluated before starting dofetilide therapy and supplemented if < 4.0 mEq/mL. Hypokalemia increases the risk of torsades de pointes. The initial dose of dofetilide is determined by creatinine clearance. A baseline electrocardiogram should be obtained before starting dofetilide therapy. If the baseline QTc or QT interval is greater than 440 msec, dofetilide is contraindicated. Dofetilide is not affected by serum albumin or hemoglobin A1C.

24. A, C. Warfarin is metabolized by multiple hepatic CYP450 isoenzymes, including CYP2C9, CYP1A2, and CYP3A4. Amiodarone inhibits these enzymes, resulting in reduced warfarin clearance and the need to reduce the dose. The sulfamethoxazole component of trimethoprim-sulfamethoxazole inhibits CYP2C9, resulting in the need to reduce the warfarin dose. Neither sotalol nor lisinopril affects hepatic CYP450 enzymes. Rifampin induces multiple hepatic CYP450 enzymes, resulting in increased warfarin dose requirements.

25. C. Apixaban inhibits clotting factor Xa. It does not affect synthesis of the vitamin K–dependent clotting factors or platelet activity.

 **14-10** **Additional Resources**

Al-Khatib SM, Stevenson WG, Ackerman MJ, et al. 2017 AHA/ACC/HRS guideline for the management of patients with ventricular arrhythmias and the prevention of sudden cardiac death: a report of the American College of Cardiology Foundation/American Heart Association Task Force on Clinical Practice Guidelines and the Heart Rhythm Society. *J Am Coll Cardiol* 2018;72:e91–220.

Epstein AE, Olshansky B, Nacarelli GV, et al. Practical management guide for clinicians who treat patients with amiodarone. *Am J Med.* 2016;129(5):468–475.

January CT, Wann LS, Alpert JS, et al. 2014 AHA/ACC/HRS guideline for the management of patients with atrial fibrillation: a report of the American College of Cardiology/American Heart Association Task Force on Practice Guidelines and the Heart Rhythm Society. *Circulation.* 2014;130:e199–e267.

January CT, Wann LS, Calkins H, et al. 2019 AHA/ACC/HRS focused update of the 2014 AHA/ACC/HRS guideline for the management of patients with atrial fibrillation: a report of the American College of Cardiology/American Heart Association Task Force on clinical practice guidelines and the Heart Rhythm Society with the Society of Thoracic Surgeons. *Circulation* 2019;140:e125–e151.

Kovacs RJ, Flaker GC, Saxonhouse SJ, et al. Practical management of anticoagulation in patients with atrial fibrillation. *J Am Coll Cardiol.* 2015;65(13):1340–1360.

Lip GY, Banerjee A, Boriani G, et al. Antithrombotic therapy for atrial fibrillation: CHEST guideline and expert panel report. *Chest* 2018;4:1121–1201.

Page RL, Joglar JA, Caldwell MA, et al. 2015 ACC/AHA/HRS guideline for the management of adult patients with supraventricular tachycardia: a report of the American College of Cardiology/American Heart Association Task Force on Clinical Practice Guidelines and the Heart Rhythm Society. *J Am Coll Cardiol.* 2016;67(13):e27–115.

Steffel J, Verhamme P, Potpara TS, et al. The 2018 European Heart Rhythm Association Practical Guide on the use of non-vitamin K antagonist oral anticoagulants in patients with atrial fibrillation. *Eur Heart J* 2018;39:1330–1393.

Tilton JJ, Sanoski CA, Bauman JL. The Arrhythmias. In: Dipiro JT, Yee GC, Posey LM, et al., eds. *Pharmacotherapy: A Pathophysiologic Approach.* 11th ed. New York, NY: McGraw-Hill; 2019:193–230.

Wiggins BS, Dixon DL, Neyens RR, et al. Select drug-drug interactions with direct oral anticoagulants. *J Am Coll Cardiol* 2020;75:1341–1350.

Ischemic Heart Disease and Acute Coronary Syndrome

15

SHANNON W. FINKS   KELLY C. ROGERS

15-1 KEY POINTS

- Address primary prevention before atherosclerotic cardiovascular disease (ASCVD) development.
- Patients with stable ischemic heart disease (SIHD) should receive **aspirin**, beta blockers, and statin therapy. Additional anginal control can be achieved with concomitant nitrates, calcium channel blockers, or ranolazine.
- Angiotensin-converting enzyme inhibitors (ACEIs) should be prescribed to SIHD patients with reduced left ventricular ejection fraction (LVEF) ≤ 40%, hypertension (HTN), diabetes, or chronic kidney disease. Angiotensin II receptor blockers (ARBs) can be used as alternatives to ACEIs.
- Acute coronary syndrome presents as ST-segment elevation myocardial infarction (STEMI) or non-ST-segment elevation acute coronary syndrome (NSTE-ACS), which includes unstable angina (UA) and non-ST-segment elevation myocardial infarction (NSTEMI), and requires immediate evaluation for reperfusion and administration of antiplatelets, anticoagulants and other supportive care therapies.
- Patients presenting with STEMI undergoing primary percutaneous coronary intervention (PCI) should receive anticoagulation with either unfractionated heparin (UFH) or bivalirudin. If thrombolytic therapy is the chosen reperfusion strategy, anticoagulation options include UFH, enoxaparin, or fondaparinux.
- NSTE-ACS patients treated medically should receive anticoagulation with UFH, enoxaparin, or fondaparinux. If PCI is planned, acceptable options include UFH, enoxaparin, or bivalirudin.
- The majority of patients post–acute coronary syndrome (ACS) will receive dual antiplatelet therapy (DAPT) with **aspirin** and a $P2Y_{12}$ inhibitor whether treated medically or with percutaneous coronary intervention (PCI). The duration of therapy depends on the clinical scenario, type of stent placed, and risk factors for bleeding.
- First-line anti-ischemic therapy for the treatment of ACS is a beta blocker given orally within the first 24 hours.
- Secondary prevention of ACS should include DAPT, beta blockers, ACEIs (or ARB if intolerant), and statin therapy in all patients without contraindications.
- Patients with pulmonary congestion or an LVEF ≤ 40% should receive an ACEI within 24 hours unless contraindicated. Therapy should be continued indefinitely for patients with heart failure (HF), LVEF ≤ 40%, HTN, diabetes, or chronic kidney disease. Aldosterone blockade should be considered post–myocardial infarction (MI) in patients with an LVEF ≤ 40% and either symptomatic HF or diabetes.
- Nonsteroidal anti-inflammatory drugs (NSAIDs) should be discontinued in any patient with stable ischemic heart disease or who presents with ACS.

15-2 STUDY GUIDE CHECKLIST

The following topics may guide your study of this subject area:

- ☐ Appropriate use of **aspirin** and statin therapy for the primary prevention of coronary artery disease.
- ☐ Optimal acute and chronic medical treatment for SIHD and ACS.
- ☐ Actions of medications used to treat patients with SIHD, ACS, and PCI.
- ☐ Indications for medications used to treat SIHD, NSTE-ACS, and STEMI.
- ☐ Trade names, available dosage forms, and dosing frequency.
- ☐ Major adverse drug effects of medications used to treat SIHD and ACS.
- ☐ Clinically significant drug interactions of medications used to treat SIHD and ACS.
- ☐ Differences in therapy between NSTE-ACS and STEMI.
- ☐ Secondary prevention strategies and post-ACS discharge medications.
- ☐ Any relevant counseling points for patients discharged with SIHD, ACS, or post-PCI.

15-3   Introduction

Definitions

- *Atherosclerotic cardiovascular disease (ASCVD):* General overarching term involving development of atherosclerotic diseases.
- *Ischemic heart disease (IHD):* Disease caused most frequently by atherosclerosis. IHD may present as silent ischemia, chest pain (at rest or on exertion), or MI.
- *Angina:* Syndrome classically described as discomfort or pain in the chest, arm, shoulder, back, or jaw. Angina is frequently worsened by physical exertion or emotional stress and is usually relieved by sublingual (SL) nitroglycerin (NTG) or rest. It, however, can occur at rest in a patient experiencing an ACS. Patients with angina usually have coronary artery disease (CAD).
- *Acute coronary syndrome (ACS):* Syndrome encompassing the following:
  - Unstable angina (UA) and non-ST-segment elevation myocardial infarction (NSTEMI); referred to as non-ST-segment elevation ACS (NSTE-ACS)
  - ST-segment elevation myocardial infarction (STEMI)
- *Coronary artery disease (CAD):* Atherosclerotic disease of the coronary arteries that typically cycles in and out of the clinically defined phases of ACS and asymptomatic, stable, or progressive angina.
- *Percutaneous coronary intervention (PCI):* Procedure to reopen a partially or completely occluded coronary vessel to restore blood flow.
- *Coronary artery bypass graft (CABG):* Surgical procedure in which an artery such as the left internal mammary or a vein from the leg is attached to the diseased coronary vessel to create a bypass of the atherosclerotic plaque.

15-4   Primary Prevention: Risk Factor Modification

- The majority of the causes of ASCVD are known and modifiable, therefore, worth prevention efforts.
- Risk factor screening should begin at age 20 with focus on modifying risk.
- Pooled Cohort Equations (which account for modifiable and nonmodifiable risk factors) should be used to calculate 10-year and lifetime risks for atherosclerotic events and are useful in determining selected drug therapy approaches for primary prevention of heart disease. See Chapter 16 for more details on ASCVD risk calculation.

Therapy for Primary Prevention of Heart Disease

Aspirin

Recent studies have shown conflicting results for the use of **aspirin** for primary prevention of disease in patients with varying risk categories and disease states. Standard guidelines have downgraded the use of **aspirin** for the primary prevention of heart disease due to an increased risk for bleeding with only modest benefit in low- to moderate-risk patients. However, high-risk patients (e.g., ASCVD 10-year risk of > 20%) have not been included adequately in these trials. The decision to use **aspirin** for primary prevention should be made on an individual basis, depending upon underlying risk for both ischemic and bleeding events.

- The 2019 American College of Cardiology/American Heart Association guidelines state **aspirin** can be considered for primary prevention among select adults aged 40 to 70 years who are at a higher ASCVD risk but recommends avoiding **aspirin** in patients older than age 70 and in those at increased bleeding risk.

■ The American Diabetes Association (2021) states low-dose **aspirin** therapy (75 to 162 mg/day) may be considered to prevent cardiovascular events in at-risk patients with diabetes after a comprehensive discussion with the patient on the benefits versus increased risk of bleeding.

■ The 2016 United States Preventive Services Task Force supports low-dose **aspirin** use for the primary prevention of heart disease and colorectal cancer only in patients aged 50 to 70 years with a 10-year ASCVD risk of ≥ 10% who are not at high risk for bleeding.

Lipid-lowering therapy

■ Statin therapy for the primary prevention of ASCVD is most beneficial in those with the highest risk.

■ A risk discussion with the patient is appropriate when ASCVD risk > 5% with risk enhancers or when 10-year ASCVD risk > 7.5%.

■ Moderate- (when risk is 7.5% to 20%) to high-intensity (when risk > 20%) statin therapy is favored, depending upon baseline ASCVD risk.

■ See Chapter 16 for more information on lipid-lowering therapy.

15-5 Stable Ischemic Heart Disease

Clinical Presentation

Symptoms of stable ischemic heart disease (SIHD) are caused by decreased oxygen (O_2) supply secondary to reduced flow in a setting of increased O_2 demand. Angina is considered stable if symptoms have been occurring for several weeks without worsening and lasts less than 20 minutes and is relieved by rest or sublingual nitroglycerin.

Pharmacologic Management

Goals of therapy are as follows:

■ Prevent MI and death
■ Reduce symptoms of angina and occurrence of ischemia to improve quality of life (Figure 15-1)
■ Modify risk factors including smoking cessation; control of HTN, diabetes, and HLD; weight and exercise; and influenza vaccination

Antiplatelets

■ Aspirin
■ P2Y$_{12}$ receptor antagonists:
  ◦ These agents include **clopidogrel** ⚠, prasugrel ⚠, and ticagrelor ⚠.
  ◦ Neither prasugrel nor ticagrelor have been studied as a single antiplatelet agent in the setting of SIHD.
■ Indications for therapy:
  ◦ **Aspirin** (acetylsalicylic acid [ASA]) (81 to 162 mg daily) is recommended in all patients with SIHD in the absence of contraindications.
  ◦ **Clopidogrel** (75 mg daily) is chosen when ASA is absolutely contraindicated due to an allergy to ASA. If ASA is contraindicated due to a bleeding risk, **clopidogrel** should be avoided as well.
  ◦ The combination of **clopidogrel** or ticagrelor plus ASA is reasonable in certain high-risk patients and in patients who have received a stent.

FIGURE 15-1. Therapy for Patients with SIHD

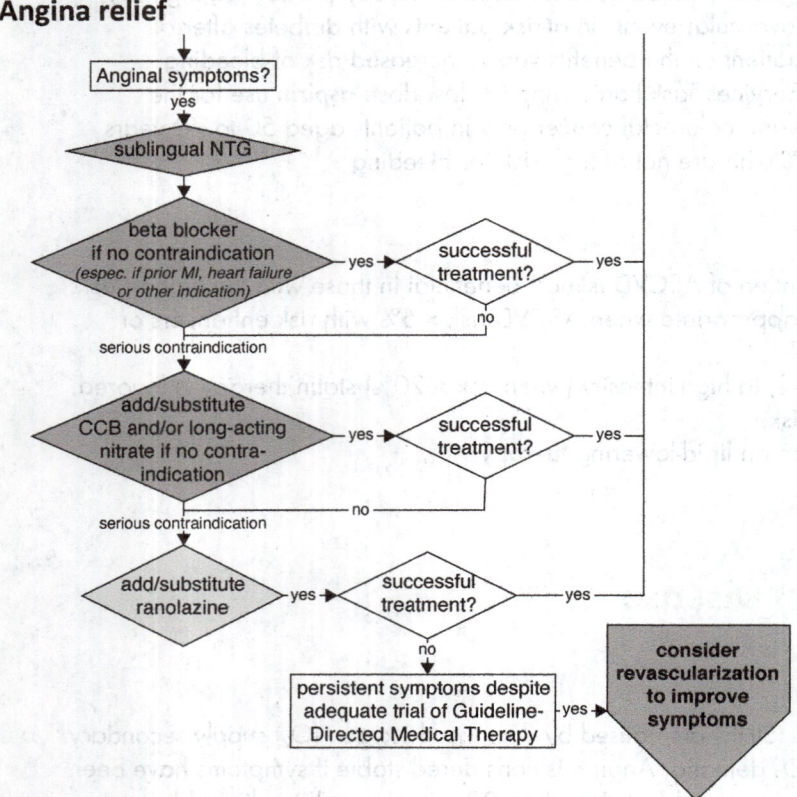

Angina relief

Guideline Directed Medical Therapy or Treatment Recommendations

- patients with established ASCVD should receive antiplatelet therapy
- all patients should be screened for HTN control
  - ACEIs/ARBs are considered first line additions to beta-blocker therapy with goal BP < 130/80 mmHg
- all patients should receive statin therapy with high-intensity statin if tolerated
- screen for other modifiable risk factors
  - smoking cessation, weight management, glucose control, and influenza vaccination

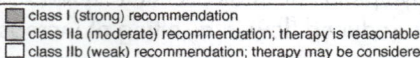

class I (strong) recommendation
class IIa (moderate) recommendation; therapy is reasonable
class IIb (weak) recommendation; therapy may be considered

 Clopidogrel *FDA BOXED WARNING*

The effectiveness of **clopidogrel** hydrogen sulfate results from its antiplatelet activity, which is dependent on its conversion to an active metabolite by the cytochrome P450 (CYP) system, principally CYP2C19. **Clopidogrel** hydrogen sulfate at recommended doses forms less of the active metabolite and so has a reduced effect on platelet activity in patients who are homozygous for nonfunctional alleles of the CYP2C19 gene, (termed "CYP2C19 poor metabolizers"). Tests are available to identify patients who are CYP2C19 poor metabolizers. Consider use of another platelet P2Y$_{12}$ inhibitor in patients identified as CYP2C19 poor metabolizers.

 Prasugrel *FDA BOXED WARNING*

Prasugrel can cause significant and sometimes fatal bleeding. Do not use prasugrel in patients with active pathological bleeding or a history of transient ischemic attack or stroke. Risk factors for bleeding include body weight of less than 60 kg, propensity to bleed, and concomitant use of medications that increase the risk of bleeding (e.g., **warfarin**, heparin, fibrinolytics, chronic use of NSAIDs). Prasugrel is not recommended in patients 75 years of age or older, except for high-risk situations (diabetes, history of prior myocardial infarction). Do not start prasugrel in patients likely to undergo urgent CABG, and discontinue at least 7 days prior to any surgery. If possible, manage bleeding without discontinuing prasugrel, as discontinuation in the first few weeks after ACS may increase risk for subsequent cardiovascular events.

Ticagrelor *FDA BOXED WARNING*

Ticagrelor can cause significant, sometimes fatal, bleeding. Do not use in patients with active pathological bleeding or history of intracranial hemorrhage. Do not start in patients undergoing urgent CABG. If possible, manage bleeding without discontinuing ticagrelor. Stopping ticagrelor increases the risk of subsequent cardiovascular events. Maintenance doses of **aspirin** above 100 mg in patients with ACS reduce the effectiveness of ticagrelor and should be avoided.

Anti-ischemic therapy

The main medication classes for anti-ischemic therapy include beta blockers, nitrates and nitroglycerin, calcium channel blockers, and ranolazine.

Beta blockers

- Effects on myocardial O_2 demand:
  - Beta blockers inhibit catecholamine effects.
  - Use may decrease heart rate (HR), blood pressure (BP), and contractility.
- Effects on O_2 supply:
  - Indirectly, beta blockers increase the time the heart is in diastole by slowing HR, which allows improved blood flow into the coronary arteries and subendocardium.
  - Negatively, the unopposed alpha stimulation may lead to coronary vasoconstriction.
- Dosing recommendations:
  - Start low, go slow.
  - Titrate to resting HR of 55 to 60 bpm, maximal exercise HR ≤ 100 bpm.
  - Avoid abrupt withdrawal, which can precipitate more severe ischemic episodes and MI; taper over 1 to 3 weeks using SL NTG or calcium channel blockers (CCBs) to control angina during the withdrawal period.
- Selection of beta blockers is based on the following factors:
  - Beta blockers with cardioselectivity have fewer adverse effects; they lose cardioselectivity at higher doses.
  - Lipophilicity is associated with more central nervous system side effects.
- Indications for therapy:
  - Beta blockers are used as first-line therapy in patients with prior MI, ACS, or a history of heart failure (HF) if not contraindicated.
  - They are often used as initial therapy in SIHD patients without prior MI.
  - They are more effective than nitrates and CCBs in silent ischemia.
  - Avoid in vasospastic angina and in patients with cocaine-induced angina due to unopposed alpha receptor vasoconstriction.
  - They are effective as monotherapy or with nitrates, CCBs, ranolazine, or a combination thereof.

Nitrates and Nitroglycerin

- Effects on myocardial O_2 demand:
  - Peripheral vasodilation leads to decreased preload and wall stress, and ultimately decreased O_2 demand.
  - Arterial vasodilation (with high doses) leads to decreased afterload and systolic BP, and ultimately decreased O_2 demand.
  - Nitrates can cause a reflex tachycardia and lead to an increase in O_2 demand in some patients. This problem can be overcome with the use of a beta blocker.

- Effects on O_2 supply: Dilation of large epicardial coronary arteries and collateral vessels in areas with or without stenosis leads to increased O_2 supply.
- Indications for therapy:
  - SL nitroglycerin (NTG) or NTG spray can be used for the immediate relief of angina.
  - Long-acting nitrates in combination with beta blockers can be used when initial treatment with beta blockers or CCBs are ineffective.
  - Long-acting nitrates should be used as initial therapy to reduce symptoms if beta blockers or CCBs are contraindicated.
  - Nitrates are preferred in patients with vasospastic angina.

Calcium channel blockers

- Effects on myocardial O_2 demand:
  - Decrease BP, HR (verapamil and **diltiazem**), and contractility (all CCBs exert varying degrees of negative inotropic effects): verapamil effects are greater than those of **diltiazem**, which are greater than those of nifedipine.
  - Dihydropyridines (**amlodipine**, nifedipine) may cause a reflex tachycardia, which can increase O_2 demand.
- Effects on O_2 supply are as follows:
  - Similar to beta blockers, CCBs (verapamil and **diltiazem**) increase the time the heart is in diastole by slowing HR, which allows improved blood flow into the coronary arteries and subendocardium.
  - CCBs decrease coronary vascular resistance and increase coronary blood flow by vasodilation of coronary arteries.
  - CCBs prevent or relieve vasospastic angina by dilation of the epicardial coronary arteries.
- Indications for therapy:
  - CCBs can be used as initial therapy for reduction of symptoms when beta blockers are not tolerated or contraindicated.
  - CCBs may be used in combination with beta blockers, nitrates, or ranolazine for ongoing anginal symptoms or if further BP reduction is needed. Use caution when combining nondihydropyridines with beta blockers because effects on lowering HR may be additive.
  - Slow-release, long-acting dihydropyridines and nondihydropyridines are effective for stable angina.
- Dihydropyridine CCBs are preferred in patients with vasospastic angina.
  - Avoid verapamil and **diltiazem** in patients with LVEF ≤ 40%.
  - Avoid using short-acting dihydropyridines as they may exacerbate angina.

Ranolazine

- Unlike beta blockers and CCBs, ranolazine's anti-anginal and anti-ischemic effects occur without causing any significant hemodynamic changes in BP or HR.
- The mechanism of action of ranolazine is not clearly understood but appears to inhibit the late sodium (Na) current (INa), preventing calcium (Ca) overload and ultimately blunting the effects of ischemia by improving myocardial function and perfusion.
- Ranolazine is indicated for the treatment of chronic angina and can be used in combination with beta blockers, CCBs, or nitrates.
- Ranolazine is beneficial in patients whose BP or HR are too low to add or increase doses of beta blockers or CCBs.

Angiotensin-converting enzyme inhibitors ⚠

- Angiotensin-converting enzyme inhibitors (ACEIs) reduce the incidence of MI, cardiovascular death, and stroke in patients at high risk for vascular disease.

- Indications for therapy:
  - ACEIs should be used in patients with SIHD who also have LVEF ≤ 40%, HTN, diabetes, or chronic kidney disease (CKD) unless contraindicated.
  - It is reasonable to consider ARBs in patients who are intolerant of ACEIs.

 Angiotensin-Converting Enzyme Inhibitors *FDA BOXED WARNING*

Discontinue ACE inhibitors as soon as possible when pregnancy is detected, as drugs that act directly on the renin-angiotensin system can cause injury and death to the developing fetus.

Lipid-lowering therapy

- Lipid-lowering therapy is recommended for all patients with established CAD.
  - Moderate- to high-intensity statins are indicated in all patients without contraindications.
  - A combination of statins with other lipid-lowering therapy is indicated when there is an inadequate response to statins or in cases of severe hypertriglyceridemia.
  - Ezetimibe is a first-line adjunct in an ACS patient when nonstatin therapy is indicated or when patients are intolerant to statins. Other nonstatin therapies may also be used in patients who cannot tolerate statins.

15-6   Acute Coronary Syndrome

Clinical Presentation and Risk Stratification

Acute coronary syndrome (ACS) is most commonly caused by an acute rupture of an atherosclerotic plaque (Figure 15-2). ACS is subdivided into STEMI and NSTE-ACS, with STEMI representing an acute total occlusion and NSTE-ACS representing an acute partial occlusion of the coronary artery. Treatment

FIGURE 15-2. Pathophysiology of Stable Ischemic Heart Disease vs. Acute Coronary Syndromes

Atherosclerosis and CAD

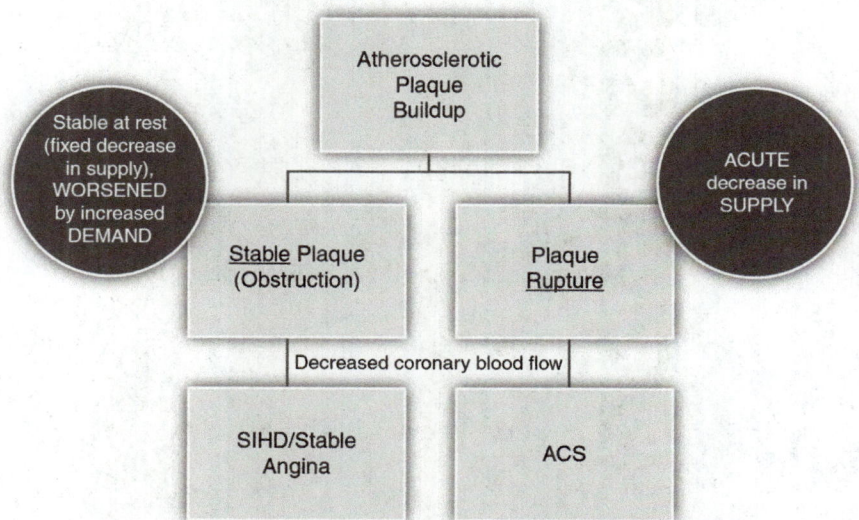

decisions are based on initial and ongoing risk stratification. Figure 15-3 provides a mnemonic to help one remember the main medication classes in the treatment of ACS.

Reperfusion/Revascularization

Early restoration of blood flow to the infarct-related artery can decrease morbidity and mortality. Reperfusion is the priority, especially in STEMI (an intervention called "primary PCI"), as cell tissue death progresses without efforts to open up the affected artery. Revascularization during NSTE-ACS is beneficial in those with ongoing or elevated risk.

Percutaneous coronary intervention (PCI)

Most common reperfusion strategy utilized during ACS including coronary stenting with either a bare metal stent (BMS) or drug-eluting stent (DES).

FIGURE 15-3. Treatment Priorities for ACS

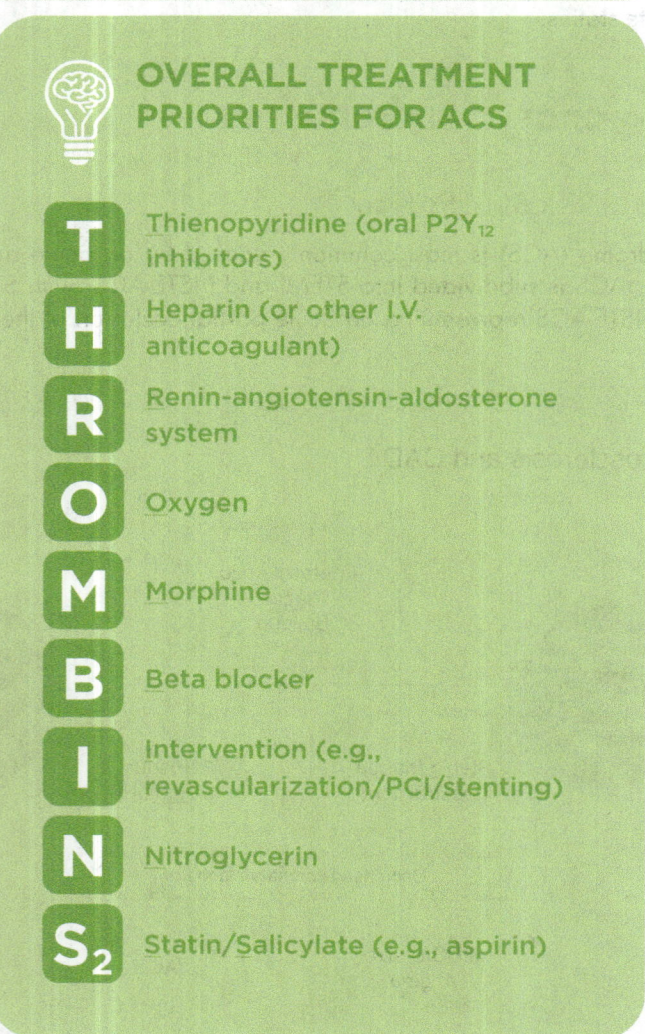

OVERALL TREATMENT PRIORITIES FOR ACS

T — Thienopyridine (oral P2Y$_{12}$ inhibitors)

H — Heparin (or other I.V. anticoagulant)

R — Renin-angiotensin-aldosterone system

O — Oxygen

M — Morphine

B — Beta blocker

I — Intervention (e.g., revascularization/PCI/stenting)

N — Nitroglycerin

S$_2$ — Statin/Salicylate (e.g., aspirin)

- DESs have pharmacologic agents, such as sirolimus, zotarolimus, or everolimus, coated on the stent that are released over time.
- DESs carry a higher risk of late-onset stent thrombosis than BMSs and DAPT is necessary to reduce incidence of acute and late stent thrombosis.
- Considerations for use of longer duration DAPT after stenting may be made on the basis of stent type, clinical presentation, and the patient's risk of bleeding.

Coronary artery bypass graft (CABG) surgery

CABG is another reperfusion strategy indicated in patients with multivessel disease, severe left main coronary artery disease, or significant disease of a major coronary vessel that is not amenable to PCI. $P2Y_{12}$ receptor antagonists should be discontinued for a minimum of 5 days (**clopidogrel** and ticagrelor) or 7 days (prasugrel) before CABG surgery to reduce the risk of bleeding.

Fibrinolytic therapy (also known as thrombolytic therapy)

Thrombolytics are a pharmacological reperfusion strategy for patients who present with STEMI when transfer to a PCI-capable facility is not feasible within 120 minutes or the patient is not a candidate for PCI. Primary PCI, however, is preferred to fibrinolytic therapy where possible.

- Agents include the following (Table 15-1):
  - Alteplase
  - Reteplase
  - Tenecteplase
- Concomitant anticoagulation is needed for at least 48 hours and up to 8 days after fibrinolytic therapy or until revascularization is performed.
- First medical contact-to-needle time of less than 30 minutes is a targeted goal.
- Indication for fibrinolytic therapy:
  - ST-segment elevation > 1 mm in 2 or more contiguous leads; left bundle branch block is present (obscuring ST observational changes); if presentation is within 12 hours and primary PCI is not feasible within 120 minutes.

Inpatient Management of ACS

Early management of ACS

Commonly, the initial 24 hours of care are focused on reperfusion, antiplatelet and anti-coagulant therapy, and acute supportive measures. Supportive care therapies such as morphine, oxygen, and nitrates may be used adjunctively, particularly as the patient is being evaluated for reperfusion, but do not reduce mortality. Indications for acute supportive care therapy are shown in Table 15-2.

TABLE 15-1. Fibrinolytic Doses

Drug	Dose
Alteplase (tPA, Activase)	15 mg I.V. bolus, followed by 0.75 mg/kg I.V. infusion over 30 minutes (not to exceed 50 mg); then 0.5 mg/kg I.V. infusion over 1 hour (not to exceed 35 mg)
Reteplase (rPA, Retavase)	10 units I.V. push over 2 minutes, followed in 30 minutes by a repeat 10 units I.V. bolus over 10 minutes
Tenecteplase (TNKase)	If patient weighs < 60 kg, give 30 mg I.V. bolus; 60 to 69.9 kg, give 35 mg I.V. bolus; 70 to 79.9 kg, give 40 mg I.V. bolus; 80 to 89.9 kg, give 45 mg I.V. bolus; > 90 kg, give 50 mg I.V. bolus; each bolus to be given over 5 seconds

TABLE 15-2. Acute Supportive Care Therapy for Acute Coronary Syndrome

Medication	Details
Morphine	Pain relief decreases tachycardia, along with vasodilatory properties on both arterial and venous sides decreasing preload and afterload; all work to decrease MVO_2.
	Increments of 2 to 4 mg I.V. are given every 5 to 15 minutes until pain is relieved.
	Nausea, vomiting, hypotension, sedation, and respiratory depression may occur.
	Morphine produces a vagotonic effect that may be contraindicated in patients with bradycardia. Monitor for hypotension, respiratory depression, and allergic reactions. Literature suggests that morphine may delay the absorption of $P2Y_{12}$ inhibitors and should not be given concomitantly.
Oxygen	Supplemental O_2 2 to 4 L/min by nasal cannula is recommended to correct and avoid hypoxia, if O_2 saturation falls below 90%.
Nitrates	All patients should receive NTG as a sublingual tablet or spray 0.4 mg, if not contraindicated. If pain is unrelieved after one dose, call 911. Patient may take an additional 2 doses every 5 minutes for unrelieved pain.
	I.V. NTG may be used in the first 48 hours of ongoing chest pain, pulmonary congestion, or hypertension.
	NTG should not be administered to patients with hypotension (SBP less than 90 mmHg), severe bradycardia, or suspected right ventricular infarction. Patients with right ventricular infarction are dependent on preload to maintain cardiac output, and the use of NTG could cause profound hypotension.
	Long-acting nitrates should be used as secondary prevention in patients who do not tolerate beta blockers and CCBs or in combination with ongoing chest pain. Nitrates are contraindicated with use of PDE-5 inhibitors including avanafil (Stendra), sildenafil (Viagra), tadalafil (Cialis), or vardenafil (Levitra).

CCBs, calcium channel blockers; I.V., intravenous; NTG, nitroglycerin; MVO_2, myocardial oxygen demand; PDE-5, phosphodiesterase-5; SBP, systolic blood pressure.

Antiplatelet therapy

Antiplatelet pharmacotherapy recommendations will vary slightly, depending upon ACS presentation (STEMI vs. NSTE-ACS) and the reperfusion strategy chosen (e.g., PCI, CABG, or conservative medication management without intervention).

See Table 15-3 for specific differences in antiplatelet recommendations.

Dual antiplatelet therapy

- **Aspirin** plus a $P2Y_{12}$ receptor antagonist reduces rates of atherothrombotic events in patients with ACS and reduces risk of stent thrombosis after PCI.
- The mechanism of platelet aggregation inhibition for the $P2Y_{12}$ receptor antagonists and **aspirin** differ; therefore, their effects are additive. Bleeding risk is higher with DAPT over **aspirin** alone.

DAPT is started early and given for at least 12 months after ACS event.

Early discontinuation or extended duration decisions regarding DAPT therapy are dependent upon bleeding and ischemic risk, respectively.

$P2Y_{12}$ inhibitors

Agents are preferred based on efficacy results from clinical studies and safety. In general, both ticagrelor and prasugrel have been shown to be superior to **clopidogrel** and are preferred in terms of efficacy. **Clopidogrel** has the least bleeding associated with its use and may be preferred for safety reasons in those at risk for bleeding and those patients who may also require oral anticoagulation.

Thienopyridines (**clopidogrel**, prasugrel)

- Inhibition of platelet aggregation is irreversible.
- **Clopidogrel** should be held 5 days before major surgery and prasugrel for 7 days to reduce the risk of bleeding.
- Therapy is initiated with a loading dose for a more rapid effect.

TABLE 15-3. **Evidence-Based Antiplatelet and Anticoagulant Therapies for the Management of Acute Coronary Syndrome**

ACS presentation	NSTE-ACS (no PCI)	NSTE-ACS or STEMI managed by PCI	STEMI managed with fibrinolytic therapy
Antiplatelet therapy			
Aspirin	Chew and swallow nonenteric-coated **aspirin** 162 to 325 mg at the onset of chest pain in all patients unless contraindicated.		
	Pre-PCI, if patient is already on **aspirin** therapy, give additional 81 to 325 mg. If not, give 325 mg before procedure.		
	Aspirin 81 to 162 mg should be continued indefinitely after ACS (with or without stenting).		
Oral P2Y$_{12}$ inhibitors	**Clopidogrel** (600 mg LD/75 mg daily MD) or ticagrelor (180 mg LD/90 mg twice daily MD)	**Clopidogrel** (600 mg LD/75 mg daily MD), ticagrelor (180 mg LD/90 mg twice daily MD), or prasugrel (60 mg LD/10 mg daily MD) 5 mg MD recommended for prasugrel in body weight < 60 kg	**Clopidogrel** preferred, 300 mg LD if within 24 hours of event; 600 mg LD if > 24 hours after the event.
	DAPT with **aspirin** and an oral P2Y$_{12}$ receptor antagonist is recommended after ACS (with or without PCI) and after PCI (with or without ACS indication).		
	Prasugrel is not recommended in ACS patients who do not undergo PCI.		
	Do not exceed 100 mg **aspirin** daily with ticagrelor.		
	It may be reasonable to choose ticagrelor or prasugrel (in those who are not at high bleeding risk) over **clopidogrel** in patients treated with PCI.		
I.V. P2Y$_{12}$ inhibitor	Cangrelor is not recommended in ACS patients who do not undergo PCI.		
	Administer 30 mcg/kg I.V. bolus, then 4 mcg/kg/min I.V. infusion. Bolus should be given before start of PCI. Infusion should continue for the duration of PCI or 2 hours, whichever is longer.		
	Transitioning to an oral P2Y$_{12}$ inhibitor: administer ticagrelor 180 mg anytime during the cangrelor infusion or immediately after discontinuation; prasugrel 60 mg or **clopidogrel** 600 mg cannot be administered until AFTER discontinuation of cangrelor.		
I.V. GP IIb/IIIa inhibitors	Greatest benefit during PCI when given to patients with high-risk features (e.g., elevated troponin) not adequately pretreated with **clopidogrel** or ticagrelor. See Table 15-4 for dosing.		
Anticoagulant therapy			
Unfractionated heparin	Give 60 unit/kg I.V. bolus (maximum 4000 units), 12 units/kg/h (maximum 1000 units/h) IV for 48 hours or until time of PCI with a goal aPTT of 50 to 70 seconds.	With GPI, give 50 to 70 units/kg IV bolus. If no GPI, give 70 units/kg IV. Give supplemental doses to target goal ACT. Discontinue at end of PCI.	Give 60 units/kg I.V. bolus (maximum 4000 units), 12 units/kg/h (maximum 1000 units/h) I.V. for 48 hours or until time of PCI, with a goal aPTT of 50 to 70 seconds.
Enoxaparin	Give 1 mg/kg subcutaneous every 12 hours for duration of hospitalization (up to 8 days).	Administer an additional 0.3 mg/kg IV dose at time of PCI if fewer than 2 therapeutic subcutaneous doses received or if last dose is more than 8 hours prior.	If patient is under 75 years of age, give 30 mg IVP, followed immediately by 1 mg/kg subcutaneous every 12 hours (first 2 doses maximum of 100 mg). If patient is over 75 years of age, give no bolus, 0.75 mg/kg subcutaneous every 12 hours (first 2 doses maximum of 75 mg). Discontinue at end of PCI.
	If CrCl is less than 30 mL/min, dose at 1 mg/kg subcutaneous daily.		
	Avoid if history of heparin-induced thrombocytopenia.		
	Therapy is continued for the duration of the hospitalization (up to 8 days) or until revascularization.		
	An initial 30 mg IV loading dose has been used in selected patients.		

(continued)

TABLE 15-3. Evidence-Based Antiplatelet and Anticoagulant Therapies for the Management of Acute Coronary Syndrome *(Continued)*

ACS Presentation	NSTE-ACS (no PCI)	NSTE-ACS or STEMI managed by PCI	STEMI managed with fibrinolytic therapy
Bivalirudin		Give 0.75 mg/kg IVP, then 1.75 mg/kg/h I.V. Reduce infusion to 1 mg/kg/h for CrCl less than 30 mL/min and 0.25 mg/kg/h for hemodialysis. Discontinue at end of PCI or continue for up to 4 hours.	
Fondaparinux	Give 2.5 mg subcutaneous daily.	Fondaparinux should not be used as the sole anticoagulant for PCI. Add UFH or bivalirudin at time of PCI if fondaparinux was given before PCI.	Give 2.5 mg IVP, then 2.5 mg subcutaneous daily.
	Fondaparinux is contraindicated in patients with CrCl < 30 mL/min.		
	Therapy is continued for the duration of the hospitalization (up to 8 days) or until revascularization.		

Boldface indicates one of top 100 drugs for 2020 by prescription volume.
ACT, activated clotting time; aPTT, activated partial thromboplastin time; BMS, bare metal stent; CrCl, creatinine clearance; DAPT, dual antiplatelet therapy; DES, drug-eluting stent; GP, glycoprotein; GPI, glycoprotein inhibitor; IVP, I.V. push; LD, loading dose; MD, maintenance dose; NSTE-ACS, non-ST-segment elevation acute coronary syndrome; PCI, percutaneous coronary intervention; STEMI, ST-segment elevation myocardial infarction; UFH, unfractionated heparin.

Cyclopentyltriazolopyrimidine (ticagrelor)

- Inhibition of platelet aggregation is reversible, although it should still be held 5 days before major surgery to reduce the risk of bleeding.
- Ticagrelor has a unique side effect profile compared to the other $P2Y_{12}$ receptor antagonists because of inhibition of adenosine reuptake.
- Therapy is initiated with a loading dose for a more rapid effect.
- Twice-daily dosing is different from other $P2Y_{12}$ receptor antagonists and is an important consideration for patient adherence.
- The dose of **aspirin** in combination with ticagrelor should not exceed 100 mg daily.

Intravenous antiplatelet therapy
$P2Y_{12}$ receptor antagonists

- Cangrelor is an I.V. $P2Y_{12}$ receptor antagonist approved as adjunct to PCI in patients not previously administered oral $P2Y_{12}$ inhibitors or planned administration of glycoprotein IIb/IIIa receptor inhibitors (GPIs).
- Transitioning to an oral $P2Y_{12}$ inhibitor: administer ticagrelor 180 mg anytime during the cangrelor infusion or immediately after discontinuation; prasugrel 60 mg or **clopidogrel** 600 mg cannot be administered until AFTER discontinuation of cangrelor.

Glycoprotein IIb/IIIa receptor inhibitors

- Agents
  - Eptifibatide
  - Tirofiban

Indications for therapy

- GPIs are considered adjuvant therapy during PCI for NSTE-ACS patients who have high-risk features such as elevated cardiac biomarkers and can be used during primary PCI for patients presenting with STEMI.

TABLE 15-4. Indications and Doses of Glycoprotein IIb/IIIa Receptor Inhibitors

Drug	Indication	Dose
Eptifibatide (Integrilin)	Adjunct to PCI	180 mcg/kg I.V. bolus twice 10 minutes apart; 2 mcg/kg/min infusion (CrCl < 50 mL/min; 1 mcg/kg/min) started after the first bolus and continued for 18 to 24 hours post procedure (minimum of 12 hours)
Tirofiban (Aggrastat)	Adjunct to PCI	25 mcg/kg I.V. bolus over 3 minutes, followed by 0.15 mcg/kg/min infusion for 12 to 24 hours (CrCl < 30 mL/min; bolus and infusion reduced by 50%)

- Special attention should be focused on proper dosage adjustments of renally cleared agents, especially in elderly patients, women, and those with renal insufficiency (Table 15-4).

Anticoagulant therapy

Anticoagulant pharmacotherapy recommendations will vary slightly, depending upon ACS presentation (STEMI vs. NSTE-ACS) and the reperfusion strategy chosen (e.g., PCI, CABG, or conservative medication management without intervention).

See Table 15-3 for specific differences in anticoagulant recommendations.

- Anticoagulant therapy should be added to antiplatelet therapy as soon as possible following presentation of ACS. Acceptable options include unfractionated heparin (UFH), enoxaparin, bivalirudin, and fondaparinux (see Table 15-3).
- Agent selection depends on type of ACS, management strategy (invasive vs. medical), and need for a surgical procedure (CABG).
- Indications for therapy
  - Medical management: enoxaparin, UFH, or fondaparinux
  - Planned PCI procedure: UFH, enoxaparin, or bivalirudin

Anti-ischemic therapy

Beta adrenergic blockade
- Any agent can be used, although agents with beta-1 selectivity are preferred in patients with bronchoconstrictive or reactive airway disease.
- Initial choices often include **metoprolol** and atenolol.
- Indications for therapy are as follows:
  - Beta blockers should be used in all patients without contraindications.
  - The first dose should be given orally within the first 24 hours unless contraindications exist, including signs of HF, symptoms of low output state, increased risk of cardiogenic shock, or other relative contraindications (e.g., bradycardia, hypotension, heart block, active asthma, reactive airway disease). In patients who are hypertensive at the time of presentation, the I.V. route may be used.

Additional Analgesia Issues in Patients with ACS

- Discontinue nonsteroidal anti-inflammatory drugs (NSAIDs) except for **aspirin** at time of ACS presentation.
- NSAIDs should not be started during hospitalization for ACS.

- If pain management is required at discharge, a stepped-care approach should be taken, starting with **acetaminophen**, small doses of narcotics, nonacetylated salicylates, or nonselective NSAIDs (e.g., **naproxen**).

Secondary Prevention of ACS

Specific agents proven to decrease mortality, HF, reinfarction, stroke, and stent thrombosis should be initiated in all without contraindications. Prior to patient discharge, the patient should be evaluated for appropriateness of the following secondary prevention medications that include anti-ischemic, antiplatelet, anti-lipid, and antihypertensive agents. See Figure 15-4 for a mnemonic to assist with remembering these medication classes.

Antiplatelet therapy

Use of DAPT for all patients post-ACS is covered in Table 15-3.

- Post ACS, DAPT with **aspirin** plus a P2Y$_{12}$ inhibitor is generally continued for at least 12 months duration.
- Early discontinuation or extended duration decisions regarding DAPT therapy are dependent upon bleeding and ischemic risk, respectively.

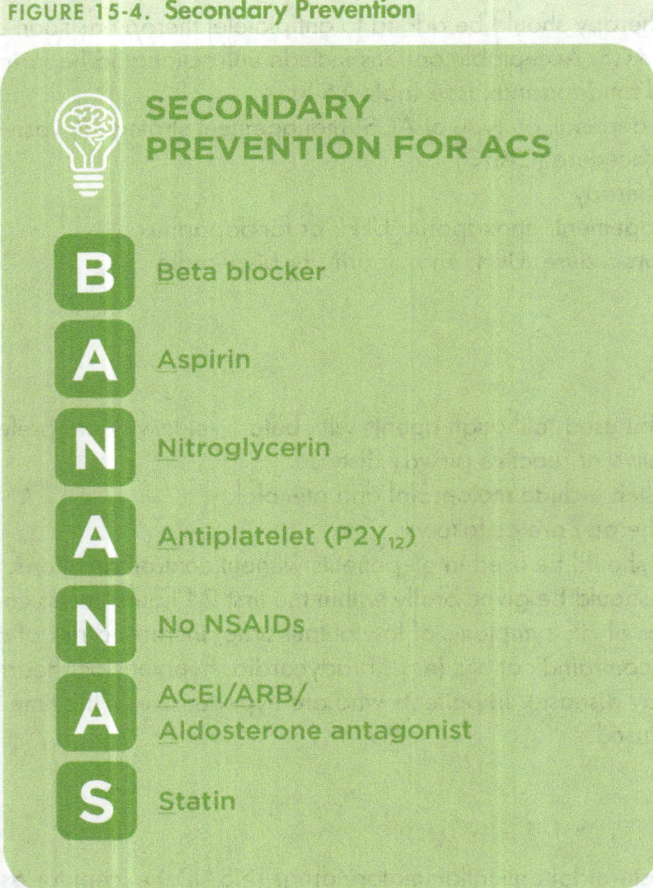

FIGURE 15-4. Secondary Prevention

SECONDARY PREVENTION FOR ACS

B — Beta blocker

A — Aspirin

N — Nitroglycerin

A — Antiplatelet (P2Y$_{12}$)

N — No NSAIDs

A — ACEI/ARB/Aldosterone antagonist

S — Statin

Beta blockers

- Beta blockers are recommended for 3 years post-MI in patients with normal LVEF. Evidence indicates treatment beyond 3 years may be reasonable in some patients who continue to experience symptoms of angina or need additional control of blood pressure.
- Beta blockers are indicated long term following ACS in patients with LVEF ≤ 40% with HF, unless contraindicated.
- Preferred beta blockers in patients with LVEF ≤ 40% are bisoprolol, **carvedilol**, and **metoprolol** succinate.

Inhibition of the RAA system

- ACEIs should be prescribed long term for patients with LVEF ≤ 40%, HTN, CKD, or DM, unless contraindicated.
- ACEIs should be considered in patients without LV dysfunction, DM, or HTN, unless contra-indicated.
- ARBs are recommended in patients who are intolerant of ACEIs.
- Unless contraindicated, long-term aldosterone blockade should be prescribed for patients who are already receiving therapeutic doses of ACEIs and beta blockers and who have an LVEF ≤ 40% and either symptomatic HF or diabetes. Creatinine clearance (CrCl) should be > 30 mL/min, and potassium should be < 5 mEq/L.

Lipid-lowering therapy

- High-intensity statin therapy is indicated for all patients post-ACS unless contraindicated.
- Ezetimibe is considered a first-line adjunct to statin therapy after ACS in select individuals where clinically indicated.
- PCSK9 inhibitors may be added in instances where desired low-density lipoprotein (LDL) reduction is difficult to achieve with combined statin plus ezetimibe therapy.

Nitroglycerin

Upon discharge from the hospital for an ACS event, patients should receive a prescription for SL NTG and be instructed on its proper use.

Protease activated receptor-1 (PAR-1) antagonism

- Vorapaxar ⚠ is indicated for the reduction of thrombotic cardiovascular events in select individuals with a history of MI or peripheral artery disease.
- It is used in combination with **aspirin** or **clopidogrel**.
- Here is limited clinical experience in combination with other P2Y$_{12}$ inhibitors.
- Vorapaxar is not widely used clinically due to increased rates of bleeding.

> ⚠ **Vorapaxar** *FDA BOXED WARNING*
>
> Antiplatelet agents increase the risk of bleeding, including intracranial hemorrhage (ICH) and fatal bleeding. Do not use vorapaxar in patients with active pathological bleeding or a history of stroke, TIA, or ICH.

15-7 Pharmacology

Anti-ischemic Drug Therapy

Beta blockers

See Chapter 12 for specific pharmacology information about beta blockers.

Nitrates

Mechanism of action

- Organic nitrates are prodrugs that must be transformed to exert pharmacological effect.
- Denitration of NTG leads to liberation of nitric oxide (NO), which results in guanylate cyclase stimulation, leading to an increase in cyclic guanosine monophosphate, and ultimately causing vasodilation.
- NO also reduces platelet adhesion and aggregation and affects endothelial function and vascular growth.

Properties

- *Oral:* Isosorbide dinitrate and NTG undergo extensive first-pass metabolism when given orally. Isosorbide mononitrate does not undergo this metabolism; it is completely bioavailable. Oral NTG requires a nitrate-free interval of 8 to 12 hours between doses to prevent tolerance.
- *I.V.:* I.V. use achieves the highest concentrations. Usually, I.V. is used for only 24 to 48 hours to avoid developing tolerance.
- *SL tablet or spray for immediate release:* Unlike tablets, spray does not degrade when exposed to air. The half-life is 1 to 5 minutes regardless of route.

Dose

See Table 15-5 for dosing information.

Monitoring parameters

Blood pressure and heart rate should be monitored.

Common adverse drug effects

Tolerance (if dosing does not allow for a nitrate-free interval of 10 to 12 hours), headache (up to 50%), hypotension, nausea, vomiting, and blurred vision are common.

Drug–drug interactions

Nitrate drug–drug interactions are described in Table 15-6.

Drug–disease interactions

Use with caution in patients with glaucoma, because nitrates may increase intraocular pressure.

Contraindications

- PDE-5 inhibitors including Avanafil, Sildenafil, Tadalafil, or Vardenafil
- Riociguat
- Hypersensitivity to nitrates

Patient instructions and counseling

- General instructions:
  - Avoid alcohol consumption.
  - May cause dizziness; use caution when driving or engaging in hazardous activities until drug effect is known.

TABLE 15-5. Pharmacologic Dosing and Properties of Nitrates

Drug	Route	Onset	Duration of action	Dose
Nitroglycerin sublingual tablet (Nitrostat)	Sublingual	1 to 3 minutes	30 to 60 minutes	0.2 to 0.6 mg every 5 minutes. Seek emergency treatment if chest pain is unrelieved after 1 dose.
Nitroglycerin spray (Nitrolingual)	Translingual	2 minutes	30 to 60 minutes	0.4 mg every 5 minutes. Seek emergency treatment if chest pain is unrelieved after 1 spray.
Nitroglycerin ointment	Topical	30 to 60 minutes	2 to 12 hours	1 to 2 inches every 8 hours up to 4 to 5 inches every 4 hours. Allow a 10 to 12-hour nitrate-free interval.
Nitroglycerin transdermal patches (Nitro-Dur)	Topical	30 to 60 minutes	Up to 24 hours	Starting dose: 0.2 to 0.4 mg/h. Apply and allow patch to stay in place for 12 hours. Remove patch after 12 hours to allow a nitrate-free interval.
Nitroglycerin sustained-release tablets or capsules	Oral	20 to 45 minutes	3 to 8 hours	Starting dose: 2.5 mg 3 to 4 times a day. Increase the dose by 2.5 mg 2 to 4 times daily to reach effective dose. Allow a 10 to 12-hour nitrate-free interval.
Nitroglycerin I.V.	I.V.	1 to 2 minutes	3 to 5 minutes	Starting dose: 5 mcg/minutes. Titrate every 3 to 5 minutes to response. Tachyphylaxis will develop within 24 hours.
Isosorbide mononitrate (Ismo, Monoket)	Oral	30 to 60 min	No data	20 mg twice a day (given 7 hours apart). Low-weight patients may need to start with 5 mg twice a day.
Isosorbide mononitrate, extended-release (Imdur)	Oral	30 to 60 min	No data	Starting dose: 30 to 60 mg daily. Maximum dose: 240 mg daily.
Isosorbide dinitrate (Isordil)	Oral	20 to 40 min	4 to 6 hours	Starting dose: 5 to 20 mg every 6 hours. Maintenance dose: 10 to 40 mg every 6 hours. Allow a 10 to 12-hour nitrate-free interval.
Isosorbide dinitrate, sustained-release tablets or capsules (Dilatrate-SR)	Oral	Up to 4 hours	6 to 8 hours	Initial dose: 40 mg every 8 hours. Maintenance dose: 40 to 80 mg every 8 to 12 hours. Allow a 10 to 12-hour nitrate-free interval.

TABLE 15-6. Nitrate Drug–Drug Interactions

Interacting medication	Effect
Avanafil (Stendra), Sildenafil (Viagra), Vardenafil (Levitra), Tadalafil (Cialis)	Significant reduction of blood pressure may occur with concomitant use with PDE-5 inhibitors and their use is contraindicated.
Other antihypertensives (e.g., beta blockers, calcium channel blockers, ACE inhibitors)	Symptomatic hypotension may occur.
Alcohol	Symptomatic hypotension may occur.
Riociguat	Symptomatic hypotension may occur and concomitant use is contraindicated

- When standing from a sitting position, rise slowly to avoid an abrupt drop in blood pressure.
- Notify physician of acute headache, dizziness, or blurred vision.
- Instructions for SL tablets:
  - Keep tablets in their original container.
  - Dissolve tablet under the tongue. Lack of tingling does not indicate a lack of potency.
  - Take 1 tablet at the first sign of chest pain. If chest pain is unrelieved after 1 tablet, seek emergency medical attention. The patient can continue to take 2 additional tablets 5 minutes apart if continued pain.
- Instructions for translingual spray:
  - Spray under tongue or onto tongue.
  - Hold spray nozzle as close to the mouth as possible, and spray medicine onto or under the tongue.
  - Do not inhale the spray, use near heat or open flame, or use while smoking.
  - Close mouth immediately after spraying.
  - Avoid eating, drinking, or smoking for 5 to 10 minutes.
  - If the pain does not go away after 1 spray, seek emergency medical attention. The patient can continue to take 2 additional tablets 5 minutes apart if continued pain.
- Instructions for ointment:
  - Measure the correct amount using the papers provided with the product.
  - Use papers for the application, not fingers.
  - Apply to the chest or back.
  - Wipe off any residual ointment before applying another dose.
- Instructions for transdermal patches:
  - Carefully tear open the wrapper. Never cut the wrapper or patch with scissors. Do not use any patch that has been cut by accident.
  - Apply to a hairless area, and rotate sites to avoid irritation.
  - Do not put the patch over burns, cuts, or irritated skin.
  - Remove the patch approximately 12 to 14 hours after placing it on every day. This removal prevents tolerance to the beneficial effects of NTG.
  - Used patches may still contain residual medication; use caution when disposing around children and pets.
  - Store the patches at room temperature in a closed container, away from heat, moisture, and direct light. Do not refrigerate.
- Instructions for sustained-release tablets:
  - Take at the same time each day as directed.
  - Do not chew or crush tablets or capsules.

Calcium channel blockers

See Chapter 12 for specific pharmacology information about CCBs.

Ranolazine

Mechanism of action

The mechanism of action of ranolazine is not clearly understood but appears to inhibit the late sodium (Na) current (I_{Na}), preventing calcium (Ca) overload and ultimately blunting the effects of ischemia by improving myocardial function and perfusion.

Dose

- Initiate at 500 mg orally twice a day and titrate to a maximum dose of 1 g orally twice a day as tolerated.
- Take without regard to meals. Do not crush, break, or chew tablet.

Monitoring parameters

- Monitor anginal symptoms.
- Perform baseline and follow-up electrocardiograms (ECGs) to evaluate QT interval.
- Monitor BP regularly in patients with severe renal insufficiency.
- Monitor renal function periodically in patients with moderate to severe renal impairment (CrCl < 60 mL/min).

Common adverse drug effects

Constipation, dizziness, headache, and nausea are common.

Drug–drug interactions

Drug–drug interactions are described in Table 15-7.

Contraindications

- Use with strong cytochrome P450 (CYP) 3A4 inhibitors (ketoconazole, clarithromycin, nelfinavir, etc.) or inducers (rifampin, phenobarbital, St. John's Wort, etc.).
- Use in patients with clinically significant hepatic impairment.

Patient instructions and counseling

- Ranolazine is not for use with acute anginal symptoms.
- Notify physician if you take any other medications, including over-the-counter medications.
- Notify physician if you have any history or family history of corrected QT (QTc) prolongation or congenital long-QT syndrome or if you are receiving drugs that prolong the QTc interval, such as antiarrhythmic agents, erythromycin, and certain antipsychotics (thioridazine, ziprasidone).
- Ranolazine may cause dizziness or light-headedness; therefore, notify physician if you experience fainting spells, and know how you react to this drug before operating heavy machinery.

TABLE 15-7. Ranolazine (Ranexa) Drug–Drug Interactions

Interacting medication	Effect
Strong CYP3A inhibitors	Concomitant use is contraindicated.
Moderate CYP3A inhibitors (**diltiazem**, verapamil, erythromycin, fluconazole, grapefruit juice, etc.)	Limit the dose of ranolazine to 500 mg twice a day.
P-glycoprotein inhibitors (e.g., cyclosporin)	Increased ranolazine concentrations can occur; titrate dose on the basis of clinical response.
CYP3A inducers (e.g., rifampin, phenobarbital, phenytoin, carbamazepine, St. John's wort)	Concomitant use is contraindicated.
CYP3A substrates: **simvastatin** (Zocor), **lovastatin,** cyclosporine, tacrolimus, sirolimus	Ranolazine may increase plasma concentrations. Do not exceed 20 mg of **simvastatin**. Dose adjustment of other substrates may be necessary.
Drugs transported by P-glycoprotein: digoxin	Concomitant use may result in increased digoxin concentrations.
CYP2D6 substrates: TCAs, antipsychotics	Concomitant use may result in increased concentration of these substrates, and lower doses may be required.
Drugs transported by OCT2: **Metformin**	Increased levels of **metformin** can occur. Do not exceed **metformin** 1700 mg daily when ranolazine 1000 mg bid is coadministered. Monitor blood glucose carefully.

Boldface indicates one of top 100 drugs for 2020 by prescription volume.
CYP, cytochrome; OCT2, organic cation transporter 2; TCA, tricyclic antidepressant.

Inhibition of the RAA system

See Chapter 12 for specific pharmacology information about ACEIs, ARBs, and aldosterone antagonists.

Antiplatelet Drug Therapy

Aspirin

Mechanism of action

Aspirin blocks prostaglandin synthesis, which prevents the formation of thromboxane A_2.

Dose

Dose information is provided in Table 15-3.

Monitoring parameters

Monitor for signs of bleeding, gastrointestinal intolerance, and tinnitus.

Adverse drug effects

Rash, urticaria, angioedema, dyspepsia, gastrointestinal ulceration, gastric erosion, duodenal ulcers, hearing loss, tinnitus, asthma, bronchospasm, dyspnea, and tachypnea may occur.

Drug–drug interactions

Antiplatelet agents, anticoagulants, and NSAIDs may all increase the risk of bleeding if used in combination with **aspirin**.

Drug–disease interactions

- Peptic ulcer disease (PUD): **Aspirin** may cause gastric ulceration or gastritis.
- **Aspirin** may cause active bleeding.

Patient instructions and counseling

- Avoid additional over-the-counter products containing **aspirin**, NSAIDs, or salicylate ingredients without the direction of a physician.
- Notify physician of dark, tarry stools; persistent stomach pain; difficulty breathing; unusual bruising or bleeding; or skin rash.
- Do not crush an enteric-coated product.
- Enteric coated tablets may reduce gastrointestinal intolerance.

P2Y$_{12}$ receptor antagonists

Mechanism of action

Both oral and I.V. P2Y$_{12}$ receptor antagonists inhibit platelet activation and aggregation mediated by the P2Y$_{12}$ adenosine diphosphate receptor.

Dose

Dose information is provided in Table 15-3.

Monitoring parameters

Monitor for signs of bleeding.

Adverse drug effects

Adverse effects are described in Table 15-8.

Drug–drug interactions

Drug–drug interactions are described in Table 15-9.

TABLE 15-8. P2Y$_{12}$ Receptor Antagonist Adverse Reactions

Drug	Reaction
Cangrelor (Kengreal)	Bleeding
Clopidogrel (Plavix)	Bleeding, blood dyscrasias, rash, thrombotic thrombocytopenic purpura
Prasugrel (Effient)	Bleeding, rash, nausea, anemia, thrombocytopenia, leucopenia, thrombotic thrombocytopenic purpura
Ticagrelor (Brilinta)	Bleeding, fatigue, syncope, ventricular pauses, dyspnea, cough, dizziness, nausea, diarrhea, elevated serum creatinine, elevated uric acid levels, blood dyscrasias

Boldface indicates one of top 100 drugs for 2020 by prescription volume.

Drug–disease interactions

PUD or other active bleeding may occur.

Contraindications

- Hypersensitivity to an individual product
- Active bleeding (e.g., gastrointestinal or intracranial hemorrhage)
- Prasugrel only: History of stroke or transient ischemic attack (TIA); use in patients ≥ 75 years of age generally is not recommended unless considered high risk (history of diabetes or prior MI)
- Ticagrelor only: **Aspirin** dose above 100 mg; severe liver disease

Doses of ASA above 100 mg may diminish the effectiveness of ticagrelor and should be avoided.

TABLE 15-9. P2Y$_{12}$ Receptor Antagonist Drug–Drug Interactions

Interacting medication	Effect
Antiplatelet agents, anticoagulants, and NSAIDs	Combination may increase the risk of bleeding.
Cangrelor (Kengreal)	
Clopidogrel, prasugrel	Cangrelor may occupy the receptor binding site. Do not administer clopidogrel or prasugrel until infusion has ended.
Clopidogrel (Plavix)	
CYP2C19 inhibitors such as proton pump inhibitors (**omeprazole** [Prilosec], **esomeprazole** [Nexium])	Avoid combination with either **omeprazole** or **esomeprazole**.
Ticagrelor (Brilinta)	
Strong CYP3A inhibitors	Increased serum concentrations of ticagrelor may occur, which may increase risk of adverse events. Avoid combination.
Strong CYP3A inducers	Decreased serum concentrations of ticagrelor may occur, which may result in a reduction in platelet inhibition. Avoid combination.
Simvastatin (Zocor), **lovastatin**	Increased concentration of simvastatin or **lovastatin** may occur, which may increase the risk of myopathy with statin therapy. Maximum dose of these statins is 40 mg.
Digoxin	Inhibition of the P-glycoprotein transporter may occur, which may result in increased digoxin serum concentration. Monitor digoxin levels closely during initiation or discontinuation of ticagrelor.
Aspirin	Doses of aspirin > 100 mg result in reduced effectiveness of ticagrelor. Maximum dose of aspirin is 100 mg.

Boldface indicates one of top 100 drugs for 2020 by prescription volume.

Patient instructions and counseling: Oral P2Y$_{12}$ agents

- Follow instructions regarding duration of therapy; do not stop without consulting physician.
- Avoid additional **aspirin**, salicylates, and NSAIDs unless under the direction of a physician.
- Notify physician for unusual bleeding or bruising; blood in the urine, stool, or emesis; skin rash; or yellowing of the skin or eyes.
- Patients taking ticagrelor should notify their physician if they experience new or unexpected shortness of breath.
- Discontinue **clopidogrel** and ticagrelor at least 5 days and prasugrel at least 7 days before major surgery.

Glycoprotein IIb/IIIa receptor inhibitors

Mechanism of action

Blockade of the glycoprotein IIb/IIIa receptor prevents fibrinogen binding, thus inhibiting platelet aggregation, the final common pathway for platelet aggregation.

Properties of individual agents

See Table 15-10 for properties of GPIs.

Indications and doses

Tables 15-3 and 15-4 provide information about indications and doses.

Monitoring parameters

- Signs and symptoms of bleeding
- Laboratory monitoring: hematocrit and hemoglobin, platelet count, activated clotting time (ACT) (during PCI), serum creatinine

Adverse drug effects

Adverse drug effects include bleeding, thrombocytopenia, and hypotension.

Drug–drug interactions

Antiplatelet agents, anticoagulants, and NSAIDs may all increase the risk of bleeding if used in combination with GPIs.

Drug–disease interactions

PUD or other active bleeding may occur.

Contraindications

- Active bleeding
- Platelet count < 100,000
- History of intracranial hemorrhage, neoplasms, atrioventricular malformations, or aneurysm
- History of stroke within the past 30 days or any history of hemorrhage stroke

TABLE 15-10. Pharmacologic Properties of Glycoprotein IIb/IIIa Receptor Inhibitors

Drug	Chemical nature	Duration of effect (hours)	Renal elimination	Renal dosing adjustment
Eptifibatide (Integrilin)	Nonpeptide	4 to 8	Yes	Yes
Tirofiban (Aggrastat)	Peptide fragment	4	Yes	Yes

- Severe HTN (BP > 180/110 mmHg)
- Major surgery within past 6 weeks
- Dialysis dependent (eptifibatide only)

PAR-1 antagonists (Vorapaxar)

Mechanism of action
Platelet activation is blocked through the PAR-1 receptor, the major thrombin receptor on platelets.

Dose
1 tablet (2.08 mg) daily

Monitoring parameters
Monitor for signs and symptoms of bleeding.

Adverse drug effects
Bleeding, including serious bleeding such as gastrointestinal and intracranial hemorrhage, depression, anemia, and rash may occur.

Drug–drug interactions
- Antiplatelet agents, anticoagulants, and NSAIDs may all increase the risk of bleeding if used in combination with vorapaxar.
- Avoid use with strong CYP3A inhibitors or inducers.
- No reversal agent exists to ameliorate effects of vorapaxar.

Drug–disease interactions
- Active bleeding may occur.
- Use with caution in patients of older age or with low body weight or reduced renal or hepatic function.

Contraindications
- Active bleeding
- History of stroke, TIA, or intracranial hemorrhage

Anticoagulants

Unfractionated heparin

Mechanism of action
Unfractionated heparin (UFH) enhances the action of antithrombin, thereby inactivating thrombin and preventing the conversion of fibrinogen to fibrin.

Dose
See Table 15-3 for information on dosing.

Monitoring parameters
Monitor activated partial thromboplastin time (aPTT) or heparin anti-Xa level, platelet count, hemoglobin and hematocrit, signs of bleeding, and ACT (during PCI).

Adverse drug effects
Bleeding, thrombocytopenia, hemorrhage, epistaxis, allergic reactions, and osteoporosis may occur. Protamine can be used to reverse the effects of UFH; 1 mg of protamine neutralizes 100 units of UFH.

Drug–drug interactions

Antiplatelet agents, anticoagulants, and NSAIDs may all increase the risk of bleeding if used in combination with UFH. Switching from UFH to low molecular weight heparin (LMWH) without an appropriate washout period may increase the risk of bleeding.

Drug–disease interaction

PUD or other active bleeding may occur.

Contraindications

- History of heparin-induced thrombocytopenia
- Severe thrombocytopenia
- Active bleeding
- Suspected intracranial hemorrhage

LMWH (enoxaparin) ⚠

Mechanism of action

The mechanism of action is similar to that of UFH; however, molecules are smaller and have a stronger affinity for factor Xa than thrombin. Advantages of LMWH over UFH include better bioavailability, more predictable response, ease of administration, fewer side effects, and no recommended routine monitoring.

Dose

See Table 15-3 for information on dosing.

Monitoring parameters

Serum creatinine, platelet count, hemoglobin and hematocrit, anti-Xa levels, signs of bleeding, and neurologic functions should be monitored.

Adverse drug effects

Adverse effects include bleeding, thrombocytopenia (decreased incidence compared to UFH), hemorrhage, and epistaxis.

Drug–drug interactions

- Antiplatelet agents, anticoagulants, and NSAIDs may all increase the risk of bleeding if used in combination with LMWH.
- Switching from LMWH to UFH without an appropriate washout period may increase the risk of bleeding.

Drug–disease interactions

PUD or other active bleeding may occur.

Warnings

Patients with recent or anticipated epidural or spinal anesthesia are at risk of hematoma and subsequent paralysis. Neurological impairment requires immediate treatment.

Contraindications

- Severe thrombocytopenia
- Active bleeding
- Suspected intracranial hemorrhage

Fondaparinux ⚠

Mechanism of action

Direct inhibition of factor Xa occurs, thereby inhibiting thrombin formation.

Dose

See Table 15-3 for information on dosing.

Monitoring parameters

Serum creatinine, platelet count, hemoglobin and hematocrit, anti-Xa levels, and signs of bleeding should be monitored.

Adverse drug effects

Adverse effects include bleeding, thrombocytopenia (decreased incidence compared to UFH), hemorrhage, and epistaxis.

Drug–drug interactions

Antiplatelet agents, anticoagulants, and NSAIDs may all increase the risk of bleeding if used in combination with fondaparinux.

Drug–disease interactions

- PUD or any active bleeding
- Not an appropriate anticoagulant when PCI is planned

Warnings

Patients with recent or anticipated epidural or spinal anesthesia are at risk of hematoma and subsequent paralysis.

Contraindications

- Severe thrombocytopenia
- Active bleeding
- Suspected intracranial hemorrhage
- CrCl (creatinine clearance) < 30 mL/min

 Enoxaparin, Fondaparinux *FDA BOXED WARNING*

Spinal or epidural hematoma
Patients receiving neuraxial anesthesia or undergoing spinal puncture are at risk for the development of epidural or spinal hematomas, which may result in long-term or permanent paralysis. Risk factors include the use of indwelling epidural catheters, the concomitant use of medications that increase the risk of bleeding (NSAIDs, antiplatelet agents, other anticoagulants), a history of traumatic or repeated spinal or epidural punctures, and a history of spinal surgery or deformity.

Bivalirudin

Mechanism of action

Bivalirudin is a direct thrombin inhibitor, which differs from UFH in that bivalirudin inhibits both bound and free thrombin.

Dose

See Table 15-3 for information on dosing.

Monitoring parameters

ACT (during PCI), aPTT, and signs of bleeding should be monitored.

Adverse drug effects

Adverse effects include bleeding, back pain, hypotension, and nausea.

Drug–drug interactions

Antiplatelet agents, anticoagulants, and NSAIDs may all increase the risk of bleeding if used in combination with bivalirudin.

Drug–disease interactions

PUD or other active bleeding may occur.

Contraindications

Severe, active bleeding may occur.

Fibrinolytic Therapy

Mechanism of action

See Chapter 11 for information on mechanism of action.

Dose

See Table 15-1 for information on dosing.

Monitoring parameters

CBC (complete blood count), ECG, aPTT, signs of bleeding, BP, and signs of reperfusion should be monitored.

Adverse drug effects

Adverse effects include bleeding, intracranial hemorrhage (less than 1%), stroke (less than 2%), and epistaxis.

Drug–drug interactions

Antiplatelet agents, anticoagulants, and NSAIDs may all increase the risk of bleeding if used in combination with fibrinolytics.

Contraindications

See Chapter 11 for information on contraindications.

15-8   Pharmacist's Role

Primary prevention efforts should be encouraged in all patients over 20 years of age. Modifiable risk factors are to be addressed such as blood pressure control, blood glucose control, and appropriate use of statin and antiplatelet therapies. In prescribed preventative medications, the pharmacist should educate and provide reminder tools to help the patient with long-term adherence. Inpatient and outpatient pharmacists should assist in the identification and prevention of drug-related problems; designing patient-specific, evidence-based medication regimens; and promote medication adherence for both SIHD and ACS. Before a patient is discharged from the hospital after having an ACS, the pharmacist should ensure appropriate secondary prevention medications are initiated and should provide counseling on the benefits and risks of each agent. Pharmacists should address cultural, ethnic, gender, and socioeconomic treatment disparities when appropriate. Finally, annual influenza vaccination should be encouraged for all patients with ASCVD.

NAPLEX Competency Statements

The questions in this chapter cover the following 2021 NAPLEX Competency Statements: **AREA 1**: 1.1; 1.2; 1.4; 1.5; 1.6 **AREA 2**: 2.1; 2.2; 2.3; 2.4 **AREA 3**: 3.2; 3.4; 3.5; 3.6; 3.7; 3.8; 3.9.

15-9 **Questions**

Use this patient profile for Questions 1 and 2.

Patient Name: Gregory Show   **Height:** 72 inches

Age: 69   **Weight:** 200 pounds

Sex: Male   **Allergies:** NKDA

Chief Complaint: Intermittent chest pain for the past 2 weeks

Diagnosis: Hypertension

                        Asthma

                        Peptic ulcer disease with GI bleed (6 months ago)

Family History: Father died age 86 years (stroke); Mother died age 82 years (diabetes and HF)

Social History: Smokes 1 pack per day x 40 years and uses alcohol 1 to 2 times weekly

Laboratory and Diagnostic Tests

ECG was normal.

Vital signs are BP 138/90 mmHg, HR 82 bpm, RR 18 breaths/min.

Initial laboratory results were all within normal limits.

Total cholesterol 240 mg/dL and HDL 38 mg/dL.

Medication Record

Date	Rx	Physician	Drug and Strength	Quantity	Sig	Refills
5/1	03456	Danes	Proventil MDI	1	2 puffs as needed	3
5/1	03457	Danes	Flovent 44 mcg	1	2 puffs twice daily	3
4/15	03299	Terry	Prilosec 20 mg	30	1 tab orally daily	2
3/20	02973	Watkins	HCTZ 25 mg	30	1 tab orally daily	1

1. A 69-year-old male presents to his primary physician with complaints of intermittent chest pain for the past few weeks. He described the pain as sharp, aching, and nonradiating, occurring mainly during his daily walk and usually relieved when he stops to rest. His 10-year atherosclerotic cardiovascular disease (ASCVD) risk is 33%. Which of the following medications is most important to initiate for primary prevention of an atherosclerotic cardiovascular event?

   A. Bupropion
   B. Rosuvastatin
   C. Lisinopril
   D. Aspirin
   E. Vitamin E

2. Which of the following interventions is best to initiate to address this man's angina symptoms?

   A. SL NTG as needed
   B. Inderal and SL NTG as needed
   C. Zestril and SL NTG as needed
   D. Cardizem and SL NTG as needed
   E. Coreg and SL NTG as needed

3. Which of the following effects on myocardial oxygen demand is affected by beta blockers? (Mark all that apply.)

A. Decreased HR
B. Decreased BP
C. Decreased contractility
D. Peripheral vasodilation
E. Arterial vasodilation

4. Which of the following statements is most accurate regarding the mechanism of action of antianginal medications in IHD?

A. Amlodipine and felodipine reduce oxygen demand by decreasing conduction through the AV node.
B. Diltiazem improves oxygen supply by dilating coronary and peripheral vessels.
C. Ranolazine increases myocardial oxygen supply by vasodilation of coronary arteries.
D. Nitrates increase myocardial oxygen demand by dilating coronary vessels.
E. Metoprolol increases myocardial oxygen supply by vasodilation of coronary arteries.

5. Which of the following patients would benefit from the addition of ranolazine therapy? (Mark all that apply.)

A. A 48-year-old man with SIHD without complaints with a BP 130/80 mmHg and HR 78 bpm
B. A 68-year-old man with severe angina symptoms on maximally tolerated beta blocker and nitrate; BP 120/80 mmHg and HR 70 bpm
C. A 72-year old-woman with angina on beta blocker and nitrate; BP 110/70 mmHg and HR 60 bpm
D. A 55-year-old man with severe angina and depression receiving fluvoxamine
E. A 62-year-old woman with angina receiving maximal doses of diltiazem with a past medical history of long QT syndrome

6. A 64-year-old male with stable ischemic heart disease complains of angina that occurs after walking 2 to 3 blocks. No lesions detected on his coronary angiogram are amenable to intervention (stent or CABG). His HR is 58 to 62 bpm and BP is 130/68 mmHg. Current medications include aspirin 81 mg daily, rosuvastatin 40 mg at bedtime, metoprolol 50 mg twice daily, ramipril 10 mg daily, and tadalafil as needed. Which of the following interventions will be most beneficial in treating this patient's angina?

A. Isosorbide mononitrate 60 mg daily
B. Diltiazem 180 mg every morning
C. Increase metoprolol to 100 mg twice daily
D. Amlodipine 5 mg daily
E. Ranolazine 1000 mg twice daily

7. Which of the following represents a DAPT strategy for a 76-year-old man with history of TIA and gastroesophageal reflux disease being discharged after an ACS with DES placement? Other medications include metoprolol, lisinopril, atorvastatin, hydrochlorothiazide, and pantoprazole. (Mark all that apply.)

A. Aspirin 81 mg daily plus clopidogrel 75 mg daily
B. Aspirin 81 mg daily plus prasugrel 10 mg daily
C. Aspirin 81 mg daily plus ticagrelor 90 mg twice daily
D. Aspirin 325 mg daily plus ticagrelor 60 mg twice daily
E. Aspirin 325 mg daily plus vorapaxar 2.08 mg daily

8. Which of the following represent benefits of LMWH over UFH? (Mark all that apply.)

A. Predictable response
B. Ease of administration
C. No recommended routine monitoring
D. Lower incidence of heparin-induced thrombocytopenia
E. No renal adjustment necessary

9. Which of the following medications is contraindicated with use of a nitrate? (Mark all that apply.)

A. Metoprolol
B. Tadalafil
C. Verapamil
D. Sildenafil
E. Felodipine

10. A 65-year-old male presents to the emergency department with chest pain and shortness of breath. ECG shows ST-segment depression in 2 leads, and the first 2 troponin values are positive. On examination, the patient is found to have pulmonary edema. His HR is 68 to 75 bpm and BP is 167/94 mmHg. Initial therapy included SL NTG, metoprolol tartrate 25 mg, and aspirin 325 mg chew and swallow. Which of the following is the preferred therapy to treat ongoing chest pain?

A. Oral meperidine
B. Oral ibuprofen
C. I.V. morphine
D. I.V. NTG
E. I.V. diltiazem

11. A 54-year-old male presents to the hospital with crushing substernal chest pain and radiation to his left arm. He is treated for acute coronary syndrome. His patient profile is as shown. Before discharge, an echocardiogram reveals a left ventricular ejection fraction of 35%. Which of the following are appropriate evidenced-based beta blockers for this patient? (Mark all that apply.)

A. Metoprolol tartrate
B. Carvedilol
C. Labetalol
D. Metoprolol succinate
E. Nebivolol

12. Which of the following therapies should be avoided in this patient?

A. Reteplase
B. Clopidogrel
C. Enalapril
D. Atorvastatin
E. Unfractionated heparin

Use this patient profile for Questions 11 and 12.

Patient Name: Donnie Land
Age: 54
Sex: Male
Chief Complaint: R/O ACS
Diagnosis: Hypertension
Gout

Height: 70 inches
Weight: 186 pounds
Allergies: Sulfa

Family History: Noncontributory
Social History: Smokes 1 pack per day x 30 years and uses alcohol occasionally

Laboratory and diagnostic tests

ECG shows ST-segment depression and T-wave changes in leads II, III, and aVF. Troponins are positive x 3.

BP 170/85 mmHg, pulse 72 bpm, RR 18 breaths/min, and temperature 97°F.

ECHO: ejection fraction 35%.

Total cholesterol 240 mg/dL and HDL 38 mg/dL.

Medication Record

Date	Rx	Physician	Drug and Strength	Quantity	Sig	Refills
6/23	094	Jabbour	EC ASA 81 mg	30	1 tab orally daily	3
8/15	135	Jabbour	Chlorthalidone 12.5 mg	30	1 tab orally daily	5
8/15	136	Jabbour	Allopurinol 300 mg	30	1 tab orally daily	5

Use this patient profile for Questions 13 and 14.

Patient Name: Suzanne Adia

Age: 56

Sex: Female

Admitting diagnosis: R/O ACS

Past Medical History:
Hypertension
T2DM
TIA x 2
Hypercholesterolemia
Metabolic syndrome

Height: 64 inches

Weight: 146 pounds

Allergies: Sulfa

Family History: Noncontributory

Social History: Smokes 1 pack per day x 30 years and uses alcohol occasionally

Laboratory and diagnostic tests

ECG shows ST-segment elevation greater than 1 mm in leads II, III, and aVF.

CrCl = 63 mL/min

BP 184/119 mmHg, pulse 100 bpm, RR 32 breaths/min, and temperature 97°F.

---

13. A 56-year-old female presents to the local emergency department complaining of crushing, substernal chest pain for 3 hours, which has been unrelieved by SL NTG. Heart rate and rhythm are regular, and no S_3 or S_4 sounds are present. She is immediately admitted to the chest pain center and started on oxygen. Her home medications are unknown at this time. The catheterization lab personnel have been notified that she is being transported to the catheterization lab for primary PCI. Which of the following regimens is most appropriate for this patient at this time?

A. Aspirin 81 mg, clopidogrel 600 mg, and enoxaparin 1 mg/kg subcutaneous twice daily

B. Aspirin 81 mg, clopidogrel 600 mg, and heparin 60 unit/kg I.V. bolus followed by heparin 12 units/kg/h

C. Ticagrelor 180 mg and eptifibatide 180 mg/kg I.V. bolus followed by eptifibatide 2 mcg/kg/h infusion

D. Aspirin 325 mg, prasugrel 60 mg, and bivalirudin 0.75 mg/kg I.V. bolus followed by bivalirudin 1.75 mg/kg/h

E. Aspirin 325 mg, ticagrelor 180 mg, and bivalirudin 0.75 mg/kg I.V. bolus followed by bivalirudin 1.75 mg/kg/h

14. Which of the following agents would be beneficial to this patient?

A. Alteplase 100 mg I.V. over 90 minutes

B. Subcutaneous fondaparinux

C. I.V. lidocaine

D. Metoprolol 50 mg orally

E. Diltiazem 240 mg orally

15. Which of the following medication regimens is the best choice for discharge therapy in a 65-year-old patient weighing 70 kg who is post-ACS with DES placement and preserved LVEF?

A. Aspirin 325 mg daily, clopidogrel 75 mg daily, diltiazem 240 mg daily, and simvastatin 40 mg daily

B. Aspirin 81 mg daily, atorvastatin 80 mg daily, ticagrelor 90 mg bid, and metoprolol tartrate 50 mg bid

C. Prasugrel 5 mg daily, enalapril 10 mg bid, metoprolol succinate 100 mg daily, and simvastatin 40 mg daily

D. Aspirin 81 mg daily, metoprolol tartrate 100 mg twice daily, prasugrel 10 mg daily, and SL NTG

E. Aspirin 325 mg daily, metoprolol tartrate 50 mg twice daily, and SL NTG

16. Which of the following antiplatelets should be held for 5 days before surgery to reduce the risk of CABG-related bleeding? (Mark all that apply.)

   A. Clopidogrel
   B. Prasugrel
   C. Ticagrelor
   D. Cangrelor
   E. Eptifibatide

17. A 65-year-old male presents to the emergency department with complaints of chest pain while he was watching television. His past medical history is positive for angina, hyperlipidemia, diabetes, chronic kidney disease, and hypertension. His current medications include aspirin, rosuvastatin, metformin, amlodipine, and sildenafil. His ECG is consistent with acute ischemia. His HR is 52 bpm and BP is 170/100 mmHg. Laboratory tests show SCr 1.7 mg/dL and estimated CrCl < 30 mL/min. Which of the following interventions should be avoided in this patient at this time? (Mark all that apply.)

   A. Enoxaparin 1 mg/kg subcutaneous twice daily
   B. UFH 60 units/kg bolus (maximum 4000 units), then 12 units/kg/h infusion (maximum 1000 units/h)
   C. Fondaparinux 2.5 mg subcutaneous daily
   D. Enoxaparin 1 mg/kg subcutaneous daily
   E. UFH 80 units/kg bolus, then 18 units/kg/h infusion

18. Which of the following agents are preferred in the setting of a planned PCI? (Mark all that apply.)

   A. Bivalirudin
   B. Enoxaparin
   C. UFH
   D. Alteplase
   E. Fondaparinux

19. Which of the following agents should *not* be administered at the same time as I.V. cangrelor because of a drug interaction at the site of action? (Mark all that apply.)

   A. Clopidogrel
   B. Ticagrelor
   C. Prasugrel
   D. Vorapaxar
   E. Aspirin

20. Which of the following statements about the GPIs are accurate? (Mark all that apply.)

   A. Eptifibatide, and tirofiban are both administered as a bolus followed by a continuous infusion.
   B. A patient might experience an allergic reaction after repeated exposure to eptifibatide.
   C. Eptifibatide and tirofiban can both be reversed by a platelet infusion.
   D. Tirofiban and eptifibatide are renally eliminated; therefore, dosage adjustment is required for patients with renal dysfunction.
   E. Both eptifibatide and tirofiban are both indicated as adjuncts to PCI.

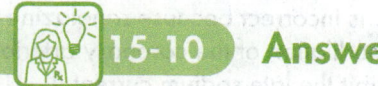 **15-10   Answers**

1. **B.** Based on this patient's calculated 10-year risk, high-intensity statin therapy (rosuvastatin) should be considered. The appropriate dose of rosuvastatin should be 20 to 40 mg to be considered high-intensity. Although smoking cessation is an optimal goal, this can be accomplished through behavioral or drug therapy, and, therefore, Answer A is not the most important agent to initiate. Answer C is not the best choice because ACEIs (lisinopril) provide the most cardiovascular benefit in risk reduction when blood pressure is not under control. Answer D is not the best choice because the benefit of aspirin in primary prevention comes after years of therapy and poses risk in patients who are prone to bleeding. His age and history of PUD with recent GI bleeding would be of concern for long-term aspirin use. Answer E is not the best choice because no vitamin therapy has been shown to reduce cardiovascular mortality.

2. **D.** All patients with chronic chest pain need SL NTG for acute use; however, SL NTG alone is not appropriate anti-anginal therapy (Answer A is incorrect). A CCB regimen (Answer D) will help control his angina and lower his HR. Although beta blockers should be considered first-line therapy in patients with stable angina for anti-ischemic effects, both Answers B and E are incorrect because Inderal (propranolol) and Coreg (carvedilol) are not beta-1 selective and could worsen his asthma. In this case, the CCB regimen in Answer D will avoid beta-2 blocking effects in this asthmatic patient. CCBs can be used in settings where a contraindication to a beta blocker exists and will help control his angina as well as lower his HR. Answer C is incorrect because this patient needs an agent to control anginal symptoms, and ACEIs are not effective as anti-anginal agents.

3. **A, B, C.** Beta blockers decrease heart rate (Answer A), blood pressure (Answer B), and contractility (Answer C). Beta blockers do not cause peripheral or arterial vasodilation (Answers D and E).

4. **B.** Diltiazem, a nondihydropyridine CCB, increases oxygen supply through vasodilation of coronary and peripheral vessels. Answer A is incorrect, because a dihydropyridine CCB, such as amlodipine and felodipine, does not affect AV nodal conduction. Answer C is incorrect because ranolazine does not cause vasodilation of the coronary arteries but appears to inhibit the late sodium current (I_{Na}), preventing Ca overload and ultimately blunting the effects of ischemia by improving myocardial function and perfusion. Answer D is incorrect because nitrates increase oxygen supply through venous and arterial vasodilation. Answer E is incorrect because Toprol XL is not a beta blocker with vasodilatory properties.

5. **B, C.** Answers B and C represent patients who require additional angina symptom control, but their BP and HR would not tolerate further dose titration of their current regimen. Ranolazine has the advantage of not affecting BP or HR and would be appropriate in these scenarios. Answer A is incorrect because this patient is without anginal symptoms, and other anti-anginals should be initiated as first-line therapy when symptoms occur. Answer D is incorrect because ranolazine is contraindicated in combination with fluvoxamine (strong CYP3A4 inhibitor). Answer E is incorrect because the patient has a history of long QT syndrome, which is a contraindication to ranolazine therapy because of its ability to prolong the QT interval.

6. **D.** Adding a calcium channel blocker will give additional anti-anginal effects, and using amlodipine rather than a nondihydropyridine CCB (Answer B) is appropriate to avoid additional HR lowering (Answer D is correct). Adding nitrates (Answer A) to this patient who occasionally takes tadalafil is contraindicated because concomitant use can cause dangerously low BP. Beta blockers (Answer C) should be titrated for anti-anginal effects, but this

patient's HR and BP are marginal and may not tolerate a doubling of dose. Ranolazine (Answer E) is an option in patients with low HR and BP who need additional anti-anginal effects, but the starting dose should be initiated at 500 mg twice daily.

7. **A, C.** Answers A and C are both correct in that they both employ low-dose aspirin with an appropriately dosed P2Y$_{12}$ inhibitor for a patient with recent ACS following stent placement (clopidogrel 75 mg daily, ticagrelor 90 mg twice daily). Answers B and E are inappropriate because they both include an agent that is contraindicated in a patient with a history of TIA (prasugrel, vorapaxar). Answers D and E are incorrect because the dose of aspirin is too high (325 mg). Ticagrelor 60 mg twice daily (in Answer D) would be the appropriate dose only after 1 year following ACS for continued thromboembolic risk reduction.

8. **A, B, C, D.** LMWH has several advantages over UFH including more predictable therapeutic response (Answer A), ease of administration (Answer B), lack of required monitoring (Answer C), and reduced incidence of heparin-induced thrombocytopenia (Answer D). Renal adjustment is necessary with LMWH in patients with a CrCl less than 30 mL/min, whereas UFH does not require dosage adjustment (Answer E is incorrect).

9. **B, D.** Tadalafil and sildenafil are PDE-5 inhibitors and all agents in this class are contraindicated with use of a nitrate. Beta blockers (metoprolol) (Answer A) and CCBs (verapamil and felodipine) (Answers C and E) can be safely combined with nitrates.

10. **D.** The appropriate therapy for ongoing chest pain is IV NTG given the fact that the patient is hypertensive and has pulmonary edema. Both meperidine and morphine (Answers A and C) are not the preferred initial choices because they may mask the signs of ongoing chest pain, and, furthermore, morphine may delay absorption of antiplatelet agents. Answer B is not correct because NSAIDs like ibuprofen are not indicated in any patient presenting with ACS and should not be resumed in patients taking them as home medications. Answer E is not preferred because there is no role for I.V. CCB in the management of ACS.

11. **B, D.** Both carvedilol (Answer B) and metoprolol succinate (Answer D) are appropriate beta blockers in patients with an ejection fraction of ≤ 40% based

on guideline recommendations. Metoprolol tartrate (Answer A), labetalol (Answer C), and nebivolol (Answer E) are not guideline-recommended beta blockers for patients with a decreased EF.

12. **A.** Reteplase is a thrombolytic agent, which does not have a role in the treatment of NSTEMI. Thrombolytic therapy is indicated for the treatment of STEMI when PCI is not possible within 120 minutes. Clopidogrel (Answer B) should be considered in all patients with NSTEMI. This patient has a clear indication for an ACEI (enalapril) (Answer C) because of his ejection fraction of ≤ 40%. High-intensity statin therapy (e.g., atorvastatin 40 to 80 mg or rosuvastatin 20 to 40 mg) should be initiated in all patients with a diagnosis of ACS (Answer D). An anticoagulant should be started on presentation (UFH) (Answer E).

13. **E.** An appropriate PCI regimen includes aspirin, a P2Y$_{12}$ receptor antagonist, and an anticoagulant agent (UFH, enoxaparin, bivalirudin). In some cases, a GPI may also be added. Answer C is incorrect because it does not include aspirin. The appropriate dose of aspirin for ACS is at least 162 mg; therefore, Answers A and B are incorrect because the dose of aspirin is not high enough. History of TIA or stroke is an absolute contraindication for prasugrel (Answer D).

14. **D.** Beta blockers are first-line therapy in patients with STEMI. Because this patient does not have any contraindications to beta blockade, Answer D is the correct choice. This patient is going immediately to the catheterization lab where primary PCI is preferred over fibrinolytic therapy for STEMI. In centers where PCI is not available within 120 minutes, fibrinolytics should be considered. However, one of the relative contraindications to fibrinolytic therapy is severe uncontrolled hypertension (BP > 180/110 mmHg). Answer A is not appropriate in this patient for these reasons. Answer B is incorrect because fondaparinux cannot be used as an anticoagulant during PCI owing to risk of catheter thrombosis. Prophylactic lidocaine (Answer C) is not part of routine management for STEMI. Calcium channel blockers do not have a role in STEMI when a beta blocker can be given (Answer E).

15. **B.** A beta blocker, a statin, and DAPT for at least 12 months should be given to all patients without contraindications post-MI. Answer A is not correct because although CCBs can be given if a patient

has contraindications to beta blockade, they are not recommended as first-line treatment. In addition, the dose of aspirin is too high and the statin dose is not high intensity. Answer C is incorrect because aspirin is omitted and the dose of prasugrel is incorrect given that the patient weighs more than 60 kg. Answer D is incorrect because high-intensity statin therapy is not included. Answer E would be a correct choice for the immediate treatment of someone who presents with ACS but not as discharge therapy because the dose of aspirin is too high and a statin is omitted.

16. **A, C.** Antiplatelet therapy should be held before surgery to reduce surgery-related bleeding. The duration of holding antiplatelet therapy depends on the agent prescribed. Both clopidogrel (Answer A) and ticagrelor (Answer C) are recommended to be held for 5 days preoperatively. Prasugrel (Answer B) should be held for 7 days preoperatively. Cangrelor (Answer D) should be held for 1 to 2 hours before surgery. Eptifibatide (Answer E) should be held for 2 to 4 hours before surgery.

17. **A, C, E.** Both enoxaparin and fondaparinux are renally eliminated and require dosage adjustment (enoxaparin, Answer A) or avoidance (fondaparinux, Answer C) when CrCl < 30 mL/min. The appropriate dose of UFH for ACS is 60 units/kg (maximum 4000 units) bolus, then 12 units/kg/h (maximum 1000 units/h). Answer E reflects the dose for venous thromboembolism treatment and is not appropriate for this patient. Answer B is the appropriate dose of heparin for this indication, and Answer D is the appropriate renally adjusted dose of enoxaparin.

18. **A, B, C.** Bivalirudin (Answer A), enoxaparin (Answer B), and UFH (Answer C) are all guideline-recommended choices in the setting of planned PCI. Answer D is a fibrinolytic and, therefore, not appropriate outside of STEMI management. Fondaparinux (Answer E) is not indicated for PCI because of the risk of catheter-related thrombosis.

19. **A, C.** Both clopidogrel (Answer A) and prasugrel (Answer C) should not be given with cangrelor until the end of the infusion because their binding site is the same. Ticagrelor (Answer B) does not have a drug interaction with cangrelor because it has an alternative binding site. Vorapaxar (Answer D) and aspirin (Answer E) have a different site of action on the platelet and, therefore, do not have an interaction with cangrelor.

20. A, D, E. All of the available GPIs are administered as a bolus and infusion (Answer A). Epitibatide is not a monoclonal antibody, therefore, development of an allergic reaction upon rechallenge is not expected (Answer B is incorrect). The only GPI that was reversed by a platelet infusion was abciximab, but it is no longer on the US market (C is an incorrect response). Both commercially available GPIs are renally eliminated and require dosage adjustment of the infusion with renal dysfunction: eptifibatide and tirofiban (Answer D). Both of the agents are indicated as adjuncts to PCI (Answer E).

15-11 Additional Resources

Amsterdam EA, Wenger NK, Brindis RG, et al. 2014 ACC/AHA guideline for the management of patients with non-ST-elevation acute coronary syndromes: a report of the American College of Cardiology/American Heart Association Task Force on Practice Guidelines. *J Am Coll Cardiol*. 2014;64(24):e139–e228.

Arnett DK, Blumenthal RS, Albert MA, et al. 2019 ACC/AHA guideline on the primary prevention of cardiovascular disease: a report of the American College of Cardiology/American Heart Association Task Force on Clinical Practice Guidelines. *J Am Coll Cardiol*. 2019;74(10):e177–232.

Fihn SD, Blankenship JC, Alexander KP, et al. 2014 ACC/AHA/AATS/PCNA/SCAI/STS focused update of the guideline for the diagnosis and management of patients with stable ischemic heart disease: a report of the American College of Cardiology/American Heart Association Task Force on Practice Guidelines, and the American Association for Thoracic Surgery, Preventive Cardiovascular Nurses Association, Society for Cardiovascular Angiography and Interventions, and Society of Thoracic Surgeons. *J Am Coll Cardiol*. 2014;64:1929–1949.

Fihn SD, Gardin JM, Abrams J, et al. 2012 ACCF/AHA/ACP/AATS/PCNA/SCAI/STS guideline for the diagnosis and management of patients with stable ischemic heart disease: a report of the American College of Cardiology Foundation/American Heart Association Task Force on Practice Guidelines, and the American College of Physicians, American Association for Thoracic Surgery, Preventive Cardiovascular Nurses Association, Society for Cardiovascular Angiography and Interventions, and Society of Thoracic Surgeons. *J Am Coll Cardiol*. 2012;60:e44–e164.

Grundy SM, Stone NJ, Bailey AL, et al. 2018 AHA/ACC/AACVPR/AAPA/ABC/ACPM/ADA/AGS/APhA/ASPC/NLA/PCNA guideline on the management of blood cholesterol: a report of the American College of Cardiology/American Heart Association Task Force on Clinical Practice Guidelines. *Circulation*. 2019;139:e1082–e1143.

Levine GN, Bates ER, Bittl JA, et al. 2016 ACC/AHA guideline focused update on duration of dual antiplatelet therapy in patients with coronary artery disease: a report of the American College of Cardiology/American Heart Association Task Force on Clinical Practice Guidelines: an update of the 2011 ACCF/AHA/SCAI guideline for percutaneous coronary intervention, 2011 ACCF/AHA guideline for coronary artery bypass graft surgery, 2012 ACC/AHA/ACP/AATS/PCNA/SCAI/STS guideline for the diagnosis and management of patients with stable ischemic heart disease, 2013 ACCF/AHA guideline for the management of ST-elevation myocardial infarction, 2014 ACC/AHA guideline for the management of patients with non-ST-elevation acute coronary syndromes, and 2014 ACC/AHA guideline on perioperative cardiovascular evaluation and management of patients undergoing noncardiac surgery. *J Am Coll Cardiol*. 2016;68:1082–1115.

Levine GN, Bates ER, Blankenship JC, et al. 2011 ACCF/AHA/SCAI guideline for percutaneous coronary intervention: a report of the American College of Cardiology Foundation/American Heart Association Task Force on Practice Guidelines and the Society for Cardiovascular Angiography and Interventions. *J Am Coll Cardiol*. 2011;58:e44–e122.

Lloyd-Jones DM, Morris PB, Ballantyne CM, et al. 2017 focused update of the 2016 ACC expert consensus decision pathway on the role of non-statin therapies for LDL-cholesterol lowering in the management of atherosclerotic cardiovascular disease risk: a report of the American College of Cardiology Task Force on Clinical Expert Consensus Decision Pathways. *J Am Coll Cardiol*. 2017;70:1785–1822.

O'Gara PT, Kushner FG, Ascheim DD, et al. 2013 ACCF/AHA guideline for the management of ST-elevation myocardial infarction: a report of the American College of Cardiology Foundation/American Heart Association Task Force on Practice Guidelines. *J Am Coll Cardiol*. 2013;61:e78–e140.

Smith SC Jr, Benjamin EJ, Bonow RO, et al. AHA/ACCF secondary prevention and risk reduction therapy for patients with coronary and other atherosclerotic vascular disease: 2011 update: a guideline from the American Heart Association and American College of Cardiology Foundation. *Circulation*. 2011;124:2458–2473.

Dyslipidemia

16

NANCY D. BORJA-HART

16-1 KEY POINTS

- Dyslipidemia is a lipid metabolism disorder causing an elevation of total cholesterol, low-density lipoprotein (LDL) cholesterol, or triglycerides, or a decrease in high-density lipoprotein (HDL).
- Disorders of lipid metabolism can lead to atherosclerotic cardiovascular disease (ASCVD).
- Dyslipidemia can be caused by genetic or environmental factors.
- Screening is recommended every 4 to 6 years in patients over 20 years old without ASCVD or diabetes.
- Lifestyle modifications are recommended for all patients with dyslipidemia.
- Though target LDL levels have historically been the mainstay of goal-directed therapy, the 2013 American College of Cardiology/American Heart Association (ACC/AHA) guidelines recommend fixed-dose statins for primary and secondary prevention of ASCVD.
- High-intensity statins are those that reduce LDL by ≥ 50%; moderate-intensity statins are those that lower LDL by 30% to 49%.
- The 2013 ACC/AHA guidelines suggest treatment with statins within 4 major groups for whom the benefit outweighs the risk (adverse effect risk, medication interactions) and when patient preference is considered.
  - High-intensity statins are recommended for all patients < 75 years of age with existing ASCVD; moderate-intensity statins can be used if high intensity is not tolerated.
  - High-intensity statins are recommended for all patients ≥ 21 years of age with an LDL ≥ 190 mg/dL; moderate-intensity statins can be used if high intensity is not tolerated.
  - Both moderate- and high-intensity statins are recommended for all diabetic patients aged 40 to 75 years; consider a high-intensity statin when the ASCVD risk is ≥ 7.5%.
  - In adults 40 to 75 years without diabetes with an LDL ≥ 70 but < 190 consider a moderate intensity statin if ASCVD risk is ≥ 7.5%, and a high intensity statin if ASCVD risk is ≥ 20%.
- The Pooled Cohort Equations are used to calculate 10-year ASCVD risk.
- Secondary causes of dyslipidemia can include medications (atypical antipsychotics, glucocorticoids), diseases (biliary obstruction, nephrotic syndrome, hypothyroidism), and altered metabolic states (obesity, pregnancy).
- The 2018 ACC/AHA guidelines suggest non-statin medications (ezetimibe, PCSK9 inhibitors) for patients unable to tolerate any statin or when high-risk patients have less than the expected response to the recommended statin doses.

16-2 STUDY GUIDE CHECKLIST

The following topics may guide your study of this subject area:

- ☐ Pathophysiology of atherosclerosis and lipid metabolism.
- ☐ Risk factors for atherosclerotic cardiovascular disease.
- ☐ Lifestyle modifications recommended for risk reduction (Dietary Approaches to Stop Hypertension [DASH] diet, exercise).
- ☐ Mechanism of action and adverse effects of drugs for dyslipidemia.
- ☐ High- and moderate-intensity statin doses.
- ☐ Combinations of medications for dyslipidemia including benefit and risk.
- ☐ Unique counseling points for medications used in dyslipidemia.
- ☐ Purpose of the 2018 ACC/AHA guidelines and their role in dyslipidemia management.
- ☐ Lipid goal setting via the National Lipid Association recommendations.

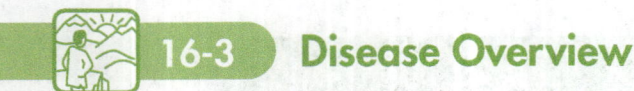

16-3   Disease Overview

Pathophysiology and Classification

Lipoproteins transport lipids through the blood. The three major forms of lipoproteins are low-density lipoprotein (LDL), high-density lipoprotein (HDL), and VLDL (very-low-density lipoprotein). The VLDL can be equated with the triglyceride (TG) content divided by 5. A simplified way to view total cholesterol (TC) is TC = LDL + HDL + VLDL. If VLDL can be estimated as TG/5, the Friedewald equation for calculating LDL is more easily understood:

$$LDL = TC - (HDL + TG/5)$$

This calculated formula is most accurate when TG < 200 mg/dL and should not be used when TG > 400 mg/dL. A direct LDL or non-HDL measurement most accurately represents LDL when TG > 200 mg/dL. See Table 16-1 for lipid classification. This is the common criteria utilized for regular lab work; however, other factors are considered to determine the need for drug therapy, which will be discussed later.

Lipids enter the bloodstream though either the exogenous or endogenous pathway. The exogenous pathway involves ingestion of dietary fat, emulsification by bile acids, and absorption via chylomicrons (TG and cholesterol esters). Triglycerides are hydrolyzed to free fatty acids to be used by muscle or stored in adipose tissue. The endogenous pathway is a complex method of cholesterol production via hepatic secretion of VLDL, which is then processed to LDL and HDL. LDL and its permeation into the endothelium and subsequent oxidation to foam cells is linked to atherosclerotic cardiovascular disease (ASCVD). Endothelial inflammation also plays a role in plaque formation, and rupture may lead to coronary and cerebrovascular events. Reverse cholesterol transports cholesterol via HDL back to the liver. Several randomized controlled trials have independently associated low HDL, elevated LDL, and elevated TG with ASCVD.

TABLE 16-1. Classification of Lipids

Type	Classification
LDL cholesterol	
< 100 mg/dL	Optimal
100 to 129 mg/dL	Near optimal or above optimal
130 to 159 mg/dL	Borderline high
160 to 189 mg/dL	High
≥ 190 mg/dL	Very high
Total cholesterol	
< 200 mg/dL	Desirable
200 to 239 mg/dL	Borderline high
≥ 240 mg/dL	High
HDL cholesterol	
< 40 mg/dL	Low
≥ 60 mg/dL	High
Triglycerides	
< 150 mg/dL	Normal
150 to 199 mg/dL	Borderline high
200 to 499 mg/dL	High
≥ 500 mg/dL	Very high

Diagnostic Criteria

Screening of adults > 20 years of age is recommended every 4 to 6 years in patients with an increased risk of coronary heart disease. Based on current evidence, the United States Preventive Services Task Force cannot recommend that children and adolescents 20 years or younger be screened.

Secondary causes of dyslipidemia should be investigated. Common causes of elevated LDL are diet (excess saturated or trans fats, weight gain, anorexia), diseases (biliary obstruction, nephrotic syndrome), or disorders and altered metabolic states (hypothyroidism, obesity, pregnancy). Elevated TG may be caused by diet (weight gain, very-low-fat diets, high intake of refined carbohydrates, excessive alcohol). See Table 16-2 for some common medication-related causes of dyslipidemia.

Familial hypercholesterolemia

Familial hypercholesterolemia (FH) is associated with a mutation in the LDL receptor gene, the apolipoprotein B (Apo B) gene, or the proprotein convertase subtilisin/kexin type 9 (PCSK9) gene. Patients who are homozygous for this mutation may have LDL cholesterol > 800 mg/dL in infancy, and those with heterozygous FH often have LDL cholesterol > 160 mg/dL.

Clinical Presentation

Dyslipidemias are usually asymptomatic, except in some familial lipid disorders in which patients may develop cutaneous manifestations of lipid deposition (e.g., xanthomas).

Treatment Principles

Before November 2013, the National Cholesterol Education Program Adult Treatment Panel guidelines (ATP III and subsequent updates) served as the standard of care for lipid management. These guidelines used the Framingham Risk Score to predict 10-year coronary heart disease events, risk factors, and comorbidities to stratify dyslipidemia treatment. In 2013, the American College of Cardiology/American Heart Association (ACC/AHA) issued updated recommendations that were markedly different from previous guidelines. Though ACC/AHA explicitly stated that these were not meant to be a comprehensive guide to lipid management, they did recommend treatment of dyslipidemia using fixed-dose statins to prevent ASCVD. Clinicians struggled with the lack of lipid goals to determine progress and cardiovascular risk reduction, among other clinical controversies with the lipid guidelines. Therefore, the National Lipid

TABLE 16-2. Medications That Cause Dyslipidemia

Elevated LDL	Elevated triglycerides
Atypical antipsychotics	Atypical antipsychotics
Omega-3 fatty acids	Glucocorticoids
Rosiglitazone	Oral estrogens
Isotretinoin	Bile acid sequestrants
SGLT2 inhibitors	Protease inhibitors
	Isotretinoin
	Anabolic steroids
	Sirolimus
	Raloxifene
	Tamoxifen
	Beta blockers (except **carvedilol**)

Boldface indicates one of top 100 drugs for 2020 by prescription volume.
SGLT2, sodium-glucose cotransporter-2.

Association (NLA) created two sets of recommendations to address these issues. The NLA guidelines included lipid classifications and therapeutic targets (Part 1) together with lifestyle recommendations and treatment optimization (Part 2).

Nondrug Therapy

Lifestyle modification

All patients with dyslipidemia should undertake lifestyle modifications. For the purposes of ASCVD prevention, the 2013 ACC/AHA guidelines on lifestyle management recommended the Dietary Approaches to Stop Hypertension (DASH) diet, the U.S. Department of Agriculture (USDA) Food Pattern, or the AHA diet because evidence shows that they can reduce the risk of ASCVD. The DASH diet consists of dietary intake patterns that emphasize vegetables, fruits, whole grains, low-fat dairy products, poultry, fish, legumes, non-tropical vegetable oils, and nuts. Intake of sweets, sugar-sweetened beverages, and red meats should be limited. Daily intake from saturated fats should be 5% to 6% of total calories. Sodium in the diet should be limited to no more than 2400 mg/day, with reduction to 1500 mg sodium/day producing the maximum blood pressure reduction. Exercise should consist of moderate- to vigorous-intensity physical activity 3 to 4 times per week, lasting an average of 40 minutes per session.

Risk evaluation

The Pooled Cohort Equations (PCE) CV Risk Calculator considers age, gender, race (non-Hispanic white, Black, or other), total cholesterol, HDL cholesterol, systolic blood pressure, blood pressure medication use, presence of diabetes, and smoking status to determine a percentage risk for an atherosclerotic event within 10 years (http://tools.acc.org/ASCVD-Risk-Estimator-Plus/). The equation may be used for other ethnic groups; however, it may underestimate risk in some subgroups (Native Americans, South Asians, Puerto Ricans) and overestimate risk for East Asians and Mexican Americans. Cut-points of ≥ 7.5% or < 7.5% have been established to guide therapy. See Figure 16-1 below of the PCE CV Risk Calculator.

FIGURE 16-1. A representation of the Pooled Cohort Equations cardiovascular risk calculator form

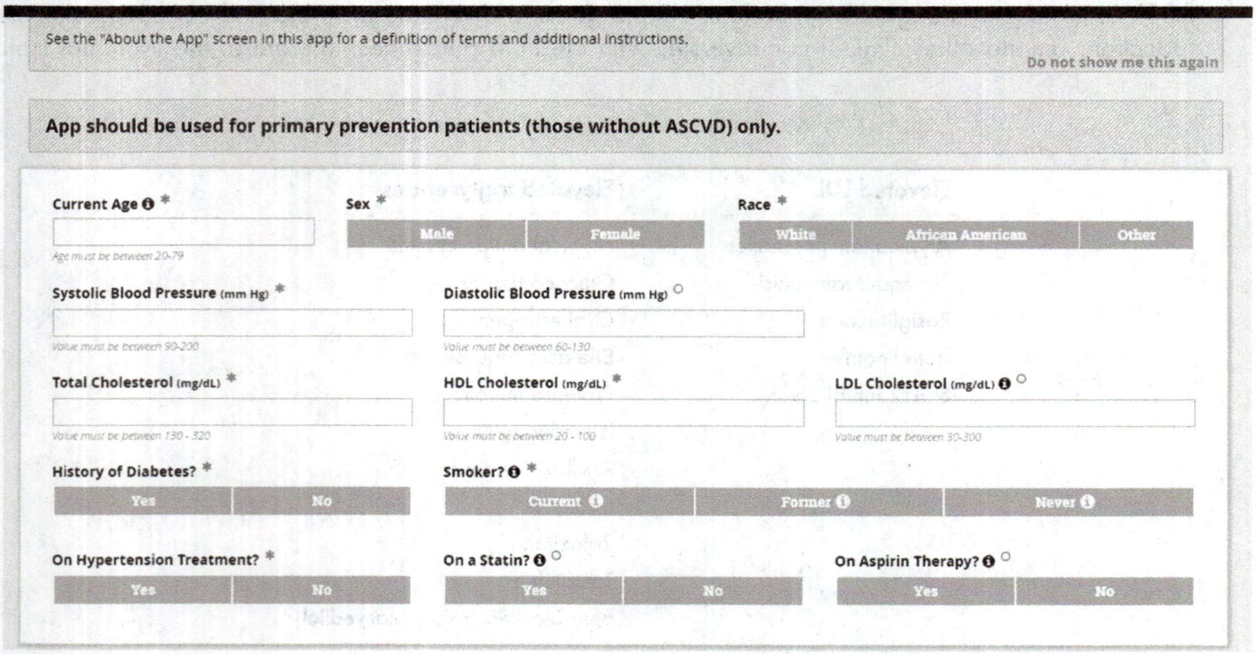

See the "About the App" screen in this app for a definition of terms and additional instructions.

Do not show me this again

App should be used for primary prevention patients (those without ASCVD) only.

Current Age *
Age must be between 20-79

Sex *
Male | Female

Race *
White | African American | Other

Systolic Blood Pressure (mm Hg) *
Value must be between 90-200

Diastolic Blood Pressure (mm Hg)
Value must be between 60-130

Total Cholesterol (mg/dL) *
Value must be between 130 - 320

HDL Cholesterol (mg/dL) *
Value must be between 20 - 100

LDL Cholesterol (mg/dL)
Value must be between 30-300

History of Diabetes? *
Yes | No

Smoker? *
Current | Former | Never

On Hypertension Treatment? *
Yes | No

On a Statin?
Yes | No

On Aspirin Therapy?
Yes | No

FIGURE 16-2. Secondary Prevention in Patients With Clinical ASCVD

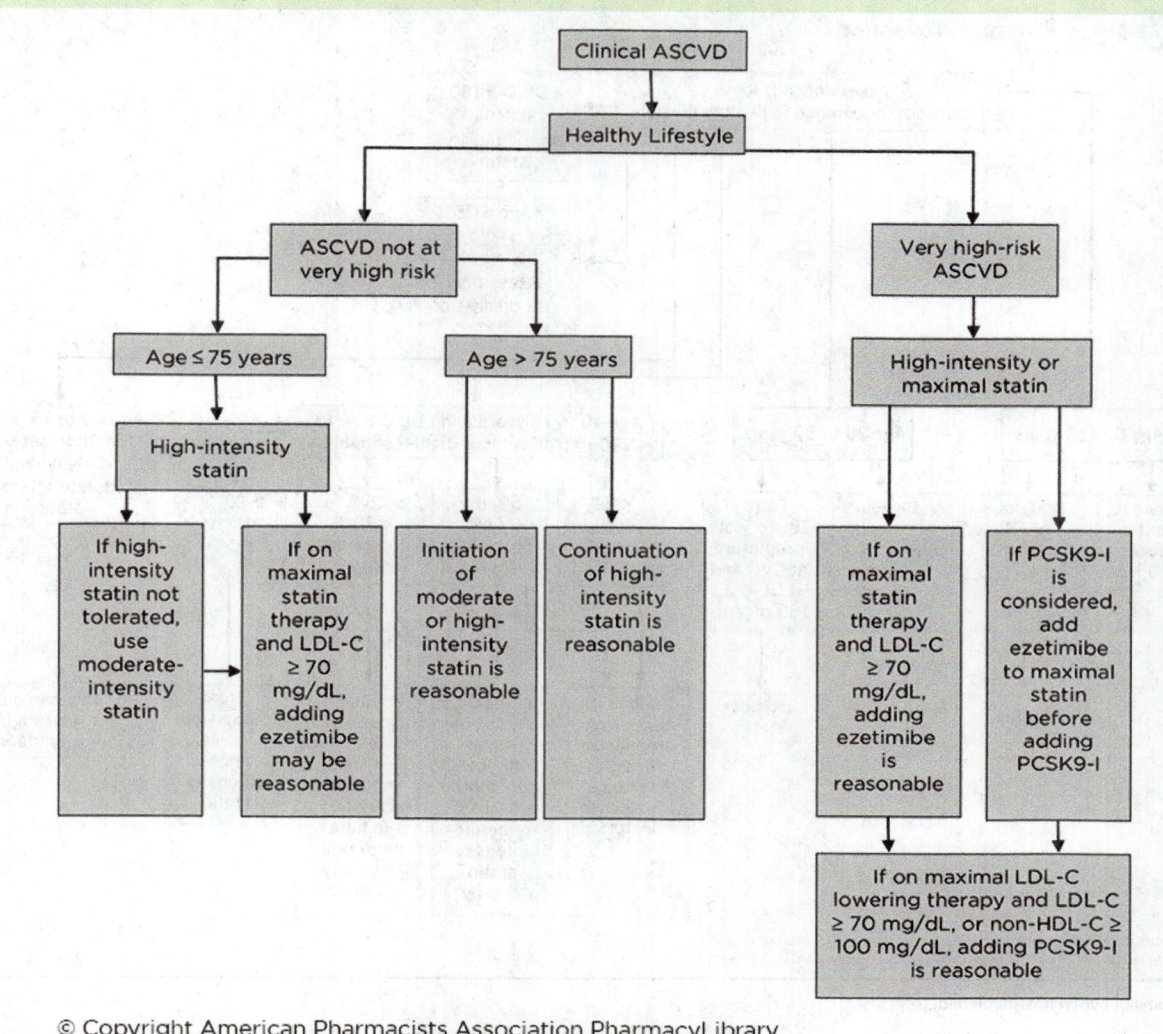

Patients are stratified by presence or absence of ASCVD, baseline LDL, diabetes, and age. Four major benefit groups are outlined, which are those patients with (1) clinical ASCVD, (2) LDL ≥ 190 mg/dL, (3) patients with diabetes, or (4) ASCVD risk ≥ 7.5% without diabetes. See Figures 16-2 and 16-3, adapted from the 2018 ACC/AHA Guidelines. See Table 16-3 for additional guidance when reviewing these figures.

Not all patients fit into one of the statin benefit groups. Risk-enhancing factors should also be considered when evaluating individual patient risk (Box 16-1).

16-4   Drug Therapy

Before initiation of therapy, a baseline fasting lipid panel (FLP) should be obtained and then reevaluated within 4 to 12 weeks to monitor therapeutic response and adherence. The NLA guidelines state goal levels should be achieved in approximately 6 months. There are a variety of medication classes available for

FIGURE 16-3. Primary Prevention

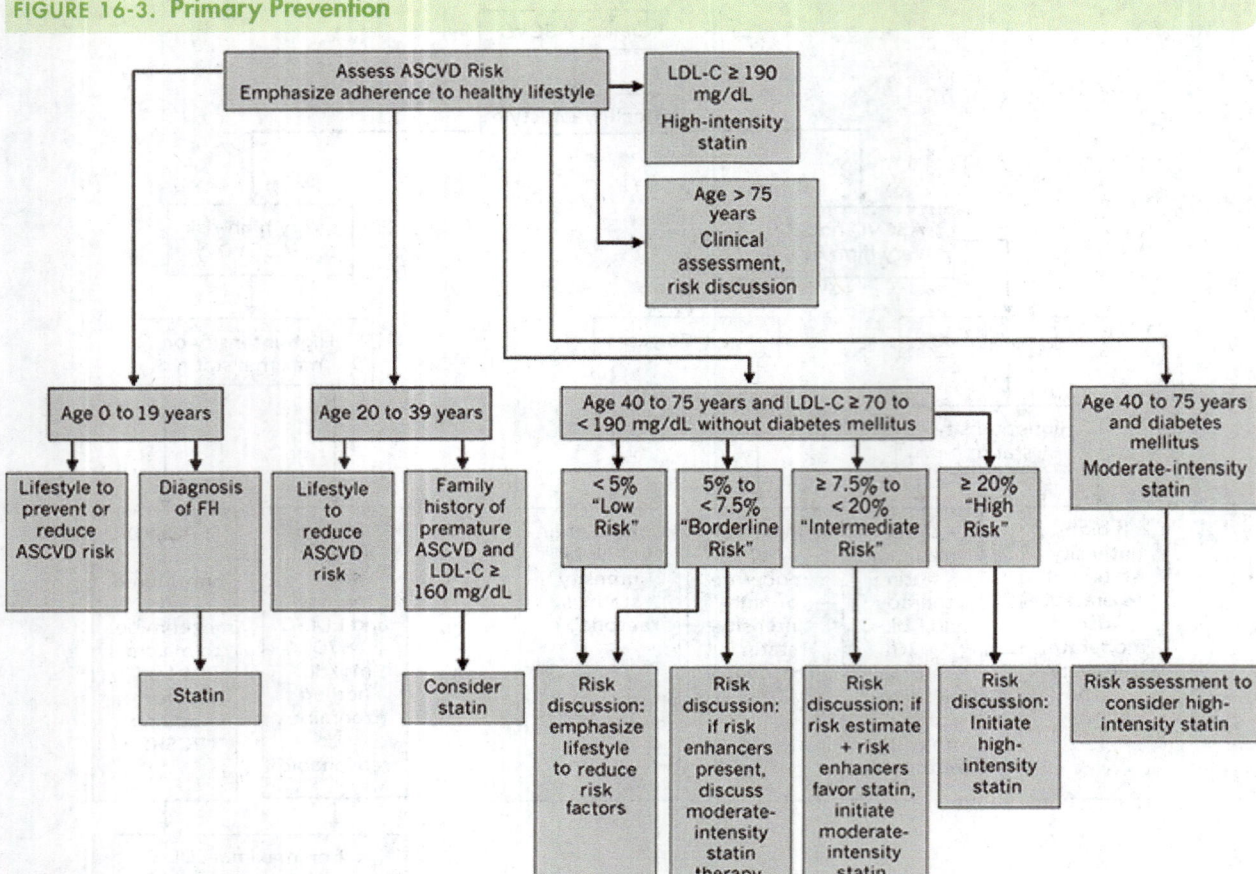

FH = familial hypercholesterolemia.

TABLE 16-3. Necessary Information for Understanding Figures 16-2 and 16-3.

Major ASCVD events	High-risk conditions	Diabetes-specific risk enhancers
Recent acute coronary syndrome	Age ≥ 65 years	Long duration of diabetes
History of myocardial infarction	Heterozygous familiar hypercholesterolemia	Albuminuria ≥ 30 mcg albumin/mg creatinine
History of ischemic stroke	History of prior coronary artery bypass surgery or PCI outside of the major ASCVD event(s)	eGFR < 60 mL/min/1.73 m²
Symptomatic peripheral arterial disease	Diabetes	Retinopathy
	Hypertension	Neuropathy
	Chronic kidney disease	ABI < 0.9
	Current smoking	
	Persistently elevated LDL-C	
	History of congestive heart failure	

Very high risk includes a history of multiple major ASCVD events or 1 major ASCVD event and multiple high-risk conditions.

BOX 16-1. Risk-Enhancing Factors for ASCVD

- LDL-C 160 to 189 mg/dL; non-HDL-C 190 to 219 mg/dL
- Family history of premature ASCVD onset (< 55 years of age in a first-degree male relative, < 65 years of age in a first-degree female relative)
- Metabolic syndrome—presence of 3 of the following factors:
  - Waist circumference ≥ 40.1 inches in males/ ≥ 34.6 inches in females
  - TG ≥ 175 mg/dL
  - HDL-cholesterol < 40 mg/dL in males < 50 mg/dL in females
  - Systolic blood pressure (BP) ≥ 130 mmHg and/or diastolic BP ≥ 85 mmHg
  - Fasting blood glucose ≥ 100 mg/dL
- Chronic kidney disease

- Chronic inflammatory conditions (e.g., psoriasis, rheumatoid arthritis, HIV/AIDS)
- History of premature menopause (before age 40) and history of pregnancy-associated conditions that increase later ASCVD risk
- High-risk ethnicities
- Lipid/biomarkers associated with increased ASCVD risk:
  - Hypertriglyceridemia ≥ 175 mg/dL
  - High-sensitivity C-reactive protein ≥ 2 mg/L
  - Lipoprotein (a) ≥ 50 mg/dL
  - Apo B ≥ 130 mg/dL
  - Ankle-brachial index < 0.9

dyslipidemia, including 3-hydroxy-3-methyl-glutaryl-coenzyme A (HMG-CoA) reductase inhibitors (statins), cholesterol-absorption inhibitors, PCSK9 inhibitors, fibric acid derivatives (fibrates), bile acid sequestrants (resins), niacin, and omega 3 fatty acids. Two drug classes primarily used in more of a specialty setting of homozygous familial hypercholesterolemia, microsomal triglyceride transfer protein (MTP) inhibitor and an antisense oligonucleotide (ASO) inhibitor directed at inhibiting the production of human apolipoprotein B-100 (Apo B) will be discussed briefly. Current guidelines prioritize the use of statins, and secondarily the use of cholesterol-absorption inhibitors and PCSK9 inhibitors. The other drug classes are still used depending on other abnormalities within the lipid profile. Figure 16-4 provides an image of the sites of action for commonly used medications in dyslipidemia. The effect of these medications on the lipid profile can be found in Table 16-4.

FIGURE 16-4. Dyslipidemia Medication Sites of Action

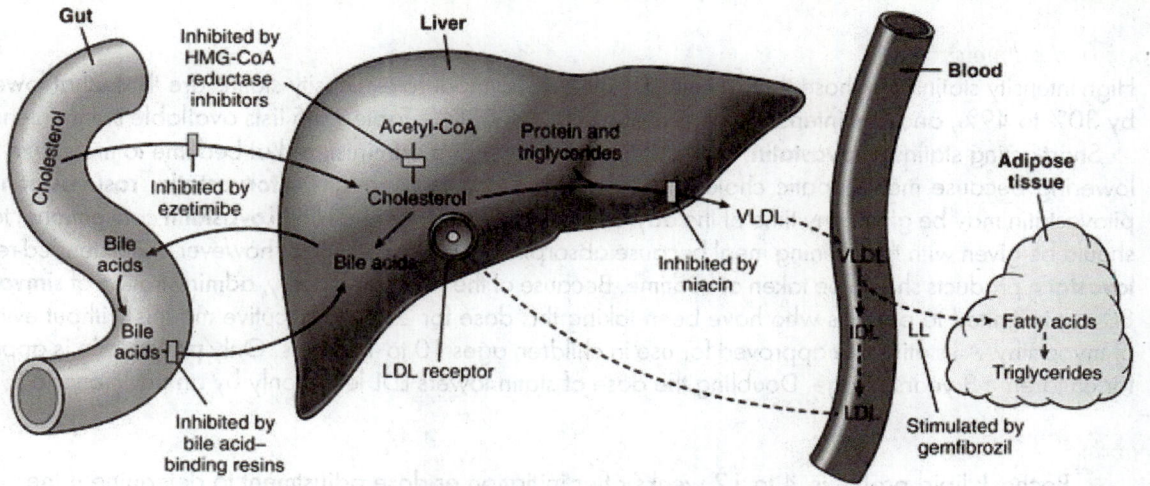

TABLE 16-4. Efficacy of Drugs Used to Treat Dyslipidemia

Drug class	Lipid and lipoprotein effect
Statins	LDL ↓18% to 55%
	HDL ↑5% to 15%
	TG ↓7% to 30%
Resins	LDL ↓15% to 30%
	HDL ↑3% to 5%
	TG (no change)
Nicotinic acid	LDL ↓5% to 25%
	HDL ↑15% to 35%
	TG ↓20% to 50%
Fibric acids	LDL ↓5% to 20%
	HDL ↑10% to 20%
	TG ↓20% to 50%
Cholesterol inhibitors	LDL ↓17%
	HDL ↓1.3%
	TG ↓6%
Omega-3 fatty acid	LDL ↑25% to 31%
	HDL ↑4% to 13%
	TG ↓45%
PCSK9 inhibitors	LDL ↓43% to 71%

↑, increase; ↓, decrease.

HMG-CoA Reductase Inhibitors (Statins)

These agents competitively inhibit HMG-CoA reductase, which is the enzyme responsible for conversion of HMG-CoA to mevalonate. Mevalonate is an early precursor to and a rate-limiting step in cholesterol synthesis. This reduction in liver cholesterol synthesis results in upregulation of liver LDL receptors and increased clearance of LDL and VLDL particles in the blood.

Dosage and administration

High-intensity statins are those that reduce LDL by ≥ 50%; moderate-intensity statins are those that lower LDL by 30% to 49%, and low-intensity statins reduce LDL by < 30%. Table 16-5 lists available statin intensities.

Short-acting statins (**pravastatin**, **simvastatin**, fluvastatin) are administered at bedtime to maximize LDL-C lowering because most hepatic cholesterol production occurs overnight. **Atorvastatin**, **rosuvastatin**, and pitavastatin may be given any time of the day because of their longer half-life. **Lovastatin** conventional tablets should be given with the evening meal because absorption is better with food; however, the extended-release **lovastatin** products should be taken at bedtime. Because of the risk of myopathy, administration of **simvastatin** 80 mg is limited to patients who have been taking this dose for ≥ 12 consecutive months without evidence of myopathy. All statins are approved for use in children ages 10 to 18 years. Only **pravastatin** is approved for children ≥ 8 years of age. Doubling the dose of statin lowers LDL levels only by an additional 6%.

Monitoring

- Recheck lipid profile in 4 to 12 weeks after initiation or dose adjustment to determine if the desired LDL-C level has been achieved, repeat every 3 to 12 months thereafter

TABLE 16-5. Statin Intensity

Major statin benefit group		
High-intensity statin (lowers LDL ≥ 50)	**Moderate-intensity statin** (lowers LDL ~ 30% to 49%)	**Low-intensity statin** (lowers LDL < 30%)
Atorvastatin 40 to 80 mg	**Atorvastatin** 10 to 20 mg	Fluvastatin 20 to 40 mg
Rosuvastatin 20 to 40 mg	Fluvastatin 40 mg twice a day	**Lovastatin** 20 mg
	Fluvastatin XL 80 mg	
	Lovastatin 40 mg	**Pravastatin** 10 to 20 mg
	Pitavastatin 1 to 4 mg	**Simvastatin** 10 mg
	Pravastatin 40 to 80 mg	
	Rosuvastatin 5 to 10 mg	
	Simvastatin 20 to 40 mg	

Boldface indicates one of top 100 drugs for 2020 by prescription volume.

- Conduct baseline liver function tests (LFTs), A1C, thyroid function tests (thyroid-stimulating hormone [TSH]), serum creatinine (SCr), and creatinine phosphokinase (CPK) in patients with a personal or family history of muscle side effects from statins.
- LFTs should be repeated only when clinically indicated.
- CPK needs to be monitored only if the patient has suspected muscle damage.
- Patients with LDL cholesterol < 40 mg/dL on 2 separate readings should have their statin dose decreased.

Adverse effects

- Myopathy (muscle damage) may occur.
- Myalgia (muscle pain, soreness, or tenderness) may occur.
- Myositis occurs in 0.2% of patients. Myositis is myalgia combined with CPK elevated 3 to 10 times the upper limit of normal (ULN).
- Rhabdomyolysis occurs rarely, but it can cause acute kidney injury. The statin or other offending drug should be discontinued immediately. Rhabdomyolysis is the combination of severe muscle symptoms and CPK elevated 10 times the ULN with increased serum creatinine and urine myoglobin.
- Elevated liver enzymes occur in 0.1% to 2.3% of patients.
- Statins may be associated with a slightly increased rate of type 2 diabetes; however, this has been seen in patients with diabetes risk factors or metabolic syndrome.
- Flu-like symptoms, headache, or mild gastrointestinal (GI) complaints may occur.
- Active liver disease is a contraindication to statin therapy; caution should be used in patients with chronic liver disease or unexplained elevations in transaminases (> 3× ULN). Statins may be beneficial in fatty liver disease.
- Statins are contraindicated in pregnant or breastfeeding women.

Drug–drug interactions

Because of their metabolism via CYP450 enzymes, prescribers should be aware of dosing considerations with statins (Table 16-6). **Atorvastatin, lovastatin**, and **simvastatin** undergo CYP3A4 metabolism, and fluvastatin, **rosuvastatin**, and pitavastatin undergo CYP2C9 metabolism. **Pravastatin** is unique in that it is not metabolized via CYP450.

SIDE EFFECTS OF STATINS (HMG-COA REDUCTASE INHIBITORS): "HMG-COA RI"

 H **H**epatotoxicity

 M **M**yopathy (myalgia, myositis)

 G **G**astrointestinal upset (nausea, vomiting, diarrhea)

 C **C**ataracts

 R **R**habdomyolysis

 I **I**ncrease risk of diabetes

Reference: Hoxha S. Statins Mnemonics. http://pharmwarthegame. blogspot.com/2019/04/statins-mnemonics.html. Published April 30, 2019. Accessed February 26, 2020.

TABLE 16-6. Statin Dosing Considerations

Statin	Drug–drug interactions	Dosing considerations
Atorvastatin	Amiodarone, boceprevir, clarithromycin	Maximum dose is 20 mg if administered with clarithromycin, itraconazole, and some ritonavir-boosted regimens.
Fluvastatin	Cyclosporine, danazol, delavirdine	Dose adjust if CrCl < 30 mL/min. Drug is not recommended in patients with hepatic impairment.
Lovastatin	Erythromycin, **fluoxetine**, fluvoxamine, verapamil	Maximum dose is 20 mg if administered with danazol or **diltiazem**. Maximum dose is 40 mg if administered with amiodarone.
Pitavastatin	Indinavir, itraconazole	Dose adjust if CrCl < 60 mL/min. Maximum dose is 1 mg if administered with erythromycin.
Simvastatin	Strong CYP450 3A4 inhibitors (ketoconazole, nefazodone, nelfinavir) contraindicated	Maximum dose is 20 mg if administered with amiodarone, **amlodipine,** or ranolazine. Maximum dose is 10 mg if administered with verapamil, **diltiazem**, or dronedarone. Dose adjust if CrCl < 30 mL/min. Avoid grapefruit juice.
Rosuvastatin	Nicardipine, pimozide, posaconazole, quinidine, ritonavir, saquinavir, sildenafil, tacrolimus, telaprevir, testosterone, verapamil, zafirlukast	Initiate at 5 mg daily in Asian patients. Dose adjust if CrCl < 30 mL/min.
Pravastatin	Metabolized by CYP450 2D6	Maximum dose is 40 mg if administered with clarithromycin and 20 mg if administered with cyclosporine.

Boldface indicates one of top 100 drugs for 2020 by prescription volume.
CrCl, creatinine clearance.

Cholesterol Inhibitor (Ezetimibe)

Cholesterol inhibitors selectively inhibit intestinal absorption of dietary and biliary cholesterol at the brush border of the small intestine, decreasing cholesterol absorption and decreasing cholesterol in the blood.

Dosing and administration

Cholesterol inhibitors are dosed once daily without regard to food. They can be taken simultaneously in combination with statins.

Monitoring

When combined with a statin, ezetimibe provides an additional 15% reduction in LDL. Monitor lipid panel periodically to evaluate efficacy. Liver function testing should occur when combined with statin, at baseline and as needed.

Adverse effects

- Diarrhea may occur.
- Use with caution in moderate to severe hepatic disease.

Drug–drug interactions

Combination with a resin may decrease absorption. Combination with a fibric acid may predispose to gallbladder disease. Cyclosporine may increase ezetimibe concentrations.

PCSK9 Inhibitors

PCSK9 inhibitors are the latest drug class to be approved for dyslipidemia. Currently, there are 2 drugs approved by the U.S. Food and Drug Administration (FDA): evolocumab and alirocumab. Both medications are indicated for use in patients with heterozygous familial hypercholesterolemia or in patients with clinical ASCVD receiving maximally tolerated statin therapy and still requiring further LDL lowering. Evolocumab has another indication in patients with homozygous familial hypercholesterolemia (HoFH). PCSK9 inhibitors are monoclonal antibodies that bind to PCSK9 and increase the number of LDL receptors available to clear circulating LDL.

Dosing and administration

Evolocumab is dosed at 140 mg subcutaneous every 2 weeks or 420 mg subcutaneous once monthly, except in patients with HoFH who receive only the monthly dose regimen. Alirocumab is initiated at 75 mg subcutaneous every 2 weeks and can be increased to 150 mg or 300 mg monthly.

Monitoring

These medications can reduce LDL by ~ 60%. LDL levels should be measured within 4 to 8 weeks after starting therapy or changing the dose.

Adverse effects

- Nasopharyngitis
- Upper respiratory infection (URI)
- Injection site reactions
- Influenza

Drug-drug interactions

There are no known drug interactions with this medication class.

Fibric Acids (Fibrates)

Fibrates lower TG by reduction of apolipoproteins B, C-III, and E. They increase HDL cholesterol by increasing apolipoproteins A-I and A-II.

Monitoring

Evaluate baseline renal and liver function because fibrates are contraindicated in severe renal or severe hepatic disease.

Patient counseling

Gemfibrozil should be taken twice daily 30 minutes before meals. **Fenofibrate** and fenofibric acid can be taken with or without food once daily.

Reduce the dose in patients with renal insufficiency, and monitor for muscle toxicity, especially when used in combination with statins or niacin.

Adverse effects

- Dyspepsia may occur.
- Gallstones have been reported.
- Risk for myopathy increases when combined with statins.

Drug–drug interactions

- These agents are highly protein bound, and they are metabolized by the cytochrome P450 (CYP450) 3A4 enzyme system.
- The effect of **warfarin** may be increased.
- Cyclosporine may increase gemfibrozil concentrations.
- Compared with other fibric acid derivatives, **fenofibrate** may have less interaction potential with **warfarin** and cyclosporine.
- Bile acid sequestrants (resins) decrease fibrate absorption.
- Combinations with statins and niacin may increase the risk of myopathy. Gemfibrozil is contraindicated to use in combination with **simvastatin**.

Bile Acid Sequestrants (Resins)

Nonabsorbable anion exchange resins exchange chloride ions for bile acids and other anions in the intestine. This action inhibits enterohepatic recycling, which results in bile excretion and a decrease in the cholesterol pool in the liver. LDL receptors are upregulated, increased LDL is cleared, and LDL is lowered. Resins may exacerbate hypertriglyceridemia and should be used with caution in patients with triglycerides above 300 mg/dL. Within the 2018 ACC/AHA guidelines this drug class has been recommended as an alternative to ezetimibe if a higher-risk, primary-prevention patient does not want to take a statin or cannot tolerate the recommended intensity of a statin.

Dosing and administration

Cholestyramine and colestipol should be titrated slowly to avoid GI side effects. They may be started with 1 dose daily with the largest meal and increased (to 2 doses daily with the largest meals or divided between breakfast and dinner). Powdered doses can be mixed with food such as soup, oatmeal, nonfat yogurt, or applesauce. The mixture can also be chilled overnight to improve palatability. To prevent constipation, a patient may mix psyllium with resins; however, this mixture should be ingested immediately after mixing to prevent gel formation. Counsel the patient to rinse the glass and drink the remains to ensure ingestion of all resin. Colesevelam (Welchol) is a tablet formulation, which may be easier for some patients to self-administer. However, the tablets are large, and some patients have difficulty swallowing them. Separate other medications 1 hour before and 4 hours after administration to prevent binding of medications.

Adverse effects

- Abdominal discomfort, constipation, flatulence, nausea, and vomiting may occur.
- Patients may experience palatability problems with the resin slurry.
- Constipation may occur that increases with the dose and in the elderly.
- Decreased absorption of other drugs may occur. Dose other drugs 1 hour before or 4 hours after ingestion of resin.
- Absolute contraindications include history of bowel obstruction, hypertriglyceridemia-induced pancreatitis, or TG > 500 mg/dL.

Drug–drug interactions

Avoid concurrent administration with all other drugs, especially digoxin, **levothyroxine**, tetracycline, **warfarin**, fat-soluble vitamins, and minerals.

Niacin

Niacin, also known as nicotinic acid or vitamin B$_3$, reduces LDL cholesterol and TG and increases HDL cholesterol. It may decrease VLDL synthesis, thereby leading to decreased LDL cholesterol and TG. It may inhibit metabolism of apolipoprotein A-I, which increases HDL cholesterol.

Monitoring

- Evaluate baseline fasting glucose, LFTs, and serum uric acid levels.
- For immediate-release niacin, repeat these tests 4 to 6 weeks after each dose titration.
- For sustained-release niacin, evaluate monthly LFTs while dosage is titrated; then every 12 weeks for the first year; and then periodically.

Patient counseling

- Immediate-release niacin should be started at a low dose and slowly titrated upward:
  - Start with 100 mg three times daily and titrate upward the second week to 200 mg three times daily. The next week, increase to 350 mg three times daily; and the following week, increase to 500 mg three times daily. When 1500 mg/day is reached and maintained for 4 weeks, assess efficacy before further increasing the dose.
  - The usual dose is 1000 to 2000 mg three times daily. The dose should not exceed 6 g/day.
- Extended-release niacin should be started with 500 mg at bedtime and titrated weekly to a maximum dose of 2000 mg/day.
  - Take with food to minimize GI upset.
  - Avoid alcohol, hot drinks, or spicy foods at time of ingestion to minimize flushing and pruritus.

Adverse effects

- Flushing is common. Pretreat with aspirin (325 mg) or **ibuprofen** 200 mg 30 minutes before the first niacin dose of the day.

- Use cautiously in patients with diabetes as niacin may cause hyperglycemia.
- Hyperuricemia or gout may occur.
- Upper GI distress has been reported.
- Hepatotoxicity may occur.
- Absolute contraindication: active liver disease, active peptic ulcer, arterial bleeding
- Relative contraindications: diabetes, hyperuricemia, or severe gout

Use caution in combination with resins. Combination therapy with statins and gemfibrozil may cause an increased risk of myopathy.

Omega-3 Fatty Acids

The mechanism of action for omega-3 fatty acids is not completely understood; however, these medications may reduce hepatic VLDL-triglyceride synthesis and increase triglyceride clearance from circulating VLDL particles. There are 2 prescription-only fish oils on the market, icosapent ethyl (Vascepa) and omega 3-acid ethyl esters (Lovaza).

Dosing and administration

The daily dose (4 g) can be taken in a single or divided dose (2 g twice daily). These agents should be taken with meals.

Monitoring

- Patients with history of fish allergy or sensitivity should not take omega-3 fatty acids.
- Assess effectiveness at 2 months. Discontinue use if the decrease in TG level is not adequate.
- Periodic monitoring of AST and ALT levels is recommended in patients with hepatic impairment.
- Periodic monitoring is recommended for increase in LDL cholesterol levels.

Adverse effects

- Burping (may complain of "fishy" burps)
- Indigestion
- Taste sense alteration
- Possible prolonged bleeding time when used with anticoagulants

Other Agents

Mipomersen

Mipomersen is an antisense oligonucleotide (ASO) inhibitor of apo B synthesis via binding to mRNA (messenger ribonucleic acid). Apo B is the principal lipoprotein associated with VLDL and LDL; therefore, inhibition of production results in lower VLDL and LDL levels.

> ⚠️ **Mipomersen** *FDA BOXED WARNING*
>
> Mipomersen sodium can cause elevations in transaminases and also increases hepatic fat (with or without concomitant increases in transaminases).

Dosage and administration

For adults with HoFH, mipomersen is to be used as an adjunct to lipid-lowering medications: 200 mg subcutaneous once weekly on the same day every week.

Monitoring

- Mipomersen is contraindicated in moderate or severe hepatic impairment.
- Monitor lipid levels every 3 months during the first year of therapy.
- Check LDL cholesterol after 6 months to weigh benefit of LDL reduction versus risk of hepatotoxicity.
- Monitor baseline ALT and aspartate aminotransferase (AST), alkaline phosphatase, and total bilirubin, and then monitor ALT and AST monthly during first year of therapy, then every 3 months or more often if clinically indicated.

Adverse effects

- ALT and AST may be elevated
- Injection site reactions can include pain, erythema, hematoma, edema, and pruritus.
- Fatigue, flu-like illness, shivering, or fever may occur
- Antibodies may develop to injection.

Lomitapide

Lomitapide is a microsomal triglyceride transfer protein inhibitor, which prevents the assembly of apo B–containing lipoproteins in hepatocytes and enterocytes. This in turn inhibits the synthesis of chylomicrons and VLDL, leading to reduced levels of LDL. This medication has an orphan drug designation and is intended for use in patients with HoFH.

Table 16-7 lists the medications described above along with dosing and availability.

> ⚠️ **Lomitapide** *FDA BOXED WARNING*
>
> Lomitapide can cause elevations in transaminases.

TABLE 16-7. Drug Products and Dosage

Generic name	Trade name	Dosage range and schedule	Dosage form and strength
Statins			
Atorvastatin	Lipitor	10 to 80 mg/day	10, 20, 40, 80 mg tablets
Fluvastatin	Lescol	20 to 80 mg nightly	20, 40 mg capsules; 80 mg XL tablet
Lovastatin	Mevacor	20 to 80 mg nightly	10, 20, 40 mg tablets
Lovastatin extended-release	Altoprev	10 to 60 mg nightly	10, 20, 40, 60 mg tablets
Pitavastatin	Livalo	1 to 4 mg/day	1, 2, 4 mg tablets
Pravastatin	Pravachol	10 to 80 mg nightly	10, 20, 40, 80 mg tablets
Rosuvastatin	Crestor	5 to 40 mg/day	5, 10, 20, 40 mg tablets
Simvastatin	Zocor	20 to 80 mg nightly	5, 10, 20, 40, 80 mg tablets

(continued)

TABLE 16-7. Drug Products and Dosage *(Continued)*

Generic name	Trade name	Dosage range and schedule	Dosage form and strength
Bile acid sequestrants			
Cholestyramine	Questran/Questran Light	8 to 16 g/day divided	Powder
Colestipol	Colestid	5 to 30 g/day divided (powder); 2 to 16 g/day (tablet)	Powder or tablet
Colesevelam	Welchol	1.875 g twice daily to 3.75 g/day	625 mg tablet
Nicotinic acid			
Immediate release	Niacor	1.5 to 3 g/day (divided three times a day)	500 mg tablet
Sustained release	Slo-Niacin	1 to 2 g nightly	250, 500, 750 mg tablets
Extended release	Niaspan	1 to 2 g nightly	500, 750, 1000 mg tablets
Fibric acids			
Fenofibrate	Tricor	48 to 145 mg/day	48, 145 mg tablets
Fenofibric acid	Fibricor	35 to 105 mg/day	35, 105 mg tablets
	Trilipix	45 to 135 mg/day	45, 135 mg capsules
Gemfibrozil	Lopid	600 mg before meals twice daily	600 mg tablet
Cholesterol inhibitors			
Ezetimibe	Zetia	10 mg/day	10 mg tablet
Omega-3 fatty acids			
Icosapent ethyl	Vascepa	2 g twice daily with food	1 g capsule
Omega-3 ethyl esters	Lovaza	4 g daily or 2 g twice daily	1 g capsule
Combinations			
Ezetimibe + **simvastatin**	Vytorin	10/10 to 10/80 mg nightly	10/10, 10/20, 10/40, 10/80 mg tablets
Ezetimibe + **atorvastatin**	Liptruzet	10/10 to 10/80 mg/day	10/10, 10/20, 10/40, 10/80 mg tablets
PCSK9 Inhibitors			
Alirocumab	Praluent	75 to 150 mg subcutaneous every 2 weeks	150 mg/mL prefilled syringe
Evolocumab	Repatha	140 mg subcutaneous every 2 weeks or 420 mg subcutaneous once monthly	140 mg/mL prefilled syringe, 420 mg/3.5 mL single-use system
Other			
Lomitapide	Juxtapid	5 to 60 mg with evening meal	5, 10, 20, 30, 40, 60 mg capsules
Mipomersen	Kynamro	200 mg subcutaneous once weekly	200 mg/mL prefilled syringe

Boldface indicates one of top 100 drugs for 2020 by prescription volume.

16-5 ## Pharmacist's Role

Pharmacists can have an impact on dyslipidemia management in all settings. Within the acute care setting, patients can be identified easily if admitted due to clinical ASCVD warranting high-intensity statins. Pharmacists that practice in the community pharmacy setting can identify patients with diabetes by reviewing their diabetic medications and determining whether these patients meet the conditions for moderate-intensity statin. Lastly, those pharmacists working in ambulatory care settings can identify any patient meeting the criterion for dyslipidemia management and then monitor progress and adherence.

NAPLEX Competency Statements

The questions in this chapter cover the following 2021 NAPLEX Competency Statements: **AREA 1:** 1.1; 1.2; 1.3; 1.4; 1.5; 1.6; 1.7 **AREA 2:** 2.1; 2.2; 2.4 **AREA 3:** 3.2; 3.4; 3.6; 3.7; 3.9; 3.11; 3.12 **AREA 4:** 4.1 **AREA 6:** 6.1; 6.3.

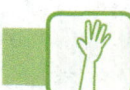 **16-6** ## Questions

Use the patient profile below to answer the following 4 questions.

1. A FLP today reveals the following: total cholesterol = 250 mg/dL, HDL = 40 mg/dL, and TG = 145 mg/dL. What is the patient's LDL cholesterol?

   A. 130 mg/dL
   B. 153 mg/dL
   C. 162 mg/dL
   D. 178 mg/dL
   E. 181 mg/dL

2. The patient above comes to your pharmacy for cholesterol and medication monitoring. He has a new prescription today for atorvastatin 10 mg/day. What medication changes, if any, are recommended for this patient?

   A. No changes should be made.
   B. Change atorvastatin to 40 mg daily.
   C. Add niacin to atorvastatin 10 daily.
   D. Discontinue hydrochlorothiazide.

PATIENT PROFILE

Patient Name: Michael Hart

Age: 50

Sex: Male   **Ethnicity:** White

PMH: hypertension, type 2 diabetes, dyslipidemia

SHx: Never smoker, no EtOH

FHx: Noncontributory

Current medications: Tylenol PRN headaches

                            Hydrochlorothiazide 25 mg/day

Vital signs: BP 144/90 mmHg

                            Pulse 70 bpm

Labs: HbA1C 7.3%

                            TC 250 mg/dL, HDL = 40 mg/dL, LDL 181 mg/dL, TG = 145 mg/dL

Height: 5'9"

Weight: 185 lb

Allergies: NKDA

3. After initiating a statin in this patient, how often should you assess the effectiveness of therapy?

   A. 3 weeks
   B. 4 to 12 weeks
   C. 6 months
   D. Only if adverse events are noted
   E. Annually

4. Which of the following baseline labs would be optimal to assess before initiating statin therapy? (Mark all that apply.)

   A. CBC
   B. Serum creatinine
   C. LFTs
   D. TSH
   E. CPK

5. His LDL decreased from 181 mg/dL to 115 mg/dL after 12 weeks of atorvastatin 10 mg once daily. What is your assessment?

   A. Stop the statin because the patient has achieved optimal LDL levels.
   B. The expected LDL reduction for this patient has been achieved.
   C. The optimal LDL reduction for this patient has not been achieved.
   D. Add fenofibrate.
   E. Add cholestyramine.

6. Which of the following statins must be given at bedtime? (Mark all that apply.)

   A. Atorvastatin
   B. Simvastatin
   C. Pitavastatin
   D. Lovastatin
   E. Rosuvastatin

7. Which of the following can cause dyslipidemia? (Mark all that apply.)

   A. ACE inhibitors
   B. Hypothyroidism
   C. Diabetes
   D. Renal disease
   E. Beta blockers

8. Cholesterol biosynthesis can be decreased by which of the following?

   A. Statins
   B. Oat bran
   C. Bile acid sequestrants (resins)
   D. Zetia
   E. Aspirin

9. Which of the following medications has the greatest efficacy in raising HDL levels?

   A. Lovastatin
   B. Pravastatin
   C. Gemfibrozil
   D. Nicotinic acid
   E. Colesevelam

10. Which of the following has the most potent LDL-lowering effect?

    A. Nicotinic acid
    B. Fibric acids
    C. Omega-3 fatty acids
    D. Cholesterol inhibitors
    E. Statins

11. Which of the following is absolutely contraindicated as an adjunct medication to maximally tolerated statin in a patient with a triglyceride level of 860 mg/dL?

    A. Welchol
    B. Niaspan
    C. Zetia
    D. Vascepa
    E. Repatha

12. Which of the following most accurately describes a medication and its corresponding effect?

    A. Diabetes is an absolute contraindication to the use of nicotinic acid.
    B. Aspirin is dosed three times per day to prevent flushing from niacin.
    C. Gemfibrozil may reduce triglycerides by as much as 50%.
    D. Colesevelam has similar patient tolerability problems as cholestyramine.
    E. Ezetimibe frequently causes muscle toxicity.

13. A 45-year-old patient has a past medical history of diabetes, hypertension, depression, and tobacco abuse. He had a history of TIA 3 years ago, and his LDL cholesterol is 140 mg/dL. The decision is made to initiate statin therapy. Which of the following doses of statin would be most appropriate?

   A. Lipitor 10 mg
   B. Crestor 40 mg
   C. Zocor 40 mg
   D. Pravachol 80 mg
   E. Lescol XL 80 mg

14. Which of the following agents would be most likely to produce myopathy when combined with a statin?

   A. Fenofibric acid
   B. Aspirin
   C. Lisinopril
   D. Levothyroxine
   E. Colesevelam

15. Which of the following patient conditions would affect the decision to initiate therapy with nicotinic acid?

   A. Concomitant therapy with a diuretic
   B. Triglycerides > 300 mg/dL
   C. Active liver disease
   D. Baseline elevation of serum creatinine
   E. Uncontrolled hypertension

16. Rank the following statins from highest to lowest intensity.

Unordered options	Ordered response
Pravastatin 40 mg	
Simvastatin 10 mg	
Rosuvastatin 20 mg	

17. Using the image below, identify the site of action for bile acid sequestrants (resins) _____.

18. Identify the drug interaction that involves the CYP450 system.

   A. Ezetimibe + niacin
   B. Colestipol + simvastatin
   C. Gemfibrozil + cholestyramine
   D. Fenofibrate + ezetimibe
   E. Lovastatin + itraconazole

19. Which of the following agents produces an additional 15% LDL reduction when combined with a statin?

   A. Colesevelam
   B. Nicotinic acid
   C. 15 grams of soluble fiber
   D. Fenofibrate
   E. Ezetimibe

20. A 57-year-old patient new to your clinic is currently taking the following medications: amlodipine 10 mg, losartan 50 mg with hydrochlorothiazide 12.5 mg, and Lantus 10 units at bedtime. His past medical history includes hypertension and diabetes. His ASCVD score today is 6%. The physician would like to initiate simvastatin therapy. Which dose would be most appropriate?

   A. 5
   B. 10
   C. 20
   D. 40
   E. 80

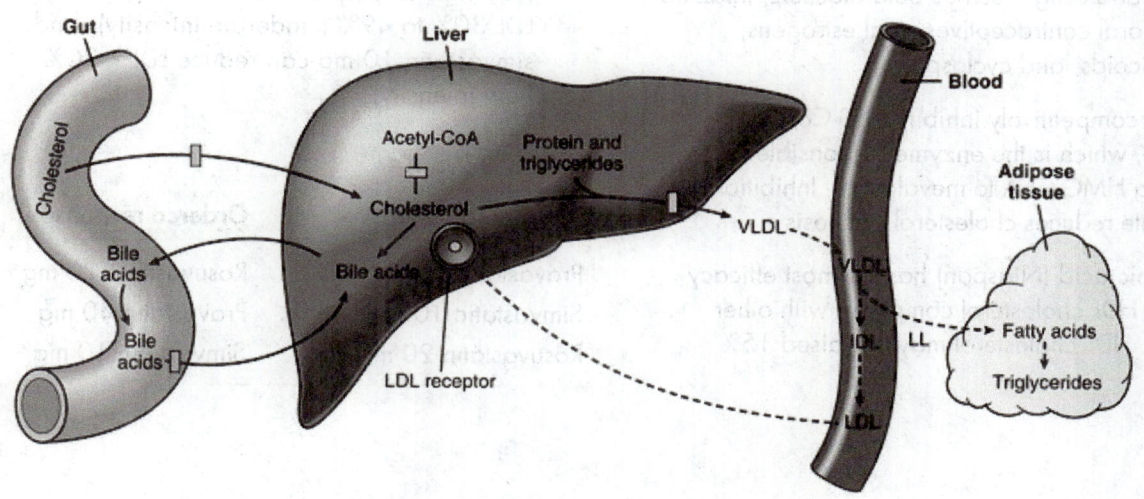

16-7   Answers

1. E. Use the Friedewald equation to calculate LDL:

$$LDL = total\ cholesterol - (HDL + TG/5)$$

$$LDL = 250 - (40 + 145/5) = 181$$

2. B. The 2013 ACC/AHA guidelines recommend a moderate-dose statin in a diabetic patient between the ages of 40 and 75 years unless the ASCVD risk > 7.5%. Because his ASCVD score is 15.8% he should be on a high-intensity statin.

3. B. A repeat FLP should be drawn to assess adherence to statin therapy within 4 to 12 weeks after initiation.

4. B, C, D, E. In addition to baseline SCr (for renally adjusted statins), CPK, and LFTs, measuring TSH is optimal because hypothyroidism is a factor in statin-induced myalgias.

5. B. The dose of statin has achieved a 36% reduction in LDL cholesterol. The expected reduction for atorvastatin 10 mg daily would approximate 30% to 49%. Had that LDL-level reduction not been achieved, a recommendation would have been to investigate possible nonadherence to therapy with the patient. In this case, however, consider adding ezetimibe as the goal LDL would be < 70 mg/dL or increasing the statin dose.

6. B, D. Simvastatin and Lovastatin must be given at bedtime due to their short half-life.

7. B, C, D, E. Causes of dyslipidemia must be ruled out. The common secondary causes are renal failure; hypothyroidism; obstructive liver disease; diabetes; and drugs such as beta blockers, thiazide diuretics, oral contraceptives, oral estrogens, glucocorticoids, and cyclosporine.

8. A. Statins competitively inhibit HMG-CoA reductase, which is the enzyme responsible for converting HMG-CoA to mevalonate. Inhibition of mevalonate reduces cholesterol synthesis.

9. D. Nicotinic acid (Niaspan) has the most efficacy in raising HDL cholesterol compared with other therapies. HDL cholesterol may be raised 15% to 35%.

10. E. From the options listed, statins are the most effective in lowering LDL cholesterol. LDL cholesterol may be lowered 18% to 55%.

11. A. Bile acid sequestrants (cholestyramine, colestipol, and colesevelam) are absolutely contraindicated in patients with triglyceride levels over 500 mg/dL.

12. C. Gemfibrozil can reduce TG by 20% to 50%. Diabetes is a relative contraindication to the use of nicotinic acid. Aspirin is dosed once daily, before the first nicotinic acid dose of the day. Colesevelam is a tablet and avoids most of the palatability problems of other resins. Ezetimibe does not cause muscle toxicity.

13. B. The patient has a history of TIA; therefore, he has existing ASCVD. He is under 75 years of age, so a high-intensity statin is preferred.

14. A. Use of fibrates in combination with statins increases the risk for myopathy. Though hypothyroidism can also contribute to myalgias, treatment with levothyroxine would not have any effect.

15. C. Active liver disease would be a contraindication to initiating therapy with nicotinic acid. Because nicotinic acid is hepatically metabolized, baseline elevations of creatinine and other renally toxic medications would not affect a decision to initiate therapy. Because of niacin's effect on blood glucose, uncontrolled diabetes may warrant consideration of use of another medication.

16. Rosuvastatin 20 mg can reduce LDL ≥ 50% (high intensity), pravastatin 40 mg can reduce LDL 30% to 49% (moderate intensity), and simvastatin 10 mg can reduce LDL < 30% (low intensity).

Unordered options	Ordered response
Pravastatin 40 mg	Rosuvastatin 20 mg
Simvastatin 10 mg	Pravastatin 40 mg
Rosuvastatin 20 mg	Simvastatin 10 mg

17. Because bile acid sequestrants (resins) work in the gut, the correct location to highlight would be the squared area below.

18. E. Lovastatin is metabolized by CYP450 3A4 enzymes, and itraconazole inhibits this enzyme system. Inhibition causes lovastatin blood and tissue concentrations to rise, thus predisposing the patient to muscle or liver toxicity.

19. E. Ezetimibe, when used in combination with a statin, produces an additional 15% reduction in LDL cholesterol.

20. C. Based on this patient's age, diabetes condition, and ASCVD score, he qualifies for moderate-intensity statin therapy, a dose of 20 to 40 mg. Because he is currently taking amlodipine, however, the maximum dose of simvastatin would be 20 mg.

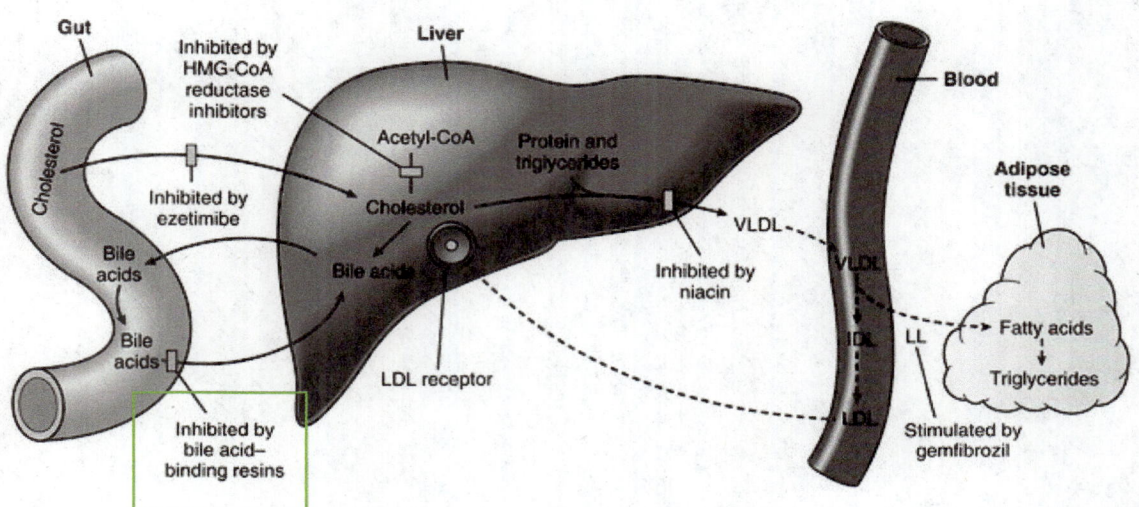

 **16-8   Additional Resources**

Grundy SM, Stone NJ, Bailey AL, et al. 2018 AHA/ACC/AACVPR/AAPA/ABC/ACPM/ADA/AGS/APhA/ASPC/NLA/PCNA Guideline on the Management of Blood Cholesterol: A Report of the American College of Cardiology/American Heart Association Task Force on Clinical Practice Guidelines. *J Am Coll Cardiol.* 2019 Jun 25;73(24):e285–e350.

Jacobson TA, Ito MK, Maki KC, et al. National Lipid Association recommendations for patient-centered management of dyslipidemia: part 1—full report. *J Clin Lipidol.* 2015;9(2):129–169.

Jacobson TA, Maki KC, Orringer C, et al. National Lipid Association recommendations for patient-centered management of dyslipidemia: part 2. *J Clin Lipidol.* 2015;9(6 suppl):S1–S122.e1.

Lloyd-Jones DM, Morris PB, Ballantyne CM, et al. 2016 ACC Expert Consensus Decision Pathway on the role of non-statin therapies for LDL-cholesterol lowering in the management of atherosclerotic cardiovascular disease risk: a report of the American College of Cardiology Task Force on Clinical Expert Consensus Documents. *J Am Coll Cardiol.* 2016;68(1):92–125.

Diabetes

17

MICHELLE Z. FARLAND

17-1 KEY POINTS

- The principal treatment goals for diabetes include maintaining blood glucose levels in the normal or near-normal range and preventing acute and chronic complications.
- Glycemic goals (A1C) should be individualized to each patient, considering factors such as past glucose control, length of time with diabetes, concomitant diseases, and psychosocial issues, as well as available support for the patient, cost for medications and supplies, and the level of risk for acute and chronic complications.
- Multiple studies have shown that improved glycemic control delays the onset, slows the progression, and lowers the risk of long-term microvascular complications.
- **Metformin** should be the backbone of pharmacotherapy for patients with type 2 diabetes unless contraindicated (severe or unstable renal dysfunction, uncontrolled heart failure) or not tolerated.
- Combination therapy of 2 or more oral medications, oral medications *plus* insulin, or oral medications *plus* glucagon-like peptide-1 (GLP-1) analogs, is required in most patients to maintain continued type 2 diabetes control.
- Selection of pharmacotherapy agents for management of type 2 diabetes should be individualized to the patient's needs. Elements to consider when selecting appropriate agents include history of atherosclerotic cardiovascular disease (ASCVD), chronic kidney disease, or heart failure; risk of hypoglycemia, changes to weight, cost, administration method and frequency, and side effects specific to each agent.
- Patients with type 1 diabetes require basal/bolus insulin for glycemic management.
- Patient education is essential for the management of diabetes because it provides a means for persons with this chronic disease to become empowered, cope effectively, and engage in appropriate self-care.
- Recommended lifestyle modifications include weight management, increased physical activity, and smoking cessation.

17-2 STUDY GUIDE CHECKLIST

The following topics may guide your study of this subject area:

- ☐ Summarize diagnostic criteria for prediabetes and diabetes.
- ☐ Differentiate mechanism of action, adverse events, efficacy, and contraindications for noninsulin antihyperglycemic agents for type 2 diabetes.
- ☐ Differentiate the pharmacokinetics of available insulin products.
- ☐ Design an initial insulin regimen for patients with type 1 and type 2 diabetes.
- ☐ Identify patient counseling points for specific antihyperglycemic agents.
- ☐ Identify components of diabetes self-management education to assist patients with lifestyle modifications to improve glycemic control.

17-3   Disease Overview

Diabetes is a group of chronic metabolic diseases caused by defects in insulin secretion, insulin action, or both that result in hyperglycemia. Diabetes is associated with long-term macrovascular and microvascular complications.

Pathophysiology and Etiology

Type 1 diabetes

Pancreatic beta-cell destruction leads to absolute insulin deficiency. Peak onset occurs at the time of puberty but may occur at any age. Patients are prone to ketoacidosis because of a lack of insulin secretion.

Type 2 diabetes

Insulin resistance and progressive pancreatic beta-cell dysfunction occur. Insulin resistance may be present for years before the onset of type 2 diabetes. Initially, normal glucose concentrations are maintained by increased insulin secretion by beta cells. Increasing insulin resistance or a failure of pancreatic beta cells to maintain insulin secretion eventually leads to the development of type 2 diabetes. It is usually diagnosed in adulthood, but it can occur at any age with recent increases in diagnosis in children and adolescents. Incidence is higher among certain ethnic populations (American Indians/Alaska Natives, non-Hispanic Blacks, Hispanics, Asian Americans, and Pacific Islanders).

Clinical Presentation

Classic signs and symptoms include polydipsia, polyuria, and polyphagia. Other common findings include fatigue, blurred vision, and frequent infections (Figure 17-1). Patients with type 1 diabetes typically experience a rapid onset of symptoms and may present with ketonuria or ketoacidosis. Patients with type 2 diabetes have a gradual onset of disease and can be asymptomatic or experience the classic symptoms of diabetes. This patient population has a high risk of obesity. Patients with type 2 diabetes can also present with established microvascular and macrovascular complications when first diagnosed. Type 2 diabetes is a progressive disease with worsening of disease control expected the longer the time since diagnosis.

Classification

See Table 17-1 for a comparison of type 1 and type 2 diabetes mellitus.

Type 1 diabetes

Type 1 diabetes comprises 5% to 10% of all diagnosed cases and requires exogenous insulin for survival.

Type 2 diabetes

Type 2 diabetes comprises 90% to 95% of all diagnosed cases.

Gestational diabetes mellitus

Gestational diabetes mellitus (GDM) involves glucose intolerance with onset of pregnancy or first recognition during pregnancy (second and third trimesters). Approximately 7% of pregnant women develop GDM, which is more than 200,000 annually. Women with GDM have a 40% to 60% chance of developing type 2 diabetes later.

FIGURE 17-1. Symptoms of Diabetes

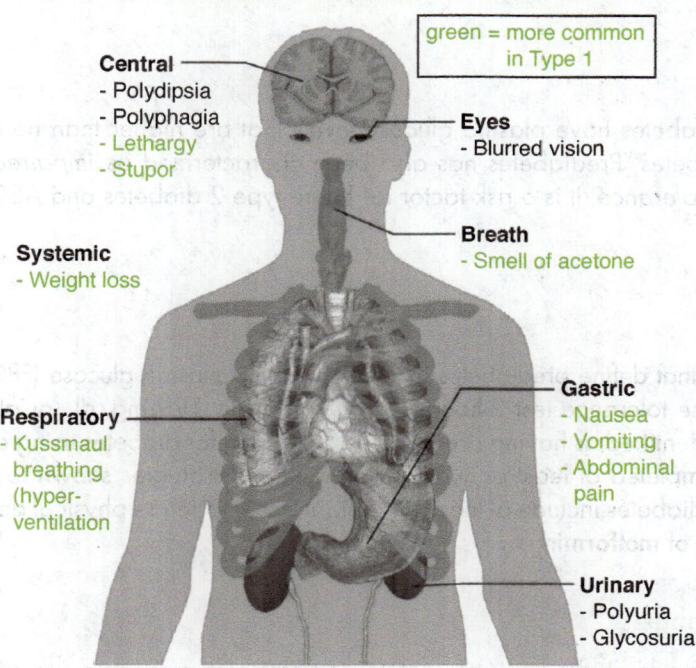

Central
- Polydipsia
- Polyphagia
- Lethargy
- Stupor

green = more common in Type 1

Eyes
- Blurred vision

Systemic
- Weight loss

Breath
- Smell of acetone

Respiratory
- Kussmaul breathing (hyper-ventilation

Gastric
- Nausea
- Vomiting
- Abdominal pain

Urinary
- Polyuria
- Glycosuria

An overview of the most significant symptoms of diabetes.

Adapted from: Häggström, Mikael (2014). "Medical gallery of Mikael Häggström 2014". WikiJournal of Medicine 1 (2). DOI:10.15347/wjm/2014.008. ISSN 2002-4436. Public Domain.

TABLE 17-1. Comparison of Type 1 and Type 2 Diabetes

	Type 1 diabetes	Type 2 diabetes
Share of diabetes cases	5% to 10%	90% to 95%
Age of occurrence	<30 years (usually childhood or adolescence); at any age following autoimmune stimulus (e.g., virus)	>30 years; increasing in childhood and adolescence in association with obesity and inactivity
Onset	Rapid	Gradual
Primary etiology	Autoimmune-mediated mechanism with genetic predisposition	Genetic and environmental (e.g., family history, ethnicity, obesity, inactivity)
Pathogenesis	Destruction of beta cells resulting in absolute insulin deficiency and abnormal glucose control	Increasing resistance of tissue (liver and skeletal muscle) to insulin; impaired insulin secretion resulting in relative deficiency of insulin; increased hepatic glucose production
Signs and symptoms	Polyuria, polydipsia, polyphagia, unexplained weight loss, fatigue, blurred vision, possibly ketoacidosis	Polyuria, polydipsia, polyphagia, obesity, fatigue, blurred vision, possibly asymptomatic
Ketoacidosis	Ketosis prone (DKA)	Not ketosis prone because of residual insulin (hyperglycemic hyperosmolar nonketotic syndrome)
Treatment:		
Nondrug therapy	Medical nutrition therapy (MNT) and physical activity approved by physician	Essential adjunct to oral antidiabetic therapy; may be sufficient as monotherapy to control blood glucose
Drug therapy	Insulin monotherapy or, rarely, oral antidiabetic drugs as adjunct to insulin therapy (if accompanied by insulin resistance)	MNT monotherapy or oral antidiabetic drugs or oral antidiabetic drugs in combination therapy or insulin monotherapy or insulin and oral antidiabetic drugs in combination therapy

DKA, diabetic ketoacidosis.

Prediabetes

Patients with prediabetes have plasma glucose levels that are higher than normal but lower than those diagnostic for diabetes. Prediabetes has also been characterized as *impaired fasting glucose* and/or *impaired glucose tolerance*. It is a risk factor for future type 2 diabetes and ASCVD.

Diagnostic Criteria

Prediabetes

Objective findings that define prediabetes includes a fasting plasma glucose (FPG) of 100 to 125 mg/dL, a 75 g oral glucose tolerance test 2-hour glucose of 140 to 199 mg/dL, or an A1C of 5.7% to 6.4%. Once a patient is identified as having prediabetes, screening for diabetes using one of the aforementioned tests should be completed at least annually. Management strategies shown to decrease the risk of progressing to type 2 diabetes include at least 7% weight loss, moderate physical activity at least 150 minutes per week, and use of **metformin**.

Type 1 and type 2 diabetes

Diagnosis can be made on the basis of an A1C, an FPG test, a random plasma glucose test, or an oral glucose tolerance test. The A1C may be more convenient because fasting is not required, and daily changes are possible during stress or illness in an FPG. The A1C may not be as accurate with certain forms of anemia (e.g., iron deficiency, hemolysis), hemoglobinopathies (e.g., sickle cell trait), and recent blood loss. The A1C should not be used to diagnose and monitor diabetes during pregnancy. Recommendations for the diagnosis of gestational diabetes can be found in the classification and diagnosis section of the American Diabetes Association Standards of Medical Care in Diabetes. Box 17-1 shows the criteria for the diagnosis of diabetes.

Treatment Principles and Goals

The primary treatment goal is to maintain glycemic control. In general, the glycemic goals include A1C < 7%, preprandial capillary plasma glucose 80 to 130 mg/dL, and 1- to 2-hour postprandial capillary plasma glucose < 180 mg/dL. Treatment goals should be individualized to be more or less stringent than these on the basis of patient characteristics such as duration of diabetes, age, life expectancy, comorbid conditions, known ASCVD, presence of microvascular complications, risk of severe hypoglycemia, and other individual patient considerations.

BOX 17-1. Criteria for the Diagnosis of Diabetes

Hemoglobin A1C ≥6.5%[a]

OR

Fasting plasma glucose ≥126 mg/dL (7.0 mmol/L). Fasting is defined as no caloric intake for at least 8 hours.[a]

OR

Two-hour plasma glucose ≥200 mg/dL (11.1 mmol/L) during an oral glucose tolerance test using a glucose load containing the equivalent of 75 g anhydrous glucose dissolved in water.[a]

OR

In a patient with classic symptoms of hyperglycemia or hyperglycemic crisis, a random plasma glucose ≥200 mg/dL (11.1 mmol/L).

American Diabetes Association, 2020.
a. In the absence of unequivocal hyperglycemia, the first three criteria should be confirmed by repeat testing of the same test.

Additional treatment goals include modifying the patient's lifestyle to promote general health and achieve weight management goals, preventing or slowing the progression of chronic microvascular and macrovascular complications, and preventing or resolving acute diabetes complications. In addition, the effect of diabetes management on quality of life should be considered.

Prevention of complications

The following activities can prevent DM complications from arising:

- Cessation of tobacco use
- **Aspirin** or antiplatelet therapy:
  - Use **aspirin** (75 to 162 mg/d), or **clopidogrel** (75 mg/d) if the patient is allergic to **aspirin**, as secondary prevention for patients with diabetes with a history of ASCVD.
  - Consider **aspirin** (75 to 162 mg/d) in men and women ≥50 years of age with one additional ASCVD risk factor (e.g., hypertension, dyslipidemia, smoking, chronic kidney disease [CKD], albuminuria, family history of premature ASCVD) and who have low bleeding risk. Risk of bleeding outweighs the potential benefit in patients 70 years of age and older.
- Immunizations: Recommended immunizations for patients with diabetes include influenza, pneumococcal polysaccharide, and hepatitis B. Refer to Chapter 36 (Immunization) for details regarding eligibility criteria for each of these immunizations.
- Foot care: Patients should be instructed to self-inspect their feet daily including the bottoms of their feet. Health care providers should also perform a visual foot inspection at each office visit and an annual comprehensive foot exam (i.e., pedal pulses, sensation).
- Skin care: Patients should inspect their skin daily and report cuts and wounds that appear to not be healing.
- Dental care: Patients should have an annual dental examination.
- Eye care: Patients should have an annual dilated eye examinction to assess for retinopathy starting at the time of diagnosis of type 2 diabetes or 5 years after the diagnosis of type 1 diabetes.
- Nephropathy screening: Patients should have an annual evaluation of serum creatinine for estimated glomerular filtration rate (eGFR) and an annual evaluation of urine albumin excretion starting at the time of diagnosis of type 2 diabetes or 5 years after the diagnosis of type 1 diabetes.

Chronic complications of diabetes (Figure 17-2)

Macrovascular complications include coronary heart disease, stroke, and peripheral arterial disease. Patients with DM have increased incidence of ASCVD. In 2008, the U.S. Food and Drug Administration (FDA) mandated medications used to treat diabetes also be evaluated for cardiovascular risk. Evidence is now emerging regarding medication treatment effect on ASCVD.

Microvascular complications include retinopathy, nephropathy, and neuropathies. Retinopathy as a result of diabetes is the leading cause of new cases of blindness in adults 20 to 74 years of age. Retinopathy can develop without symptoms. Treatment includes glycemic control, blood pressure control, and laser photocoagulation. Nephropathy occurs in 20% to 40% of patients with diabetes and is the leading cause of end-stage renal disease. Treatment includes glycemic and blood pressure control. Patients with diabetes should be prescribed an angiotensin-converting enzyme inhibitor or angiotensin II receptor blocker if they have elevated blood pressure or evidence of elevated urinary albumin excretion. Refer to Chapter 12 (Hypertension) for additional discussion. Published reports of secondary outcome measures support the use of certain sodium-glucose cotransporter-2 (SGLT-2) inhibitors and glucagon-like peptide-1 (GLP-1) agonists to reduce risk of worsening nephropathy or to decrease incidence of nephropathy. These medications include empagliflozin, canagliflozin, dapagliflozin, liraglutide, semaglutide, and dulaglutide. Diabetic peripheral neuropathy (DPN) is a dysfunction of the sensorimotor nervous system. It is characterized by pain or diminished sensation and is most commonly present in the feet and hands. Presence of DPN increases

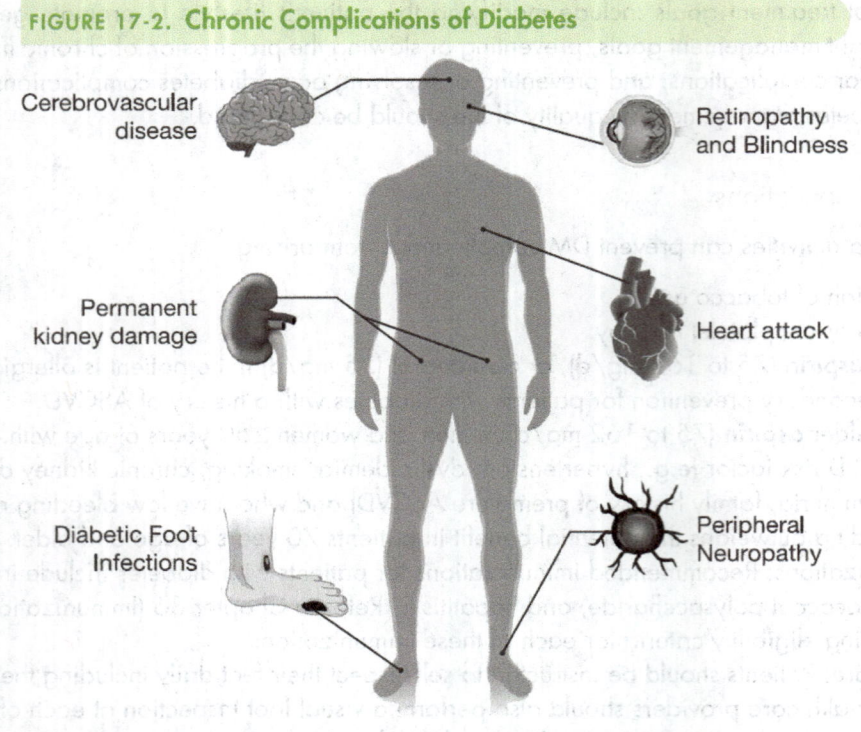

FIGURE 17-2. Chronic Complications of Diabetes

Cerebrovascular disease

Retinopathy and Blindness

Permanent kidney damage

Heart attack

Diabetic Foot Infections

Peripheral Neuropathy

risk of ulceration and infection. See Chapter 27 (Pain Management and Migraines) for information about treatment of neuropathic pain. Autonomic neuropathies can manifest in the gastrointestinal tract (e.g., gastroparesis, constipation, diarrhea), genitourinary system (e.g., neurogenic bladder, sexual dysfunction in men), and cardiovascular system (e.g., orthostatic hypotension, resting tachycardia). Treatment is limited to glycemic control and symptomatic management.

Acute complications of diabetes

Acute complications of diabetes include hypoglycemia, diabetic ketoacidosis (DKA), and hyperglycemic hyperosmolar state (HHS). Hypoglycemia is defined as plasma glucose <70 mg/dL. Symptoms can be mild (tremor, palpitations, sweating) to severe (unresponsiveness, unconsciousness, or convulsions). Treatment includes 15 to 20 g glucose tablets/gel or other carbohydrate (e.g., 4 oz fruit juice, 4 oz regular soda, 8 oz low-fat milk, 3 teaspoons granulated sugar). Plasma glucose should improve in approximately 15 minutes, but symptoms may continue for hours. Severe hypoglycemia may require assistance from another individual for treatment with glucagon (subcutaneous injection or intranasal) or intravenous glucose.

Patients with type 1 diabetes are at increased risk for DKA as a result of insulin deficiency. It can be caused by omission of insulin doses, major stress, infection, or trauma. DKA is characterized by glucose >250 mg/dL, elevated ketones, arterial pH >7.2, and plasma bicarbonate <15 mEq/L. Kussmaul respirations (deep and rapid) are commonly observed as a mechanism to compensate for metabolic acidosis. Ketone bodies are formed in excess because of fatty acid metabolism in the liver, leading to ketonuria and ketonemia and ultimately DKA. Treatment requires prompt intervention with insulin, fluids, and electrolytes to prevent coma and death.

HHS is a complication of type 2 diabetes characterized by elevated plasma glucose (typically >500 mg/dL), dehydration, and hyperosmolarity without significant ketoacidosis. HHS can be triggered by infection or other stressors such as stroke or myocardial infarction. Treatment includes insulin, fluids, and electrolytes.

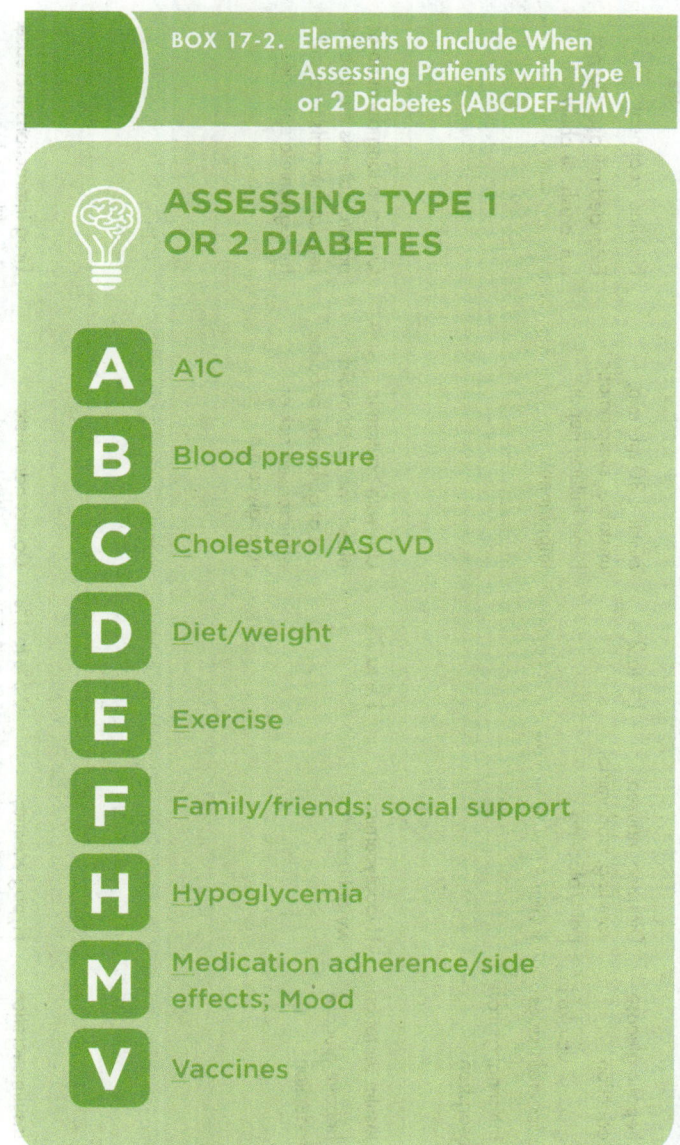

BOX 17-2. Elements to Include When Assessing Patients with Type 1 or 2 Diabetes (ABCDEF-HMV)

ASSESSING TYPE 1 OR 2 DIABETES

A A1C

B Blood pressure

C Cholesterol/ASCVD

D Diet/weight

E Exercise

F Family/friends; social support

H Hypoglycemia

M Medication adherence/side effects; Mood

V Vaccines

Patient assessment

The management of type 1 and 2 diabetes requires a multifactorial approach because of the impact the diseases have on various organ systems. The treatment of type 1 and 2 diabetes is also complex as it involves both drug therapy and nondrug therapy interventions to assist patients in achieving their goals. The mnemonic in Box 17-2 will help to recall all aspects of a patient with type 1 or 2 diabetes that should be considered.

17-4 Drug Therapy

Oral Antihyperglycemic Agents

Table 17-2 provides an overview of oral antihyperglycemic agents.

TABLE 17-2. Oral and Noninsulin Injectable Antihyperglycemic Agents[a]

Drug (trade name)	Daily dose	Mechanism of action	Common adverse drug effects	A1C reduction	Contraindications	Comments
Biguanide						
Metformin (Glucophage, Riomet)	500 mg orally daily to 1000 mg orally twice daily; no added clinical benefit from doses higher than 2000 mg daily	↓ hepatic glucose production ↑ glucose uptake in peripheral tissues ↓ intestinal glucose absorption	Diarrhea, nausea, vomiting, abdominal pain/bloating ↓ vitamin B_{12}	1% to 2%	eGFR < 30 mL/min; unstable, symptomatic heart failure; hepatic impairment	First-line treatment
Metformin extended release (Glucophage XR, Glumetza, Fortamet)						Extended release: Do *not* cut, crush, or chew.
Sulfonylureas, second generation						
Glimepiride (Amaryl)	1 to 8 mg orally daily	↑ insulin secretion ↓ hepatic glucose production	Hypoglycemia, weight gain	1% to 2%	Use with caution in elderly patients; avoid use of glyburide because of increased risk of hypoglycemia.	Owing to long duration of action, patients must eat in regular intervals to avoid hypoglycemic episodes.
Glipizide (Glucotrol, Glucotrol XL)	5 to 40 mg orally daily 5 to 20 mg orally daily (extended release)					
Glyburide (Diabeta, Micronase)	1.25 to 20 mg orally daily to twice daily					
Glyburide, micronized (Glynase)	1.5 to 12 mg orally daily					
Meglitinides						
Nateglinide (Starlix)	60 to 120 mg orally before each meal	↑ insulin secretion ↓ hepatic glucose production	Hypoglycemia, weight gain	0.5% to 1% 1% to 1.5%	Do not administer repaglinide with gemfibrozil.	Drug interactions increase risk of hypoglycemia; see text for details.
Repaglinide (Prandin)	0.5 to 4 mg orally before each meal; maximum 16 mg/d					Meglitinides have a shorter duration of action versus sulfonylureas. Skip dose if not eating a meal. Do not use in combination with sulfonylureas.

Drug	Dosage	Action	Adverse effects		Precautions	Special considerations
Thiazolidinediones						
Pioglitazone (Actos)	15 to 45 mg orally daily	↑ insulin sensitivity	Weight gain, edema	1% to 2%	Bladder cancer (pioglitazone), heart failure, hepatic impairment, ischemic heart disease, myocardial infarction (rosiglitazone), risk of bone fracture	Dispense with medication guide.
Rosiglitazone (Avandia)	4 to 8 mg orally daily or 2 to 4 mg orally twice daily	↓ hepatic glucose production				
Dipeptidyl peptidase-4 (DPP4) inhibitors						
Alogliptin (Nesina)	25 mg orally daily	↓ breakdown of endogenous GLP-1	Nasopharyngitis, upper respiratory tract infections, headache, urinary tract infections (saxagliptin)	0.5% to 1%	Pancreatitis	CrCl 30 to < 60 mL/min: 12.5 mg daily; CrCl < 15 mL/min or requiring hemodialysis: 6.25 mg daily without regard to timing of hemodialysis
Linagliptin (Tradjenta)	5 mg orally daily					No dose adjustment is needed for renal impairment.
Saxagliptin (Onglyza)	2.5 to 5 mg orally daily					eGFR < 45 mL/min/1.73 m²: 2.5 mg daily ESRD requiring hemodialysis: 2.5 mg daily (postdialysis)
Sitagliptin (Januvia)	100 mg orally daily					eGFR 30 to 45 mL/min/ 1.73 m²: 50 mg daily; eGFR < 30 mL/min/1.73 m²: 25 mg daily; ESRD requiring hemodialysis or peritoneal dialysis: 25 mg daily
Sodium-glucose cotransporter-2 (SGLT2) inhibitors						
Canagliflozin (**Invokana**)	100 to 300 mg orally daily	Inhibit SGLT2 ↑ urinary glucose excretion	Hypotension, dehydration, weight loss, genital mycotic infections, urinary tract infections, hyperkalemia (canagliflozin) ↑ LDL ↑ hematocrit (dapagliflozin, empagliflozin)	0.7% to 1%	Renal insufficiency (empagliflozin and ertuliflozin eGFR < 30 mL/min/1.73 m²; canagliflozin eGFR < 25 to 30 mL/min/1.73 m² and urinary albumin excretion ≤ 300 mg/day or hemodialysis or peritoneal dialysis; dapagliflozin hemodialysis or peritoneal dialysis)	Use with caution in patients taking diuretics and in elderly patients.
Dapagliflozin (Farxiga)	5 to 10 mg orally daily					
Empagliflozin (Jardiance)	10 to 25 mg orally daily					
Ertugliflozin (Steglatro)	5 to 15 mg orally daily					

(continued)

TABLE 17-2. Oral and Noninsulin Injectable Antihyperglycemic Agents[a] (Continued)

Drug (trade name)	Daily dose	Mechanism of action	Common adverse drug effects	A1C reduction	Contraindications	Comments
Alpha-glucosidase inhibitors						
Acarbose (Precose)	25 to 100 mg orally three times daily	Delay digestion of carbohydrates	Flatulence, GI upset, abdominal pain/bloating, diarrhea ↑ LFTs and bilirubin (acarbose)	0.5% to 1%	Inflammatory bowel disease, ulcerative colitis, Crohn's disease, partial intestinal obstruction, short bowel syndrome, renal impairment (SCr >2 mg/dL, CrCl ≤25 mL/min)	General use is not recommended by the American Diabetes Association Standards of Medical Care—2020.
Miglitol (Glyset)	25 to 100 mg orally three times daily					
Glucagon-like peptide-1 (GLP-1) agonists						
Dulaglutide (Trulicity)	0.75 to 1.5 mg subcutaneous weekly	Stimulate GLP-1 receptors resulting in glucose-dependent insulin secretion ↓ postprandial glucagon secretion ↓ gastric emptying rate Early satiety	Nausea, vomiting, diarrhea, headache, weight loss	0.5% to 2%	Gastroparesis, pancreatitis, multiple endocrine neoplasia syndrome type 2, personal or family history of medullary thyroid carcinoma	No renal dose adjustment is needed.
Exenatide (Byetta)	5 to 10 mcg subcutaneous twice daily, 2 mg subcutaneous weekly					Use is not recommended with CrCl <30 mL/min.
Exenatide extended release (Bydureon)						
Liraglutide (Victoza)	0.6 to 1.8 mg subcutaneous daily					No renal dose adjustment is needed.
Lixisenatide (Adlyxin)	10 to 20 mcg subcutaneous daily					Use is not recommended with eGFR < 15 mL/min/ 1.73 m².
Semaglutide (Ozempic)	0.25 to 1 mg subcutaneous weekly					No renal dose adjustment is needed.
Semaglutide (Rybelsus)	3 to 14 mg orally daily					No renal dose adjustment is needed.
Amylin mimetic						
Pramlintide (SymlinPen)	Type 1 diabetes: 15 to 60 mcg three times daily immediately before meals type 2 diabetes: 60 to 120 mcg three times daily immediately before meals	Amylin analog resulting in: ↓ postprandial glucagon secretion, ↓ gastric emptying rate, early satiety	Hypoglycemia, nausea, vomiting, diarrhea, headache, anorexia	0.5% to 1%	Severe, recurrent hypoglycemia, hypoglycemic unawareness, gastroparesis, ESRD, poor adherence to insulin regimen, poor adherence to self-monitoring blood glucose	Do not mix with insulin for administration. Reduce mealtime insulin dose 50% when initiating to avoid hypoglycemia.

Boldface indicates one of top 100 drugs for 2020 by prescription volume.

CrCl, creatinine clearance; eGFR, estimated glomerular filtration rate; ESRD, end-stage renal disease; LDL, low-density lipoprotein; SCr, serum creatinine; ↑, increase; ↓, decrease.

a. Numerous combination products are available in the United States. Please refer to the Additional Resources section for the WebMD resource page, which lists each product available.

Biguanide

Metformin is the only agent currently FDA approved in this class. It is considered a first-line treatment for patients with type 2 diabetes because of its efficacy, tolerable adverse event profile, low risk of hypoglycemia, effects on weight loss or weight neutrality, potential to decrease risk of ASCVD, and cost. It is indicated for use in patients ≥10 years of age. Off-label uses include prevention of type 2 diabetes, gestational diabetes, and polycystic ovary syndrome. **Metformin** lowers the A1C approximately 1% to 2%.

> ### ⚠ Metformin *FDA BOXED WARNING*
>
> Lactic acidosis has been associated with metformin use in patients with renal impairment, age ≥ 65 years, recent use of contrast for a radiologic study, surgery, hypoxemia, excessive alcohol consumption, hepatic impairment, and when used with carbonic anhydrase inhibitors (e.g., **Topiramate**).

Mechanism of action

Mechanism of action includes inhibition of hepatic glucose production, enhanced glucose uptake in peripheral tissues, and decreased intestinal absorption of glucose.

Adverse drug effects

The most common adverse drug effects include gastrointestinal (GI) symptoms such as diarrhea, nausea, vomiting, and abdominal pain and bloating. **Metformin** can also cause anorexia and metallic taste. Hypoglycemia is rare when used as monotherapy. Long-term use of **metformin** can reduce vitamin B_{12} concentrations. Vitamin B_{12} deficiency may cause symptoms similar to DPN, but each condition is treated differently. The most severe, though rare, adverse drug effect is lactic acidosis (FDA boxed warning).

Monitoring for safety and efficacy

Recommendations for safety monitoring include eGFR at least annually with increased frequency of monitoring with declining eGFR (every 6 months when eGFR is 45 to 60 mL/min/1.73 m²; every 3 months when eGFR is 45 to 60 mL/min/1.73 m²). The maximum daily dose of **metformin** should not exceed 1 g when eGFR < 45 mL/min/1.73 m². Discontinue use when eGFR < 30 mL/min/1.73 m². For patients using **metformin** more than 1 year, especially patients with symptoms of DPN, checking vitamin B_{12} concentration regularly is recommended.

Cautions and contraindications

Most of the cautions and contraindications for the use of **metformin** are in regard to the increased risk of lactic acidosis. **Metformin** should be used with caution in patients with impaired renal function. **Metformin** should also be avoided in patients with unstable symptomatic heart failure and hepatic impairment. **Metformin** should be discontinued temporarily in patients with acute myocardial infarction, heart failure exacerbation, severe respiratory disease, shock, and septicemia. **Metformin** should also be discontinued for procedures that require iodinated contrast media and major surgeries (resume 2 to 3 days after renal function has returned to baseline and remains stable).

Significant drug interactions

Medications that increase the risk of lactic acidosis are contraindicated with **metformin** (e.g., **topiramate**, zonisamide, dichlorphenamide, acetazolamide).

Patient instructions and counseling

- To minimize stomach upset, take with food and titrate dose no more often than weekly.
- GI effects are transient and improve in most patients with continued use.
- Glumetza contains an insoluble tablet shell that may be visible in stool.
- Fortamet and Glucophage XR may appear as a soft mass in stool.

Secretagogues

Secretagogues include first- and second-generation sulfonylureas and meglitinides. Second-generation sulfonylureas are preferred over first-generation sulfonylureas because of safety concerns. First-generation sulfonylureas will not be discussed in this chapter because of their limited clinical use. Second-generation sulfonylureas and meglitinides are considered second-line treatment options in patients with type 2 diabetes who have not achieved blood glucose control with **metformin** and lifestyle interventions. Use is not recommended in children, during pregnancy, or while breastfeeding. However, glyburide can be used during pregnancy and while breastfeeding. Second-generation sulfonylureas have a longer duration of action than meglitinides and lower the A1C approximately 1% to 2%. Meglitinides are typically used to control prandial blood glucose and lower the A1C 0.5% to 2%. Loss of efficacy has been observed in patients with progressive beta-cell destruction. Because of overlap of mechanism of action, use of sulfonylureas and meglitinides in combination together is not recommended.

Mechanism of action

These agents prompt release of insulin from pancreatic beta cells through the stimulation of sulfonylurea receptor 1. This effect is diminished for the meglitinides when serum glucose concentrations are low. Insulin secretion may in turn cause a decrease in hepatic gluconeogenesis and a slight decrease in insulin resistance at the muscle level. Effectiveness depends on pancreatic beta cell function.

Adverse drug effects

The most common adverse drug effects include hypoglycemia and weight gain. Glyburide poses the highest risk of hypoglycemia and should be avoided in elderly patients. Risk of hypoglycemia is reduced with meglitinides because of their shorter duration of action. Clinical trials with sulfonylureas have observed mean weight gain of 5 kg.

Cautions and contraindications

Renal and hepatic impairment can lead to increased risk of hypoglycemia. **Glipizide** and **glimepiride** are preferred over glyburide. Elderly, malnourished, and debilitated patients have a higher risk of developing hypoglycemia. Repaglinide should not be used in combination with gemfibrozil. Risk of hypoglycemia increases with repaglinide when it is co-administered with sulfonamides, cyclosporine, chloramphenicol, probenecid, and beta blockers. Risk of hypoglycemia increases with nateglinide when it is co-administered with cytochrome P450 (CYP) 2C9 inhibitors.

Patient instructions and counseling

- Take before meals (sulfonylureas 1 to 2 times daily; meglitinides before each meal).
- Sulfonylureas: eat meals spaced 4 to 6 hours apart to avoid hypoglycemia.
- Meglitinides: if a meal is skipped, do not administer the dose for that meal.
- Avoid alcohol as consumption increases risk of hypoglycemia.
- Carry a fast-acting oral carbohydrate to treat hypoglycemia if it occurs.

Thiazolidinediones ⚠

Thiazolidinediones (TZDs) are considered second-line treatment options in patients with type 2 diabetes who have not achieved blood glucose control with **metformin** and lifestyle interventions. Recently, there has been controversy regarding cardiovascular safety of rosiglitazone, increased risk of bladder cancer with pioglitazone, and fractures with both agents. They have been used to treat and prevent type 2 diabetes and treat nonalcoholic fatty liver disease. TZDs lower the A1C approximately 1% to 2%.

Mechanism of action

TZDs are agonists of the PPARγ (peroxisome proliferator-activated receptor γ) receptor, which, when stimulated, improves peripheral muscle and adipose tissue insulin sensitivity and suppresses hepatic glucose output.

Adverse drug effects

The most common adverse drug effects include weight gain and edema. Typical weight gain is 5 kg or more when used in combination with insulin or secretagogues. Edema may be dose related and can be observed in patients without a history of cardiovascular disease. When TZDs are used in combination with insulin, there is a higher incidence of edema. Edema may best be treated by aldosterone antagonists. Severe adverse drug effects include heart failure, hepatotoxicity, bone fractures, and bladder cancer (pioglitazone).

Cautions and contraindications

TZDs should not be used in patients with New York Heart Association class III/IV heart failure , ischemic heart disease, hepatic impairment (alanine aminotransferase [ALT] >2.5 × upper limit normal [ULN] before initiation or ALT >3 × ULN while on therapy), bladder cancer (pioglitazone), or presence of fracture risk factors.

> ⚠️ **Thiazolidinediones (TZDs)** *FDA BOXED WARNING*
>
> Congestive heart failure. Rosiglitazone and pioglitazone have been shown to cause or exacerbate congestive heart failure in some patients. Rosiglitazone and pioglitazone are contraindicated in patients with NHYA class III or IV heart failure

Patient instructions and counseling

- Hypoglycemia is rare unless taken with other medications known to cause hypoglycemia.
- Notify the prescribing provider if you notice new or worsening edema, shortness of breath, bone fractures, blood in the urine or red urine, or pain when urinating.
- An FDA-approved medication guide must be dispensed with TZD-containing products.
- TZDs can decrease effectiveness of oral contraceptives.

Dipeptidyl peptidase-4 inhibitors

Dipeptidyl peptidase-4 (DPP4) inhibitors are considered second-line treatment options in patients with type 2 diabetes who have not achieved blood glucose control with **metformin** and lifestyle interventions. Agents in this class are generally well tolerated and weight neutral and do not cause hypoglycemia when used as monotherapy. DPP4 inhibitors lower the A1C approximately 0.5% to 1%.

Mechanism of action

DPP4 inhibitors inhibit the degradation of endogenous glucagon-like peptide-1 (GLP-1) and glucose-dependent insulinotropic polypeptide, which in turn causes increased insulin production in a glucose-dependent fashion and decreased production of glucagon.

Adverse drug effects

The most common adverse drug effects include nasopharyngitis, upper respiratory tract infections, headache, and urinary tract infections. There have also been reports of pancreatitis and increased risk of hospitalizations for heart failure (saxagliptin). Hypersensitivity reactions (urticarial, angioedema, anaphylaxis, Stevens–Johnson syndrome, vasculitis) have been observed.

Cautions and contraindications

Dose adjustments are needed for renal insufficiency, with the exception of linagliptin (Tradjenta). Avoid use in patients with history of pancreatitis while taking a DPP4 inhibitor.

Co-administration with CYP 3A4/5 inhibitors (ketoconazole, atazanavir, clarithromycin, indinavir, itraconazole, nefazodone, nelfinavir, ritonavir, saquinavir, telithromycin) significantly increases saxagliptin concentrations. Limit dose to 2.5 mg daily.

Patient instructions and counseling

- Hypoglycemia is rare unless taken with other medications known to cause hypoglycemia.
- Notify the prescribing provider if you notice severe abdominal pain or back pain, new or worsening edema, shortness of breath, weight gain of more than 5 pounds in 24 hours, skin blisters or breakdown, or persistent joint pain.

Sodium-glucose cotransporter-2 inhibitors

Sodium-glucose cotransporter-2 (SGLT2) inhibitors are considered second-line treatment options in patients with type 2 diabetes who have not achieved blood glucose control with **metformin** and lifestyle interventions. Agents in this class induce weight loss and do not cause hypoglycemia when used as monotherapy. SGLT2 inhibitors lower the A1C approximately 0.7% to 1%. In addition to glycemic control, SGLT2 inhibitors decrease risk of major adverse cardiovascular events in patients with type 2 diabetes and ASCVD. They also reduce risk of heart-failure-related hospitalization and progression of renal disease in patients with type 2 diabetes.

Mechanism of action

These medications inhibit SGLT2 in the proximal renal tubule, which reduces reabsorption of glucose filtered in the tubular lumen and lowers the renal threshold for glucose. This results in increased urinary glucose excretion and decreased plasma glucose.

Adverse drug effects

The most common adverse drug effects include hypotension (~3 to 5 mmHg reduction in systolic blood pressure and 1 to 2 mmHg reduction in diastolic blood pressure), dehydration, weight loss (1.4 to 3.4 kg), genital mycotic and urinary tract infections, increased low-density lipoprotein (LDL) cholesterol, and elevated hematocrit (dapagliflozin and empagliflozin). Canagliflozin also causes hyperkalemia. Hypersensitivity reactions have also been observed.

Rare but serious adverse drug effects include euglycemic ketoacidosis, acute kidney injury, bone fractures, lower limb amputations (canagliflozin), and bladder cancer (dapagliflozin).

Cautions and contraindications

Efficacy of SGLT2 inhibitors declines and risk of adverse drug effects increase with impaired renal function. Avoid use in patients with renal insufficiency and those taking empagliflozin or ertugliflozin (eGFR < 30 mL/min/1.73 m²), canagliflozin (eGFR < 25 to 30 mL/min/1.73 m² and urinary albumin excretion ≤ 300 mg/day or hemodialysis or peritoneal dialysis), and dapagliflozin (hemodialysis or peritoneal dialysis).

Use with caution in patients who have low blood pressure or impaired renal function, currently use diuretics, or are elderly. Canagliflozin should also be used with caution in patients with or who are predisposed to elevated potassium.

Canagliflozin can be used concomitantly with digoxin, but digoxin levels need to be monitored. Canagliflozin doses may need to be increased when used with uridine diphosphate glucuronosyltransferase (UDPGT) 1A9 inducers (e.g., ritonavir, rifampin, phenytoin).

Patient instructions and counseling

- These medications can cause dehydration that may result in orthostatic hypotension.
- Report symptoms of genital mycotic infections and urinary tract infections to a health care provider.

Alpha-glucosidase inhibitors

Alpha-glucosidase inhibitors have fallen out of favor because of tolerability and relatively low effect on A1C reduction. The American Diabetes Association Standards of Medical Care in Diabetes—2020 do not include this class in their treatment algorithm for type 2 diabetes. Alpha-glucosidase inhibitors primarily target reduction of postprandial hyperglycemia, have minimal risk of hypoglycemia when used as monotherapy, and have minimal effect on weight. They lower the A1C approximately 0.5% to 1%.

Mechanism of action

Alpha-glucosidase inhibitors delay the digestion of carbohydrates into simple sugars and their subsequent absorption in the small intestine.

Adverse drug effects

The most common adverse drug effects include GI symptoms including flatulence, GI upset, abdominal pain, diarrhea, and bloating. Those effects dissipate with continued use. Doses should be titrated weekly to reduce adverse drug effects. Acarbose can increase liver function tests (LFTs) and bilirubin depending on the dose (>300 mg/d).

Cautions and contraindications

Alpha-glucosidase inhibitors are contraindicated in patients with inflammatory bowel disease, ulcerative colitis, Crohn's disease, partial intestinal obstruction, and short bowel syndrome. Avoid use in patients with serum creatinine >2 mg/dL. Acarbose can increase LFTs with doses >300 mg/d. Alpha-glucosidase inhibitors decrease the bioavailability of digoxin and **propranolol**.

Patient instructions and counseling

- Hypoglycemia should be treated with glucose (tablets or gel). Use fructose (100% fruit juice) or lactose (milk) if glucose is not available. Do not use sucrose (soft drinks, candy, table sugar).
- Increase complex carbohydrate intake and limit intake of simple sugars to assist in reducing common GI adverse drug effects.

Miscellaneous antihyperglycemic agents

Colesevelam and bromocriptine are also approved for use in patients with type 2 diabetes. Because of their limited efficacy (lower A1C 0.1% to 0.5%), the American Diabetes Association Standards of Medical Care—2020 do not include this class in the treatment algorithm for type 2 diabetes. For more information on these agents, refer to the American Diabetes Association Standards of Medical Care—2020 Section 9, Pharmacologic Approaches to Glycemic Treatment.

Combination oral antihyperglycemic agents

Many combination oral antihyperglycemic agents are currently marketed in the United States. WebMD provides an online resource describing oral and injectable medications, including the available combinations. This resource is listed in the Additional Resources section of this chapter.

Injectable Antihyperglycemic Agents

Table 17-2 also provides an overview of injectable antihyperglycemic agents.

Glucagon-like peptide-1 agonists ⚠

GLP-1 agonists are considered second-line treatment options in patients with type 2 diabetes who have not achieved blood glucose control with **metformin** and lifestyle interventions. GLP-1 agonists target both fasting and postprandial glucose. Agents in this class induce weight loss (0.2 to 4 kg) and do not cause hypoglycemia when used as monotherapy. GLP-1 agonists lower the A1C approximately 0.5% to 2%. There is one agent in this class (semaglutide) that can be administered subcutaneously or orally. All other agents require subcutaneous administration.

> ⚠️ **Glucagon-like Peptide-1 Agonists** *FDA BOXED WARNING*
>
> Dulaglutide, Exenatide extended release, Liraglutide, Semaglutide (subcutaneous injection and oral tablet). Animal models demonstrated increased risk of thyroid C-cell tumors. It is not currently known if these agents cause thyroid C-cell tumors (e.g., medullary thyroid carcinoma) in humans. These agents are contraindicated for use in patients with a personal or family history of medullary thyroid carcinoma and patients with history of multiple endocrine neoplasia type 2.

Mechanism of action

Incretin mimetics are receptor agonists of endogenous GLP-1 that cause (1) increased insulin production in a glucose-dependent fashion, (2) decreased postprandial release of glucagon, (3) slowing of gastric emptying, and (4) early satiety and weight loss.

Adverse drug effects

Common adverse drug effects include nausea and vomiting (dose-related), diarrhea, headache, and weight loss. Incidence of nausea is ~30% to 50% and most common during initiation and dose titration. Nausea can be reduced by educating patients to eat more slowly. Frequency and severity of nausea and vomiting dissipate with continued use. Injection-site reactions are also common and occur at higher rates with exenatide extended release. Hypersensitivity reactions have also been reported.

Rare, but serious adverse drug effects include pancreatitis, pancreatic cancer, thyroid cancer, acute renal failure, and exacerbation of chronic renal failure. Hypersensitivity reactions have also been reported. Dulaglutide has also been associated with tachycardia, PR interval prolongation, and first-degree atrioventricular block.

Cautions and contraindications

Avoid use in patients with gastroparesis, pancreatitis, multiple endocrine neoplasia syndrome type 2, or personal or family history of medullary thyroid carcinoma. There is an FDA boxed warning for the risk of thyroid C-cell tumors. GLP-1 agonists slow gastric emptying time and have the potential to alter absorption of oral medications. Use with caution in patients taking medications that have a narrow therapeutic index.

Patient instructions and counseling

- Nausea is the most common adverse drug effect. Eating more slowly can help reduce the severity of nausea. Frequency and severity may decrease with continued use.
- Injection-site reactions are also common. Report these to health care providers.
- If a dose is missed, refer to product-specific instructions for information on when the next dose should be taken.
- Administration technique and timing is product specific. Be sure to provide the correct administration technique and timing information to patients.
- Review of proper subcutaneous injection technique.
- Review storage instructions specific to each product.

Amylin mimetic

Pramlintide is the only FDA-approved agent in this class. It is considered a third-line agent for patients with type 1 diabetes and a fourth-line agent for patients with type 2 diabetes who use mealtime insulin and have not achieved glycemic control. Pramlintide cannot be mixed with insulin for administration. During initiation of pramlintide, the mealtime insulin dose should be reduced by 50% to avoid severe hypoglycemia. Pramlintide lowers the A1C 0.5% to 1%.

 Pramlintide *FDA BOXED WARNING*

Hypoglycemia. Pramlintide increases the risk of severe hypoglycemia, especially in patients with type 1 diabetes. Severe hypoglycemia is typically observed within 3 hours of pramlintide administration. To prevent risk of severe hypoglycemia, mealtime (bolus) insulin dose should be reduced.

Mechanism of action

Pramlintide is an analog of endogenous amylin that when dosed at therapeutic levels (1) decreases production of glucagon, (2) slows gastric emptying, and (3) promotes early satiety and weight loss.

Adverse drug effects

Common adverse drug effects include severe hypoglycemia (8% to 15%), nausea and vomiting (dose-related), diarrhea, headache, and anorexia. Incidence of nausea is ~30% to 50% and most common during initiation and dose titration. Nausea can be reduced by educating patients to eat more slowly. Frequency and severity of nausea and vomiting dissipate with continued use.

Rare but serious adverse drug effects include pancreatitis and hypersensitivity reactions.

Cautions and contraindications

Avoid use in patients with history of severe, recurrent hypoglycemia, hypoglycemic unawareness, gastroparesis, end-stage renal disease, or poor adherence to insulin regimen or self-monitoring of blood glucose.

Pramlintide slows gastric emptying time and has the potential to alter absorption of oral medications. Use with caution in patients taking medications that have a narrow therapeutic index.

Patient instructions and counseling

- Decrease the dose of mealtime insulin by 50% when initiating pramlintide to reduce the risk of hypoglycemia.
- Nausea is the most common adverse drug effect. Eating more slowly can help reduce the severity of nausea. Frequency and severity may decrease with continued use.
- Review proper subcutaneous injection technique.
- Review storage instructions.

Insulin

Table 17-3 provides an overview of available insulin products.

Insulin is indicated for use in patients with type 1 or type 2 diabetes. Insulin is required for treatment of patients with type 1 diabetes and can be used as combination therapy or monotherapy in patients with type 2 diabetes. A typical starting dose for patients with type 1 diabetes is 0.4 to 0.5 units/kg/d, divided as 50% basal and 50% bolus/mealtime (bolus is then divided between meals). A typical starting dose for patients with type 2 diabetes is 0.1 to 0.2 units/kg/d of basal insulin when added to a regimen that includes one or more oral or non-insulin injectable antihyperglycemic agents. The dose of basal insulin for patients with type 2 diabetes will be titrated to response on the basis of fasting blood glucose (typical basal insulin dose for fasting blood glucose control is 0.4 to 0.6 units/kg/d). Bolus insulin may also need to be initiated in patients with type 2 diabetes. The average daily dose used to obtain glycemic control in patients with type 2 diabetes on a basal/bolus insulin regimen is 1 unit/kg/d (50% basal, 50% bolus). There is no upper limit, however, to doses of insulin in patients with type 1 or type 2 diabetes. Insulin doses

TABLE 17-3. Insulin Products

Insulin type	Trade name	Device availability	Onset of action	Time of peak	Duration of action
Rapid acting					
Glulisine	Apidra	SoloStar	25 min	1.6 to 2.8 hours	3 to 4 hours
Aspart	NovoLog	FlexPen, PenFill	10 to 20 min	1 to 3 hours	3 to 5 hours
Lispro	Humalog	KwikPen	15 to 30 min	0.5 to 2.5 hours	≤5 hours
Lispro U-200	Humalog U-200	KwikPen	15 to 30 min	0.5 to 2.5 hours	≤5 hours
Inhaled insulin	Afrezza	4-unit, 8-unit, and 12-unit cartridges	15 to 30 min	0.5 to 1 hour	1.5 to 4.5 hours
Short acting					
Regular	Novolin R, Novolin R/ReliOn, Humulin R		0.5 to 1 hour	2.5 to 5 hours	4 to 12 hours
Intermediate acting					
Human NPH	Novolin N		1 to 2 hours	4 to 12 hours	10 to 18 hours
	Humulin N	KwikPen	1 to 2 hours	3 to 13 hours	16 to 24 hours
Regular U-500	Humulin R U-500	KwikPen	30 min	4 to 8 hours	13 to 24 hours
Long acting					
Glargine U-100	Lantus	SoloStar	3 to 4 hours	No significant peak	10.8 to >24 hours
Glargine U-300	Toujeo	SoloStar	Develops over 6 hours	No significant peak	>24 hours
Detemir	Levemir	FlexTouch	3 to 4 hours	3 to 9 hours	6 to 23 hours (dose dependent)
Ultra-long acting					
Degludec U-100; U-200	Tresiba	FlexTouch	1 hour	12 hours	Up to 42 hours
Premixed[a]					
NPH + regular	Novolin 70/30	FlexPen			
	Humulin 70/30	KwikPen			
Insulin protamine + analogs	NovoLog Mix 70/30	FlexPen			
	Humalog Mix 75/25	KwikPen			
	Humalog Mix 50/50	KwikPen			

Boldface indicates one of top 100 drugs for 2020 by prescription volume. Product concentration = 100 units per mL, unless otherwise noted.
NPH, neutral protamine Hagedorn.
a. The onset of action, time to peak, and duration of action for mixed insulin is a combination of the two agents included in the mixture. Refer to information on individual agents to assess approximate onset of action, time to peak, and duration of action.

⚠ **Inhaled Insulin** *FDA BOXED WARNING*

Acute bronchospasms have been observed in patients with asthma and COPD who are using inhaled insulin. Prior to initiation of therapy with inhaled insulin, patients should have pulmonary function testing to identify undiagnosed chronic lung disease.

should be individualized to patients accounting for glucose readings, renal function, patient schedule and preferences, patient education, health literacy and numeracy level, intensity of glucose control desired, and cost. Insulin pharmacokinetics are detailed in Table 17-3. Noting that insulin pharmacokinetics can be altered by site of administration, total dose administered, concentration of insulin, and increased blood flow to site of injection (e.g., rubbing, exercising, heat application) is important.

Mechanism of action

At low levels, insulin causes suppression of endogenous hepatic glucose production. At higher levels, insulin promotes glucose uptake by muscle tissue.

Adverse drug effects

Common adverse drug effects include hypoglycemia, weight gain, injection-site reactions, and lipohypertrophy (bulging of the injection site). Hypoglycemia can range from mild to severe. Lipohypertrophy can be avoided by rotating the injection site for administration. Insulin is able to lower the A1C more than any other antihyperglycemic agents, on average approximately 2.5%.

Cautions and contraindications

Insulin dose response should be monitored closely in patients with renal and hepatic insufficiency. Dose titrations in this population should be more conservative than in patients without renal or hepatic insufficiency.

Patient instructions and counseling

- Patients should clearly understand the dose and administration timing of each insulin product they use.
- Review signs, symptoms, and management of hypoglycemia.
- Review proper subcutaneous injection technique.
- Review storage instructions specific to each product.

17-5   Nondrug Therapy

Lifestyle changes through diet and exercise should be emphasized. Weight loss is recommended for all patients with diabetes who are overweight or obese. Modest weight loss (5% to 10%) has been shown to improve insulin resistance in type 2 diabetes.

Diabetes self-management education and support is an essential component of successful diabetes management.

Medical Nutrition Therapy

Medical nutrition therapy should be individualized to achieve treatment goals with consideration of usual dietary habits, metabolic profile, and lifestyle. Emphasis should be placed on nutrient-dense healthful food choices such as whole grains, vegetables, fruits, legumes, low-fat dairy, lean meats, and nuts and seeds.

There is no established optimal amount of daily carbohydrate intake. Carbohydrate intake can be monitored by exchanges, carbohydrate counting, or experience-based estimation (e.g., plate method, Figure 17-3). The mix of carbohydrates, protein, and fat should be adjusted to meet the weight and metabolic goals of the patient.

Protein intake may need to be modified if renal function is reduced. Saturated fat should be < 7% of total daily calories. Fiber intake should be encouraged, but there is no reason to recommend a greater

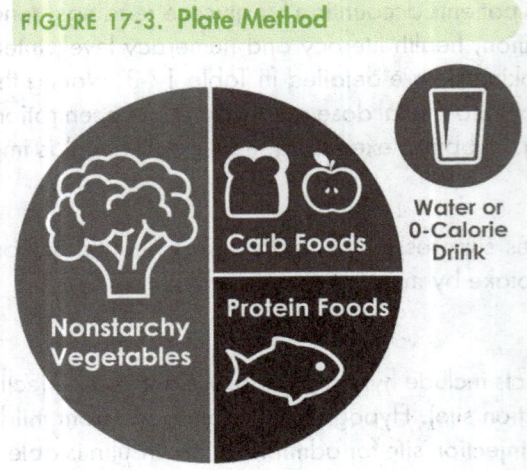

FIGURE 17-3. Plate Method

Carb Foods

Water or
0-Calorie
Drink

Nonstarchy
Vegetables

Protein Foods

The plate method is a 9-inch diameter plate with half the plate
filled with nonstarchy vegetables, a quarter of the plate filled
with lean protein, and a quarter of the plate filled with starchy
foods (e.g., grains, rice, pasta, bread, legumes, potato).
Materials Developed by CDC.

amount than that recommended for persons without diabetes (14 g fiber/1000 kcal). Alcohol can cause both hypoglycemia and hyperglycemia. Alcohol intake should be limited (adult females: one drink or fewer per day; adult males: two drinks or fewer per day).

Physical Activity and Exercise

Regular exercise improves blood glucose control, reduces cardiovascular risk factors, and contributes to weight loss. An exercise regimen should be individualized. The patient's history and a detailed medical examination are essential.

For most patients, a program of 150 min/week of moderate-intensity aerobic exercise is recommended. The program should be adjusted in the presence of macro- and microvascular complications that may be worsened:

- *Retinopathy:* Vigorous exercise may be contraindicated because of the risk of triggering vitreous hemorrhage or retinal detachment.
- *Peripheral neuropathy:* Nonweight-bearing activities may be best because decreased pain sensation in the extremities increases the risk of skin breakdown and infection.
- *Autonomic neuropathy:* Patients should undergo cardiac evaluation before increasing physical activity, which may lead to decreased cardiac responsiveness to exercise or postural hypotension.

Blood glucose monitoring may be necessary before, during, and after exercise. Fast-acting oral carbohydrates (e.g., glucose tablets, gel) should be available during and after exercise.

Diabetes Self-Management Education and Support

Diabetes self-management education and support (DSMES) provide a means for those with diabetes to become empowered with the knowledge of self-care. The Association of Diabetes Care & Education Specialists' 7 self-care behaviors are healthy eating, being active, monitoring, taking medication, problem solving, reducing risk, and healthy coping.

DSMES should be offered in a variety of settings, typically by a multidisciplinary team.

17-6   Pharmacist's Role

Type 1 and type 2 diabetes are complex diseases that require an interprofessional approach to care. Pharmacists play a vital role to assist patients to achieve their glycemic targets and maintain their quality of life. Most notably, pharmacists assist with ensuring that pharmacotherapy regimens include medications with complementary mechanisms of action and minimize adverse drug reactions. Pharmacists also educate patients on proper medication administration and techniques for self-monitoring blood glucose. In addition, pharmacists can encourage patients to implement and continue healthy lifestyle choices (e.g., selecting nutrient dense foods, balancing carbohydrate intake, and engaging in physical activity).

NAPLEX Competency Statements

The questions in this chapter cover the following 2021 NAPLEX Competency Statements: **AREA 1:** 1.1; 1.2; 1.4; 1.5; 1.6 **AREA 2:** 2.1; 2.2; 2.4 **AREA 3:** 3.2; 3.4; 3.5; 3.7; 3.8 **AREA 6:** 6.3.

17-7   Questions

1. A 76-year-old male was recently diagnosed with type 2 diabetes. His medical history includes heart failure with frequent exacerbations, hypertension, dyslipidemia, and COPD with frequent exacerbations. His A1C is 8.3%, and he is asymptomatic. What is the best medication to use as first-line treatment for this patient?

   A. Metformin
   B. Pioglitazone
   C. Dapagliflozin
   D. Insulin glargine
   E. Saxagliptin

2. Which glucagon-like peptide-1 agonist has the highest incidence of injection-site reactions?

   A. Byetta
   B. Bydureon
   C. Victoza
   D. Ozempic
   E. Trulicity

3. What insulin products are available in a concentration that is not U-100? (Mark all that apply.)

   A. Insulin glargine
   B. Insulin degludec
   C. Insulin aspart
   D. NPH insulin
   E. Regular insulin

4. A 56-year-old male has uncontrolled type 2 diabetes while taking metformin 1000 mg twice daily and following initiation of lifestyle modifications. His medical history includes HTN. His A1C is 7.6% and CrCl is 86 mL/min. Medication affordability is his primary concern. Which medication is the best agent to add to this patient's treatment regimen?

   A. Nesina 12.5 mg daily
   B. Tradjenta 5 mg daily
   C. Jardiance 10 mg daily
   D. Actos 15 mg daily
   E. Lantus 10 units every night

5. Patients using insulin should rotate inject sites to reduce the risk of _____.

   A. infection
   B. lipoatrophy
   C. lipohypertrophy
   D. generalized myalgia
   E. injection site pain

6. What is the most appropriate treatment for a severe hypoglycemic episode when a patient is unconscious?

   A. 1/2 cup of regular soda
   B. 5 hard candies containing sugar
   C. 3 glucose tablets
   D. Glucagon injection
   E. 1 cup of low-fat milk

7. Insulin therapy is recommended for which of the following situations?

    A. Newly diagnosed patient with type 2 diabetes, A1C 8.5%
    B. Patient with type 2 diabetes taking metformin 1000 mg twice daily, A1C 7.3%
    C. Patient with type 2 diabetes not able to tolerate metformin, currently using linagliptin 5 mg daily, A1C 6.8%.
    D. Newly diagnosed patient with type 1 diabetes, A1C 7.9%
    E. Patient with type 2 diabetes taking glipizide extended-release 10 mg daily, A1C 7.8%

8. Which of the following oral antidiabetic agents has been associated with euglycemic ketoacidosis?

    A. Acarbose
    B. Canagliflozin
    C. Linagliptin
    D. Metformin
    E. Glipizide

9. Which of the following scenarios can alter the pharmacokinetics of insulin products?

    A. Rotating of injection site around the abdomen
    B. Rubbing the injection site
    C. Needle size and length
    D. Administration time of day
    E. Insulin product container (pen versus vial)

10. What antihyperglycemic agents should be avoided in patients with a history of pancreatitis? (Mark all that apply.)

    A. Glucotrol XL
    B. Actos
    C. Tradjenta
    D. Jardiance
    E. Trulicity

11. Which of the following lifestyle recommendations should be made for patients with type 2 diabetes? (Mark all that apply.)

    A. Decrease weight 5% to 10%.
    B. Increase fiber intake to 50 g/1000 kcal daily.
    C. Restrict carbohydrate intake to less than 100 g daily.
    D. Engage in moderate-intensity exercise at least 150 minutes weekly.
    E. Increase protein to 2 g/kg daily.

12. A 12-year-old male was recently diagnosed with type 1 diabetes. His current weight is 87 lb. Which of the following is the most appropriate starting dose for his basal insulin?

    A. Insulin aspart 15 units daily
    B. Insulin glargine 20 units daily
    C. Insulin detemir 10 units daily
    D. Insulin degludec 5 units daily
    E. Insulin lispro 10 units daily

13. Which of the following secretagogues (sulfonylurea or meglitinide) should be avoided in elderly patients because of the risk of hypoglycemia? (Mark all that apply.)

    A. Repaglinide
    B. Glipizide
    C. Glyburide
    D. Glimepiride
    E. Nateglinide

14. A 68-year-old female with type 2 diabetes calls the pharmacy with reports of diarrhea following initiation of metformin 500 mg orally daily. Which of the following counseling points assist with management of this adverse drug effect? (Mark all that apply.)

    A. Take metformin on an empty stomach.
    B. Take metformin with food.
    C. Diarrhea will improve with continued use.
    D. Titrate the dose of metformin more quickly, because diarrhea is more common with lower doses.
    E. Eat meals and snacks more slowly.

15. Metformin should be withheld for 48 hours before any procedure requiring the use of parenteral iodinated contrast medium because of the potential for which adverse drug effect?

    A. Optic neuritis
    B. Metabolic alkalosis
    C. Lactic acidosis
    D. Purple-toe syndrome
    E. Diabetic peripheral neuropathy

16. Which of the following sodium-glucose cotransporter-2 inhibitors should not be initiated in patients with an eGFR of 35 mL/min/1.73 m²? (Mark all that apply.)

 A. Apagliflozin
 B. Canagliflozin
 C. Dapagliflozin
 D. Empagliflozin
 E. Ertugliflozin

17. Which of the following is a common adverse effect of Tradjenta when used as monotherapy?

 A. Upper respiratory infection
 B. Weight gain
 C. Hypoglycemia
 D. Angioedema
 E. Myopathy

18. Which of the following antidiabetic agents require LFTs for monitoring? (Mark all that apply.)

 A. Insulin glargine
 B. Miglitol
 C. Rosiglitazone
 D. Acarbose
 E. Metformin

19. Which of the following are adverse drug effects reported for pioglitazone? (Mark all that apply.)

 A. Heart failure
 B. Myocardial infarction
 C. Angioedema
 D. Bone fractures
 E. Atrial fibrillation

20. What is the pharmacologic class of pramlintide (Symlin)?

 A. Basal insulin
 B. Insulin analog
 C. Inhaled insulin
 D. Glucagon-like peptide-1 agonist
 E. Amylin analog

21. Order the insulin products below from shortest duration of action to longest duration of action.

 A. Insulin NPH
 B. Insulin glargine U-300
 C. Insulin aspart
 D. Insulin regular
 E. Insulin degludec

22. Select the proper locations to administer insulin subcutaneously.

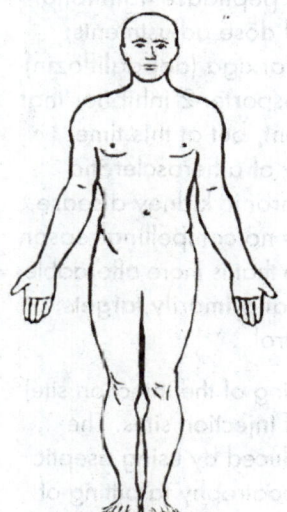 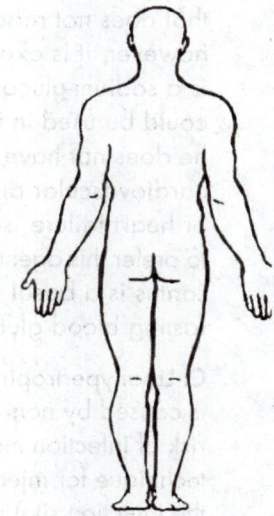

 **17-8**   **Answers**

1. **C.** Dapagliflozin is the best agent because of the balance of efficacy and decreased risk of heart failure hospitalization. Adverse drug effects include hypotension, dehydration, and weight loss; therefore, the patient should be educated regarding these. Metformin, pioglitazone, and saxagliptin should not be used in this patient because of frequent exacerbations of heart failure. Basal insulin is not indicated as first-line therapy in this patient because his A1C < 10% and he is asymptomatic.

2. **B.** Exenatide extended release (Bydureon) is associated with a higher incidence of injection-site reactions, including nodules, compared with the other agents in the same class.

3. **A, B, E.** Insulin glargine is available as a U-300 concentration product (Toujeo). Insulin degludec is available as a U-200 concentration product (Tresiba). Regular insulin is available as a U-500 concentration product (Humulin R U-500).

4. **D.** Based on the request by the patient to make his treatment regimen affordable, Actos (pioglitazone) is the best medication at this time. Pioglitazone improves glycemic control without increasing risk of hypoglycemia. Tradjenta (linagliptin) is a dipeptidyl peptidase-4 inhibitor that does not require renal dose adjustments; however, it is expensive. Farxiga (dapagliflozin) is a sodium-glucose cotransporter-2 inhibitor that could be used in this patient, but at this time he does not have a history of atherosclerotic cardiovascular disease, chronic kidney disease, or heart failure, so there is no compelling reason to prefer this agent over one that is more affordable. Lantus is a basal insulin that primarily targets fasting blood glucose control.

5. **C.** Lipohypertrophy (a bulging of the injection site) is caused by nonrotation of injection sites. The risk of infection may be reduced by using aseptic technique for injections. Lipoatrophy (a pitting of the injection site) may be caused by an antigenic response to insulin. Injection site pain and generalized myalgia are not reduced with injection site rotation.

6. **D.** Glucagon, a pancreatic hormone that is given parenterally, is the most appropriate treatment for a severe hypoglycemic episode because the patient may be unconscious and not able to take a fast-acting carbohydrate by mouth. The other items represent appropriate treatment for mild to moderate hypoglycemia.

7. **D.** Patients with type 1 diabetes require insulin for management. Patients with type 2 diabetes can also use insulin, however, the case situations described do not indicate the need for insulin at this time. Patients with newly diagnosed type 2 diabetes with A1C < 10% should first be treated with lifestyle modifications and metformin (if able to tolerate). Combination oral therapy would be indicated next with failure of monotherapy. Then, following the failure of oral therapy, insulin monotherapy or insulin therapy in combination with oral agents is indicated.

8. **B.** Canagliflozin is a sodium-glucose cotransporter-2 inhibitor. This class of medications has been associated with euglycemic ketoacidosis.

9. **B.** Insulin pharmacokinetics can be altered by temperature at the site of administration. Activities such as rubbing the area will alter the temperature and, therefore, the pharmacokinetics. Rotating the administration site between the abdomen, arm, and leg can alter the pharmacokinetics, but rotation in the same general area does not significantly change the onset, peak, and duration. The needle size and length, timing of administration, and insulin product container do not alter the pharmacokinetics of insulin.

10. **C, E.** There has been controversy regarding the association of pancreatitis with dipeptidyl peptidase-4 inhibitors and glucagon-like peptide-1 agonists. However, use of these agents should be avoided in patients with history of pancreatitis.

11. **A, D.** Modest weight loss (5% to 10%) can improve insulin resistance. Moderate-intensity exercise of 150 minutes per week should be recommended, similar to the general population. Scientific evidence does not support an ideal amount of carbohydrates that should be consumed by patients with type 2 diabetes. Fiber and protein intake should be the same as the general population (fiber 14 g/1000 kcal daily; protein intake is individualized based on current eating patterns).

12. **C.** Patients with type 1 diabetes should be initiated at a dose of 0.4 to 0.5 unit/kg/d of total daily insulin use. Basal insulin should make up 50% of the total daily dose. The patient's current weight of 87 lb is equivalent to 40 kg. A dosage of 0.5 unit/kg/d would calculate to a total daily insulin dose of 20 units, and 50% (10 units) should be initiated as basal insulin.

13. **C, D.** Glyburide and glimepiride are on the American Geriatrics Society's Beers list of medications to avoid in elderly owing to significantly increased risk for hypoglycemic events.

14. **B, C.** Diarrhea is a common adverse drug effect for metformin. To decrease frequency and severity of diarrhea, patients should take metformin with food, change to the extended release formulation, and titrate the medication more slowly than once weekly. Patients should be reassured that frequency and severity of diarrhea will decline with continued use.

15. C. Lactic acidosis can result if metformin is given in this situation, and it can be potentially fatal. Renal function must be evaluated following such a procedure, and it must be stabilized before metformin may be resumed.

16. C, E. SGTL2 inhibitors require renal function for efficacy. Dapagliflozin and ertuglifozin should not be initiated with eGFR less than 45 mL/min/1.73 m² and 60 mL/min/1.73 m², respectively. For patients who were already taking the agents prior to decline in eGFR, experts recommend use may be continued, though efficacy may be limited. Apagliflozin is not an FDA-approved medication.

17. A. Tradjenta is a dipeptidyl peptidase-4 inhibitor. This class of medications can increase a patient's risk for upper respiratory tract infections. When used as monotherapy, agents in this class do not cause hypoglycemia, weight gain, or myopathy. Angioedema can occur but is very rare.

18. B, C, D, E. The alpha-glucosidase inhibitors (acarbose and miglitol), biguanide (metformin), and thiazolidinediones (e.g., rosiglitazone) all require LFTs for monitoring. Insulin glargine, a long-acting insulin, does not require LFTs for monitoring; rather, it requires blood glucose monitoring.

19. A, D. Pioglitazone is a thiazolidinedione and has been associated with exacerbation of heart failure, which led to an FDA boxed warning against use in patients with this condition. Pioglitazone has also been associated with bone fractures. Rosiglitazone has been associated with heart failure, bone fractures, and myocardial infarction. Neither drug in the TZD class has been associated with angioedema or atrial fibrillation.

20. E. Pramlintide (Symlin) was approved in March 2005 as the first new type 1 diabetes treatment in more than 80 years. It is an injectable synthetic version of the human hormone amylin.

21. C, D, A, B, E. Insulin aspart is a rapid-acting insulin with a duration of action of 3 to 5 hours. Insulin regular is a short-acting insulin with a duration of action of 4 to 12 hours. Insulin NPH is an intermediate-acting insulin with a duration of action of 10 to 24 hours. Insulin glargine U-300 is a long-acting insulin with a duration of action >24 hours. Insulin degludec is an ultra-long-acting insulin with a duration of action of up to 42 hours.

22. The correct locations to administer insulin subcutaneously include the back of the upper arm, abdomen (avoiding the umbilicus; extending to the sides), and outer thigh. Administration should be in the subcutaneous tissue, not intradermal or intramuscular.

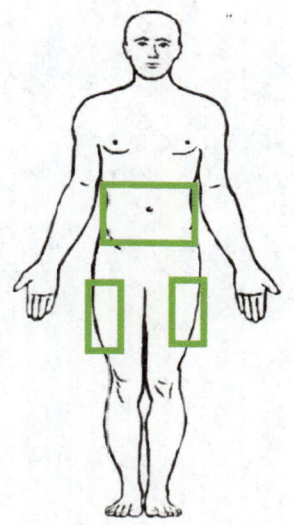 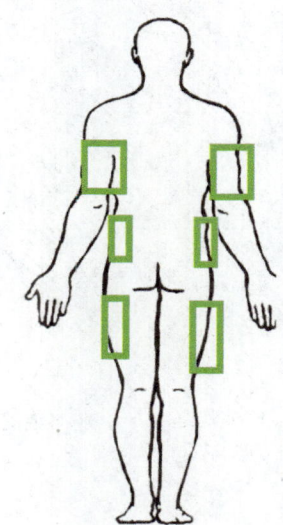

 **17-9 Additional Resources**

American Diabetes Association. Standards of medical care in diabetes—2020. *Diabetes Care.* 2020;43(suppl 1):S1–S212.

Battelino T, Danne T, Bergenstal RM, et al. Clinical targets for continuous glucose monitoring data interpretation: recommendations from the International Consensus on Time in Range. *Diabetes Care.* 2019;42(8):1593–1603.

Beck J, Greenwood DA, Balnton L, et al. 2017 National standards for diabetes self-management education and support. *Diabetes Care.* 2017;40(10):1409–1419.

Diabetes medicines you don't inject. WebMD Web site. Available at: http://www.webmd.com/diabetes/guide/oral-medicine-pills-treat-diabetes#4. Accessed June 6, 2020.

Evert AB, Dennison M, Gardner CD, et al. Nutrition therapy for adults with diabetes or prediabetes: a consensus report. *Diabetes Care.* 2019;42(5):731–754.

Endocrine Disorders

JOYCE E. BROYLES

18-1 KEY POINTS

- **Levothyroxine** is the drug of choice for hypothyroidism.
- Lower doses of **levothyroxine** are used in elderly and cardiac patients.
- Antacids, bile acid sequestrants, calcium, and iron supplements decrease absorption of **levothyroxine** and must be separated by at least 4 hours.
- Propylthiouracil and methimazole are thioamide derivatives used to treat hyperthyroidism.
- Thioamides may cause life-threatening agranulocytosis or hepatitis, so patients must report to their health care provider if they experience fever, sore throat, abdominal pain, or jaundice.
- Corticosteroids should be used at the lowest dose for the shortest time to reduce the risk of hypothalamic-pituitary-adrenocortical axis suppression and adrenal insufficiency.

18-2 STUDY GUIDE CHECKLIST

The following topics may guide your study of this subject area:

- [ ] Regulation of endocrine system.
- [ ] Signs and symptoms of thyroid disease.
- [ ] Monitoring parameters for thyroid replacement.
- [ ] Etiology of Cushing's disease.
- [ ] Symptoms of Addison's disease.
- [ ] Treatment strategies for Addison's disease, including those for an Addisonian crisis.

18-3   Thyroid

Hypothyroidism

Definition and epidemiology

- Hypothyroidism is a syndrome of deficient thyroid hormone production that results in a decrease of all metabolic functions.
- Retardation of growth occurs in infants and children.
- Prevalence of hypothyroidism is greater in women and increases with age; it affects 1.5% to 2% of women and 0.2% of men.

Types

- Primary hypothyroidism is caused by direct thyroid gland failure or injury.
- Other causes of hypothyroidism include thyroidectomy, iodine deficiency, or increasing age.

Hypothyroidism clinical presentation

- Symptoms include cold intolerance, fatigue, somnolence, constipation, menorrhagia, myalgia, and hoarseness.
- Signs include thyroid gland enlargement or atrophy, bradycardia, edema, dry skin, and weight gain.
- Myxedema coma is an end stage of hypothyroidism characterized by weakness, confusion, hypothermia, hypoventilation, hypoglycemia, hyponatremia, coma, and shock.

Pathophysiology

- Thyroxine (T4) is the major hormone secreted by the thyroid; T4 is converted to the more potent triiodothyronine (T3) in tissues.
- Thyroxine secretion is stimulated by the thyroid-stimulating hormone (TSH).
- TSH secretion is inhibited by T3, forming a negative feedback loop.
- Hashimoto's disease is an autoimmune-mediated disease resulting from cell- and antibody-mediated thyroid injury.

Diagnosis

- Plasma TSH assay is the initial test of choice if hypothyroidism is suspected clinically.
- TSH levels are elevated in primary hypothyroidism.
- Low plasma-free T4 (or T4 index) confirms the diagnosis of hypothyroidism.

Treatment principles

- Synthetic thyroxine (**levothyroxine**) is the drug of choice for hypothyroidism because it is chemically stable, inexpensive, free of antigenicity, and uniformly potent.
- Typical maintenance dose is 125 mcg orally once daily.
  - The starting dose in the elderly and in patients with coronary artery disease is reduced to 25 mcg daily to decrease the risk of precipitating cardiac symptoms.
  - Replacement dose should be based on ideal body weight rather than actual body weight.
  - Most adult patients will reach a **levothyroxine** dose of 1.7 mcg/kg/d at steady state.
- The goal of therapy is to maintain plasma TSH in the normal range.
- Dose changes are made at 6 to 8-week intervals until TSH is normalized.
- Overtreatment is detected by subnormal TSH and is associated with symptoms of hyperthyroidism.

- Failure to respond to appropriate doses is most often due to poor compliance.
- Patient compliance may be assessed by monitoring T4 levels.
- Thyroid hormones have a narrow therapeutic index; careful monitoring of clinical condition is required.

Drug therapy for hypothyroidism

Thyroid preparations for the treatment of hypothyroidism are described in Table 18-1.

Mechanism of action

Thyroid hormones enhance oxygen consumption by most tissues and increase basal metabolic rate and metabolism of carbohydrates, lipids, and proteins.

Patient instructions and counseling

- Take once daily, 30 minutes before breakfast, because food may decrease absorption.
- Replacement therapy is usually for life; do not discontinue without advice of the prescriber.
- Notify the prescriber if rapid or irregular heartbeat, chest pain, shortness of breath, nervousness, irritability, tremors, heat intolerance, or weight loss is experienced.

Adverse effects

- *Cardiovascular:* Tachycardia, arrhythmia, angina, myocardial infarction
- *Central nervous system (CNS):* Tremor, headache, nervousness, insomnia, irritability, hyperactivity
- *Gastrointestinal (GI):* Diarrhea, vomiting, cramps
- *Miscellaneous:* Weight loss, fatigue, menstrual irregularities, excessive sweating, heat intolerance, fever, muscle weakness, hair loss, decreased bone mineral density, hypersensitivity

 Thyroid Hormone Medications *FDA BOXED WARNING*

Though thyroid hormone medications can cause weight loss, a U.S. Food and Drug Administration (FDA) boxed warning states that these medications should not be used for treatment of obesity or for weight loss.

TABLE 18-1. **Thyroid Preparations for the Treatment of Hypothyroidism**

Trade name	Generic name	Dosage forms	Usual dosage range
Synthroid, Levothroid, Levoxyl, Unithroid, Thyro-Tabs	Levothyroxine sodium (T4)	Tablet: 0.025, 0.05, 0.075, 0.088, 0.1, 0.112, 0.125, 0.137, 0.15, 0.175, 0.2, 0.3 mg Injection: 200, 500 mcg	0.1 to 0.15 mg orally daily for hypothyroidism (dosage is individualized); higher doses used in treating thyroid cancer
Armour Thyroid, Nature-Throid, Westhroid	Desiccated thyroid USP	Tablet: 15, 30, 32.4, 60, 64.8, 65, 90, 120, 129.6, 130, 180, 194.4, 195, 240, 300 mg	60 to 120 mg orally daily for hypothyroidism (dosage is individualized); higher doses used in treating thyroid cancer
Cytomel, Triostat	Liothyronine (T3)	Tablet: 5, 25, 50 mcg Injection: 10 mcg	25 mcg orally daily for hypothyroidism
Thyrolar	Liotrix (T4 and T3 in a 4:1 ratio)	Tablet: 3.1/12.5, 6.25/25, 12.5/50, 25/100, 37.5/150 mcg	60 to 120 mg orally daily for hypothyroidism

Boldface indicates one of top 100 drugs for 2020 by prescription volume.

Drug–drug interactions

- Use of amiodarone may cause hypothyroidism or hyperthyroidism in euthyroid patients.
- Antidiabetic agents may be less effective with **levothyroxine**. An increase in the antidiabetic therapy may be needed.
- Antacids, calcium, bile acid sequestrants, sucralfate, and iron supplements decrease absorption of **levothyroxine**. Do not take these medications within 4 hours of **levothyroxine**.
- Lithium commonly causes hypothyroidism.
- **Levothyroxine** may enhance **warfarin's** effect and warfarin dosages may need to be decreased.
- **Levothyroxine** supplementation may reduce digoxin levels.
- Soybean enteral formulas decrease **levothyroxine** absorption.
- Sympathomimetic drugs may potentiate the effects of **levothyroxine**.

Monitoring parameters

- Plasma TSH should be evaluated every 6 to 8 weeks until normalization.
- Signs and symptoms of hypothyroidism should improve within a few weeks.
- Once the optimum replacement dose is attained, TSH level should be monitored every 6 to 12 months.
- Patients at risk for coronary artery disease should be closely monitored for signs and symptoms of angina during therapy.

Pharmacokinetics

- The FDA states that all **levothyroxine** products should be considered therapeutically inequivalent unless equivalence (AB rating) has been established and noted in its *Orange Book: Approved Drug Products with Therapeutic Equivalence Evaluations*.
- Because of the narrow therapeutic index of **levothyroxine**, many experts recommend rechecking TSH concentrations 6 to 8 weeks after any change in formulation, even when bioequivalent.
- Oral absorption is improved by fasting but decreased by dietary fiber and foods.
- A half-life of 7 days allows once-daily dosing.
- Average bioavailability of **levothyroxine** products ranges from 40% to 80%. When a switch is made from oral to intravenous (I.V.) **levothyroxine**, the dosage should be reduced by 25% to 50%.

Other

- Use of natural thyroid hormones such as desiccated thyroid USP (United States Pharmacopeia) is discouraged because their potency and stability are less predictable than those of synthetic **levothyroxine**.
- Synthetic T3 (liothyronine) has a shorter half-life than **levothyroxine**, has a higher incidence of cardiac side effects, and is more difficult to monitor.

Hyperthyroidism

Definition and epidemiology

- Hyperthyroidism (thyrotoxicosis) is the clinical syndrome that results when tissues are exposed to high levels of thyroid hormone.
- Thyrotoxicosis is more common in women than men, occurring in 3 per 1000 women.

Types

- Graves' disease is the most common cause of hyperthyroidism.
- Exogenous thyroid hormone ingestion may also cause hyperthyroidism.
- Thyroid storm is a life-threatening, sudden exacerbation of all the symptoms of thyrotoxicosis, characterized by fever, tachycardia, delirium, and coma.
  - Hyperthyroidism clinical presentation
  - Symptoms include heat intolerance, weight loss, weakness, palpitations, and anxiety.

- Signs include tremor; tachycardia; weakness and eyelid lag; and warm, moist skin.
- Other manifestations include atrial fibrillation and congestive heart failure in patients with documented cardiac history.

Pathophysiology

Graves' disease is an autoimmune disease in which thyroid-stimulating antibodies are produced. These antibodies mimic the action of TSH on thyroid tissue.

Diagnosis

Elevated T4 or T3 in the presence of a decreased TSH confirms the diagnosis of hyperthyroidism.

Treatment principles

- The 3 primary methods for controlling hyperthyroidism are surgery, radioactive iodine (RAI), and antithyroid (thioamide) drugs.
- The goals are to minimize symptoms and eliminate excess thyroid hormone.
- RAI is often considered the treatment of choice in Graves' disease.
- Propylthiouracil ⚠ is no longer preferred in pregnancy because of the increased risk of hepatotoxicity; RAI is contraindicated in pregnancy.
- Thioamide drugs (propylthiouracil and methimazole) have no permanent effect on thyroid function; RAI selectively destroys thyroid cells and decreases the ability to produce hormone.
- Adjunctive treatments for hyperthyroidism include beta-adrenergic receptor blockers or nondihydropyridine calcium channel blockers to control tachycardia associated with hyperthyroidism.

Drug therapy for hyperthyroidism

Antithyroid medications are summarized in Table 18-2.

Thioamides

Mechanism of action

- Propylthiouracil and methimazole inhibit the synthesis of thyroid hormones by preventing the incorporation of iodine into iodotyrosines and by inhibiting the coupling of monoiodotyrosine and diiodotyrosine to form T4 and T3, respectfully.
- Propylthiouracil inhibits the peripheral conversion of T4 to T3.

TABLE 18-2. Antithyroid Medications

Drug name	Drug contains	Dosage forms	Usual dosage range
PTU	Propylthiouracil	Tablet: 50 mg	150 to 300 mg orally daily at 8-hour intervals
Tapazole	Methimazole	Tablet: 5, 10 mg	5 to 40 mg orally in single daily dose or divided
Lugol's solution	Strong iodine solution	Solution: 5% iodine and 10% **potassium** iodide; delivers 6.3 mg iodine per drop	0.1 to 0.3 mL (3 to 5 drops) orally three times daily
SSKI	Saturated solution of **potassium** iodide	Solution: 1 g/mL; delivers 38 mg iodine per drop of saturated solution	1 to 5 drops orally three times daily in water or juice

Boldface indicates one of top 100 drugs for 2020 by prescription volume.

Propylthiouracil *FDA BOXED WARNING*

Severe liver injury and acute liver failure, in some cases fatal, have been reported in patients treated with propylthiouracil. These reports of hepatic reactions include cases requiring liver transplantation in adult and pediatric patients. Propylthiouracil should be reserved for patients who cannot tolerate methimazole and in whom radioactive iodine therapy or surgery are not appropriate treatments for the management of hyperthyroidism. Propylthiouracil may be the treatment of choice when an antithyroid drug is indicated during or just prior to the first trimester of pregnancy.

Patient instructions and counseling

- This medication prevents excessive thyroid hormone production and must be taken regularly to be effective.
- Do not discontinue use without first consulting a physician.
- Notify a health care provider if fever, sore throat, unusual bleeding, rash, abdominal pain, or yellowing of the skin occurs.

Adverse effects associated with antithyroid therapy

- **CNS:** Fever, headache, paresthesias
- **General:** Rash, arthralgia, urticaria
- **GI:** Jaundice, hepatitis
- **Hematologic:** Agranulocytosis, leukopenia, bleeding

Drug–drug interactions

Potentiation of **warfarin's** effect may occur, requiring adjustment of dose.

Monitoring parameters

- Monitor for improvement in signs and symptoms of hyperthyroidism.
- Perform thyroid function tests with periodic blood counts; watch for signs and symptoms of agranulocytosis (fever, malaise, sore throat).

Pharmacokinetics

Propylthiouracil and methimazole are typically dosed 3 to 4 times daily, but evidence exists that both drugs may be given once daily.

Iodides

Mechanism of action

- Iodine blocks hormone release and inhibits thyroid hormone synthesis.
- Iodide may be used to rapidly reduce thyroid hormone secretion when desired, such as in thyroid storm, or to decrease glandular vascularity before thyroidectomy.
- Because of its harsh taste and tachyphylaxis with prolonged use, iodides are not used for long-term thyroid suppression.

Patient instructions

- Dilute with water or fruit juice to improve taste.
- Notify a health care provider if fever, skin rash, metallic taste, swelling of the throat, or burning of the mouth occurs.

Adverse effects

Adverse effects include rash, swelling of salivary glands, metallic taste, burning of the mouth, GI distress, hypersensitivity, and goiter.

Drug–drug interactions

Lithium potentiates the antithyroid effect of iodides.

Monitoring parameters

Monitor for improvement in signs and symptoms of hyperthyroidism and for adverse effects.

18-4 Adrenals

Cushing's Syndrome and Cushing's Disease

Definition and epidemiology

- Cushing's syndrome results from chronic glucocorticoid excess.
- The incidence rate is 2 to 4 persons per million population each year.

Types

- Cushing's syndrome is usually iatrogenic, caused by therapy with glucocorticoid drugs.
- Endogenous Cushing's syndrome is usually caused by overproduction of adrenocorticotropic hormone (ACTH) by pituitary gland adenomas.

Clinical presentation

Patients may present with obesity involving the face, neck, trunk, and abdomen; hypertension; hirsutism; acne; amenorrhea; depression; thin skin; easy bruising; diabetes; and osteopenia.

Pathophysiology

The hypothalamus produces a corticotropin-releasing hormone, which stimulates the anterior pituitary gland to release ACTH (corticotropin). Circulating ACTH stimulates the adrenal cortex to produce cortisol.

Diagnosis

- Diagnosis is usually based on signs and symptoms of hypercortisolism.
- Dexamethasone suppression test or 24-hour urine cortisol measurement may be used to determine etiology.

Treatment principles

- If the etiology is iatrogenic, minimization of corticosteroid exposure is essential.
- Pharmacotherapy of Cushing's disease is aimed at reducing cortisol production or activity with drugs, radiation, or surgery.

Drug therapy for Cushing's syndrome

Drugs for Cushing's syndrome are described in Table 18-3.

TABLE 18-3. Drugs for Cushing's Syndrome

Trade name	Generic name	Dosage forms	Usual dosage range
Nizoral	Ketoconazole	Tablet: 250 mg	800 to 1200 mg orally daily
Lysodren	Mitotane	Tablet: 500 mg	9 to 10 g/d orally in divided doses
Metopirone	Metyrapone	Capsule: 250 mg	1 to 6 g/d orally in 4 to 6 divided doses

Mechanism of action
- Drugs used to treat Cushing's disease suppress synthesis of cortisol.
- Ketoconazole inhibits cytochrome P450 (CYP450)–dependent enzymes and cortisol synthesis.
- Mitotane ⚠ is a cytotoxic drug that suppresses ACTH secretion and reduces synthesis of cortisol.
- Metyrapone decreases cortisol synthesis by inhibition of 11-hydroxylase activity.

Patient instructions and counseling
- Ketoconazole should be taken with food.
- Separate from antacids by at least 2 hours.
- Notify a health care provider if abdominal pain, yellow skin, or pale stool occurs.

Adverse effects
- Ketoconazole causes nausea, vomiting, headache, impotence, and hepatotoxicity.
- Metyrapone causes nausea, vomiting, dizziness, and sedation.
- Mitotane may cause nausea, vomiting, diarrhea, and tiredness.

 Mitotane *FDA BOXED WARNING*

In patients taking mitotane, adrenal crisis occurs in the setting of shock or severe trauma and response to shock is impaired. Administer hydrocortisone, monitor for escalating signs of shock, and discontinue mitotane until recovery.

Drug–drug interactions
Ketoconazole is a CYP450 3A4 enzyme inhibitor. Drugs that lower gastric acidity will decrease ketoconazole absorption.

Monitoring parameters
Cortisol monitoring is required with mitotane.

Adrenal Insufficiency

Definition and epidemiology
- Primary adrenocortical deficiency (Addison's disease) is caused by autoimmune-mediated destruction of the adrenal cortex and results in glucocorticoid and mineralocorticoid deficiency.
- Addison's disease occurs in 5 to 6 persons per million population per year.

Types
- Primary adrenal insufficiency (Addison's disease) involves autoimmune destruction of the adrenal cortex.
- Secondary adrenal insufficiency occurs after cessation of chronic exogenous corticosteroid use.
- Acute adrenal insufficiency, or Addisonian crisis, is an endocrine emergency precipitated by severe stress.

Clinical presentation

- *Glucocorticoid deficiency:* Weight loss, malaise, abdominal pain, depression
- *Mineralocorticoid deficiency:* Dehydration, hypotension, hyperkalemia, salt craving

Pathophysiology

- Cortisol is synthesized in the adrenal cortex when cholesterol is converted to pregnenolone by ACTH stimulation.
- The adrenal cortex secretes aldosterone, cortisol, and androgenic hormones.
- Mineralocorticoids (e.g., aldosterone) enhance reabsorption of sodium and water from the distal tubule of the kidney and increase urinary potassium excretion.
- Glucocorticoids affect glucose, carbohydrate, and fat metabolism; produce anti-inflammatory and immunosuppressive effects; and affect other physiologic processes.
- Chronic administration of corticosteroids results in inhibition of pituitary ACTH secretion and reduced cortisol production (hypothalamic-pituitary-adrenocortical [HPA] axis suppression).
- Abrupt cessation of steroids may precipitate adrenal insufficiency.

Diagnosis

A cosyntropin (ACTH) stimulation test may be used to assess hypocortisolism.

Treatment principles

- Addison's disease requires lifelong glucocorticoid and mineralocorticoid replacement.
- Hydrocortisone 100 mg I.V. every 8 hours is the drug of choice for acute adrenal crisis.
- *Stress doses* of corticosteroids may be given for minor illness, injury, or surgery.
- Gradual tapering of exogenous corticosteroids reduces the risk of adrenal insufficiency in patients with HPA axis suppression.
- Fludrocortisone has minimal anti-inflammatory activity and is used only when mineralocorticoid activity is needed, such as when increased blood pressure is desired.

Drug therapy for adrenal insufficiency

Information about corticosteroids is provided in Table 18-4.

Mechanism of action

- Glucocorticoids increase blood glucose by stimulating gluconeogenesis and glycogenolysis; fat deposition is increased.
- Catabolic effects occur in lymphoid and connective tissue, bone, muscle, fat, and skin.
- Glucocorticoids may inhibit of inflammation and immunosuppression by reducing prostaglandin and leukotriene synthesis, decreasing neutrophils at sites of inflammation, and inhibiting macrophage function.

Patient instructions and counseling

- Steroids may cause stomach upset, so take them with food.
- Taking the dose before 9:00 AM is preferable.
- Wear or carry medication identification if on chronic steroid therapy.
- Therapy may mask signs of infection.
- Drugs may increase insulin or oral hypoglycemic requirements if diabetic.
- Notify a health care provider if weight gain, muscle weakness, sore throat, or infection occurs.
- Report tiredness, stomach pain, weakness, and high or low blood sugar to a health care provider.
- Do not discontinue abruptly if taking long term.

TABLE 18-4. Corticosteroids and Dose Equivalents

Trade name	Generic name	Anti-inflammatory potency	Sodium-retaining potency	Equivalent dose (mg)	Half-life
Cortone	Cortisone	0.8	2	25	Short
Cortef, Hydrocortone, Solu-Cortef	**Hydrocortisone**	1	2	20	Short
Deltasone, Liquid Pred	**Prednisone**	4	1	5	Medium
Prelone, Pediapred, Delta-Cortef	**Prednisolone**	4	1	5	Medium
Medrol, Solu-Medrol, Depo-Medrol, A-Methapred	**Methylprednisolone**	5	0	4	Medium
Aristocort, Kenacort, Kenalog	**Triamcinolone**	5	0	4	Medium
Decadron, Dexameth, Dexone, Hexadrol	Dexamethasone	30	0	0.75	Long
Celestone	Betamethasone	25	0	0.75	Long
Florinef	Fludrocortisone	15	150	2	Medium

Boldface indicates one of top 100 drugs for 2020 by prescription volume.

Adverse effects
- *Cardiac:* Hypertension, sodium and fluid retention, atherosclerosis
- *CNS:* Insomnia, anxiety, depression, psychosis
- *Metabolic:* Obesity, hyperglycemia, hypokalemia, amenorrhea, impotence
- *Ophthalmic:* Cataracts, glaucoma
- *Immunologic:* Infections, impaired wound healing, leukocytosis
- *Musculoskeletal:* Myopathy, osteoporosis

Drug–drug interactions
- Rifampin and other enzyme-inducing drugs increase metabolism of corticosteroids and decrease their effectiveness.
- Corticosteroids may impair immunologic response to vaccines in some patient populations.
- Estrogen therapy may increase corticosteroid clearance.
- Concurrent use with nonsteroidal anti-inflammatory drugs may increase the possibility of peptic ulcers.
- Ketoconazole, macrolides, and other CYP450 3A4 enzyme–inhibiting drugs may decrease clearance of corticosteroids.
- Corticosteroids increases blood glucose, increasing insulin and oral hypoglycemic drug requirements.

Monitoring parameters
Patients should be monitored for weight gain, edema, increased blood pressure, abnormal electrolytes, blood glucose, and infection.

Pharmacokinetics
Many doses, schedules, and dosage forms are used, including tablets, topicals, enemas, oral liquids, injections, as well as depot injection forms for intra-articular or intramuscular use.

18-5   Miscellaneous Endocrine Drugs

ACTH and Cosyntropin

Table 18-5 provides information about ACTH and cosyntropin.

TABLE 18-5. ACTH and Cosyntropin

Trade name	Generic name	Dosage forms	Usual dosage range
Cortrosyn	Cosyntropin	Injection: 0.25 mg	0.25 to 0.75 mg for testing
Acthar (ACTH)	Corticotropin	Injection: 25, 40 units	10 to 25 units for testing
H.P. Acthar Gel		Repository injection: 40, 80 units/mL	40 to 80 units of repository injection every 1 to 3 days

Therapeutic uses

ACTH and cosyntropin are used for diagnosis of adrenal insufficiency.

Mechanism of action

- ACTH stimulates the adrenal cortex to secrete adrenal hormones.
- If ACTH fails to elicit an appropriate cortisol response, adrenal insufficiency is present.
- Cosyntropin is a synthetic peptide that is similar to human ACTH but less allergenic.

Patient instructions and counseling and adverse effects

Patients should receive the same counseling as for corticosteroids (see Section 18-4). Adverse effects are the same (see Section 18-4).

Drug–drug interactions

The effects of cosyntropin may be decreased by corticosteroids, estrogen, and **spironolactone**.

Monitoring parameters

Monitoring parameters are the same as for corticosteroids.

Vasopressin

Table 18-6 describes the dosages for vasopressin.

Therapeutic uses

Vasopressin is used to treat diabetes insipidus, variceal hemorrhage, shock, and ventricular fibrillation.

Mechanism of action

- Vasopressin is also known as antidiuretic hormone; it increases water resorption.
- Vasopressin causes vasoconstriction in portal and splanchnic vessels (GI tract).

Adverse effects

Adverse effects of vasopressin include angina, myocardial infarction, vasoconstriction, hyponatremia, gangrene, abdominal cramps, tissue necrosis (if extravasation occurs), and hypersensitivity.

TABLE 18-6. Vasopressin

Trade name	Generic name	Dosage forms	Usual dosage range
Pitressin	Vasopressin	Injection: 20 units/mL	10 to 20 units intramuscular, subcutaneous, or I.V. daily at 3- to 4-hour intervals or as a continuous infusion

Drug–drug interactions

Vasopressin may enhance effects of other pressors.

Monitoring parameters

- With diabetes insipidus, monitor urine volume and plasma osmolality.
- When I.V. vasopressin is used, monitor blood pressure and pulse.

Androgens and Anabolic Steroids

Table 18-7 provides information about androgens and anabolic steroids.

Therapeutic uses

- Androgens ⚠ and anabolic steroids are used to treat hypogonadism, delayed puberty, metastatic breast cancer, anemia, corticosteroid-induced hypogonadism and osteoporosis, and moderate to severe vasomotor symptoms associated with menopause (when combined with estrogen). See Chapter 38.
- They are schedule C-III controlled substances because they are intentionally misused by individuals seeking performance-enhancing effects and enhanced muscular development and endurance.

Mechanism of action

- Androgens promote growth and development of male sex organs and maintenance of secondary sex characteristics.

TABLE 18-7. Androgens and Anabolic Steroids

Trade name	Generic name	Dosage forms	Usual dosage range
AndroGel 1.62%	Testosterone	Gel: 1.62%	40.5 mg once daily
Axiron	Testosterone	Solution: 30 mg/1.5 mL	30 mg once daily
Fortesta	Testosterone	Gel: 10 mg/0.5 g	40 mg once daily
Testoderm	Testosterone transdermal system	Patch: 2.5, 4, 5, 6 mg	Patch: 2.5 to 6 mg for 24 hours
Androderm	Testosterone transdermal system	Patch: 2, 2.5, 4, 5 mg	Patch: 2 to 7.5 mg for 24 hours
AndroGel 1%, Testim	Testosterone	Gel: 1%	5 g once daily
Depo-Testosterone	Testosterone cypionate (in oil)	Injection in oil: 100, 200 mg/mL	50 to 400 mg every 2 to 4 weeks
Delatestryl	Testosterone enanthate (in oil)	Injection in oil: 100, 200 mg/mL	50 to 400 mg every 2 to 4 weeks
Testopel	Testosterone	Pellet for subcutaneous implantation: 75 mg	150 to 450 mg every 3 to 6 months
Striant	Testosterone	Buccal tablet: 30 mg	30 mg every 12 hours
Methitest	Methyltestosterone	Tablet: 10, 25 mg	10 to 50 mg once daily
Testred, Android	Methyltestosterone	Capsule: 10 mg	10 to 50 mg once daily
Halotestin, Androxy	Fluoxymesterone	Tablet: 2, 5, 10 mg	5 to 10 mg once daily
Anadrol-50	Oxymetholone	Tablet: 50 mg	50 to 100 mg once daily
Winstrol	Stanozolol	Tablet: 2 mg	2 mg daily three times daily
Oxandrin	Oxandrolone	Tablet: 2.5, 10 mg	2.5 to 10 mg daily
Deca-Durabolin	Nandrolone decanoate	Injection: 100, 200 mg/mL (in oil)	100 to 200 mg once weekly

- Androgens also cause retention of nitrogen, sodium, potassium, and phosphorus; increase protein anabolism; and decrease protein catabolism.
- Androgens are responsible for the growth spurt of adolescence and termination of linear growth by fusion of epiphyseal growth centers.
- Exogenous androgens stimulate production of red blood cells, suppress endogenous testosterone release through feedback inhibition of luteinizing hormone, and suppress spermatogenesis through feedback inhibition of follicle-stimulating hormone.

 Androgen *FDA BOXED WARNING*

SECONDARY EXPOSURE TO TESTOSTERONE: Virilization has been reported in children who were secondarily exposed to testosterone gel. Children should avoid contact with unwashed or unclothed application sites in men using testosterone gel. Health care providers should advise patients to strictly adhere to recommended instructions for use.

Patient instructions and counseling

- Medication may cause stomach upset.
- Notify a health care provider if swelling of the ankles or persistent erections occur.
- This product is a controlled substance; do not misuse or abuse it.
- For females, notify a health care provider if deepening of the voice, increased facial hair, or menstrual irregularities occur.
- Patients receiving transdermal testosterone should be provided with the manufacturer's patient instructions and carefully counseled on use and disposal of the system.

Adverse effects

- **General:** Jaundice, hepatitis, edema, high abuse potential in an effort to enhance athletic performance, hypercholesterolemia and atherosclerosis, increased aggression, and libido
- **Women:** Hirsutism, voice deepening, acne, decreased menses, clitoral enlargement
- **Men:** Acne, sleep apnea, gynecomastia, azoospermia, prostate enlargement, decreased testicular size

18-6 Pharmacist's Role

Patient education is key to successful treatment of many endocrine conditions, because therapy is dependent upon excellent patient compliance and the need for frequent laboratory monitoring. Because these are often lifetime conditions, the pharmacist should make periodic assessment of the patient's knowledge. Pharmacists may also actively manage many endocrine conditions in the outpatient setting.

NAPLEX Competency Statements

The questions in this chapter cover the following 2021 NAPLEX Competency Statements: **AREA 1:** 1.1; 1.2; 1.3; 1.4; 1.5 **AREA 2:** 2.1; 2.2 **AREA 3:** 3.2; 3.3; 3.4; 3.6; 3.7; 3.8; 3.9 **AREA 5:** 5.1.

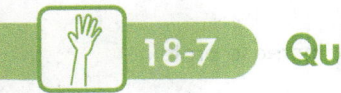

18-7   Questions

Use Patient Profile 18-1 to answer Question 1.

1. The Synthroid prescription dispensed to the patient on 3/21 requires advising her to _____.

A. take 4 hours before or 4 hours after Questran
B. take with food
C. watch for signs of infection
D. take as needed to keep her desired level of energy
E. discontinue if she experiences nausea

2. Which of the following conditions could Synthroid exacerbate?

A. Hypercholesterolemia
B. Anemia
C. Coronary artery disease
D. Hypertension
E. Constipation

3. Excessive doses of **levothyroxine** may cause _____.

A. weight gain
B. osteoporosis
C. cold intolerance
D. bradycardia
E. sedation

PATIENT PROFILE 18-1. Corn State Community Pharmacy

Patient: 78-year-old female   **Height:** 4'8"
Race: Hispanic   **Weight:** 103 lb
Allergies: Cats

Pharmacist notes

Diagnosis	Date	Comment
1. Hypercholesterolemia	2/23	Reminded patient to continue taking aspirin 325 mg for CAD
2. Anemia		Advised patient to take OTC ferrous sulfate 325 mg daily for 3 months for anemia
3. Coronary artery disease		Advised patient to begin docusate 100 mg daily if constipation occurs
4. Hypertension		

Medication orders

Date	Rx No.	Physician	Drug and strength	Quantity	Sig	Refills
2/23	88768	Hooper	Zocor 40 mg	30	1 orally nightly	5
2/23	88769	Hooper	Questran 4 g	60	1 packet twice a day, mix with juice	5
2/23	88770	Hooper	Tenormin 50 mg	30	1 orally daily	5
2/23	88771	Hooper	Enalapril 5 mg	60	1 orally twice a day	5
3/21	89995	Stubie	Synthroid 0.025 mg	30	1 orally daily	0

4. Which of the following drugs may produce hypothyroidism?

   A. Amitriptyline
   B. Sertraline
   C. Cholestyramine and ACTH
   D. Lithium and amiodarone
   E. Levothyroxine

5. Which of the following is *not* likely to decrease the effect of thyroid hormone supplementation?

   A. Antacids
   B. Bile acid sequestrants
   C. Estrogens
   D. Sucralfate
   E. Theophylline

6. A patient who is suffering from heat intolerance, weight loss, tachycardia, tremor, and anxiety may be treated with _____.

   A. acetaminophen
   B. mitotane
   C. cyproheptadine
   D. propylthiouracil
   E. diazepam

7. A patient with atrial fibrillation may require a decreased warfarin dosage when which of the following drugs is initiated?

   A. Liothyronine
   B. Propylthiouracil
   C. Methimazole
   D. ACTH
   E. Diphenhydramine

8. Which of the following drugs is used to treat Cushing's disease?

   A. Clotrimazole
   B. Propylthiouracil
   C. Mitotane
   D. Vasopressin
   E. Prednisone

9. Which of the following drugs works by decreasing cortisol synthesis?

   A. Cortrosyn
   B. ACTH
   C. Oxandrolone
   D. Prednisone
   E. Metyrapone

10. Decreased ketoconazole absorption may occur if it is administered concomitantly with which of the following?

    A. Antacids
    B. Food
    C. Warfarin
    D. Cyclosporine
    E. CYP450 3A4 inhibitors

11. Close monitoring of adrenal hormone secretion may be required when administering which of the following?

    A. Methyltestosterone
    B. Mitotane
    C. Desmopressin
    D. Iodides
    E. Propylthiouracil

12. Which of the following is used to treat adrenal crisis?

    A. Cosyntropin
    B. Levothyroxine
    C. Fluoxymesterone
    D. Vasopressin
    E. Hydrocortisone

13. Which of the following is *not* an effect of glucocorticoids?

    A. Immunosuppression
    B. Decreased prostaglandin synthesis
    C. Inhibition of glycogenolysis
    D. Decreased neutrophils at sites of infection
    E. Inhibition of macrophages

Use Patient Profile 18-2 to answer Question 14.

14. Which of the following is least likely to contribute to the increased blood glucose seen in this patient?

    A. Dextrose 5%/NaCl 0.9% solution
    B. Captopril
    C. Epinephrine
    D. Methylprednisolone
    E. Anaphylaxis

PATIENT PROFILE 18-2. Big Sky Hospital

Patient: 28-year-old male
Race: White

Date of admission: 4/21 at 15:26
Height: 5'8"
Weight: 178 lb
Allergies: Aspirin

Diagnosis
Admit diagnosis
Secondary

1. Anaphylactic reaction to aspirin
1. Type 2 diabetes mellitus
2. Hypertension

Laboratory

Date	Time	Lab	Result	(Normal range)
4/21	15:29	Glucose	144	(60 to 110 mg/dL)
4/21	19:20	Glucose	181	(60 to 110 mg/dL)
4/22	06:00	Glucose	240	(60 to 110 mg/dL)
4/22	12:21	Glucose	289	(60 to 110 mg/dL)
4/22	19:15	Glucose	352	(60 to 110 mg/dL)
4/23	06:20	Glucose	391	(60 to 110 mg/dL)
4/23	12:32	Glucose	443	(60 to 110 mg/dL)

Active medication orders

Date	Time	Drug and strength	Route	Frequency or schedule
4/21	15:30	Solu-Medrol 125 mg	I.V.	Every 6 hours
4/21	15:30	Dextrose 5%/NaCl 0.9%	I.V.	200 mL/h
4/21	15:30	Diphenhydramine 50 mg	I.V.	Every 6 hours
4/21	17:03	Glipizide 5 mg	Oral	Twice daily
4/21	17:03	Glucophage 850 mg	Oral	Twice daily
4/21	17:03	Captopril 50 mg	Oral	Twice daily

Discontinued medication orders

Date	Time	Drug and strength	Route	Frequency or schedule
4/21	15:30	Epinephrine 0.1 mg	Subcutaneous	Stat
4/21	15:30	Diphenhydramine 50 mg	I.V.	Stat

Dietary

Date	Comment
4/21	1800 kcal American Diabetes Association diet

15. A diabetic patient is given a new prescription for Deltasone 40 mg orally daily for 7 days. He should be instructed to _____.

   A. check feet closely for wounds
   B. take ibuprofen for musculoskeletal pain
   C. take Deltasone on an empty stomach
   D. take Deltasone at bedtime
   E. wear identification for steroid therapy

16. Chronic administration of glucocorticoids predisposes patients to which of the following?

   A. Arthritis
   B. Obesity
   C. Alzheimer's disease
   D. Osteoporosis
   E. Hepatitis

17. A patient is taking prednisone 40 mg daily for 6 months. On abrupt cessation, which of the following may occur?

   A. Myopathy
   B. Diabetes
   C. Infection
   D. Adrenal crisis
   E. Psychosis

18. An increased risk of peptic ulcer disease occurs when nonsteroidal anti-inflammatory drugs are combined with which of the following?

   A. Ranitidine
   B. Ferrous sulfate
   C. Dexamethasone
   D. Carbamazepine
   E. Acetaminophen

19. Which of the following drugs may be used to diagnose adrenal insufficiency?

   A. Desmopressin
   B. Clemastine
   C. Captopril
   D. Cosyntropin
   E. Aminoglutethimide

20. Which of the following hormones is secreted by the pituitary gland?

   A. Adrenocorticotropic hormone
   B. Testosterone
   C. Cortisol
   D. Thyroxine
   E. Corticotropin-releasing hormone

21. Chronic administration of testosterone is *not* likely to produce which of the following complications?

   A. Prostate enlargement
   B. Increased testicular size
   C. Gynecomastia in men
   D. Accelerated atherosclerosis
   E. Decreased menses in women

22. Androderm is administered _____.

   A. once daily
   B. 3 times per week
   C. once weekly
   D. every 2 weeks
   E. monthly

23. Which of the following is *not* an acceptable indication for testosterone?

   A. Anemia
   B. Hypogonadism
   C. Delayed puberty
   D. Body building
   E. Metastatic breast cancer

 18-8   Answers

1. **A.** Bile acid sequestrants reduce levothyroxine absorption and must be separated from levothyroxine administration by at least 4 hours. Levothyroxine should be administered before a meal on an empty stomach to maximize absorption.

2. **C.** Thyroid hormones enhance oxygen consumption and increase the oxygen demand. They should be used with caution in patients with coronary artery disease.

3. **B.** Levothyroxine decreases bone mineral density and, when given in supratherapeutic doses, may cause osteoporosis. For this reason, the lowest possible replacement dose should be administered.

4. **D.** Lithium and amiodarone both have been associated with hypothyroidism. Amiodarone contains iodine and may cause hypo- or hyperthyroidism.

5. **E.** Numerous drugs are known to decrease thyroid hormone absorption, including antacids that contain divalent and trivalent cations, calcium salts, magnesium, sucralfate, and bile acid sequestrants. Estrogens and enzyme-inducing drugs may decrease circulating thyroid hormone levels and necessitate a dose increase of thyroxine.

6. **D.** Heat intolerance, weight loss, tachycardia, tremor, and anxiety are cardinal features of hyperthyroidism. Propylthiouracil is effective at reducing the excessive thyroxine level.

7. **A.** Liothyronine (Cytomel) is T3, a potent thyroid hormone. In states of hypothyroidism, metabolism is decreased. However, if thyroid hormone is supplemented, blood clotting factors will be metabolized more quickly, leading to decreased warfarin requirements.

8. **C.** Mitotane is used to treat Cushing's disease. Propylthiouracil is used to treat hyperthyroidism. Clotrimazole is a topical antifungal, vasopressin is used to treat diabetes insipidus, and prednisone is a steroid.

9. **E.** Metyrapone (Metopirone) inhibits 11-hydroxylase activity and, thus, decreases cortisol synthesis.

10. **A.** Ketoconazole requires the presence of stomach acid to be absorbed. Any drug that decreases gastric acidity will decrease the extent of ketoconazole absorption. Food increases ketoconazole absorption because food stimulates release of gastric acid.

11. **B.** Mitotane is cytotoxic to adrenal cells and, thus, reduces cortisol synthesis and release. ACTH increases cortisol release. Close monitoring of cortisol levels is important when mitotane is used.

12. **E.** Hydrocortisone is the drug of choice for adrenal crisis because it possesses both mineralocorticoid and glucocorticoid properties. Although cosyntropin increases cortisol release, patients with adrenal crisis may not have enough adrenal reserve to meet their increased demand.

13. **C.** Glucocorticoids have potent effects on glucose and carbohydrate metabolism. They promote glycogen breakdown, rather than inhibit it.

14. **B.** Captopril increases insulin sensitivity and would not be expected to contribute to increased blood glucose. This patient's blood glucose began rising shortly after admission. His I.V. fluids contain glucose; epinephrine increases blood glucose by increasing glycogen breakdown, methylprednisolone (Solu-Medrol) promotes glycogenolysis, and anaphylaxis would be expected to increase stress response, thereby leading to increased epinephrine release and increased blood glucose.

15. **A.** The patient has diabetes and will be given prednisone (Deltasone), which would be expected to increase blood glucose. When diabetes is poorly controlled, infections are more likely to occur. For this reason, he should monitor more closely for wounds that may become infected. He will not be taking prednisone long enough to develop adrenal insufficiency, so he does not need to wear identification for steroid therapy.

16. **D.** Glucocorticoids have catabolic effects on several tissues, including muscle, fat, skin, and bone. Chronic administration leads to osteopenia and osteoporosis.

17. **D.** Chronic administration of glucocorticoids such as prednisone will lead to feedback inhibition of pituitary ACTH release and atrophy of the adrenal cortex. When prednisone is abruptly stopped, the adrenals will not be able to meet the body's demand for cortisol during severe stress, and adrenal crisis may occur.

18. **C.** Corticosteroids such as dexamethasone (Decadron) are known to increase the risk of peptic ulcers when used in combination with NSAIDs.

19. **D.** Cosyntropin (Cortrosyn) is a synthetic analogue of ACTH that is used to diagnose adrenal insufficiency. It works by stimulating the adrenal cortex to secrete cortisol. If cosyntropin administration does not result in an appropriate increase in cortisol release, adrenal insufficiency is present.

20. **A.** Adrenocorticotropic hormone, or ACTH, is released by the pituitary and acts on the adrenal glands to increase cortisol release. Corticotropin-releasing hormone is released by the hypothalamus and acts on the pituitary to stimulate ACTH release.

21. **B.** Stanozolol (Winstrol) is an androgen that would be expected to promote growth and development of male sex organs. However, chronic administration leads to feedback inhibition of testosterone secretion, which leads to testicular atrophy.

22. **A.** Testosterone transdermal systems (Androderm, Testoderm) are applied once daily for 24 hours. Longer-acting androgens are available, such as nandrolone decanoate (Deca-Durabolin), for once-weekly administration.

23. **D.** Anabolic steroids may be abused by those who are seeking enhanced muscular development and endurance, such as athletes. For this reason, all these agents are subject to the Controlled Substances Act.

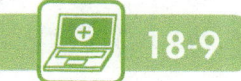 **18-9** ## Additional Resources

Baskin HJ, Cobin RH, Duick DS, et al. American Association of Clinical Endocrinologists medical guidelines for clinical practice for the evaluation and treatment of hyperthyroidism and hypothyroidism (AACE Thyroid Task Force). *Endocr Pract.* 2002;8(6):457–469.

Dietrich E, Smith SM, Gums JG. Adrenal gland disorders. In: DiPiro J, Talbert R, Yee G, et al., eds. *Pharmacotherapy: A Pathophysiologic Approach.* 9th ed. New York, NY: McGraw-Hill; 2014:1217–1236.

Garber JR, Cobin RH, Gharib H, et al. Clinical practice guidelines for hypothyroidism in adults: cosponsored by the American Association of Clinical Endocrinologists and the American Thyroid Association. *Endocr Pract.* 2012;18(6):988–1028.

Jonklaas J, Kane MP. Thyroid disorders. In: DiPiro J, Talbert R, Yee G, et al., eds. *Pharmacotherapy: A Pathophysiologic Approach.* 10th ed. New York, NY: McGraw-Hill; 2017:1183–1206.

Smith SM, Gums JG. Adrenal gland disorders. In: DiPiro J, Talbert R, Yee G, et al., eds. *Pharmacotherapy: A Pathophysiologic Approach.* 8th ed. New York, NY: McGraw-Hill; 2011:1327–1344.

U.S. Food and Drug Administration. *Orange Book: Approved Drug Products with Therapeutic Equivalence Evaluations.* 36th ed. Silver Spring, MD: U.S. Food and Drug Administration; 2016. Available at: https://www.accessdata.fda.gov /scripts/cder/ob/default.cfm.

Geriatrics and Gerontology

SHANNON L. STEWART

19-1 KEY POINTSS

ALZHEIMER'S DISEASE

- Alzheimer's disease is a progressive neurologic disease that results in impaired memory and intellectual functioning and altered behavior.
- Alzheimer's disease has no cure, but therapies exist to decrease memory impairment and to improve behavior and patient functioning.
- Other forms of dementia that are potentially reversible should be identified and treated accordingly.
- New drug therapies may slow the progression of Alzheimer's disease and allow patients to remain in the least restrictive environment possible.

PARKINSON'S DISEASE

- Parkinson's disease is a chronic, progressive neurologic disease for which no cure exists; medications are available to slow the progression of symptoms.
- The etiology of Parkinson's disease is unknown but may involve genetic susceptibility combined with environmental toxins and age-related changes in the brain.
- Dopamine, the central neurotransmitter, is decreased in Parkinson's disease, and current drug therapy is primarily directed at increasing dopamine levels.
- Drug therapy monitoring in Parkinson's disease requires an understanding of a variety of different medications that may cause significant adverse effects.

GLAUCOMA

- Glaucoma, a group of eye diseases, is characterized by increased intraocular pressure resulting in damage to the optic nerve and possible blindness.
- Open-angle glaucoma is the most common form of this disease; angle-closure glaucoma can be a medical emergency.
- The goal of therapy is to reduce intraocular pressure with the simplest medication regimen possible.
- Drug therapy for glaucoma usually begins with a topical beta-adrenergic antagonist; patients often require combination therapy.

URINARY INCONTINENCE

- Urinary incontinence is a significant issue with social and functional implications for geriatric patients.
- Urge incontinence is the most common complaint in older women whereas overflow incontinence is the most frequent issue for geriatric men.
- Drug therapy can improve symptoms but may not completely resolve urinary incontinence.
- Correctly identifying the type of urinary incontinence is important because the drug therapy for one type can worsen another type of incontinence.

Editor's Note: This chapter is based on the 11th edition chapter written by William Nathan Rawls.

19-2 STUDY GUIDE CHECKLIST

The following topics may guide your study of this subject area:

- ☐ Risks associated with taking multiple medications.
- ☐ Pharmacokinetic changes associated with aging.
- ☐ Proposed mechanism of action of drugs used for Alzheimer's disease.
- ☐ Trade names and available dosage forms of drugs used for Alzheimer's disease.
- ☐ Significant drug interactions of drugs used for Alzheimer's disease.
- ☐ Actions of medications used for Parkinson's disease.
- ☐ Considerations for selection of medications for Parkinson's disease.
- ☐ The role of medications in treating glaucoma.
- ☐ Actions of medications used for glaucoma.
- ☐ Trade names and available dosage forms of medications used for glaucoma.
- ☐ Patient instructions for the use of medications for glaucoma.
- ☐ Types of urinary incontinence and medication treatment selection.
- ☐ Actions of medications used for urinary incontinence.
- ☐ Trade names and available dosage forms of drugs used for urinary incontinence.
- ☐ Drug interactions that can worsen urinary incontinence.

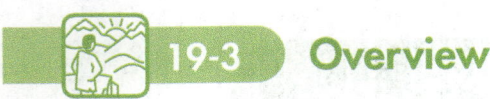

19-3   Overview

Gerontology is the study of the problems of aging and all its aspects. *Geriatrics* focuses on the diseases associated with aging and the treatments for those conditions.

More than 12% of the U.S. population is older than 65 years of age. By 2050, the percentage is expected to increase to over 20%.

Persons older than 65 years of age have more chronic illnesses and take more prescription and non-prescription drugs than persons in younger age groups.

Age-related physiologic changes and increased medication use contribute to a greater risk of adverse drug events. Changes in vision, hearing, and mental functioning can result in increased problems with medication compliance.

Adverse Drug Events in the Older Adult

Drug-related hospitalizations occur four times more often for older adults than for younger adults. Nearly 100,000 older adults are hospitalized each year because of adverse drug effects; insulin, oral hypo-glycemic agents, and **warfarin** are the most often implicated medications. Other drugs of concern and selected issues are documented in Table 19-1.

Older adults receiving multiple medications are at risk of a "prescribing cascade" that occurs when an unrecognized adverse effect of a medication is treated as a new illness and additional medications are prescribed.

Older adults are at increased risk of drug–drug interactions when taking multiple medications, and this potential is decreased by medication simplification.

Changes in Pharmacokinetics Associated with Aging

Decreased absorption of various drugs occurs secondary to decreased stomach acidity and changes in blood flow to the stomach (the least altered by aging). Absorption is also altered by co-administration of medications that either bind or compete for absorption.

Altered drug distribution is caused by a decrease in total body water, increased lipid storage, and decreased serum albumin in malnourished elderly persons. These factors can contribute to increased serum levels of drugs. With increased body fat as seen in many older adults, greater storage of lipid-soluble drugs occurs. Benzodiazepines such as diazepam ⚠ will accumulate with repeated doses and have a prolonged effect. Hydrophilic drugs are distributed in lean body mass and can accumulate in older persons with increased blood levels that can prove excessive.

Drug metabolism is necessary to allow the elimination of most drugs; however, decreased hepatic blood flow and reduced hepatic enzyme activity slow drug metabolism. Increased levels of drugs require

TABLE 19-1. Drugs of Concern

Drugs causing ADE and hospitalizations	Drugs causing psychiatric symptoms	Drugs causing anxiety	Drugs causing nutritional deficiencies
Warfarin	Narcotics	Theophylline	Diuretics
Insulin	Tricyclic antidepressants	Nasal decongestants	Digoxin, digitalis
Oral hypoglycemic agents	CNS stimulants	Beta agonists	Laxatives (overuse)
Oral antiplatelet agents	Antiparkinson drugs	Antiparkinson drugs	Sedatives (overuse)
	Anticholinergic drugs	Appetite suppressants	

ADE, adverse drug effect; CNS, central nervous system.

Diazepam *FDA BOXED WARNING*

Concomitant use of benzodiazepines and opioids may result in profound sedation, respiratory depression, coma, and death. Limit use to lowest possible dose and shortest possible duration if must be used.

increased metabolism by the liver, but a decrease in liver size and function is associated with aging. The resulting increase in drug levels can produce adverse effects.

Elimination of drugs by the kidneys is slowed because of decreased renal blood flow and lowered glomerular filtration; thus, drug accumulation develops.

In dosing the elderly, the general rule is to start with doses lower than those used in younger patients and to increase doses at a slower rate.

19-4   Alzheimer's Disease and Related Dementias

Dementia is the decline in intellectual abilities (e.g., impairment of memory, judgment, and abstract thinking) coupled with changes in personality. Dementia patients tend to be described as cognitively impaired.

Cognition is the mental process by which people become aware of objects of thought and perception, including all aspects of thinking and remembering.

Types of Dementia

Alzheimer's disease accounts for approximately 70% of dementias. Vascular dementias account for approximately 15% of dementias. Patients may have both Alzheimer's disease and vascular dementia. Table 19-2 lists other causes of dementia.

Clinical Presentation

Alzheimer's disease is a progressive neurologic disease that results in impaired memory and intellectual functioning and altered behavior. Alzheimer's disease is characterized by the slow onset of symptoms leading to loss of ability to function independently. Symptoms may include psychoses with hallucinations, illusions, and delusional thinking. As Alzheimer's disease progresses, the brain continues to deteriorate.

Depression can cause cognitive impairment similar to that of Alzheimer's disease and should be identified and treated.

TABLE 19-2. Other Causes of Dementia

Cause	Example
Vascular	Vascular disease, cerebrovascular accidents
Neurologic disorders	Parkinson's disease, frontotemporal dementia, dementia with Lewy bodies, Huntington's chorea
Metabolic disorders	Hypothyroidism, alcoholism, anemia
Infectious diseases	Meningitis, AIDS, syphilis

Pathophysiology

Hallmark pathologic changes in the brain are linked to Alzheimer's disease (i.e., neuritic plaques and neurofibrillary tangles increase). Neuritic plaques are composed of amyloid proteins deposited on neurons. Neurofibrillary tangles exist within neurons and disrupt normal function.

Neurotransmitters are also altered in Alzheimer's disease. Acetylcholine concentrations decrease significantly.

Diagnostic Criteria

Diagnostic criteria are described in Box 19-1.

Treatment Principles

When evaluating a patient for treatment of dementia and Alzheimer's disease, review the patient's medications and consider any that might cause mental confusion or worsen underlying disease states. Drugs that block activity of acetylcholine can worsen dementia and decrease the effectiveness of medications used to treat Alzheimer's disease.

Anticholinergic drugs are used for a variety of conditions, ranging from depression to incontinence. Anticholinergic effects can be additive (i.e., a combination of anticholinergic drugs can result in toxicity even when each is given at low doses (Table 19.3).

Other goals are to provide support to caregivers and to treat the patient's behavioral and mood symptoms.

Providers may consider a trial of a cholinesterase inhibitor. Benefits to memory and cognitive functioning should be monitored.

Monitoring

Monitor memory and cognitive functions every 6 to 12 months.

Routinely assess behaviors and ability to perform activities of daily living (e.g., bathing, feeding, toileting, dressing).

Monitor for focal neurologic signs and symptoms that may suggest other causes of changes in cognitive function.

Drug Therapy

The pharmacologic approach to treatment falls into two categories:

- Medications used to control behavioral and emotional symptoms
- Medications used to slow or reverse the disease process

Symptomatic therapy

Medications used to control behavioral and emotional symptoms are used to provide symptomatic improvement and do not affect the outcome of the disease.

> BOX 19-1. Diagnostic Criteria

Diagnosis of Alzheimer's disease requires the presence of memory impairment and one or more of the following:

- Aphasia (language disturbance)
- Apraxia (impaired motor abilities)
- Agnosia (failure to recognize objects)
- Disturbance of executive function (e.g., planning, organizing)

TABLE 19-3. Anticholinergic Drugs that Can Worsen Alzheimer's Disease

Class	Drugs
Antidepressants	*Highest effects:* **amitriptyline** ⚠, amoxapine ⚠, clomipramine ⚠, protriptyline ⚠ *Moderate effects:* **bupropion** ⚠, doxepin ⚠, imipramine ⚠, maprotiline ⚠, trimipramine ⚠
Antiparkinson agents	Benztropine, trihexyphenidyl
Antipsychotics	*Highest effects:* clozapine ⚠, mesoridazine ⚠, olanzapine ⚠, triflupromazine, thioridazine ⚠ *Moderate effects:* chlorpromazine ⚠, chlorprothixene, pimozide
Antispasmodics	Atropine, belladonna alkaloids, dicyclomine, glycopyrrolate, hyoscyamine, methscopolamine, propantheline, **oxybutynin**, flavoxate
Antihistamines	*Highest effects:* carbinoxamine, clemastine, diphenhydramine, promethazine *Moderate effects:* azatadine, brompheniramine, chlorpheniramine, cyproheptadine, dexchlorpheniramine, triprolidine, **hydroxyzine**
Antiemetic–antivertigo agents	Meclizine, scopolamine, dimenhydrinate, trimethobenzamide, prochlorperazine ⚠
Other agent with some anticholinergic activity	**Paroxetine** ⚠

Boldface indicates one of top 100 drugs for 2020 by prescription volume.

 FDA BOXED WARNINGS

Amitriptyline
Antidepressants increased the risk of suicidal thinking in children, adolescents, and young adults, in short-term studies of major depressive disorder and other psychiatric disorders. No increased risk beyond age 24, and there was a reduction in risk with antidepressants compared to placebo in adults aged 65 and older.

Amoxapine
Antidepressants increased the risk of suicidal thinking in children, adolescents, and young adults, in short-term studies of major depressive disorder and other psychiatric disorders. No increased risk beyond age 24, and there was a reduction in risk with antidepressants compared to placebo in adults aged 65 and older.

Clomipramine
Antidepressants increased the risk of suicidal thinking and behavior in children, adolescents, and young adults in short-term studies with major depressive disorder and other psychiatric disorders. No increased risk beyond age 24, and there was a reduction in risk with antidepressants compared to placebo in adults aged 65 and older.

Protriptyline
In short-term studies, antidepressants increased the risk of suicidal thinking and behavior compared with placebo in children, adolescents, and young adults with psychiatric disorders, including major depressive disorder (MDD); there was not an increased risk of suicidality with antidepressants in adults older than 24 years, and there was a decreased risk of suicidality in adults aged 65 years or older.

Bupropion
Antidepressants increased the risk of suicidal thoughts and behavior in children, adolescents, and young adults in short-term trials. These trials did not show an increase in the risk of suicidal thoughts and behavior with antidepressant use in subjects aged 65 and older.

Doxepin
Antidepressant use has been associated with an increased risk of suicidal thinking and behavior in children, adolescents, and young adults. Short-term studies did not show an increase in the risk of suicidality with antidepressants compared with placebo in adults beyond age 24, and there was a reduction in risk with antidepressants compared with placebo in adults aged 65 or older.

(continued)

FDA BOXED WARNINGS *(Continued)*

Imipramine

Antidepressant use has been associated with an increased risk of suicidal thinking and behavior in children, adolescents, and young adults. Short-term studies did not show an increase in the risk of suicidality with antidepressants compared with placebo in adults beyond age 24, and there was a reduction in risk with antidepressants compared with placebo in adults aged 65 or older.

Maprotiline

Antidepressants increased the risk of suicidal thinking in children, adolescents, and young adults in short-term studies of major depressive disorder and other psychiatric disorders. No increased risk beyond age 24, and there was a reduction in risk with antidepressants compared to placebo in adults aged 65 and older.

Trimipramine

Antidepressants increased the risk of suicidal thoughts and behaviors in pediatric and young adult patients in short-term studies. These studies did not show any increased risk of suicidality with antidepressants compared to placebo in adults beyond age 24; there was a reduction in risk with antidepressants compared to placebo in adults aged 65 and older.

Clozapine

May cause severe neutropenia, which can lead to serious and fatal infections. Patients initiating and continuing treatment with clozapine must have a baseline blood absolute neutrophil count (ANC) measured before treatment initiation and regular ANC monitoring during treatment. Orthostatic hypotension, bradycardia, and syncope: risk is dose related. Starting dose is 12.5 mg. Titrate gradually and use divided dosages. Seizure: Risk is dose-related. Titrate gradually and use divided doses. Use with caution in patients with history of seizure or risk factors for seizure. Myocarditis, cardiomyopathy, and mitral valve Incompetence: Can be fatal. Discontinue and obtain cardiac evaluation if findings suggest these cardiac reactions. Increased mortality in Elderly patients with dementia-related psychosis.

Mesoridazine

Mesoridazine has been shown to prolong the QTc interval in a dose related manner, and drugs with this potential have been associated with torsades de pointes–type arrhythmias and sudden death.

Olanzapine

Increased risk of death in elderly patients with dementia-related psychosis treated with antipsychotic medications.

Thioridazine

May prolong the QT interval in a dose-related manner, and drugs with this potential have been associated with torsades de pointes–type arrhythmias and sudden death. Elderly patients with dementia-related psychosis treated with antipsychotic drugs are at an increased risk of death.

Chlorpromazine

Elderly patients with dementia-related psychosis treated with antipsychotic drugs are at an increased risk of death compared to placebo.

Prochlorperazine

Elderly patients with dementia-related psychosis treated with antipsychotic drugs are at an increased risk of death compared to placebo.

Paroxetine

Antidepressants increased the risk of suicidal thoughts and behaviors in pediatric and young adult patients in short-term studies. These studies did not show any increased risk of suicidality with antidepressants compared to placebo in adults beyond age 24; there was a reduction in risk with antidepressants compared to placebo in adults aged 65 and older.

Anxiolytics are used to decrease anxiety and possibly agitation, motor restlessness, and insomnia. Such medications include **lorazepam** ⚠ (Ativan), oxazepam ⚠ (Serax), and **buspirone** (Buspar). Benzodiazepines can increase the risk of falls and injury.

Antidepressants improve depression, which can worsen the cognitive functioning of a patient with Alzheimer's disease. Common antidepressants in the elderly include **sertraline** ⚠ (Zoloft) and **citalopram** ⚠ (Celexa).

Antipsychotics are used to decrease psychotic symptoms such as hallucinations and delusions. Antipsychotics such as haloperidol ⚠ (Haldol), risperidone ⚠ (Risperdal), and aripiprazole ⚠ (Abilify) may reduce agitation and aggressiveness in dementia patients. A U.S. Food and Drug Administration (FDA) boxed warning concerning the risk of increased mortality (cardiac events and infections) is associated with the use of antipsychotics in demented elderly patients.

Sedative hypnotics are used for the short-term treatment of insomnia but can increase confusion and memory impairment. These medications include **trazodone** ⚠ (Desyrel), **zolpidem** ⚠ (Ambien), and temazepam ⚠ (Restoril).

⚠ FDA BOXED WARNINGS

Lorazepam
Concomitant use of benzodiazepines and opioids may result in profound sedation, respiratory depression, coma, and death. Limit doses and durations to the minimum required. Use of benzodiazepines expose users to risks of abuse, misuse, and addiction, which can lead to overdose and death. Continued use of benzodiazepines for several days to weeks may led to significant physical dependence.

Oxazepam
Concomitant use of benzodiazepines and opioids may result in profound sedation, respiratory depression, coma, and death. Limit doses and durations to the minimum required. Use of benzodiazepines expose users to risks of abuse, misuse, and addiction, which can lead to overdose and death. Continued use of benzodiazepines for several days to weeks may led to significant physical dependence.

Sertraline
Antidepressants increased the risk of suicidal thoughts and behaviors in pediatric and young adult patients in short-term studies. These studies did not show any increased risk of suicidality with antidepressants compared to placebo in adults beyond age 24; there was a reduction in risk with antidepressants compared to placebo in adults aged 65 and older.

Citalopram
Antidepressants increased the risk of suicidal thoughts and behaviors in pediatric and young adult patients in short-term studies. These studies did not show any increased risk of suicidality with antidepressants compared to placebo in adults beyond age 24; there was a reduction in risk with antidepressants compared to placebo in adults aged 65 and older.

Haloperidol
Elderly patients with dementia-related psychosis treated with antipsychotics are at an increased risk of death compared to placebo.

Risperidone
Elderly patients with dementia-related psychosis treated with antipsychotic medications are at in increased risk of death.

Aripiprazole
Increased mortality in patients with dementia related psychosis; increased risk of suicidal thoughts and behavior in children, adolescents, and young adults with antidepressants shown in short-term studies. No increased risk beyond age 24, and there was a reduction in risk with antidepressants compared to placebo in adults aged 65 and older.

Trazodone
Increased risk of suicidality. Not approved for use in pediatric patients.

Zolpidem
Complex sleep behaviors including sleep-walking, sleep-driving, and engaging in other activities while not fully awake may occur following use. Some of these events may result in serious injuries, including death.

Temazepam
Concomitant use of benzodiazepines and opioids may result in profound sedation, respiratory depression, coma, and death. Limit dosages and durations to the minimum required in patients who must receive the combination. The use of benzodiazepines exposes users to risks of abuse, misuse, and addiction. The continued use of benzodiazepines may lead to clinically significant physical dependence.

Cholinesterase inhibitors

Medications used to slow or reverse the symptoms of Alzheimer's (Table 19-4) affect acetylcholine activity in the brain. Acetylcholine levels may be decreased by as much as 90% in Alzheimer's disease. These levels can be increased by inhibiting the enzyme acetylcholinesterase.

Acetylcholinesterase inhibitors increase acetylcholine but do not replace lost cholinergic neurons or change the underlying pathology. This class of medications is used to prevent or slow deterioration in cognitive functioning. Currently, three acetylcholinesterase inhibitors are available:

- Donepezil (Aricept) is selective for acetylcholinesterase in the brain (i.e., not in peripheral tissues) and is approved for mild-to-moderate and moderate-to-severe dementia. A 23 mg tablet is now approved for moderate-to-severe dementia, but additional benefits of this higher dose are modest at best, and it has an increased incidence of adverse effects.
- Rivastigmine (Exelon), a nonselective cholinesterase inhibitor, decreases acetylcholinesterase. It is approved for mild-to-moderate Alzheimer's disease and dementia associated with Parkinson's disease.
- Galantamine (Razadyne) is a selective acetylcholinesterase inhibitor that activates nicotinic receptors, which may increase acetylcholine. It is approved for mild-to-moderate Alzheimer's disease dementia.

Patient instructions and counseling
Donepezil (Aricept)

- Give orally, 5 mg daily at bedtime for 4 to 6 weeks. Increase dosage to 10 mg daily at bedtime.
- Take with or without food.
- A 23 mg dose is available that has shown statistical significance but less clear observable benefits. This higher dose causes increased adverse effects, and there is limited research to support clinical benefits.

Rivastigmine (Exelon)

- Oral doses are given with a gradual dosage increase. Begin at 1.5 mg twice daily and then 3 mg twice daily, 4.5 mg twice daily, and 6 mg twice daily, with a minimum of 2 weeks between dose increases.

TABLE 19-4. Drugs Used to Treat Alzheimer's Disease

Generic name	Trade name	Usual dosage	Dosage forms	Adverse effects
Donepezil	Aricept	5 to 23 mg at bedtime	5, 10, 23 mg tablets; 5 mg/5 mL oral solution; 5, 10 mg disintegrating tablets	Nausea and vomiting, GI upset
Rivastigmine	Exelon	1.5 to 6 mg twice daily	1.5, 3, 4.5, 6 mg capsules; 4.6 mg/24 h, 9.5 mg/24 h, 13.3 mg/24 h transdermal patches; 2 mg/mL oral solution	Nausea and vomiting, GI upset, anorexia, weight loss
Galantamine	Razadyne	4 to 12 mg twice daily	4, 8, 12 mg tablets; 8, 16, 24 mg extended-release capsules; 4 mg/mL oral solution	Nausea and vomiting, GI upset
Memantine	Namenda	5 to 10 mg twice daily	5, 10 mg tablets	Headache, constipation, dizziness, hypertension
Donepezil/ Memantine	Namzaric	7 to 28 mg daily 10 mg to 7 mg to 10 mg to 28 mg	7, 14, 21, 28 mg extended-release capsules; 5, 10 mg tablets; 2 mg/mL oral solution 10 mg to 7 mg; 10 mg to 14 mg; 10 mg to 21 mg; 10 mg to 28 mg	Nausea, vomiting, diarrhea, loss of appetite, headache, dizziness, insomnia, syncope

GI, gastrointestinal.

- If rivastigmine is discontinued because of adverse effects, restart at beginning dose.
- Take with meals in divided doses.
- Transdermal patch dosing begins with 4.6 mg every 24 hours, once daily for 4 weeks. It then increases to 9.5 mg every 24 hours, once daily. It may be increased to a maximum of 13.3 mg every 24 hours.

Galantamine (Razadyne)

- Doses begin with 4 mg twice daily for 4 weeks, 8 mg twice daily for 4 weeks, and then 12 mg twice daily.
- If galantamine is discontinued for more than a few days, restart at the beginning dose.
- In hepatic or renal dysfunction, doses should not exceed 16 mg/d. Do not use in instances of severe dysfunction.
- Take with meals in divided doses.
- Initiate therapy with extended-release capsules at 8 mg daily with a morning meal for 4 weeks. Increase the dose to 16 mg daily for 4 weeks and then 24 mg daily.

N-methyl-D-aspartate–receptor antagonists

Blocking the excitotoxicity effects of the neurotransmitter glutamate at N-methyl-D-aspartate (NMDA) receptors has been reported to be beneficial in Alzheimer's disease. Memantine (Namenda) is an NMDA-receptor antagonist with FDA approval for moderate-to-severe Alzheimer's disease dementia. There is no evidence to support memantine use in mild Alzheimer's disease, and efficacy is modest at best in moderate Alzheimer's dementia. Immediate release dosing starts with 5 mg daily and is increased in 5 mg increments at weekly intervals up to a target dose of 10 mg twice daily. Sustained release formulation doses begin with 7 mg daily for 1 week, with weekly increases to 28 mg daily, if tolerated. The dose should be reduced to 14 mg daily in patients with renal impairment (creatinine clearance [CrCl] less than 30 mL/min).

Drug–Drug Interactions

Anticholinergic drugs reduce the effectiveness of cholinesterase inhibitors and cause dry mouth, blurred vision, constipation, and mental confusion (i.e., conditions that are more problematic in the elderly).

Cytochrome P450 (CYP) enzyme inhibitors of 2D6 and 3A4 increase levels of galantamine and donepezil by inhibiting their metabolism.

Dextromethorphan (Robitussin DM), a potent NMDA-receptor antagonist, should be used cautiously with memantine. This caution also includes co-administration with amantadine and ketamine. Smoking and nicotine products may alter levels of memantine. Concurrent use of amantadine increases the potential for adverse effects.

Parameters to monitor

- Monitor cognitive function (e.g., poor results on mini–mental state exam, decline in performance of activities of daily living, incidence of behaviors that indicate cognitive decline).
- Watch for signs and symptoms of toxicity.
- Discontinue treatment with active peptic ulcer disease, severe bradycardia, and acute medical illness.
- Perform periodic complete blood cell count and basic chemistries.
- Look for expected benefits with the use of cholinesterase inhibitors and NMDA-receptor antagonists. Such benefits include improvement in memory, some stabilization of behaviors or mood, and possible slowing of the progression of the disease.

Nonprescription agents

High-dose vitamin E (2000 units daily) has been recommended as an antioxidant to slow progression of Alzheimer's disease. Vitamin E may interfere with vitamin K absorption and result in increased risk of bleeding. Increased mortality has been reported with high-dose vitamin E. The potential toxicity of high-dose vitamin E may outweigh the benefits.

Ginkgo biloba, an herb, has been used to treat symptoms of Alzheimer's disease with reports of modest benefits. Ginkgo biloba is associated with an increased risk of bleeding and hemorrhage, especially when combined with daily **aspirin** use, and is not recommended. There is growing evidence that ginkgo biloba does not provide any benefits over a placebo.

19-5 Parkinson's Disease

Parkinson's disease (PD) is a chronic, progressive neurologic disorder with symptoms that present as a variable combination of rigidity, tremor, bradykinesia, and changes in posture and ambulation. Approximately 60,000 new cases are diagnosed each year.

The risk of developing PD increases with age, and a substantial increase in the U.S. population of persons over 60 years of age is predicted.

Classification

The two classes of PD are primary parkinsonism and secondary parkinsonism. Primary parkinsonism has no identified cause. Secondary parkinsonism can be the result of drug use (e.g., reserpine, metoclopramide, antipsychotics), infections, trauma, or toxins.

Clinical Presentation

Clinical signs and symptoms of PD (Table 19-5) develop insidiously, progress slowly, may fluctuate, and worsen with time despite pharmacologic therapy.

Pathophysiology

PD involves a progressive degeneration of the substantia nigra in the brain with a decrease in dopaminergic cells (more than the typical decrease that accompanies normal aging). The most significant neurotransmitter in PD is dopamine, but other neurotransmitters may play a role (e.g., acetylcholine, glutamate, GABA [gamma-aminobutyric acid], serotonin, norepinephrine).

TABLE 19-5. Symptoms of Parkinson's Disease

Symptom	Description/examples
Tremors	Begin unilaterally; present in 70% of PD patients; may worsen with stress
Rigidity	Usually in limbs and trunk; difficulty dressing or standing from seated position; face may have mask-like expression
Movement disorders	Akinesia (absence of movement); bradykinesia (slowed movement); postural instability; abnormal gait; increased falls
Mood disorders	Depression; dementia
Other	Micrographia (small writing), drooling, decreased blinking, constipation, incontinence, dysphagia (difficulty swallowing), dysarthria (difficulty speaking)

The etiology is unknown, but genetic susceptibility is possible. Environmental toxins combined with aging may also be responsible for the development of PD.

Diagnostic Criteria

Clinical diagnosis is based on the presence of bradykinesia and either rest tremor or rigidity.

Treatment Principles and Goals

The goal for treating PD is to relieve symptoms and maintain or improve quality of life for the patient. Treatment should be initiated when functional impairment and discomfort for the patient or caregiver occurs.

Drug Therapy

Mechanism of action

Medications increase dopamine or dopamine activity by directly stimulating dopamine receptors or by blocking acetylcholine activity, which results in increased dopamine effects (Table 19-6).

Selection of an initial medication to treat PD may vary with the prescriber. Most therapy will begin with levodopa or with a direct dopamine agonist. Medications that increase dopamine activity should not be discontinued abruptly because of the risk of sudden onset of Parkinson's symptoms.

TABLE 19-6. Drugs for Treating Parkinson's Disease

Generic Name	Trade Name	Mechanism of Action	Dosage (mg), schedule, available strengths
Carbidopa-levodopa	Sinemet	Increases dopamine (levodopa); prevents metabolism (carbidopa)	300 to 2000; up to 8 times daily; 10 to 100 mg; 25 to 100 mg; 25 to 250 mg
Carbidopa-levodopa Orally Disintegrating Tablet	Parcopa	Increases dopamine (levodopa); prevents metabolism (carbidopa)	300 to 2000; up to 8 times daily; 10 to 100 mg; 25 to 100 mg; 25 to 250 mg
Carbidopa-levodopa Controlled Release	Sinemet Controlled Release	Increases dopamine (levodopa); prevents metabolism (carbidopa)	400 to 2000; twice daily; 25 to 100 mg; 50 to 200 mg
Carbidopa-levodopa Immediate Release/ Extended Release	Rytary	Increases dopamine (levodopa); prevents metabolism (carbidopa)	435 to 2450; 3 times daily; 23.75 to 95 mg; 36.25 to 145 mg; 48.75 to 195; 61.25 to 245 mg
Carbidopa-levodopa enteral suspension	Duopa	Increases dopamine (levodopa); prevents metabolism (carbidopa)	1000 to 2000; given over 16 hours via pump; 4.6 mg/1 mL; 20 mg/1 mL
Carbidopa-levodopa-entacapone	Stalevo	Increases dopamine (levodopa); prevents metabolism (carbidopa); inhibits COMT (entacapone)	600 to 1600; up to 8 times daily (only 6 times daily with maximum dose) 12.5 to 200 to 50 mg; 18.75 to 200 to 75 mg; 25 to 200 to 100 mg; 31.25 to 200 to 125 mg; 37.25 to 200 to 150 mg; 50 to 200 to 200 mg
Carbidopa	Lodosyn	Prevents metabolism	25 to 75; up to 4 times daily; 25 mg
Bromocriptine	Parlodel	Directly stimulates dopamine receptors	2.5 to 100 mg; twice daily; 2.5 mg and 5 mg
Pramipexole	Mirapex	Directly stimulates dopamine receptors	1.5 to 4.5 mg; 3 times daily; 0.125 mg, 0.25 mg, 0.5 mg, 0.75 mg, 1 mg; 1.5 mg; ER is 0.375 mg, 0.75 mg, 1.5 mg; 22.5 mg, 3 mg, 3.75 mg, 4.5 mg given daily

(continued)

TABLE 19-6. Drugs for Treating Parkinson's Disease *(Continued)*

Generic Name	Trade Name	Mechanism of Action	Dosage (mg), schedule, available strengths
Ropinirole	Requip	Directly stimulates dopamine receptors	IR 1.5 to 24 mg; 3 times daily; 0.25 mg, 0.5 mg, 1 mg, 2 mg, 3 mg, 4 mg, 5 mg; ER 2 to 24 mg; daily; 2 mg, 4 mg, 6 mg, 12 mg
Rotigotine	Neupro	Directly stimulates dopamine receptors	2 to 8 mg; daily patch; 1 mg/24 h, 2 mg/24 h, 3 mg/24 h, 4 mg/24 h, 6 mg/24 h, and 8 mg/24 h
Apomorphine	Apokyn	Directly stimulates dopamine receptors	2 to 6 mg; 0.2 to 0.6 mL) subcutaneous for acute attacks; oral antiemetic (trimethobenzamide) is given concurrently; 10 mg/1 mL solution
Selegiline ⚠	Eldepryl; Zelapar (Orally Disintegrating Tablet)	Inhibits MAO-B; increases dopamine and serotonin	5 to 10 mg; twice daily; 5-mg tablets and capsules; ODT 1.25 to 2.5; daily; 1.25 mg ODT tablets
Rasagiline	Azilect	Inhibits MAO-B; increases dopamine and serotonin	0.5 to 1 mg; daily; 0.5- and 1 mg tablets
Safinamide	Xadago	Inhibits MAO-B; increases dopamine and serotonin (only approved as adjunct therapy)	50 to 100 mg; daily; 50 mg; 10 mg tablets
Entacapone	Comtan	Inhibits COMT; increases dopamine	200 to 1600 mg; up to 8 times daily; 200 mg tablets
Tolcapone ⚠	Tasmar	Inhibits COMT; increases dopamine	100 to 300 mg; 3 times daily; 100 mg tablets
Amantadine	Symmetrel	May increase presynaptic release of dopamine; blocks reuptake	100 to 400 mg; twice daily; 100 mg tablets, 100 mg capsules, and 50 mg/50 mL syrup.
Amantadine Extended Release capsule	GoCovri	May increase presynaptic release of dopamine; blocks reuptake	137 to 274 mg; daily; 68.5 mg, 137 mg
Amantadine Extended Release tablet	Osmolex Extended Release	May increase presynaptic release of dopamine; blocks reuptake	129 to 322 mg; daily; 129 mg, 193 mg, 258 mg; (not interchangeable with other amantadine formulations)
Benztropine	Cogentin	Blocks acetylcholine may balance dopamine	0.5 to 6 mg; daily or divided 2 to 4 doses; 0.5 mg, 1 mg, 2 mg, 1 mg/mL
Trihexyphenidyl	Artane	Blocks acetylcholine; may balance dopamine	1 to 10 mg; up to 4 times daily; 2 mg, 5 mg, 2 mg/5 mL

MAO-B, monoamine oxidase B; COMT, catechol-O-methyl transferase.

 Selegiline Patch *FDA BOXED WARNING*

Antidepressants increased the risk of suicidal thoughts and behaviors in pediatric and young adult patients in short-term studies.

Tolcapone *FDA BOXED WARNING*

Potentially fatal, acute fulminant hepatic failure risk; reserve for patients on levodopa-carbidopa with symptom fluctuations who are not candidates or not responding to alternative adjunct treatment. Discontinue treatment if no substantial benefit after 3 weeks.

Levodopa (Sinemet when combined with carbidopa)

Levodopa is the most effective drug in the treatment of PD and is converted to dopamine in the body. It is given with carbidopa, a decarboxylase inhibitor that prevents the peripheral conversion of levodopa to dopamine, thereby reducing nausea and vomiting while allowing more drug to pass through the blood–brain barrier.

Generally, doses are increased gradually to minimize the risk of side effects with the goal of improving symptoms with the lowest dose possible. In maintenance therapy or advanced disease, doses are given before meals to facilitate absorption. Carbidopa effectively inhibits peripheral conversion of levodopa at doses of 100 mg/d.

Levodopa provides benefits to all stages of PD, but chronic use is associated with adverse effects. Patients may have periods of good mobility alternating with periods of impaired motor function.

Dopamine agonists

Dopamine agonists work directly on dopamine receptors and do not require metabolic conversion. They may be used as monotherapy or as adjunctive therapy, allowing lower doses of carbidopa-levodopa. Some clinicians will initiate therapy with a direct dopamine agonist in younger newly diagnosed patients. Pramipexole (Mirapex), bromocriptine (Parlodel), and ropinirole (Requip) are available orally, and rotigotine (Neupro) is administered as a transdermal patch.

Apomorphine (Apokyn) is a direct-acting dopamine agonist that is administered by subcutaneous injection. It causes significant nausea and vomiting, and an antiemetic (e.g., trimethobenzamide) is given concurrently. Apomorphine is reserved for the treatment of "freezing" episodes associated with advanced disease. Monitor for orthostatic hypotension after initial doses and with dose escalation.

Selective monoamine oxidase type B inhibitors

Monoamine oxidase (MAO)-B inhibitors may be used as initial therapy in early PD and as adjunct treatment for more advanced disease. Although neuroprotective properties have been seen in animal models, benefits as monotherapy are modest.

With doses used for PD, adverse effects from consuming tyramine-containing foods would not be expected.

Catechol-O-methyl transferase inhibitors

Catechol-O-methyl transferase (COMT) inhibitors impair the secondary pathway that is responsible for the peripheral conversion of levodopa to dopamine and are ineffective when given alone. These medications should always be prescribed in conjunction with carbidopa-levodopa (Sinemet). They are most often used to treat patients during end-of-dose wearing-off periods and patients experiencing motor fluctuations. Treatment complications and strategies for improving patient response are listed in Table 19-7.

TABLE 19-7. Strategies for Improving Patient Response to Treatment

Complication	Strategy
No initial response	No initial response to carbidopa-levodopa combination; gradually increase the dose to 1000 to 1500 mg of levodopa.
Suboptimal response	After increasing levodopa, add another drug (dopamine agonist, MAO-B inhibitor, or COMT inhibitor).
"On and off" phenomenon	Associated with advancing disease; use more frequent doses or sustained release levodopa.
Acute intermittent hypomobility "freezing" episodes	These episodes are seen with advancing disease; treat with subcutaneous injections of apomorphine.
End-of-dose or wearing-off period	Due to a decreased duration of benefit, levodopa wanes after less than 4 hours. Use combination therapy, give levodopa more frequently, or use sustained-release carbidopa-levodopa.

MAO-B, monoamine oxidase B; COMT, catechol-O-methyl transferase.

Patient instructions and counseling

- Usually take medications on an empty stomach. Eat shortly afterward to avoid upset stomach.
- Take a missed dose as soon as possible. Skip the missed dose if the next scheduled dose is within 2 hours. Parkinson medications should not be abruptly discontinued because of the risk of rapid worsening of symptoms.
- Dizziness, drowsiness, and stomach upset may occur; therefore, use caution when operating equipment.
- Report any confusion, mood changes, and uncontrolled movements to the prescriber as soon as possible.
- Do not crush a sustained-release product.

Adverse effects and drug–drug interactions

Adverse effects of medications used to treat PD are described in Table 19-8. Table 19-9 contains information on drug–drug interactions.

As PD progresses, increasing dopamine levels can result in hallucinations and delusions. Psychotic symptoms can also be associated with advanced PD. Treatment of psychoses with antipsychotic medications can result in worsening motor symptoms secondary to dopamine D_2 receptor antagonism. Clozapine (Clozaril) has proved effective in decreasing hallucinations and delusions, but its use is complicated by the need for frequent blood monitoring to detect possible blood dyscrasias. Low doses of other antipsychotics are sometimes used with the goal of titrating between worsening motor function and improvement of psychotic symptoms. Pimavanserin ⚠ (Nuplazid) is an antipsychotic specifically approved for the treatment of hallucinations and delusions associated with PD. Mechanism of action is thought to be through inverse agonist and antagonist activity at serotonin 5-HT (2A) and serotonin 5-HT (2C) receptors. The dose

 Pimavanserin *FDA BOXED WARNING*

Elderly patients with dementia-related psychosis treated with antipsychotics are at an increased risk of death.

TABLE 19-8. Adverse Effects of Medications Used to Treat Parkinson's Disease

Drug	Adverse effects
Dopaminergics	
Levodopa, pramipexole, bromocriptine, ropinirole, amantadine	Nausea and vomiting, agitation, confusion, depression, psychoses, orthostatic hypotension, dyskinetic movements, "sleep attacks," "pathologic gambling" (dopamine agonists), possible heart failure (pramipexole)
MAO-B inhibitors	
Selegiline, rasagiline	Nausea and vomiting, insomnia, dizziness, agitation, confusion, dyskinetic movements, anorexia
Amantadine	Confusion, dizziness, depression, anxiety, psychoses, insomnia
COMT inhibitors	
Tolcapone, entacapone	Nausea and vomiting, diarrhea, dyskinesia, urine coloration, possible liver toxicity (tolcapone)
Anticholinergics	
Benztropine, trihexyphenidyl	Dry mouth, blurred vision, constipation, urinary retention, confusion, agitation, psychoses

is 34 mg (two 17 mg tablets) daily. No dose adjustment is needed in mild-to-moderate renal impairment or hepatic insufficiency; however, it should be used with caution in severe renal impairment or end stage kidney disease (CrCl < 30 mL/min). Decrease dose to 10 mg daily when given with strong CYP3A4 inhibitors. Avoid use with moderate to strong CYP3A4 inducers.

Parameters to monitor

- Liver function, complete blood count, basic chemistries (periodically)
- Blood pressure, pulse, electrocardiogram (periodically)
- Reduction of rigidity, tremor, slowed movements
- Examination for mental confusion, mood changes, psychotic thinking

TABLE 19-9. Drug–Drug Interactions with Medications Used to Treat Parkinson's Disease

Medication	Interacting drug	Outcome
Dopamine agonists (e.g., bromocriptine, ropinirole)	Dopamine antagonists (e.g., haloperidol, metoclopramide)	Inhibition of benefits with worsening parkinsonism
Levodopa	Dopamine antagonists	Inhibition of benefits with worsening parkinsonism
Apomorphine	**Ondansetron**, other serotonin-receptor antagonists, dopamine antagonists	Severe hypotension and loss of consciousness; inhibition of benefits with worsening parkinsonism
Selegiline	Serotonergics, selective serotonin reuptake inhibitors, **buspirone**, mirtazapine	Serotonin syndrome (confusion, agitation, tremor, seizures, coma)
COMT inhibitors	Nonselective MAO inhibitors: phenelzine	Serotonin syndrome; hypertensive crisis secondary to increased catecholamines

Boldface indicates one of top 100 drugs for 2020 by prescription volume.

19-6 Glaucoma

Glaucoma is a group of eye diseases characterized by an increase in intraocular pressure (IOP), which causes pathologic changes in the optic nerve and typical visual-field defects. Glaucoma affects more than 4 million Americans, and as many as 15 million more people may have increased IOP but no clinical signs and symptoms of glaucoma.

The prevalence of glaucoma increases with age and is most often seen in those 65 years of age or older. The number of persons with glaucoma is expected to increase with the aging U.S. population. With improved screening programs to identify those with increased IOP, an increase in the number of those diagnosed with glaucoma is expected.

Classification

Open-angle glaucoma is a form of primary glaucoma. The angle of the anterior chamber remains open in an eye, but filtration of aqueous humor is gradually diminished because of the tissues of the angle. Open-angle glaucoma accounts for approximately 80% to 90% of cases.

Angle-closure (narrow-angle) glaucoma is a form of primary glaucoma in an eye characterized by a shallow anterior chamber and a narrow angle. The filtration of aqueous humor is compromised because of the iris blocking the angle.

Congenital glaucoma results from defective development of the structures in and around the anterior chamber of the eye and results in impairment of aqueous humor.

Clinical Presentation

Clinical signs and symptoms of open-angle glaucoma develop slowly and may present with only minor symptoms, such as headache and mild eye pain. Optic nerve damage results from chronic elevations in IOP; therefore, early and consistent treatment is important to prevent loss of vision.

Acute angle-closure glaucoma presents with blurred vision, severe ocular pain, and possible nausea and vomiting. It should be considered a medical emergency, and immediate care should be recommended.

Chronic angle-closure glaucoma may have symptoms similar to those of open-angle glaucoma.

Tonometry is used to screen for IOP, but direct ophthalmoscopy (slit-lamp examination) is necessary to accurately evaluate the eye for changes in the optic nerve.

Pathophysiology

The pathogenesis of glaucoma results from changes in aqueous humor (the fluid filling the eye and in front of the lens) outflow that result in increased IOP. This increase in pressure leads to optic nerve atrophy and progressive loss of vision.

Increased IOP can result from decreased elimination or increased production of aqueous humor. Aqueous humor is secreted by the ciliary processes into the posterior chamber of the eye. It then flows through the trabecular meshwork and the canal of Schlemm.

Open-angle glaucoma is the result of decreased elimination of aqueous humor as it passes through the trabecular meshwork, thereby resulting in elevated IOP.

Angle-closure glaucoma is caused by papillary blockage of aqueous humor outflow. This blockage can result when a patient has a narrow anterior chamber in the eye or a dilated pupil where the iris comes into greater contact with the lens. With the blocking of outflow, aqueous humor accumulates in the posterior chamber, presses the lens forward, and further decreases drainage, with possible complete blockage as the outcome.

Diagnostic Criteria

- Elevated IOP as determined by tonometry
- Funduscopic assessment to identify characteristic changes in the optic disc and retina

Treatment Principles

Figure 19-1 illustrates the treatment of open-angle glaucoma. Treatment principles of glaucoma are as follows:

- Reduce IOP to prevent optic nerve damage and visual field loss.
- Use topical medications as first-line treatment.
- Consider acute angle-closure glaucoma as a medical emergency.

Monitoring

Periodic screening for increased IOP should be done, with yearly examinations for those over 65 years of age and as part of a routine eye examination.

Drug Therapy

Mechanism of action

Medications are considered the mainstay of therapy for the treatment of glaucoma (Table 19-10). Topical medications treat glaucoma by increasing aqueous humor outflow or by decreasing aqueous humor production. Prostaglandins, alpha-adrenergic agonists, and cholinergics all reduce IOP by increasing aqueous humor outflow. Beta-adrenergic antagonists, alpha-adrenergic agonists, and carbonic anhydrase inhibitors decrease aqueous humor formation (Table 19-11).

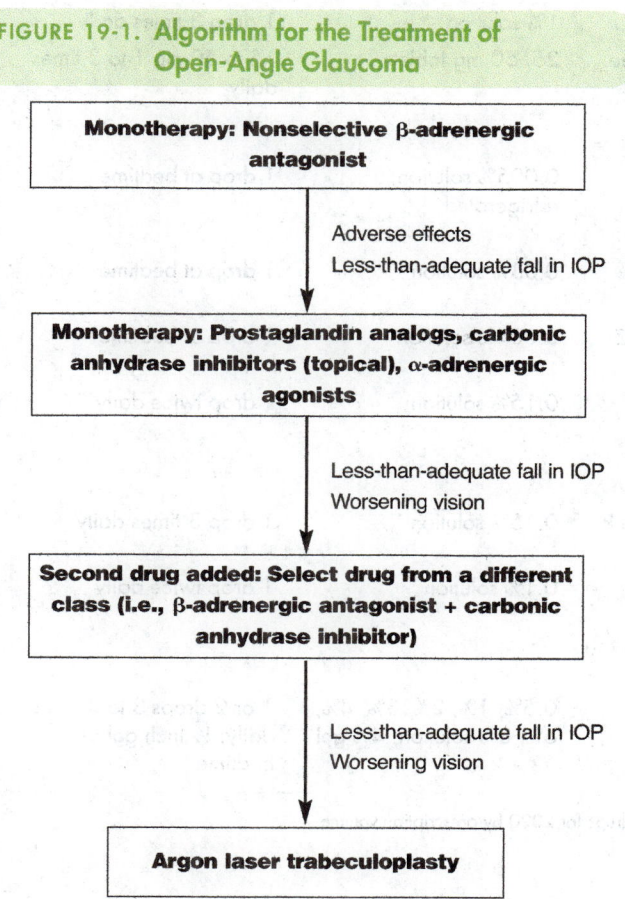

FIGURE 19-1. Algorithm for the Treatment of Open-Angle Glaucoma

TABLE 19-10. Medications for the Treatment of Glaucoma

Generic name	Trade name	Form	Usual dosage	Comments
Nonselective beta antagonists				
Timolol	Timoptic	0.25%, 0.50% solution and gel-forming solution	1 drop twice daily; gel solution used once daily	
Carteolol	Ocupress	1% ophthalmic solution	1 drop twice daily	
Levobunolol	Betagan	0.25%, 0.50% solution	1 or 2 drops 1 to 4 times daily	
Metipranolol	OptiPranolol	0.3% solution	1 drop twice daily	
Selective beta-1 antagonists				
Betaxolol	Betoptic	0.25%, 0.50% solution	1 or 2 drops twice daily	Drug is cardioselective. It has less effect on heart rate and blood pressure.
Carbonic anhydrase inhibitors				
Acetazolamide	Diamox	125, 250 mg tablets; 500 mg extended-release capsules	250 mg 1 to 4 times daily; extended-release 1 or 2 times daily	Do not use with sulfa allergy.
Dorzolamide	Trusopt	2% solution	1 drop 3 times daily	Do not use with sulfa allergy.
Brinzolamide	Azopt	1% solution	1 drop 3 times daily	Do not use with sulfa allergy.
Methazolamide	Neptazane	25, 50 mg tablets	15 to 50 mg 1 to 3 times daily	Do not use with sulfa allergy.
Prostaglandin analogs				
Latanoprost	Xalatan	0.005% solution, refrigerated	1 drop at bedtime	Drug can change blue eyes to brown; drug can cause darkening of eyelids and eyelashes.
Bimatoprost	Lumigan	0.03% solution	1 drop at bedtime	Drug can cause darkening of eyelids and eyelashes.
Travoprost	Travatan Z	0.004% solution	1 drop at bedtime	Ocular hyperemia frequently occurs.
Unoprostone	Rescula	0.15% solution	1 drop twice daily	If used with another drop, wait 5 minutes.
Alpha-2-adrenergic agonists				
Brimonidine	Alphagan P	0.15% solution	1 drop 3 times daily	Wait at least 15 minutes after using before placing soft contacts.
Dipivefrin	Propine	0.1% solution	1 drop twice daily	Dipivefrin is a prodrug of epinephrine.
Cholinergics (miotics)				
Pilocarpine	Pilocar	0.5%, 1%, 2%, 3%, 4%, 6%, 8% solution; 4% gel	1 or 2 drops 3 to 4 times daily; ½ inch gel at bedtime	A once weekly dose form (Ocuserts) is available.

Boldface indicates one of top 100 drugs for 2020 by prescription volume.

TABLE 19-11. Classification, Mechanism of Action, and Adverse Effects of Glaucoma Medications

Medication class	Mechanism of action	Adverse effects
Beta-adrenergic antagonists (timolol, metipranolol, carteolol, levobunolol, etc.)	Decrease in aqueous humor formation with slight increase in outflow (beta selective)	Adverse cardiac effects, worsening pulmonary disease, depression, dizziness
Miotics (cholinergics) (pilocarpine, carbachol)	Increase in aqueous humor outflow	Miosis, brow ache, dizziness, nausea, flushing, itching, sweating, confusion
Carbonic anhydrase inhibitors (dorzolamide, brinzolamide)	Decrease in aqueous humor formation	Lethargy, decreased appetite, GI upset, urinary frequency
Prostaglandin analogs (**latanoprost** [Xalatan], travoprost [Travatan Z], bimatoprost [Lumigan])	Increased uveoscleral outflow without effect on aqueous humor formation	Iris pigmentation, eyelid darkening, macular edema
Alpha-2-adrenergic agonists (apraclonidine [Iopidine], brimonidine [Alphagan P])	Decrease in aqueous humor formation	Tachycardia, dry mouth, eyelid elevation, central nervous system effects in elderly and very young persons
Other alpha-adrenergic agonists (epinephrine, dipivefrin [Propine])	Increase in aqueous humor outflow	Tachycardia, increased blood pressure, allergic responses

Boldface indicates one of top 100 drugs for 2020 by prescription volume.
GI, gastrointestinal.

Prostaglandins

Prostaglandin analogs are used as first-line treatment (or in combination with beta blockers).
Prostaglandins are dosed once daily, which is a significant advantage in managing glaucoma.

Beta adrenergic antagonists

Beta-adrenergic antagonists are also used as initial therapy and can be nonselective (i.e., they block both beta-1 and beta-2 receptors) or selective (i.e., they block only beta-1 receptors). Drugs that block only beta-1 receptors are considered cardioselective and cause less decrease in blood pressure and heart rate. Nonselective beta antagonists include timolol (Timoptic), carteolol (Ocupress), levobunolol (Betagan), and metipranolol (OptiPranolol). Beta-1-selective antagonists include betaxolol (Betoptic) and levobetaxolol (Betaxon).

Therapy is initiated with a single topical ophthalmic solution, and additional agents are added if the decrease in IOP is less than acceptable. The effects of therapy on IOP should be apparent after a week of treatment.

Topical carbonic anhydrase inhibitors and alpha-2 agonists may be used in treatment.

Medications such as epinephrine, pilocarpine, and oral carbonic anhydrase inhibitors are prescribed less often, but they are considered to be effective adjunctive drugs.

Patient instructions and counseling

Multiple factors present obstacles that can interfere with good compliance. Patients are often asymptomatic and do not feel treatment is necessary. Because decreased vision is associated with glaucoma, patients may have difficulty with written instructions.

Adequate glaucoma therapy often requires 2 or more types of eye drops that may have to be given more than once daily. Correct administration of eye drops requires coordination and reasonable cognitive functioning.

BOX 19-2. Glaucoma Drug–drug Interactions

Drug interactions between topical medications and systemic drugs are unlikely. Acetazolamide (Diamox) interacts with the following:

- *Aspirin:* Causes increased **aspirin** levels and possible toxicity
- *Cyclosporine* ⚠: Causes increased cyclosporine levels
- *Lithium* ⚠: Causes either increased or decreased lithium levels
- *Phenytoin* ⚠: Causes an increased risk of osteomalacia

Boldface indicates one of top 100 drugs for 2020 by prescription volume.

Patient guidelines concerning the use of eye drops to treat glaucoma follow:

- Wash hands before administering eye drops, and avoid touching the dropper tip.
- Confirm that the medication is not outdated and has been stored properly.
- Looking upward, pull the lower lid down and instill the correct number of drops.
- Close the eye to allow the medication to have maximal effect.
- In most cases, wait 5 or more minutes between administration of different medications.

Adverse drug effects

Table 19-11 describes the adverse effects that may be seen with glaucoma medications. Drug-drug interactions for glaucoma medications are listed in Box 19-2.

Other aspects

Combination products are available: timolol 0.5% and dorzolamide 2% (Cosopt), and brimonidine 0.2% and timolol 0.5% (Combigan). These combinations effectively lower IOP and require only twice daily doses. This simplified dosing should improve compliance with treatment. Combinations (i.e., using 2 drugs from different categories) represent a sound treatment approach. Poor response to therapy may result in the prescribing of multiple medications, which may negatively affect the patient's ability to successfully use the more complex regimen.

⚠ FDA BOXED WARNINGS

Cyclosporine

Only physicians experienced in the management of systemic immunosuppressive therapy for the indicated disease should prescribe cyclosporine. OK to administer with adrenal corticosteroids but not with other immunosuppressive agents. Increased susceptibility to infection and the possible development of lymphoma may result from immunosuppression. Cyclosporine and cyclosporine-modified are not bioequivalent. Cyclosporine absorption is erratic during chronic administration. Monitor blood levels.

Lithium

Lithium toxicity is closely related to lithium levels and can occur at doses close to therapeutic levels.

Phenytoin

The rate of I.V. phenytoin sodium administration should not exceed 50 mg/min in adults and 1 to 3 mg/kg/min (or 50 mg/min, whichever is slower) in pediatric patients because of the risk of severe hypotension and cardiac arrhythmias.

19-7 Urinary Incontinence

Urinary incontinence in older adults often results in functional limitations and medical complications; it negatively affects social activities. Urinary incontinence is more common in elderly women than men and more common in institutionalized patients.

Types of Urinary Incontinence

Transient incontinence is common in elderly adults and can be the result of a variety of causes such as infections, delirium, stool impaction, restricted mobility, and pharmaceuticals. Medications prescribed for other conditions can cause urinary incontinence (Table 19-12). Sedative-hypnotic and opioid use may result in decreased alertness and inability to respond in a timely manner to the urge to urinate. Diuretics increase urine flow and urinary frequency and challenge older adults in reaching the toilet in a timely manner. Anticholinergic drugs, used to treat certain types of urinary incontinence, can impair the bladder's contractility and result in incomplete voiding. Alpha-adrenergic receptor agonists can result in urinary retention by increasing internal urethral sphincter tone.

Urge incontinence (detrusor hyperactivity) is more common in older women than men and is the result of a sudden bladder contraction that often results in complete bladder emptying before reaching a toilet.

Overflow incontinence is more common in elderly men and often relates to prostatic enlargement. Common symptoms include frequent urinations of small amounts, and this frequency may interfere with sleep.

Stress incontinence is more common in women and may be caused by pelvic floor laxity and inadequate sphincter contractility.

Functional incontinence in elderly persons is the result of decreased mobility and decreased manual dexterity, environmental barriers, and lack of motivation to remain continent of urine.

Pathophysiology

In simple terms, urination occurs when the detrusor muscle contracts the bladder and the internal and external urethral sphincters relax. Urinary incontinence in older adults may be the result of a variety of factors. The prevalence of uninhibited detrusor contractions may increase with age, and urethral closure pressure may decrease. In males, prostate enlargement may obstruct urine flow and result in residual urine remaining in the bladder, which can result in urinary tract infections. In addition, the ability to be able to successfully control urination requires adequate cognitive functioning so that there is proper response to the urge to urinate. Patients with dementia or delirium may not be able to control bowel and bladder functions.

TABLE 19-12. **Medications that Can Worsen or Cause Urinary Incontinence**

Class	Effect
Diuretics	Increased urine output
Sedative hypnotics	Sedation interfering with response to body's signal
Anticholinergics	Altered alertness, decreased bladder contractility
Opiates	Sedation, decreased bladder contractility
Alpha-adrenergic receptor agonists	Excessive internal urethral sphincter tone
Alpha-adrenergic receptor blocking agents	Decreased internal urethral sphincter tone
Combination OTC products containing antihistamine/decongestants	Combined effect with decreased urine flow (in males)

OTC, over-the-counter.

Clinical Presentation

The classic presentation of urinary incontinence is either sudden, uncontrolled release of large amounts of urine (urge incontinence) or the frequent release of small amounts of urine ("dribbling" associated with overflow incontinence). Stress incontinence is the loss of bladder control associated with physical stresses such as coughing or sneezing. Treatment is complicated by the fact that older adults may present with mixed incontinence, as seen when an older woman may have stress incontinence while developing urge incontinence.

Diagnostic Criteria

An accurate history of urinary frequency and the amount voided is critical to determining the most likely type of urinary incontinence. In addition, to determine the extent of overflow incontinence, the amount of urine remaining in the bladder after voiding can be evaluated by the use of a catheter or ultrasound. More than 100 to 120 mL of urine remaining in the bladder would indicate abnormal urinary retention. A urinalysis also provides information to determine whether a urinary tract infection is present.

Treatment Principles

When evaluating a patient for treatment of urinary incontinence, review the patient's prescription and over-the-counter and herbal medications for agents that could cause or worsen urinary incontinence. Be prepared to suggest alternative medications that would be less likely to worsen incontinence and would not interact with potential drug therapies. Although symptoms should improve with treatment, complete resolution may not be achieved.

Drug Therapy

The pharmacologic approach to treatment is based on the type of incontinence and the patient's other medical conditions (Table 19-13). Treatment is complicated by the fact that the treatment for one type of urinary incontinence may worsen symptoms in other types.

Urge incontinence

Anticholinergic drugs are prescribed to decrease detrusor hyperactivity. A variety of agents are available that decrease urinary frequency and improve control. Sustained-release **oxybutynin** (Ditropan) is effective and produces fewer adverse effects than immediate-release **oxybutynin**. Newer agents such as tolterodine (Detrol) and solifenacin (VESIcare) are reported to be more selective for the bladder, but all can cause anticholinergic adverse effects similar to those of **oxybutynin** and other first-generation anticholinergics. Mirabegron (Myrbetriq) is a selective beta-3-adrenergic agonist that causes bladder relaxation and provides modest benefit for urge incontinence. It may be an alternative for patients who cannot tolerate anticholinergic therapy.

Overflow incontinence

Alpha-adrenergic receptor-blocking agents improve symptoms of overflow incontinence by decreasing internal urethral sphincter contractility. The internal sphincter is controlled by alpha-adrenergic receptors; stimulation causes contraction, and alpha-blocking agents allow this sphincter to remain open longer during urination with more complete voiding. Newer alpha-adrenergic receptor blockers such as **tamsulosin** (Flomax) are more selective for bladder function and may have less risk of adverse effects but have the potential to cause similar events as seen with earlier drugs such as terazosin (Hytrin). All alpha-receptor blocking agents have similar efficacy.

TABLE 19-13. Medications Used to Treat Urinary Incontinence

Generic name	Trade name	Used to treat	Dosage and available strengths and forms
Alpha-adrenergic receptor blockers			
Terazosin	Hytrin	Overflow	1 mg at bedtime, slow increase up to 10 mg; 1, 2, 5, 10 mg tablets
Doxazosin	Cardura	Overflow	Immediate release: 1 mg daily, titrate up to 8 mg if needed; 1, 2, 4, 8 mg tablets
	Cardura XL		Extended release: 4 mg daily, increase to 8 mg daily after 3 to 4 weeks; 4, 8 mg tablets
Prazosin	Minipress	Overflow	2 mg twice daily; 1, 2, 5 mg capsules
Tamsulosin	Flomax	Overflow	0.4 mg daily before a meal, increase to 0.8 mg daily after 2 to 4 weeks if needed; 0.4 mg tablets
Alfuzosin	Uroxatral	Overflow	Extended release: 10 mg daily; 10 mg tablets
Silodosin	Rapaflo	Overflow	8 mg daily with a meal; 4, 8 mg tablets
5-α-reductase inhibitors			
Finasteride	Proscar	Overflow	5 mg daily with up to 6 months for response; 5 mg tablets
Dutasteride	**Avodart**	Overflow	0.5 mg daily with up to 6 months for response; 0.5 mg gel capsules
Anticholinergics			
Oxybutynin	Ditropan	Urge	Immediate release: 2.5 mg 2 to 3 times daily, increase to 5 mg 2 to 3 times daily; 5 mg tablets, 5 mg/5 mL syrup
	Ditropan XL		Extended release: 5 to 10 mg daily, increase weekly by 5 mg to maximum 30 mg daily; 5, 10, 15 mg tablets
	Oxytrol	Urge	Transdermal patch, 1 patch every 3 days (3.9 mg/day)
	Gelnique	Urge	Transdermal gel once daily; 3% gel, 100 mg/g gel packets
Tolterodine	Detrol	Urge	Immediate release: 1 to 2 mg twice daily; 1, 2 mg tablets
	Detrol LA		Extended release: 2 to 4 mg once daily; 2, 4 mg tablets
Trospium	Sanctura	Urge	Immediate release: 20 mg twice daily (once daily for age > 75 years); 20 mg tablets
	Sanctura XR		Extended release: 60 mg daily; 60 mg capsules
Darifenacin	Enablex	Urge	Extended release: 7.5 mg once daily, after 2 weeks may increase to 15 mg daily; 7.5, 15 mg tablets
Solifenacin	VESIcare	Urge	5 mg daily, may increase to 10 mg daily; 5, 10 mg tablets
Fesoterodine	Toviaz	Urge	Extended release: 4 mg daily, may increase to 8 mg daily; 4 mg tablets
Beta-3-adrenergic agonist			
Mirabegron	Myrbetriq	Urge	Extended release: 25 mg once daily, may increase to 50 mg once daily; 25, 50 mg tablets

Boldface indicates one of top 100 drugs for 2020 by prescription volume.

In older males, overflow incontinence is usually associated with prostate enlargement, and the addition of a 5-alpha-reductase inhibitor may be necessary. Drugs such as **finasteride** (Proscar) and dutasteride (Avodart) inhibit the conversion of testosterone to a more active form and treat benign prostatic hyperplasia by reducing prostate enlargement. This in combination with an alpha-blocking agent improves urine flow to a greater extent than either drug used alone. 5-Alpha-reductase inhibitors are usually added if a trial of an alpha-blocker is not successful because the reduction of testosterone activity can negatively affect libido and cause impotence.

Stress incontinence

Several nonpharmacologic approaches are used to treat stress incontinence, but if not contraindicated, alpha-adrenergic agonists are often prescribed. The use of drugs such as pseudoephedrine, ephedrine, and midodrine (ProAmatine, Orvaten) stimulate the urethral sphincter and may improve bladder control. These drugs are associated with the risk of hypertension, anxiety, and insomnia and should be used with caution. The antidepressant **duloxetine** (Cymbalta) has been shown to be more effective than a placebo for stress incontinence, but its usefulness is limited because of frequent adverse effects.

⚠ **Duloxetine** *FDA BOXED WARNING*

Antidepressant use has been associated with an increased risk of suicidal thinking and behavior in children, adolescents, and young adults. Short-term studies did not show an increase in the risk of suicidality with antidepressants compared with placebo in adults beyond age 24, and there was a reduction in risk with antidepressants compared with placebo in adults aged 65 or older.

Patient Counseling

Adverse drug effects (Box 19-3) should be reviewed with the patient or caregiver with instructions to communicate with the prescriber or pharmacist for possible dosage adjustment or medication change. Patients should be advised to keep a record of changes in urination patterns, such as frequency of loss of control, as well as how often they need to urinate during the night.

Drug–Drug Interactions

Anticholinergics can worsen overflow incontinence by weakening bladder contractions and decreasing urine flow while alpha-adrenergic-receptor agonists can cause increased internal urethral sphincter pressure and further decrease flow. Antihistamine–decongestant combinations have the ability to significantly decrease urine flow in older males.

The concurrent use of alpha-adrenergic-receptor agonists and alpha-adrenergic blockers should be avoided.

> **BOX 19-3. Adverse Drug Effects**

- *Anticholinergics:* Adverse effects include dizziness, dry mouth, blurred vision, confusion, significant risk of falls, and a risk of worsening dementia.
- *Alpha-adrenergic-receptor blocking agents:* Side effects include lower blood pressure, orthostatic hypotension, dizziness, headache, and somnolence.
- *Alpha-adrenergic-receptor agonists:* Hypertension, anxiety, and insomnia are side effects.

19-8   Pharmacist's Role

Pharmacists play vital roles in assisting geriatric patients with medication management. Drug regimen review should be the first step for pharmacists who assist geriatric patients with their medication. This review allows the pharmacist an opportunity to identify potential drug–drug interactions, medication adverse effects, and medications without an indication. The review is also a chance to determine if any potentially inappropriate medications (based on the Beer's List) have been prescribed. Through careful profile review and patient counseling, pharmacists are often able to stop the "prescribing cascade" (prescribing a medication to treat a side effect of another medication) from becoming a reality. Counseling on medication side effects as well as goals of therapy are especially important for patients with Alzheimer's disease or Parkinson's disease. Pharmacists may also help to devise medication administration schedules for patients with complex drug regimens.

NAPLEX Competency Statements

The questions in this chapter cover the following 2021 NAPLEX Competency Statements: **AREA 1:** 1.1; 1.2; 1.3; 1.4; 1.5; 1.6; 1.7 **AREA 2:** 2.1; 2.2 **AREA 3:** 3.1; 3.2; 3.3; 3.4; 3.5; 3.6; 3.7; 3.8; 3.9; 3.10; 3.11; 3.12 **AREA 5:** 5.4 **AREA 6:** 6.4.

 ## 19-9   Questions

1. Of the following pharmacokinetic processes, which is the least altered by aging?

   A. Absorption
   B. Distribution
   C. Metabolism
   D. Elimination
   E. Excretion

2. Based on pharmacokinetic changes associated with aging, which of the following medications would be most likely to accumulate with repeated doses?

   A. Alprazolam
   B. Diazepam
   C. Donepezil
   D. Penicillin
   E. Selegiline

3. Galantamine increases levels of which neurotransmitter?

   A. Acetylcholine
   B. Dopamine
   C. Melatonin
   D. Norepinephrine
   E. Serotonin

4. Weight loss is most often associated with which of the following?

   A. Donepezil
   B. Galantamine
   C. Mirtazapine ⚠
   D. Rivastigmine
   E. Memantine

⚠ **Alprazolam** *FDA BOXED WARNING*

Concomitant use of benzodiazepines and opioids may result in profound respiratory depression, coma and death. Reserve combination for patients without other treatment options. Limit dosages and durations to the minimum required and follow patients for signs and symptoms of respiratory depression.

Mirtazapine *FDA BOXED WARNING*

Increased risk of suicidal thoughts and behavior in pediatric and young adult patients taking antidepressants.

5. Of the following medications, which has FDA approval only for moderate-to-severe Alzheimer's disease?

   A. Donepezil
   B. Exelon
   C. Galantamine
   D. Namenda
   E. Aricept

6. Of the following medications used to treat behavioral and emotional symptoms in Alzheimer's patients, which has an FDA boxed warning of increased mortality?

   A. Buspirone
   B. Citalopram
   C. Lorazepam
   D. Risperidone
   E. Zolpidem

7. The maximum daily dose of galantamine in patients with renal impairment is _____.

   A. 8 mg/d
   B. 12 mg/d
   C. 16 mg/d
   D. 24 mg/d
   E. 32 mg/d

8. Which of the following drugs is *not* likely to worsen cognition in Alzheimer's disease patients?

   A. Dicyclomine
   B. Dimenhydrinate
   C. Meclizine
   D. Trazodone
   E. Trihexyphenidyl

9. Memantine's reported benefit in treating the symptoms of Alzheimer's disease is thought to be the result of _____.

   A. increasing serotonin receptor activity
   B. blocking the effect of glutamate on receptors
   C. directly blocking acetylcholine receptors
   D. decreasing intracellular dopamine activity
   E. decreasing amyloid deposits in the brain

10. Which of the following works by direct stimulation of dopamine receptors?

    A. Amantadine
    B. Benztropine
    C. Entacapone
    D. Ropinirole
    E. Selegiline

11. Urge urinary incontinence secondary to detrusor hyperactivity is most effectively treated with which of the following medications?

    A. Avodart
    B. Sanctura
    C. Tamsulosin
    D. Midodrine
    E. Proscar

12. What would be the most likely outcome if a patient with Parkinson's disease taking levodopa were also prescribed haloperidol?

    A. Excessive nausea and vomiting
    B. Hypertensive crisis
    C. Tachycardia and possible chest pain
    D. Worsening symptoms of Parkinson's disease
    E. Excessive somnolence

13. Which of the following inhibits MAO?

    A. Benztropine
    B. Bromocriptine
    C. Pramipexole
    D. Rasagiline
    E. Tolcapone

14. How does carbidopa affect levodopa?

    A. It slows the release from presynaptic neurons.
    B. It prevents the excretion of dopamine.
    C. It increases stimulation of dopamine receptors.
    D. It decreases tolerance to normal doses.
    E. It inhibits the peripheral conversion to dopamine.

15. C. H. is an 82-year-old male with a history of falls related to low blood pressure and now reports urinary incontinence. Which of the following would have the greatest potential for worsening his orthostatic hypotension?

    A. Alfuzosin
    B. Darifenacin
    C. Doxazosin
    D. Dutasteride
    E. Tamsulosin

16. Which of the following statements is true concerning the treatment of Parkinson's disease? (Mark all that apply.)

    A. Entacapone is not used as monotherapy except for patients with end-of-dose wearing-off periods and for those experiencing motor fluctuations.
    B. Pramipexole has been reported to cause "sleep attacks."
    C. Food–drug interactions would not be expected with selegiline when given at doses of 10 mg daily.
    D. Nuplazid is indicated for hallucinations and delusions associated with Parkinson's disease.
    E. Apomorphine is reserved for treatment of "off" episodes in advanced disease.

17. Timolol ophthalmic drops would be more likely to cause which of the following adverse effects as compared to levobetaxolol ophthalmic drops?

    A. Agitation and restlessness
    B. Nausea and vomiting
    C. Confusion
    D. Change in heart rate and blood pressure
    E. Altered intraocular pressure

18. Which of the following would *not* be considered for monotherapy of glaucoma?

    A. Latanoprost
    B. Dorzolamide
    C. Carteolol
    D. Methazolamide
    E. Brimonidine

19. Which of the following can cause iris pigmentation changes?

    A. Acetazolamide
    B. Betaxolol
    C. Brimonidine
    D. Latanoprost
    E. Pilocarpine

20. Which of the following is available as a fixed combination product?

    A. Dorzolamide and timolol
    B. Betaxolol and bimatoprost
    C. Bimatoprost and levobunolol
    D. Latanoprost and timolol
    E. Methazolamide and latanoprost

21. Which of the following is *not* available as an ophthalmic solution?

    A. Brimonidine
    B. Dipivefrin
    C. Dorzolamide
    D. Methazolamide
    E. Metipranolol

22. Which of the following should *not* be used if a patient has a sulfa allergy?

    A. Betaxolol
    B. Bimatoprost
    C. Brimonidine
    D. Brinzolamide
    E. Unoprostone

23. Which of the following is true about prostaglandin analogs?

A. They cause an increase in aqueous humor synthesis.

B. They cause a decrease in aqueous humor formation.

C. They cause an increase in uveoscleral outflow without effect on aqueous humor formation.

D. They cause pupil contraction resulting in aqueous humor outflow.

E. They cause a decrease in uveoscleral outflow.

24. During a recent visit to his pharmacy, 79-year-old R. H. is recommended a combination antihistamine/decongestant for his runny nose and congestion. He says he is currently taking Proscar and Flomax. What would be the potential effect of taking these medications?

A. Increased drowsiness when combining Flomax with an antihistamine/decongestant

B. Decreased urine output and more frequent urinations

C. Decreased absorption of Proscar, resulting in fewer benefits

D. Increase in bladder spasms and sudden discharge of urine

E. Dry mouth and blurred vision secondary to taking Proscar with a decongestant

25. Use the following profile to answer the question.

PATIENT PROFILE	
Name: Bill Smith	**Height:** 6'1"
Age: 70	**Weight:** 185 lbs
Sex: male	**Allergies:** none
Dx: BPH, HTN, HLD	**Vitals:** BP 127/69, Pulse 72, RR 16, Temp 98.7
Medications: multivitamin 1 daily; atorvastatin 40 mg daily; amlodipine 10 mg daily; Flomax 0.8 mg daily	

Mr. Smith has been receiving Flomax for BPH. About a month ago, the Flomax was increased to 0.8 mg daily due to continued symptoms. Patient continues to have frequent urinary symptoms at night. He still awakens 5 to 6 times a night to urinate. He also continues with weak flow and dribbling. Which medication change would be appropriate at this time?

A. Increase Flomax to 1.2 mg daily
B. Change to Rapaflo 8 mg daily
C. Start Vesicare 5 mg daily
D. Add Proscar 5 mg daily
E. Add oxybutynin 2.5 mg twice daily

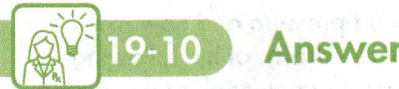 **19-10** **Answers**

1. A. Of all the age-related changes of the pharmacokinetic process, absorption is the least altered, perhaps because most drugs are passively absorbed.

2. B. Diazepam is a lipid-soluble drug and will accumulate in older adults secondary to increased storage in body fat. The potential for accumulation is much less with the other medications listed.

3. A. Galantamine is a cholinesterase inhibitor, and all cholinesterase inhibitors increase levels of acetylcholine, the neurotransmitter that appears to be involved with memory function.

4. D. Weight loss, probably because of nausea and vomiting, is a warning for rivastigmine. In controlled trials, approximately 26% of women on doses of 9 mg/d or greater had weight loss of equal to or greater than 7% of their baseline weight. There is less reported weight loss with donepezil, galantamine, and memantine. The antidepressant mirtazapine is associated with weight gain in the elderly.

5. D. Namenda did not show benefit in mild-to-moderate Alzheimer's disease and is only FDA approved for moderate-to-severe disease. The others listed are all acetylcholinesterase inhibitors and are approved for mild-to-moderate Alzheimer's disease. Donepezil is also approved for moderate-to severe-disease.

6. **D.** Risperidone, as well as other atypical antipsychotics, increases mortality risk when given to patients with dementia who have agitation or aggressive behaviors. This is probably a class effect, and any antipsychotic should be used only if no alternative medication is effective.

7. **C.** With renal or hepatic dysfunction, galantamine doses should not exceed 16 mg/d. With severe renal or hepatic dysfunction, galantamine should not be used.

8. **D.** All of the drugs listed—with the exception of trazodone—have anticholinergic activity. Decreasing the activity of acetylcholine could worsen dementia and block benefits of cholinesterase inhibitors. Trazodone is an antidepressant with sedating properties but little anticholinergic activity. It may be given at bedtime to help with sleep. Trazodone has a side effect of orthostatic hypotension.

9. **B.** Glutamate is the main excitatory neurotransmitter in the central nervous system, and one theory states that blocking the effects of glutamate on NMDA receptors will block neurotoxic effects and decrease symptoms of Alzheimer's disease.

10. **D.** Ropinirole directly stimulates dopamine receptors; the other drugs treat Parkinson's disease by different mechanisms.

11. **B.** Sanctura (trospium) is an anticholinergic that decreases acetylcholine-mediated contractions of the detrusor muscle. This improves bladder control in urge incontinence. Avodart (dutasteride) and Proscar (finasteride) are used to treat overflow incontinence by reducing prostate enlargement. Tamsulosin, an alpha-adrenergic antagonist, would decrease bladder control in urge incontinence. Midodrine, an alpha-adrenergic agonist, is used for stress incontinence and is less beneficial for urge incontinence than the use of an anticholinergic.

12. **D.** Haloperidol and other antipsychotics block dopamine activity and can worsen PD. They can also block the benefits of PD medications, which increase dopamine activity.

13. **D.** Rasagiline is an MAO inhibitor that is selective for MAO-B, which decreases the potential for drug–drug and drug–food interactions. At higher doses, this selectivity lessens.

14. **E.** Carbidopa inhibits the peripheral conversion of levodopa to dopamine, thus allowing more levodopa to cross the blood–brain barrier, and decreases adverse effects from dopamine.

15. **C.** Doxazosin, an alpha-adrenergic antagonist, could improve urine flow but has the potential to induce orthostatic hypotension and falls with geriatric patients being at greater risk. Alfuzosin and tamsulosin have a similar mechanism of action but may produce less orthostatic hypotension because of greater selectivity to bladder function.

16. **B, C, D, E.** Entacapone should always be given with carbidopa-levodopa because benefits depend on carbidopa inhibiting the peripheral conversion of levodopa.

17. **D.** Timolol is a nonselective beta-adrenergic antagonist that causes a reduction in heart rate and blood pressure. There is enough absorption from eye drops to produce cardiac effects.

18. **D.** All of the other choices could be considered as monotherapy for glaucoma. Methazolamide is an oral carbonic anhydrase inhibitor and is used in conjunction with ophthalmic drops.

19. **D.** Latanoprost, a prostaglandin analog, is known to change iris pigmentation.

20. **A.** Dorzolamide plus timolol is a combination ophthalmic solution for treating glaucoma. An advantage for using a combination product would be increased compliance.

21. **D.** Methazolamide and acetazolamide are both available only as oral tablets or capsules. Topical carbonic anhydrase inhibitors are brinzolamide and dorzolamide.

22. **D.** Patients with sulfa allergy should not be given a carbonic anhydrase inhibitor.

23. **C.** Prostaglandin analogs increase outflow without changing aqueous humor formation. Beta-adrenergic antagonists decrease formation with only a slight increase in outflow.

24. **B.** R. H.'s current medications indicate that he has overflow incontinence and that a decongestant would counter the benefits of tamsulosin and an antihistamine could decrease bladder contractions. The result would be urinary retention and more frequent release of small amounts of urine.

25. **D.** Because we have maximized the alpha-blocker (maximum dose of Flomax is 0.8 mg daily), the next step would be to add a 5-alpha-reductase inhibitor. Proscar is the only one listed. Rapaflo is another alpha-blocker. Vesicare and oxybutynin are anticholinergics.

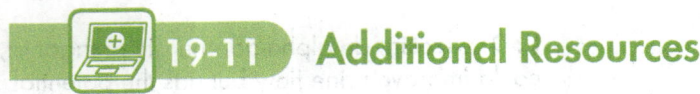

19-11   Additional Resources

American Geriatrics Society 2015 Beers Criteria Update Expert Panel. American Geriatrics Society updated Beers Criteria for potentially inappropriate medication use in older adults. *J Am Geriatr Soc.* 2015;63(11):2227–2246.

2019 American Geriatrics Society Beers Criteria Update Expert Panel. American Geriatrics Society 2019 Updated AGS Beers Criteria for potentially inappropriate medication use in older adults. *J Am Geriatr Soc.* 2019; 67(4):674–694.

Boland MV, Ervin AM, Friedman DS, et al. Comparative effectiveness of treatments for open-angle glaucoma: a systematic review for the U.S. Preventive Services Task Force. *Ann Intern Med.* 2013;158(4):271–279.

Cho S, Lau SW, Tandon V, et al. Geriatric drug evaluation: where we are now and where should we be in the future? *Arch Intern Med.* 2011;171(10):937–940.

Farlow MR, Cummings JL. Effective pharmacologic management of Alzheimer's disease. *Am J Med.* 2007;120(5):388–397.

Fernandez HH. Updates in the medical management of Parkinson disease. *Cleve Clin J Med.* 2012;79(1):28–35.

Griebling TL. Urinary incontinence in the elderly. *Clin Geriatr Med.* 2009;25(3):445–457.

Kwon YH, Fingert JH, Kuehn MH, et al. Primary open-angle glaucoma. *N Engl J Med.* 2009;360:1113–1124.

Qato DM, Alexander GC, Conti RM, et al. Use of prescription and over-the-counter medications and dietary supplements among older adults in the United States. *JAMA.* 2008;300(24):2867–2878.

Rawls WN. Alzheimer's disease. In: Herfindal ET, Gourley DR, eds. *Textbook of Therapeutics.* 8th ed. Philadelphia, PA: WB Saunders; 2006:1811–1828.

Stacy M. Medical treatment of Parkinson disease. *Neurol Clin.* 2009;27(3):605–631.

Kidney Diseases

JOANNA Q. HUDSON

20-1 KEY POINTS

ACUTE KIDNEY INJURY

- Acute kidney injury (AKI) is classified on the basis of changes in serum creatinine or glomerular filtration rate (GFR) and urine output.
- Types of AKI include prerenal, intrinsic, and postrenal.
- Prevention of kidney dysfunction in high-risk patients is the most effective strategy to address AKI.
- Conditions that increase the risk of AKI include decreased perfusion of the kidney and administration of nephrotoxic agents.
- Early recognition and treatment of AKI may prevent irreversible kidney damage.
- Goals of treatment for patients with AKI are achievement of baseline kidney function and prevention of both chronic kidney disease (CKD) and the need for renal replacement therapy.
- Supportive care includes maintaining hemodynamic stability, providing nutritional support, avoiding nephrotoxic agents, and using renal replacement therapy if indicated.
- Diuretics are often used in patients with AKI to maintain fluid balance and hemodynamic stability.
- A review of medications is necessary to ensure appropriate dose adjustments based on kidney function.
- Kidney function estimation equations that depend on stable kidney function should not be used to assess kidney function in patients with AKI.

CHRONIC KIDNEY DISEASE

- CKD is classified on the basis of cause, GFR, and the level of proteinuria.
- Screening for proteinuria and assessment of kidney function in individuals at high risk for kidney disease are important to identify patients with kidney disease and to monitor progression of the disease.
- Therapy to delay progression of kidney disease is based on the underlying cause, but typically includes initiation of therapy with angiotensin-converting enzyme inhibitors or angiotensin II receptor blockers.
- Sodium-glucose cotransporter-2 (SGLT2) inhibitors have shown benefits in delaying progression of kidney disease in individuals with type 2 diabetes with albuminuria.
- Common secondary complications of CKD include fluid and electrolyte abnormalities, anemia, CKD–mineral and bone disorder (CKD-MBD), and metabolic acidosis.
- Therapeutic management of anemia includes erythropoiesis-stimulating agents and iron supplementation to achieve target hemoglobin while preventing iron deficiency.
- Hyperphosphatemia associated with CKD-MBD is managed by dietary phosphorus restriction, phosphate-binding agents, and dialysis in patients with end-stage kidney disease.
- Management of secondary hyperparathyroidism associated with CKD-MBD includes control of serum calcium, phosphorus, and parathyroid hormone. Therapeutic management includes vitamin D therapy and the calcimimetic agents cinacalcet (Sensipar) and etelcalcetide (Parsabiv), which are approved only for patients with end-stage kidney disease on dialysis.

20-2 STUDY GUIDE CHECKLIST

The following topics may guide your study of AKI:

- ☐ Risk factors for AKI.
- ☐ Considerations for drug dosing in AKI.
- ☐ Mechanism of action of diuretics.
- ☐ Common drug-induced causes of AKI.
- ☐ Kidney Disease: Improving Global Outcomes (KDIGO) guideline for AKI.
- ☐ Indications for renal replacement therapy.
- ☐ Drug removal by renal replacement therapy.

The following topics may guide your study of CKD:

- ☐ Risk factors for CKD.
- ☐ Estimating equations to assess kidney function.
- ☐ American Diabetes Association guidelines for management of diabetes.
- ☐ Review of antihypertensive agents.
- ☐ KDIGO guidelines for CKD, CKD-MBD, and anemia.

20-3   Acute Kidney Injury

Disease Overview

Definition and classification of acute kidney injury

Acute kidney injury (AKI) is defined as rapid (hours to days) deterioration of kidney function resulting in azotemia (retention of nitrogenous waste products such as urea) and failure of the kidney to maintain fluid, electrolyte, and acid–base homeostasis. A reduction in urine output frequently occurs, but normal urine output does not rule out AKI (i.e., reduction in urine output is not a specific marker of AKI). Urine output is classified as nonoliguric (urine output > 400 mL/d), oliguric (urine output < 400 mL/d), or anuric (urine output < 50 mL/d).

One classification system proposed to distinguish between mild or severe and early or late cases of AKI is known as RIFLE: *R*isk of kidney dysfunction, *I*njury to the kidney, *F*ailure or *L*oss of kidney function, and *E*nd-stage kidney disease (ESKD):

- **Risk:** A 1.5-fold increase in the serum creatinine or a decrease in glomerular filtration rate (GFR) by 25% or urine output < 0.5 mL/kg/h for 6 hours
- **Injury:** A twofold increase in the serum creatinine or a decrease of GFR by 50% or urine output < 0.5 mL/kg/h for 12 hours
- **Failure:** A threefold increase in the serum creatinine, a decrease of GFR by 75% or urine output of < 0.3 mL/kg/h for 24 hours, or anuria for 12 hours
- **Loss:** Complete loss of kidney function (e.g., need for renal replacement therapy) for more than 4 weeks
- **ESKD:** Complete loss of kidney function (e.g., need for renal replacement therapy) for more than 3 months

A modification of RIFLE that includes slightly adapted diagnostic criteria and a staging system was proposed by the Acute Kidney Injury Network (AKIN). The classification or staging system corresponds to risk (stage 1), injury (stage 2), and failure (stage 3) of the RIFLE criteria. Because loss and ESKD were removed from the AKIN staging system and defined as outcomes, stage 3 of AKIN includes those individuals requiring renal replacement therapy.

To provide one definition of AKI, the Kidney Disease: Improving Global Outcomes (KDIGO) clinical practice guideline for AKI was developed. KDIGO defines AKI as (1) an increase in serum creatinine by at least 0.3 mg/dL within 48 hours, (2) an increase in serum creatinine by at least 1.5 times baseline within the prior 7 days, or (3) a urine volume less than 0.5 mL/kg/h for 6 hours. The KDIGO stages of AKI are based on changes in serum creatinine and urine output:

- **Stage 1:** Increase in serum creatinine by ≥ 0.3 mg/dL or 1.5 to 1.9 times from baseline; urine output of < 0.5 mL/kg/h for 6 to 12 hours
- **Stage 2:** Increase in serum creatinine > 2 to 2.9 times from baseline; urine output of < 0.5 mL/kg/h for ≥ 12 hours
- **Stage 3:** One of the following—(1) an increase in serum creatinine of three times from baseline, (2) an increase in serum creatinine to ≥ 4 mg/dL, (3) the need for renal replacement therapy, or (4) in patients < 18 years, a decrease in estimated GFR to < 35 mL/min/1.73 m^2. Urine output < 0.3 mL/kg/h for ≥ 24 hours or anuria for ≥ 12 hours.

[Note: KDIGO recently suggested the terminology *acute kidney disease* (AKD) to describe patients with AKI for ≤ 3 months who cannot yet be declared as ESKD and replacement of the term ESKD with *kidney failure with replacement therapy* (KFRT)].

Epidemiology

- Community-acquired AKI accounts for approximately 1% of hospital admissions.
- Hospital-acquired AKI occurs in 2% to 20% of hospitalized patients, and the highest incidence occurs in patients in intensive care units.

> **BOX 20-1. Clinical Presentation of AKI**
>
> - Decreased urine output
> - Signs of hypovolemia (prerenal causes), such as tachycardia, decreased blood pressure, and orthostasis
> - Unique color and composition of urine: Cola-colored urine (suggesting bleeding) and foaming (indicating proteinuria)
> - Symptoms of uremia (a clinical syndrome resulting from azotemia), including weakness, shortness of breath, fatigue, mental status changes, nausea and vomiting, bleeding, loss of appetite, and edema
>
> - Flank pain
> - Increased weight (suggesting fluid accumulation)
> - Increased blood pressure (suggesting fluid accumulation)
> - Signs and symptoms of electrolyte abnormalities (hyperkalemia) and metabolic acidosis (see Chapter 21 on fluids and electrolytes)
> - Bladder distention or prostate enlargement (postrenal causes)
> - Other findings specific to the cause of AKI (see section on pathophysiology)

Types

AKI is classified according to the area of the kidney affected:

- *Prerenal AKI* is characterized by a decrease in perfusion to the kidney with or without systemic arterial hypotension. It is the most common type of AKI and is usually reversible.
- *Intrinsic* or *intrarenal AKI* is the result of structural damage to the parenchymal tissue of the kidney. It is divided into vascular, glomerular, interstitial, and tubular disorders (most common).
- *Postrenal AKI* is an obstruction of urine flow occurring at any level of the urinary outflow tracts.

Clinical Presentation

Box 20-1 describes the signs and symptoms of AKI.

Pathophysiology and Etiologies

Prerenal AKI

Prerenal AKI is caused by conditions that decrease glomerular hydrostatic pressure, leading to a decrease in GFR. Hypoperfusion leads to increased sodium and water reabsorption by the kidney and stimulates compensatory mechanisms.

The following compensatory mechanisms (also known as autoregulation) aid in increasing glomerular hydrostatic pressure and GFR (Figure 20-1).

- Vasodilation of the afferent arteriole (mediated primarily by prostaglandins)
- Vasoconstriction of the efferent arteriole (mediated primarily by angiotensin II)

FIGURE 20-1. Autoregulation in the Nephron

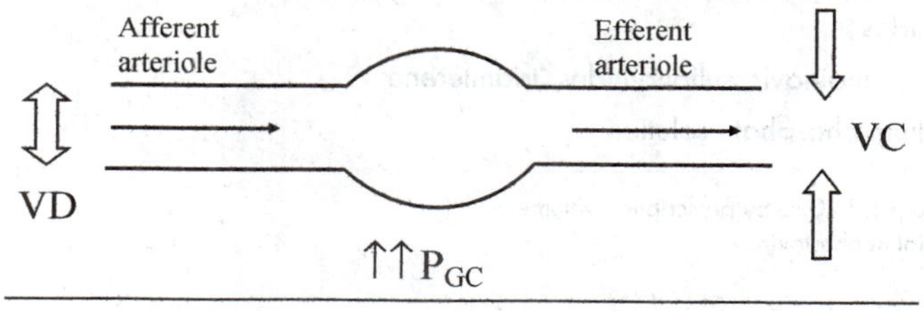

BOX 20-2. Etiologies of Prerenal AKI

Intravascular volume depletion related to excessive diuresis, vomiting, excessive gastrointestinal (GI) fluid loss, and bleeding

Severe hypotension

Decreased effective blood volume (volume sensed by arterial baroreceptors) as occurs with congestive

heart failure, cirrhosis, nephrotic syndrome, and hepatorenal syndrome

Systemic vasodilation that can occur with sepsis, liver failure, and anaphylaxis

Large-vessel renal vascular disease, including renal artery thrombosis or embolism and renal artery stenosis

Alterations in afferent and efferent arteriolar tone can affect compensatory mechanisms. Nonsteroidal anti-inflammatory drugs (NSAIDs) and cyclooxygenase-2 (COX-2) inhibitors can prevent compensatory vasodilation of the afferent arteriole. Angiotensin-converting enzyme inhibitors (ACEIs), angiotensin II receptor blockers (ARBs), and renin inhibitors (aliskiren) can prevent compensatory vasoconstriction of the efferent arteriole. See Box 20-2 for a list of the etiologies of prerenal AKI.

Medications (Table 20-1)

Intrinsic AKI

The primary anatomic sites of the kidney are prone to structural damage from prolonged ischemia and direct toxicity because of the high metabolic activity and concentrating ability of the kidney.

TABLE 20-1. Drug-Induced Causes of AKI

Type of AKI	Causative drugs[a]
Prerenal AKI	ACEIs, ARBs, COX-2 inhibitors, cyclosporine, diuretics, NSAIDs, radiocontrast media, renin inhibitors, SGLT2 inhibitors, tacrolimus
Intrinsic AKI	
Vascular	Vasculitis and thrombosis: Adalimumab, bevacizumab, cisplatin, cyclosporine, gemcitabine, hydralazine, methamphetamines, mitomycin C, propylthiouracil, tacrolimus
	Cholesterol emboli: **Warfarin**, thrombolytic agents
Glomerular	COX-2 inhibitors, gold, heroin, Interferon-alpha and -beta, lithium, NSAIDs, pamidronate, phenytoin, sirolimus, tyrosine kinase inhibitors
Interstitial nephritis	Allergic interstitial nephritis: Ciprofloxacin, COX-2 inhibitors, NSAIDs, penicillins, proton pump inhibitors
	Chronic interstitial nephritis: Aristolochic acid (Chinese herbs), cyclosporine, lithium
	Papillary necrosis: Analgesic combinations (phenacetin, **aspirin**, caffeine), NSAIDs
Tubular epithelial cell damage	Acute tubular necrosis: Adefovir, aminoglycosides, amphotericin B, carboplatin, cidofovir, cisplatin, cocaine, cyclosporine, foscarnet, ifosfamide, pentamidine, radiocontrast media, tacrolimus, tenofovir, zoledronate
	Osmotic nephrosis: Dextran, hydroxyethyl starch solutions, mannitol, sucrose-containing intravenous immunoglobulin
Postrenal AKI	
Obstructive	Acyclovir, ascorbic acid, atazanavir, ethylene glycol, foscarnet, indinavir, methotrexate, oxalate, sulfonamides
Nephrolithiasis	Atazanavir, indinavir, sulfonamides, triamterene
Nephrocalcinosis	Oral sodium phosphate solution

Boldface indicates one of top 100 drugs for 2020 by prescription volume.
a. This list does not include all potential nephrotoxins.

Select etiologies of intrinsic AKI by anatomic site are as follows:

- *Vascular:* Inflammation and emboli
- *Glomerular (glomerulonephritis):* Systemic lupus erythematosus (SLE), immune-mediated causes, and medications (see Table 20-1)
- *Interstitial:* Ischemia, allergic interstitial nephritis, infections, and medications (see Table 20-1). Clinical presentation of acute allergic interstitial nephritis may include fever, rash, and eosinophilia; however, these findings may be absent in patients with this type of injury.
- *Tubular—accounts for 90% of intrinsic cases:* Intrarenal vasoconstriction, direct tubular toxicity, and intratubular obstruction; prolonged ischemia from prerenal causes; and toxins that may be endogenous or exogenous:
  - *Endogenous:* Myoglobin, hemoglobin, and uric acid
  - *Exogenous:* Medications (see Table 20-1; aminoglycosides are common nephrotoxins leading to nonoliguric acute tubular necrosis after 5 to 7 days of therapy) and other exogenous substances such as ethylene glycol and pesticides

Postrenal AKI

This disorder is characterized by an obstruction of urinary flow at any level from the urinary collecting system to the urethra. Medications associated with postrenal AKI are identified in Table 20-1.

Etiologies of postrenal AKI by anatomic site are as follows:

- *Renal pelvis or tubules:* Crystal deposition
- *Ureteral:* Tumor, stricture, and stones
- *Bladder neck obstruction:* Prostatic hypertrophy and bladder carcinoma

Diagnostic Criteria

Table 20-2 shows the diagnostic tests and the findings associated with AKI. A diagnosis requires the following:

- *Evaluate physical findings:* Assess for signs and symptoms listed in clinical presentation.
- *Take medication history (including over-the-counter medications and herbals):* Identify potentially nephrotoxic agents (see Table 20-1). *Note:* Patients with contrast-induced nephrotoxicity (CIN) may have received the dose 24 to 72 hours before the rise in serum creatinine is noted.
- *Estimate GFR:* Normal is generally in the range of 90 to 125 mL/min/1.73 m^2.

TABLE 20-2. Laboratory Findings to Help Differentiate Prerenal and Intrinsic AKI*

Diagnostic test	Prerenal AKI	Intrinsic AKI
BUN:Cr ratio	> 20:1	≤ 15:1
Urinalysis	Normal with few cells or casts (hyaline casts normal)	Granular casts with tubular epithelial cells
Urine osmolality	> 500 mOsm/kg	≤ 300 to 350 mOsm/kg
Urinary Cr:Plasma Cr ratio	> 40:1	< 20:1
Specific gravity	> 1.018	< 1.012
Urine sodium	< 20 mEq/L	> 40 mEq/L
FE$_{Na}$	< 1%	> 2%
Urinary RBCs and WBCs	Absent	2 to 4+

BUN, blood urea nitrogen; Cr, creatinine; FE$_{Na}$, fractional excretion of sodium; RBC, red blood cell; WBC, white blood cell.
*Use in conjunction with clinical presentation.

Consider limitations in using serum creatinine as a marker of kidney function (e.g., conditions of poor muscle mass) and in using equations to estimate GFR in patients with unstable kidney function. See discussion of assessment of kidney function in Section 20-4. Changes in serum creatinine are generally evaluated in individuals with AKI as opposed to calculating a GFR as a result of the unstable kidney function (see section above on Definition and Classification of AKI).

Other assessment equations and methods (e.g., Jelliffe and Jelliffe equation) are available to estimate GFR in patients with unstable kidney function but are not used often in clinical practice.

Blood tests

- *Elevated:* Serum creatinine, blood urea nitrogen (BUN), and electrolytes (potassium and phosphorus). The BUN:serum creatinine ratio may be elevated in prerenal AKI.
- *Decreased:* Calcium (consider albumin concentration to correct calcium), bicarbonate

Urinalysis

A low urine sodium and an elevated specific gravity and osmolality are indicative of prerenal causes and stimulation of sodium and water retention.

Proteinuria includes the following:

- *Albuminuria:* See Table 20-3
- *Proteinuria (includes albumin and other proteins):* Moderately increased (category A2: > 150 to 500 mg/d) and severely increased (category A3: > 500 mg/d) proteinuria and nephrotic range proteinuria > 3.5 g/d
- Hematuria is indicated by red blood cells.
- Glucose and ketones may be present.
- Urine sediment consisting of granular casts and cellular debris suggests structural damage (hyaline casts are normal).
- White blood cells suggest inflammation.
- Eosinophils are associated with acute allergic interstitial nephritis.

Consider whether fluids or diuretics were previously administered when interpreting urinalysis.

TABLE 20-3. KDIGO Classification of CKD Based on GFR and Albuminuria

GFR category	GFR description	GFR (mL/min/ 1.73 m²)	Albuminuria category	Albuminuria description	Albumin excretion rate (mg/24 h)	Albumin: creatinine ratio (mg/g)
G1	Normal or high	≥ 90	A1	Normal to mildly increased	< 30	< 30
G2	Mildly decreased	60 to 89	A2	Moderately increased[a]	30 to 300	30 to 300
G3a	Mildly to moderately decreased	45 to 59	A3	Severely increased[b]	> 300	> 300
G3b	Moderately to severely decreased	30 to 44				
G4	Severely decreased	15 to 29				
G5	Kidney failure	< 15				

Adapted from KDIGO Chronic Kidney Disease Work Group, 2012.
a. Also referred to as *microalbuminuria,* although KDIGO does not advocate this terminology.
b. Also referred to as *albuminuria* (or overt *proteinuria* if proteins other than albumin are measured), although KDIGO does not advocate this terminology.

Urine chemistries

Evaluate urine sodium, potassium, chloride, creatinine, and urinary anion gap. The fractional excretion of sodium (FE_{Na}) is useful to differentiate prerenal AKI from intrinsic AKI. A low value (< 1%) suggests retention of sodium and water (prerenal etiology) versus intrinsic cause.

Other tests

Radiographic procedures include ultrasound, plain film radiograph, radioisotope scan, and computed tomography.

Renal biopsy may be indicated when other diagnostic tests have not identified the cause of a patient's AKI.

Treatment Principles and Goals

Prevention

Identify the following risk factors:

- Volume depletion
- Exposure to nephrotoxic medications
- Preexisting kidney or hepatic disease
- Surgical procedures

Diagnostic tests requiring radiocontrast media can put patients at risk of AKI. Contrast agents are hyperosmolar compared to plasma osmolality and may cause osmotic diuresis, dehydration, and renal ischemia. Risk factors for CIN include diabetes, heart failure, age > 75 years, hypotension, and an estimated GFR < 60 mL/min/1.73 m². Hydration with either intravenous (I.V.) isotonic sodium chloride or sodium bicarbonate solutions is strongly recommended to prevent CIN in high-risk patients. Guidelines suggest that N-acetylcysteine (Mucomyst) given before and following exposure to radiocontrast dye may be beneficial to prevent CIN; however, because of the lack of supportive evidence, this approach is not strongly recommended.

Treatment goals

- Correct underlying causes of AKI to allow for return of baseline kidney function or highest function possible (e.g., discontinue nephrotoxic agents, correct fluid status, treat underlying infection, address cause of urinary tract obstructions).
- Prevent development of chronic kidney disease and the need for chronic renal replacement therapy.
- Avoid and reduce exposure to nephrotoxic agents when possible.
- Adjust doses of medications based on kidney function. As kidney function recovers, drug doses may need to be increased.
- Avoid agents contraindicated in patients with kidney disease, such as **metformin** (Glucophage) and gadolinium-based contrast dyes used for magnetic resonance imaging (MRI) procedures.
- Address complications of AKI (i.e., hyperkalemia, hyperphosphatemia, fluid overload, metabolic acidosis).

Drug Therapy

Diuretics

Loop diuretics are recommended only for management of fluid overload in patients with AKI (Table 20-4).

TABLE 20-4. Loop Diuretics for Fluid Overload in AKI

Generic name	Trade name	Daily dosage range	Dosage forms	Frequency of administration[a]
Furosemide	**Lasix**	20 to 400 mg	Oral	Every 6 to 12 hours
		20 to 200 mg (up to 1 to 3 g/d in AKI)	I.V.	
Bumetanide	Bumex	0.5 to 10 mg	Oral, I.V.	Every 12 to 24 hours
Torsemide	Demadex	10 to 200 mg	Oral, I.V.	Every 24 hours
Ethacrynic acid	Edecrin	50 to 400 mg	Oral	Every 8 to 12 hours
		50 to 100 mg	I.V.	

Boldface indicates one of top 100 drugs for 2020 by prescription volume.
a. Loop diuretics are also administered as a continuous infusion. Higher dose ranges for intermittent dosing are reserved for patients who are unresponsive to initial smaller doses.

Mechanism of action

Loop diuretics are delivered to the tubular lumen of the kidney by active secretion from the blood into the urine at the proximal tubule. Once at the site of action, loop diuretics cause inhibition of sodium and chloride reabsorption in the thick ascending limb of the loop of Henle to promote water excretion.

Thiazide and thiazide-like diuretics inhibit the Na^+-Cl^- cotransporter in the early distal convoluted tubules. They are generally used in combination with loop diuretics for resistant edema and fluid overload, particularly metolazone (Zaroxolyn, Mykrox), which is effective at a GFR < 30 mL/min/1.73 m². Other thiazide diuretics are generally not effective when GFR < 30 mL/min/1.73 m².

Adverse effects of loop diuretics

- Hypokalemia, hypomagnesemia, hyponatremia, hypovolemia, hyperuricemia, hyperglycemia
- Hypercalciuria, hypocalcemia
- Orthostatic hypotension, dehydration
- Metabolic alkalosis (partly attributable to extracellular fluid volume contraction)
- Ototoxicity
- Diarrhea, nausea

Furosemide (Lasix), bumetanide (Bumex), and torsemide (Demadex) have a sulfonamide substituent lending to a potential for hypersensitivity reactions. Ethacrynic acid (Edecrin) is generally reserved for patients with a true allergy to sulfa compounds.

Adverse effects of thiazide diuretics

- Hypokalemia, hyponatremia, hypercalcemia, hyperuricemia
- Hypovolemia, orthostatic hypotension
- Hyperglycemia, hypochloremic alkalosis, hyperlipidemia
- Hypersensitivity reactions from sulfonamide substituents
- Chest pain (metolazone; more common with Mykrox, which is more rapidly and extensively absorbed than Zaroxolyn)

Drug–drug and drug–disease interactions

- Loop diuretics and aminoglycosides have an increased potential for ototoxicity.
- Diuretics and other nephrotoxins have an increased risk of nephrotoxicity if hypovolemia occurs.
- Diuretics and lithium (Lithane, Lithobid) used concomitantly may result in decreased renal clearance of lithium. Monitor lithium concentrations more closely.
- For diuretics and digoxin (Lanoxin, Digox), hypokalemia from diuretic use may increase risk of toxicity with digoxin. Monitor **potassium** and digoxin.

- Loop and thiazide diuretics may increase gout attacks because of hyperuricemia.
- For thiazide diuretics and diabetes, hyperglycemia may result from thiazides. Increase glucose monitoring.
- Loop diuretics may alter the interpretation of the FE_{Na} as they alter sodium reabsorption (and, thus, elimination).

Monitoring parameters for diuretics

- Blood pressure (sitting and standing)
- Pulse
- Urine output
- Fluid intake
- Serum creatinine
- Serum electrolytes
- BUN
- Bicarbonate
- Calcium
- Glucose
- Uric acid

Pharmacokinetics
Loop diuretics

- *Oral bioavailability:* **Furosemide** (60%), bumetanide (85%), torsemide (85%)
- *Oral:I.V. dose ratios:* **Furosemide** (2:1), bumetanide (1:1), torsemide (1:1)
- *Equivalent doses:* 40 mg **Furosemide** = 1 mg bumetanide = 20 mg torsemide
- *Elimination route:* **Furosemide** (primarily renal), bumetanide (hepatic and renal), torsemide (primarily hepatic), ethacrynic acid (hepatic and renal)

Other factors

Patients with kidney disease generally require larger doses of diuretics to achieve adequate concentrations of the drug at the site of action in the kidney. Loop diuretics also must be bound to albumin to be delivered to the site of action and are actively secreted into the loop of Henle.

Dopamine

Low-dose dopamine is a potent vasodilator that increases renal blood flow and has been associated with an increase in urine output in AKI, but evidence does not support its use and KDIGO guidelines do not currently advocate dopamine for AKI treatment.

Nondrug Therapy

Fluid management

Fluid intake and output should be evaluated, and adjustments made to maintain hemodynamic stability (consider sensible and insensible losses).

Fluid selection (e.g., crystalloids, colloids, or normal saline) and rate of correction depend on the clinical condition of the patient. Isotonic crystalloids are recommended over colloids for intravascular volume expansion. *Note:* Hetastarch has been associated with worsening kidney function and increased risk of mortality and should be avoided in patients with or at risk of acute kidney injury.

Nutritional therapy

A high-calorie diet is generally required (patient specific), but restriction of sodium, potassium, and phosphorus should be considered in all patients.

Renal replacement therapies

Renal replacement therapies are procedures by which the blood is artificially cleared of waste and some essential metabolic products to augment the function of failed or failing kidneys. These procedures include hemodialysis and hemofiltration, in which the semipermeable membrane is a dialyzer, and peritoneal dialysis, in which the peritoneal cavity serves as this membrane. Procedures may be intermittent or continuous. Hemodialysis and hemofiltration are the modalities used for patients with AKI. Continuous renal replacement therapies (CRRTs) require lower blood and dialysate flow rates, remove fluid more gradually than intermittent procedures, and are used often for patients with AKI who are hemodynamically unstable. Common terminologies used for CRRT include continuous venovenous hemofiltration, continuous venovenous hemodialysis, and continuous venovenous hemodiafiltration.

The potential for drug removal by dialysis must be considered, particularly for CRRT procedures that are performed over a prolonged period (e.g., > 24 hours). Drug doses may need to be increased to account for removal by CRRT (e.g., certain antibiotics). Drug characteristics that make a drug more likely to be removed by dialysis are small molecular weight, low protein binding, and low volume of distribution.

Indications for renal replacement therapy

Any of the following conditions refractory to conservative measures are an indication for renal replacement therapy. These are sometimes referred to as the AEIOUs for renal replacement therapy indications:

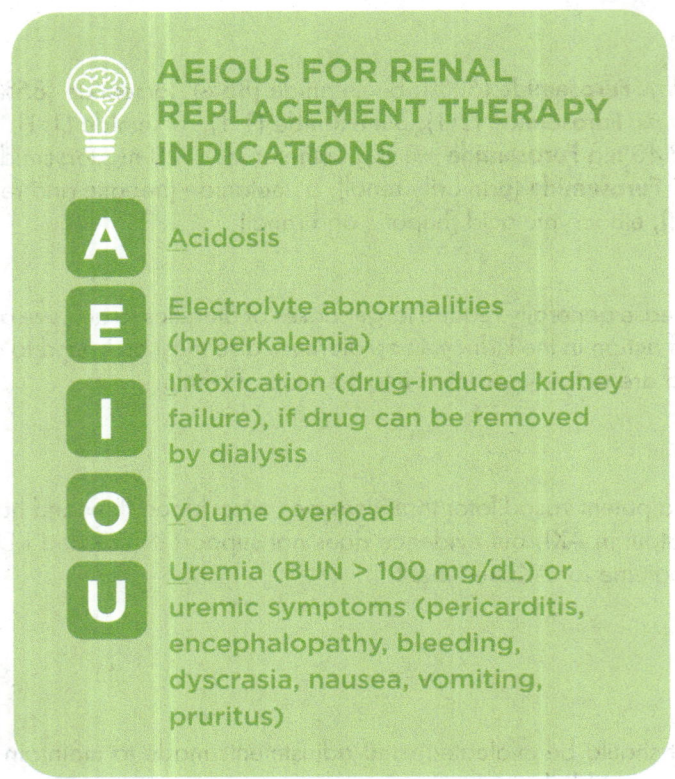

AEIOUs FOR RENAL REPLACEMENT THERAPY INDICATIONS

A — Acidosis

E — Electrolyte abnormalities (hyperkalemia)

I — Intoxication (drug-induced kidney failure), if drug can be removed by dialysis

O — Volume overload

U — Uremia (BUN > 100 mg/dL) or uremic symptoms (pericarditis, encephalopathy, bleeding, dyscrasia, nausea, vomiting, pruritus)

20-4   Pharmacist's Role

AKI is a preventable condition and pharmacists in any practice setting should be able to identify individuals at risk for AKI and recommend that they avoid medications that may contribute to AKI (e.g., NSAIDS in patients with pre-existing kidney disease or who are prone to be hypotensive). The role of the pharmacist for patients with AKI is to work with other members of the health care team to provide supportive care for these patients. This may include determining appropriate fluid administration, measures to correct electrolyte abnormalities, and selection and monitoring of diuretic therapy. Another key component is to identify nephrotoxic medications that may have contributed to AKI and to avoid the use of agents that may be nephrotoxic in individuals with existing AKI. Pharmacists are also well qualified to make recommendations regarding drug dosing in response to changes in kidney function (e.g., as kidney function worsens or as kidney function improves) and when patients are receiving renal replacement therapy.

20-5 Chronic Kidney Disease

Disease Overview

Definition and classification of chronic kidney disease

Chronic kidney disease (CKD) is defined as at least a 3-month period of kidney damage with or without a decrease in GFR or a GFR < 60 mL/min/1.73 m² for longer than 3 months, with implications for health. Kidney damage is defined as pathologic abnormalities or markers of damage, including abnormalities in blood or urine tests or in imaging studies.

The KDIGO guidelines classify CKD by cause of kidney disease, GFR category, and albuminuria level (i.e., CGA [cause, GFR, and albuminuria] staging) (Table 20-3). Patients are considered to have ESKD when renal replacement therapy (either dialysis or transplantation) is required to sustain life. *Note:* KDIGO recently suggested replacement of the term *ESKD* with *kidney failure with replacement therapy* (KFRT)].

Epidemiology

Approximately 26 million American adults have CKD and in 2016 approximately 726,000 individuals had ESKD with approximately 509,000 requiring dialysis (the remainder being transplant patients). The number of patients with CKD continues to increase, with the percent of patients with CKD expected to increase from the current 15% to 17% by 2030. The incidence of CKD is approximately 4 times higher in the Black population. The incidence is greatest in individuals over 65 years of age.

Clinical presentation of CKD

Box 20-3 describes the signs and symptoms of CKD.

> ### BOX 20-3. Clinical Presentation of CKD

- Changes in urine output (may not occur in earlier stages of CKD)
- Foaming of urine (suggesting proteinuria).
  - Table 20-3 shows levels of albuminuria. If total protein levels are measured (including albumin and other proteins), different thresholds apply. A protein excretion ratio (PER) of < 50 mg/24 h and a protein-to-creatinine ratio (PCR) of < 150 mg/g are considered normal. A PER or PCR of > 150 is considered moderately increased, whereas levels > 500 are considered severely increased.
  - *Note: Nephrotic syndrome* is a clinical syndrome associated with total protein in the urine in amounts > 3.5 g/d (referred to as nephrotic range proteinuria), hypoalbuminemia, edema, and hyperlipidemia.
- Hypertension (common etiology of CKD)
- Diabetes (common etiology of CKD)

- Fluid and electrolyte abnormalities (e.g., hyperkalemia, fluid overload; see Chapter 21 on fluids and electrolytes)
- Development of secondary complications of CKD:
  - *Anemia:* Decreased hemoglobin and hematocrit, iron deficiency also common
  - *CKD mineral and bone disorder:* Hyperphosphatemia, hypocalcemia (may develop hypercalcemia as kidney disease progresses), increased parathyroid hormone, vitamin D deficiency, increased fibroblast growth factor 23
  - *Metabolic acidosis:* Decreased serum bicarbonate, increased anion gap
  - *Malnutrition:* Decreased albumin and prealbumin (see Chapter 22 on nutrition)
- Signs of uremia (see Section 20-3) in later stages of CKD (CKD categories G4 and G5)

Pathophysiology of Progressive Kidney Disease and Selected Secondary Complications

Progressive kidney disease

Progressive loss of nephron function results in adaptive changes in remaining nephrons to increase single-nephron glomerular filtration pressure (see Figure 20-1). Over time, the compensatory increase in single-nephron GFR leads to hypertrophy from sustained increases in pressure and loss of individual nephron function.

Proteinuria, one of the initial diagnostic signs, may also contribute to the progressive decline and irreversible loss of kidney function.

Each of the following may result in damage to the kidney that over time leads to a decrease in functioning nephrons and total GFR:

- Diabetes (accounts for primary cause in 45% of patients with ESKD)
- Hypertension (accounts for primary cause in 29% of patients with ESKD)
- Glomerulonephritis (multiple causes, e.g., systemic lupus erythematosus)
- Polycystic kidney disease
- Human immunodeficiency virus (HIV) nephropathy
- Other contributing factors (smoking, obesity, genetic factors, gender differences)

Anemia of CKD

The primary etiology is a decrease in production of the hormone erythropoietin by the kidney as kidney disease progresses. More than 90% of erythropoietin production occurs in the kidney and approximately 10% in the liver.

CKD results in a normochromic, normocytic anemia. Red blood cell lifespan is also decreased from 120 days to approximately 60 days in patients with kidney failure. Other contributors include iron deficiency and blood loss (e.g., from uremic bleeding, dialysis).

CKD mineral and bone disorder

CKD mineral and bone disorder (CKD-MBD) includes abnormalities in parathyroid hormone (PTH), calcium, phosphorus, vitamin D, fibroblast growth factor 23 (FGF23), and bone turnover. Patients with CKD-MBD are also at risk for calcifications as kidney disease progresses.

As kidney function declines, phosphorus elimination decreases. Hyperphosphatemia causes a reciprocal decrease in serum calcium concentrations (hypocalcemia). Hypocalcemia stimulates the release of PTH by the parathyroid glands. Conversion of the vitamin D precursor (25-hydroxyvitamin D) to the active form (1,25-dihydroxyvitamin D_3) occurs in the kidney. As kidney disease progresses, there is a decline in the 1-alpha-hydroxylase enzyme that promotes the final hydroxylation step in the kidney, resulting in a deficiency in active vitamin D. Deficiencies in the precursor form of vitamin D also occur in CKD. Active vitamin D (1,25-dihydroxyvitamin D_3) promotes increased intestinal absorption of calcium and suppresses production of parathyroid hormone by the parathyroid gland; therefore, vitamin D deficiency leads to worsening secondary hyperparathyroidism (Box 20-4).

As kidney disease progresses, the following occurs:

- Hyperphosphatemia and subsequent hypocalcemia progressively worsen, and secondary hyperparathyroidism becomes more severe.

BOX 20-4. Consequences of Increased PTH

Decreased phosphorus reabsorption within the kidney

Increased calcium reabsorption by the kidney

Increased calcium mobilization from bone

Stimulated production of active vitamin D

- The renal effects of PTH on phosphorus and calcium are no longer maintained, and PTH predominantly stimulates calcium resorption from bone.
- Hyperphosphatemia (and active vitamin D) also promotes an increase in FGF23, produced and secreted primarily from osteocytes in bone, which reduces phosphorus by decreasing renal tubular reabsorption of phosphate and decreasing production of active vitamin D.
- Decreased production of active vitamin D worsens hypocalcemia and secondary hyperparathyroidism.
- In more severe CKD, category G5 and ESKD, patients are prone to develop hypercalcemia, because of decreased renal elimination and use of calcium-containing phosphate binders.
- Patients with CKD G5 are at risk for calcifications and calciphylaxis.
- Uncontrolled secondary hyperparathyroidism leads to hyperplasia of the parathyroid gland and renal osteodystrophy (a high bone turnover disease that results from sustained effects of PTH on bone).

Metabolic acidosis

Metabolic acidosis results from the following:

- Decreased excretion of acid by the kidney
- Accumulation of endogenous acids attributable to impaired kidney function (e.g., phosphates, sulfates)

Diagnostic Criteria

Progressive kidney disease

There is a progressive increase in serum creatinine: > 1.1 to 1.2 mg/dL for females and > 1.2 to 1.3 mg/dL for males. Consider factors that may alter serum creatinine, such as decreased muscle mass and nutritional status.

There is a decreased GFR (see Table 20-3 for CKD classification). Consider the assessment method used to estimate creatinine clearance or GFR. There are several equations available to assess kidney function in patients with stable kidney function (Table 20-5). Because GFR cannot be directly measured, it is assessed by clearance of either exogenous or endogenous markers that are primarily filtered by the kidney. Creatinine is produced from creatine in muscle tissue proportionally to muscle mass. It is released at a constant rate into the general circulation and is distributed to total body water. The glomerulus passively filters creatinine, making this a reasonable endogenous filtration marker; however, active tubular secretion accounts for up to 10% to 40% of the total creatinine found in urine.

Cystatin C is also being used for assessment of kidney function. Cystatin C is a cysteine proteinase inhibitor protein produced by all nucleated cells at a fairly constant rate, which has been shown to correlate with measured GFR. It is freely filtered at the glomerulus with 99% of the filtered load being reabsorbed in the proximal tubule where it is catabolized. Cystatin C has been used in several GFR estimating equations, either alone or in combination with creatinine (see Table 20-2).

Other diagnostic criteria for CKD include the following:

- Proteinuria as assessed by the extent of albuminuria (see Table 20-3) or proteinuria
- Abnormal serum chemistries, such as increased SCr and BUN:
  - Abnormalities that may indicate development of secondary complications of CKD: increased potassium, decreased serum bicarbonate, increased phosphorus, decreased calcium (may have hypercalcemia in later stages of CKD)

Anemia of CKD

Testing for anemia is recommended in all patients with CKD. Guidelines for anemia management in patients with CKD recommend further evaluation for anemia when hemoglobin < 12 g/dL in females and < 13.5 g/dL in males.

TABLE 20-5. Methods to Assess Kidney Function

Equation	Estimate of:	Formula
Cockcroft and Gault	CrCl (mL/min)	$CrCl = \dfrac{(140) - age \times W}{Cr \times 72} \times 0.85$ if female where Cr is serum creatinine in mg/dL; W is weight (kg)
MDRD	GFR (mL/min/1.73 m²)	$GFR = 175 \times (S_{cr})^{-1.154} \times (age)^{-0.203} \times 0.742$ (if female) $\times 1.21$ (if black)
CKD-EPI	GFR (mL/min/1.73 m²)	$GFR = 141 \times min(Scr/\kappa, 1)^{\alpha} \times max(Scr/\kappa, 1)^{-1.209} \times 0.993^{Age} \times 1.018$ [if female] $\times 1.159$ [if black] *where κ is 0.7 for females and 0.9 for males; α is -0.329 for females and -0.411 for males; min indicates minimum of Scr/κ or 1, and max indicates maximum of Scr/κ or 1*
CKD-EPI Cr-Cystatin C	GFR (mL/min/1.73 m²)	$eGFR_{Creat-Cyst} = 135 \times min(Scr/\kappa, 1)^{\alpha} \times max(Scr/\kappa, 1)^{-0.601} \times min(SCysC/0.8, 1)^{-0.375} \times max(SCysC/0.8, 1)^{-0.711} 0.995^{Age} \times 0.969$ [if female] $\times 1.108$ [if black] *where κ is 0.7 for females and 0.9 for males; α is -0.248 for females and -0.207 for males; min indicates minimum of Scr/κ or 1, and max indicates maximum of Scr/κ or 1*
CKD-EPI, Cystatin C	GFR (mL/min/1.73 m²)	$eGFR = 133 \times min(CysC/0.8, 1)^{-0.499} \times max(CysC/0.8, 1)^{-1.328} \times 0.996^{Age} \times 0.932$ [if female] *where min indicates minimum of CysC/0.8 or 1, and max indicates maximum of CysC/0.8 or 1*
Urine Collection Method	Measured CrCl (mL/min)	$CrCl = \dfrac{Ucr \times Volume}{Cr \times time}$ Where Ucr = urine creatinine; Cr = serum creatinine

CKD-EPI, chronic kidney disease Epidemiology Collaboration equation; Cr, serum creatinine in mg/dL; CrCl, creatinine clearance; Cys, cystatin C; GFR, glomerular filtration rate; MDRD, Modification of Diet in Renal Disease.

For iron deficiency, evaluate red blood cell indices and iron indices to identify iron deficiency as a contributing factor. Iron deficiency manifests as a microcytic anemia.

Evaluate for folate and vitamin B_{12} deficiencies (manifests as a macrocytic anemia), sources of blood loss (e.g., GI bleeding), and confounding disease states (e.g., cancer and HIV).

CKD-MBD

- Serum phosphorus above normal range
- Calcium abnormalities:
  - *Hypocalcemia:* Corrected serum calcium < 8.5 mg/dL
  - *Hypercalcemia:* Corrected calcium above the normal range (a concern in CKD G5 and ESRD).
    Note: Corrected calcium = measured serum calcium + 0.8 × (normal serum albumin − measured serum albumin); normal serum albumin = 4 g/dL
- Elevated PTH: Normal PTH ~ 10 to 60 pg/mL
- Radiographic evidence of bone abnormalities (e.g., osteitis fibrosa cystica)

Metabolic acidosis

Metabolic acidosis is indicated by a serum bicarbonate (HCO_3^-) < 20 mEq/L.

Typically, the anion gap is increased: anion gap = $[Na^+] - ([Cl^-] + [HCO_3^-])$.

Signs and symptoms of chronic metabolic acidosis that develop as CKD progresses are generally not of the same magnitude as those of acute metabolic acidosis (e.g., hyperventilation, cardiovascular system manifestations, and central nervous system manifestations).

Treatment Goals and Strategies

Progressive kidney disease

Treatment goals

- Control underlying cause of progressive CKD (e.g., hypertension and diabetes; see Chapters 12 and 17, respectively) and slow the rate of progression.
- Meet blood pressure goals: < 140/90 mmHg in patients with CKD if albumin excretion rate (AER) < 30 mg/24 h or < 130/80 mmHg for patients with CKD and AER > 30 mg/24 h (*Note:* the lower blood pressure goal for AER > 30 is a KDIGO suggestion based on a relatively low level of evidence).
- Prevent or minimize albuminuria or proteinuria.
- Prevent drug-induced causes of kidney disease (see Table 20-1).
- Manage secondary complications of CKD (anemia, MBD, electrolyte abnormalities).
- Control hyperlipidemia.
- Address cardiovascular risk factors (cardiovascular disease is the leading cause of death in the CKD population).
- Adjust drug doses based on kidney function.
- Avoid medications contraindicated in patients with reduced kidney function. For example, **metformin** (Glucophage) is contraindicated in patients with GFR < 30 mL/min/1.73 m² because of the increased risk of lactic acidosis. Gadolinium-based contrast dyes used for MRI procedures should not be used in individuals with CKD G4 or G5 because of the risk of nephrogenic systemic fibrosis.
- Avoid NSAIDs for pain management and combination analgesic agents (associated with papillary necrosis; see Table 20-1).
- Start dialysis if baseline GFR < 15 mL/min/1.73 m² and if other indications are present (see Section 20-3 on indications for renal replacement therapy).
- Recommend smoking cessation.

Treatment strategies

- ACEIs and ARBs are used to delay progression of kidney disease (recommended for patients with diabetes and individuals with hypertension and an AER > 300 mg/24 h). Combination therapy with both an ACEI and an ARB is not recommended because of the risk of hyperkalemia and hypotension that outweighs any added benefit. The renin inhibitor aliskiren (Tekturna) also has an "unlabeled/investigational" indication for treatment of persistent proteinuria in patients with type 2 diabetes, hypertension, and nephropathy despite optimized renoprotective therapy (e.g., ARB therapy). In April 2012, the U.S. Food and Drug Administration (FDA) warned of possible risks when using aliskiren in combination with ACEIs and ARBs in patients with diabetes or reduced kidney function. The drug labels for aliskiren-containing products include a contraindication against the use of aliskiren with ACEIs or ARBs in patients with diabetes because of the risk of worsening kidney function, hypotension, and hyperkalemia and a warning to avoid use of these combinations in patients with reduced kidney function (i.e., eGFR < 60 mL/min/1.73 m²).
- The sodium-glucose transport-2 inhibitors (SGLT2 inhibitors) canagliflozin (Invokana) may be used in patients with type 2 diabetes mellitus and diabetic nephropathy (AER > 300 mg/d) to reduce the risk of ESKD, cardiovascular death, and hospitalization for heart failure. Other SGLT2 inhibitors are being studied for this purpose. See Chapter 17 for more information on use of SGLT-2 inhibitors.

- Consider use of diuretics for fluid balance and management of hypertension.
- Consider use of antihypertensives with diet and lifestyle modifications for control of blood pressure (see Chapter 12 on hypertension).
- Consider use of antidiabetic agents with diet and lifestyle modifications for control of blood glucose (see Chapter 17 on diabetes).
- Protein restriction to 0.8 g/kg/d:
  - Use only in adults with a GFR < 25 mL/min/1.73 m² because of the risk of malnutrition from prolonged protein restriction.
  - Consider for patients with > 1 g/d proteinuria despite optimal blood pressure control with a regimen that includes an ACEI or ARB.
- Be cautious about maintaining adequate caloric intake, and avoid malnutrition.
- Renal replacement therapy:
  - Consider plans for dialysis therapy (hemodialysis or peritoneal dialysis) during CKD G4.
  - Evaluate candidacy for kidney transplantation.

Anemia of CKD

Treatment goals

An FDA boxed warning for erythropoiesis-stimulating agents warns that target hemoglobin should not exceed 11 g/dL. This warning is based on studies showing a greater risk for death, serious adverse cardiovascular reactions, and stroke when erythropoiesis-stimulating agents (ESAs) (Table 20-6) were used to target a hemoglobin level above this threshold. *Note:* The FDA labeling for all ESAs states that initiation of therapy is recommended in patients with CKD on dialysis when the hemoglobin level < 10 g/dL and in patients with CKD not on dialysis when the hemoglobin < 10 g/dL and the following apply: (1) the rate of hemoglobin decline indicates the likelihood of requiring a red blood cell transfusion and (2) a goal is to reduce the risk of alloimmunization and the risks of other red blood cell transfusions. A dose reduction or interruption of the ESA dose is recommended if the hemoglobin > 11 g/dL in patients with CKD on dialysis or > 10 g/dL in CKD patients not on dialysis. Using the lowest ESA dose necessary to reduce the need for red blood cell transfusions is recommended.

Transferrin saturation (TSat) and serum ferritin should be maintained at higher values for CKD patients with anemia. KDIGO recommends iron supplementation when the TSat ≤ 30% and ferritin ≤ 500 ng/mL when the goal is to improve hemoglobin, reduce use of ESAs, or both. Consider the risk of iron overload

TABLE 20-6. Erythropoiesis-Stimulating Agents

Generic name	Trade name	Starting dose	Route of administration	Frequency of administration
Epoetin alfa	Epogen, Procrit	50 to 100 units/kg	I.V. or subcutaneously	1 to 3 doses per week
Epoetin alfa-epbx*	Retacrit			
Darbepoetin alfa	Aranesp	0.45 mcg/kg once every 4 weeks for patients with CKD not on dialysis; 0.45 mcg/kg once weekly or 0.75 mcg/kg once every 2 weeks for patients on dialysis	I.V. or subcutaneously	Once weekly or once every other week (may prolong interval to every 3 to 4 weeks)
Methoxy PEG-epoetin beta	Mircera	0.6 mcg/kg	I.V. or subcutaneously	Every 2 weeks

PEG, polyethylene glycol.
* Biosimilar of epoetin alfa.

if TSat and serum ferritin are elevated (e.g., TSat > 50%). *Note:* Ferritin is an acute phase reactant and may be elevated during conditions of infection or inflammation and not truly reflect iron status under these conditions.

Treatment strategies
ESAs

ESAs stimulate red blood cell production in the bone marrow. Available ESAs and initial doses are listed in Table 20-6.

ESAs may be administered subcutaneously or intravenously. Subcutaneous administration is generally preferred for patients not on hemodialysis (i.e., peritoneal dialysis, early-stage CKD patients who do not have I.V. access).

Recommendations for dose conversion from epoetin alfa (units/wk) to darbepoetin alfa (mcg/wk) are provided in the prescribing information. The darbepoetin package insert states that for patients receiving epoetin alfa 2 to 3 times per week, darbepoetin alfa should be administered weekly. For patients receiving epoetin alfa once per week, darbepoetin alfa should be administered once every 2 weeks. In this situation, the weekly epoetin dose should be multiplied by 2, and that dose should be used in the conversion table to determine the appropriate darbepoetin dose. There is also a dose conversion table in the labeling for methoxy PEG-epoetin beta for patients converting from epoetin alfa or darbepoetin to this agent.

For dose titration, allow at least 2 to 4 weeks before making a change in the ESA dose based on the change in hemoglobin. If a change in hemoglobin < 1 g/dL in a 4-week period and iron stores are adequate, increase the ESA dose by 25%. If a change in hemoglobin > 1 g/dL in a 2-week period, reduce the ESA dose by 25%.

 FDA BOXED WARNINGS

Cardiovascular events
Erythropoiesis-stimulating agents (ESAs) increase the risk of death, MI, stroke, venous thromboembolism, thrombosis of vascular access.

Chronic kidney disease
In controlled trials, patients experienced greater risks for death, serious adverse cardiovascular reactions, and stroke when administered ESAs to target a hemoglobin level > 11 g/dL. No trial has identified a hemoglobin target level, ESA dose, or dosing strategy that does not increase these risks. Use the lowest ESA dose sufficient to reduce the need for red blood cell (RBC) transfusions.

Iron supplementation

Iron supplementation prevents iron deficiency as a cause of resistance to therapy with ESAs. Iron deficiency should be corrected before making changes in the dose of the ESA. Common oral iron agents and all I.V. iron agents available in the United States are listed in Table 20-7.

Oral iron supplementation is limited by poor absorption and is often inadequate to achieve goal iron indices. I.V. iron supplementation is preferred for treatment of absolute iron deficiency and in hemodialysis patients with regular I.V. access. The route of administration for CKD patients not on dialysis (nondialysis CKD) should be based on the severity of iron deficiency, response to prior oral iron therapy, side effects with prior oral or I.V. therapy, and adherence. The recommended dose of oral iron is 200 mg elemental iron per day. Ferric maltol is approved at a dose of 30 mg twice daily. A full course of I.V. iron for absolute iron deficiency is typically 1 g administered in divided doses. Weekly maintenance doses of iron (e.g., 25 to 125 mg) may be administered in hemodialysis patients to prevent absolute iron deficiency.

TABLE 20-7. Iron Supplements

Generic name	Trade name[a]	For oral formulations: Commonly prescribed unit size (amount elemental iron in mg) — For IV formulations: Dose[b]	Dosage forms	Frequency of administration[c]
Carbonyl iron	Feosol Carbonyl iron, Ferralet (combination with ferric gluconate, docusate)	45 (45)	Oral	Twice a day to 3 times a day
Ferric maltol	Accufer	30 (30)	Oral	Twice a day
Ferrous fumarate	Femiron, Vitron-C	200 (66)	Oral	Twice a day to 3 times a day
Ferrous gluconate	Fergon	325 (38)	Oral	Twice a day to 3 times a day
Ferrous sulfate	Fer-In-Sol, Feosol, Slow FE	325 (65)	Oral	Twice a day to 3 times a day
Heme iron polypeptide	Proferrin	11 mg elemental iron per tablet	Oral	Twice a day to 4 times a day
Polysaccharide iron	Ferrex, Niferex, Nu-Iron	150 (150)	Oral	Every day to twice a
Ferric carboxymaltose	Injectafer	If ≥ 50 kg: give up to 750 mg as a single dose. Give 2 doses separated by at least 7 days for a total cumulative dose of 1500 mg per treatment course.	I.V.	As needed to treat iron deficiency in nondialysis CKD patients
Ferumoxytol	Feraheme	510 mg × 1 followed by second 510 mg dose 3 to 8 days after first dose	I.V.	As needed to treat iron deficiency in CKD
Iron dextran	INFeD, Dexferrum	25 to 1000 mg	I.V.	Weekly, 3 times per week, or monthly[b]
Iron sucrose	Venofer	100 to 400 mg	I.V.	Weekly, 3 times per week, or monthly[b]
Sodium ferric gluconate	Ferrlecit	62.5 to 125 mg	I.V.	Weekly, 3 times per week, or monthly[c]

Boldface indicates one of top 100 drugs for 2020 by prescription volume.
a. Not all trade names are included in table for oral agents.
b. Target dose for oral administration is typically 200 mg elemental iron per day (may start with lower doses and titrate as tolerated). Ferric maltol is approved at a dose of 30 mg twice daily. Approved single dose regimens for each I.V. iron agent are listed in the text. Iron dextran and ferumoxytol carry an FDA boxed warning regarding the risk of anaphylactic and hypersensitivity reactions.
c. For oral formulations, frequency of administration depends on the amount of elemental iron per unit; 200 mg elemental iron per day is recommended.

Approved doses for the available I.V. iron formulations are listed below. Higher dose infusions are administered but must be done so cautiously and over a more prolonged infusion period to minimize the risk of adverse events.

■ *Iron sucrose:* The 100 mg dose may be diluted in 100 mL of 0.9% NaCl (sodium chloride) administered intravenously over at least 15 minutes or administered undiluted over 2 to 5 minutes. The approved dosing regimen in nondialysis CKD patients is 200 mg over 2 to 5 minutes on 5 different occasions within a 14-day period. Peritoneal dialysis patients may receive 300 mg in 0.9% NaCl administered intravenously over 1.5 hours, followed by a second infusion of 300 mg 14 days later and then by a 400 mg dose administered over 2.5 hours 14 days later.

- *Iron dextran* ⚠️*:* The 100 mg dose may be administered over 2 minutes I.V. push. Administer a 25 mg test dose because of the risk of anaphylactic reactions. Higher total dose infusions are administered in clinical practice, but the risk of reactions must be considered.
- *Sodium ferric gluconate:* The 125 mg dose may be diluted in 100 mL of 0.9% NaCl and administered intravenously over 1 hour or administered undiluted as an I.V. injection at a rate up to 12.5 mg/min. Dosing in pediatric patients is 1.5 mg/kg in 25 mL of 0.9% NaCl over 60 minutes (maximum dose 125 mg).
- *Ferumoxytol (Feraheme)* ⚠️*:* The approved dosing regimen is 510 mg (17 mL) as a single dose, followed by a second 510 mg dose 3 to 8 days after the initial dose. Administer over a minimum of 15 minutes.
- *Ferric carboxymaltose (Injectafer):* Up to 1500 mg as a total cumulative dose is administered as two 750 mg doses separated by at least 7 days. The dose may be given by either slow I.V. push (100 mg/min) or infused over at least 15 minutes.
- Administration of iron via the dialysate during hemodialysis is another option for iron supplementation in ESKD patients requiring chronic hemodialysis. Soluble ferric pyrophosphate citrate (Triferic) is the dialysate iron formulation that allows iron to diffuse from the dialysate into the blood during the hemodialysis procedure.

For patients with more severe anemia or when blood loss is a major contributing factor, blood transfusions may be required.

 Iron Dextran *FDA BOXED WARNING*

Anaphylactic-type reactions, including fatalities, have followed the parenteral administration of iron dextran injection.

 Ferumoxytol (Feraheme) *FDA BOXED WARNING*

Fatal and serious hypersensitivity reactions including anaphylaxis have occurred in patients receiving ferumoxytol.

CKD-MBD

Treatment goals

The following are goals for phosphorus, calcium, and PTH based on KDIGO guidelines by CKD category. Goal serum phosphorus:

- Normal range for CKD categories G3a, G3b, and G4; "toward normal" for ESKD patients

Goal serum calcium:

- Normal range for all CKD categories

Goal PTH:

- Upper limit of the normal range for CKD categories G3a, G3b, and G4; 2 to 9 times the upper limit of normal for ESKD patients (upper limit of normal range for PTH is approximately 60 pg/mL; therefore, target in ESKD patients is approximately 120 to 550 pg/mL)
- A 25-hydroxyvitamin D level below 30 ng/mL indicates a deficiency in the precursor form of vitamin D (25-hydroxyvitamin D is converted to the active form by the kidney). Supplementation is recommended when there is a deficiency in the precursor form.

Treatment strategies

- Restrict dietary phosphorus to 800 to 1000 mg/d phosphorus (consult with dietitian).
- Use phosphate-binding agents—elemental (calcium, lanthanum, sucroferric oxyhydroxide, ferric citrate) and nonelemental (sevelamer):
  - Titrate doses based on phosphorus level.
  - Limit use of calcium-containing phosphate binders if hypercalcemia occurs.
  - Aluminum- and magnesium-containing agents also work to bind phosphorus, but they are not first-line agents because of the potential for accumulation in kidney disease and adverse effects. Aluminum products should be prescribed for short-term use (< 30 days) to minimize the risk of accumulation.
- Remove phosphorus by dialysis for patients with ESRD. Continue phosphorus restriction and use of phosphate-binding agents with dialysis.
- Maintain goal calcium, phosphorus, and PTH.
- Provide vitamin D supplementation depending on the CKD category. Supplementation with the active form (calcitriol) or a vitamin D analog (doxercalciferol or paricalcitol) is necessary in more severe CKD (category G5 and ESKD). Supplementation with a vitamin D precursor (e.g., **ergocalciferol**) may be required in earlier stages, especially when 25-hydroxyvitamin D levels are below 30 ng/mL.
- Use a calcimimetic agent (cinacalcet [Sensipar] or etalcalcetide [Parsabiv]) to help control PTH in patients with ESKD.
- Control metabolic acidosis (which causes bone demineralization if not controlled).

Metabolic acidosis

Treatment goals

- Decrease in serum bicarbonate: Normal value = 22 to 26 mEq/L
- Decrease in blood pH: Normal value = 7.35 to 7.45

Treatment strategies

- Administration of sodium bicarbonate or other alkali preparation: Gradual correction (over days to weeks) is usually appropriate for asymptomatic patients with mild to moderate acidosis (serum bicarbonate 12 to 20 mEq/L and pH 7.2 to 7.4).
- Dialysis: Bicarbonate or lactate contained within the dialysate solution diffuses from dialysate to plasma and effectively treats metabolic acidosis.

Monitoring

Patients at high risk for CKD (e.g., patients with diabetes or hypertension) or patients diagnosed with CKD should have regular monitoring of parameters listed in Box 20-5.

BOX 20-5. Monitoring for CKD Progression

- *Serum creatinine:* Consider limitations. *Note:* Patients started on ACEIs or ARBs may have an initial rise in serum creatinine. A 25% to 30% increase is generally acceptable. Increases higher than this may indicate AKI caused by the medications.

- *Estimated GFR:* Assess rate of progression (the decline in GFR in mL/min/1.73 m² per year).

- *Proteinuria:* Monitor annually in patients with type 1 diabetes with diabetes duration of ≥ 5 years and at diagnosis for patients with type 2 diabetes.

- *Serum electrolytes*
- *Blood pressure*
- *Blood glucose:* Assess in individuals with diabetes.
- *Medication regimens:* Evaluate and adjust on the basis of kidney function.

Anemia of CKD

- Monitor hemoglobin every 1 to 2 weeks after initiation of ESAs or following a dose change and every 2 to 4 weeks once a stable target hemoglobin level is achieved.
- Monitor iron indices (TSat and serum ferritin).
- Evaluate patient for signs and symptoms of anemia.

CKD-MBD

- Phosphorus
- Calcium
- Parathyroid hormone
- Vitamin D: Measure precursor levels, 25-hydroxyvitamin D, in patients with CKD G3a, G3b, and G4

Metabolic acidosis

- Serum bicarbonate
- Potassium

Drug Therapy

Progressive kidney disease

- ACEIs and ARBs (see Chapter 12 on hypertension and Chapter 17 on diabetes): ACEIs and ARBs decrease intraglomerular pressure by preventing vasoconstriction of the efferent arteriole mediated by angiotensin II. This and other mechanisms independent of the effects on renal hemodynamics lead to a decrease in proteinuria and delay progression of CKD. The renin inhibitor (aliskiren) may also be used to delay progression, but not in combination with ACEIs or ARBs.
- Sodium-glucose transport-2 inhibitors (SGLT2 inhibitors) reduce glucose and sodium reabsorption in the proximal tubule of the kidney. This results in more sodium detected at the macula densa (as part of tubuloglomerular feedback), which promotes vasoconstriction of the afferent arteriole leading to decreased glomerular pressure and decreased hyperfiltration (protective to delay progressive kidney disease). Canagliflozin (Invokana) was approved for patients with type 2 diabetes and diabetic nephropathy (AER > 300 mg/d) to reduce the risk of ESKD, cardiovascular death, and hospitalization for heart failure. This agent, when added with therapy to block the renin-angiotensin-aldosterone system (i.e., ACEIs), slowed progression of CKD in patients with eGFRs in the range of 30 to < 90 mL/min/1.73 m². Other SGLT2 inhibitors are being studied for this purpose. See Chapter 17 for more information on use of SGLT2 inhibitors.
- Antihypertensive agents (see Chapter 12 on hypertension)
- Antidiabetic agents (see Chapter 17 on diabetes)

Anemia of CKD

ESAs

Anemia is treated with ESAs (Table 20-6).

Mechanism of action

These agents stimulate the division and differentiation of erythroid progenitor cells and induce the release of reticulocytes from the bone marrow into the bloodstream, where they mature into erythrocytes.

Adverse effects of ESAs

- Hypertension
- Red blood cell aplasia (rare)
- Seizures (rare)

- Polycythemia
- Thrombocytosis

Note: ESAs when dosed to achieve a higher hemoglobin level (> 11 g/dL) have been shown to cause an increased risk of death, serious cardiovascular events, and stroke in patients with CKD. Using the lowest ESA dose necessary to reduce the need for red blood cell transfusions is recommended.

Drug–drug and drug–disease interactions

Causes of ESA resistance

- Iron deficiency
- Secondary hyperparathyroidism
- Inflammatory conditions
- Aluminum accumulation
- Other disease states causing anemia (e.g., cancer, HIV)

Monitoring parameters

- Hemoglobin
- Iron indices
- Blood pressure

Pharmacokinetics

The half-life of ESAs is as follows:

- **Epoetin alfa and epoetin alfa-epbx:** Approximately 8.5 hours intravenously and 24 hours subcutaneously
- **Darbepoetin alfa:** Approximately 25 hours intravenously and 48 hours subcutaneously
- **Methoxy PEG-epoetin beta:** Approximately 134 hours intravenously and 139 hours subcutaneously

Iron supplementation

Iron supplements are described in Table 20-7.

Mechanism of action

Iron supplements supply a source of elemental iron necessary for the function of hemoglobin, myoglobin, and specific enzyme systems and allow transport of oxygen via hemoglobin.

Patient instructions and counseling

- Oral iron may cause stools to be dark in color.
- Take between meals to increase absorption.
- Oral iron may be taken with food if GI upset occurs.
- Do not take with dairy products or antacids.

Adverse effects of iron

- Oral iron may cause stomach cramping, constipation, nausea, vomiting, and dark stools.
- In the case of I.V. iron, anaphylactic reactions have occurred with iron dextran (INFeD), and there is an FDA boxed warning about this risk; administer a 25 mg test dose before administration of the full dose. If no signs or symptoms of anaphylactic-type reactions follow the test dose, administer the full dose and continue to observe the patient.
- Ferumoxytol carries an FDA boxed warning about the risk of fatal and serious hypersensitivity reactions, including anaphylaxis, which have also occurred in patients in whom a previous dose of ferumoxytol was tolerated.
- Patients should be closely observed for signs of hypersensitivity during and for at least 30 minutes after administration of I.V. iron.

- For all I.V. iron preparations, observe patients for diaphoresis, nausea, vomiting, lower back pain, dyspnea, and hypotension.
- Iron overload may be treated with deferoxamine (Desferal).

Drug–drug and drug–disease interactions of iron

- GI absorption of oral iron is decreased when given with antacids, quinolones, and tetracycline and increased when administered with vitamin C.
- I.V. iron has a potential to increase risk of infection. Administration to patients with severe systemic infections is not recommended.
- Ferumoxytol is a superparamagnetic iron oxide, and administration may alter MRI studies for up to 3 months following administration.

Monitoring parameters

- Ferritin and TSat
- Hemoglobin
- Anaphylactic or hypersensitivity reactions after I.V. administration

CKD-MBD

Phosphate-binding agents

Phosphate-binding agents are used to treat CKD-MBD (Table 20-8).

TABLE 20-8. Phosphate-Binding Agents[a]

Generic name	Trade name	Dosage form(s)	Starting dosage or range[b]
Calcium containing			
Calcium acetate (25% elemental calcium)	PhosLo	Capsule	1334 to 2001 mg
	Phoslyra	Liquid	
	Calphron (OTC)	Tablet	
Calcium carbonate (40% elemental calcium)	$CaCO_3$ (multiple preparations), Caltrate, Os-Cal, Rolaids, Tums	Multiple formulations OTC, including chewable tablet	0.8 to 2 g elemental calcium
Non-calcium containing			
Lanthanum carbonate	Fosrenol	Chewable tablet	250 to 500 mg
Sevelamer carbonate	Renvela	Tablet, powder	800 to 1600 mg
Sevelamer hydrochloride	Renagel	Tablet	800 to 1600 mg
Iron containing			
Ferric citrate	Auryxia	Tablet	420 mg
Sucroferric oxyhydroxide	Velphoro	Chewable tablet	500 mg
Nonpreferred binders			
Aluminum hydroxide[c]	AlternaGel, Alu-Cap, Alu-Tab, Amphojel, Basaljel	Multiple formulations OTC	300 to 600 mg
Magnesium carbonate[c]	Mag-Carb	Multiple formulations OTC	70 mg
Magnesium hydroxide (milk of magnesia)[c]	Various	Multiple formulations OTC	300 to 400 mg

OTC, over-the-counter.
a. All agents are taken orally and should be taken with meals.
b. Dose per meal.
c. Not preferred because of the risk of accumulation and adverse effects.

Mechanism of action

These agents combine with dietary phosphate in the GI tract to form an insoluble complex that is excreted in the feces.

Patient instructions and counseling

- Take with meals and snacks.
- For drug interactions, see the section on drug–drug and drug–disease interactions.
- Lanthanum carbonate (Fosrenol) and sucroferric oxyhydroxide (Velphoro) are chewable tablets (do not swallow whole). Some forms of calcium carbonate can also be chewed.
- Sevelamer carbonate (Renvela) is also available as a powder that should be mixed with the appropriate amount of water (1 oz for the 0.8 g packet; 2 oz for the 2.4 g packet). The powder does not dissolve and should be stirred vigorously before drinking. Drink within 30 minutes of preparation.
- Use in conjunction with dietary phosphorus restriction.

Adverse drug effects of phosphate binders

- Calcium products can result in hypercalcemia, nausea, vomiting, abdominal pain, and constipation.
- Ferric citrate may cause darkened stools, nausea, and diarrhea. It contains iron and may increase iron indices.
- Lanthanum carbonate may cause nausea, vomiting, diarrhea, dyspepsia, abdominal pain, and constipation.
- Sevelamer carbonate and sevelamer hydrochloride may cause nausea, vomiting, diarrhea, dyspepsia, abdominal pain, flatulence, and constipation. They are contraindicated in patients with bowel obstruction. *Note:* Sevelamer carbonate has less risk of metabolic acidosis than does sevelamer hydrochloride.
- Sucroferric oxyhydroxide may cause darkened stools, nausea, and diarrhea.
- Aluminum may cause constipation, aluminum toxicity, chalky taste, cramps, nausea, and vomiting. There is a risk of accumulation in patients with kidney disease.
- Magnesium products may cause diarrhea, hypermagnesemia, cramps, and muscle weakness. There is a risk of accumulation in patients with kidney disease.
- All products may cause hypophosphatemia.

Drug–drug and interactions

In general, to minimize the risk of the drug interactions in the following list, administer the interacting drug at least 1 to 2 hours before or 3 to 4 hours after the phosphate binder. Specific drug interactions with phosphate binders are described in Box 20-6.

Monitoring parameters

- Phosphorus, calcium, PTH, and 25-hydroxyvitamin D levels (in CKD G3a-G4)
- Aluminum and magnesium levels (if receiving aluminum- or magnesium-containing products)
- Serum bicarbonate with sevelamer

Vitamin D therapy

Vitamin D therapy is described in Table 20-9.

Mechanism of action (active vitamin D)

Active vitamin D binds to and activates the vitamin D receptor in the kidney, parathyroid gland, intestine, and bone. This causes suppression of parathyroid hormone synthesis, an increase in intestinal calcium (and phosphorus) absorption, and an increase in tubular reabsorption of calcium by the kidney (in patients with sufficient kidney function). *Note:* **Ergocalciferol** (vitamin D$_2$), calcifediol (vitamin D$_3$), and

> ### BOX 20-6. Phosphate Binder Drug Interactions
>
> **Calcium-containing binders:** Mycophenolate, oral iron salts, quinolone antibiotics, tetracycline derivatives (not inclusive of all potential drug interactions)
>
> **Ferric citrate:** Bisphosphonate derivatives, **levothyroxine**, methyldopa, quinolone antibiotics, tetracycline derivatives
>
> **Lanthanum carbonate:** ACEIs, 3-hydroxy-3-methyl-glutaryl-coenzyme A (HMG-CoA) reductase inhibitors, **levothyroxine**, quinolone antibiotics, tetracycline derivatives
>
> **Sevelamer carbonate and hydrochloride:** Cyclosporine, **levothyroxine**, mycophenolate, quinolone antibiotics, tacrolimus. These drugs may decrease absorption of vitamins D, E, and K and **folic acid**.
>
> **Sucroferric oxyhydroxide:** **Levothyroxine**, tetracycline derivatives
>
> **Boldface** indicates one of top 100 drugs for 2020 by prescription volume.

cholecalciferol (vitamin D_3) are precursor forms that require conversion to the active form by the kidney. Therefore, an active form of vitamin D or a vitamin D analog (i.e., calcitriol, doxercalciferol, or paricalcitol) must be used in advanced CKD (CKD G5 or ESKD). Paricalcitol and doxercalciferol are vitamin D_2 analogs. Paricalcitol is active and requires no conversion by the liver or kidney. Doxercalciferol requires conversion to the active form by the liver.

Patient instructions and counseling

- Use in conjunction with dietary phosphorus restriction and phosphate-binding agents; vitamin D therapy may need to be discontinued temporarily if calcium and phosphorus are elevated.
- Notify health care provider of any of the following signs of hypercalcemia: weakness, headache, decreased appetite, and lethargy.

Adverse drug effects of vitamin D

- **Hypercalcemia:** Decreased incidence with vitamin D_2 analogs (paricalcitol, doxercalciferol) compared to calcitriol
- **Hyperphosphatemia:** Decreased incidence with vitamin D_2 analogs
- **Adynamic bone disease:** Caused by oversuppression of PTH

TABLE 20-9. Vitamin D Agents

Generic name	Trade name	Dosage range	Dosage forms	Frequency of administration
Vitamin D precursors				
Calcifediol (vitamin D_3)	Rayaldee	30 to 60 mcg	Oral	Daily
Cholecalciferol (vitamin D_3)	Multiple agents	600 to 50,000 units	Oral	Daily or weekly
Ergocalciferol (vitamin D_2)	Calciferol, Calcidol	400 to 50,000 units	Oral	Daily, weekly, or monthly
Active vitamin D and vitamin D analogs[a]				
Calcitriol	Calcijex	0.5 to 5 mcg	I.V.	3 times per week
	Rocaltrol	0.25 to 5 mcg	Oral	Daily, every other day, or 3 times per week
Doxercalciferol	Hectorol	5 to 20 mcg	Oral	Daily or 3 times per week
		2 to 8 mcg	I.V.	3 times per week
Paricalcitol	Zemplar	1 to 4 mcg	Oral	Daily or 3 times per week
		2.5 to 15 mcg	I.V.	3 times per week

Boldface indicates one of top 100 drugs for 2020 by prescription volume.

a. Calcitriol is a vitamin D_3 agent. Paricalcitol and doxercalciferol are vitamin D_2 agents and are less likely to cause hypercalcemia and hyperphosphatemia.

Drug-drug interactions

- Active vitamin D may increase levels and effects of aluminum hydroxide, cardiac glycosides, and magnesium.
- Levels of active vitamin D may be increased by cytochrome P450 (CYP) 3A4 inhibitors.
- Levels of active vitamin D may be decreased by bile acid sequestrants, CYP3A inducers, orlistat, and sevelamer.

Monitoring parameters

- PTH
- Calcium
- Phosphorus
- Alkaline phosphatase
- Signs of vitamin D intoxication and hypercalcemia (e.g., weakness, headache, somnolence, nausea, vomiting, bone pain, polyuria)

Pharmacokinetics

- Calcitriol (Calcijex):
- Half-life: 3 to 8 hours
- Protein binding: 99.9%
- Paricalcitol (Zemplar):
- Half-life: Healthy subjects, 4 to 6 hours (oral); CKD categories G3 and G4, 17 to 20 hours (oral); CKD category G5, 14 to 15 hours (IV)
- Protein binding: >99%
- Doxercalciferol (Hectorol):
- Half-life of active metabolite: 32 to 37 hours

Ergocalciferol and cholecalciferol require hydroxylation within the liver and kidney to form active vitamin D. Doxercalciferol requires conversion to its active form 1-alpha, 25-dihydroxyvitamin D_2 in the liver.

Calcimimetics: cinacalcet (Sensipar) and etelcalcetide (Parsabiv)

Cinacalcet is an oral calcimimetic, and etelcalcetide is an I.V. formulation. Both are approved only for patients with ESKD. They may be used in conjunction with phosphate binders and vitamin D therapy. The dose range for cinacalcet is 30 to 180 mg/day; initial dose is 30 mg titrated every 4 weeks on the basis of PTH levels. The dose range for etelcalcetide is 2.5 to 15 mg I.V. 3 times per week. Both agents should not be initiated if the corrected serum calcium < 8.4 mg/dL.

Mechanism of action

Calcimimetics bind with the calcium-sensing receptor on the parathyroid gland and increase sensitivity of the receptor to extracellular calcium, thereby decreasing the stimulus for PTH secretion.

Dosing, instructions, and counseling
Cinacalcet

- Starting dose of cinacalcet is 30 mg orally daily.
- The dose of cinacalcet should be titrated no more frequently than every 4 weeks through sequential doses of 60, 90, 120, and 180 mg once daily.
- Should be taken with food or shortly after a meal.
- Tablets should be taken whole and should not be divided.

Etelcalcetide

- The starting dose of etelcalcetide is 5 mg I.V. 3 times per week with hemodialysis.
- The dose of etelcalcetide should be titrated every 4 weeks in 2.5 to 5 mg increments to a maximum dose of 15 mg I.V. 3 times per week.

- If switching to etelcalcetide from cinacalcet, discontinue cinacalcet for at least 7 days before starting etelcalcetide.
- Administer at the end of hemodialysis (during rinse back) to avoid removal of this agent by hemodialysis.
- Protect from light and keep refrigerated.
- If doses are missed for more than 2 weeks, reinitiate at the recommended starting dose of 5 mg 3 times per week (or 2.5 mg if that was the patient's last dose).

Adverse effects of calcimimetics

- Hypocalcemia (use these agents with caution in patients with seizure disorder)
- Hypophosphatemia
- Nausea, vomiting
- Diarrhea
- Myalgias

Drug–drug interactions

Cinacalcet is metabolized by multiple CYP enzymes, primarily CYP3A4, CYP2D6, and CYP1A2. Adjustments in dose may be required for patients taking agents that inhibit metabolism of cinacalcet (e.g., ketoconazole). Dose reductions of drugs with a narrow therapeutic range and with a metabolism dependent on these enzymes may also be required (e.g., tricyclic antidepressants, flecainide, thioridazine).

Monitoring parameters

Serum calcium and serum phosphorus should be measured within 1 week, and PTH should be measured 1 to 4 weeks after initiation or dose adjustment.

Pharmacokinetics

Cinacalcet

- The maximum concentration is achieved in approximately 2 to 6 hours following administration and is increased with food.
- Half-life is 30 to 40 hours.
- Volume of distribution is approximately 1000 L.
- Cinacalcet is approximately 93% to 97% bound to plasma proteins.
- Cinacalcet is metabolized primarily by CYP3A4, CYP2D6, and CYP1A2.

Etelcalcetide

- Half-life in patients with normal kidney function is 18 to 20 hours; half-life in patients with ESKD is 3 to 4 days
- Volume of distribution is approximately 800 L
- Removed extensively by hemodialysis (administer after hemodialysis)

Metabolic acidosis

See Chapter 21 on critical care.

Metabolic acidosis is frequently corrected once a patient begins chronic dialysis treatments (either hemodialysis or peritoneal dialysis). If the patient required sodium bicarbonate, this medication may be discontinued once dialysis is initiated and the serum bicarbonate levels correct to the normal range.

Vitamin supplementation (specific to the dialysis population)

A select list of water-soluble vitamins for dialysis patients is included in Table 20-10.

Mechanism of action

Vitamin supplementation replaces water-soluble vitamins lost during dialysis without providing supratherapeutic amounts of fat-soluble vitamins.

TABLE 20-10. Water-Soluble Vitamin Supplements for Dialysis Patients[a]

Generic name	Trade name[b]
Vitamin B complex, vitamin C, and **folic acid**	Nephrocaps, Nephro-Vite, Nephro-Vite Rx, Rena-Vite
Vitamin B complex, vitamin C, **folic acid**, and iron	Nephro-Vite Rx + Iron
Vitamin B complex	Allbee with C

Boldface indicates one of top 100 drugs for 2020 by prescription volume.
a. All these supplements are taken orally, 1 capsule or tablet once per day.
b. Not all trade names are included in the table.

Patient instructions and counseling
- Take daily to replace water-soluble vitamins.
- Hemodialysis patients should take after dialysis.

Adverse drug effects of recommended vitamins
- *General:* Nausea, headache, pruritus, flushing (depending on specific vitamin)
- *Vitamin B$_6$ (pyridoxine):* Neuropathy, increased aspartate transaminase
- *Vitamin C (ascorbic acid):* Hyperoxaluria, dizziness, diarrhea, fatigue, nausea
- *Folic acid:* Headache, rash, pruritus

Drug–drug and drug–disease interactions
Folic acid may decrease phenytoin concentrations by increasing the metabolism.

Nondrug Therapy

When patients reach CKD category G4, prepare them for chronic dialysis by choosing the most appropriate type of renal replacement therapy (in-center hemodialysis, home hemodialysis, or peritoneal dialysis) and dialysis access site. The patient should also be evaluated for transplantation (see Chapter 42 for information on transplantation).

Renal replacement therapies

Hemodialysis
The intermittent hemodialysis procedure is generally performed 3 times per week for 3 to 5 hours for patients with ESKD (with in-center dialysis). It requires a viable permanent access site (fistula or graft) or a temporary site for patients requiring immediate dialysis or experiencing failed permanent access sites. Fistulas are the preferred access for chronic hemodialysis.

Complications include infection, hypotension during dialysis, clotting, and dialyzer reactions. Drug removal by hemodialysis is most likely to occur for drugs with small molecular weight, low protein binding, and small volume of distribution.

Peritoneal dialysis
Peritoneal dialysis requires insertion of a catheter into the peritoneum. Types include continuous ambulatory peritoneal dialysis and automated peritoneal dialysis (which includes continuous cycling, nocturnal tidal, and nightly intermittent peritoneal dialysis). Several complications are possible including peritonitis, hyperglycemia from glucose content of dialysate solution, and malnutrition from increased protein loss.

20-6   Pharmacist's Role

A multidisciplinary team structure is ideal to address CKD progression and the secondary complications presented in this chapter. Pharmacists are involved in the care of individual with CKD at all stages including outpatient and inpatient. Working through the pharmacist patient care process to identify medication-related problems and address such problems is a critical part of caring for individuals with CKD who are taking many different medications and have multiple providers because of the complexity of their disease states. The pharmacist reconciles medications during transitions from one care giver to another to provide accurate medication lists and to identify medication-related problems. Patients also require extensive counseling as changes are made to their medication regimens and to avoid drug interactions and minimize potential adverse effects.

NAPLEX Competency Statements

The questions in this chapter cover the following 2021 NAPLEX Competency Statements: **AREA 1:** 1.1; 1.2; 1.3; 1.4; 1.5; 1.6; 1.7 **AREA 2:** 2.1; 2.2; 2.3 **AREA 3:** 3.1; 3.2; 3.3; 3.4; 3.6; 3.7; 3.8; 3.9; 3.10; 3.11 **AREA 4:** 4.1; 4.9 **AREA 5:** 5.1.

 **20-7** **Questions**

1. A 45-year-old female is admitted to the hospital after fainting at work. Her medical history includes type 2 diabetes and rheumatoid arthritis. Her only complaint is that she has had difficulty over the past 5 days keeping down anything she eats or drinks. She has also noticed a decrease in urination over the past 24 hours. Regular medications include aspirin 325 mg daily, ibuprofen 600 mg daily for arthritis, metformin 500 mg daily, glyburide 5 mg daily, and acetaminophen as needed for headache. Laboratory values in the emergency department showed a serum creatinine of 2 mg/dL and BUN of 56 mg/dL, consistent with AKI. Her lab tests from 1 month ago at a regular checkup were normal. The most likely etiology of this patient's AKI is _____.

   A. dehydration from poor oral intake
   B. age-related decreases in kidney function
   C. kidney failure caused by diabetes
   D. obstruction of urine outflow
   E. inflammation of the kidney caused by rheumatoid arthritis

2. A 45-year-old female is admitted to the hospital after fainting at work. Her medical history includes type 2 diabetes and rheumatoid arthritis. Her only complaint is that she has had difficulty over the past 5 days keeping down anything she eats or drinks. She has also noticed a decrease in urination over the past 24 hours. Regular medications include aspirin 325 mg daily, ibuprofen 600 mg daily for arthritis, metformin 500 mg daily, glyburide 5 mg daily, and acetaminophen as needed for headache. Laboratory values in the emergency department showed a serum creatinine of 2 mg/dL and BUN of 56 mg/dL, consistent with AKI. Her lab tests from 1 month ago at a regular checkup were normal. Which medication most likely contributed to her AKI?

   A. Aspirin
   B. Ibuprofen
   C. Metformin
   D. Glyburide
   E. Acetaminophen

3. Which diuretic is known to retain its effectiveness for diuresis at a glomerular filtration rate < 30 mL/min?

   A. Hydrochlorothiazide
   B. Chlorothiazide
   C. Metolazone
   D. Spironolactone
   E. Aldactone

4. Which abnormality typically occurs in patients with severe kidney dysfunction (i.e., creatinine clearance < 15 mL/min)?

A. Metabolic acidosis
B. Metabolic alkalosis
C. Hypophosphatemia
D. Hypernatremia
E. Respiratory acidosis

5. A 55-year-old female patient presents to the outpatient pharmacy asking for a recommendation for a pain medication for headaches. You learn that she also has heart failure and receives an ACEI. She has just been discharged from the hospital where she was diagnosed with AKI associated with a heart failure exacerbation and ACEI. She did recover kidney function and is back to her baseline (eGFR 43 mL/min/1.73 m²). Which medication is most appropriate to suggest for this patient?

A. Naproxen
B. Acetaminophen
C. Ibuprofen
D. Aspirin/caffeine (BC Powder) with ibuprofen
E. Pain medications are not recommended for individuals with kidney disease.

6. Which diuretic (as single-drug therapy) would be most appropriate for the initial treatment of a patient with AKI and significant volume overload?

A. Metolazone
B. Spironolactone
C. Mannitol
D. Bumetanide
E. Acetazolamide

7. A patient with nephrotoxicity caused by gentamicin would likely present with an increase in serum creatinine _____.

A. within 2 days after starting therapy and with anuria
B. immediately after starting therapy and with nonoliguria
C. immediately after starting therapy and with oliguria
D. 5 to 7 days after starting therapy and with oliguria
E. 5 to 7 days after starting therapy and with nonoliguria

8. Lisinopril may cause hemodynamically mediated AKI by preventing which compensatory mechanism by the kidney?

A. Vasodilation of the afferent arteriole
B. Vasoconstriction of the afferent arteriole
C. Vasodilation of the efferent arteriole
D. Vasoconstriction of the efferent arteriole
E. Vasodilation of both the afferent and efferent arterioles

9. The estimated creatinine clearance for a 47-year-old male patient with an ideal body weight of 176 lb (slightly less than actual body weight) and a serum creatinine of 2.2 mg/dL is _____.

A. 20 mL/min
B. 32 mL/min
C. 40 mL/min
D. 47 mL/min
E. 93 mL/min

10. A 53-year-old Black female (body weight = 65 kg; close to her ideal body weight) with hypertension and hypercholesterolemia is seen in the outpatient nephrology clinic for evaluation of kidney disease progression. Her current blood pressure is 156/82 mmHg, SCr is 2.6 mg/dL (stable for the past 4 months), BUN is 44 mg/dL, and urinary albumin excretion rate < 30 mg/d. Her medications are enalapril 20 mg/d × 1 year and simvastatin 20 mg daily × 2 years. According to this patient's estimated creatinine clearance, she would be classified in which of the following KDIGO categories of chronic kidney disease?

A. G1
B. G2
C. G3a
D. G4
E. G5

11. A 53-year-old Black female (body weight = 65 kg; close to her ideal body weight) with hypertension and hypercholesterolemia is seen in the outpatient nephrology clinic for evaluation of kidney disease progression. Her current blood pressure is 156/82 mmHg, SCr is 2.6 mg/dL (stable for the past 4 months), BUN is 44 mg/dL, and urinary albumin excretion rate < 30 mg/day. Her medications are enalapril 20 mg/d × 1 year and simvastatin 20 mg daily × 2 years. The recommended target blood pressure for this patient is _____.

A. < 110/70 mmHg
B. < 125/90 mmHg
C. < 130/80 mmHg
D. < 140/90 mmHg
E. < 150/90 mmHg

12. Which is the most appropriate agent to add to delay progression of kidney disease in a patient with CKD category G3a, type 2 diabetes, and an albumin-to-creatinine ratio of 600 mg/g who has been receiving lisinopril for the past year?

A. Losartan
B. Aliskiren
C. Spironolactone
D. Canagloflozin
E. Enalapril

13. Erythropoietin stimulating agents (ESAs) stimulate erythropoiesis by which of the following?

A. Prevent excessive red blood cell destruction
B. Prevent degradation of bone marrow stem cells
C. Differentiation of peritubular interstitial cells of the kidney
D. Differentiation of erythroid progenitor stem cells in the bone marrow
E.

14. When administered intravenously, epoetin alfa-epbx has a terminal half-life approximately _____ that of epoetin alfa.

A. 2 times shorter than
B. 2 times longer than
C. 3 times longer than
D. 3 times shorter than
E. equal to

15. One of the most commonly reported adverse reactions with epoetin alfa and darbepoetin alfa is _____.

A. nausea
B. hypertension
C. constipation
D. anaphylaxis
E. bleeding

16. At least how much time should be allowed to lapse before a change in dose of an erythropoiesis stimulating agent is made on the basis of a change in hemoglobin and hematocrit?

A. 1 week
B. 2 to 4 weeks
C. 6 to 8 weeks
D. 2 months
E. 3 months

17. A 42-year-old male (body weight = 70 kg) on hemodialysis 3 times per week receives epoetin alfa for treatment of anemia. He has been stable on an epoetin dose of 4000 units I.V. 3 times per week with an average hemoglobin of 11 g/dL (hematocrit of 33%). Over the past 3 months, his hemoglobin has dropped to 9 g/dL. Iron indices reveal the following: serum ferritin 78 ng/mL and TSat 12%. The best initial treatment for this patient is to _____.

A. increase the dose of epoetin alfa to maintain a hemoglobin of 11 to 12 g/dL (hematocrit of 33% to 36%)
B. administer I.V. iron (sodium ferric gluconate) at a maintenance dose of 125 mg/wk
C. administer a 1-g total dose of I.V. iron in divided doses
D. begin oral ferrous sulfate 325 mg 3 times daily
E. begin oral ferric maltol 30 mg twice daily

18. In the GI tract, calcitriol promotes _____.

A. absorption of calcium and inhibits absorption of phosphorus
B. absorption of both calcium and phosphorus
C. decreased binding of calcium and phosphorus
D. increased elimination of calcium and phosphorus
E. absorption of phosphorus and inhibits absorption of calcium

19. A 63-year-old female with end-stage kidney disease is receiving peritoneal dialysis. Her most recent laboratory analysis reveals the following: BUN 58 mg/dL, SCr 5.2 mg/dL, phosphorus 7.4 mg/dL, calcium 9 mg/dL, albumin 2.5 g/dL, and iPTH 360 pg/mL. In addition to dietary restriction of phosphorus, which agent is best for initial management of this patient's hyperphosphatemia?

   A. Lanthanum carbonate
   B. Calcium acetate
   C. Aluminum hydroxide
   D. Calcium carbonate
   E. Etelcalcetide

20. A 63-year-old female with end-stage kidney disease is receiving peritoneal dialysis. Her most recent laboratory analysis reveals the following: BUN 58 mg/dL, SCr 5.2 mg/dL, phosphorus 7.4 mg/dL, calcium 9 mg/dL, albumin 2.5 g/dL, and iPTH 360 pg/mL. This patient should be instructed to take her phosphate binder _____.

   A. with meals to enhance systemic absorption of phosphorus
   B. with meals to minimize systemic absorption of phosphorus
   C. between meals to avoid food–drug interactions
   D. between meals to minimize GI side effects
   E. at any time in relation to food intake

21. Which agent is most appropriate for a patient with ESKD on hemodialysis, secondary hyperparathyroidism (PTH 800 pg/mL), and hypercalcemia (corrected calcium 10.5 mg/dL) who requires treatment to reduce PTH?

   A. Cinacalcet
   B. Paricalcitol
   C. Calcitriol
   D. Ergocalciferol
   E. Calcifediol

22. Etelcalcetide is a calcimimetic that works by which of the following mechanisms?

   A. Decreases the sensitivity of the calcium-sensing receptors on the parathyroid gland to calcium, which prevents secretion of PTH
   B. Increases the sensitivity of the calcium-sensing receptors on the parathyroid gland to calcium, which prevents secretion of PTH
   C. Stimulates the breakdown of PTH and prevents the effects of PTH on bone turnover
   D. Increases calcium concentrations, which suppresses secretion of PTH from the parathyroid gland
   E. Binds with circulating PTH to inactivate PTH and promote elimination by dialysis

23. A drug with which of the following characteristics is most likely to be removed by hemodialysis (f_u = fraction unbound in plasma; Vd = volume of distribution)?

   A. f_u 0.05, Vd 2 L/kg
   B. f_u 0.05, Vd 0.2 L/kg
   C. f_u 0.50, Vd 0.6 L/kg
   D. f_u 0.95, Vd 2 L/kg
   E. f_u 0.95, Vd 0.2 L/kg

24. Which iron agent has an FDA boxed warning regarding the risk of anaphylactic reactions?

   A. Ferumoxytol
   B. Sodium ferric gluconate
   C. Iron sucrose
   D. Ferric carboxymaltose
   E. Ferric maltol

25. Which of the following supplements should be recommended daily for a patient with ESKD?

   A. Multivitamin
   B. Nephrocaps
   C. Vitamin A
   D. Nephrocaps + vitamin A
   E. Vitamin supplements are not recommended because of the variability in formulations

20-8   Answers

1. A. Dehydration is the most likely cause of AKI in this patient because she has had a decrease in oral intake over the past 5 days. Dehydration would be classified as a prerenal cause of AKI. A serum creatinine of 2 mg/dL would not be considered normal in a person age 45 years, eliminating age as a rationale for kidney disease. Diabetes would be more likely to cause a chronic decrease in her kidney function as opposed to an acute change (lab tests from 1 month ago were normal, ruling out evidence of chronic kidney disease). She has had some urine output in the past 24 hours, which rules out obstruction. Rheumatoid arthritis is not known to cause acute kidney injury.

2. B. NSAIDs are associated with hemodynamic changes (in particular, they prevent the compensatory vasodilation of the afferent arteriole that occurs in conditions of prerenal acute kidney disease). Metformin is not a cause of AKI in this case but would need to be discontinued at this time because of the risk of lactic acidosis in a patient with decreased kidney function (serum creatinine > 1.4 mg/dL in females and > 1.5 mg/dL in males).

3. C. There is evidence that metolazone is beneficial for diuresis in patients with a GFR < 30 mL/min/1.73 m². This is not the case with other thiazide or thiazide-like diuretics or with potassium-sparing diuretics. Metolazone is frequently used in combination with loop diuretics for this reason.

4. A. Metabolic acidosis is a common secondary complication of AKI. Other electrolyte abnormalities include hyperkalemia and hyperphosphatemia. Sodium disorders are usually caused by other concomitant disorders but not by AKI alone. Primary respiratory disorders such as respiratory acidosis are not associated with AKI.

5. B. The preferred pain medication for patients with reduced kidney function is acetaminophen. This patient has a baseline GFR of approximately 48 mL/min indicating reduced kidney function and should not receive any agents associated with worsening kidney function, especially because she had a recent AKI event. She also takes an ACEI for her heart failure. This medication in addition to other agents such as NSAIDs can negatively affect autoregulation in conditions of decreased renal per-

fusion (e.g., heart failure exacerbation and/or low blood pressure). All NSAIDs such as naproxen and ibuprofen should be avoided. Combination therapy with agents that include aspirin and caffeine are also associated with papillary necrosis (particularly when they were combined with phenacetin in previous formulations) and are not generally recommended.

6. D. A patient with AKI generally requires aggressive diuresis (while avoiding dehydration). Bumetanide is a loop diuretic that is more potent than a thiazide-like diuretic (metolazone) or a potassium-sparing diuretic (spironolactone) and would be a rational choice for initial therapy of AKI. Spironolactone may cause hyperkalemia in a patient with AKI. Mannitol is an osmotic diuretic that may cause volume depletion and requires more aggressive monitoring and is not indicated. Acetazolamide is a carbonic anhydrase inhibitor primarily used as adjunctive treatment of edema and metabolic alkalosis (off label use) and is not used to promote aggressive diuresis as would be needed in a patient with AKI.

7. D. Aminoglycoside-induced nephrotoxicity is characterized by a delay in changes in serum creatinine (approximately 5 to 7 days) and relatively normal urine output (nonoliguria). While these agents can induce kidney injury very quickly after initiating therapy, there is a lag time for creatinine elevations to reflect the degree of kidney damage. This is the downside to using creatinine as a marker of kidney function.

8. D. Angiotensin-converting enzyme inhibitors may contribute to development of AKI in patients with conditions resulting in prerenal kidney disease (e.g., conditions resulting in decreased perfusion of the kidney, hypovolemia, heart failure, liver disease). ACEIs (and ARBs) prevent the compensatory vasoconstriction of the efferent arteriole mediated by angiotensin II that occurs in an attempt to increase GFR.

9. D. Using the Cockcroft–Gault equation to estimate creatinine clearance, this patient has an estimated creatinine clearance of 47 mL/min. For females, multiply the calculated value by 0.85.

$$CrCl = \frac{(140 - age)(BW\ in\ kg)}{SCr \times 72}$$

$$BW\ (kg) = 176\ lb/2.2 = 80\ kg$$

$$SCr = 2.2\ mg/dL$$

10. D. This patient's estimated creatinine clearance determined using the Cockcroft–Gault equation is 26 mL/min, classified as category G4 CKD (GFR 15 to 29 mL/min/1.73 m^2), with the result multiplied by 0.85 for a female. *Note:* The estimated GFR determined using the CKD-EPI equation is 23 mL/min/1.73 m^2.

$$CrCl = \frac{(140 - age)(BW \text{ in kg})}{SCr \times 72}$$

11. C. The recommended blood pressure for this patient with CKD G4 is < 130/80 mmHg. If her AER exceeded 300 mg/d the KDIGO guidelines would support a lower blood pressure of < 130/80 mmHg; however, this is somewhat controversial and based more on opinion than evidence.

12. A. Among the agents listed, canagliflozin has been shown to further delay progression of kidney disease in individuals with diabetic kidney disease with albumin excretion ratios (AER) above 300 mg per day when added with other renin-angiotensin-aldosterone system (RAAS) blockers (i.e., ACEIs, ARBs). Canagliflozin (Invokana) was approved for patients with type 2 diabetes and diabetic nephropathy (AER > 300 mg/d) to reduce the risk of ESKD, cardiovascular death and hospitalization for heart failure. This patient has diabetic kidney disease and stage 3a CKD with an AER of 600 mg per day and would qualify for addition of an SGLT2 inhibitor. Combination therapy with other RAAS blockers has not consistently shown added benefit and significantly increases the risk of hyperkalemia and hypertension. Therefore, combination therapy with ACEIs and ARBs is not recommended. A warning also exists of the possible risks when using aliskiren in combination with ACEIs and ARBs in patients with diabetes or kidney disease. Spironolactone has not proved beneficial in delaying progression of kidney disease when added to RAAS inhibitors and may increase the risk of hyperkalemia.

13. D. ESAs including epoetin alfa, darbepoetin alfa, and methoxy PEG-epoetin beta work in the bone marrow to stimulate differentiation of erythroid progenitor stem cells and result in an increase in red blood cell production (increase in erythrocytes).

14. C. The half-life of darbepoetin alfa is 3 times longer than that of epoetin alfa, giving this agent the added benefit of reduced frequency of administration.

15. B. Hypertension is the most common adverse effect in patients receiving ESAs.

16. B. Stimulation of erythropoiesis by epoetin alfa and darbepoetin alfa occurs immediately; however, at least 2 to 4 weeks will pass before substantial changes in hemoglobin are observed as a result of any change in dose of ESA therapy.

17. C. This patient is iron deficient, as indicated by his low serum ferritin (< 100 ng/mL) and TSat (< 20%). No change in epoetin alfa should be made until the iron deficiency is corrected (this is the leading cause of resistance to ESAs). This patient will require a full course of iron (1 g administered intravenously in divided doses with each dialysis session) as opposed to a maintenance dose, which should be administered once the patient is iron replete. Sodium ferric gluconate may be administered in doses of 125 mg per dialysis session for 8 sessions to give the total 1 g dose (iron sucrose would be administered in 100 mg increments over 10 hemodialysis sessions). Ferumoxytol would be administered as two 510 mg doses given 3 to 8 days apart. Absorption of oral iron is poor, making I.V. iron preferred in this hemodialysis patient.

18. B. Active vitamin D (calcitriol) promotes absorption of both calcium and phosphorus in the GI tract. For this reason, therapy with calcitriol or a vitamin D analog may need to be withheld if the calcium or phosphorus is elevated.

19. A. Lanthanum carbonate or sevelamer carbonate (Renvela) is preferred over a calcium-containing binder for initial management because this patient has a corrected calcium of 10.2 mg/dL (corrected calcium = measured serum calcium + 0.8 × [normal serum albumin – measured serum albumin]). The elevated calcium and phosphorus increase the risk of metastatic calcifications. She requires a phosphorus-binding agent without calcium to minimize calcium absorbed in the GI tract. Aluminum is not preferred because of the risk of accumulation and adverse effects. Etelcalcetide is a I.V. calcimimetic agent approved for individuals with ESKD. While it will lower calcium and phosphorus, its primary indication is to lower PTH, and this patient does not need aggressive lowering of PTH because she is at goal (2 to 9 times the upper limit of normal; approximately 120 to 600 pg/mL). This patient would also need to have regular I.V. access to receive etelcalcetide (the reason it is used in hemodialysis patients).

20. B. Phosphate binders should be taken with meals to minimize systemic absorption of phosphorus from the GI tract.

21. A. Active vitamin D (calcitriol) and vitamin D analogs (paricalcitol and doxercalciferol) may worsen hypercalcemia in this patient through increased GI absorption and are not recommended until the calcium levels are lowered. Cinacalcet works to decrease secretion of PTH and does not cause hypercalcemia (there is a risk of hypocalcemia). This agent is approved only in patients with ESKD, so it would be appropriate in this case. Of note, etelcalcetide would also be appropriate. Vitamin D should be considered when this patient's calcium levels are within the normal range. Ergocalciferol and calcifediol are vitamin D precursors that require activation by the kidney and would not be recommended as the sole vitamin D agent for a patient with ESKD without the necessary activity of the enzyme in the kidney (1-alpha-hydroxylase) responsible for final conversion to the active form.

22. B. The calcimimetic agent etelcalcetide (Parsabiv) works by binding with the calcium-sensing receptor on the parathyroid gland and increases the sensitivity of this receptor to calcium, thereby suppressing secretion of PTH.

23. E. Drug characteristics that make an agent more likely to be removed by dialysis include low protein binding, small volume of distribution, and low molecular weight. Among the choices given, the agent that best meets these criteria is choice E, which has a high fraction unbound in the plasma (unbound fraction is 95% as indicated by the f_u of 0.95) and a low volume of distribution (Vd 0.2 L/kg).

24. A. In addition to iron dextran, ferumoxytol carries an FDA boxed warning about the risk of fatal and serious hypersensitivity reactions, including anaphylaxis, which have also occurred in patients in whom a previous dose of ferumoxytol was tolerated. The other I.V. agents listed (sodium ferric gluconate and ferric carboxymaltose) do not have this warning. Ferric maltol is an oral agent and not associated with anaphylaxis.

25. B. Nephrocaps include water-soluble vitamins (vitamin B complex + vitamin C + folic acid) recommended for a patient with kidney failure. Supplementation with fat-soluble vitamins is not recommended in patients with kidney failure because of toxicities associated with accumulation.

20-9 Additional Resources

Hudson JQ, Wazny LD, Komenda P. Chronic kidney disease. In: DiPiro J, Yee CG, Posey LM, et al., eds. *Pharmacotherapy: A Pathophysiologic Approach*. 11th ed. New York, NY: McGraw-Hill; 2020:647–676.

KDIGO (Kidney Disease: Improving Global Outcomes) Acute Kidney Injury Work Group. KDIGO clinical practice guideline for acute kidney injury. *Kidney Int Suppl*. 2012;2(1):1–138.

KDIGO Anemia Work Group. KDIGO clinical practice guideline for anemia in chronic kidney disease. *Kidney Int Suppl*. 2012;2(4):279–335.

KDIGO Chronic Kidney Disease–Mineral and Bone Disorder Update Work Group. KDIGO 2017 clinical practice guideline for the diagnosis, evaluation, prevention, and treatment of chronic kidney disease–mineral and bone disorder (CKD-MBD). *Kidney Int Suppl*. 2017;7:1–59.

KDIGO Chronic Kidney Disease Work Group. KDIGO 2012 clinical practice guideline for the evaluation and management of chronic kidney disease. *Kidney Int Suppl*. 2013;3:1–150.

Maker JH, Roller L, Dager WE, Acute kidney injury. In: DiPiro J, Yee CG, Posey LM, et al., eds. *Pharmacotherapy: A Pathophysiologic Approach*. 11th ed. New York, NY: McGraw-Hill; 2020:625–646.

National Kidney Foundation. KDOQI clinical practice guidelines for anemia of chronic kidney disease: 2007 update of hemoglobin target. *Am J Kidney Dis*. 2007;50(3):471–530.

Nolin TD, Perazella MA. Drug-induced kidney disease. In: DiPiro J, Yee CG, Posey LM, et al., eds. *Pharmacotherapy: A Pathophysiologic Approach*. 11th ed. New York, NY: McGraw-Hill; 2020:697–714.

Critical Care

G. CHRISTOPHER WOOD

 ## 21-1 KEY POINTS

- The widely used mnemonic FAST HUG outlines routine care issues for intensive care unit (ICU) patients that should be addressed every day.
- Appropriate sedation and analgesia are essential because pain and agitation are common in critically ill patients. Drug selection should be based on clinical guidelines and patient parameters.
- Opioids are still widely used in critically ill patients; however, there is an increasing emphasis on multimodal analgesia with nonopioid therapies.
- For sedation, propofol or dexmedetomidine are generally preferred to benzodiazepines.
- For ICU delirium, there is no clearly effective therapy though newer antipsychotics such as **quetiapine** (Seroquel) are generally preferred over older agents such as haloperidol (Haldol).
- Pain, agitation, and delirium should be monitored using the recommended assessment tools.
- Neuromuscular blocking (NMB) agents should be used only after sedation and analgesia have been maximized.
- NMB agents should be monitored using peripheral nerve stimulation in addition to observation of clinical signs and symptoms.
- Appropriate stress ulcer prophylaxis is recommended for patients with one or more risk factors for a stress ulcer.
- Sepsis and septic shock are systemic progressions of infection. Therapy includes hemodynamic stabilization, appropriate antimicrobial agents, and removal of infectious foci, if possible.
- Key recommendations in the Surviving Sepsis Guidelines include resuscitation goals and a timeline for monitoring patient progress, the selection and use of resuscitation fluids and catecholamine vasopressors, and the use of vasopressin and corticosteroids.
- Maintaining adequate fluid status is vital to maintaining tissue perfusion and organ function; however, many clinical factors can affect fluid and electrolyte status in critically ill patients. Finding and treating underlying causes of fluid and electrolyte abnormalities are essential.
- Fluid and electrolyte abnormalities are generally asymptomatic unless severe.
- Fluid and electrolyte therapy should be monitored closely because of patient instability and the risk of iatrogenic abnormalities (e.g., cardiac arrhythmias, fluid overload).

 ## 21-2 STUDY GUIDE CHECKLIST

The following topics may guide your study of this subject area:

- ☐ Appropriate assessment tools for pain, agitation, and delirium.
- ☐ Appropriate drug selection for pain, agitation, and delirium based on patient factors.
- ☐ Risk factors for stress ulcers and appropriate prophylaxis.
- ☐ Major points regarding initial therapy in sepsis or septic shock.
- ☐ Appropriate selection of vasopressors or inotropes in sepsis or septic shock.
- ☐ Appropriate use of corticosteroids in sepsis or septic shock.
- ☐ Severe, life-threatening electrolyte disorders and appropriate treatments.

21-3   Routine Care Issues in Critically Ill Patients: FAST HUG

This chapter will focus on some of the most common pharmacotherapeutic issues in critically ill patients. The widely used mnemonic FAST HUG outlines a number of routine care issues in the ICU that should be addressed in every patient every day (Figure 21-1). Some of these issues are addressed in other chapters as noted.

"F" – Feeding

See Chapter 22 on nutrition support.

"A" – Analgesia and "S" – Sedation

Disease Overview

Pathophysiology

Pain is extremely common in critically ill patients and comes from a variety of sources. Many states can lead to pain, agitation, or delirium including (1) injuries, (2) medical procedures and equipment (e.g., mechanical ventilation equipment or catheters), (3) mental status changes (e.g., fear, infection, hypoxia, sleep deprivation, adverse drug effects, withdrawal), or (4) preexisting medical conditions (e.g., chronic pain).

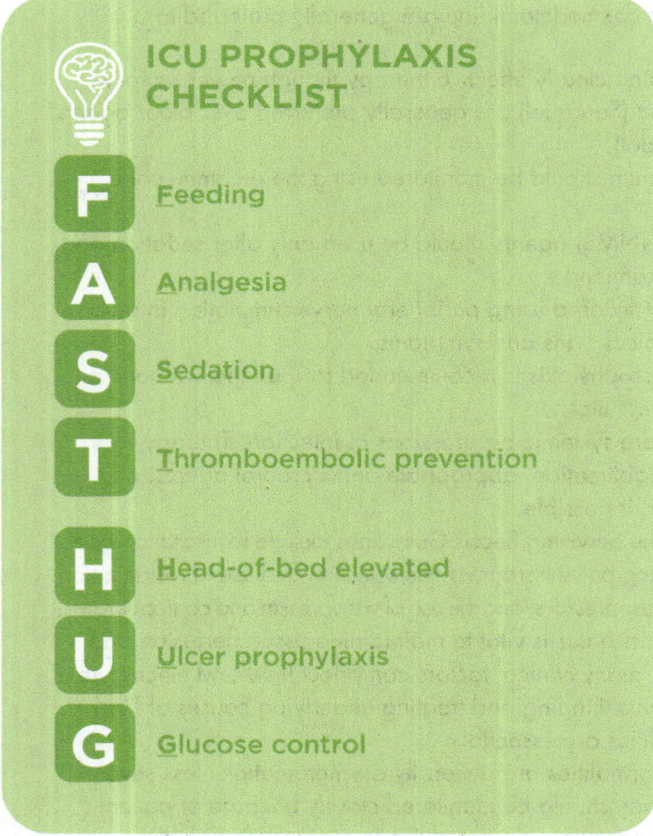

FIGURE 21-1. Routine Care Issues in the ICU to be Addressed Daily

ICU PROPHYLAXIS CHECKLIST

F Feeding

A Analgesia

S Sedation

T Thromboembolic prevention

H Head-of-bed elevated

U Ulcer prophylaxis

G Glucose control

Clinical Presentation

The presentation of pain, agitation, or both in patients with impaired consciousness may include the patient's pulling of tubes or lines, writhing, kicking, restlessness, hypertension, tachycardia, tachypnea, diaphoresis, or moaning.

The presentation of delirium is an acute change or fluctuation of mental status with any of the following: (1) inattention, (2) disorganized thinking, or (3) an altered level of consciousness. Patients may be hyperactive (agitated) or hypoactive (lethargic), or they may fluctuate between both states.

Diagnostic Criteria

In patients who can communicate, pain can be self-reported. In patients who cannot communicate, pain should be assessed using the Behavioral Pain Scale (BPS) or the Critical-Care Pain Observation Tool (CPOT).

Agitation should be assessed using the Richmond Agitation-Sedation Scale (RASS) or the Riker Sedation–Agitation Scale (SAS).

Delirium should be assessed using the Confusion Assessment Method for the ICU (CAM-ICU) scale or the Intensive Care Delirium Screening Checklist (ICDSC).

Treatment Principles and Goals

Treatment goals include (1) finding and removing the cause of pain, agitation, or delirium; and (2) achieving a balance between patient comfort, adverse effects, and ability to provide care. The risk of ICU delirium and the duration of mechanical ventilation might be decreased by avoiding benzodiazepines in favor of analgesia-only therapy or by using dexmedetomidine or propofol for sedation.

A major focus of analgesia management recently has been a desire to minimize opioid use by employing multimodal therapy with nonopioid agents. These can include **acetaminophen (Tylenol)**, nonsteroidal anti-inflammatory drugs (NSAIDs), treating neuropathic pain with drugs such as **pregabalin** (Lyrica) or **gabapentin (Neurontin)** (see Chapter 17 on diabetes), and localized pain control such as nerve blocks or epidural anesthesia when indicated.

The treatment of delirium is unclear. The Society of Critical Care Medicine (SCCM) guidelines changed their recommendations in 2018. Dexmedetomidine (Precedex) can be used to help facilitate extubation from mechanical ventilation in agitated patients with delirium. Neither newer antipsychotics (e.g., **quetiapine**) nor haloperidol are recommended for routine treatment of ICU delirium. Only nondrug measures are recommended for preventing delirium such as establishing sleep–wake cycles and early mobilization.

- Neuromuscular blocking (NMB) agents induce muscle paralysis and can be used in the ICU for short-term procedures, such as facilitating endotracheal intubation, or for longer-term use, such as allowing better patient compliance with mechanical ventilation. This is often done in patients with acute respiratory distress syndrome (ARDS). NMBs can also be used in patients whose agitation is not controlled with maximum doses of sedation and analgesia.

Drug Therapy

Selected drug therapy is described in Table 21-1.

- Ideally, many ICU patients will have their pain reasonably controlled and will not become agitated. Agitation in the ICU, however, is extremely common and may require treatment with sedatives. Overall goals including finding a balance between efficacy, adverse drug events, and other common treatment goals such as minimizing the duration of mechanical ventilation.
- Minimizing dosing is preferred when possible and may start with dosing as needed before progressing to continuous infusions if necessary.

TABLE 21-1. Selected Drug Therapy Based on Guidelines for Use in ICU Patients

Generic name	Trade name	Dosage range	Forms[a]	Schedule[b]	Notes on usage
Morphine sulfate		0.5 to 10 mg	I.V., I.M., oral	Continuous; every 6 hours	General-use opiate
Hydromorphone	Dilaudid	0.3 to 1.5 mg	I.V.	Continuous; every 6 hours	Used in morphine intolerance, hemodynamic instability, renal dysfunction
Fentanyl	Sublimaze	50 to 200 mcg/h	I.V.	Continuous	Used in morphine intolerance, hemodynamic instability, renal dysfunction, when more rapid titration is needed
Acetaminophen	Ofirmev, **Tylenol**	Up to 4 g/d	Oral, rectal, I.V.	Every 4 to 6 hours	Can be added to opiates
Ibuprofen	Advil, Caldolor	100 to 800 mg	Oral, I.V.	Every 4 to 6 hours	Maximum 3200 mg/d
Ketorolac	Toradol	10 to 30 mg	I.V., I.M., oral	Every 6 hours	Maximum use 5 days
Lorazepam	Ativan	0.5 to 4 mg	I.V., oral	Continuous; every 6 hours	Longer acting than midazolam
Midazolam	Versed	1 to 5 mg	I.V.	Continuous; every 2 hours	Shorter acting than lorazepam
Propofol	Diprivan	1 to 5 mg/kg/h	I.V.	Continuous	Used when rapid awakening needed; rapid onset; very short half-life; highly titratable
Dexmedetomidine	Precedex	0.2 to 0.7 mcg/kg/h	I.V.	Continuous	Must monitor for hypotension, bradycardia; good titratability
Pancuronium	Pavulon	0.05 to 0.1 mg/kg	I.V.	Continuous; every 2 hours	Causes tachycardia; is longer acting
Vecuronium	Norcuron	0.05 to 0.1 mg/kg	I.V.	Continuous; very hour	Used in hemodynamic instability, renal dysfunction, cardiac disease
Rocuronium	Zemuron	0.6 to 1.2 mg/kg	I.V.	Continuous; every 30 minutes	Used if a shorter acting agent is needed
Cisatracurium	Nimbex	0.05 to 0.1 mg/kg	I.V.	Continuous; every hour	Used in renal and hepatic dysfunction (elimination is not organ-dependent)

Boldface indicates one of top 100 drugs for 2020 by prescription volume.
I.M., intramuscular; I.V., intravenous.
a. Long-acting drugs and dosage forms generally are not used in ICU (e.g., fentanyl patch, controlled-release morphine, doxacurium).
b. Continuous analgesia and sedation with frequent titration (patient-controlled analgesia pump, I.V. infusion, or scheduled) are preferred to as-needed therapy alone. NMB agents used as needed are preferred over continuous use.

■ In general, either propofol or dexmedetomidine is preferred over benzodiazepines (usually midazolam (Versed)) because some studies show a decreased incidence of ICU delirium and shorter time on mechanical ventilation.

Mechanism of action
■ **Opiates, NSAIDs:** See Chapter 27 on pain management.
■ **Benzodiazepines, antipsychotics:** See Chapter 29 on psychiatric disease.
■ **Propofol (Diprivan):** Unclear but may involve gamma-aminobutyric acid (GABA) receptors.
■ **Dexmedetomidine (Precedex):** Centrally acting alpha-2-adrenergic agonist.
■ **NMB agents:** Cholinergic receptor antagonists (these do not provide analgesia or sedation).

Patient counseling
If a patient-controlled analgesia (PCA) pump is used, ensure the patient understands how to activate the device.

Adverse drug effects
■ **Opiates, NSAIDs:** See Chapter 27 on pain management.
■ **Benzodiazepines, antipsychotics:** See Chapter 29 on psychiatric disease.
■ **Propofol (Diprivan):** Respiratory depression, hypotension, and hypertriglyceridemia may occur. Propofol infusion syndrome (e.g., metabolic acidosis, rhabdomyolysis, cardiac dysfunction) may occur at high doses (> 5 mg/kg/h for > 48 h). Thus, the maximum dose is 5 mg/kg/h.
■ **Dexmedetomidine (Precedex):** Hypotension and bradycardia may occur. Respiratory depression is less likely than with other agents.
■ **NMB agents:** Respiratory depression, prolonged weakness or paralysis after discontinuation, and tachycardia (pancuronium) have been reported.

Drug–drug interactions
■ **Opiates, NSAIDs:** See Chapter 27 on pain management.
■ **Benzodiazepines, antipsychotics:** See Chapter 29 on psychiatric disease.
■ **Propofol (Diprivan), dexmedetomidine (Precedex):** Actions are potentiated by other sedatives.
■ **NMB agents:** Actions are potentiated by corticosteroids, aminoglycosides, clindamycin, calcium channel blockers, and anesthetics; actions are inhibited by anticholinesterase inhibitors (e.g., neostigmine).

Monitoring parameters
■ **Opiates, NSAIDs:** Use BPS or CPOT if the patient is unable to communicate. Monitor vital signs, but do not use alone for assessment. See Chapter 27 on pain management.
■ **Sedative agents:** Use RASS or SAS. Monitor vital signs. See Chapter 29 on psychiatric disease. For propofol (Diprivan), avoid overfeeding from calories in the lipid vehicle (1 kcal/mL) and monitor triglycerides 1 to 2 times a week. Maximum hang time for 1 bottle is 12 hours. Propofol is contraindicated in patients with egg or soy allergy.
■ **Antipsychotics:** Use CAM-ICU or ICDSC. See Chapter 29 on psychiatric disease.
■ **NMB agents:** Monitor movement, breathing, blood pressure (BP), heart rate (HR), and intracranial pressure along with peripheral nerve stimulation ("train of four" monitoring).

Note: In patients with continuous sedation, using light sedation goals, a daily awakening and assessment period, or both, results in decreased sedative use and a shorter ICU length of stay.

Nondrug Therapy

Nondrug therapies for pain may include music, massage therapy, relaxation therapy, or cold therapy.

"T" – Venous Thromboembolism Prophylaxis

Note: See Chapter 30 on thromboembolic disease.

"H" – Elevate the Head of Bed

Critically ill patients should have the head of their bed elevated 30 to 45 degrees whenever possible to minimize the risk of pneumonia and aspiration of enteral feedings or stomach contents.

"U" – Stress Ulcer Prophylaxis

Definition

Stress ulcer prophylaxis refers to gastrointestinal (GI) mucosal damage related to metabolic stress in the ICU.

Clinical Presentation

Presentation is similar to that of peptic ulcer disease (see Chapter 25 on GI diseases).

Pathophysiology

Shunting of blood from the GI tract to vital organs during critical illness results in breakdown of gastric mucosal defenses (e.g., bicarbonate and mucus production, epithelial cell turnover).

Risk Factors

The primary risk factors for stress ulcers are mechanical ventilation > 48 hours and coagulopathy.

Other risk factors include disease states or organ dysfunction where GI perfusion may be compromised (e.g., sepsis, burns, severe trauma, renal failure, ICU stay > 7 days, other organ dysfunction).

Diagnostic Criteria

Diagnosis is based on signs and symptoms and can be confirmed with endoscopy.

Treatment Goals

The goal is to prevent stress ulcers.

- See Chapter 25 on GI diseases for full drug information and treatment of ulcers (stress ulcers are treated similarly to peptic ulcers). Patients in the ICU should be given stress ulcer prophylaxis if they have a risk factor listed above.
- Proton pump inhibitors (PPIs) are a primary option in many ICUs (e.g., **esomeprazole [Nexium]**, **omeprazole [Prilosec]**, **pantoprazole [Protonix]**). Some recent analyses suggest that PPIs might be more effective than histamine 2–receptor antagonists (H2RAs), but these findings remain controversial. PPIs may be associated with higher rates of *Clostridium difficile*–associated diarrhea than H2RAs, but this also is unclear.
- H2RAs (e.g., famotidine [Pepcid], **ranitidine [Zantac]**) still are considered by many to be a primary option.

- Sucralfate (Carafate) is a secondary option that has fallen out of favor. It is less effective than H2RAs, is not available in intravenous (I.V.) form, and has significant drug-binding interactions.
- Antacids are not recommended. They are less effective, have higher aspiration risk, and require frequent dosing.
- Optimal duration of therapy is unknown. A reasonable approach is to discontinue prophylaxis when risk factors have resolved or upon transfer from the ICU.

"G" – Glucose Control

The SCCM recommends keeping critically ill patients' serum glucose < 180 mg/dL. Intensive glucose control (i.e., goal 80 to 110 mg/dL) is no longer recommended due to worse outcomes. See Chapter 17 on diabetes for more information.

21-4   Sepsis and Septic Shock

Definition and Classifications

See Chapter 33 on infectious diseases.

Sepsis is dysfunction of one or more major organs (e.g., respiratory insufficiency, hypotension, renal dysfunction, acute mental status change, coagulopathy) caused by a suspected or proven infection. Organ dysfunction is identified using the sequential organ failure assessment (SOFA) score; alternatively, patients can be screened rapidly using the abbreviated quick SOFA (qSOFA) score (both widely available online).

Septic shock is sepsis plus hypotension that requires vasopressors to maintain mean arterial pressure (MAP) ≥ 65 mmHg and a serum lactate ≥ 2 mmol/L (18 mg/dL) despite adequate fluid resuscitation.

Clinical Presentation

See Chapter 33 on infectious diseases.

Pathophysiology

Progression is seen in the systemic manifestations of sepsis. Imbalances in the inflammatory, immune, and coagulation systems lead to organ hypoperfusion and organ dysfunction with or without refractory hypotension. See Chapter 33 on infectious diseases for typical causative organisms by site of infection.

Diagnostic Criteria

See Chapter 33 on infectious diseases.

Treatment Goals

- A primary treatment goal is to stabilize hemodynamic parameters rapidly (MAP > 65 mmHg) and to reverse organ dysfunction and elevated serum lactate within 6 hours.
- Concurrently, collect appropriate cultures based on the suspected site of infection, start appropriate antimicrobial therapy within 1 hour, and eliminate the source of infection if applicable (e.g., vascular or urinary catheter, abscess). The duration of antimicrobial therapy typically is 7 to 10 days depending on the site of infection and type of organism.
- Modulate inflammatory, coagulation, and hormonal derangements if applicable.

Drug and Nondrug Therapy

See Chapter 33 on infectious diseases for antimicrobial information (mechanism of action, dosing, adverse effects, etc.) and empiric antimicrobial selection. Definitive therapy should be streamlined to a narrower spectrum agent, if possible, on the basis of the final culture and sensitivity reports.

See Section 21-5 for details on fluid therapy. Initial fluid therapy for severe sepsis and septic shock should be 30 mL/kg of isotonic crystalloids (e.g., 0.9% NaCl or lactated Ringer's [LR] solution). Albumin can be given as a secondary fluid in patients requiring high doses of crystalloids. Other colloids (e.g., hetastarch [Hespan]) no longer are recommended because of the risk of acute kidney insufficiency. Vasopressors should be used only after appropriate fluid therapy fails to normalize BP adequately (Table 21-2). Inotropes can be used if cardiac index is poor following adequate fluid resuscitation.

Mechanism of action

Vasopressors and inotropes are adrenergic-receptor agonists.

Adverse drug effects

Adverse effects for vasopressors and inotropes include tachycardia, arrhythmias, organ and extremity ischemia, and hypertension.

Drug–drug interactions

There are no drug–drug interactions among vasopressors and inotropes.

Monitoring parameters

For vasopressors and inotropes, monitor BP, HR, cardiac output, urine output, and extremity perfusion on physical exam.

TABLE 21-2. Vasopressors[a] and Inotropes Used in Severe Sepsis and Septic Shock

Name	Dosage range	Adrenergic-receptor activity	Comments
Dopamine	< 5 mcg/kg/min	Increased renal perfusion (dopaminergic receptors)	Use of low-dose "renal tonic" dopamine is not recommended; only use if increased beta-1 activity is needed.
	5 to 10 mcg/kg/min	Increased cardiac output/HR (beta 1) > increased BP (alpha 1)	
	10 to 20 mcg/kg/min	Increased cardiac output/HR and BP	
Norepinephrine	0.01 to 3 mcg/kg/min	Increased BP (alpha-1) > increased cardiac output/HR (beta 1)	Preferred agent; fewer arrhythmias occur than with dopamine.
Epinephrine	0.01 to 0.5 mcg/kg/min	Increased cardiac output/HR and BP (all receptors)	Second-line agent
Phenylephrine	0.01 to 5 mcg/kg/min	Increased BP only (alpha 1)	Use only in selected patients.
Dobutamine	5 to 20 mcg/kg/min	Increased cardiac output/HR (beta 1)	
Vasopressin	0.01 to 0.03 units/min	None; acts on vasopressin receptors	Add to catecholamine vasopressor in nonresponsive patients; do not exceed maximum dose.

a. All catecholamine vasopressors are given as continuous I.V. infusions and are titrated to effect.

Other aspects
Vasopressin

Vasopressin infusion (0.03 units/min) may be used to increase BP in patients refractory to high doses of traditional vasopressors. Doses > 0.04 units/min are associated with severe adverse effects (e.g., cardiac arrest). Patients receiving lower doses of catecholamine vasopressors (i.e., < 15 mcg/min of norepinephrine) may benefit more from vasopressin than do patients on higher doses of norepinephrine.

Hydrocortisone

Low-dose hydrocortisone (200 mg/day I.V. infusion for approximately 7 days) is recommended for patients with septic shock who are not responsive to fluids and vasopressors. Several studies have shown that low-dose hydrocortisone (with or without fludrocortisone) can decrease the duration of vasopressor use and might decrease mortality in some patients. Hydrocortisone may be tapered sooner than day 7 of treatment if vasopressors are discontinued.

Miscellaneous therapies

The following therapies are not recommended for treating sepsis: selenium, immunoglobulins, sodium bicarbonate (unless pH < 7.15), or erythropoietin (unless already being used for another indication).

21-5   Fluid and Electrolyte Abnormalities in Critically Ill Patients

See Chapter 20 on kidney disease (for hyperphosphatemia), Chapter 22 on nutrition, and Chapter 23 on oncology (for hypercalcemia).

Disease Overview

Definition

Fluid and electrolyte abnormalities are pathologic alterations in fluid and electrolyte homeostasis.

Classifications

Fluid and electrolyte abnormalities are classified by electrolyte (see the discussion on clinical presentation).

Clinical Presentation

In all cases, mild-to-moderate abnormalities usually are asymptomatic.

Sodium (normal range: 135 to 145 mEq/L)

In cases of hyponatremia or hypernatremia, conditions including lethargy, nausea, headache, dry mucous membranes, poor skin turgor (dependent on hydration status), and confusion may occur.

Coma, seizures, or central pontine myelinolysis may occur in severe hyponatremia or if sodium increases or decreases rapidly (> 12 mEq/L/day).

Chloride (normal range: 96 to 106 mEq/L)

Symptoms are related to acid–base or fluid abnormalities, not chloride itself.

Water (moves osmotically with sodium)

In cases of dehydration, conditions including dry mucous membranes, poor skin turgor, lethargy, nausea, headache, hypotension, and tachycardia occur. Seizures, coma, or death can result if dehydration is severe. Decreased urine output, metabolic acidosis, and hypotension also are found.

For edema or fluid overload, see Chapter 13 on heart failure.

Potassium (normal range: 3.5 to 5 mEq/L)

In cases of hypokalemia, conditions including confusion, muscle cramps, weakness, and cardiac arrhythmias occur.

In cases of hyperkalemia, conditions including muscle cramps, weakness, and cardiac arrhythmias occur.

Magnesium (normal range: 1.5 to 2.2 mEq/L)

With hypomagnesemia, presentation is similar to that of hypocalcemia.

In cases of hypermagnesemia, conditions including lethargy, weakness, and cardiac arrhythmias occur. Coma is possible in severe cases.

Phosphorus (normal range: 2.6 to 4.5 mg/dL)

In cases of hypophosphatemia, conditions including confusion, anxiety, weakness, respiratory depression, paresthesias, and lethargy occur. Seizures and coma are possible if hypophosphatemia is severe.

For hyperphosphatemia, see Chapter 20 on kidney disease.

Calcium (normal range: 8.5 to 10.5 mg/dL)

In cases of hypocalcemia, conditions including confusion, anxiety, paresthesias, muscle cramps, and tetany occur. Coma and cardiac arrhythmias may occur in severe cases.

For hypercalcemia, see Chapter 23 on oncology.

Pathophysiology

Normal distribution of fluids and electrolytes

Electrolytes with high serum concentrations primarily are extracellular (Na, Cl); those with low serum concentrations mostly are intracellular or in bone (K, P, Mg, Ca).

Total body water is approximately 60% to 70% of total body weight (differs by age, gender, disease states):

- Of all body water, approximately two-thirds is intracellular; approximately one-third is extracellular.
- Of extracellular water, approximately three-fourths is interstitial; approximately one-fourth is intravascular (plasma).

Typical fluid requirements for adults are approximately 35 mL/kg/d; they can be much higher in patients with critical illness because of extrarenal losses (GI tract, wounds) and fluid shifts (trauma, sepsis).

Primary hormonal controls are aldosterone (sodium retention) and antidiuretic hormone (water retention).

Hyponatremia

The first three forms of hyponatremia listed below are hypotonic:

- ***Hypovolemic (sodium and water loss):*** This condition is characterized by high urine osmolality. It is related to extrarenal fluid losses (GI, wounds), diuretics, and adrenal insufficiency.

■ *Euvolemic (moderate water retention):* This condition occurs with syndrome of inappropriate antidiuretic hormone (SIADH) release, renal failure, carbamazepine, NSAIDs, and chlorpropamide.

■ *Hypervolemic (sodium and water retention):* This condition occurs with congestive heart failure, cirrhosis, nephrotic syndrome, and glucocorticoids.

■ *Hypertonic:* This condition is the dilutional effect of abnormal osmotic agents in the vasculature (severe hyperglycemia).

Hypernatremia

Hypernatremia occurs in cases of water loss or excessive sodium intake (e.g., from I.V. fluids). It is related to extrarenal fluid losses (GI, wounds) and diabetes insipidus.

Hypochloremia

Hypochloremia occurs with GI losses.

Hypokalemia

Hypokalemia is related to diuretics, beta-2 agonists, amphotericin B, glucocorticoids, cisplatin, and GI losses.

Hyperkalemia

Hyperkalemia is related to renal dysfunction, acidosis, angiotensin-converting enzyme inhibitors, potassium-sparing diuretics, trimethoprim, salt substitutes taken orally, and adrenal insufficiency.

Hypomagnesemia

Hypomagnesemia occurs with GI losses, diuretics, amphotericin B, alcohol, and cisplatin. It should be treated before treating hypokalemia; Na+K+-ATPase pumps require magnesium to work.

Hypermagnesemia

Hypermagnesemia is related to renal dysfunction, magnesium-containing antacids, adrenal insufficiency, and hyperparathyroidism.

Hypophosphatemia

Hypophosphatemia is related to refeeding syndrome, phosphate binders, diuretics, hypercalcemia, vitamin D deficiency, and glucocorticoids.

Hyperphosphatemia

See Chapter 20 on kidney disease for information about hyperphosphatemia.

Hypocalcemia

Hypocalcemia occurs with hypoparathyroidism, hypomagnesemia, vitamin D deficiency, and loop diuretics. Total calcium is artificially low in hypoalbuminemia (calcium is highly albumin bound).

Diagnostic Criteria

- Criteria include serum concentration, signs, and symptoms.
- Sodium analysis may use urine sodium and urine osmolality.

Treatment Goals

- Find and treat the underlying cause of abnormality.
- Treat abnormality to avoid sequelae.

Drug and Nondrug Therapy

Fluid replacement

Administer fluids as follows:

- *Crystalloids:* Salt solutions—½ or ¼ normal saline (NS) ± dextrose 5% ± KCl 20 mEq/L (approximates urine electrolytes), NS (154 mEq/L of Na), LR solution, ¼ NS, or dextrose 5%—are chosen on the basis of sodium and fluid needs. NS or LR typically are used for fluid resuscitation (sodium is the major osmotic cation in plasma).
- *Colloids:* Albumin 5% to 25% can be used to provide fluid resuscitation or to raise oncotic pressure (e.g., cirrhosis).
- *Vasopressors ± isotropic activity:* After fluids are optimized, vasopressors ± isotropic activity may be used (see Chapter 13 on heart failure).

Edema

Fluid restriction ± diuretics may be used. See Chapter 13 on heart failure and Chapter 20 on kidney disease.

Hyponatremia

If the case is severe, titrate 3% NaCl to maximum serum sodium increase of 12 mEq/d. Treat specific forms as follows:

- *Hypovolemic:* Replace fluid losses with I.V. NS (0.9% NaCl, 154 mEq/L).
- *Euvolemic (SIADH):* Use fluid restriction ± demeclocycline. Newer vasopressin antagonists conivaptan (Vaprisol) or tolvaptan (Samsca) also can be used.
- *Hypervolemic:* Use fluid restriction ± diuretics.
- *Hypertonic:* Correct hyperglycemia.

Hypernatremia

Titrate low-sodium fluids (e.g., dextrose 5%, ¼ NS) to a normal serum sodium. In cases of diabetes insipidus, use DDAVP (desmopressin).

Hyperchloremia

Give sodium acetate or LR instead of NS, especially if acidemic (acetate is converted to bicarbonate by the liver).

Hypokalemia

Administer IV (KCl) or oral **potassium** (KCl, K phosphate, or K acetate). Each 10 mEq dose increases serum potassium by about 0.1 mEq/L. I.V. administration faster than 10 mEq/h requires electrocardiogram monitoring for arrhythmias.

Hyperkalemia

Treat hyperkalemia as follows:

- *Potassium removal (slower onset of action):* Use Na polystyrene sulfonate (Kayexalate) orally or rectally, loop diuretics, or hemodialysis (if severe).
- *Intracellular potassium shifting (rapid onset of action):* Administer regular insulin + dextrose I.V., **albuterol**, or Na bicarbonate.
- *Potassium antagonism of cardiac effects (rapid onset of action):* Administer I.V. calcium.

Hypomagnesemia

Dosages are described below. A large percentage of the dose is renally wasted. Repletion requires 3 to 5 days of treatment.

- *I.V.:* Administer 0.5 to 1 mEq/kg/d (8 mEq = 1 g); administration rate = 8 mEq/h.
- *I.M.:* Intramuscular (I.M.) administration is possible but is painful.
- *Oral:* Administer magnesium-containing antacid or laxative 3 to 4 times a day as tolerated or magnesium oxide 300 to 600 mg 2 to 4 times a day.

Hypermagnesemia

Treat with diuretics, I.V. calcium, or hemodialysis (similar to hyperkalemia).

Hypophosphatemia

If the case is severe, use I.V. sodium or **potassium** phosphate 0.16 to 0.64 mmol/kg at 7.5 mmol/h to avoid potassium overdose (if potassium phosphate is used), calcium precipitation, or both.

Administer orally 1 to 2 g/d (5 to 60 mmol/d), for example, Neutra-Phos, Neutra-Phos-K, or Fleet Phospho-soda.

Hyperphosphatemia

See Chapter 20 on kidney disease for information about hyperphosphatemia.

Hypocalcemia

If patient is symptomatic, administer I.V. calcium gluconate (2 to 3 g) or I.V. calcium chloride (1 g) over 10 minutes. In addition, the following may be administered:

- I.V. infusion of 0.5 to 2 mg/kg/h of elemental calcium
- Calcium salts such as calcium carbonate (oral 1 to 3 g elemental calcium/d ± vitamin D)

Patient Counseling

In cases of oral administration, advise patient about potential adverse effects.

Adverse Drug Effects

- *Sodium:* Edema or central pontine myelinolysis can occur if serum Na changes rapidly (> 12 mEq/d).
- *Crystalloids:* Vein irritation is possible with hypotonic (¼ NS, ½ NS) or hypertonic (3% NaCl) fluids. Dextrose 5% is approximately isotonic and often is added to low-sodium fluids.

- *Potassium:* Events include cardiac arrhythmias (> 10 mEq/h), vein irritation (I.V.), GI upset (oral; worse with wax matrix controlled-release tablets), and bad taste (oral liquid). With sodium polystyrene sulfonate, constipation may occur (medication usually is mixed with sorbitol).
- *Magnesium:* Events include diarrhea (oral), flushing, sweating (I.V.), and vein irritation (I.V.).
- *Phosphorus:* Events include diarrhea (oral) and calcium phosphate precipitation (I.V.).
- *Calcium:* I.V. calcium gluconate is less irritating than calcium chloride. Cardiac dysfunction can occur if medication is administered > 60 mg/min (elemental calcium). Effects also include calcium phosphate precipitation (I.V.) and constipation (oral).

Drug–drug interactions

- Hypokalemia and hypomagnesemia can predispose the patient to digoxin toxicity.
- Binding of drugs in the GI tract by calcium or magnesium is possible (see Chapter 22 on nutrition).

Monitoring Parameters

- Serum concentrations
- Resolution of signs and symptoms
- With fluid replacement, normalization of the following: BP, HR, urine output (goal > 0.5 mL/kg/h), skin turgor, mucous membrane hydration, edema, cardiac output, pulmonary artery wedge pressure (see Chapter 13 on heart failure), serum lactate/base deficit

21-6   Pharmacist's Role

Pharmacists have a huge role to play as part of the ICU team in the care of critically ill patients. Much of the routine care of critically ill patients (e.g., FAST HUG) can be made better and more consistent by working with physicians, nurses, and others to develop clinical pathways (protocols) for issues such as stress ulcer and venous thromboembolism (VTE) prophylaxis, sedation/analgesia/delirium management, sepsis management, and antibiotic selection. Then, pharmacists are often the point people for educating other ICU staff about pathways. A number of studies have shown that when multidisciplinary teams (including pharmacists) implement pathways drug therapy can be optimized and patient outcomes improved. This is perhaps most notable in the realm of analgesia/sedation. Readers are also referred to the joint ACCP/SCCM statement on the role of pharmacists in the ICU.

Pharmacists can help the team with appropriate selection, titration, and monitoring of agents based on patient parameters. Some examples include transitioning patients between continuous and as-needed regimens, helping the team balance analgesia and sedation needs with the desire to get patients off mechanical ventilation as soon as possible, counterbalanced by adverse events such as respiratory depression and hypotension. Ideally, many of the FAST-HUG processes will be protocolized in the unit; however, in the real world things can get missed and pharmacists are ideally positioned to "poke, prod, and remind" the team to make sure these essential measures are started, restarted (e.g., after surgery), and discontinued (e.g., before the patient leaves the ICU) appropriately.

Pharmacists can also work with the team to hit critical time goals for the initial management of sepsis and septic shock including rapid initiation of appropriate antimicrobial therapy, appropriate fluid resuscitation, and vasopressors and hydrocortisone, if needed. Pharmacists can also help ensure that attention is paid to achieving physiologic goals such as normalization of MAP and serum lactate. Depending on the hospital, pharmacists may also play a critical role in procuring and distributing fluids and medications in emergent situations. Lastly, dealing with electrolyte abnormalities could begin with clinical pathways. Pharmacists can help teams to individualize dosing (e.g., in renal dysfunction) and have roles here in making sure that computerized order-entry procedures include safe limits on administration rates.

NAPLEX Competency Statements

The questions in this chapter cover the following 2021 NAPLEX Competency Statements: **AREA 1:** 1.1; 1.2; 1.3; 1.4; 1.5; 1.6; 1.7 **AREA 2:** 2.1; 2.2 **AREA 3:** 3.1; 3.2; 3.4; 3.5; 3.6; 3.7; 3.8; 3.9; 3.10; 3.11; 3.12 **AREA 4:** 4.3 **AREA 5:** 5.5.

 **21-7   Questions**

1. Which of the following is the most easily titratable opioid for use in the ICU?

A. Morphine
B. Hydromorphone
C. Fentanyl
D. Acetaminophen
E. Dexmedetomidine

2. In which situations should hydromorphone or fentanyl be used instead of morphine for analgesia in critically ill patients? (Mark all that apply.)

A. Morphine allergy
B. Renal dysfunction
C. Hemodynamic instability
D. Need for longer acting agent
E. Desire for less respiratory depression

3. What is the maximum duration of therapy for ketorolac?

A. 5 days
B. 7 days
C. 14 days
D. 30 days
E. There is no restriction on the length of use.

4. Which of the following nonopioid agents would be best to add in a critically ill patient with neuropathic pain in his legs from a spinal cord injury?

A. Acetaminophen
B. Ibuprofen
C. Ketamine
D. Gabapentin
E. Midazolam

5. Which of the following is a concern when using ketamine as a nonopioid agent for treating pain in the ICU?

A. Hypotension
B. Bradycardia
C. Hallucinations
D. Respiratory depression
E. Propylene glycol toxicity

6. Which of the following sedative agents is least likely to cause respiratory depression?

A. Lorazepam
B. Propofol
C. Dexmedetomidine
D. Midazolam
E. Fentanyl

7. Which of the following sedative agents are recommended to minimize the risk of ICU delirium? (Mark all that apply.)

A. Midazolam
B. Lorazepam
C. Propofol
D. Dexmedetomidine
E. Diazepam

8. Based on current evidence, which of the following is the best agent for treating ICU delirium in an agitated patient when extubation from mechanical ventilation is desired?

A. Propofol
B. Dexmedetomidine
C. Haloperidol
D. Quetiapine
E. Ziprasidone

9. A critically ill patient with moderate renal and hepatic dysfunction will require a continuous infusion of a neuromuscular blocker to facilitate ventilation because of ARDS. Which of the following is the best option?

A. Succinylcholine
B. Vecuronium
C. Cisatracurium
D. Pancuronium
E. Rocuronium

10. Which of the following is recommended for monitoring the use of NMBs?

A. Behavioral pain scale (BPS)
B. Critical-care pain observation tool (CPOT)
C. Clinical signs alone (e.g., movement and breathing)
D. Serum triglycerides 1 to 2 times per week
E. Peripheral nerve stimulation plus clinical signs

11. Which of the following are risk factors for the development of stress ulcers? (Mark all that apply.)

A. Sepsis
B. Coagulopathy
C. Mechanical ventilation > 48 hours
D. Age > 40 years
E. ICU stay > 3 days

12. Which of the following is correct regarding stress ulcer prophylaxis?

A. H2RAs or sucralfate are equally effective and considered drugs of choice.
B. PPIs and H2RAs generally are considered the drugs of choice.
C. Antacids have the most direct effect on gastric pH and are considered drugs of choice.
D. Sucralfate is more effective than H2RAs and PPIs.
E. All agents (H2 antagonists, sucralfate, PPIs, antacids) are equally effective.

13. Which of the following is the most appropriate initial resuscitation fluid choice in sepsis or septic shock?

A. Either crystalloids or colloids are acceptable
B. Starch colloids are recommended first
C. Albumin is recommended first
D. Crystalloids and albumin should be started together
E. Crystalloids are recommended first

14. Which of the following describes the appropriate use of hydrocortisone in sepsis or septic shock?

A. Use in all patients with severe sepsis or septic shock.
B. Use in all patients on vasopressors (i.e., in septic shock).
C. Use only in patients with documented adrenal insufficiency.
D. If started, treat until the patient is discharged from the ICU.
E. Use only if BP is refractory to fluids and vasopressors.

15. How soon after the onset of sepsis or septic shock should antibiotic therapy be administered?

A. 1 hour
B. 3 hours
C. 4 hours
D. 6 hours
E. 12 hours

16. Which of the following describes appropriate use of vasopressin in septic shock?

A. It is an option if a first-line vasopressor is failing.
B. It is recommended as a first-line vasopressor.
C. It should be titrated similarly to a catecholamine vasopressor.
D. It should be used only if hydrocortisone is used.
E. It can be used to increase cardiac output more than BP.

17. Which of the following is the general vasopressor of choice in septic shock?

A. Dopamine
B. Epinephrine
C. Phenylephrine
D. Norepinephrine
E. Vasopressin

18. A critically ill patient with a serum potassium of 3.3 mEq/L is prescribed I.V. potassium chloride 40 mEq x 1 dose. Over what time period should this dose be administered?

A. 5 minutes
B. 30 minutes
C. 1 hour
D. 2 hours
E. 4 hours

19. M.W. is a 25-year-old pregnant female who is admitted to the medical ICU following several days of severe nausea and vomiting. She is hypotensive, tachycardic, and confused, and her urine output is very low. Her serum sodium is 128 mEq/L. Which of the following should be given to treat her fluid and sodium abnormality?

A. I.V. NS or LR solution
B. I.V. 5% dextrose in water
C. Oral water
D. I.V. furosemide
E. Desmopressin

20. Which of the following electrolyte abnormalities is common with loop diuretics (e.g., furosemide)?

A. Hypokalemia
B. Hyperkalemia
C. Hypermagnesemia
D. Hypernatremia
E. Hypercalcemia

21. R.T. is a 40-year-old male admitted to the medical ICU following a severe asthma exacerbation. R.T.'s serum phosphorus is 0.9 mEq/L, and his body weight is 70 kg (100% of ideal). Which of the following acute phosphorus supplementation regimens is most appropriate?

A. 45 mmol of sodium phosphate I.V. over 6 hours
B. 45 mmol of sodium phosphate I.V. over 10 minutes
C. 15 mmol of oral phosphorus (e.g., Neutra-Phos) over the next 24 hours
D. 15 mmol of I.V. sodium phosphate over 2 hours
E. No acute phosphorus therapy is required.

22. The most common electrolyte abnormality associated with angiotensin-converting enzyme inhibitors is

_____.

A. hypomagnesemia
B. hypokalemia
C. hyperkalemia
D. hyperphosphatemia
E. hypernatremia

23. Which of the following acts the slowest when rapid treatment of severe hyperkalemia is needed?

A. Potassium restriction
B. I.V. calcium
C. I.V. regular insulin and dextrose
D. I.V. sodium bicarbonate
E. Oral Kayexalate

24. Which of the following electrolyte abnormalities are most commonly associated with amphotericin B? (Mark all that apply.)

A. Hyponatremia
B. Hypokalemia
C. Hypomagnesemia
D. Hypocalcemia
E. Hypophosphatemia

25. Which of the following best describes GI side effects of antacids containing magnesium and calcium salts?

A. Mg causes constipation; Ca causes diarrhea.
B. Mg causes diarrhea; Ca causes constipation.
C. Both cause diarrhea.
D. Both cause constipation.
E. Neither has GI side effects.

 **21-8   Answers**

1. **C.** Fentanyl is used as a continuous infusion and is more titratable than morphine or hydromorphone. Acetaminophen and dexmedetomidine are not opiates.

2. **A, B, C.** Morphine may cause more hemodynamic instability than hydromorphone or fentanyl because of more histamine release. In addition, morphine has a renally excreted, partially active metabolite that may accumulate in renal dysfunction. Hydromorphone and fentanyl do not have such a metabolite. The reason for using these agents in morphine allergy is self-explanatory. D is incorrect because hydromorphone and fentanyl are shorter acting. E is incorrect because respiratory depression is common with all opiates.

3. **A.** According to the manufacturer, ketorolac should not be used longer than 5 days because of the high risk of GI bleeding with this drug.

4. **D.** Gabapentin (or pregabalin) can be used for neuropathic pain in the ICU. Acetaminophen, ibuprofen, and ketamine are acceptable nonopioid agents but are not preferred when neuropathic pain is being treated. Midazolam is a sedative and doesn't control pain.

5. **C.** A dissociative syndrome including hallucinations can occur with ketamine, especially at higher doses. Advantages of ketamine compared to other agents include the lack of hypotension, bradycardia, and respiratory depression. Lorazepam can cause propylene glycol toxicity, not ketamine.

6. **C.** Dexmedetomidine does not cause respiratory depression. All the other agents can do so.

7. C, D. Propofol and dexmedetomidine cause less ICU delirium than benzodiazepines in some studies and are recommended to decrease the risk of delirium.

8. B. The SCCM guidelines state that dexmedetomidine can be used in ICU delirium if the patient is agitated and extubation is desired. Newer (atypical) antipsychotics and haloperidol are no longer recommended for routine treatment of ICU delirium.

9. C. Cisatracurium is metabolized by nonspecific plasma esterases (i.e., not organ dependent), whereas pancuronium, vecuronium, and rocuronium have varying degrees of hepatic or renal elimination. This patient has hepatic and renal dysfunction, so cisatracurium avoids those issues. Succinylcholine is only for one-time procedural use (e.g., intubation) and not continuous infusion.

10. E. NMB monitoring requires clinical signs plus peripheral nerve stimulation. BPS and CPOT are for pain monitoring, not specifically for NMB usage. Triglyceride monitoring is needed for propofol.

11. A, B, C. Increased age is not an independent risk factor for stress ulcers. An ICU stay > 3 days is not a risk factor (> 7 days is a risk factor).

12. B. PPIs and H2RAs are considered by most clinicians to be the drugs of choice. PPIs have pros and cons: they may be more effective, but they also may have other disadvantages based on outpatient use. Sucralfate is a secondary option for a number of reasons described in the text, and antacids are not used for this indication.

13. E. The Surviving Sepsis Guidelines recommend crystalloids first, then albumin is acceptable if the patient's hypotension is refractory. Nonalbumin colloids cause more renal dysfunction and are not recommended.

14. E. The Surviving Sepsis Guidelines recommend using hydrocortisone only in patients who are refractory to fluids and vasopressors. The typical duration is 7 days.

15. A. The Surviving Sepsis Guidelines recommend administering antibiotics within 1 hour.

16. A. Vasopressin is recommended in the Surviving Sepsis Guidelines for use as a second vasopressor if a first-line agent (e.g., catecholamine) is failing. It is not titrated, its use is not related to hydrocortisone use, and it improves only BP (not cardiac output).

17. D. Norepinephrine is the preferred vasopressor recommended in the Surviving Sepsis Guidelines. Compared to dopamine, it causes less arrhythmias and is more effective.

18. E. IV potassium chloride should be given no faster than 10 eEq/h except in emergency situations because of the risk of arrhythmias.

19. A. M.W. is hyponatremic, and her clinical signs and symptoms indicate severe dehydration from GI losses of water and sodium. She requires rapid fluid resuscitation with a fluid that has an approximately physiologic amount of sodium (either NS 154 mEq/L or LR 130 mEq/L). This amount of sodium will increase her serum sodium into the normal range over time, and the osmotic effect will hold water in the extracellular compartment (the vasculature and interstitium) to help restore organ perfusion.

20. A. Loop diuretics enhance renal excretion of potassium (hypokalemia), magnesium (hypomagnesemia), and calcium (hypocalcemia).

21. A. R.T. is severely hypophosphatemic and requires high-dose I.V. therapy (0.64 mmol/kg × 70 kg = 44.8 mmol). The dose should be infused at 7.5 mmol/h (total time: 6 hours) to avoid precipitation with calcium.

22. C. ACE inhibitors cause hyperkalemia because of aldosterone inhibition.

23. E. Oral Kayexalate (sodium polystyrene sulfonate) does not act very quickly. It requires transit time through the intestines to bind potassium and create a gradient that pulls more potassium into the lumen of the GI tract.

24. B, C. Amphotericin B causes renal wasting of potassium and magnesium.

25. B. Magnesium salts (e.g., milk of magnesia) often are used as osmotic laxatives and may cause diarrhea. Calcium salts may cause constipation.

21-9   Additional Resources

Barletta JF, Bruno JJ, Buckley MS, et al. Stress ulcer prophylaxis. *Crit Care Med.* 2016;44(7):1395–1405.

Chessman KH, Haney J. Disorders of sodium and water homeostasis. In: DiPiro JT, Yee GC, Posey, ML, et al., eds. *Pharmacotherapy: A Pathophysiologic Approach.* 11th ed. New York, NY: McGraw-Hill; 2020:755–778.

Devlin JW, Skrobik Y, Gelinas C, et al. Clinical practice guidelines for the prevention and management of pain, agitation, delirium immobility, and sleep disruption in adult patients in the ICU. *Crit Care Med.* 2018;46:e825–e873.

Flurie RW. Disorders of potassium and magnesium homeostasis. In: DiPiro JT, Yee GC, Posey, ML, et al., eds. *Pharmacotherapy: A Pathophysiologic Approach.* 11th ed. New York, NY: McGraw-Hill; 2020:797–812.

Murray MJ, DeBlock H, Erstad B, et al. Clinical practice guidelines for sustained neuromuscular blockade in the adult critically ill patient. *Crit Care Med.* 2016;44(11):2079–2103.

Pai AB. Disorders of calcium and phosphorus homeostasis. In: DiPiro JT, Yee GC, Posey, ML, et al., eds. *Pharmacotherapy: A Pathophysiologic Approach.* 11th ed. New York, NY: McGraw-Hill; 2020:779–796.

Rhodes A, Evans LE, Alhazzani W, et al. Surviving Sepsis Campaign: International guidelines for management of sepsis and septic shock: 2016. *Crit Care Med.* 2017;45:486–552.

Singer M, Deutschman CS, Seymour CW, et al. The third international consensus definitions for sepsis and septic shock (Sepsis-3). *JAMA.* 2016;315(8):801–810.

SCCM/ACCP. Position paper on critical care pharmacy services. *Pharmacotherapy* 2000;11:1400–1406.

Nutrition

JOSEPH M. SWANSON   EDWARD T. VAN MATRE

22-1 KEY POINTS

- Malnutrition can present as either undernutrition or obesity.
- The components of a nutritional assessment include a history and physical exam, anthropometric measurements, and biochemical tests.
- An increase in energy expenditure (energy needs) is defined as *hypermetabolism,* and an increase in nitrogen excretion (protein needs) is defined as *hypercatabolism.*
- Most patients receiving specialized nutrition support (parenteral or enteral nutrition) require 25 to 30 kcal/kg/d and 1 to 2 g protein/kg/d.
- The water requirement for most adult patients without substantial extrarenal losses is 30 to 40 mL/kg/d.
- Parenteral nutrition (PN) should be reserved for patients whose gastrointestinal tracts are not functional or accessible (e.g., severe short bowel syndrome).
- Total nutrient admixtures (TNAs) contain dextrose, amino acids, lipid emulsion, electrolytes, vitamins, and trace elements in 1 container, while 2-in-1 PNs lipid emulsion is administered separately from the other ingredients.
- For PN calculations: 1 g hydrated dextrose = 3.4 kcal, 1 g amino acids = 4 kcal, and 1 g lipid = 9 kcal. (Intravenous [I.V.] fat emulsion actually provides 10 kcal/g because it includes calories provided as glycerol and phospholipid.)
- All PN formulations should be filtered during administration (0.22-micron filter for 2-in-1 PN formulations and 1.2-micron filter for TNAs).
- Enteral nutrition support is generally used in patients who cannot or will not eat but have a functional and accessible gastrointestinal tract.
- Enteral tube feeding can be provided by one of the following methods: nasogastric, nasoduodenal, nasojejunal, gastrostomy, or jejunostomy.
- Diarrhea associated with enteral tube feeding is often caused by pharmacotherapy (e.g., sorbitol in liquid drug preparations as a vehicle).
- Patients receiving phenytoin or **warfarin** concurrently with enteral tube feeding should have the tube feeding held at least 1 hour before and after each dose.
- Pharmacists are involved in all aspects of the provision of nutrition support to patients.

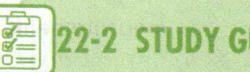

22-2 STUDY GUIDE CHECKLIST

The following topics may guide your study of this subject area:

- ☐ General understanding of macronutrient and micronutrient requirements.
- ☐ Factors incorporated into a nutritional assessment.
- ☐ Patient factors that influence the nutrition support route.
- ☐ Assessment of nutrition support tolerance and efficacy.
- ☐ Management of electrolytes and trace elements.
- ☐ Identification of nutrition-support complications.
- ☐ Major drug–nutrient interactions.

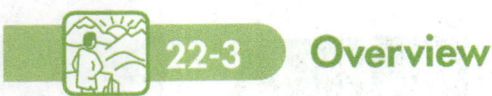

22-3 Overview

Definition

Nutrition is defined as the process of obtaining the food necessary to maintain health and growth. The Dietary Guidelines for Americans 2015–2020 suggest that all forms of foods can be included in healthy eating and that these foods should be nutrient-dense, containing essential vitamins, minerals, and dietary fiber.

Pharmacists involved in the provision of appropriate nutrition to patients will most likely interact with patients unable to consume food needed to provide health. These patients will need to receive nutrition through alternative routes such as direct enteral or parenteral administration.

Malnutrition

Malnutrition is the inadequate provision of food required to maintain health and growth and can be classified by 3 different pathophysiologic states:

- *Starvation-related malnutrition:* Features depleted fat and muscle stores and normal biochemical measurements (e.g., classic starvation without inflammation)
- *Chronic disease-related malnutrition:* Features mild-to-moderate inflammation (e.g., congestive heart failure, chronic kidney disease, sarcopenic obesity)
- *Acute disease or injury-related malnutrition:* Features severe and acute inflammation (e.g., major infection, trauma)

Nutritional assessment components

History and physical examination

- Dietary intake (anorexia, bulimia, hyperphagia, taste alterations)
- Underlying pathology affecting nutrition (cancer, burns)
- End-organ effects (diarrhea, constipation)
- Gastrointestinal surgery (bariatric surgery, gastrectomy, bowel resection)
- General appearance (edema, cachexia)
- Skin appearance (scaling skin, decubitus ulcers)
- Musculoskeletal effects (depressed muscle mass, growth retardation)
- Neurologic effects (depressed sensorium, encephalopathy)
- Hepatic effects (jaundice, hepatomegaly)

Anthropometrics

- Skinfold measurements for assessment of fat (triceps, calf)
- Arm muscle circumference for assessment of skeletal muscle
- Waist circumference for assessment of abdominal fat (metabolic syndrome)
- Weight for height to determine undernutrition or obesity
  - Change in weight over time is one of the best indicators of nutritional status.
- Head circumference in infants to document appropriate growth
- Percentage of ideal body weight (IBW) after calculation of IBW for patient:
  - IBW of males (kg) = 50 + (2.3 × height in inches over 5 feet)
  - IBW of females (kg) = 45.5 + (2.3 × height in inches over 5 feet)
- Body mass index (BMI) for assessment of undernutrition or obesity calculated from body weight (kg) and height (m): BMI = weight (kg)/height^2 (m^2)

Biochemical assessment
Serum albumin concentration

- Good prognostic indicator and good for assessment of long-term nutritional status
- Poor for repletion marker because of long half-life (21 days) and large body pool

Serum prealbumin concentration

Serum prealbumin concentration
- Good for short-term assessment of nutrition support because of short half-life (2 days) and small body pool
- Possible increase in serum prealbumin concentrations in patients with kidney disease because of impaired excretion

Serum transferrin concentration
- Good for short-term assessment of nutrition support because of short half-life (7 days) and small body pool
- Elevated in iron-deficiency anemia

Other methods of nutritional assessment
- Muscle strength testing
- Bioelectrical impedance (i.e., a low-grade electrical current is sent through the body to identify body protein stores and fat stores)

Selected definitions

- *Hypermetabolism:* An increase in energy expenditure above normal (usually > 10% above normal)
- *Hypercatabolism:* An increase in protein losses above normal (usually via urinary excretion of urea nitrogen)
- *Obesity:* Demonstrated as elevated body weight to at least 120% of IBW or BMI > 30
  - Class I obesity: BMI ≥ 30 and < 35
  - Class II obesity: BMI ≥ 35 and < 40
  - Class III obesity: BMI > 40
- *Nutrition support therapy:* parenteral nutrition (PN) or enteral nutrition (EN)
- *Basal energy expenditure (BEE):* A calculation of the normal energy needs of healthy adult men or women using sex, age, height, and weight
- *Harris–Benedict equations for BEE and Mifflin St. Jeor (sometimes listed only as Mifflin) equations for energy expenditure:* The most commonly used equations for estimating the BEE of patients and can be found in any nutrition resource or online
- *Resting energy expenditure (REE):* A measured value of energy expenditure (generally ~ 10% above BEE or Mifflin St. Jeor in health but can be 100% above BEE in severe burns)
- *Indirect calorimetry:*
  - Indirect calorimetry is the most accurate method to determine energy requirements.
  - It is a noninvasive procedure that measures VO_2 (oxygen consumption) and VCO_2 (carbon dioxide production), and resting energy requirements are then calculated using the Weir equation: metabolic rate (kcal/d) = $1440(3.94 VO_2 + 1.11 VCO_2)$
- *Body cell mass:* Lean, metabolically active tissue (skeletal muscle, body organs)
- *Lean body mass:* Body cell mass, extracellular fluid, and extracellular solids (bone, serum proteins)

22-4   Nutritional Requirements

Calorie Requirements

- Most clinicians dose nutrition support therapies in total calories (i.e., using carbohydrate, fat, and protein-calorie contributions to obtain the desired dose).
- Caloric goals can be determined by measuring the REE via indirect calorimetry.

- Boxes 22-1 and 22-2 show different methods to estimate caloric goals based on a patient's clinical conditions, degree of stress, and certain equations.
- Box 22-3 depicts the calories supplied from different macronutrients, while Box 22-4 provides protein dosing recommendations based on a patient's condition.

Recommended Daily Allowance of Protein Based on Patient Condition
- 0.8 g/kg/day is the adult recommended daily allowance (RDA) for protein in the United States.
- 1 g/kg/d is the adult RDA for patients with minor stress (elective operations).
- 1.5 g/kg/d is the adult RDA for patients with major trauma or infection.
- 2 g/kg/d is the adult RDA for patients with severe head injury, sepsis, or severe thermal injury.
- 2.5 g/kg/d is the adult RDA for patients receiving continuous renal replacement therapy.

Measurement of Nutritional Efficacy Using Nitrogen Balance (NB)

- NB = nitrogen in − nitrogen out
- Nitrogen in (grams) is determined by dividing the grams of protein taken in on the day of balance by 6.25.
- Nitrogen out (grams) is determined by measuring the grams of urea nitrogen excreted during a 24-hour urine collection and then adding a factor of 2 or 4 g for insensible nitrogen loss or stool loss.

> ### BOX 22-1. Caloric Goals Based Only On Patient Condition

- 25 kcal/kg/d for adults with little stress (e.g., elective surgery)
- 30 kcal/kg/d for patients with infections and skeletal trauma
- 35 kcal/kg/d for patients with major trauma (head injury, long-bone fractures)
- 40 kcal/kg/d for patients with major thermal injury (burn covers >50% total body surface area)

> ### BOX 22-2. Caloric Goals Based on BEE Calculation and Patient Condition

- 1 × BEE for patients with little stress
- 1.3 × BEE for patients with infections or skeletal trauma
- 1.5 × BEE for patients with major trauma
- 2 × BEE for patients with severe thermal injury

> ### BOX 22-3. Caloric Contribution of the Major Macronutrients

Kilocalories From Glucose, Fat, and Protein

- *Glucose:* 3.4 kcal/g because hydrated glucose is used in PN (glucose powder would be 4 kcal/g)
- *Fat:* 9 kcal/g
- *Protein:* 4 kcal/g
  - Protein requirements are usually dosed in grams per kilogram per day.

BOX 22-4. Other Requirements during Nutrition Support

Water

- Recommended Water Volumes
  - 30 to 40 mL/kg/d for average-sized adults
  - 40 mL/kg/d for smaller adults and adolescents
  - >40 mL/kg/d for patients with extrarenal losses (e.g., gastrointestinal drains)

Electrolytes

- Daily Electrolyte Intake Recommendations
  - Sodium requirements:
    - 60 to 100 mEq/d in adults
    - 26 mEq/kg/d in children
  - Chloride requirements:
    - 60 to 100 mEq/d in adults
    - 2 to 6 mEq/kg/d in children
  - Potassium requirements:
    - 60 to 100 mEq/d in adults
    - 2 to 5 mEq/kg/d in children
  - Calcium requirements:
    - 5 to 15 mEq/d in adults
    - 2 to 3 mEq/kg/d in children
  - Phosphorus requirements:
    - 20 to 45 mmol/d in adults
    - 1 to 2 mmol/kg/d in children
  - Magnesium requirements:
    - 10 to 20 mEq/d in adults
    - 0.25 to 1 mEq/kg/d in children

Vitamins

- Vitamins are provided daily in both PN (added) and EN (endogenous).
- Most enteral formulations provide the dietary reference intakes (DRI) for vitamins in a volume of 1000 to 1500 mL.
- For parenteral vitamin products:
  - Adult products contain 12 (Multi Vitamin Infusion without vitamin K (M.V.I.-12®)) or 13 vitamins (Infuvite® Adult, M.V.I. Adult™); vitamin K is added separately when the product with 12 vitamins is used.
  - Pediatric products (M.V.I. Pediatric®, Infuvite® Pediatric) contain all 13 vitamins.

Trace elements

- Trace Element Doses in Adults and Children
  - *Zinc:* 3 to 5 mg/d in adults with PN; 50 to 250 mcg/kg/d in children with PN
  - *Copper:* 0.5 to 1.2 mg/d in adults with PN; 20 mcg/kg/d in children with PN (maximum of 300 mcg/d)
  - *Chromium:* 10 to 15 mcg/d in adults with PN; monitored but not given to children
  - *Manganese:* 50 to 100 mcg/d in adults with PN; monitored but not given to children
  - *Selenium:* 40 to 80 mcg/d in adults with PN; 1.5 to 3 mcg/kg/d in children with PN

- Positive NB can be used to document adequacy of nutritional support:
  - In undernourished patients, + 4 to + 6 g/d is desired.
  - Nitrogen equilibrium (− 2 to + 2 g/d) is usually adequate in critically ill patients.

22-5   Nutrition Support Therapies

Parenteral Nutrition

Indications

PN is generally used for patients who cannot be fed via the gastrointestinal tract. PN should begin after 5 to 7 days of lack of bowel function.

Short bowel syndrome

This condition requires PN from a few weeks to lifelong, as needed.

Ileus

This condition is secondary to lack of bowel function (e.g., postoperative after gastrointestinal surgery). Box 22-5 provides the recommended volumes of water required in various patients.

Components of parenteral nutrition

Protein

- Protein should be included in all PN formulations.
- Standard amino acids from 10%, 15%, or 20% stock solutions can be used for most patients.
- Final concentrations in the PN formulation vary from 2% to 7%.

Fat

- Fat is provided as I.V. lipid emulsion either as a separate infusion or as an admixture with the rest of the PN formulation, making a TNA.
- Products are manufactured as 10%, 20%, and 30% lipid emulsions. (In the United States, 30% can be used only for TNAs, not for direct infusion.)
- Fat provides essential fatty acids to the patient who is most likely not eating by mouth.
- Fat provides nonprotein calories other than glucose.

> **BOX 22-5. Other Indications for Parenteral Nutrition**
>
> - Bowel obstruction
> - Bowel ischemia
> - Neonates who cannot eat in the first day of life
> - Preoperatively for undernourished patients who are undergoing an elective operation and for whom there is no direct access to the gastrointestinal tract (e.g., partial small bowel obstruction from cancer)
> - Pregnancy with severe hyperemesis gravidarum (i.e., an inability to tolerate oral or enteral nutrition)
> - Gastrointestinal fistulae where oral or EN should be restricted

- Common doses used in adults are ~ 1 g/kg/d (9 to 10 kcal/kg/d) but should not exceed 2.5 g/kg/d.
- I.V. lipid emulsions contain a phospholipid to emulsify the product and a glycerol to make the emulsion isotonic. (Both of these components provide modest calories that result in supplying 10 kcal/g equivalent of fat.)

Dextrose

- Common doses of dextrose in critically ill patients are 3 to 4 mg/kg/min (~15 to 20 kcal/kg/d).
- Dextrose is in all PN formulations for obligate needs (central nervous system, renal medulla, white blood cells, red blood cells, wound healing).
- PN formulations are usually made from 50% to 70% dextrose in water.
- Final concentrations in the PN formulation vary from D10W (10% dextrose in water) to D35W (35% dextrose in water).
- Dextrose should never exceed a dose of 5 mg/kg/min (~25 kcal/kg/d).

Sodium

- Sodium can be provided as chloride, acetate, or phosphate salts in PN.
- After phosphate addition, the remaining anions are added on the basis of acid–base status. They are split between chloride and acetate with a normal pH, predominantly acetate with metabolic acidosis, and predominantly chloride with metabolic alkalosis.
- Requirements can be increased when the patient has extrarenal losses from nasogastric suction, abdominal drains, or ostomy losses.

Potassium

- **Potassium** can be provided as chloride, acetate, or phosphate salts in PN.
- Requirements can be increased with administration of potassium-wasting drugs (diuretics, steroids) or in severe undernutrition.
- Like sodium, the remaining potassium can be added as acetate or chloride on the basis of acid–base status after the proper dose of phosphate is determined.

Calcium

- Most practitioners add calcium as the gluconate salt.
- Higher doses of calcium (~20 to 25 mEq/d) are needed in patients receiving long-term PN to help prevent metabolic bone disease.
- Addition of calcium is limited in PN formulations because of the potential to precipitate with phosphate salts, which ultimately results in insoluble calcium phosphate.

Phosphate

- Phosphate is added as the sodium or **potassium** salt.
- Higher doses of phosphorus (e.g., 30 mmol/L) are needed to prevent refeeding syndrome in severely undernourished patients.
- Phosphorus should be decreased or removed in patients with renal failure.
- Most practitioners prefer sodium phosphate over **potassium** phosphate because of the higher concentration of aluminum in the latter product, especially in chronic use of PN.
- Addition of phosphorus is limited in PN formulations because of the potential to precipitate with calcium or magnesium salts to form an insoluble compound.

Magnesium

- Most practitioners add magnesium as the sulfate salt.
- Higher doses should be used in patients with alcoholism or large bowel losses or in patients receiving drugs causing renal wasting of magnesium (cisplatin, amphotericin B, aminoglycosides, loop diuretics).
- Magnesium should be restricted or eliminated in patients with renal failure.

Multivitamins

- Multivitamins are given daily as part of PN.
- Additional thiamine and **folic acid** are often given to patients with alcoholism who are receiving PN.
- Additional **folic acid** (at least 600 mcg/d) should be given to pregnant patients receiving PN.

Trace elements

- Trace elements are given daily as a cocktail of 4 or 5 trace metals.
- Extra zinc should be given to patients with ostomy or diarrhea losses.
- Copper and manganese should be reduced or eliminated in patients with cholestasis.
- Extra selenium is usually needed in homebound PN patients.

Total nutrient admixtures versus 2-in-1 admixtures

Box 22-6 provides reasons for and against the use of TNAs.
Box 22-7 describes the benefits and limitations of using a central vein or peripheral vein for PN.

Parenteral nutrition calculations

D20W (final concentration of PN formulation)

- D20W = 20% dextrose = 20 g/100 mL = 200 g/L × 3.4 kcal/g = 680 dextrose kcal/L
- 2 L/d of D20W (final concentration of PN formulation) = 1360 dextrose kcal/d

Amino acids 5% (final concentration of PN formulation)

- 5% amino acids = 5 g/100 mL = 50 g/L × 4 kcal/g = 200 protein kcal/L
- 2 L/d of 5% amino acids = 100 g/d = 400 protein kcal/d

Lipid 2% (final concentration of TNA formulation)

- 2% lipid will deliver 200 kcal/L (includes calories from glycerol/phospholipid)
- 2 L/d of lipid 2% = 400 fat kcal/d

Lipid 20% infused at 20 mL/h × 24 h (separate infusion given with 2-in-1 PN formulations)

- 20% lipid = 2 kcal/mL
- 20 mL/h × 24 h = 480 mL/d
- 480 mL/d × 2 kcal/mL = 960 fat kcal/d

> ### BOX 22-6. **Advantages and Disadvantages of TNAs**

- Advantages
  - Nursing time for administration is decreased.
  - Potentially touch contamination is decreased.
  - Less pharmacy preparation time is needed (assuming a 24-hour hang time).
  - Financial savings are possible (use of only 1 pump and 1 I.V. administration set).
- Disadvantages of TNAs
  - TNAs are better media for bacterial growth than are 2-in-1 admixtures.
  - Visualizing particulate matter is impossible.
  - Filter formulation with a 0.22-micron filter is not possible.
  - Some additives like calcium and phosphorus are less compatible in TNAs.

> **BOX 22-7. Benefits and Limitations of Using a Central Vein PN versus Peripheral Vein PN**

- Advantages of Central Vein PN
  - Central vein PN can maximize caloric intake.
  - Volume restriction of patients is possible.
  - Long-term catheter can be maintained.
- Disadvantages of Central Vein PN
  - Mechanical complications can occur during catheter placement (e.g., pneumothorax).
  - Potential hyperosmolar complications are possible (e.g., from use of hypertonic dextrose).
  - Potential septic catheter complications are possible.
- Advantages of Peripheral Vein PN
  - The catheter (i.e., peripheral vein stick) is placed more easily.
  - Hyperosmolar complications are avoided because dilute formulations must be used.
- Disadvantages of Peripheral Vein PN
  - Incidence of thrombophlebitis is high.
  - Frequent vein rotation is necessary.
  - Energy intake is limited.
  - Volume restriction is not possible (using dilute formulations).
  - Cost is higher because more lipid calories are generally used. (Lipids are isotonic.)

Example: D30W; amino acids 4%; lipid 3%; at 60 mL/h
- 60 mL/h × 24 h/d = 1440 mL/d (1.44 L/d)
- D30W = 30% dextrose = 300 g/L × 3.4 kcal/g = 1020 kcal/L × 1.44 L = 1469 dextrose kcal
- 4% amino acids = 40 g/L = 160 kcal/L × 1.44 L = 230 protein kcal
- 3% lipid = 300 kcal/L × 1.44 L = 432 fat kcal
- 1469 kcal + 230 kcal + 432 kcal = 2131 total kcal/d from the above PN formulation

Example: dextrose 400 g; amino acids 100 g; lipids 40 g; at 85 mL/h
- Dextrose 400 g × 3.4 kcal/g = 1360 kcal/d
- Amino acids 100 g × 4 kcal/g = 400 kcal/d
- Lipids 40 g × 10 kcal/g (includes phospholipid and glycerol) = 400 kcal/d

TNA Macronutrient Compounding Calculations Example: dextrose 400 g; amino acids 100 g; lipids 40 g; at 85 mL/h
- 85 mL/h × 24 h/d = 2040 mL/day (2.04 L/d)
- Dextrose 70% (D70W) = 70 g/100 mL
  - 400 g of 70 g/100 mL solution = 571.43 mL to PN
- Amino acids 15% = 15 g/100 mL
  - 100 g of 15 g/100 mL solution = 666.67 mL added to PN
- Lipid 20% = 20 g/100 mL
  - 40 g of 20 g/100 mL solution = 200 mL added to PN

2-in-1 Macronutrient Compounding Calculations Example: dextrose 400 g; amino acids 100 g; lipids 40 g; at 85 mL/h
- The same calculations as above would be used for the dextrose and amino acids
- Lipid 10% = 10 g/100 mL would be run separately
  - 40 g of 10 g/100 mL solution = 400 mL run separately

General principles of compounding parenteral nutrition

- Each component of the PN prescription should be reviewed to ensure a balanced PN formulation is provided.
- Each component should be assessed for dose and potential compatibility programs.
- All compounded PN formulations should be visually inspected to ensure no gross contamination or precipitation is present.
- Manufacturers of automated compounders should provide the additive sequence to ensure safety in PN preparation.

General principles of stability and compatibility of parenteral nutrition

- Parenteral multivitamins should be added shortly before dispensing and administering the PN formulation because vitamins A and C degrade fairly quickly.
- Preparation of TNAs using dual-chambered bags (lipid is kept in a separate compartment until administration) can enhance the shelf life of a PN formulation.
- Dibasic calcium phosphate can precipitate in PN formulations if the amounts of calcium gluconate and sodium or **potassium** phosphate are excessive.
- Generally, phosphate should be added first to the PN formulation.
- Generally, calcium should be added last to the PN formulation.
- Calcium chloride should not be used in PN because it is highly reactive with phosphate.
- Iron dextran can be added to 2-in-1 PN formulations but should not be added to TNAs.

Parenteral nutrition filtration

- Filters are used to prevent administration of particulate matter, microorganisms, and air.
- Use a new 0.22-micron filter each day with 2-in-1 PN formulations. (0.22-micron filters with positive charged nylon can be used for up to 72 hours in 2-in-1 PN formulations.)
- Use a new 1.2-micron filter each day with TNAs.

Complications of parenteral nutrition

Metabolic
Hyperglycemia

- Patients with stress of trauma or infection or those with diabetes often need regular **human insulin** added to the PN formulation to control hyperglycemia.
- Regular insulin continuous infusions are often needed to control hyperglycemia.

Electrolyte disorders
Hypokalemia

Patients often require extra **potassium** in PN (e.g., 60 mEq/L).

Hypophosphatemia

Patients often require extra phosphorus in PN (e.g., 30 mmol/L).

Hypomagnesemia

Patients often require extra magnesium in PN (e.g., 16 mEq/L).

Hyponatremia

Diagnosis of sodium disorders must include an assessment of extracellular fluid status (i.e., volume status):

- *Volume depleted:* Add sodium and water to PN or increase I.V. fluid administration.
- *Volume overloaded:* Remove sodium from PN and concentrate the formulation.
- *Euvolemic:* Generally, water restriction is first-line therapy (concentrate the PN formula).

Acid–base disorders

- Increase acetate and decrease chloride anions if the patient has metabolic acidosis.
- Increase chloride and decrease acetate anions if the patient has metabolic alkalosis.

Essential fatty acid deficiency

During PN, at least 4% of total calories need to be provided as I.V. lipid (easily attained when lipid is used daily as a calorie source).

Trace element disorders

- Patients with increased ostomy output or chronic diarrhea need extra zinc.
- Copper and manganese should be withheld in patients with cholestasis.

Hepatic steatosis

- Fatty infiltration of the liver has been reported with long-term PN and is thought to be primarily caused by administration of excessive dextrose calories.
- The key to prevention is through administration of an appropriate dose of dextrose (e.g., <5 mg/kg/min).

Mechanical complications

- Pneumothorax (punctured lung) can occur during central vein cannulation.
- Subclavian artery injury can occur when the artery is cannulated instead of the vein.
- Subclavian vein thrombosis can occur with long-term central vein access. (Heparin is used in some PN patients to prevent this condition.)

Infectious complications

- Such complications are usually due to catheter-related breakdown in sterile technique.
- They are rarely solution related.

Monitoring of PN

Frequency and intensity of monitoring is based on the patient's condition, as assessed by the following:

- Electrolyte balance and glucose control
- Acid–base status via arterial blood gases
- Intake and output for assessment of fluid balance
- Serum prealbumin concentrations, nitrogen balance, or both to document efficacy

Enteral Nutrition

Indications

- EN is generally used in patients who cannot or will not eat but have a functional and accessible gastrointestinal tract.
- Neonates should begin EN as early as possible, even if receiving PN.
- Cardiac patients may need fluid-restricted EN with fluid overload.
- In short bowel syndrome, EN is used to enhance small bowel hypertrophy after major bowel resection.
- In inflammatory bowel syndrome, EN is the preferred method of nutrition support.

Types of Enteral Nutrition Access

- Oral route (by drinking supplements)
- Nasal tubes are used for short-term EN.
  - Nasogastric, nasoduodenal, or nasojejunal tubes are used.
  - Nasogastric, nasoduodenal, or nasojejunal tubes are placed manually or using endoscopy.

- Feeding enterostomies are used for long-term EN.
- Percutaneous endoscopic gastrostomy (PEG), gastrostomy (G-tube), or jejunostomy (J-tube) are used.
- A PEG requires endoscopy for placement.
- A G-tube or J-tube requires a laparotomy for placement.

Products for enteral nutrition

- Polymeric, nutritionally complete oral supplements are used to supplement an insufficient oral diet (e.g., 1 or 1.5 kcal/mL).
- Polymeric, nutritionally complete tube feeding is used for patients with normal digestive processes (e.g., 1 kcal/mL).
- Concentrated, nutritionally complete tube feeding is used for patients who need significant fluid restriction (e.g., 2 kcal/mL).
- Chemically defined, nutritionally complete tube feeding is used for patients with impaired digestive processes such as short bowel syndrome or pancreatic insufficiency (e.g., 1 kcal/mL).
- Fiber-containing, nutritionally complete tube feeding is beneficial in patients who receive long-term tube feeding (can prevent diarrhea and constipation; e.g., 1 or 1.2 kcal/mL).
- Concentrated, low-protein, low-electrolyte tube feeding is generally used for patients with kidney dysfunction.
- High-fat, low-carbohydrate, nutritionally complete tube feeding is helpful in the management of patients who have diabetes or are glucose-intolerant (e.g., 1 or 1.2 kcal/mL).

Complications of enteral nutrition

Pulmonary (e.g., aspiration pneumonia)

- Pulmonary complications are caused by regurgitation of gastric contents into the lung (with or without tube feeding).
- Prevention is important:
  - Elevate the head of the bed to 30° to 45° if possible.
  - Frequently assess the patient's abdomen to ensure tolerance.
  - Frequently assess the placement of the feeding tube (especially nasally placed tubes).

Gastrointestinal

Diarrhea is associated with the administration of EN, but all causes of diarrhea should be investigated.

Increased frequency or volume of stools

- Pharmacotherapy is often the cause due to sorbitol in liquid vehicles.
- Lack of fiber and excessive infusion rate advancements can also be causes.
- *Clostridium difficile* colitis can be a cause, especially if the patient has recently received antibiotics.
- Decreasing (or at least not advancing) the infusion rate is appropriate.
- Change to a fiber-containing formulation if the patient is not receiving one.
- Use pharmacotherapeutic treatment if the above factors are ruled out (bismuth subsalicylate, loperamide , or diphenoxylate).

⚠ **Loperamide** *FDA BOXED WARNING*

Loperamide hydrochloride has been associated with cases of torsades de pointes, cardiac arrest, and death. Avoid using higher than recommended dosages of loperamide hydrochloride in adults and pediatric patients due to risk of serious adverse cardiac reactions.

Constipation (decrease in stool frequency)

- Lack of fiber can be a cause.
- Lack of water can be a cause.
- Poor mobility and drugs with anticholinergic activity can contribute.
- Keep patient well hydrated and use a fiber-containing EN formulation.

Mechanical

- To prevent esophageal injury or nasal necrosis, use a small-bore feeding tube.
- To prevent the feeding tube from clogging, frequently flush it with warm water.

Metabolic

Hyperglycemia

- Use regular **human insulin**.
- Consider a high-fat, low-carbohydrate EN formulation.
- Regular insulin continuous infusions are sometimes necessary.

Hypokalemia

- Provide additional **potassium** as an I.V. or per tube supplement.
- Some institutions allow the addition of **potassium** salts to the EN formulation.

Hypophosphatemia

- Provide additional phosphorus as an I.V. supplement (e.g., **potassium** phosphate).
- Some institutions allow the addition of phosphorus salts to the EN formulation (e.g., injectable sodium or **potassium** phosphate).

Monitoring of enteral nutrition

- The condition of the patient will dictate the intensity of the monitoring of the following:
  - Electrolyte balance and glucose control
  - Acid–base status via arterial blood gases (critical care only)
  - Intake and output for assessment of fluid balance
  - Assessment of the patient's abdomen:
    - The abdomen should be soft, nontender, and nondistended in most cases.
    - A profoundly distended abdomen usually requires the EN to be decreased or discontinued temporarily while the etiology is investigated.

Gastric residual volumes may be monitored in some institutions to help assess intolerance and delayed gastric emptying

- Metoclopramide ⚠ 10 to 20 mg I.V. every 6 hours can be used to decrease gastric emptying time.
- Erythromycin in I.V. doses of 3 to 7 mg/kg/d has been used to decrease gastric emptying time.

Serum prealbumin concentrations, nitrogen balance, or both should be assessed to document efficacy.

 Metoclopramide *FDA BOXED WARNING*

Metoclopramide can cause tardive dyskinesia (TD), a serious movement disorder that is often irreversible. There is no known treatment for TD. The risk of developing TD increases with duration of treatment and total cumulative dosage. Discontinue metoclopramide in patients who develop signs or symptoms of TD. In some patients, symptoms may lessen or resolve after metoclopramide is stopped. Avoid treatment with metoclopramide for longer than 12 weeks because of the increased risk of developing TD with longer-term use.

Home Nutrition Support

Parenteral nutrition

- PN can be given from weeks to a lifetime (e.g., severe short bowel syndrome).
- PN is usually cycled at night over 10 to 16 hours for convenience and for a decrease in incidence of hepatic complications.
- Patient must be monitored closely for iron deficiency because iron supplementation is not routinely added to PN.
  - Regular assessment of hemoglobin, hematocrit, and mean corpuscular volume is required.
  - Serum iron, total iron-binding capacity, and ferritin are commonly used in the diagnosis of iron deficiency.
- Metabolic bone disease is another long-term complication of home PN.
  - Supplemental calcium in the PN formulation is usually required (15 to 25 mEq/d).
  - Adequate vitamin K for osteocalcin is important on a long-term basis.

Enteral nutrition

- EN can be given indefinitely as full nutrition support or as a supplement to an oral diet.
- Permanent feeding ostomies are used almost exclusively in home EN.
- Patients in nursing homes and extended care facilities usually receive EN as a continuous (24 hours) or intermittent (e.g., 12 hours) infusion.
- Patients who receive home EN via gastrostomy usually receive bolus feeding (e.g., two 240 mL cans 3 times a day via PEG).
- Patients who receive home EN as a supplement to oral intake are often cycled at night (e.g., 1000 mL at 85 mL/h from 7:00 PM to 7:00 AM each night).

22-6   Major Drug–Nutrient Interactions

Phenytoin and Enteral Tube Feeding

Enteral feeding has been demonstrated to bind to phenytoin, thus impairing the absorption dramatically, possibly because of the protein component of EN (caseinates).

Management of Phenytoin–Enteral Nutrition Interaction

- Hold the EN 2 hours before and after the daily dose of phenytoin capsules.
- Hold the EN 1 hour before and after each dose of phenytoin suspension (usually given twice daily or 3 times a day).
- Increase the EN infusion rate to allow the desired nutritional dose of EN to be given (i.e., to make up for the lost time while the EN is being held for drug administration).

Warfarin and Enteral Tube Feeding

Adequate anticoagulation with **warfarin** has been reported to be very difficult to achieve with concurrent EN (low international normalized ratios).

Management of Warfarin–Enteral Nutrition Interaction

Hold EN 1 hour before and after the daily **warfarin** dose. If this is done, the EN rate should be increased to attain the desired nutritional dose.

Management of Grapefruit Juice–Drug Interaction

- Grapefruit juice interacts with many drugs (e.g., **amlodipine**, carbamazepine, cyclosporine).
- Grapefruit juice from frozen concentrate has been reported to inhibit gastrointestinal cytochrome P450 3A4, resulting in enhancement of oral absorption of some drugs (toxicity).
- When taking drugs that are known to interact with grapefruit juice, patients should be advised to avoid grapefruit products (i.e., substitute another fruit juice such as apple or orange juice).

22-7   Pharmacist's Role

There is considerable variability in the role pharmacists play in providing nutrition support to patients. These roles can be divided into 2 major categories.

Compounding

- Pharmacists are often responsible for following steps in compounding PN, which includes activities such as
  - Review and verification of the PN order
  - Preparation and inspection of the PN (see various steps in the Parenteral Nutrition Section of this chapter)
  - Proper labeling of the final product
  - Proper delivery of the PN to the patient

Direct Patient Care

- Pharmacists can provide direct patient care as part of a nutrition support multidisciplinary service or as an individual consultant for parenteral nutrition. In this role, pharmacists are often responsible for activities such as
  - Patient caloric and protein needs assessment
  - Determination and calculation of patient-specific goals
  - Monitoring response to EN or PN administration
  - Monitoring for adverse effects, drug–drug and drug–nutrient interactions
  - Modification of EN or PN as patient requirements change
  - Transition from EN or PN to oral diet

NAPLEX Competency Statements

The questions in this chapter cover the following 2021 NAPLEX Competency Statements: **AREA 1:** 1.1; 1.2; 1.3; 1.4; 1.5; 1.6; 1.7 **AREA 2:** 2.1; 2.2; 2.4 **AREA 3:** 3.1; 3.2; 3.4; 3.5; 3.6; 3.7; 3.8; 3.9; 3.11; 3.12 **AREA 4:** 4.2; 4.3; 4.6 **AREA 5:** 5.1; 5.4.

22-8 Questions

1. What is the most appropriate daily protein intake for a healthy adult male weighing 80 kg?

A. 64 g
B. 80 g
C. 96 g
D. 120 g
E. 160 g

Use the following case study to answer Questions 2 and 3.

A patient presents for a comprehensive nutritional assessment. She is 35 years old, is 5 feet 8 inches, and weighs 52 kg. She has a history of Crohn's disease involving both the small bowel and the colon. She has had no surgeries but has intermittent diarrhea.

Medications

- Prednisone 5 mg every other day
- Mesalamine 1 g 3 times a day
- Loperamide 2 mg every 6 hours and as needed for diarrhea

Measurements

- Triceps skinfold = 3 mm (normal, 10 to 14 mm)
- Calf skinfold = 4 mm (normal, 10 to 15 mm)
- Serum albumin concentration = 2.5 g/dL
- Serum prealbumin concentration = 13 mg/dL (normal, 15 to 45 mg/dL)

2. The triceps skinfold measurement for this patient is an anthropometric measurement for assessment of _____.

A. somatic protein stores
B. fat stores
C. visceral protein stores
D. immune competence
E. body cell mass

3. What type of malnutrition does this patient have?

A. Starvation-related
B. Acute disease–related
C. Obesity
D. Chronic disease–related
E. Injury-related

4. A patient with a bone fracture and gram-negative pneumonia excretes 15 g (normal, 6 to 8 g/d) of urea nitrogen during a 24-hour urine collection. On the basis of these data, the patient is _____.

A. hypercatabolic
B. hypermetabolic
C. hypocatabolic
D. hypometabolic
E. euvolemic

5. During nutritional assessment, the measurement of body cell mass includes _____.

A. bone
B. interstitial fluid
C. skeletal muscle
D. intravascular fluid
E. extracellular fluid solids

Use the following case study to answer Questions 6–9.

Following major gastrointestinal resection, a patient with severe short bowel syndrome is started on PN. It is anticipated that this patient may need this therapy for 6 months to 1 year. The PN prescription for this patient includes the following:

Dextrose 300 g, amino acids 125 g, lipid emulsion 55 g to be run at 75 mL/h (1800 mL/day)

0.45% sodium chloride injection at 50 mL/h × 24 h (1200 mL/d)

6. How many calories from dextrose will this patient receive each day?

A. 1020
B. 1120
C. 1220
D. 1450
E. 1550

7. How many calories from protein will this patient receive each day?

A. 300
B. 400
C. 500
D. 600
E. 125

8. How many calories from I.V. lipid emulsion will this patient receive each day?

A. 175
B. 250
C. 360
D. 495
E. 527

9. Calculate the daily nitrogen balance (grams per day) in this patient if she excretes 12 g of urea nitrogen during the urine collection and 4 g are used as insensible and stool loss each day.

A. −4
B. −2
C. 0
D. 2
E. 4

10. What would be an appropriate water or fluid requirement for a 70-kg patient with no extrarenal fluid losses? (Mark all that apply.)

A. 1750 mL
B. 2000 mL
C. 2250 mL
D. 2500 mL
E. 2750 mL

11. Which of the following disease states or clinical conditions would usually require the administration of parenteral nutrition?

A. Postoperative ileus
B. Motor vehicle crash resulting in femur fracture and head injury
C. 20% body surface area burn from a house fire
D. Laparoscopic cholecystectomy
E. Acute exacerbation of hepatic encephalopathy

12. What is the maximum dose (in milligrams per kilogram per day) of dextrose in PN for adult patients?

A. 1
B. 2
C. 5
D. 10
E. 15

13. In a patient with metabolic acidosis, what anion salt would you use to add the majority of sodium and potassium to a PN formulation?

A. Chloride
B. Gluconate
C. Phosphate
D. Acetate
E. Sulfate

14. If excessive amounts of calcium are added to a standard PN formulation, it will likely precipitate with _____.

A. phosphate
B. gluconate
C. magnesium
D. chloride
E. sodium

15. Which vitamin should be supplemented above standard amounts during nutrition support of a pregnant patient?

A. Cyanocobalamin
B. Folic acid
C. Biotin
D. Chromium
E. Pantothenic acid

16. Which of the following is an advantage of central vein PN over peripheral vein PN? (Mark all that apply.)

A. Allows easier catheter placement
B. Does not require a pump for administration
C. Allows for fluid restriction
D. Does not have to be filtered
E. Maximizes caloric intake

17. Which component of a total nutrient admixture should be added last before storing it in a refrigerator?

A. Phosphorus
B. Magnesium
C. Trace elements
D. Calcium
E. Intravenous fat emulsion

18. Which of the following are advantages of using a 0.22-micron filter compared to a 1.2-micron filter?

A. Traps particulate matter
B. Prevents precipitates from entering the patient
C. Filters bacteria
D. Allows uninterrupted flow of lipid emulsion
E. Can be used for over 96 hours

19. Which trace element should be reduced or removed in patients with cholestasis who are receiving PN?

A. Zinc
B. Chromium
C. Selenium
D. Copper
E. Iodine

20. A 70-year-old female who has mild congestive heart failure, gastroesophageal reflux disease (GERD), type II diabetes, and rheumatoid arthritis had a recent cerebral vascular accident. She will not regain her premorbid degree of mental status, so a decision is made to give her long-term nutritional support. Which method would be most appropriate for this patient?

A. Central parenteral nutrition
B. Nasogastric tube feeding
C. Peripheral parenteral nutrition
D. Jejunostomy tube feeding
E. Nasoduodenal tube feeding

21. A common cause of diarrhea in patients receiving EN is from the _____.

A. osmotic load of the EN formulation
B. liquid medications with sorbitol as a vehicle
C. addition of fiber to the EN formulation
D. solute load from the protein component of the EN formulation
E. improper placement of a nasogastric feeding tube

22. What is the drug of choice for enhancing gastric emptying in a patient receiving EN support?

A. Bismuth subsalicylate
B. Azithromycin
C. Metoclopramide
D. Loperamide
E. Acyclovir

23. A patient is receiving phenytoin capsules 300 mg each day for seizure control. She requires tube feeding with a 1 kcal/mL formulation at 85 mL/h (2000 mL/d). What would be the most appropriate intervention to maintain a therapeutic drug concentration and maintain the required nutrition support?

A. Increase the dose of phenytoin to 600 mg/d.
B. Hold the EN 2 hours before and after the dose, and increase the rate to 100 mL/h.
C. Hold the EN 2 hours before and after the dose, and maintain the rate of 85 mL/h.
D. Increase the frequency of phenytoin to 100 mg every 8 hours.
E. Increase the dose and frequency of phenytoin to 200 mg every 8 hours.

24. What is the mechanism for grapefruit juice to inhibit the metabolism of some drugs that can result in drug toxicity?

A. Decreased renal excretion of drug
B. Inhibition of gastrointestinal cytochrome P450 3A4
C. Decreased systemic clearance of drug
D. Inhibition of hepatic cytochrome P450 3A4
E. Expanded apparent volume of distribution

 **22-9 Answers**

1. **A.** The adult RDA for protein in the United States is 0.8 g/kg/d. For an adult who weighs 80 kg, the total daily protein intake would be 80 kg × 0.8 g/kg/d = 64 g/d.

2. **B.** Skinfold measurements measure body fat stores, which assess the lipid component of the body. Visceral protein stores are serum proteins. Body cell mass and somatic protein stores assess skeletal muscle and visceral organs. Immune competence assessment requires a skin test with a common antigen.

3. **D.** Measurements of nutritional assessment are depressed, and the patient has a chronic disease that is contributing to inflammation (i.e., weight for height, anthropometric measurements, and biochemical serum markers of protein status).

4. **A.** Catabolism is related to loss of body protein. Because urea nitrogen output is increased, the patient would be considered hypercatabolic in this case.

5. **C.** Lean body mass includes bone, skeletal muscle, visceral organs, and extracellular solids. Body cell mass includes only the lean, metabolically active tissue such as skeletal muscle and visceral organs (e.g., liver).

6. **A.** Dextrose 300 g/d × 3.4 kcal/g = 1020 kcal/d.

7. **C.** Amino acids 125 g/d × 4 kcal/g = 500 kcal/d.

8. **D.** Lipid emulsion 55 g × 9 kcal/g = 495 kcal/d.

9. **E.** The nitrogen intake is calculated by dividing the protein intake (125 g) by 6.25, which results in 20 g. The nitrogen output would be the sum of the urinary urea nitrogen and insensible losses (12 g + 4 g = 16 g/d). Therefore, the nitrogen balance would be 20 g − 16 g = 4 g. A nitrogen balance of 4 would be suggestive of nutritional adequacy with this PN formulation.

10. **C, D,** and **E.** Water requirements for average size adults is 30 to 40 mL/kg/d in patients without extrarenal fluid losses: 70 kg × 30 mL/kg/d = 2100 mL/d; 70 kg × 40 mL/kg/d = 2800 mL/d. C. 2250 mL, D. 2500 mL, and E. 2750 mL all fall within the 2100 mL to 2800 mL range.

11. **A.** Feeding a patient with postoperative ileus enterally or orally is inappropriate. The other clinical conditions, such as trauma and burns, would occur in patients in whom the gastrointestinal tract could and should be used for nutrition support. A patient receiving laparoscopic cholecystectomy would not need nutrition support. Most patients with hepatic encephalopathy can be fed enterally if they require nutrition support.

12. **C.** The dose of dextrose in PN should never exceed 5 mg/kg/min in adult patients. This dose can be converted to 25 kcal/kg/d.

13. **D.** Acetate is converted to bicarbonate in the liver and would, thus, help or at least not exacerbate the metabolic acidosis.

14. **A.** Calcium phosphate is a relatively insoluble compound, so manufacturer guidelines for the concentrations of these 2 elements must be followed closely to prevent precipitation. The order of mixing these components in the PN formulation is also important.

15. **B.** Folic acid should be given at a dose of at least 600 mcg/d during pregnancy. Many practitioners administer 1 mg/d above what the patient is eating or receiving via nutrition support. This practice has been shown to prevent neural tube defects in the newborn.

16. **C** and **D.** Hyperosmolar nutrients (dextrose, amino acids) can be used to concentrate the PN formulation, but the PN would have to be administered via a central vein. Providing full caloric requirements using central vein PN (to maximize caloric intake) is also possible.

17. **D.** If calcium is added last, the PN formulation will contain the final volume, including all other nutrients. The chance of calcium causing a precipitate will be decreased because all other components (e.g., phosphorus) are diluted in the entire volume of the PN.

18. **C.** A 1.2-micron filter (used with TNAs) will not filter most bacteria. Both filters trap particulate matter and prevent precipitates from entering the patient. The 0.22-micron filter cannot be used in TNAs because lipids cannot freely pass through the smaller pore size.

19. **D.** Copper is excreted via the biliary tract. Patients with severe cholestasis should have copper removed during short-term PN. In long-term PN, copper may be required in reduced doses to prevent anemia. Serum copper concentrations should be monitored regularly in long-term patients who have cholestasis.

20. **D.** She is not a candidate for long-term PN because her gastrointestinal tract would be accessible and functional. Nasogastric and nasoduodenal methods are used only for short-term EN. A jejunostomy tube would be ideal because she also has GERD and perhaps gastroparesis from her diabetes.

21. **B.** Several liquid preparations for drugs contain sorbitol as a pharmaceutical vehicle. These liquid preparations are commonly used in patients with tubes because the drugs can be given easily this way, especially if the patient cannot swallow. Most EN formulations are close to being isotonic (i.e., the osmotic load or solute load is not a major factor causing diarrhea). Fiber will prevent or improve diarrhea in most cases.

22. C. Metoclopramide enhances gastric emptying and is commonly used in patients with gastrointestinal intolerance. This is true in patients with and without diabetes.

23. B. Absorption of phenytoin is markedly impaired when it is given concurrently with enteral tube feeding. The enteral tube feeding should be held 2 hours before and after the daily dose of phenytoin capsules. To maintain the current dose of EN, the rate of feeding should be increased to 100 mL/h (2000 mL/d).

24. B. Drugs such as amlodipine, carbamazepine, and cyclosporine are profoundly metabolized in the gastrointestinal tract before absorption. Grapefruit juice from frozen concentrate has been shown to inhibit gastrointestinal cytochrome P450 3A4 and, thus, allows more of the drug to be absorbed, thereby causing drug toxicity for drugs with a narrow therapeutic index.

 **22-10** **Additional Resources**

American Society for Parenteral and Enteral Nutrition Board of Directors and Clinical Guidelines Task Force. Guidelines for the use of parenteral and enteral nutrition in adult and pediatric patients. *J Parenter Enteral Nutr.* 2002;26(suppl 1): 1SA–138SA.

Brown RO, Dickerson RN. Drug–nutrient interactions. *Am J Managed Care.* 1999;5:345–351.

Chessman KH, Kumpf VJ. Assessment of nutrition status and nutrition requirements. In: DiPiro JT, Talbert RL, Yee GC, et al., eds. *Pharmacotherapy: A Pathophysiologic Approach.* 11th ed. New York, NY: McGraw-Hill; 2017:2323–2344.

Cohen MR. Safe Practices for Compounding of Parenteral Nutrition. *J Parenter Enteral Nutr.* 2012;36(2 Suppl):14S–19S.

Kumpf VJ, Mulherin DW. Enteral nutrition. In: DiPiro JT, Talbert RL, Yee GC, et al., eds. *Pharmacotherapy: A Pathophysiologic Approach.* 11th ed. New York, NY: McGraw-Hill; 2017:2367–2384.

Mattox TW, Crill CM. Parenteral nutrition. In: DiPiro JT, Talbert RL, Yee GC, et al., eds. *Pharmacotherapy: A Pathophysiologic Approach.* 11th ed. New York, NY: McGraw-Hill; 2017:2345–2366.

McClave SA, Taylor BE, Martindale RG, Warren MM, et al. Guidelines for the provision and assessment of nutrition support therapy in the adult critically ill patient: Society of Critical Care Medicine (SCCM) and American Society for Parenteral and Enteral Nutrition (A.S.P.E.N.). *J Parenter Enteral Nutr.* 2016;40(2):159–211.

Task Force for the Revision of Safe Practices for Parenteral Nutrition. Safe practices for parenteral nutrition. *J Parenter Enteral Nutr.* 2004;28(suppl):S39–S70.

Ukleja A, Freeman KL, Gilbert K, et al. Standards for nutrition support: adult hospitalized patients. *Nutr Clin Pract.* 2010;25:403–414.

Oncology

23

GREGORY T. SNEED

23-1 KEY POINTS

- Oncology includes more than 100 diverse diseases that share properties of abnormal and detrimental cell growth.
- Diseases are classified on the basis of the tissue in which they originate (e.g., breast cancer metastasized to the brain is classified as breast cancer).
- Signs and symptoms of cancer often do not follow a specific pattern. A health care provider should evaluate any unusual or persistent change in body appearance or function.
- Before a diagnosis of cancer can be made and systemic treatment can begin, a positive biopsy or blood examination must confirm the presence of the disease.
- Further imaging and laboratory workup should be done to evaluate the extent of the disease (i.e., determine the stage of disease).
- Cancer therapy must be individualized to each patient on the basis of the type and severity of disease, patient characteristics, and patient and family preferences.
- Surgery, radiation, chemotherapy, and biologic therapy are all cancer treatment modalities. They are often used in combination.
- Chemotherapy is often used in combinations to take advantage of different mechanisms of action, prevent resistance, and minimize toxicities.
- Most chemotherapy is aimed at rapidly proliferating cancerous cells. Many chemotherapy-related adverse effects occur, however, in normal highly proliferative cells of the body, such as hair follicles, the gastrointestinal tract lining, and blood cell progenitors.
- Patients should be aware of expected toxicities of chemotherapy, which include alopecia, diarrhea, nausea and vomiting, infertility, myelosuppression, neurotoxicity, nephrotoxicity, hepatotoxicity, stomatitis, and pulmonary toxicity.
- All prophylactic and posttreatment medications for chemotherapy-related complications should be made available to the patient. Counsel the patient to keep a diary of events that occur before and after treatments. Use this record to make interventions and monitor the patient's quality of life.
- All pharmacists should be aware of the accepted cancer screening recommendations and should discuss these with patients. Many cancers can be cured if they are caught early enough.

23-2 STUDY GUIDE CHECKLIST

The following topics may guide your study of this subject area:

- ☐ General symptoms of malignant diseases.
- ☐ General goals of therapy for malignant diseases.
- ☐ Definitions of response goals to therapy for solid tumors.
- ☐ First-line antineoplastic medications for each type of cancer.
- ☐ Dominant adverse effects of various classes of chemotherapy agents.
- ☐ Medications used to prevent and treat chemotherapy-induced nausea and vomiting.
- ☐ Screening recommendations for major cancers (e.g., breast, cervical, colorectal, and prostate).

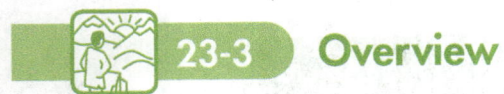

23-3   Overview

Definition

Oncology can be defined as the science dealing with the etiology, pathogenesis, and treatment of cancers. It encompasses more than 100 different diseases that share characteristics of uncontrollable cell proliferation, invasion of local tissues, sustained angiogenesis, defective programmed cell death, and metastasis (e.g., spread from original site).

Incidence and Mortality

In the United States, people have roughly a 40% cumulative lifetime risk of developing cancer. In 2021, an estimated 1,898,160 new cases of cancer were diagnosed, and an estimated 608,570 cancer deaths occurred. It is estimated that about 16.9 million people in the United States have a current or past history of cancer. The most common types of cancer are prostate, lung, and colorectal in men and breast, lung, and colorectal in women. The leading cause of cancer death in men and women is lung cancer, followed by prostate and colorectal in men and breast and colorectal in women.

Clinical Presentation

The American Cancer Society developed an acronym, CAUTION, denoting warning signs of cancer (see Box 23-1). The first signs and symptoms of cancer (solid tumors) develop when a tumor has grown to approximately 10^9 cells (1 cm in diameter or 1 g in mass). The type of cancer determines the presentation of signs and symptoms, which vary widely across tumor types. Positive screening tests (see Table 23-11) or generalized signs of anorexia, fatigue, fever, weight loss, and anemia should also be evaluated.

Pathophysiology and Etiology

The following factors promote cancer:

- *External factors:* Tobacco, chemicals, radiation, infectious organisms, and diet
- *Internal factors:* Genetics, hormones, and immune conditions

Development of cancer is genetically regulated and is a multistage process:

- *Initiation:* Normal cells are exposed to chemical, physical, or biological carcinogens. Such exposure results in irreversible damage, genetic mutations, and selective growth advantages.
- *Promotion:* Reversible environmental changes favor the growth of the mutated cells.
- *Transformation:* The cells become cancerous.
- *Progression:* Additional genetic changes occur, resulting in increased cancerous proliferation. Tumors invade local tissues, and metastasis occurs.

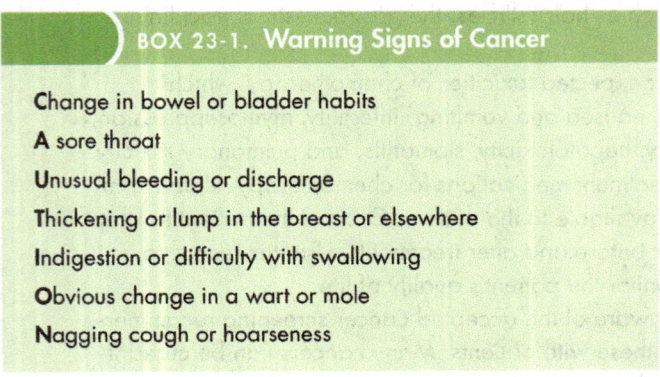

BOX 23-1. Warning Signs of Cancer

Change in bowel or bladder habits

A sore throat

Unusual bleeding or discharge

Thickening or lump in the breast or elsewhere

Indigestion or difficulty with swallowing

Obvious change in a wart or mole

Nagging cough or hoarseness

Malignant tumor cells do not resemble their tissue of origin (in contrast to benign tumors). They are unstable and are incapable of performing normal cellular functions.

Treatment Principles and Goals

Treatment regimens are based on the type of cancer, its stage, the age of the patient, and other prognostic factors (e.g., presence of a tumor marker, poor performance status, and ethnicity). The 4 main goals of cancer therapy are cure, adjuvant/neoadjuvant effect, life extension, and palliation.

Primary therapy is the initial and mainstay approach to treat cancer. It usually consists of removal of the tumor or debulking through surgery but may also include chemotherapy, radiation, or both.

Neoadjuvant therapy is given before the primary therapy. The goal is to reduce the size of the tumor, thereby increasing the efficacy of the primary treatment. Examples include chemotherapy or radiation.

Adjuvant therapy is additional therapy given after the primary treatment, which is usually surgery. The goal is to ensure that all the residual disease has been eradicated. Adjuvant therapy usually consists of chemotherapy, radiation therapy, or both.

The 4 main cancer treatments are surgery, radiation, chemotherapy, and biologic therapy. Most regimens are a combination of these modalities.

23-4 ▶ Drug Therapy

Drug Classes

There are numerous chemotherapy agents. Drugs are grouped by class. Refer to the corresponding table in this chapter for each drug class. The first 5 described below (alkylating agents, antimetabolites, antitumor antibiotics, plant alkaloids, and platinum analogs) make up what is generally accepted as *traditional* chemotherapy. These chemotherapy agents have a very narrow therapeutic index and a toxic adverse effect profile. They are generally more effective in combination because of synergism through biochemical interactions. Choosing drugs with different mechanisms of action, resistance, and toxicity profiles to gain the full benefit of combination therapy is important. Traditional chemotherapy has the greatest effect on rapidly dividing cells because most of the potent chemotherapy drugs act by damaging deoxyribonucleic acid (DNA). A therapeutic effect is seen on cancer cells, but adverse effects also are seen on human cells that rapidly divide (e.g., hair follicles, gastrointestinal [GI] tract, and blood cell progenitors). Agents can be cell cycle phase–specific or cell cycle phase–nonspecific in their pharmacologic action.

Alkylating Agents

See Table 23-1 for summary information about alkylating agents.

Mechanism of action

Alkylating agents cause covalent bond formation of drugs to nucleic acids and proteins, which results in the cross-linking of 1 or 2 DNA strands and inhibition of DNA replication. These agents are cell cycle phase–nonspecific.

Adverse drug effects

Adverse effects include myelosuppression (manifested by low platelet and neutrophil counts and anemia), mucosal ulceration, pulmonary fibrosis and interstitial pneumonitis (carmustine ⚠, cyclophosphamide), fever, fatigue, alopecia, nausea and vomiting, amenorrhea and azoospermia, hemorrhagic cystitis (cyclophosphamide and ifosfamide ⚠), encephalopathy (ifosfamide), seizures (carmustine), and syndrome of inappropriate antidiuretic hormone secretion (SIADH) (cyclophosphamide).

TABLE 23-1. Alkylating Agents

Generic name	Trade name	Dosage range	Dosage form	Frequency	Cancer type*
Nitrogen mustards					
Cyclophosphamide	Cytoxan	500 to 2000 mg/m²	I.V.	Varies	ALL, AML, breast, BL, CLL, CML, HL, MCL, MM, neuroblastoma, NHL, ovarian, retinoblastoma, SLL
	Neosar	40 to 100 mg/m²	Oral	Varies	
Ifosfamide	Ifex	1.2 g/m²	I.V.	Daily for 5 days every 3 weeks	Testicular
Melphalan	Alkeran	16 to 100 mg/m²	I.V.	Varies	MM, ovarian
		2 to 6 mg/m²	Oral	Varies	
Chlorambucil	Leukeran	0.03 to 0.2 mg/kg	Oral	Daily for 3 to 6 weeks	CLL, HL, NHL
Bendamustine	Bendeka Treanda	90 to 120 mg/m²	I.V.	Days 1 and 2 every 21 to 28 days	CLL, NHL
Imidazole	Dacarbazine	150 to 375 mg/m²	I.V.	Varies	HL, melanoma
Ethylenimines and methylmelamines					
Altretamine	Hexalen	260 mg/m²	Oral	Daily for 14 to 21 days every 28 days	Ovarian
Thiotepa	Thioplex	0.3 to 0.4 mg/kg	I.V.	Every 1 to 4 weeks	Bladder, breast, ovarian
Alkyl sulfonates					
Busulfan	Myleran	1 to 8 mg	Oral	Daily	CML
	Busulfex	0.8 mg/kg	I.V.	Every 6 hours for 4 days	
Nitrosoureas					
Carmustine	BiCNU	150 to 200 mg/m²	I.V.	Every 6 weeks	Brain tumors, HL, MM, NHL

ALL, acute lymphocytic leukemia; AML, acute myeloid leukemia; BL, Burkitt's lymphoma; CLL, chronic lymphoid leukemia; CML, chronic myeloid leukemia; HL, Hodgkin's lymphoma; I.V., intravenous; MCL, mantle cell lymphoma; MM, multiple myeloma; NHL, non-Hodgkin's lymphoma; SLL, small lymphocytic lymphoma.
*Appearance of cancer type in the list indicates U.S. Food and Drug Administration approval for the drug's use in treatment of that cancer type.

Drug–drug interactions

Drugs with specific interactions include the following:

- *Bendamustine:* Strong cytochrome P450 (CYP) 1A2 inhibitors
- *Busulfan* ⚠: Itraconazole, phenytoin, and **acetaminophen**
- *Carmustine:* Cimetidine, ethyl alcohol, phenytoin, and amphotericin B
- *Cyclophosphamide:* **Allopurinol**, barbiturates, digoxin, phenytoin, and **warfarin**
- *Ifosfamide:* **Allopurinol**, phenytoin, and **warfarin**
- *Streptozocin* ⚠: Nephrotoxic agents

Antimetabolites

See Table 23-2 for summary information about antimetabolites.

Busulfan *FDA BOXED WARNING*

Busulfan is a potent drug. Busulfan oral tablets should not be used unless a diagnosis of chronic myelogenous leukemia (CML) has been adequately established and the responsible health care provider is knowledgeable in assessing response to chemotherapy. (2) Busulfan tablets can induce severe bone marrow hypoplasia. Reduce or discontinue the dosage of oral busulfan immediately at the first sign of any unusual depression of bone marrow function as reflected by an abnormal decrease in any of the formed elements of the blood. A bone marrow examination should be performed if the bone marrow status is uncertain. Busulfan injection causes severe and prolonged myelosuppression at the recommended dosage. Hematopoietic progenitor cell transplantation is required to prevent potentially fatal complications of the prolonged myelosuppression.

 Streptozocin *FDA BOXED WARNING*

(1) Streptozocin should be administered under the supervision of a physician experienced in the use of cancer chemotherapeutic agents. A patient need not be hospitalized but should have access to a facility with a laboratory and supportive resources sufficient to monitor drug tolerance and to protect and maintain a patient compromised by drug toxicity. The physician must judge the possible benefit to the patient against the known toxic effects of this drug in considering the advisability of therapy with streptozocin. The physician should be familiar with the following text before making a judgment and beginning treatment. (2) Renal toxicity is dose-related and cumulative and may be severe or fatal. Other major toxicities are nausea and vomiting, which may be severe and at times treatment-limiting. In addition, liver dysfunction, diarrhea and hematological changes have been observed in some patients. (3) Streptozocin is mutagenic. When administered parenterally, it has been found to be tumorigenic or carcinogenic in some rodents.

TABLE 23-2. Antimetabolites

Generic name	Trade name	Dosage range	Dosage form	Frequency	Cancer type*
Folic acid antagonists					
Pralatrexate	Folotyn	30 mg/m²	I.V.	Weekly for 6 weeks every 7 weeks	PTCL
Pemetrexed	Alimta	500 mg/m²	I.V.	Every 3 weeks	Mesothelioma, NSCLC
Methotrexate	Rheumatrex	10 to 12 mg	IT	Varies	ALL, breast, head and neck, NHL, osteosarcoma
		1 to 12 g/m²	I.V.		
		25 mg/m²	I.M.		
		10 to 25 mg	Oral		
Pyrimidine analogs					
Azacitidine	Vidaza	75 to 100 mg/m²	SQ (I.V.)	Daily for 7 days every 4 weeks	MDS
Fluorouracil (5-FU)	Adrucil	425 to 500 mg/m²	I.V.	Varies	Breast, CRC, gastric, pancreatic, BCC
Cytarabine	Cytosar-U	100 to 200 mg/m²	I.V.	Every 12 hours for 7 days	AML, CML
	DepoCyt	30 mg/m²	IT	Every 4 days	
Capecitabine	Xeloda	2500 mg/m²	Oral	Daily for 14 days every 3 weeks	Breast, CRC

(continued)

TABLE 23-2. **Antimetabolites** *(Continued)*

Generic name	Trade name	Dosage range	Dosage form	Frequency	Cancer type*
Gemcitabine	Gemzar	1000 to 1250 mg/m^2	I.V.	Weekly	Breast, NSCLC, ovarian, pancreatic
Decitabine	Dacogen	15 mg/m^2	I.V.	Q8H x 3D Q6W	MDS
Purine analogs					
Clofarabine	Clolar	52 mg/m^2	I.V.	Daily for 5 days every 2 to 6 weeks	ALL
Mercaptopurine	Purinethol	1.5 to 2.5 mg/kg	Oral	Daily	ALL
Thioguanine	Tabloid	2 to 3 mg/kg	Oral	Daily	AML
Fludarabine	Fludara	25 mg/m^2	I.V.	Daily for 5 days every 28 days	B-CLL
Guanosine analogs					
Nelarabine	Arranon	1500 mg/m^2	I.V.	Days 1, 3, and 5 every 21 days	T-ALL

ALL, acute lymphocytic leukemia; AML, acute myeloid leukemia; BCC, basal cell carcinoma; B-CLL, B-cell chronic lymphoid leukemia; CML, chronic myeloid leukemia, CRC: colorectal cancer, I.M., intramuscular; I.V., intravenous; IT, intrathecal; MCL, mantle cell lymphoma; MDS, myelodysplastic syndrome; NHL, non-Hodgkin's lymphoma; NSCLC, non–small cell lung cancer; PTCL, primary t-cell lymphoma; SQ, subcutaneous; T-ALL, T-cell acute lymphocytic leukemia.
*Appearance of cancer type in the list indicates U.S. Food and Drug Administration approval for the drug's use in treatment of that cancer type.

Mechanism of action

Antimetabolites are structural analogs of natural metabolites and act by falsely inserting themselves in place of a pyrimidine or purine ring, causing interference in nucleic acid synthesis. Cell cycle phase–specific agents are most active in the S phase and in tumors with a high growth fraction. They are subdivided into 3 groups: folate, purine, and pyrimidine antagonists.

Adverse drug effects

Adverse effects include hand-foot syndrome and stomatitis (painful inflammation and ulceration of the mucous membranes of the mouth) (continuous infusion 5-fluorouracil [5-FU] and capecitabine ⚠, which is an oral 5-FU prodrug); severe diarrhea, GI mucosal damage, nausea, vomiting, fatigue, myelosuppression (manifested by low platelet and neutrophil counts and anemia), alopecia, and neurotoxicity (nelarabine ⚠, cytarabine ⚠, fludarabine ⚠, and methotrexate ⚠); rash, fever, and flu-like symptoms (gemcitabine); renal toxicity (methotrexate) and mucositis (painful inflammation and ulceration of the

 Nelarabine *FDA BOXED WARNING*

Severe neurologic adverse reactions have been reported with the use of nelarabine. These reactions have included altered mental states, including severe somnolence; CNS effects, including convulsions; and peripheral neuropathy, ranging from numbness and paresthesias to motor weakness and paralysis. There have also been reports of adverse reactions associated with demyelination and ascending peripheral neuropathies similar in appearance to Guillain-Barré syndrome. Full recovery from these reactions has not always occurred with cessation of therapy with nelarabine. Monitor frequently for signs and symptoms of neurologic toxicity during treatment with nelarabine. Discontinue nelarabine for neurologic reactions of National Cancer Institute (NCI) Common Toxicity Criteria for Adverse Events (CTCAE) grade 2 or greater.

mucous membranes lining the digestive tract) (5-FU); conjunctivitis (high-dose cytarabine); hemolytic uremic syndrome (gemcitabine); opportunistic infections (cladribine and fludarabine); and tumor lysis syndrome, systemic inflammatory response syndrome, or capillary leak (clofarabine).

Drug–drug interactions

Drugs with specific interactions include the following:

- *Capecitabine:* **Warfarin** and phenytoin
- *Cytarabine:* Digoxin
- *Fluorouracil:* **Warfarin**
- *Mercaptopurine:* **Warfarin** and **allopurinol**
- *Methotrexate:* Nonsteroidal anti-inflammatory drugs (NSAIDs), amiodarone, **amoxicillin**, sulfasala-zine, doxycycline, erythromycin, **hydrochlorothiazide**, mercaptopurine, **omeprazole**, phenytoin, and **folic acid**

Other factors

When high-dose methotrexate (typically 1 to 12 g/m^2) is administered, methotrexate levels are followed daily for several days after the dose. Leucovorin rescue is administered after the end of the high-dose methotrexate infusion and continued until the methotrexate level falls below 0.05 to 0.1 mcmol/L.

Antitumor Antibiotics

See Table 23-3 for summary information about antitumor antibiotics.

Mechanism of action

Anthracyclines block DNA and ribonucleic acid (RNA) transcription through the intercalation (insertion) of adjoining nucleic acid pairs in DNA, which results in DNA strand breakage. They also inhibit the topoisomerase II enzyme. Mitomycin is an alkylating-like agent that cross-links DNA. Dactinomycin blocks RNA synthesis. Bleomycin inhibits DNA synthesis in mitosis and G$_2$ stages of growth. Bleomycin is the only cell cycle–specific antitumor antibiotic.

Adverse drug effects

Adverse effects include severe nausea and vomiting, alopecia, and stomatitis. Anthracyclines may cause acute or chronic cardiac toxicity (doxorubicin ⚠ = daunorubicin ⚠ > idarubicin ⚠ > epirubicin ⚠ > mitoxantrone ⚠). All anthracyclines have limits on cumulative lifetime dosing, are vesicants, and are associated with secondary acute myelogenous leukemia—avoid in patients with a cardiac history. Myelosuppression (manifested by low platelet and neutrophil counts and anemia) exists with all agents, although mitomycin demonstrates a delayed effect. Dactinomycin may cause renal toxicity, leukopenia, and increased pigmentation of previously radiated skin. Bleomycin ⚠ may cause pulmonary fibrosis and interstitial pneumonitis. Mitomycin ⚠ may cause hemolytic uremic syndrome.

Drug–drug interactions

Drugs with specific interactions include the following:

- *Bleomycin:* Phenytoin and digoxin
- *Doxorubicin:* Cisplatin, digoxin, paclitaxel, phenytoin, phenobarbital, trastuzumab, and zidovudine
- *Epirubicin:* Cimetidine and trastuzumab
- *Idarubicin:* Probenecid and trastuzumab

TABLE 23-3. Antitumor Antibiotics

Generic name	Trade name	Dosage range	Dosage form	Frequency	Cancer type*
Anthracyclines					
Doxorubicin	Adriamycin	60 to 75 mg/m²	I.V.	Every 3 weeks	ALL, AML, breast, HL, nephroblastoma, neuroblastoma, NHL, NSCLC, osteosarcoma, ovarian, STS, thyroid
Doxorubicin (liposomal)	Doxil	20 to 50 mg/m²	I.V.	Varies	AIDS-related Kaposi's sarcoma, MM, ovarian
Daunorubicin	Cerubidine	45 mg/m²	I.V.	Daily for 3 days	ALL, AML, NHL
Epirubicin	Ellence	60 to 120 mg/m²	I.V.	Every 3 weeks	Breast
Idarubicin	Idamycin	12 to 13 mg/m²	I.V.	Daily for 3 days	AML
Mitoxantrone	Novantrone	12 to 14 mg/m²	I.V.	Every 3 weeks	AML, prostate
Alkylating-like					
Mitomycin	Mutamycin	10 to 20 mg/m²	I.V. Intravesical	Every 6 to 8 weeks	Gastric, pancreatic, urothelial
Chromomycin					
Dactinomycin	Cosmegen	12 to 15 mcg/kg	I.V.	Daily for 5 days	Ewing's sarcoma, nephroblastoma, rhabdomyosarccma
Miscellaneous					
Bleomycin I.V. SQ	Blenoxane	10 to 20 USP units/m²/wk	I.M.	Weekly	HL, NHL, SCC, testicular

AIDS, acquired immune deficiency syndrome; ALL, acute lymphocytic leukemia; AML, acute myeloid leukemia; HL, Hodgkin's lymphoma; I.M., intramuscular; I.V., intravenous; MM, multiple myeloma; NHL, non-Hodgkin's lymphoma; NSCLC, non–small cell lung cancer; SCC, squamous cell carcinoma; STS, soft tissue sarcoma; SQ, subcutaneous.
*Appearance of cancer type in the list indicates U.S. Food and Drug Administration approval for the drug's use in treatment of that cancer type.

Other factors

Lifetime doses of doxorubicin should not exceed 450 to 550 mg/m², taking into account other anthracycline agents received. The lifetime maximum for epirubicin is 900 mg/m²; for idarubicin, it is 150 mg/m².

Plant Alkaloids

See Table 23-4 for summary information about plant alkaloids.

Mechanism of action

Plant alkaloids inhibit the replication of cancerous cells. Taxanes and vincas interfere with microtubule assembly in the M phase. Camptothecins and epipodophyllotoxins inhibit topoisomerase I and II enzymes, respectively, causing DNA strand breaks. Topoisomerase I and II affect G_2 and S phases, respectively.

Adverse drug effects

Adverse effects include myelosuppression (manifested by low platelet and neutrophil counts and anemia); mucositis; nausea and vomiting; alopecia; edema and hand–foot syndrome (docetaxel ⚠); hypotension or hypersensitivity on administration (paclitaxel ⚠); neurotoxicity (vincristine ⚠ and paclitaxel);

TABLE 23-4. Plant Alkaloids

Generic name	Trade name	Dosage range	Dosage form	Frequency	Cancer type*
Taxanes					
Docetaxel	Taxotere	60 to 100 mg/m²	I.V.	Every 3 weeks	Breast, gastric, NSCLC, prostate, SCC
Paclitaxel	Taxol	135 to 175 mg/m²	I.V.	Every 3 weeks	AIDS-related Kaposi's sarcoma, breast, NSCLC, ovarian
Paclitaxel (protein-bound)	Abraxane	260 mg/m²	I.V.	Every 3 weeks	Breast, NSCLC, pancreatic
Cabazitaxel	Jevtana	25 mg/m²	I.V.	Every 3 weeks	Prostate
Halichondrin B analog					
Eribulin	Halaven	1.4 mg/m²	I.V.	Days 1 and 8 every 21 days	Liposarcoma, breast
Epothilones					
Ixabepilone	Ixempra	40 mg/m²	I.V.	Every 3 weeks	Breast
Epipodophyllotoxins					
Etoposide	Toposar	50 to 100 mg/m²	I.V.	Varies	SCLC, testicular
		100 to 200 mg/m²	Oral		
Camptothecins					
Irinotecan	Camptosar	100 to 125 mg/m²	I.V.	Weekly	CRC
Topotecan	Hycamtin	1.5 mg/m²	I.V.	Daily for 5 days every 21 days	Cervical, ovarian, SCLC
Vinca alkaloids					
Vincristine	Oncovin	1.4 mg/m²	I.V.	Weekly	ALL, HL, MCL, nephroblastoma, neuroblastoma, NHL, rhabdomyosarcoma
Vinblastine	Velban	6 mg/m²	I.V.	Every 2 to 3 weeks	Breast, HL, Kaposi's sarcoma, NHL, SLL, testicular
Vinorelbine	Navelbine	25 to 30 mg/m²	I.V.	Weekly	NSCLC

AIDS, acquired immune deficiency syndrome; ALL, acute lymphocytic leukemia; CRC, colorectal cancer; HL, Hodgkin's lymphoma; I.V., intravenous; MCL, mantle cell lymphoma; NHL, non-Hodgkin's lymphoma; NSCLC, non–small cell lung cancer; SCC, squamous cell carcinoma; SCLC, small cell lung cancer; SLL, small lymphocytic lymphoma.

*Appearance of cancer type in the list indicates U.S. Food and Drug Administration approval for the drug's use in treatment of that cancer type.

peripheral neuropathy and myalgia or arthralgia (vincristine and paclitaxel); diarrhea, headache, and secondary malignancies (topoisomerase II inhibitors); and SIADH (vinca alkaloids).

Drug–drug interactions

Drugs with specific interactions include the following:

- *Docetaxel:* CYP3A4 inducers and inhibitors
- *Etoposide* ⚠: Cyclosporine, St. John's wort, and **warfarin**
- *Irinotecan* ⚠: St. John's wort
- *Paclitaxel:* CYP3A4 inducers and inhibitors
- *Vinblastine* ⚠: Phenytoin, erythromycin, mitomycin, and zidovudine

- *Vinca alkaloids:* CYP3A4 inhibitors, itraconazole, and voriconazole
- *Vincristine:* Phenytoin, l-asparaginase, carbamazepine, digoxin, filgrastim, nifedipine, and zidovudine

Platinum Analogs

See Table 23-5 for summary information about platinum analogs.

Mechanism of action

Platinum analogs have the ability to cross-link with the purine bases on DNA, interfering with DNA repair mechanisms, causing DNA damage, and subsequently inducing apoptosis in cancer cells. These agents are cell cycle phase–nonspecific.

Adverse drug effects

Adverse effects include myelosuppression (manifested by low platelet and neutrophil counts and anemia), acute kidney failure (cisplatin ⚠), neurotoxicity, laryngospasm (oxaliplatin ⚠), ototoxicity, hypersensitivity reactions (especially after about 10 doses), electrolyte abnormalities (cisplatin), hepatotoxicity (oxaliplatin), severe nausea and vomiting (cisplatin), and moderate nausea and vomiting (carboplatin ⚠, oxaliplatin).

Drug–drug interactions

Drugs with specific interactions include the following:

- *Cisplatin:* Amiodarone and clozapine
- *Carboplatin:* Clozapine and leflunomide
- *Oxaliplatin:* Amiodarone, dolasetron, sotalol, and clozapine

Other factors

Carboplatin is the only traditional chemotherapy drug that is pharmacokinetically dosed. It is dosed in units of area under the curve (AUC) using what is commonly known as the Calvert formula. The typical dose is AUC 2 every 7 days or AUC 5/6 every 21 to 28 days. The dose in milligrams is calculated by multiplying the AUC dose by the sum of a constant of 25 plus the patient's glomerular filtration rate (determined by nuclear medicine methods or approximated by 24-hour creatinine clearance or the Cockcroft–Gault formula).

Cisplatin administration must be accompanied by vigorous hydration with saline-based intravenous (I.V.) fluids to avoid nephrotoxicity.

TABLE 23-5. Platinum Analogs

Generic name	Trade name	Dosage range	Dosage form	Frequency	Cancer type*
Cisplatin	Platinol-AQ	50 to 100 mg/m²	I.V.	Every 3 to 4 weeks	Bladder, testicular, ovarian
Carboplatin	Paraplatin	300 to 400 mg/m² AUC 6	I.V.	Every 3 to 4 weeks	Ovarian
Oxaliplatin	Eloxatin	85 to 130 mg/m²	I.V.	Every 2 weeks	CRC

CRC, colorectal cancer; I.V., intravenous.
*Appearance of cancer type in the list indicates U.S. Food and Drug Administration approval for the drug's use in treatment of that cancer type.

Hormones and Antagonists

See Table 23-6 for summary information about hormones and antagonists.

Mechanism of action

This diverse group of compounds acts on hormone-dependent tumors by inhibiting or decreasing the production of the disease-causing hormone.

TABLE 23-6. Hormones and Antagonists

Generic name	Trade name	Dosage range	Dosage form	Frequency	Cancer type*
Progestins					
Megestrol acetate	Megace	40 to 320 mg	Oral	Varies	Breast, endometrial
Medroxyprogesterone	Depo-Provera	400 to 1000 mg	I.M.	Weekly	Endometrial, RCC
Antiestrogens					
Tamoxifen	Nolvadex	20 to 40 mg	Oral	Daily	Breast
Fulvestrant	Faslodex	500 mg	I.M.	Every 2 weeks for 4 weeks, then monthly	Breast
Toremifene	Fareston	60 mg	Oral	Daily	Breast
Third-generation aromatase inhibitors					
Exemestane	Aromasin	25 mg	Oral	Daily	Breast
Anastrozole	Arimidex	1 mg	Oral	Daily	Breast
Letrozole	Femara	2.5 mg	Oral	Daily	Breast
Androgens					
Fluoxymesterone	Halotestin	10 to 40 mg	Oral	Daily	Breast
Antiandrogens					
Flutamide	Eulexin	250 mg	Oral	Every 8 hours	Prostate
Bicalutamide	Casodex	50 mg	Oral	Daily	Prostate
Nilutamide	Nilandron	150 to 300 mg	Oral	Daily	Prostate
Abiraterone acetate	Zytiga	1000 mg	Oral	Daily	Prostate
Apalutamide	Erleada	240 mg	Oral	Daily	Prostate
Enzalutamide	Xtandi	160 mg	Oral	Daily	Prostate
LHRH agonists					
Triptorelin	Trelstar	3.75 to 22.5 mg	I.M.	Varies	Prostate
Leuprolide	Lupron	7.5 to 45 mg	I.M.	Varies	Prostate
	Eligard	7.5 to 45 mg	SQ	Varies	
	Viadur	65 mg	SQ	Yearly	
Goserelin	Zoladex	3.6 to 10.8 mg	SQ	Varies	Breast, prostate
GNRH antagonist					
Degarelix	Firmagon	80 to 240 mg	SQ	Every 28 days	Prostate

GNRH, gonadotropin-releasing hormone; I.M., intramuscular; LHRH, luteinizing hormone–releasing hormone; RCC, renal cell carcinoma; SQ, subcutaneous.
*Appearance of cancer type in the list indicates U.S. Food and Drug Administration approval for the drug's use in treatment of that cancer type.

Adverse drug effects

Adverse effects include edema, menstrual disorders, hot flashes, transient muscle or bone pain, tumor flare, and transient increase in serum testosterone (luteinizing hormone–releasing hormone [LHRH] agonists); thromboembolic events, gynecomastia, elevated liver enzymes, nausea and vomiting, diarrhea, erectile impotence, decreased libido, endometrial cancers with tamoxifen, and bone loss (LHRH agonists, aromatase inhibitors); seizures (enzalutamide); and risk of ventricular arrhythmias and QT prolongation.

Drug–drug interactions

Drugs with specific interactions include the following:

- *Anastrozole:* Estrogens and antiestrogens
- *Bicalutamide:* **Warfarin**
- *Degarelix:* Amiodarone, procainamide, quinidine, and sotalol
- *Apalutamide:* Strong CYP2C8 or CYP3A4 inhibitors and CYP314, CYP2C9, CYP2C19, or UGT substrates
- *Enzalutamide:* Strong CYP2C6 inhibitors and strong or moderate CYP3A4/2C8 inducers
- *Exemestane:* CYP3A4 inducers (such as carbamazepine and phenytoin), estrogens, and antiestrogens
- *Fluoxymesterone:* Cyclosporine, anticoagulants, and valerian
- *Flutamide* : **Warfarin**
- *Letrozole:* Estrogens and antiestrogens
- *Medroxyprogesterone acetate* : Aminoglutethimide and rifampin
- *Megestrol:* Dofetilide contraindication
- *Nilutamide* : Alcohol
- *Tamoxifen* : Anticoagulants and cyclophosphamide
- *Toremifene* : CYP3A4 inducers (such as carbamazepine and phenytoin)

Monitoring parameters

Note any weight changes, abnormal vaginal bleeding, body or bone pain, galactorrhea, or decreased libido. Monitor for embolic disorders and uterine cancer in females. Check prostate-specific antigen

---

 Medroxyprogesterone acetate *FDA BOXED WARNING*

Estrogen plus Progestin Therapy: Do not use for the prevention of cardiovascular disease or dementia. Increased risk of DVT, PE, and MI in postmenopausal women. Increased risk of invasive breast cancer. Should be used at lowest dose possible for the least amount of time that is necessary.

 Toremifene *FDA BOXED WARNING*

Toremifene has been shown to prolong the QTc interval in a dose- and concentration-related manner. Prolongation of the QT interval can result in a type of ventricular tachycardia called torsades de pointes, which may result in syncope, seizure, and/or death. Toremifene should not be prescribed to patients with congenital/acquired QT prolongation, uncorrected hypokalemia, or uncorrected hypomagnesemia. Avoid drugs known to prolong the QT interval and strong CYP3A4 inhibitors.

(PSA) and testosterone levels in males. Monitor bone mineral density for LHRH agonists and aromatase inhibitors.

Pharmacokinetics

The majority of agents are available orally with longer half-lives, allowing for once-daily dosing.

Patient instructions and counseling

- Avoid use in pregnant women; several agents may cause weight gain and menstrual irregularities in women.
- Be aware of leg swelling or tenderness (e.g., signs of a deep-vein thrombosis), breathing problems, and sweating.
- Transient muscle or bone pain, problems urinating, and spinal cord compression may occur initially in patients receiving LHRH agonists.

Biologic Response Modifiers and Monoclonal Antibodies

See Table 23-7 for summary information about biologic response modifiers and monoclonal antibodies.

Mechanism of action

Biologic response modifiers activate the body's immune-mediated host defense mechanisms to malignant cells. In contrast to immunotherapy, these agents have direct biological effects on malignancies. Monoclonal antibodies bind to specific antigens and kill malignant cells through the activation of apoptosis, antibody-mediated toxicity, or complement-mediated lysis.

Adverse drug effects

Adverse effects include hypotension and hypersensitivity during infusion; cardiac, pulmonary, and renal impairment; mental status changes (e.g., depression), fever, chills, nausea, and musculoskeletal pain. Other events include tumor lysis syndrome (rituximab ⚠); bleeding, hemorrhage, hypertension, proteinuria, and skin rash (bevacizumab); cutaneous and severe infusion reactions and interstitial lung disease (cetuximab ⚠); neurotoxicity (thalidomide ⚠); and neutropenia, deep-vein thrombosis, and pulmonary embolism (lenalidomide ⚠, pomalidomide ⚠, and thalidomide).

Drug–drug interactions

Drugs with specific interactions include the following:

- *Aldesleukin* ⚠: Glucocorticoids, NSAIDs, and antihypertensives
- *Brentuximab vedotin* ⚠: CYP3A4 inhibitors and inducers
- *Ibritumomab tiuxetan* ⚠: Antiplatelet and anticoagulant agents
- *Interferon alfa-2 b* ⚠: Zidovudine, theophylline, phenytoin, and phenobarbital
- *Trastuzumab* ⚠: Anthracyclines, cyclophosphamide, and **warfarin**

Monitoring parameters

Monitor baseline and follow-up pulmonary, cardiac, and renal function tests. Check complete blood counts with differential, liver function tests, thyroid-stimulating hormone, electrolytes, and glucose regularly. Premedicate with **acetaminophen** and diphenhydramine for monoclonal antibodies, especially chimeric monoclonal antibodies. Observe blood pressure during infusion (hypotension concerns) for all agents.

TABLE 23-7. Biologic Response Modifiers and Monoclonal Antibodies

Generic name	Trade name	Dosage range	Dosage form	Frequency	Cancer type*
Immune therapies					
Aldesleukin	Proleukin	600,000 units/kg	I.V.	Every 8 hours	Melanoma, RCC
Peginterferon alfa-2b	PEG-Intron	1.5 mcg/kg	SQ	Weekly	Melanoma
Sipuleucel-T	Provenge	Varies	I.V.	Every 2 weeks for 3 doses	Prostate
Thalidomide	Thalomid	200 mg	Oral	Daily	MM
Lenalidomide	Revlimid	10 to 25 mg	Oral	Varies	FL, MCL, MDS, MZL, MM
Monoclonal antibodies					
Rituximab	Rituxan	375 mg/m²	I.V.	Varies	CLL, NHL
Trastuzumab	Herceptin	2 to 6 mg/kg	I.V. SubQ	Weekly	Breast, gastric
Ado-trastuzumab emtansine	Kadcyla	3.6 mg/kg	I.V.	Every 3 weeks	Breast
Pertuzumab	Perjeta	420 to 840 mg	I.V.	Varies	Breast
Bevacizumab	Avastin	5 to 15 mg/kg	I.V.	Every 3 weeks	Cervical, CRC, glioblastoma, NSCLC, ovarian, RCC
Cetuximab	Erbitux	250 to 500 mg/m²	I.V.	Every 1 to 2 weeks	CRC, SCC
Ofatumumab	Arzerra	300 to 2000 mg	I.V.	Varies	CLL
Ipilimumab	Yervoy	1 to 3 mg/kg	I.V.	Varies	CRC, HCC, melanoma, NSCLC, RCC
Panitumumab	Vectibix	6 mg/kg	I.V.	Every 1 to 2 weeks	CRC
Ibritumomab tiuxetan	Zevalinᶜ	0.3 to 0.4 mCi/kg	I.V.	Once	NHL
Brentuximab vedotin	Adcetris	1.8 mg/kg	I.V.	Every 3 weeks	HL, PTCL
Nivolumab	Opdivo	1 to 3 mg/kg 240 to 480 mg	I.V.	Varies	CRC, HCC, HL, melanoma, NSCLC, RCC, SCC, SCLC, urothelial
Pembrolizumab	Keytruda	200 to 400 mg	I.V.	Varies	Cervical, CRC, endometrial, gastric, HCC, head and neck, HL, melanoma, NSCLC, RCC, SCLC, urinary, urothelial
Atezolizumab	Tecentriq	840 to 1680 mg	I.V.	Varies	Breast, NSCLC, urothelial, SCLC
Avelumab	Bavencio	800 mg	I.V.	Every 2 weeks	RCC, urothelial
Durvalumab	Imfinzi	10 to 20 mg/kg 1500 mg	I.V.	Varies	NSCLC, SCLC, urothelial
Ramucirumab	Cyramza	8 to 10 mg/kg	I.V.	Varies	CRC, gastric, HCC, NSCLC
Olaratumab	Lartruvo	15 mg/kg	I.V.	Days 1 and 8 every 3 weeks	STS

CLL, chronic lymphocytic leukemia; CRC, colorectal cancer; FL, follicular lymphoma; HCC, hepatocellular carcinoma; HL, Hodgkin's lymphoma; I.V., intravenous; MDS, myelodysplastic syndrome; MM, multiple myeloma; MZL, marginal zone lymphoma; NHL, non-Hodgkin's lymphoma; NSCLC, non–small cell lung cancer; PTCL, primary t-cell lymphoma; RCC, renal cell carcinoma; SCC, squamous cell carcinoma; SCLC, small cell lung cancer; SQ, subcutaneous; STS, soft tissue sarcoma.

*Appearance of cancer type in the list indicates U.S. Food and Drug Administration approval for the drug's use in treatment of that cancer type.

Aldesleukin *FDA BOXED WARNING*

Risk of capillary leak syndrome (CLS); disseminated infection, including sepsis and bacterial endocarditis; and coma.

 Ibritumomab tiuxetan *FDA BOXED WARNING*

Serious infusion reactions, prolonged and severe cytopenias, and severe cutaneous and mucocutaneous reactions have been reported.

 Interferon alfa-2 b *FDA BOXED WARNING*

Alpha interferons, including interferon alfa-2b, cause or aggravate fatal or life-threatening neuropsychiatric, autoimmune, ischemic, and infectious disorders. Patients should be monitored closely with periodic clinical and laboratory evaluations. Patients with persistently severe or worsening signs or symptoms of these conditions should be withdrawn from therapy. In many but not all cases, these disorders resolve after stopping interferon alfa-2b therapy.

Perform blood pressure monitoring (hypertensive concerns) and urine dipstick analysis (bevacizumab). Monitor for vital signs, itching, and swelling. Check for trouble breathing (cetuximab, ibritumomab, and daratumumab).

Patient instructions and counseling
- Inform a health care provider if severe fatigue, trouble breathing, or irregular heart rhythms occur.
- Chills, fever, depression, and flu-like symptoms are common.
- Monoclonal antibodies can cause infusion-related reactions such as fever and chills.
- If receiving bevacizumab, have blood pressure checked regularly and have tests that check for protein in the urine.
- Wear sunscreen and avoid excessive sunlight if receiving cetuximab.
- For both men and women, do not try to conceive until 12 months after finishing therapy.
- Do not get pregnant while using lenalidomide, pomalidomide, or thalidomide. For those on 1 of these drugs, 2 forms of birth control must be used by both women of childbearing age and men who have sexual contact with women of childbearing age.

Tyrosine Kinase Inhibitors

See Table 23-8 for summary information about tyrosine kinase inhibitors (TKIs).

Mechanism of action

Tyrosine kinases are enzymes responsible for the activation of a wide variety of proteins by signal transduction cascades. TKIs inhibit phosphorylation, a process in which a protein is activated by the addition of a phosphate group. There has been an explosion in the number of TKIs approved by U.S. Food and

TABLE 23-8. Tyrosine Kinase Inhibitors

Generic name	Trade name	Dosage range	Dosage form	Frequency	Cancer type*
Imatinib	Gleevec	400 to 600 mg	Oral	Daily	ALL, CML, GIST, MDS
Erlotinib	Tarceva	100 to 150 mg	Oral	Daily	NSCLC, pancreatic
Gefitinib	Iressa	250 mg	Oral	Daily	NSCLC
Afatinib	Giotrif	40 mg	Oral	Daily	NSCLC
Sunitinib	Sutent	50 mg	Oral	Daily for 28 days, then 2 weeks off	GIST, RCC
Dasatinib	Sprycel	100 to 180 mg	Oral	Daily	ALL, CML
Sorafenib	Nexavar	400 mg	Oral	Twice daily	HCC, RCC, thyroid
Lapatinib	Tykerb	1250 mg	Oral	Daily for 21 days	Breast
Nilotinib	Tasigna	300 to 400 mg	Oral	Twice daily	CML
Pazopanib	Votrient	800 mg	Oral	Daily	RCC, STS
Dabrafenib	Tafinlar	150 mg	Oral	Twice daily	Melanoma, NSCLC, thyroid
Vemurafenib	Zelboraf	960 mg	Oral	Twice daily	Melanoma
Crizotinib	Xalkori	250 mg	Oral	Twice daily	NSCLC
Axitinib	Inlyta	5 to 7 mg	Oral	Twice daily	RCC
Bosutinib	Bosulif	400 to 600 mg	Oral	Daily	CML
Cabozantinib	Cabometyx Cometriq	60 mg (tab) 140 mg (cap)	Oral	Daily	HCC, RCC, thyroid
Ponatinib	Iclusig	45 mg	Oral	Daily	ALL, CML
Regorafenib	Stivarga	160 mg	Oral	Daily for 21 days every 28 days	CRC, GIST, HCC
Ceritinib	Zykadia	450 mg	Oral	Daily	NSCLC
Alectinib	Alecensa	600 mg	Oral	Twice daily	NSCLC
Brigatinib	Alunbrig	90 to 180 mg	Oral	Daily	NSCLC
Lorlatinib	Lorbrena	100 mg	Oral	Daily	NSCLC
Ibrutinib	Imbruvica	420 to 560 mg	Oral	Daily	CLL, MCL, MZL, SLL
Acalabrutinib	Calquence	100 mg	Oral	Twice daily	CLL, MCL, SLL
Zanubrutinib	Brukinsa	160 mg 320 mg	Oral	Twice daily Daily	MCL
Avapritinib	Ayvakit	300 mg	Oral	Daily	GIST
Ripretinib	Qinlock	150 mg	Oral	Daily	GIST
Erdafitinib	Balversa	8 to 9 mg	Oral	Daily	Urothelial
Trametinib	Mekinist	2 mg	Oral	Daily	Melanoma, NSCLC, thyroid
Capmatinib	Tabrecta	400 mg	Oral	Twice daily	NSCLC
Osimertinib	Tagrisso	80 mg	Oral	Daily	NSCLC

ALL, acute lymphocytic leukemia; CLL, chronic lymphocytic leukemia; CML, chronic myelogenous leukemia; CRC, colorectal cancer; GIST, gastrointestinal stromal tumor; HCC, hepatocellular carcinoma; MCL, mantle cell lymphoma; MDS, myelodysplastic syndrome; MZL, marginal zone lymphoma; NHL, non-Hodgkin's lymphoma; NSCLC, non–small cell lung cancer; RCC, renal cell carcinoma; SLL, small lymphocytic lymphoma; STS, soft tissue sarcoma.
*Appearance of cancer type in the list indicates U.S. Food and Drug Administration approval for the drug's use in treatment of that cancer type.

Drug Administration (FDA) in the past 20 years. Some of the more notable and frequently encountered TKIs are described below:

Bosutinib

Bosutinib inhibits the BCR-ABL kinase that promotes chronic myelogenous leukemia (CML). Adverse effects include diarrhea, nausea, thrombocytopenia, vomiting, abdominal pain, rash, anemia, pyrexia, and fatigue. Avoid moderate or strong CYP3A4/5 inhibitors or inducers (increased or decreased bosutinib levels), P-glycoprotein inhibitors (increased bosutinib levels), and proton pump inhibitors (decreased bosutinib levels).

Crizotinib

Crizotinib is an anaplastic lymphoma kinase 4 (ALK4) TKI used to treat ALK4-positive non–small cell lung cancer (NSCLC), a type of lung cancer most often encountered in nonsmokers. Adverse effects include diarrhea, nausea, transaminitis, vomiting, abdominal pain, fatigue, decreased appetite, and constipation. Administration of crizotinib with CYP3A substrates with narrow therapeutic indices should be avoided.

Dasatinib

Dasatinib specifically targets BCR-ABL mutations (including those resistant to imatinib), thereby inhibiting leukemic cell growth. It is used for treatment of Philadelphia-chromosome-positive (Ph+) CML and Ph+ acute lymphocytic leukemia (ALL). It causes rash, neutropenia, thrombocytopenia, edema, diarrhea, nausea and vomiting, weight changes, arthralgia, myalgia, cough, shortness of breath, infection, electrolyte changes, and arrhythmias. Significant drug interactions occur with CYP3A4 inhibitors; avoid concurrent use, or reduce dose. Avoid acid reduction therapies (e.g., proton pump inhibitors and histamine H2-receptor antagonists) because they will reduce absorption. Avoid medications that prolong QT interval.

Erlotinib

Erlotinib is an HER1 and epidermal growth factor receptor (EGFR) TKI used in the treatment of NSCLC with EGFR mutations, a type of lung cancer that typically occurs in nonsmokers. For oral therapy, take 1 hour before or 2 hours after meals. Erlotinib causes rash, diarrhea, anorexia, stomatitis, and interstitial lung disease. Drug interactions occur with CYP3A4 inducers and inhibitors. Monitor hepatic function.

Gefitinib

Gefitinib is an EGFR TKI and a third-line agent for NSCLC. It causes diarrhea, rash, acne, and dry skin. Drug interactions occur with CYP3A4 inducers and inhibitors and with **warfarin**.

Imatinib

Imatinib is a selective inhibitor of the Philadelphia chromosome (biomarker in CML). It causes hepatotoxicity, fluid retention (pleural effusions, weight gain), neutropenia, GI effects, muscle cramps, nausea, and vomiting. Drug interactions occur with CYP3A4 substrates (cyclosporine, **simvastatin**, erythromycin, itraconazole) and CYP2C9 substrates (**warfarin**).

Lapatinib ⚠

Lapatinib inhibits multiple tyrosine kinases and is used in combination with capecitabine to treat human epidermal growth factor receptor–2 (HER2) positive breast cancer. Common adverse effects include fatigue, diarrhea, nausea, vomiting, myelosuppression, increased liver enzymes, and palmar-plantar erythrodysesthesia. Significant drug interactions occur with strong CYP3A4 inhibitors and inducers; avoid concurrent use, or reduce dose. These agents should be taken by mouth, on an empty stomach, 1 hour before or 2 hours after a meal.

Nilotinib ⚠

Nilotinib selectively inhibits BCR-ABL kinase and is used for the treatment of Ph+ CML. Adverse effects include headache, fatigue, rash, pruritus, constipation, nausea, vomiting, and diarrhea. Significant drug interactions occur with strong CYP3A4 inhibitors and inducers; avoid concurrent use, or reduce dose. Capsules should be taken by mouth, on an empty stomach, and swallowed whole; do not crush or open.

Ponatinib ⚠

Ponatinib is a TKI that inhibits the BCR-ABL kinase that promotes CML. Adverse effects include hypertension, neutropenia, leucopenia, thrombocytopenia, increased aspartate aminotransferase (AST), increased alanine aminotransferase (ALT), hemorrhage, peripheral edema, cardiac failure, arterial ischemic events, pancreatitis, and venous thromboembolism. Avoid strong CYP3A and CYP3A4/5 inhibitors, or reduce ponatinib dose.

Sorafenib

Sorafenib inhibits multiple tyrosine kinases and is used for treatment of advanced renal cell carcinoma (RCC). Take tablets on an empty stomach. Sorafenib causes diarrhea, fatigue, rash, hand-foot syndrome, hypertension, nausea and vomiting, neutropenia, and alopecia. It can decrease doxorubicin and irinotecan levels.

Sunitinib ⚠

Sunitinib inhibits multiple tyrosine kinases and is used for treatment of advanced RCC and gastrointestinal stromal tumors (GIST). Take it with or without food. It causes neutropenia, rash, changes in skin color, fatigue, myalgia, headaches, hypertension, nausea and vomiting, diarrhea, and increased liver enzymes. It is extensively metabolized by CYP3A4; CYP3A4 inhibitors may increase levels, and CYP3A4 inducers may decrease levels. Ketoconazole increases levels, and rifampin reduces levels.

Miscellaneous Agents

See Table 23-9 for summary information about miscellaneous agents.

Asparaginase

Asparaginase removes exogenous asparagine from leukemic cells that are required for the cells' survival. Intradermal skin testing is needed because of severe anaphylactic reactions. Adverse effects include myelosuppression, hyperuricemia, hyperglycemia, and renal problems. Drug interactions occur with methotrexate, prednisolone, **prednisone**, and vincristine.

Bortezomib

Bortezomib inhibits the 26S proteasome and stabilizes regulatory proteins, causing apoptosis and disrupting cell proliferation. Adverse effects include nausea, vomiting, thrombocytopenia, neuropathy, hypotension, and diarrhea.

TABLE 23-9. Miscellaneous Agents

Generic name	Trade name	Dosage range	Dosage form	Frequency	Cancer type*
Enzymes					
Asparaginase	Elspar	6000 IU/m^2	I.M., I.V.	3 times a week	ALL
	Erwinaze	25,000 IU/m^2	I.M., I.V.	3 times a week	
Pegaspargase	Oncaspar	2500 IU/m^2	I.M., I.V.	Every 14 days	ALL
Cell-specific					
Hydroxyurea	Hydrea	20 to 30 mg/kg	Oral	Daily	CML, SCC
Histone deacetylase inhibitor					
Romidepsin	Istodax	14 mg/m^2	I.V.	Days 1, 8, and 15 every 28 days	PTCL
Belinostat	Beleodaq	1000 mg/m^2	I.V.	Days 1 and 5 every 21 days	PTCL
Panobinostat	Farydak	20 mg	Oral	3 times a week for 2 weeks every 21 days	MM
Vorinostat	Zolinza	400 mg	Oral	Daily	CTCL
mTOR inhibitors					
Temsirolimus	Torisel	25 mg	I.V.	Weekly	RCC
Everolimus	Afinitor	10 mg	Oral	Daily	Breast, RCC
Hedgehog pathway inhibitor					
Vismodegib	Erivedge	150 mg	Oral	Daily	BCC
Multiple angiogenic factor trap					
Ziv-aflibercept	Zaltrap	4 mg/kg	I.V.	Every 2 weeks	CRC
26S Proteasome inhibitor					
Bortezomib	Velcade	1.3 mg/m^2	I.V. SQ	Varies	MCL, MM
20S Proteasome inhibitor					
Carfilzomib	Kyprolis	20 to 27 mg/m^2	I.V.	Varies	MM
PARP inhibitor					
Olaparib	Lynparza	300 mg (tab) 400 mg (cap)	Oral	Twice daily	Breast, ovarian, pancreatic, prostate
CDK4/6 inhibitor					
Abemaciclib	Verzenio	150 to 200 mg	Oral	Twice daily	Breast
Palbociclib	Ibrance	125 mg	Oral	Daily for 21 days every 28 days	Breast
Ribociclib	Kisqali	600 mg	Oral	Daily for 21 days every 28 days	Breast
Phosphatidylinositol-3-kinase (PI3K) inhibitor					
Alpelisib	Piqray	300 mg	Oral	Daily	Breast
Copanlisib	Aliqopa	60 mg	I.V.	Days 1, 8, and 15 every 28 days	FL
Duvelisib	Copiktra	25 mg	Oral	Twice daily	CLL, FL, SLL
Idelalisib	Zydelig	150 mg	Oral	Twice daily	CLL, NHL, SLL

ALL, acute lymphocytic leukemia; BCC, basal cell carcinoma; CDK, cyclin-dependent kinase; CLL, chronic lymphoid leukemia; CML, chronic myelogenous leukemia; CRC, colorectal cancer; CTC, cutaneous t-cell lymphoma; ER, estrogen receptor; FL: follicular lymphoma; IM: intramuscular; IV: intravenous; MCL: mantle cell lymphoma; MM: multiple myeloma; mTOR: mammalian target of rapamycin; NHL: non-Hodgkin's lymphoma PARP: poly ADP ribose polymerase; PO: by mouth; PTCL, primary T-cell lymphoma; RCC, renal cell carcinoma; SCC, squamous cell carcinoma; SLL, small lymphocytic lymphoma; SQ, subcutaneous.
*Appearance of cancer type in the list indicates U.S. Food and Drug Administration approval for the drug's use in treatment of that cancer type.

Carfilzomib

Carfilzomib irreversibly binds to the N-terminal threonine-containing active sites of 20S proteasome. Adverse effects include fatigue, anemia, nausea, thrombocytopenia, dyspnea, diarrhea, and pyrexia.

Hydroxyurea

Hydroxyurea inhibits DNA synthesis without interfering with RNA and protein synthesis. Adverse effects include myelosuppression (leukopenia), development of secondary leukemias, nausea, vomiting, diarrhea, constipation, mucositis, and rare but fatal hepatotoxicity and pancreatitis. Drug interactions occur with didanosine and stavudine.

Everolimus

Everolimus inhibit the mammalian target of rapamycin (mTOR) and are used for the treatment of RCC. Adverse effects include myelosuppression, anorexia, rash, mucositis, edema, hyperglycemia, dyslipidemia, and nausea. Drug interactions occur with angiotensin-converting enzyme inhibitors and strong CYP3A4 inhibitors and inducers.

Glasdegib ⚠, sonidegib ⚠, and vismodegib ⚠

Glasdegib, sonidegib, and vismodegib are selective hedgehog pathway inhibitors and are used to treat acute myeloid leukemia (glasdegib) and basal cell carcinoma [BCC] (sonidegib and vismodegib). Adverse effects include muscle spasms, alopecia, dysgeusia, decreased appetite and weight, fatigue, diarrhea, nausea and vomiting, constipation, arthralgias, and ageusia. P-glycoprotein inhibitors may increase glasdegib, sonidegib, and vismodegib concentrations. Proton pump inhibitors, histamine-2 (H2) antagonists, and antacids may reduce drug bioavailability by increasing gastric pH. Glasdegib,

> ### ⚠ Glasdegib *FDA BOXED WARNING*
>
> Glasdegib can cause embryo-fetal death or severe birth defects when administered to a pregnant woman. Glasdegib is embryotoxic, fetotoxic, and teratogenic in animals. Conduct pregnancy testing in females of reproductive potential prior to initiation of glasdegib treatment. Advise females of reproductive potential to use effective contraception during treatment with glasdegib and for at least 30 days after the last dose. Advise males of the potential risk of glasdegib exposure through semen and to use condoms with a pregnant partner or a female partner of reproductive potential during treatment with glasdegib and for at least 30 days after the last dose to avoid potential drug exposure.

> ### ⚠ Sonidegib *FDA BOXED WARNING*
>
> Sonidegib can cause embryo-fetal death or severe birth defects when administered to a pregnant woman. Sonidegib is embryotoxic, fetotoxic, and teratogenic in animals. Verify the pregnancy status of females of reproductive potential prior to initiating therapy. Advise females of reproductive potential to use effective contraception during treatment with sonidegib and for at least 20 months after the last dose. Advise males of the potential risk of exposure through semen and to use condoms with a pregnant partner or a female partner of reproductive potential during treatment with sonidegib and for at least 8 months after the last dose.

Vismodegib *FDA BOXED WARNING*

Vismodegib can cause embryofetal death or severe birth defects when administered to a pregnant woman. Vismodegib is embryotoxic, fetotoxic, and teratogenic in animals. Teratogenic effects included severe midline defects, missing digits, and other irreversible malformations. Verify pregnancy status of females of reproductive potential within 7 days prior to initiating vismodegib. Advise pregnant women of the potential risks to a fetus. Advise females of reproductive potential to use effective contraception during and after vismodegib. Advise males of the potential risk of vismodegib exposure through semen and to use condoms with a pregnant partner or a female partner of reproductive potential.

sonidegib, and vismodegib inhibit CYP2C8, CYP2C9, CYP2C19, and transporter breast cancer resistance protein in vitro.

Ziv-aflibercept

Ziv-aflibercept acts as a soluble receptor that binds to human (vascular endothelial growth factor-A [VEGF-A], vascular endothelial growth factor-B [VEGF-B], and placental growth factor [PlGF]). Adverse effects include diarrhea, neutropenia, proteinuria, thrombocytopenia, decreased weight and appetite, stomatitis, fatigue, hypertension, epistaxis, dysphonia, and increased serum creatinine.

Chemotherapy-Induced Nausea and Vomiting

The prevention and treatment of chemotherapy-induced nausea and vomiting (CINV) constitutes an important area in which pharmacists may play a role in drug selection for oncology patients. The selection of antiemetic agents should be based on the emetogenic potential of the drug regimen, prior experience with antiemetics, and patient factors. Patient risk factors that increase the risk of CINV include younger age, female sex, previous CINV history, little or no history of alcohol use, susceptibility to motion sickness, history of morning sickness during pregnancy, and anxiety. The risk for acute (≤24 hours) and delayed (>24 hours) CINV may last up to at least 3 days following the last dose of chemotherapy depending upon emetic risk of the drug regimen. All patients receiving chemotherapy agents with emetogenic potential should receive prophylactic therapy, with rescue medication readily available. Table 23-10 provides information about antiemetic drugs used for the prevention and treatment of CINV.

Antiemetic treatment for parenteral highly emetogenic chemotherapy

A 4-drug regimen is preferred for parenteral highly emetogenic chemotherapy. The 4-drug regimen should consist of a neurokinin-1 receptor antagonist (NK1 RA), a serotonin receptor antagonist (5-HT3 RA), dexamethasone, and olanzapine. A 3-drug regimen may be utilized, if desired. The 3-drug regimen should consist of (1) olanzapine, palonosetron, and dexamethasone or (2) a NK1 RA, a 5-HT3 RA, and dexamethasone.

Antiemetic treatment for parenteral moderately emetogenic chemotherapy

A 2-drug or 3-drug regimen is preferred for parenteral moderately emetogenic chemotherapy. The 3-drug regimen should consist of (1) olanzapine, palonosetron, and dexamethasone or (2) a NK1 RA, a 5-HT3 RA, and dexamethasone. The 2-drug regimen should consist of a 5-HT3 RA and dexamethasone.

Antiemetic treatment for parenteral low emetogenic chemotherapy

A single-drug regimen is preferred for parenteral low emetogenic chemotherapy. The single-drug regimen should consist of dexamethasone, prochlorperazine, metoclopramide, or an orally administered 5-HT3 RA.

TABLE 23-10. Pharmacologic Management for the Prevention of Acute Chemotherapy-Induced Nausea and Vomiting

Generic name	Trade name	Dose*	Dosage form	Frequency	Adverse effects
5-HT₃ receptor antagonists					
Dolasetron	Anzemet	100 mg	Oral	1 hour before chemotherapy	Headache, dizziness, constipation, blurred vision, elevated liver enzymes
Granisetron	Kytril	1 to 2 mg	Oral	1 hour before chemotherapy	Headache, dizziness, constipation, blurred vision, elevated liver enzymes
	Sancuso	0.01 mg/kg	I.V.		
	Sustol	10 mg	SQ		
		3.1 mg/24 h	TD		
Ondansetron	Zofran	16 to 24 mg	Oral	30 minutes before chemotherapy	Headache, dizziness, constipation, blurred vision, elevated liver enzymes
	Zuplenz	8 to 16 mg	I.V.		
Palonosetron	Aloxi	0.25 mg	I.V.	30 minutes before chemotherapy	Diarrhea, headache, fatigue, insomnia, arrhythmias
Phenothiazines					
Prochlorperazine	Compazine	10 to 25 mg	I.V., oral, rectal	Every 4 to 6 hours as needed	Sedation, hypotension, extrapyramidal effects, lethargy
Chlorpromazine	Thorazine	25 to 50 mg	Oral	Every 4 to 6 hours as needed	Sedation, hypotension, extrapyramidal effects, lethargy
Promethazine	Phenergan	12.5 to 25 mg	I.V., oral, rectal	Every 4 to 6 hours as needed	Sedation, hypotension, extrapyramidal effects, lethargy
Butyrophenones					
Droperidol	Inapsine	1.25 to 2.5 mg	I.M., slow I.V.	Every 4 hours as needed	Sedation, tachycardia, hypotension
Haloperidol	Haldol	2 mg	I.V., I.M., oral	Every 4 to 6 hours as needed	Sedation, tachycardia, hypotension
Corticosteroid					
Dexamethasone	Decadron	4 mg	I.V.	Varies	Anxiety, insomnia, GI upset, psychosis
		10 to 20 mg	Oral		
Cannabinoids					
Dronabinol	Marinol	10 to 20 mg	Oral	Every 3 to 6 hours	Drowsiness, euphoria, dry mouth
Nabilone	Cesamet	1 to 2 mg	Oral	Twice daily	Drowsiness, euphoria, dry mouth
Benzodiazepine					
Lorazepam	Ativan	2 mg	Oral	Every 6 hours	Sedation, amnesia
Benzamide					
Metoclopramide	Reglan	20 mg	Oral	3 to 4 times a day	Diarrhea, sedation, agitation

TABLE 23-10. Pharmacologic Management for the Prevention of Acute Chemotherapy-Induced Nausea and Vomiting *(Continued)*

Generic name	Trade name	Dose*	Dosage form	Frequency	Adverse effects
Neurokinin-1 antagonists					
Aprepitant	Emend	80 to 125 mg	Oral	30 min (I.V.)-1 hour (oral) before chemotherapy	Somnolence, fatigue, diarrhea
	Cinvanti	130 mg	I.V.		
Fosaprepitant	Emend	150 mg	I.V.	30 minutes before chemotherapy	Somnolence, fatigue, diarrhea
Rolapitant	Varubi	180 mg	Oral	Day 1	Hiccups, dizziness, indigestion
Combination drugs					
Netupitant/ palonosetron hydrochloride	Akynzeo	300 mg/0.5 mg	Oral	1 hour before chemotherapy	Headache, asthenia, dyspepsia, fatigue, erythema
Fosnetupitant/ palonosetron hydrochloride	Akynzeo	235 mg/0.25 mg	I.V.	30 minutes before chemotherapy	Headache, asthenia, dyspepsia, fatigue, erythema

Boldface indicates one of top 100 drugs for 2020 by prescription volume.
I.V., intravenous; SQ, subcutaneous; TD, transdermal.
*Most agents are available in more than one dosage form; oral dosing has been given preference.

Antiemetic treatment for high or moderate emetic risk oral chemotherapy

A single-drug regimen is preferred for high or moderate emetic risk oral chemotherapy. The single-drug regimen should consist of granisetron, **ondansetron**, or dolasetron.

Antiemetic treatment for low or minimal emetic risk oral chemotherapy

An as-needed drug regimen is preferred for low or minimal emetic risk oral chemotherapy. The as-needed regimen should consist of granisetron, **ondansetron**, or dolasetron, metoclopramide, or prochloperazine.

The antiemetic drug regimens preferred for the prevention and treatment of delayed CINV are dependent upon which antiemetic drug regimen was use for prevention and treatment of acute CINV. However, common agents used for delayed CINV include olanzapine (if used for acute CINV) and/or aprepitant (if used for acute CINV) and/or dexamethasone.

Traditional Chemotherapy Monitoring Parameters

All traditional chemotherapy requires laboratory value monitoring for myelosuppression. Testing for pretreatment levels of neutrophils and platelets must be performed to guide decision making in dosing and scheduling of these medications. Because of the narrow therapeutic index of these medications, renal function tests (serum creatinine, creatinine clearance) and hepatic function tests (AST, ALT, total and conjugated bilirubin) must be monitored as well to inform dosage reductions for agents that are renally or hepatically cleared.

Traditional Chemotherapy Patient Instructions and Counseling

- Take scheduled and breakthrough CINV medications as instructed; prevention of CINV is key.
- Contact an oncologist or report to emergency care for a fever following chemotherapy.
- Contact an oncologist if you develop mouth sores following chemotherapy.

- Contact an oncologist or report to emergency care for severe diarrhea, constipation, or vomiting not relieved by over-the-counter or prescription medications prescribed by the oncology team following chemotherapy.
- Contact an oncologist or report to emergency care for any unusual bruising or bleeding while on chemotherapy.
- Contact an oncologist for severe tingling, numbness, redness, or pain in extremities following chemotherapy.
- Eat smaller, more frequent meals.
- Stay well hydrated.
- Try to maintain a light exercise regimen.
- Use an electric razor instead of a blade razor.
- Use a soft-bristle toothbrush.
- Avoid use of suppositories unless instructed to do so by the oncology team.
- Avoid crowds and people who have obvious symptoms of infectious disease (e.g., fever, cough, flu symptoms, or diarrhea).
- If eating raw foods, wash them thoroughly and peel them before eating.
- Monitor weight; report weight loss to the oncology team.
- Ensure that all members of the health care team (i.e., physicians, nurses, pharmacists, dentists, etc.) know the patient is currently on chemotherapy.
- Avoid live vaccines during chemotherapy.
- Avoid becoming pregnant or breastfeeding during and immediately after chemotherapy.

23-5 FDA Boxed Warning Information for Cancer Drugs

Note: Almost all cancer drugs carry a boxed warning requiring an experienced physician.

Ado-trastuzumab Emtansine

Cardiotoxicity, hepatotoxicity, teratogenicity

Bleomycin

Idiosyncratic reaction, pulmonary toxicity (with increased risk with cumulative dose >400 units)

Brentuximab Vedotin

Progressive multifocal leukoencephalopathy

Cabazitaxel

Hypersensitivity, neutropenia

Capecitabine

Warfarin interaction

Carboplatin

Bone marrow suppression, hypersensitivity reactions, vomiting

Carmustine

Bone marrow suppression, pulmonary toxicity (with increased risk at cumulative doses > 1400 mg/m^2)

Cetuximab

Cardiopulmonary arrest, infusion reactions

Chlorambucil

Bone marrow suppression, teratogenicity

Cisplatin

Myelosuppression, nausea and vomiting, nephrotoxicity, peripheral neuropathy

Cladribine

Bone marrow suppression, malignancy, nephrotoxicity, neurotoxicity, teratogenicity

Cytarabine, Liposomal

Chemical arachnoiditis

Dacarbazine

Bone marrow suppression, hepatic necrosis, teratogenicity

Daunorubicin, Conventional

Bone marrow suppression, cardiomyopathy (with increased risk at cumulative doses >400 to 550 mg/m^2), extravasation, hepatic impairment, renal impairment

Daunorubicin, Liposomal

Bone marrow suppression, hepatic impairment, infusion reactions, myocardial toxicity

Docetaxel

Fluid retention, hepatic function impairment, hypersensitivity, increased mortality, neutropenia

Doxorubicin, Conventional

Cardiomyopathy (increased risk at cumulative doses >450 mg/m^2), extravasation, secondary malignancy, myelosuppression

Doxorubicin, Liposomal

Cardiomyopathy (increased risk at cumulative doses >450 mg/m^2), infusion-related reactions

Epirubicin

Bone marrow suppression, cardiac toxicity (increased risk after cumulative dose of 550 mg/m^2), extravasation and tissue necrosis, secondary malignancy

Etoposide

Bone marrow suppression

Everolimus

Immunosuppression, mortality in heart transplant, nephrotoxicity, renal graft thrombosis

Fludarabine

Autoimmune effects, bone marrow suppression, neurotoxicity, pulmonary toxicity (in combination with pentostatin)

Fluorouracil

Hematologic risk

Flutamide

Hepatic injury

Hydroxyurea

Bone marrow suppression, secondary malignancy

Idarubicin

Bone marrow suppression, cardiomyopathy, extravasation, hepatic impairment, renal impairment

Ifosfamide

Bone marrow suppression, CNS toxicity, hemorrhagic cystitis, nephrotoxicity

Ipilimumab

Immune-mediated adverse reactions

Irinotecan, Conventional

Bone marrow suppression, diarrhea

Ixabepilone

Hepatic impairment

Lapatinib

Hepatotoxicity

Lenalidomide

Fetal risk, hematologic toxicity, venous and arterial thromboembolism

Melphalan

Bone marrow suppression, hypersensitivity, secondary malignancy

Methotrexate

Appropriate use (due to serious toxic reactions which can be fatal), bone marrow suppression, dermatologic toxicity, gastrointestinal toxicity, hepatotoxicity, intrathecal and high-dose therapy (use preservative-free formulation in these settings), opportunistic infections, pneumonitis, pregnancy, radiotherapy (increased risk of soft tissue necrosis and osteonecrosis when used in combination), renal impairment, secondary malignancy, tumor lysis syndrome

Mitomycin

Bone marrow suppression, hemolytic uremic syndrome

Mitoxantrone

Appropriate administration (I.V. only), bone marrow suppression, cardiotoxicity (increased risk with cumulative doses > 140 mg/m²), secondary leukemia

Nilotinib

QT prolongation and sudden deaths

Nilutamide

Interstitial pneumonitis

Obinutuzumab

Hepatitis B virus reactivation, progressive multifocal leukoencephalopathy

Ofatumumab

Hepatitis B virus reactivation, progressive multifocal leukoencephalopathy

Oxaliplatin

Hypersensitivity/anaphylactic reactions

Paclitaxel

Bone marrow suppression, hypersensitivity reactions (premedication regimen required)

Paclitaxel, Protein-bound

Do not interchange, neutropenia

Panitumumab

Dermatologic toxicity

Pazopanib

Hepatotoxicity

Pertuzumab

Cardiotoxicity, pregnancy

Pomalidomide

Pregnancy, thromboembolic events

Ponatinib

Arterial occlusion, heart failure, hepatotoxicity, venous thromboembolism (VTE)

Raloxifene

Cardiovascular disease, increased risk of venous thromboembolism

Regorafenib

Hepatotoxicity

Rituximab

Hepatitis B virus reactivation, infusion-related reactions, mucocutaneous reactions, progressive multifocal leukoencephalopathy

Sunitinib

Hepatotoxicity

Tamoxifen

Uterine malignancies and thromboembolic events

Thalidomide

Pregnancy, thromboembolic events

Topotecan

Bone marrow suppression

Trastuzumab

Cardiomyopathy, infusion reactions and pulmonary toxicity, pregnancy

Vinblastine

Appropriate administration (I.V. only), extravasation

Vincristine

Appropriate administration (I.V. only), extravasation

Vinorelbine

Bone marrow suppression

Ziv-aflibercept

Compromised wound healing, GI perforation, hemorrhage

23-6 Nondrug Therapy

As mentioned previously, cancer treatment is generally a combination of modalities. Chemotherapy is an important component because most patients present with advanced disease at diagnosis. Surgery plays a role in resecting primary tumors or metastases. It can also be used for diagnostic purposes to biopsy tumors or for other exploratory purposes. Radiation is used to shrink primary tumors in local disease or metastases. It can be used in neoadjuvant therapy to reduce tumor size, in adjuvant therapy to eradicate residual disease, and in combination with chemotherapy as a primary treatment.

Screening is also an important part of cancer therapy because it can allow for the detection of disease in very early stages, when the survival rates are much higher. Table 23-11 refers to American Cancer Society screening recommendations for patients at average risk of developing cancer.

Tests can also be performed to screen and monitor tumor markers. These markers are found in the plasma, serum, or other body fluids and may be used to identify neoplastic growth. They are often not

TABLE 23-11. American Cancer Society Guidelines for the Early Detection of Cancer

Cancer type*	Gender	Age (years)	Procedure	Frequency
Breast	F	40 to 44	Mammography (if desired)	Annually
		45 to 54	Mammography	Annually
		55+	Mammography	Every 1 to 2 years
Cervical	F	21 to 29†	Pap test	Every 3 years
		30 to 65	Pap test and HPV DNA test	Every 3 years (if pap test alone)
				Every 5 years (if pap test and HPV DNA test)
Colorectal	M/F	45+‡	Fecal occult blood test	Annually
			Flexible sigmoidoscopy	Every 5 years
			CT colonography	Every 5 years
			Colonoscopy	Every 10 years
Lung	M/F	55 to 74 (current/former smokers with 30+ pack-year history)	Low-dose helical CT	Annually
Prostate	M	50+	PSA with or without DRE (if desired and 10-year life expectancy)	Dependent upon PSA level

Adapted from the American Cancer Society, 2019.
CT, computed tomography; DNA, deoxyribonucleic acid; DRE, digital rectal exam; F, female; HPV, human papilloma virus; M, male; PSA, prostate-specific antigen.
*No specific screening recommendations have been made for skin and testicular cancer in patients with average risk. After age 40 years, however, all men and women are recommended to receive health counseling and a physical exam every year.
†Screening should be done earlier if patient is sexually active.
‡Screening should be done earlier if there is a strong family history or presence of other risk factors of cancer.

sensitive enough to diagnose cancer and may produce false-positive results (i.e., falsely identify people with a disease that they do not have). They are helpful, however, in identifying the recurrence of advanced disease in patients who have elevated levels on diagnosis.

Pharmacist's Role

Pharmacists play an important role as the medication expert in oncology through:

- Completing chemotherapy calculations to verify accurate dosing of medications, serving as a double-check for these hazardous drugs.
- Assisting in the formulation of CINV treatment and prevention plans for patients receiving low/minimal-to-high emetogenic risk chemotherapy.
- Providing nonpharmacologic and pharmacologic supportive care recommendations based on known adverse effects of chemotherapeutic agents.

NAPLEX Competency Statements

The questions in this chapter cover the following 2021 NAPLEX Competency Statements: **AREA 1:** 1.1; 1.2; 1.5; 1.6; 1.7 **AREA 2:** 2.1; 2.2; 2.3 **AREA 3:** 3.1; 3.3; 3.4; 3.5; 3.6; 3.7; 3.8; 3.10; 3.11 **AREA 4:** 4.1; 4.6; 4.8; 4.9 **AREA 5:** 5.1; 5.5; 5.6 **AREA 6:** 6.3; 6.4.

Questions

Use Patient Profile 23-1 to answer Questions 1–5.

PATIENT PROFILE 23-1. Medication Profile: Community

Age: 33 years

Gender: Female

Diagnosis:
1. Stage II right breast cancer, estrogen receptor positive, and HER2-negative (diagnosed 12/01/20). Genetic testing suggests patient would not benefit from adjuvant antineoplastic chemotherapy. Right simple mastectomy with sentinel lymph node resection on 12/15/20. Sentinel lymph node was negative for breast cancer.
2. Weight loss (25 lb)
3. Seasonal allergies

Height: 5′ 8″

Weight: 150 lb

Allergies: Sulfa, penicillin

Pharmacist notes

Date	Note
01/01/21	Patient complained of soreness and swelling of right arm after sentinel lymph node resection.
02/20/21	Patient did not pick up allergy medication (desloratadine) this month on due date of 02/01/21. Called patient to remind her of importance of this medication with upcoming allergy season. Patient picked up refill on 02/16/21.
03/04/21	Patient is starting Zoladex 3.6 mg SQ every 28 days at oncology clinic; received first dose today.
03/12/21	Patient signed for pseudoephedrine 30 mg tablets.

PATIENT PROFILE 23-1. **Medication Profile: Community** *(Continued)*

Pharmacy medication record

Date	Rx #	Physician	Drug and strength	Quantity	Sig	Refills
12/16/20	12345	Buford	Percocet 5/325	30	1 to 2 every 4 hours as needed	0
02/16/21	12346	Buford	Desloratadine 5 mg	30	1 orally daily	4
03/01/21	12347	Buford	Tamoxifen 20 mg	30	—	2
03/01/21	12349	Buford	Megace 40 mg/mL	300	5 mL twice a day	2
03/01/21	12350	Charles	Celebrex 10 mg	30	1 orally daily	2
03/04/21	12351	Buford	Zoladex 3.6 mg		SQ every 28 days	
03/12/21	12352	Buford	Pseudoephedrine 30 mg			

1. Which agent can be used to treat breast and prostate cancer?

   A. Zoladex
   B. Tamoxifen
   C. Celebrex
   D. Percocet
   E. Pseudoephedrine

2. When the patient presents the tamoxifen prescription, you notice that the directions are missing. You call the health care provider to clarify the instructions for this patient. Which is a correct choice?

   A. 10 mL by mouth daily
   B. 20 mL by mouth daily
   C. 40 mg by mouth twice daily
   D. 10 mg by mouth daily
   E. 20 mg by mouth daily

3. The patient presents to your pharmacy with complaints of lower leg calf pain that is tender to the touch and red. You suspect a deep vein thrombosis. Which agent is most likely to be associated with this condition?

   A. Desloratadine
   B. Pseudoephedrine
   C. Tamoxifen
   D. Percocet
   E. Celebrex

4. The patient calls you on 05/05/17. She has been experiencing frequent hot flashes and wants to know if one of her medications might be causing this adverse effect. You tell her that the hot flashes are likely caused by _____.

   A. Tamoxifen and desloratadine
   B. Percocet and Zoladex
   C. Celebrex and tamoxifen
   D. Zoladex and tamoxifen
   E. Percocet and desloratadine

5. The patient's mother (age 59 years) is worried that she will develop breast cancer like her daughter. Which is appropriate advice for the patient's mother?

   A. Perform monthly breast self-examinations
   B. Undergo mammography annually
   C. Receive mammography once every 5 years
   D. Undergo annual bilateral breast biopsies
   E. No mammography is needed based on her age

6. Which class of agents is best known for causing infusion-related reactions, such as fever and chills?

   A. Monoclonal antibodies
   B. Tyrosine kinase inhibitors
   C. Vinca alkaloids
   D. Platinum alkylating agents
   E. Antimetabolites

7. Your patient has just received 5-FU and irinotecan for the treatment of colorectal cancer. Before he leaves the clinic, you ensure that he has a prescription to prevent or treat which adverse effect from irinotecan?

A. Nausea with Aloxi
B. Vomiting with ondansetron
C. Headache with aspirin
D. Delayed allergic reaction with epinephrine
E. Diarrhea with loperamide

8. Which drug is an oral prodrug of 5-FU?

A. Fluorouracil
B. Xeloda
C. Fludara
D. Cytoxan
E. Leucovorin

9. An elderly male patient comes to your pharmacy and is worried that he might have prostate cancer. He just had some laboratory studies done, and his health care provider told him that some level was abnormal, indicating potential prostate cancer. Which lab test might he be talking about?

A. PSA
B. Cortisol
C. ESR
D. PRR
E. DRE

10. *Stomatitis* is the clinical term for which chemotherapy-related adverse effects?

A. Nausea and vomiting
B. Inflammation of the mucosal lining of the mouth
C. Obstruction of the lower esophageal sphincter
D. Inflammation of the mucosal lining of the colon and rectum
E. Inflammation of a gastrointestinal stromal tumor

11. Which describes a known characteristic of most antineoplastic chemotherapy agents?

A. They have a narrow therapeutic index.
B. They do not interfere with DNA synthesis and replication.
C. Acute adverse effects occur primarily in slowly dividing normal cells.
D. They have largely been developed in the last 5 years.
E. They have only cell cycle phase-specific actions.

Use Patient Profile 23-2 to answer Questions 12–17.

12. A nurse would like to know if she can administer the diphenhydramine and the ranitidine to the patient in the same I.V. line simultaneously. Which resource will provide you with this information?

A. Wolters Kluwer Health's Facts & Comparisons
B. Trissel's *Handbook on Injectable Drugs* and *Drug Prescribing in Renal Failure*
C. Micromedex and *The Sanford Guide to Antimicrobial Therapy*
D. Lexicomp
E. Trissel's *Handbook on Injectable Drugs* and Micromedex

PATIENT PROFILE 23-2. Medication Profile: Institution

Age: 60 years
Gender: Male
Diagnosis:
    1. Metastatic non–small cell lung cancer (diagnosed: 02/01/21)
    2. Chronic obstructive pulmonary disease
    3. Asthma
Height: 180 cm
Weight: 200 lb
Allergies: NKDA

PATIENT PROFILE 23-2. Medication Profile: Institution *(Continued)*

Lab and diagnostic tests

Date	Test
03/01/21	WBC: 6500/mcL
03/01/21	Absolute neutrophil count: 3500/mcL
03/01/21	PLT: 67,000/mcL
03/01/21	Hgb: 13 g/dL
03/01/21	Hct: 39%

Medication record

Date	Route	Drug and strength	Sig
03/01/21	I.V.	Paclitaxel 175 mg/m^2	175 mg/m^2 over 3 hours every 3 weeks
03/01/21	I.V.	Carboplatin AUC 6	AUC 6 over 30 minutes every 3 weeks
03/01/21	Inhale	Albuterol inhaler	2 puffs as needed
03/01/21	Inhale	Advair inhaler	1 puff twice a day
03/01/21	I.V.	Dexamethasone 20 mg	Infuse 30 minutes before chemotherapy
03/01/21	I.V.	Diphenhydramine 50 mg	Infuse 30 minutes before chemotherapy
03/01/21	I.V.	Ranitidine 50 mg	Infuse 30 minutes before chemotherapy

13. Which agent requires the premedication regimen of dexamethasone, diphenhydramine, and ranitidine to prevent an anaphylactic reaction?

A. Taxotere
B. Taxol
C. Paraplatin
D. Cisplatin
E. Osimertinib

14. On the basis of the patient's weight and height, you calculate the patient's body surface area to be 2.1 m^2. Paclitaxel is supplied as 6 mg/mL in 5-mL, 16.7-mL, and 50-mL vials. Your pharmacy has all quantities available. What is the best way to correctly dose this patient?

A. 1 50-mL vial and 1 16.7-mL vial
B. 1 50-mL vial and 1 5-mL vial
C. 2 16.7-mL vials
D. 2 16.7-mL vials and 1 5-mL vial
E. 2 50-mL vials

15. You are concerned that the patient will develop nausea and vomiting from his highly emetogenic chemotherapy. Which regimen would be appropriate to prevent acute CINV?

A. Dexamethasone, granisetron, and aprepitant
B. Granisetron and prochlorperazine
C. Metoclopramide, dexamethasone, and aprepitant
D. Palonosetron and granisetron
E. Dolasetron and olanzapine

16. On the basis of the patient's laboratory values, which of the following adverse reactions appears to have occurred as a likely result of the chemotherapy?

A. Thrombocytopenia
B. Anemia
C. Neutropenia
D. Leukocytopenia
E. Hyperkalemia

17. The goal of the patient's treatment regimen is to
_____.

A. cure his disease
B. palliate his disease-related symptoms and increase his quality of life
C. provide adjuvant therapy following definitive surgery
D. increase his survival time by several years
E. provide neoadjuvant therapy before definitive surgery

18. Doxorubicin is an antineoplastic agent that _____.

A. is not related to epirubicin and daunorubicin
B. interacts with the microtubules of cells during mitosis
C. has an oral dosage form commercially available
D. is in the same drug class as Zytiga
E. causes cumulative cardiac toxicity

19. Which agent is used in cancer regimens but is *not* considered an antineoplastic agent?

A. Methotrexate
B. Leucovorin
C. Doxorubicin
D. Cyclophosphamide
E. Bosutinib

20. Methotrexate (Rheumatrex) is available in which dosage forms? (Mark all that apply)

A. An I.V. injection
B. An oral tablet or capsule
C. An intrathecal injection
D. An ointment
E. A suppository

 **23-9** Answers

1. A. Zoladex (goserelin) is an LHRH agonist that can be used to treat both breast and prostate cancer. LHRH agonists are approved by the U.S. Food and Drug Administration for premenopausal women because they inhibit estrogen production from the ovaries.

2. E. The FDA-approved dose for breast cancer therapy is 20 mg by mouth daily. The drug is not available in a liquid form.

3. C. Tamoxifen is well-known to increase the incidence of thromboembolic events. All patients on this medication should be counseled on the signs and symptoms of thromboembolic events.

4. D. Hot flashes are a common adverse effect experienced by patients taking selective estrogen receptor modifiers (e.g., tamoxifen) and gonadotropin-releasing hormone agonists (e.g., Zoladex).

5. B. Biopsies should never be performed as initial screening tests; however, if results from the mammography point to disease, a biopsy is needed to make a diagnosis. The American Cancer Society still recommends an annual mammography for a woman at normal risk for breast cancer.

6. A. Monoclonal antibodies are commonly associated with infusion-related reactions. Patients should receive premedication, such as acetaminophen and diphenhydramine to prevent this.

7. E. Diarrhea is a dose-limiting toxicity of irinotecan. Late-onset diarrhea can be life threatening. All patients should receive a prescription for loperamide to treat delayed-onset diarrhea. Patients should be instructed to take 2 mg by mouth every 2 hours while awake and 4 mg by mouth every 4 hours during the night until the diarrhea has stopped for at least 12 hours. Acute-onset diarrhea can be treated with atropine.

8. B. Xeloda (capecitabine) is an oral prodrug of 5-FU. Fluorouracil is another name for 5-FU. Fludarabine (Fludara) is used to treat chronic lymphocytic leukemia and non-Hodgkin lymphoma intravenously. Cyclophosphamide (Cytoxan) and is available in I.V. and oral dosage forms.

9. A. PSA is a lab test that is commonly done in men over age 40 years. It should be performed annually in men over age 50 years with or without a digital rectal exam (if the patient is agreeable and has a 10-year life expectancy) to check for prostate cancer.

10. B. *Stomatitis* is used to describe an irritation or ulceration of the mucosal lining. This adverse effect is common with fluorouracil and methotrexate. Having the patient hold ice chips in his or her mouth during treatment can prevent it. The cold is thought to cause vasoconstriction of the lining and prevent damage.

11. **A.** Chemotherapy agents have a very narrow therapeutic index. This is one of the main reasons these drugs have so many toxic effects. They can be cell cycle phase–specific or cell cycle phase–nonspecific in their pharmacologic action and can cause many adverse effects to normal cells that undergo rapid proliferation.

12. **E.** Both Trissel's *Handbook on Injectable Drugs* and the Micromedex IV compatibility tool can be used to assess whether diphenhydramine and ranitidine are compatible.

13. **B.** Taxol is the brand name of paclitaxel. This agent has been shown to cause hypersensitivity reactions in patients. It is unclear if these reactions are a result of the drug itself or the drug's vehicle (Cremophor). All patients receiving paclitaxel should receive a premedication regimen of dexamethasone, diphenhydramine, and ranitidine.

14. **A.** The patient requires 367.5 mg of drug. Choice A will provide 400 mg of drug, and this is the most economical way to provide the required dose.

15. **A.** This patient's regimen contains carboplatin ≥ AUC 4 and paclitaxel, making it highly emetogenic chemotherapy. A 4-drug regimen is preferred for parenteral HEC. The 4-drug regimen should consist of a neurokinin-1 receptor antagonist (NK1 RA), a serotonin receptor antagonist (5-HT3 RA), dexamethasone, and olanzapine. A 3-drug regimen may be used, if desired. The 3-drug regimen should consist of (1) olanzapine, palonosetron, and dexamethasone or (2) a NK1 RA, a 5-HT3 RA, and dexamethasone. Choice B is incorrect because it contains only 2 drugs and drug classes of 5-HT3 RA and dopamine antagonist. Choice C is incorrect because it adds dexamethasone, aprepitant, and a dopamine antagonist; aprepitant is an option

if combined with dexamethasone and a 5-HT$_3$ antagonist. Choice D is incorrect because it contains 2 5-HT$_3$ antagonists; therapy should include more than 1 drug class. Choice E is incorrect because it only contains 2 drugs.

16. **A.** Myelosuppression is a common adverse reaction to most chemotherapy agents. Both paclitaxel and carboplatin can cause anemia, thrombocytopenia, and leukopenia. In this case, thrombocytopenia is the dominant hematologic toxicity.

17. **B.** The patient has metastatic disease. When most solid tumors are diagnosed as stage IV, this finding is representative of the fact that the disease is incurable. This is true of non–small cell lung cancer. The treatment goals for these patients include relieving any disease-related symptoms, minimizing toxicity from treatments, and increasing the patient's quality of life through treatment or supportive care measures.

18. **E.** Doxorubicin is an antitumor antibiotic related to epirubicin and daunorubicin. These agents act by binding tightly to DNA through intercalation and by inhibiting the topoisomerase II enzyme. Doxorubicin does have a liposomal IV product, but it is not available orally. All anthracyclines are associated with cardiac toxicity and have recommended cumulative dosing limits.

19. **B.** Leucovorin is a reduced-folate agent that is used in combination with 5-FU to potentiate the therapeutic effects of 5-FU and as a rescue treatment for high-dose methotrexate.

20. **A, B, C.** Methotrexate is available as an I.V. or intrathecal injection and an oral tablet or capsule. It is not commercially available for topical use or as a suppository.

23-10 Additional Resources

American Cancer Society. Cancer facts & figures 2020. Available at: http://www.cancer.org.

IBM Micromedex [database]. Truven Health Analytics. Available at: http://www.micromedexsolutions.com.

Lexicomp [database]. Wolters Kluwer. Available at: http://www.online.lexi.com.

National Comprehensive Cancer Network. NCCN clinical practice guidelines in oncology—antiemesis. Version 2.2020. Available at: http://www.nccn.org.

Trissel, LA. *Handbook on Injectable Drugs.* 20th ed. Bethesda, MD: American Society of Health-System Pharmacists; 2018.

Anemias

JESSICA N. HODGE

24

24-1 KEY POINTS

- Anemia is a reduction in red cell mass that decreases the blood's oxygen-carrying capacity.
- Iron deficiency anemia (IDA) is the most common anemia, accounting for 25% of all cases. IDA presents as a microcytic, hypochromic anemia.
- Iron preparations are best absorbed on an empty stomach but usually are not tolerated without the co-administration of food.
- Certain medications and factors that induce gastric acid hyposecretion are associated with reduced absorption of oral iron.
- Megaloblastic anemias are macrocytic and result from **folic acid** or vitamin B_{12} deficiency.
- Determining whether the megaloblastic anemia is due to either folate or vitamin B_{12} deficiency is essential because folate therapy can mask the hematopoietic features of vitamin B_{12} deficiency while allowing the sometimes-irreversible neurologic sequelae to progress.
- Vitamin B_{12} requires intrinsic factor to be optimally absorbed.
- Patients with chronic kidney disease typically are anemic because of the lack of erythropoietin production.
- Anemia of chronic kidney disease is treated with subcutaneous or intravenous (I.V.) epoetin and I.V. iron therapy.
- Patients receiving epoetin must have routine monitoring of hematocrit, hemoglobin, and blood pressure.
- Darbepoetin has the same mechanism of action as epoetin, but it is longer acting and can be administered less frequently.

24-2 STUDY GUIDE CHECKLIST

The following topics may guide your study of this subject area:

- ☐ Diagnostic criteria for anemia.
- ☐ Various types of anemia and potential causes of each.
- ☐ Presenting symptoms that could lead to suspicion of anemia.
- ☐ Different available dosage forms of both oral and I.V. iron preparations and when to recommend each.
- ☐ Drug interactions that could affect oral iron administration.
- ☐ Indications for drugs other than iron preparations (i.e., **folic acid**, vitamin B_{12}, epoetin alfa, darbepoetin alfa).
- ☐ Monitoring parameters for patient response to treatment.
- ☐ Possible nondrug treatment options.
- ☐ Unique patient counseling points to maximize response to treatment while minimizing potential adverse effects.

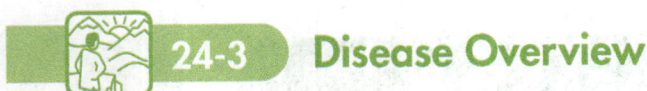

24-3 Disease Overview

Anemia is a reduction in red cell mass that decreases the oxygen-carrying capacity of the blood. The World Health Organization suggests a plasma hemoglobin (Hgb) concentration of < 12 mg/dL for non-pregnant females, < 11 mg/dL for pregnant females, and < 13 mg/dL for males as diagnostic for anemia. This chapter focuses on iron deficiency anemia (IDA), megaloblastic anemia, and anemia of chronic kidney disease.

Epidemiology

Approximately 3.4 million Americans have anemia. Anemia is more common in menstruating and pregnant women than in men. The incidence of anemia also increases with age and is more prevalent in the elderly population. Of all anemias, 75% result from iron deficiency, anemia of chronic disease, and acute bleeding. The remaining 25% of anemia cases are the result of bone marrow damage, decreased erythropoiesis, and hemolysis. IDA is the single most common form of anemia, accounting for 25% of all cases.

Kinetic Approach to Anemia

Using the kinetic methodology, one can classify anemia by 3 major mechanisms: decreased red blood cell (RBC) production (due to lack of nutrients, bone marrow disorders, or suppression), increased RBC destruction (e.g., hemolytic anemia), or blood loss.

Classification by Morphology

The most common way to classify an anemia is by the morphology (shape and structure) of the RBCs.

Macrocytic (large-sized cell) morphology (RBC size > 100 femtoliters [fL])

Anemias in this class include megaloblastic (oval cells often with hypersegmented neutrophils) and normoblastic (round cells) and may result from the following:

- Megaloblastic
  - Folic acid deficiency
  - Vitamin B_{12} deficiency or pernicious anemia (lack of intrinsic factor)
- Normoblastic
  - Alcohol
  - Liver disease
  - Hypothyroidism
  - Nucleoside reverse transcriptase inhibitors
  - Valproic acid

Normocytic (normal-sized cell) morphology (RBC size 80 to 100 fL)

Anemias in this class may result from the following:

- Acute blood loss
- Bone marrow failure (decreased RBC production)
- Hemolysis (increased RBC destruction)
- Immunologic destruction, such as that which occurs in autoimmune diseases
- Anemia of chronic disease or chronic inflammation (early onset)

Microcytic (small-sized cell) morphology (RBC size < 80 fL)

Anemias in this class include the following:

- Hypochromic (pale RBCs lacking hemoglobin with decreased mean corpuscular Hgb [MCH] and mean corpuscular Hgb concentration [MCHC])
  - IDA
  - Anemia of chronic disease or chronic inflammation (late onset)
- Normochromic (normal color RBCs)
  - Certain genetic anomalies, such as thalassemia

Clinical Presentation

The signs and symptoms of anemia depend on the amount of time during which the anemia has developed and the severity of RBC depletion. An anemia that has developed over a long period of time may be asymptomatic in the beginning stages and then progress to fatigue, malaise, headache, exertional dyspnea, angina, pallor, or loss of skin tone. A patient with acute anemia (e.g., from recent blood loss) may present with tachycardia, shortness of breath, or light-headedness. Many of the signs and symptoms of anemia are secondary to tissue hypoxia. In the case of hypoxia, blood supply is shunted to life-sustaining organs (brain, heart, kidney) and away from nonvital organs (e.g., extremities, nail beds), which results in pallor of the skin. The various types of anemia have additional signs and symptoms that will be discussed in further detail elsewhere in the chapter.

Pathophysiology

Iron deficiency anemia

IDA is the most common anemia, accounting for approximately 25% of all anemia cases. It is caused by iron store depletion resulting from the following:

- Inadequate oral intake of iron (especially animal protein)
- Increased iron demands, such as those found in
  - Pregnant or lactating women
  - Infants and adolescents who experience periods of rapid growth
  - The elderly
- Blood loss as a result of
  - Menstruation or postpartum blood loss
  - Trauma
  - Gastrointestinal (GI) ulcers
- Inadequate absorption as a result of
  - Medications (e.g., tetracyclines, antacids, histamine-2 [H2] antagonists, proton-pump inhibitors)
  - Gastrectomy
  - Enteritis or malabsorption syndrome
  - Ingestion of large amounts of tannins (tea) or phytates (brans, grains)
- Disease states, such as
  - Carcinomas
  - Rheumatoid arthritis

Hemoglobin is composed of iron (heme) and proteins (globin). Lack of iron results in reduced hemoglobin synthesis. The RBCs produced under those conditions are

- Hypochromic (decreased concentration of hemoglobin)
- Microcytic (smaller-sized cells)

Megaloblastic anemias

Megaloblastic anemias are caused by either a deficiency in or an inability to use vitamin B_{12} (cobalamin) or folic acid.

Vitamin B_{12} deficiency can result from the following:

- *Decreased intake:* This problem may occur with patients who are strict vegetarians (e.g., vegans or ovo-lacto vegetarians) or in alcoholics with a poor diet.
- *Decreased absorption:* For vitamin B_{12} to be absorbed at the terminal ileum, intragastric intrinsic factor must be attached to it. The lack of production of intrinsic factor results in pernicious anemia, which can be inherited or acquired after gastrectomy. Malabsorption can also occur in patients with gastric bypass surgery, chronic pancreatitis, and chronic diarrhea (e.g., celiac disease, short bowel syndrome, regional enteritis, inflammatory bowel disease, human immunodeficiency virus enteropathy, *Helicobacter pylori* infections), or it can result from **metformin** therapy (calcium-dependent ileal membrane antagonism).
- *Achlorhydria:* Vitamin B_{12} requires an acidic environment to be absorbed. Chronic therapy with proton-pump inhibitors and H2 antagonists may contribute to vitamin B_{12} deficiency; those with atrophic gastritis may be vitamin B_{12} deficient as well.

Folic acid deficiency can result from the following:

- *Decreased intake:* This problem is found especially in patients who are alcoholic, indigent, or elderly.
- *Decreased absorption:* This problem occurs in patients with inflammatory bowel disease or malabsorption disorders.
- *Increased demands:* For example, deficiencies may occur during pregnancy or growth spurts or could accompany malignancy or long-term hemodialysis.
- *Drugs:* Examples include trimethoprim, sulfasalazine, pyrimethamine, triamterene, methotrexate, cyclophosphamide, hydroxyurea, mercaptopurine, 5-fluorouracil, and phenytoin.

Anemia of chronic kidney disease

The primary reason that patients with chronic kidney disease are anemic is lack of erythropoietin (EPO) production. EPO is a hormone produced primarily (90%) in the kidneys that stimulates the synthesis and differentiation of erythroid progenitor cells (precursors to RBCs). The uremic environment in patients with chronic kidney disease decreases the lifespan of RBCs.

Folic acid deficiency also can develop as a result of increased folic acid demands during synthesis of RBCs. Additionally, folic acid can be removed during hemodialysis. Patients with chronic kidney disease become iron deficient as a result of the iron and blood loss during dialysis and the diseased kidneys' impaired ability to manufacture EPO in response to that loss.

Diagnostic Criteria

If anemia is suspected, a complete blood cell count (CBC) should be performed. Other tests performed for diagnostic purposes may include a stool test for presence of blood, a peripheral blood smear, and a thorough medical history and physical exam.

Iron deficiency anemia

Blood tests

Serum iron, transferrin, and total iron binding capacity (TIBC) historically have been used to confirm IDA. Serum transferrin (one of the major transport proteins for iron) concentration and TIBC (the amount of binding space left for iron on the transferrin protein) increase with iron deficiency, whereas transferrin saturation will decrease to < 15%. Unfortunately, serum iron and serum transferrin are not very sensitive markers because both are acute phase reactants that may be influenced by a variety of other conditions.

Serum ferritin (the storage form of iron) is now considered the best and most reliable initial marker of choice for assessing iron status. A patient with a serum ferritin concentration of < 45 ng/mL has a significant potential for iron deficiency; a concentration of < 25 ng/mL indicates a very high probability of iron deficiency. Unfortunately, serum ferritin also is influenced by stress, inflammation, and neoplasia, because serum ferritin concentration is increased under these conditions. As the iron deficiency progresses, Hgb decreases because iron is a component of Hgb. As a result, the RBCs become paler in color (MCH and MCHC are decreased), and the RBCs become smaller in size (decreased mean corpuscular volume [MCV]), indicating microcytosis. The blood smear will reflect a microcytic, hypochromic cell.

Specific signs and symptoms

In addition to the general signs and symptoms listed previously for anemia, the following symptoms may be present in severe IDA:

- Koilonychia (spoon-shaped nails)
- Angular stomatitis or glossitis
- Pica (appetite for nonfood substances such as chalk, soil, ice, or clay)

Megaloblastic anemias (macrocytic anemias resulting from vitamin B_{12} or folate deficiency)

Blood tests

Blood tests should show the following:

- Decreased hematocrit (Hct) and Hgb
- Decreased RBC count
- Elevated MCV, which indicates macrocytosis
- Abnormalities in serum homocysteine, methylmalonic acid, or both
- Normal ferritin

Because of the lack of sensitivity and specificity of serum vitamin B_{12} (cobalamin) and folate concentrations, many clinicians now use serum homocysteine or methylmalonic acid to ascertain if a patient has a vitamin B_{12} or folate deficiency. Those compounds are used because vitamin B_{12} or folate must be present for either their synthesis or their metabolism. A patient with macrocytic anemia and normal concentrations of homocysteine and methylmalonic acid likely has a non–vitamin deficiency macrocytic anemia from liver disease, alcohol abuse, valproic acid, nucleoside reverse transcriptase inhibitors, hypothyroidism, or increased reticulocytosis. The diagnostic utility of these metabolites is given in Table 24-1. The clinician must appropriately diagnose whether the megaloblastic anemia is the result of folate or vitamin B_{12} depletion. An incorrect diagnosis may lead to permanent neurologic sequelae if a vitamin B_{12} deficiency is misdiagnosed and treated as a folate deficiency without appropriate vitamin B_{12} supplementation.

TABLE 24-1. Vitamin-Dependent Metabolites in Patients with Vitamin B_{12} or Folate Deficiency

Serum metabolite concentrations	Vitamin deficiency
Elevated HCY, normal MMA	Folate deficiency
Elevated HCY, elevated MMA	Vitamin B_{12} deficiency or possibly a combined vitamin B_{12} and folate deficiency
Normal HCY, elevated MMA	Vitamin B_{12} deficiency
Normal HCY, normal MMA	Macrocytic anemia not due to a folate or vitamin B_{12} deficiency

HCY, homocysteine; MMA, methylmalonic acid.

Vitamin B$_{12}$ deficiency

Because of the large amount of vitamin B$_{12}$ stored in the liver, the etiology (e.g., malabsorption, drug therapy) generally must be prevalent for 3 to 5 years before the deficiency is manifested. If the etiology for the megaloblastic anemia is vitamin B$_{12}$ deficiency, serum methylmalonic acid concentration definitely will be elevated, and serum homocysteine concentration also likely will be elevated.

Additional signs and symptoms include the following:

- Loss of vibratory sensation in lower extremities
- Ataxia or vertigo
- Glossitis
- Muscle weakness
- Neuropsychiatric abnormalities (e.g., irritability or emotional instability, dementia, psychosis)

Folic acid deficiency

Folic acid deficiency results in an increased serum homocysteine concentration with a normal serum methylmalonic acid concentration. Folate deficiency can occur sooner than vitamin B$_{12}$ deficiency, with signs and symptoms of deficiency appearing within 6 months of folate depletion. Overall, signs and symptoms of folic acid deficiency anemia are very similar to those of vitamin B$_{12}$ deficiency anemia, except that the neurological symptoms that may be present with vitamin B$_{12}$ deficiency anemia are absent. **Folic acid** supplementation is given to pregnant women preemptively, because folate depletion can lead to neural tube birth defects (e.g., spina bifida) during fetal development.

Anemia of chronic kidney disease

As the name implies, this anemia occurs in patients with chronic kidney disease who require maintenance hemodialysis. The etiology for this type of anemia is multifactorial, including the effects of hemodialysis itself, which can lead to hemolysis, the removal of water-soluble vitamins (e.g., vitamin B$_{12}$ and folate), and iron deficiency. Lack of EPO production also is a major factor. EPO is a hormone released from the kidney that stimulates the bone marrow to make new RBCs. Before diagnosis, other causes must be ruled out. A CBC usually will reveal a normochromic, normocytic anemia.

Treatment Principles and Goals

Iron deficiency anemia

In IDA treatment, the first goal is to normalize Hgb and Hct:

- Hgb should increase 2 g/dL in 3 weeks.
- Hct should increase 6% in 3 weeks.
- Reticulocytosis usually will occur within 1 week.

If those indices do not improve within their respective time frames, the diagnosis should be reevaluated, and compliance with therapy should be confirmed. A second goal is to replenish iron stores. Although Hgb and Hct will return to normal within 1 to 2 months, iron therapy should be continued for 3 to 6 months after Hgb is normalized to replenish total body iron stores.

Megaloblastic anemias

Goals of vitamin B$_{12}$ replacement

Hgb should increase within 1 week. If neurologic symptoms were present, they should improve within 24 to 72 hours. However, if vitamin B$_{12}$ deficiency is longstanding, symptoms may not be relieved for several months. In some cases, some residual neurologic signs and symptoms may not resolve completely. Maintenance administration of vitamin B$_{12}$ should continue for as long as nutritional intake, increased losses, or malabsorption is a problem.

Goals of folic acid replacement

RBC morphology will correct within a few days. Hgb will start to normalize within 10 days. Hct will return to normal levels within 2 months. Maintenance administration of **folic acid** should continue for as long as nutritional intake, increased losses, or malabsorption is a problem.

24-4 Drug Therapy

Iron Deficiency Anemia

Iron supplementation

Treatment consists of iron supplementation to achieve a total elemental iron dose of about 200 mg per day (Table 24-2). The total daily dose usually is divided into 2 to 3 dosing intervals throughout the day. The **ferrous sulfate** salt, which is 20% elemental iron, is the most commonly used and inexpensive salt form for iron therapy. Treatment of IDA with **ferrous sulfate** 325 mg 3 times daily for 3 to 6 months is adequate for many patients.

Iron is best absorbed in the reduced (ferrous) form. Iron is maximally absorbed in the duodenum, primarily because of the acidic nature of the stomach. Vitamin C (ascorbic acid) may facilitate increased absorption of iron, although its clinical relevance has been questioned. Additionally, orange juice may improve absorption. High-fiber foods, tea (rich in iron-binding tannins), coffee, and milk should be avoided during the administration of iron preparations. Taking the iron product on an empty stomach is recommended; however, most patients experience significant adverse GI effects, necessitating that the drug be taken with either a snack or meal. Some patients can tolerate only a product with low elemental iron content (e.g., ferrous gluconate), a slow-release or sustained-release preparation, or an enteric-coated iron product. The sustained-release and enteric-coated products are less effective, however, because absorption is delayed owing to slower dissolution, and iron is not available for absorption until the product has reached the jejunum or ileum, where iron absorption is decreased. If the patient is selected for one of these latter therapeutic options, then clinical recovery from the IDA would be expected to occur at a slower rate, and increased duration of therapy from 3 to 6 months to 6 to 12 months would be expected.

Once the iron deficiency has been adequately treated, maintenance therapy may consist of a lower dose (e.g., **ferrous sulfate** 325 mg once daily or a multivitamin product that is enriched with iron) if the precipitating cause for the IDA is still evident (e.g., menses). Additionally, dietary intake of meat, fish, and poultry may be encouraged, because iron from vegetable, grain, and dairy sources is poorly absorbed.

Mechanism of action

Iron supplementation corrects the iron deficiency and enables Hgb to be synthesized at normal levels.

Iron dextran may be given intravenously in intermittent doses (e.g., 100 mg daily) or as a total dose infusion mixed in 250 to 1000 mL of normal saline (0.9% NaCl) over 4 to 6 hours. Iron dextran formulations

TABLE 24-2. Common Oral Iron Preparations Used to Treat IDA

Generic name	Trade name	Elemental Fe (%)	Dose (mg)	Fe content (mg)
Ferrous sulfate	Feosol, Fer-In-Sol	20	325	65
Ferrous gluconate	Fergon	12	300	35
Ferrous fumarate	Femiron, Fumerin, Feostat	33	300	99
Polysaccharide iron complex	Niferex, Ferrex	100	150	150
Carbonyl iron	Feosol Carbonyl Iron	100	45	45

Boldface indicates one of top 100 drugs for 2020 by prescription volume.

carry a U.S. Food and Drug Administration (FDA) boxed warning about fatal anaphylactic reactions. Prior to the first therapeutic infusion, a 25 mg test dose must be administered by slow intravenous (I.V.) push or intermittent infusion, and the patient must be observed for any adverse or allergic reactions for up to 1 hour after administration. This test dose is required before the patient can receive a larger therapeutic dose of iron dextran. The other I.V. iron products do not contain dextran and have a better safety profile; therefore, they do not require a test dose. Iron dextran is the only I.V. iron product approved for total dose infusion. Iron dextran also may be given intramuscularly (by Z-track injection to avoid injection or leakage into the subcutaneous tissue) at doses up to 100 mg per injection. Iron dextran can be added to lipid-free parenteral nutrition solutions; however, it cannot be added to lipid-containing parenteral nutrition solutions, because iron is a trivalent cation and can disrupt the emulsification of lipids, resulting in "oiling out" or coalescence of lipid particles. Any patient receiving I.V. iron infusion should be monitored for signs and symptoms of hypersensitivity reactions.

The I.V. iron formulations may have the following adverse effects:

- Immediate reaction (within minutes of infusion)
  - Malaise, urticaria, nausea, diaphoresis, headache
  - Anaphylactic: Anaphylactoid reaction, hypotension, circulatory collapse. Premedication with antihistamines and corticosteroids may prevent anaphylaxis but is rarely done because of the low incidence of these reactions.
- Delayed reaction (within 1 to 2 days after infusion)
  - Myalgias, arthralgias, fever, flu-like symptoms

Patient instructions (for oral supplementation)

- Take iron supplementation 1 to 2 hours before a meal (on an empty stomach if tolerable).
- If iron is intolerable on an empty stomach, take it with a small snack, but try to avoid dairy products or tea. Food can decrease the absorption of iron by 50%. Iron may be taken with an acidic fruit beverage such as orange juice to improve absorption.
- Keep out of reach of children. Iron is a major cause of ingestion deaths in children.
- Take iron 1 hour before or 3 hours after any antacids.
- Some medications interact with iron. Please ask a health care provider or pharmacist before taking any new medications in combination with iron.
- If constipation occurs, over-the-counter docusate may be taken.

Adverse drug effects

Oral iron formulations primarily have GI effects:

- Dark-colored stools
- Constipation or diarrhea
- Nausea or vomiting

Drug Interactions

- **Antibiotics (tetracyclines and quinolones):** Iron binds to these antibiotics, preventing absorption.
- **Antacids:** Iron needs an acidic environment for optimal absorption.

I.V. iron preparations should be used only in the following cases:

- Iron malabsorption with the inability to overcome the malabsorption with enteral iron supplementation
- Oral noncompliance with severe anemia
- Refusal of blood transfusion for severe anemia
- Chronic kidney disease patients or cancer patients receiving human recombinant erythropoiesis-stimulating agents

Patients with an active infection should not receive I.V. iron therapy. When iron is given intravenously, free iron concentration can easily exceed maximum transferrin saturation (unlike when given orally).

The abundant free iron is then available to be used by various microorganisms for proliferation and may actually increase the virulence of the offending organisms.

Five I.V. iron products are available in the United States:

- Iron dextran (INFeD and Dexferrum)
- Ferric gluconate (Ferrlecit)
- Iron sucrose (Venofer)
- Ferumoxytol (Feraheme)
- Ferric carboxymaltose (Injectafer)

Monitoring parameters

- Have reticulocytes, Hgb, and Hct increased?
- Is the iron tolerable? (Tolerance will influence compliance.)
- Is the patient improving symptomatically?

Megaloblastic Anemias

Vitamin B$_{12}$ supplementation

Treatment of an existing vitamin B$_{12}$ deficiency usually is done by the parenteral route; however, some clinicians have been successful with sublingual, intranasal, or high-dose oral therapy. Early and aggressive treatment is warranted, particularly if the patient has any neurologic signs and symptoms, because these adverse effects may not be completely reversible if the anemia has been allowed to persist for a substantial time.

A severe vitamin B$_{12}$ deficiency (e.g., neurologic signs or symptoms) usually is corrected through intramuscular (I.M.) or subcutaneous (SQ) vitamin B$_{12}$ (cyanocobalamin) injection, although I.V. administration, if available, also is an option. Multiple dosing schemes are published in the literature. Some typical methods are as follows:

- Initially 1000 mcg I.M., I.V., or SQ every day for 1 week, then 1000 mcg I.M., I.V., or SQ every week for 4 to 6 weeks
- 1000 mcg IM, IV, or SQ every week for 4 to 6 weeks
- 500 mcg intranasally or sublingually daily for 4 to 6 weeks (for less severe deficiency)

Once the deficiency has been corrected, various maintenance methods for prevention of recurrence exist depending on the etiology for the deficiency. If the etiology is low dietary intake such as with vegans (or ovo-lacto vegetarians), one simple maintenance solution is daily ingestion of a multivitamin that meets the Dietary Reference Intake for vitamin B$_{12}$. If the etiology is malabsorption because of achlorhydria, pernicious anemia, chronic pancreatitis, drug-induced malabsorption, or gastric bypass therapy, either sublingual or intranasal administration (500 mcg weekly) is reasonable. Hot liquids or foods should be avoided for 1 hour before and after intranasal administration in an effort to avoid rhinorrhea and potentially reducing absorption. High oral doses of vitamin B$_{12}$ may be used as maintenance therapy for some patients (e.g., 1000 to 2000 mcg daily is necessary to benefit from passive absorption). For patients with short bowel syndrome or severe malabsorption, the oral route should be avoided. The parenteral route also is an option (e.g., 1000 mcg I.M., I.V., or SQ every 1 to 3 months), although most patients would prefer sublingual or nasal administration.

Mechanism of action

Vitamin B$_{12}$ supplementation allows for normal synthesis of the ribonucleic acid (RNA) involved in RBC synthesis.

Patient instructions

If injections are given at home, the patient or caregiver should be counseled on sterile injection techniques and proper needle disposal.

Adverse drug effects

Vitamin B_{12} supplementation can cause the following adverse effects:

- Hyperuricemia or hypokalemia caused by increased synthesis of reticulocytes
- Sodium retention
- An expansion of the intravascular volume as a result of increased RBC synthesis, which can increase cardiac output and cause angina or dyspnea
- Itching in 1% to 10% of patients
- Diarrhea in 1% to 10% of patients
- Anaphylaxis in < 1% of patients

Monitoring parameters

- Monitor CBC. Is there an increase in Hgb? The hemoglobin should improve within 2 weeks. The anemia should correct within 1 to 2 months, although abnormalities in the blood smear may persist for several months.
- Is the patient improving symptomatically (especially neurologic symptoms, if present)?
- Methylmalonic acid concentrations should normalize within 1 month depending on the intensity of the repletion therapy.

Folic Acid Deficiency Anemia

Folic acid supplementation

Folic acid deficiency is corrected by administering 1 mg **folic acid** daily for 4 months. Five mg daily may be given if the patient has severe malabsorption. Once the underlying cause of the deficiency is corrected, **folic acid** supplementation may be discontinued. Long-term folate administration is necessary if the cause is not corrected, such as in hemodialysis, chronic drug therapy with sulfasalazine, or alcoholism.

Mechanism of action

Folic acid supplementation allows for normal RNA synthesis, which is involved in the synthesis of RBCs.

Patient instructions

- Stress the importance of compliance with the regimen.
- Women of childbearing age should be counseled to take a multivitamin containing **folic acid**, regardless of whether an anemia is present, to prevent neural tube birth defects.

Adverse drug effects

Fewer than 1% of patients have allergic reactions to **folic acid**.

Drug interactions

Folic acid may increase phenytoin metabolism.

Phenytoin, primidone, sulfasalazine, para-aminosalicylic acid, and oral contraceptives may decrease **folic acid** concentrations.

Chloramphenicol may blunt the response to **folic acid**.

Monitoring parameters

- Is the RBC morphology normalizing?
- Are the Hgb and Hct normalizing? An improvement in Hgb should occur within 2 weeks. The anemia should be corrected within 1 to 2 months.
- Homocysteine concentrations should normalize within 1 month.
- Is the patient complying?

Anemia of Chronic Kidney Disease

Recombinant human erythropoietin

The primary cause of anemia in chronic kidney disease is decreased EPO synthesis; therefore, the optimal drug for this type of anemia is an erythropoiesis-stimulating agent (ESA). Epoetin alfa (Procrit, Epogen) and darbepoetin alfa (Aranesp) are ESAs with similar mechanisms of action, but darbepoetin alfa has a longer half-life. Epoetin alfa-epbx (Retacrit) is newly approved biosimilar product for Procrit and Epogen. Retacrit carries the same dosing and indications as Procrit and Epogen giving an additional treatment option for ESA treatment. Prescriber approval is required before substituting Retacrit for either Procrit or Epogen.

An ESA is indicated in the treatment of anemia associated with chronic kidney disease, including dialysis and nondialysis patients. ESAs are indicated to elevate or maintain the RBCs and to decrease the need for transfusions in these patients. The goal of combined iron therapy and ESAs for anemia of chronic kidney disease is to reach a target Hgb of ≥ 10 g/dL through a slow, steady increase (usually within 2 to 4 months). Rapid increases in or overcorrection of Hgb concentrations as a result of ESA use has led to increased thrombotic vascular events, congestive heart failure, and cardiac ischemia. The FDA has removed the labeling from ESAs for a specific Hgb or Hct target range because of those safety concerns. The National Kidney Foundation–Kidney Disease Outcomes Quality Initiative (NKF-KDOQI) guidelines recommend that epoetin be administered subcutaneously, because that route of administration is as effective as, or better than, I.V. administration. However, epoetin often is administered intravenously in patients receiving hemodialysis, because the dialysis port offers easy I.V. access. Concurrent I.V. iron therapy also is recommended for effective erythropoiesis during therapy with ESAs.

Mechanism of action

Human recombinant EPO stimulates erythropoiesis (increased RBC production).

Patient instructions

Epoetin alfa is available in preservative-free, single-dose vials, multidose vials, and predrawn syringes. Epoetin afla-epbx is only available in single-dose vials. All dosage forms should be stored at 36° to 46°F (2° to 8°C) until ready for use.

Adverse drug effects

Table 24-3 shows adverse effects of epoetin alfa and the percentage of patients reporting them. The most common adverse effect is elevated blood pressure, which is associated with the rate of rise in Hgb concentration. Increased numbers of thromboembolic complications, cardiac failure, and cardiac ischemia have been associated with a rapid rise in Hgb (e.g., > 1 g/dL within 2 weeks). ESAs are contraindicated in patients with uncontrolled hypertension. Pure red cell aplasia (PRCA), in association with neutralizing antibodies to native EPO, has been reported rarely in the literature. If PRCA is suspected, epoetin should be discontinued immediately.

Drug interactions

No drug interactions have been reported.

Monitoring parameters

Before initiation of therapy, the patient's iron stores should be evaluated. Transferrin saturation should be at least 20% and ferritin at least 100 ng/mL. Monitor Hgb very closely. The dose should be titrated to maintain the lowest Hgb concentration sufficient to avoid an RBC transfusion. Once the Hct approaches the target Hgb concentration (e.g., 10 g/dL per the NKF-KDOQI guidelines), the dose of epoetin should be decreased. If Hgb increases more than 1 g/dL within 2 weeks, the dose should be decreased. The dose should be increased if Hgb has not increased 1 g/dL in 8 weeks.

Blood pressure should be adequately controlled before initiation of ESA therapy. Blood pressure must be closely monitored and controlled during therapy.

Serum chemistries should be monitored.

TABLE 24-3. Percentage of Patients Reporting Adverse Effects of Epoetin Alfa

Event	Patients treated with epoetin alfa (n = 200)	Patients on placebo (n = 135)
Hypertension	24%	19%
Headache	16%	12%
Arthralgias	11%	6%
Nausea	11%	9%
Edema	9%	10%
Fatigue	9%	14%
Vomiting	8%	5%
Chest pain	7%	9%
Skin reaction at site of administration	7%	12%
Asthenia	7%	12%
Dizziness	7%	13%
Clotted access	7%	2%
Significant adverse events[a]		
Seizure	1.1%	1.1%
Cerebrovascular accident—transient ischemic attack	0.4%	0.6%
Myocardial infarction	0.4%	1.1%
Death	0.0%	1.7%

Reproduced from Procrit package insert with permission of Ortho Biotech Products.

a. Significant adverse events of concern in patients with chronic kidney disease treated in double-blind, placebo-controlled trials occurred in the percentages of patients shown during the blinded phase of the studies.

Darbepoetin

Mechanism of action

Darbepoetin has the same mechanism of action as epoetin.

Patient instructions

Counseling points are very similar for both darbepoetin and epoetin, except that all darbepoetin vials are single use only; therefore, the patient should dispose of the vial as instructed after each dose. Darbepoetin is also available in predrawn syringes.

Adverse drug effects

The most common adverse effects are as follows:

- **Cardiovascular:** Hypertension, hypotension, edema, arrhythmia
- **GI:** Nausea, vomiting, diarrhea, constipation
- **Central nervous system:** Fatigue, fever, headache
- **Neuromuscular or skeletal:** Myalgia, arthralgia, limb pain
- **Respiratory:** Infection, dyspnea, cough

Drug interactions

No drug interactions have been reported.

Monitoring parameters

- Monitor patient's iron stores before and during therapy.
- Monitor patient's blood pressure.

■ Adjust dose by closely monitoring Hgb every week until a maintenance dose is established. Target Hgb ≥ 10 g/dL. Increase dose if Hgb increases more than 1 g/dL over a 4-week period. Decrease dose by 25% if Hgb increases more than 1 g/dL over a 2-week period.

24-5 Nondrug Therapy

Iron Deficiency Anemia

Dietary supplementation plays an important role in IDA treatment:

■ Increase intake of iron-rich foods, such as meat, fish, and poultry.
■ Orange juice may improve iron absorption.
■ Avoid tea or milk with concurrent iron administration.

Folic Acid Deficiency Anemia

Dietary supplementation also is important in treating folic acid deficiency:

■ To get as much dietary folate as possible, do not overcook vegetables. Eat them raw, microwaved, or steamed.
■ Eat a wide variety of properly prepared vegetables and fruits.

NAPLEX Competency Statements

The questions in this chapter cover the following 2021 NAPLEX Competency Statements: **AREA 1:** 1.1; 1.2; 1.5 **AREA 2:** 2.1; 2.2; 2.3 **AREA 3:** 3.1; 3.2; 3.4; 3.5; 3.6; 3.7; 3.8; 3.9; 3.10; 3.11 **AREA 4:** 4.1; 4.2 **AREA 5:** 5.1.

24-6 Questions

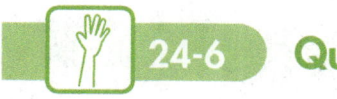

Use Patient Profile 24-1 to answer Question 1.

PATIENT PROFILE 24-1	
Patient: 62-year-old male	**Allergies:** NKDA
Weight: 193 lb	
Problem list	**OTC recommendations**
Gastroesophageal reflux disease	Maalox 1 tbsp every 2 hours as needed for "indigestion"
Iron deficiency anemia	Acetaminophen 325 mg every 4 to 6 hours as needed for headache
Hypertension	Famotidine 20 mg daily as needed for "heartburn"
Medication record	Docusate 100 mg daily for constipation
Ferrous sulfate 325 mg three times daily	
Hydrochlorothiazide 25 mg daily	

1. Which of the following medications could present a problem with this patient's iron supplement?

   A. Acetaminophen
   B. Famotidine
   C. Maalox
   D. Docusate
   E. Famotidine and Maalox

2. A patient admits to you that he is not able to take his iron tablet because it makes him nauseated. What advice can you give him?

   A. Take your iron with some crackers and milk.
   B. Take your iron with some crackers and water.
   C. Don't worry about it. It's only a vitamin.
   D. Start taking iron with the largest meal of the day.
   E. Take iron after breakfast.

3. If a patient's anemia progresses to severe stages, what effects may he experience? (Mark all that apply.)

   A. Koilonychia (spoon-shaped nails)
   B. Pica (e.g., craving ice, clay, chalk)
   C. Glossitis (sore, beefy red tongue)
   D. Extreme fatigue
   E. Constipation

4. If you were to examine a peripheral blood smear of a patient with iron deficiency anemia, you would find cells that are _____.

   A. microcytic and hypochromic
   B. macrocytic and hypochromic
   C. macrocytic and normochromic
   D. microcytic and normochromic
   E. macrocytic and megaloblastic

5. When one is examining iron study results of a patient with iron deficiency anemia, which of the following would be consistent with iron deficiency anemia?

   A. Elevated TIBC
   B. Elevated ferritin
   C. Elevated MCV
   D. Elevated Hgb
   E. Elevated Hct

6. Which iron preparation is most likely to cause an anaphylactic reaction?

   A. I.V. iron dextran
   B. I.V. iron sucrose
   C. I.V. sodium ferric gluconate
   D. Extended-release ferrous sulfate by mouth
   E. Immediate-release ferrous sulfate by mouth

7. Why are sustained-release (SR) preparations of iron *not* the ideal formulation?

   A. The incidence of nausea is higher with SR formulations.
   B. They are dosed only once daily, and goal Hgb levels are not attained.
   C. Because SR preparations are dissolved in the small intestines, the alkaline environment results in a lower bioavailability than in the acidic environment of the stomach.
   D. Dissolution in the small intestines is not bioavailable, because intrinsic factor is not present in the small intestines.
   E. SR preparations require dosing with food.

8. Which of the following options would you advise a patient to drink with meals to optimize iron absorption from meals?

   A. Orange juice
   B. Coffee
   C. Tea
   D. Milk
   E. Wine

9. The most likely regimen to supplement vitamin B_{12} is _____.

   A. 1000 mcg orally every month
   B. 1000 mcg I.V. every month
   C. 1000 mcg I.M. every month
   D. 1000 mcg I.M. every day
   E. 1000 mcg SQ every 2 months

10. To be absorbed, vitamin B_{12} requires which of the following?

    A. Pernicious factor
    B. Transcobalamin II
    C. Intrinsic factor
    D. Vitamin B_{12} absorption factor
    E. Hydrochloric acid

11. Which of the following patients probably have a diet that prevents folic acid deficiency?

    A. Strict vegetarians
    B. Alcoholics
    C. Indigents
    D. People who routinely overcook their vegetables
    E. College students whose diet consists of burgers and potato chips

12. Folic acid may interact with which of the following medications?

    A. Propranolol
    B. Propoxyphene
    C. Piroxicam
    D. Phenytoin
    E. Prednisone

13. The 2 macrocytic anemias are _____.

    A. vitamin B_{12} deficiency and iron deficiency anemias
    B. vitamin B_{12} deficiency and folic acid deficiency anemias
    C. iron deficiency and folic acid deficiency anemias
    D. sickle cell anemia and anemia of chronic kidney disease
    E. iron deficiency and pernicious anemias

14. The best regimen to replace folic acid is _____.

    A. folic acid 1 mg orally every day for 3 to 4 months
    B. folic acid 10 mg orally every day for 3 to 4 months
    C. folic acid 10 mg I.V. for 2 weeks, then 1 mg orally every day for 2 months
    D. folic acid 1 mg orally 3 times weekly for 3 to 4 months
    E. folic acid 1 mg orally once monthly for 6 months

15. The most common medication given to treat anemia of chronic kidney disease is _____.

    A. vitamin B_{12}
    B. a solution of citric acid in combination with sodium acetate
    C. epoetin alfa
    D. ferrous sulfate by mouth
    E. folic acid by mouth

16. What advantage does darbepoetin have over epoetin?

    A. Lower incidence of hypertension
    B. Fewer drug interactions
    C. Lower cost
    D. Longer half-life and less frequent administration
    E. Improved tolerability

17. The most common side effect of epoetin is _____.

    A. anaphylaxis
    B. hypertension
    C. pure red cell aplasia
    D. injection site reaction
    E. weight gain

18. Before initiation of epoetin therapy, which of the following should be evaluated?

    A. Folic acid and vitamin B_{12} levels
    B. Transferrin and ferritin levels
    C. EPO receptor level
    D. Presence or absence of intrinsic factor
    E. Stomach acid pH

19. Which of the following will be monitored when a patient starts epoetin therapy? (Mark all that apply.)

    A. Blood pressure
    B. Hematocrit
    C. Serum chemistries
    D. Iron profile

20. Which of the following medications is known to interact with epoetin?

    A. Insulin
    B. Simvastatin
    C. Atenolol
    D. Nephrocaps
    E. No medications are known to interact with epoetin.

PATIENT PROFILE 24-2. Central Dialysis Center

Patient: 44-year-old female

Weight: 148 lb

Diagnosis:

Hypertension

Diabetes mellitus

End-stage kidney disease

Hyperlipidemia

Labs:

Ferritin: 80 ng/mL (normal)

Transferrin saturation: 15% (low)

Hct: 32% (low)

Hgb: 8.6 g/dL (low)

Allergies: Penicillin (rash)

Dialysis schedule: Monday, Wednesday, Friday

Medications:

Insulin NPH 30 U twice daily

Simvastatin 20 mg nightly

Atenolol 25 mg after dialysis

Nephrocaps 1 capsule daily

Use Patient Profile 24-2 to answer Question 21.

21. What medication should be added to the patient's regimen?

   A. Oral propranolol
   B. I.V. iron
   C. Oral levothyroxine
   D. I.M. vitamin B$_{12}$
   E. Oral vitamin B$_6$

 **24-7**   **Answers**

1. E. Iron is best absorbed in an acidic environment; therefore, antacids dramatically decrease the absorption of iron. Iron supplements should be taken 1 hour before or 3 hours after antacids.

2. B. Many patients are not able to tolerate iron on an empty stomach. Those patients should take iron with a small snack. Milk would not be acceptable in this case, because dairy products decrease the absorption of iron.

3. A, B, C, D. Koilonychia, pica, extreme fatigue, and glossitis all are symptoms of severe iron deficiency anemia.

4. A. Iron deficiency produces a hypochromic (low-Hgb) anemia, given that iron is a component of the Hgb molecule. The cells also are microcytic (meaning "small cell"), because they spend a longer time in

the marrow awaiting proper Hgb synthesis and, therefore, divide more.

5. A. TIBC is elevated in IDA. TIBC is a measure of the amount of binding space left on transferrin (the transport protein of iron). Less iron in the blood means that more space is available on the transferrin molecule.

6. A. I.V. iron dextran has the highest incidence of anaphylaxis among the 5 I.V. iron preparations available.

7. C. SR preparations are left intact in the stomach and are dissolved in the small intestine. The alkaline environment of the small intestine tends to form insoluble iron complexes that cannot be absorbed.

8. A. Tea and milk can decrease the absorption of iron from a meal by more than 50%. Orange juice, however, can double the absorption of iron from food.

9. C. The most common I.M. dose of vitamin B$_{12}$ is 1000 mcg per month. However, vitamin B$_{12}$ may be supplemented by the oral route if absorption is not impaired. Additionally, it may be supplemented in very high doses, such as 1000 to 2000 mcg per day, in pernicious anemia.

10. C. Vitamin B$_{12}$ requires intrinsic factor for absorption.

11. A. Folic acid deficiency is found in alcoholics, indigents, and—rarely—people who routinely overcook their vegetables. Strict vegetarians do not develop folic acid deficiency because a folate-rich diet includes various types of vegetables.

12. D. Phenytoin increases the metabolism of folate, thereby decreasing the effectiveness of folic acid.

13. B. Both vitamin B_{12} deficiency anemia and folic acid deficiency anemia are macrocytic (large cell) anemias. Both iron deficiency anemia and sickle cell anemia are microcytic and hypochromic anemias.

14. A. Folic acid is administered orally because it is absorbed easily. The proper dose is 1 mg folic acid by mouth every day, and the deficiency should be corrected after 3 to 4 months.

15. C. Epoetin is the most common medication used to treat anemia of chronic kidney disease, because it stimulates erythropoiesis. The lack of EPO production is the primary cause of anemia of chronic kidney disease.

16. D. Darbepoetin is very similar to epoetin because it has the same mechanism of action and similar side effects. However, it has a longer half-life and can be administered less frequently.

17. B. Hypertension is the most common adverse drug effect from epoetin.

18. B. Transferrin and ferritin levels should be evaluated before epoetin therapy. IDA is a common problem in patients with end-stage kidney disease. The patient's transferrin should be at least 20% and ferritin should be at least 100 ng/mL before epoetin therapy is initiated.

19. A, B, C, D. Iron profiles need to be monitored before starting epoetin and periodically during therapy because IDA is very common in dialysis patients. Blood pressure needs to be monitored because increased blood pressure is the most common adverse effect of epoetin. Hct levels need to be checked as a measure of response to epoetin, and levels should be maintained at 30% to 36%. Serum chemistries need to be monitored regularly in any patient with end-stage kidney disease because most electrolytes are regulated by the kidneys.

20. E. No medications are known to interact with epoetin.

21. B. The patient's ferritin < 100 ng/mL, and her transferrin saturation < 20%. Most hemodialysis patients receiving epoetin need iron therapy at some point during their treatment.

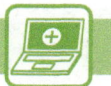 **24-8** ## Additional Resources

Alleyne M, Horne MK, Miller JL. Individualized treatment for iron deficiency anemia in adults. *Am J Med.* 2008;121(11): 943–948.

Kidney Disease: Improving Global Outcomes (KDIGO) Anemia Work Group. KDIGO clinical practice guidelines for anemia in chronic kidney disease. *Kidney Int Suppl.* 2012;2(4):279–335.

Krikorian S, Shafai G, Shamim K. Managing iron deficiency anemia of CKD with IV iron. *US Pharmacist.* 2013;38(8): 22–26.

Longo, D. Iron-deficiency anemia. *New Engl J Med.* 2015;372:1832–1843.

National Kidney Foundation. KDOQI clinical practice guideline and clinical practice recommendations for anemia in chronic kidney disease: 2007 update of hemoglobin target. *Am J Kidney Dis.* 2007;50(3):471–530.

National Kidney Foundation. KDIGO clinical practice guideline for anemia in chronic kidney disease. 2012. Available at: www.kidney.org/professionals/guidelines/guidelines_commentaries/anemia.

Unger EF, Thompson AM, Blank MJ, Temple R. Erythropoiesis-stimulating agents: time for a reevaluation. *New Engl J Med.* 2010;362:189–192.

Weiss G, Goodnough LT. Anemia of chronic disease. *New Engl J Med.* 2005;352:1011–1023.

Gastrointestinal Diseases

25

CHRISTA M. GEORGE

 25-1 KEY POINTS

- Peptic ulcer disease (PUD) is a group of disorders of the upper gastrointestinal (GI) tract characterized by ulcerative lesions that require acid and pepsin for their formation.
- The American College of Gastroenterology treatment guidelines for *Helicobacter pylori* eradication in PUD recommend initial therapy with one of several regimens consisting of combinations of antibiotics, proton pump inhibitors (PPIs), and bismuth subsalicylate.
- Treatment of PUD related to nonsteroidal anti-inflammatory (NSAID) use consists of discontinuing the NSAID and beginning therapy with a PPI or a histamine 2–receptor antagonist (H2RA) for 4 weeks.
- Gastroesophageal reflux disease (GERD) "should be defined as symptoms or complications resulting from the reflux of gastric contents into the esophagus or beyond, into the oral cavity (including larynx) or lung," according to The American College of Gastroenterology guidelines.
- For GERD, an 8-week course of once-daily PPI therapy is the treatment of choice for symptom relief and healing of erosive esophagitis in patients with typical symptoms.
- Idiopathic inflammatory bowel disease (IBD) is divided into 2 major types: ulcerative colitis and Crohn's disease.
- Treatment of IBD involves medications that target inflammatory mediators and alter immuno-inflammatory processes. These medications include anti-inflammatory, antimicrobial, immunosuppressive, and biologic agents.
- Surgery may be necessary for patients with severe ulcerative colitis or Crohn's disease.
- Irritable bowel syndrome (IBS) is abdominal pain or discomfort that occurs in association with altered bowel habits over a period of 3 months.
- Common symptoms include abdominal pain, diarrhea, and constipation.
- Numerous drugs may be used to treat IBS including anticholinergic and antimuscarinic agents, psyllium, calcium polycarbophil, polyethylene glycol, loperamide, tricyclic antidepressants, selective serotonin reuptake inhibitors, tegaserod, alosetron, lubiprostone, and linaclotide.
- Patients should be counseled on medication dosing and administration, importance of adherence to treatment regimens, side effects of medications, drug–drug interactions, monitoring of symptoms, proper nutrition (IBD), and lifestyle modifications (PUD, GERD).

 25-2 STUDY GUIDE CHECKLIST

The following topics may guide your study of PUD, GERD, IBD, and IBS:

- ☐ Definitions of PUD, GERD, ulcerative colitis, Crohn's disease, and IBS.
- ☐ Clinical signs and symptoms of PUD, GERD, ulcerative colitis, Crohn's disease, and IBS.
- ☐ Risk factors associated with NSAID-related ulcers and upper GI complications.
- ☐ Drug regimens used to eradicate *H. pylori* infection.
- ☐ For drugs used to treat PUD, GERD, ulcerative colitis, Crohn's disease, and IBS:
  - ○ Mechanism of action.
  - ○ Drug dosing frequency.
  - ○ Major adverse drug effects.
  - ○ Clinically significant drug–drug interactions.
  - ○ Major patient counseling points.
  - ○ Nonpharmacologic treatment of PUD, GERD, ulcerative colitis, Crohn's disease, and IBS.

25-3   Peptic Ulcer Disease Overview

Pathophysiology

Peptic ulcer disease (PUD) is a group of disorders of the upper gastrointestinal (GI) tract characterized by ulcerative lesions that depend on acid and pepsin for their formation. Duodenal ulcers result from the imbalance between duodenal acid load and the acid-buffering capacity of the duodenum. Duodenal ulcers are more frequently associated with an antrum-predominant gastritis.

H. pylori is a gram-negative microaerophilic bacterium that inhabits the area between the stomach's mucosal layer and epithelial cells. The bacteria can be found anywhere gastric epithelium is present. *H. pylori* causes duodenal inflammation, increases duodenal acid load, and impairs duodenal bicarbonate secretion, which leads to duodenal ulcers. It causes inflammation of gastric epithelium, particularly in the antrum-corpus area. The inflammation disrupts mucosal defense, which also leads to gastric ulcers.

NSAIDs are the leading cause of PUD in patients negative for *H. pylori* infection. They are directly toxic to gastric epithelium and inhibit the synthesis of prostaglandins. Inhibition of prostaglandin synthesis leads to decreased secretion of bicarbonate and mucus, decreased mucosal perfusion, decreased epithelial proliferation, and decreased mucosal resistance to injury.

NSAIDs may cause gastric (more frequently) or duodenal ulcers.

Clinical Presentation

Epigastric pain that occurs 1 to 3 hours after meals and is relieved by ingestion of food or antacids is the classic presentation of PUD. Pain typically occurs in episodes lasting weeks to months and may be followed by variable periods of spontaneous remission and recurrence.

Ten percent of patients with PUD present with complications and have no prior history of pain.

Classification

Ulcers are either duodenal or gastric in nature. Duodenal ulcers are more common.

The 3 common forms of duodenal and gastric ulcers are related to *Helicobacter pylori*, nonsteroidal anti-inflammatory drugs (NSAIDs), or stress.

Drug Therapy

The goals of PUD therapy include healing the ulcer and eliminating its cause. Additional considerations include preventing complications and relieving symptoms. Choice of PUD therapy is based on the etiology of the case. See Box 25-1: First-line recommendations for *H. pylori* eradication in PUD.

For *H. pylori*–related PUD, antibacterial therapy is used with antisecretory therapy:

Eradication of *H. pylori* reduces the recurrence of PUD and is of prime importance.

For NSAID-related PUD, discontinuation of the offending agent is imperative. Antisecretory therapy with a PPI, H2RA, or sucralfate should be administered for 4 weeks to promote healing and to relieve symptoms. If *H. pylori* is also present, antibacterial therapy should be initiated. Eradication of *H. pylori* does not prevent NSAID-related complications or recurrence.

PPIs, H2RAs, or misoprostol should be used to prevent PUD in patients who require chronic NSAIDs and who are at risk of developing PUD (e.g., patients who are elderly or who have concomitant cardiovascular disease, patients with a history of PUD, patients using high-dose NSAID therapy, and patients who concomitantly use corticosteroids or anticoagulants).

Sucralfate may also be used to aid in ulcer healing, but it requires multiple daily dosing and is associated with many significant drug interactions.

Non–*H. pylori*, non-NSAID-related PUD should be treated with antisecretory therapy.

BOX 25-1. First-Line Recommendations for *H. Pylori* Eradication In PUD

The American College of Gastroenterology treatment guidelines for *H. pylori* eradication in PUD recommend first-line therapy with any of the following regimens:

- *Clarithromycin triple:* PPI (standard or double-dose twice daily), clarithromycin (twice daily), and either **amoxicillin** twice daily or **metronidazole** 3 times daily for 14 days.

- *Bismuth quadruple:* PPI (standard dose twice daily), bismuth subcitrate or subsalicylate (4 times daily), tetracycline (4 times daily), and **metronidazole** (3 to 4 times daily) for 10 to 14 days.

- *Concomitant:* PPI (standard dose twice daily), clarithromycin (twice daily), **amoxicillin** (twice daily), and either **metronidazole** or tinidazole (twice daily) for 10 to 14 days.

- *Sequential:* PPI (standard dose twice daily) and **amoxicillin** (twice daily) for 5 to 7 days, followed by PPI (standard dose twice daily), clarithromycin (twice daily), and either **metronidazole** or tinidazole (twice daily) for 5 to 7 days.

- *Hybrid:* PPI (standard dose twice daily) and **amoxicillin** (twice daily) for 7 days, followed by PPI, **amoxicillin**, clarithromycin, and either **metronidazole** or tinidazole (all twice daily) for 7 days.

- *Levofloxacin triple:* PPI (standard dose twice daily), levofloxacin (daily), **amoxicillin** (twice daily) for 10 to 14 days.

- *Levofloxacin sequential:* PPI (standard or double dose twice daily) and **amoxicillin** (twice daily) for 5 to 7 days, followed by PPI (twice daily), **amoxicillin** (twice daily), levofloxacin (daily), and either **metronidazole** or tinidazole (twice daily) for 5 to 7 days.

Boldface indicates one of top 100 drugs for 2020 by prescription volume.

⚠ **Metronidazole** *DA BOXED WARNING*

Metronidazole has been shown to be carcinogenic in mice and rats. Unnecessary use of the drug should be avoided. Its use should be reserved only for conditions for which it is approved

Mechanism of action

PPIs suppress gastric acid secretion specifically by inhibiting the H^+-K^+-ATPase enzyme system of the secretory surface of the gastric parietal cell.

H2RAs suppress gastric acid secretion by reversibly blocking histamine 2–receptors on the surface of the gastric parietal cell.

Clarithromycin, **amoxicillin**, **metronidazole**, tetracycline, bismuth subsalicylate, and furazolidone exhibit antibacterial effects against *H. pylori.*

Nitazoxanide is an antiprotozoal agent that inhibits the growth of *Cryptosporidium parvum* and *Giardia lamblia.* It can be used in combination regimens to eliminate *H. pylori* infections.

When exposed to gastric acid, sucralfate forms a viscous adhesive that binds positively charged protein molecules in the ulcer crater, thus forming a protective barrier that protects against back-diffusion of hydrogen ions.

Misoprostol is a synthetic prostaglandin E1 analog that moderately inhibits acid secretion and enhances gastric mucosal defense.

See Table 25-1 for selected medications for PUD.

Common adverse effects

- Side effects occur in 15% to 20% of patients, but they are usually minor.
- PPIs and H2RAs are generally well tolerated, but headache, diarrhea, and nausea have been reported.

TABLE 25-1. Selected Medications Used in Treatment of Peptic Ulcer Disease

Generic name	Trade name	Classification	Dosage range and frequency	Dosage forms
Omeprazole	Prilosec	Proton pump inhibitor	20 to 40 mg daily	C, G
Omeprazole	Prilosec OTC	Proton pump inhibitor	20 mg daily × 14 days	T
Omeprazole + sodium bicarbonate	Zegerid	Proton pump inhibitor and antacid	20 to 40 mg daily	C, P
Omeprazole + sodium bicarbonate	Zegerid OTC	Proton pump inhibitor/ antacid	20 mg daily	C
Esomeprazole	Nexium	Proton pump inhibitor	20 to 40 mg daily	C, I.V., G
Lansoprazole	Prevacid, Prevacid SoluTab	Proton pump inhibitor	15 mg daily to 30 mg twice daily	C, ODT, L, ST
Lansoprazole	Prevacid 24 Hour	Proton pump inhibitor	15 mg daily	C
Dexlansoprazole	Dexilant	Proton pump inhibitor	30 to 60 mg daily	C
Rabeprazole	Aciphex	Proton pump inhibitor	10 to 20 mg daily	T
Pantoprazole	Protonix	Proton pump inhibitor	40 to 80 mg daily	T, G, I.V.
Cimetidine	Tagamet	H2RA	300 mg 4 times daily to 800 mg at bedtime	T, L, I.V.
Ranitidine	Zantac	H2RA	150 mg twice daily to 300 mg at bedtime	T, L, I.V., C, EfT
Nizatidine	Axid	H2RA	150 mg twice daily to 300 mg at bedtime	C, L, T
Famotidine	Pepcid	H2RA	20 mg twice daily to 40 mg at bedtime	T, C, P, I.V.
Clarithromycin	Biaxin	Antibacterial	500 mg twice daily × 10 to 14 days	T, G
Amoxicillin	Amoxil	Antibacterial	1 g twice × 10 to 14 days	C, P, CT
Metronidazole	Flagyl	Antibacterial	500 mg 3 times daily × 10 to 14 days	T, C, I.V.
Tetracycline	Various trade names	Antibacterial	500 mg 4 times daily × 10 to 14 days	C
Nitazoxanide	Alinia	Antiprotozoal	500 mg twice × 7 to 10 days	T, L
Sucralfate	Carafate	Cytoprotective	1 g 4 times daily	T, L
Misoprostol	Cytotec	Prostaglandin	200 mcg 4 times daily	T

Boldface indicates one of top 100 drugs for 2020 by prescription volume.
C, capsule; CT, chewable tablet; EfT, effervescent tablet; G, granules for oral suspension; I.V., intravenous; L, liquid; ODT, orally disintegrating tablet; P, powder for oral suspension; ST, SoluTab; T, tablet.

⚠ **Misoprostol** *FDA BOXED WARNING*

Misoprostol administration to women who are pregnant can cause birth defects, abortion, premature birth, or uterine rupture.

- PPIs may increase the risk of *Clostridium difficile*–associated diarrhea. Use the lowest effective dose for the shortest treatment duration possible.
- PPIs may increase incidences of osteoporosis-related fractures of the hip in patients who have at least 1 additional risk factor for hip fractures. The American College of Gastroenterology guidelines for the management of gastroesophageal reflux disease (GERD) state that patients with known osteoporosis and no other risk factors for hip fracture may remain on PPI therapy.
- PPIs may also lower magnesium levels when used chronically. Consider monitoring magnesium levels and using magnesium supplements in patients using PPIs for more than 3 months.
- Short-term use of PPIs may increase the risk of community-acquired pneumonia.
- Antibiotics may cause diarrhea, nausea, dysgeusia, rash, and monilial vaginitis.
- Bismuth subsalicylate may cause black, tarry stools.
- Constipation is the most common side effect of sucralfate.
- Nitazoxanide may cause nausea, vomiting, diarrhea, and headache.
- Diarrhea occurs in 10% to 30% of patients taking misoprostol. Abdominal cramping, nausea, flatulence, and headache may also occur.

Monitoring

Patients should monitor for the return of PUD symptoms and for the side effects of medications, as discussed in the earlier section.

Drug interactions

- **Omeprazole** inhibits the cytochrome P450 (CYP450) 2C19 enzyme, which decreases the elimination of **warfarin**, phenytoin, and diazepam. Some pharmacokinetic and pharmacodynamic studies show that concomitant use of **omeprazole** significantly reduces the ability of **clopidogrel** to inhibit platelet activity. This could be because **clopidogrel** is a prodrug that requires the CYP450 2C19 enzyme to be converted into its active form. Since the U.S. Food and Drug Administration (FDA) issued a warning in 2009 regarding this interaction, subsequent prospective studies have shown that concomitant PPI and **clopidogrel** therapy does not increase the incidence of cardiovascular events. The 2013 American College of Gastroenterology Guidelines for the Diagnosis and Management of Gastroesophageal Reflux Disease state that PPI therapy does not need to be altered in concomitant **clopidogrel** users.
- Lansoprazole has been reported to increase theophylline clearance by approximately 10%.
- PPIs and H2RAs may alter the bioavailability of drugs that require an acidic environment for absorption (e.g., ketoconazole, digoxin, iron).
- Cimetidine is a potent inhibitor of the CYP450 enzyme system, which decreases the elimination of numerous drugs (e.g., **warfarin**, theophylline, phenytoin).
- **Amoxicillin** may decrease the effectiveness of oral contraceptives.
- Clarithromycin is a potent inhibitor of the CYP450 enzyme system, which decreases the elimination of **warfarin**, digoxin, cyclosporine, carbamazepine, theophylline, and cisapride (no longer on the market; available for restricted special use only).
- Tetracycline may decrease the effectiveness of oral contraceptives. Antacids, iron products, and dairy products bind to tetracycline, decreasing its effectiveness. Tetracycline can also increase the therapeutic effect of **warfarin**. Tetracycline can increase or decrease lithium serum concentrations.
- **Metronidazole** produces a disulfiram-like reaction when ingested with alcohol and increases the therapeutic effect of **warfarin** and lithium.
- Sucralfate leads to the absorption of small amounts of aluminum, which may accumulate if given to patients with renal insufficiency (especially when combined with aluminum-containing antacids). Sucralfate also alters the absorption of numerous drugs, including **warfarin**, digoxin, phenytoin, ketoconazole, quinidine, and quinolones.

- Magnesium-containing antacids may increase the GI side effects of misoprostol.
- Disulfiram-like reactions have been reported with the concurrent ingestion of alcohol and furazolidone.

Patient counseling

- Educate patients about the importance of completing the entire course of therapy to ensure the eradication of *H. pylori* and to avoid bacterial resistance.
- PPIs should be taken before the first meal of the day (generally 30 to 60 minutes before).
- Lansoprazole and dexlansoprazole granules may be sprinkled onto applesauce for patients who have trouble swallowing pills. Lansoprazole orally disintegrating tablets should not be crushed or chewed. **Omeprazole** capsules should be swallowed whole. **Omeprazole** over-the-counter (OTC) tablets should not be crushed or chewed. Omeprazole–sodium bicarbonate capsules should be swallowed whole.
- If antacids are being used to control breakthrough symptoms, the dose should be taken no less than 1 to 2 hours before or after an H2RA is taken. H2RAs may be taken without regard to meals.
- **Amoxicillin**, clarithromycin, and **metronidazole** may be taken without regard to meals. Taking clarithromycin and metronidazole with meals, however, often reduces the incidence of stomach upset.
- Tetracycline is best taken on an empty stomach. Antacids, dairy products, or iron-containing products should be taken 2 hours before or after tetracycline.
- Nitazoxanide should be taken with food. The suspension should be shaken before administration.
- Sucralfate should be taken 1 hour before meals and at bedtime.
- Misoprostol should be taken with or after meals and at bedtime.

Nondrug Therapy

Patients should be counseled to decrease psychological stress and to discontinue drinking alcohol, smoking, taking NSAIDs, and ingesting food or beverages that may exacerbate PUD symptoms.

25-4   Gastroesophageal Reflux Disease Overview

Pathophysiology

The American College of Gastroenterology guidelines state that "GERD should be defined as symptoms or complications resulting from the reflux of gastric contents into the esophagus or beyond, into the oral cavity (including larynx) or lung." It may be further classified as "the presence of symptoms without erosions on endoscopic examination (nonerosive disease/NERD) or symptoms with erosions (ERD)."

The effortless movement of gastric contents into the esophagus is a physiologic process that occurs numerous times daily throughout life and does not produce symptoms. It occurs more frequently in patients with GERD.

The pathophysiology of GERD involves the prolonged contact of esophageal epithelium with refluxed gastric contents containing acid and pepsin. Prolonged contact between esophageal epithelium and gastric contents can overwhelm esophageal defense mechanisms and produce symptoms.

Higher-potency gastric refluxate may produce symptoms during times of esophageal contact of normal duration. The presence of refluxate in an esophagus with impaired defense mechanisms may also produce symptoms.

Esophageal defenses consist of the antireflux barrier, luminal clearance mechanisms, and tissue resistance:

- Components of the *antireflux barrier* are the lower esophageal sphincter (LES) and the diaphragm. The LES is a thickened ring of circular smooth muscle localized to the distal 2 to 3 cm of the esophagus. It is contracted at rest, thereby serving as a barrier to refluxate. The diaphragm encircles the LES and acts as a mechanical support, especially during physical exertion.
- *Luminal clearance mechanisms* include gravity, esophageal peristalsis, and salivary and esophageal gland secretions (which contain acid-neutralizing bicarbonate).
- The 3 areas of *tissue resistance* are preepithelial, epithelial, and postepithelial defense. Preepithelial and epithelial tissues limit the rate of diffusion of H+ between cell membranes. Postepithelial defense is provided by the blood supply, which removes hydrochloride and supplies oxygen, nutrients, and bicarbonate.

Clinical Presentation

Heartburn and regurgitation are the common characteristic symptoms of the typical reflux syndrome. *Heartburn* is defined as a burning sensation in the retrosternal area. *Regurgitation* is defined as the perception of flow of refluxed gastric content into the mouth or hypopharynx.

Symptoms usually occur shortly after having a meal, when reclining after a meal, or on lying down at bedtime. Symptoms often awaken patients from sleep. Symptoms are exacerbated by eating a large meal (especially a high-fat meal), by bending over, and occasionally by exercising.

Symptoms suggestive of complications from GERD (i.e., alarm symptoms) include continuous pain, dysphagia, odynophagia, bleeding, unexplained weight loss, and choking.

Symptom severity does not correlate with the degree of esophagitis present on endoscopy, but severity usually does correlate with the duration of reflux.

Classification

The manifestations of GERD are divided into esophageal and extraesophageal syndromes.

Esophageal syndromes

Esophageal syndromes comprise those that are only symptomatic in nature and those that are symptomatic with esophageal injury on endoscopy. Symptomatic syndromes include the typical reflux syndrome and the reflux chest pain syndrome:

- The *typical reflux syndrome* is defined by the presence of troublesome heartburn, regurgitation, or both. Patients may have other symptoms, such as epigastric pain or sleep disturbance.
- The *reflux chest pain syndrome* occurs when GERD causes chest pain that is similar to ischemic cardiac pain. This pain can occur without concurrent heartburn or regurgitation.

Symptomatic syndromes with esophageal injury include GERD complications such as reflux esophagitis, reflux stricture, Barrett's esophagus, and esophageal adenocarcinoma.

- *Reflux esophagitis* is characterized by visible breaks in the distal esophageal mucosa.
- A *reflux stricture* is defined as a persistent luminal narrowing of the esophagus caused by GERD.
- *Barrett's esophagus* occurs when esophageal squamous epithelium from the gastroesophageal junction is replaced with metaplastic columnar epithelium. It is a risk factor for the development of *esophageal adenocarcinoma*.

Extraesophageal syndromes

Extraesophageal syndromes include those syndromes that have established associations with GERD and those with proposed associations with GERD. Esophageal syndromes that have established associations with GERD include reflux cough syndrome, reflux laryngitis syndrome, reflux asthma syndrome, and reflux dental erosion syndrome. Esophageal syndromes that have proposed associations with GERD include pharyngitis, sinusitis, idiopathic pulmonary fibrosis, and recurrent otitis media.

Drug Therapy

Goals of therapy are to alleviate or eliminate symptoms, decrease frequency and duration of reflux, promote healing of the injured mucosa, and prevent the development of complications.

Therapy is aimed at increasing lower esophageal pressure, improving esophageal acid clearance and gastric emptying, protecting esophageal mucosa, decreasing the acidity of refluxate, and decreasing the amount of gastric contents being refluxed.

An 8-week course of once-daily PPI therapy is the treatment of choice for symptom relief and healing of erosive esophagitis in patients with typical symptoms. PPI therapy is associated with increased healing rates and decreased relapse rates of erosive esophagitis compared to H2RAs.

For patients who partially respond to PPI therapy, increasing the dose to twice daily or switching to a different PPI may provide additional symptom relief.

Maintenance PPI therapy should be given to patients who have symptoms when PPIs are discontinued and in patients with complications (e.g., erosive esophagitis, Barrett's esophagus) at the lowest effective dose. On-demand or intermittent therapy may also be used for maintenance.

H2RA therapy may be used as maintenance therapy in patients without erosive esophagitis if they experience symptom relief. Bedtime therapy with H2RAs may be added to daytime PPI therapy in patients with objectively confirmed nighttime reflux, but tachyphylaxis may develop after several weeks of use.

Prokinetic therapy with metoclopramide, baclofen, or both, should not be used in GERD patients without diagnostic evaluation.

See Table 25-2 for selected medications.

Mechanism of action

For information on H2RA and PPIs, see the section above on the treatment of PUD.

Antacids neutralize gastric acid (which increases LES tone) and inhibit the conversion of pepsinogen to pepsin, thus raising the pH of gastric contents. Antacids may be useful for the self-treatment of mild, infrequent heartburn.

TABLE 25-2. Selected Antacids and Absorbents

Generic name	Trade name	Classification	Dosage range and frequency	Dosage forms
Magnesium hydroxide	Milk of magnesia	Antacid	15 to 30 mL as needed	T, L
Aluminum hydroxide	Amphojel, ALternaGEL	Antacid	15 to 30 mL as needed	T, L
Magnesium hydroxide + aluminum hydroxide	Maalox	Antacid	15 to 30 mL as needed	T, L
Calcium carbonate	Tums, Titralac	Antacid	15 to 30 mL as needed	T, L
Alginic acid + aluminum hydroxide + magnesium hydroxide	Gaviscon	Absorbent + antacid	15 to 30 mL as needed; after meals	T, L

L, liquid; T, tablet.

Alginic acid reacts with sodium bicarbonate in saliva to form sodium alginate viscous solution, which floats on the surface of gastric contents. The solution acts as a barrier to protect the esophagus from the corrosive effects of gastric reflux.

Common Adverse Effects

- For information on H2RAs and PPIs, see the treatment of PUD section earlier on in this chapter.
- Magnesium-containing antacids frequently cause diarrhea. Aluminum-containing antacids frequently cause constipation and bind to phosphate in the gut, which can lead to bone demineralization. Antacids may also cause acid–base disturbances.
- Magnesium and aluminum toxicity may occur when used chronically in patients with renal insufficiency. Sodium bicarbonate may cause sodium overload, particularly in patients with hypertension, congestive heart failure, and chronic renal failure. It may also lead to systemic alkalosis. It should be used on a short-term basis, if at all.

Monitoring

Patients should monitor for the return of GERD symptoms and for the side effects of medications as discussed in the previous section.

Drug interactions

For information on H2RAs and PPIs, see the section above on the treatment of PUD.

When taken with antacids, the absorption and effectiveness of tetracycline, **ferrous sulfate**, and quinolones are reduced because the antacids form chelates with them. Antacids decrease the absorption of azoles and sucralfate by increasing gastric pH. Antacids increase urine pH, which decreases the renal clearance of quinidine. Antacids decrease the systemic absorption of digoxin and H2RAs when taken concomitantly with them. Large doses of antacid may decrease the absorption of phenytoin.

Digoxin and phenytoin serum concentrations should be monitored frequently when antacids are used concomitantly. Suspected adverse effects of antacids should be reported to a health care provider.

Patient counseling

For information on H2RA and PPIs, see the section above on the treatment of PUD.

Antacids and alginic acid are appropriate for the initial management of symptoms of GERD that are not troublesome to the patient (e.g., mild, infrequent heartburn). Symptoms persisting longer than 2 weeks require further evaluation and treatment with prescription medications.

Refrigeration of liquid antacids may aid in palatability. Chewable tablets may be more effective than liquids because of increased adherence of antacid and saliva to the distal esophagus. Antacids must be taken at least 2 hours apart from tetracyclines, iron, and digoxin. Antacids and quinolones should be taken 4 to 6 hours apart.

Alginic acid is effective for the relief of GERD symptoms, but no data indicate esophageal healing on endoscopy. Alginic acid is ineffective if the patient is in the supine position and must not be taken at bedtime.

Nondrug Therapy

- Weight loss should be recommended for GERD patients who are overweight or have had recent weight gain.
- Head-of-bed elevation and avoidance of meals 2 to 3 hours before bedtime should be recommended for patients with nocturnal GERD.

- The routine global elimination of food that may trigger GERD symptoms is not recommended. However, patients should avoid any food or beverage that triggers their own GERD symptoms (e.g., chocolate, caffeine, alcohol, acidic or spicy foods).
- Calcium channel blockers, beta blockers, nitrates, barbiturates, anticholinergics, and theophylline decrease LES pressure. Tetracyclines, NSAIDs, **aspirin**, bisphosphonates, iron, quinidine, and **potassium** chloride have direct irritant effects on the esophageal mucosa. The appropriateness of these drugs in patients with GERD should be evaluated on an individual patient basis.

Surgery is a treatment option for long-term therapy in GERD patients who desire to stop medical therapy, are noncompliant with medical therapy, have adverse effects from medical therapy, or have persistent symptoms caused by refractory GERD.

 **25-5**   # Inflammatory Bowel Disease Overview

Pathophysiology

Idiopathic inflammatory bowel disease (IBD) is divided into 2 major types:

- *Ulcerative colitis* is defined as a chronic mucosal inflammatory condition confined to the rectum and colon.
- *Crohn's disease* is defined as a transmural inflammation of the GI tract that can affect any part of the GI tract from mouth to anus.

The etiology of ulcerative colitis and Crohn's disease is unclear, but similar factors may contribute to both diseases. These factors include infectious agents, genetics, environmental factors, psychological factors, and immune factors. Major etiologic theories involve a combination of infectious and immunologic factors.

Ulcerative colitis is confined to the rectum and colon and affects only the mucosa and submucosa. The primary lesion of ulcerative colitis is a crypt abscess, which forms in the crypts of the mucosa. Crohn's disease most commonly affects the terminal ileum and involves extensive damage to the bowel wall.

Ulcerative colitis and Crohn's disease complications can be local or systemic (extraintestinal). Local complications of ulcerative colitis include hemorrhoids, anal fissures, and perirectal abscesses. Toxic megacolon can lead to perforation and is a major complication that affects 1% to 3% of patients with ulcerative colitis or Crohn's disease. Colonic strictures and hemorrhage may also occur. Small bowel strictures, obstruction, and fistulae are common in Crohn's disease.

Clinical Presentation

IBD is characterized by acute exacerbations of symptoms followed by periods of remission that are spontaneous or secondary to changes in medical therapy or concurrent illnesses.

Ulcerative colitis

The hallmark clinical symptom of ulcerative colitis is bloody diarrhea, which is often accompanied by rectal urgency and tenesmus (straining to empty an already empty bowel associated with pain and cramping).

The extent and severity of ulcerative colitis are determined by clinical and endoscopic findings. Clinical symptoms are categorized as mild, moderate, severe, and fulminant. Endoscopic findings are categorized as distal (limited to below the splenic flexure) or extensive (extending proximal to the splenic flexure).

- *Mild ulcerative colitis* is characterized by fewer than 4 stools per day with or without blood, without systemic disturbance, and with a normal erythrocyte sedimentation rate (ESR).

- *Moderate ulcerative colitis* is characterized by more than 4 stools per day with minimal signs of toxicity.
- *Severe ulcerative colitis* is characterized by more than 6 stools per day with blood, systemic disturbance (e.g., fever, tachycardia, anemia), and ESR greater than 30.
- *Fulminant ulcerative colitis* is characterized by more than 10 bowel movements per day, continuous bleeding, toxicity, abdominal tenderness and distension, blood transfusion requirement, and colonic dilation on abdominal plain films.

Crohn's disease

The hallmark symptoms of Crohn's disease are abdominal pain, diarrhea, and fatigue. Other symptoms that can occur at presentation include weight loss, fever, growth failure, anemia, recurrent fistulas, or extraintestinal manifestations. Extraintestinal symptoms include inflammation of the skin, joints, and eyes. Symptoms differ depending on the site and severity of inflammation:

- *Mild-to-moderately severe/low-risk Crohn's disease:* Patients are ambulatory and tolerate oral alimentation without dehydration, toxicity (fever, rigors, or prostration), abdominal tenderness, painful mass or obstruction, or weight loss >10%.
- *Moderate-to-severe/moderate-to-high-risk Crohn's disease:* Patients fail to respond to treatment for mild-to-moderate disease or have fever, weight loss, abdominal pain, nausea, vomiting (without obstruction), or anemia.
- *Severe/fulminant Crohn's disease:* Patients have persistent symptoms despite the outpatient use of steroids or biologic agents, or individuals present with high fever, persistent vomiting, evidence of obstruction, rebound tenderness, cachexia, or abscess.

Symptomatic remission occurs when a patient is asymptomatic or without any symptomatic inflammatory sequelae.

The ileum and colon are the most commonly affected sites. Ileitis may mimic appendicitis. Intestinal obstruction and inflammatory masses or abscesses may also develop. Patients with colonic Crohn's disease commonly have rectal bleeding, perianal lesions, and extraintestinal manifestations (e.g., spondyloarthritis, peripheral arthritis, erythema nodosum, pyoderma gangrenosum, uveitis, fatty liver, chronic active hepatitis, cirrhosis, primary sclerosing cholangitis, gallstones, cholangiocarcinoma, hypercoagulability).

Oral Crohn's disease is characterized by lesions ranging from a few aphthous ulcers to deep linear ulcers with edema and induration. Gastroduodenal involvement may mimic PUD.

Drug Therapy

Treatment of IBD involves medications that target inflammatory mediators and alter immuno-inflammatory processes. These medications include anti-inflammatory, antimicrobial, immunosuppressive, and biologic agents. See Table 25-3 for selected medications used in IBD.

Goals of therapy for ulcerative colitis (UC) and Crohn's disease include induction and maintenance of remission of symptoms, induction and maintenance of mucosal healing, improved quality of life, resolution of complications and systemic symptoms, and prevention of future complications. For patients with Crohn's disease, remission means that patients are asymptomatic or without inflammatory sequelae, including patients who have responded to medical intervention. Patients who require steroids to maintain their condition are considered steroid dependent, not in remission.

For mildly active UC, treatment options are as follows:

- Rectal 5-aminosalicylate preparations at a dose of 1 g/d should be used to induce remission and for maintenance of remission in patients with ulcerative proctitis.
- For left-sided UC, rectal 5-aminosalicylate enemas at a dose of 1 g/d may be used alone or in combination with oral 5-aminosalicylate at a dose of 2 g/d to induce remission.
- For extensive UC, oral 5-aminosalicylate at a dose of 2 g/d should be used to induce remission.

TABLE 25-3. Selected Medications Used in Treatment of Inflammatory Bowel Disease

Generic name	Trade name	Classification	Dosage range and frequency	Dosage forms
Sulfasalazine	Azulfidine	Aminosalicylate	4 to 6 g daily	T
Mesalamine	Asacol	Aminosalicylate	2.4 to 4.8 g daily	DT
Mesalamine	Pentasa	Aminosalicylate	2 to 4 g daily	DC
Mesalamine	Rowasa, Canasa	Aminosalicylate	1 to 4 g daily	EN, SU
Mesalamine	Lialda	Aminosalicylate	2.4 to 4.8 g daily	DT
Mesalamine	Canasa	Aminosalicylate	500 to 1000 mg daily	SU
Balsalazide	Colazal	Aminosalicylate	6.75 g daily	DC
Metronidazole	Flagyl	Antibacterial	10 to 20 g daily	T, I.V.
Ciprofloxacin ⚠	Cipro	Antibacterial	500 mg twice daily	T, I.V.
Prednisone	Various trade names	Corticosteroid	40 to 60 mg daily	T
Methylprednisolone	Solu-Medrol	Corticosteroid	60 mg daily	I.V.
Budesonide	Entocort EC	Corticosteroid	9 mg daily	C
Azathioprine ⚠	Imuran	Immunosuppressive	1 to 2.5 mg/kg daily	T, I.V.
6-mercaptopurine	Purinethol	Immunosuppressive	1.5 mg/kg daily	T
Methotrexate ⚠	Abitrexate	Antimetabolite	25 mg/wk	I.M., SQ
Infliximab ⚠	Remicade	Immunomodulator	Induction: 5 mg/kg at week 0, 2, and 6; maintenance: 5 mg/kg every 8 weeks	I.V.
Adalimumab ⚠	Humira	Immunomodulator	Induction: 160 mg as 4 injections over 1 to 2 days, then 80 mg 2 weeks later; maintenance: 40 mg every other week starting on day 29	SQ
Certolizumab pegol ⚠	Cimzia	Immunomodulator	Induction: 400 mg (given as 2 separate doses of 200 mg each) at week 0, 2, and 4; maintenance: 400 mg every 4 weeks	SQ
Natalizumab ⚠	Tysabri	Immunomodulator	300 mg over 1 hour every 4 weeks	I.V.
Golimumab ⚠	Symponi	Immunomodulator	200 mg at week 0; 100 mg at week 2; 100 mg every 4 weeks	SQ
Vedolizumab ⚠	Entyvio	Immunomodulator	300 mg over 30 min at week 0, 2, 6; then every 4 weeks; stop if no response by week 14	I.V.
Ustekinumab	Stelara	Immunomodulator	<55 kg: 260 mg x 1	I.V.
			55 to 85 kg: 390 mg x 1	SQ
			>85 kg: 520 mg x 1	
			Maintenance: 90 mg every 8 weeks	
Tofacitinib ⚠	Xeljanz	Janus kinase inhibitor	10 mg twice daily x 8 weeks	Oral
Cyclosporine ⚠	Neoral, Sandimmune	Immunosuppressive	4 mg/kg daily	I.V, C, L

Boldface indicates one of top 100 drugs for 2020 by prescription volume.
C, capsule; DC, delayed-release capsule; DT, delayed-release tablet; EN, enema; I.M., intramuscular; I.V., intravenous; L, liquid; SQ, subcutaneously; SU, suppository; T, tablet.

FDA BOXED WARNINGS

Ciprofloxacin

Fluoroquinolones, including ciprofloxacin, are associated with disabling and potentially irreversible serious adverse reactions that have occurred together, including tendinitis and tendon rupture, peripheral neuropathy, and CNS effects.

Azathioprine

Chronic immunosuppression with azathioprine, a purine antimetabolite increases risk of malignancy in humans. Reports of malignancy include post-transplant lymphoma and hepatosplenic T-cell lymphoma (HSTCL) in patients with inflammatory bowel disease. Physicians using this drug should be very familiar with this risk as well as with the mutagenic potential to both men and women and with possible hematologic toxicities. Physicians should inform patients of the risk of malignancy with azathioprine.

Methotrexate

Methotrexate can cause severe or fatal toxicities. Monitor closely and modify dose or discontinue for the following toxicities: bone marrow suppression, infection, renal, gastrointestinal, hepatic, pulmonary, hyper-sensitivity and dermatologic. Methotrexate can cause embryo-fetal toxicity and fetal death. Use in polyarticular juvenile idiopathic arthritis is contraindicated in pregnancy.

Hepatotoxicity, fibrosis, and cirrhosis may occur with prolonged use. Lung disease, including acute or chronic interstitial pneumonitis may occur, and has been reported at low doses. Diarrhea and ulcerative stomatitis require therapy interruption. Malignant lymphoma may occur.

Infliximab

Increased risk of serious infections leading to hospitalization or death, including tuberculosis (TB), bacterial sepsis, invasive fungal infections (such as histoplasmosis) and infections due to other opportunistic pathogens. Discontinue infliximab if a patient develops a serious infection. Lymphoma and other malignancies, some fatal, have been reported in children and adolescent patients treated with tumor necrosis factor (TNF) blockers, including infliximab. Postmarketing cases of fatal hepatosplenic T-cell lymphoma (HSTCL) have been reported in patients treated with TNF blockers including infliximab. Almost all had received azathioprine or 6-mercaptopurine concomitantly with a TNF-blocker at or prior to diagnosis. The majority of infliximab cases were reported in patients with Crohn's disease or ulcerative colitis, most of whom were adolescent or young adult males.

Adalimumab

Patients treated with adalimumab are at increased risk of infection, some of which may become serious and lead to hospitalization or death. These infections have included TB, invasive fungal infections, bacterial, viral, and those caused by opportunistic pathogens including Legionella and Listeria. Lymphoma and other malignancies, some fatal, have been reported in pediatric and adolescent patients treated with tumor necrosis factor (TNF) blockers such as adalimumab. Postmarketing cases of hepatosplenic T-cell lymphoma (HSTCL), usually fatal, have been reported in patients treated with TNF blockers including adalimumab, primarily in adolescent and young adult males with Crohn disease and ulcerative colitis. Most cases occurred in patients receiving concomitant treatment with azathioprine or 6-mercaptopurine.

Certolizumab pegol

Patients treated with certolizumab pegol are at increased risk for developing serious infections that may lead to hospitalization or death. Most patients who developed these infections were taking concomitant immuno-suppressants such as methotrexate or corticosteroids. Certolizumab pegol should be discontinued if a patient develops a serious infection or sepsis. Reported infections include:

- Active tuberculosis, including reactivation of latent tuberculosis. Patients with tuberculosis have frequently presented with disseminated or extrapulmonary disease. Patients should be tested for latent tuberculosis before certolizumab pegol use and during therapy. Treatment for latent infection should be initiated prior to certolizumab pegol use.
- Invasive fungal infections, including histoplasmosis, coccidioidomycosis, candidiasis, aspergillosis, blastomycosis, and pneumocystosis. Patients with histoplasmosis or other invasive fungal infections may present with disseminated, rather than localized disease. Antigen and antibody testing for histoplasmosis may be negative in some patients with active infection. Empiric anti-fungal therapy should be considered in patients at risk for invasive fungal infections who develop severe systemic illness.
- Bacterial, viral, and other infections due to opportunistic pathogens, including Legionella and Listeria.

(continued)

FDA BOXED WARNINGS (Continued)

The risks and benefits of treatment with certolizumab pegol should be carefully considered prior to initiating therapy in patients with chronic or recurrent infection. Patients should be closely monitored for the development of signs and symptoms of infection during and after treatment with certolizumab pegol, including the possible development of tuberculosis in patients who tested negative for latent tuberculosis infection prior to initiating therapy. Lymphoma and other malignancies, some fatal, have been reported in children and adolescent patients treated with TNF blockers, of which certolizumab pegol is a member. certolizumab pegol is not indicated for use in pediatric patients.

Natalizumab

Natalizumab increases the risk of progressive multifocal leukoencephalopathy (PML), an opportunistic viral infection of the brain that usually leads to death or severe disability. Because of the risk of PML, natalizumab is available only through a restricted distribution program called the TOUCH® Prescribing Program.

Golimumab

Serious infections leading to hospitalization or death including tuberculosis (TB), bacterial sepsis, invasive fungal (such as histoplasmosis), and other opportunistic infections have occurred in patients receiving golimumab. Lymphoma and other malignancies, some fatal, have been reported in children and adolescent patients treated with TNF blockers, of which golimumab is a member.

Tofacitinib

Serious infections leading to hospitalization or death, including tuberculosis and bacterial, invasive fungal, viral, and other opportunistic infections, have occurred. If a serious infection develops, interrupt tofacitinib until the infection is controlled.

Cyclosporine

Should be administered with adrenal corticosteroids but not with other immunosuppressive agents. Increased susceptibility to infection and the possible development of lymphoma may result from immunosuppression.

- Oral **budesonide** multimatrix (MMX) 9 mg/d may be added to therapy in patients who are intolerant of or nonresponsive to oral and rectal 5-aminosalicylate to induce remission in UC of any extent.
- Oral 5-aminosalicylate at a dose of 2 g/d should be used in left-sided or extensive UC to maintain remission.
- Systemic corticosteroids should not be used for the maintenance of remission.

For moderately to severely active UC, treatment options are as follows:

- Oral 5-aminosalicylate may be used to induce remission in moderately active UC only.
- Oral **budesonide** MMX 9 mg/d may also be used to induce remission. Once remission is achieved, **budesonide** should not be used for maintenance and should be tapered over 8 to 12 weeks.
- Thiopurines should be used for maintenance of remission in patients who achieved remission with corticosteroids.
- Infliximab, adalimumab, and golimumab may be used for induction of remission and for maintenance of remission once achieved.
- Infliximab should be combined with a thiopurine when used for the induction of remission.
- Vedolizumab may be used to induce remission, especially in patients who are intolerant of or nonresponders to infliximab, adalimumab, and golimumab. It may also be used as maintenance therapy.
- Oral tofacitinib 10 mg twice daily for 8 weeks may be used to induce remission, especially in patients who are intolerant of or nonresponders to infliximab, adalimumab, and golimumab. It may also be used as maintenance therapy.

For hospitalized patients with acute severe UC (ASUC), treatment options are as follows:

- Methylprednisolone 60 mg/d or hydrocortisone 100 mg 3 or 4 times daily should be used to induce remission.
- If the patient does not respond to I.V. corticosteroids after 3 to 5 days, rescue therapy with infliximab or cyclosporine should be used. Infliximab may also be used for maintenance therapy once remission is achieved.
- Thiopurines or vedolizumab may be used for maintenance therapy when remission is achieved with cyclosporine.

For mild-to-moderately severe Crohn's disease/low-risk disease, treatment options are as follows:

- Sulfasalazine may be used to treat colonic Crohn's disease.
- Oral mesalamine should not be used to treat active Crohn's disease as it is no more effective than placebo.
- Controlled ileal-release **budesonide** 9 mg daily should be given to induce remission in ileocecal Crohn's disease. It should not be used longer than 4 months.
- **Metronidazole** should not be used as primary therapy, though it may reduce recurrence of disease after surgery for Crohn's disease.
- Ciprofloxacin does not induce remission or heal mucosa in patients with active Crohn's disease. It may be used to treat abscesses and fistulas in patients with Crohn's disease.
- There is no role for antimycobacterial agents in the treatment of Crohn's disease.
- Some patients with mild, asymptomatic Crohn's disease may not require maintenance therapy.
- Thiopurines, infliximab, adalimumab, certolizumab pegol, vedolizumab, or ustekinumab may be used for maintenance therapy once remission is achieved. Natalizumab may be considered for maintenance therapy if the patient tests negative for the John Cunningham (JC) virus because of the risk of developing progressive multifocal leukoencephalopathy (PML).

For patients with moderate-to-severe Crohn's disease/moderate-to-high risk disease, treatment options are as follows:

- **Prednisone** 40 to 60 mg daily should be given short term to alleviate signs and symptoms.
- Steroids are not appropriate maintenance therapy and should be used sparingly in Crohn's disease.
- Azathioprine and 6-mercaptopurine (thiopurines) should not be used to induce remission as they are not more effective than placebo in this circumstance. They should be used to "spare" the use of steroids and for maintenance therapy once remission is achieved.
- Methotrexate I.M. or SQ may be used to reduce symptoms in steroid-dependent Crohn's disease and to maintain remission once it is achieved.
- Infliximab, adalimumab, and certolizumab pegol should be used in patients who do not respond to oral corticosteroids, thiopurines, or methotrexate.
- Combining infliximab and a thiopurine is more effective than either agent alone in patients without previous exposure to those agents.
- Natalizumab may be used to induce remission; however, it should only be used for maintenance of remission if the patient tests negative for antibodies to JC virus. This testing should be repeated every 6 months.
- Vedolizumab with or without a thiopurine agent should be considered for the induction of remission in Crohn's disease.
- Ustekinumab may be used in patients who do not respond to treatment with corticosteroids, thiopurines, methotrexate, vedolizumab, or natalizumab. It may also be used for patients who have not been exposed to therapy with vedolizumab or natalizumab.
- Thiopurines, infliximab, adalimumab, certolizumab pegol, vedolizumab, or ustekinumab may be used for maintenance therapy once remission is achieved. Natalizumab may be considered for maintenance therapy if the patient tests negative for the JC virus because of the risk of developing PML.

For severe/fulminant Crohn's disease, treatment options are as follows:

- I.V. methylprednisolone in doses of 40 to 60 mg/d should be administered.
- Infliximab, adalimumab, and certolizumab pegol may also be considered for severely active disease.
- In fulminant disease, infliximab may be more effective than adalimumab or certolizumab pegol.
- For perianal/fistulizing disease, treatment options are as follows:
  - Infliximab, adalimumab, certolizumab pegol, or thiopurines may be considered.
  - Tacrolimus may be used short-term for the treatment of perianal and cutaneous fistulas.
  - **Metronidazole**, ciprofloxacin, or levofloxacin may be effective in the treatment of simple fistulas.
  - Thiopurines, infliximab, adalimumab, certolizumab pegol, vedolizumab, or ustekinumab may be used for maintenance therapy once remission is achieved. Natalizumab may be considered for maintenance therapy if the patient tests negative for the JC virus because of the risk of developing PML.

Mechanism of action

Sulfasalazine is cleaved by bacteria in the gut to form sulfapyridine (excreted in the urine) and mesalamine (the active component). The sulfapyridine molecule is responsible for the many side effects associated with sulfasalazine.

Mesalamine's mechanism of action is poorly understood. Mesalamine inhibits cyclooxygenase and may also inhibit production of cyclooxygenase, thromboxane synthetase, platelet-activating factor synthetase, and interleukin-1 in macrophages. It may also act as a superoxide free-radical scavenger.

Corticosteroids have immunomodulatory effects and inhibit the production of cytokines and other inflammatory mediators.

Corticosteroids, azathioprine, 6-mercaptopurine, cyclosporine, and tacrolimus are immunosuppressive agents. For a full discussion of their mechanism of action, patient counseling, side effects, drug interactions, and pharmacokinetics, see Chapter 42 on solid organ transplantation.

The exact mechanism of action of **metronidazole** and ciprofloxacin in IBD is not known. One theory suggests that antibacterials interrupt the role of bacteria in the inflammatory process.

Methotrexate inhibits dihydrofolate reductase and purine synthesis, reduces the production of leukotriene-B$_4$ and interleukin-1 and -2, and may induce T-cell apoptosis.

Infliximab is a chimeric monoclonal antibody that inhibits human tumor necrosis factor (TNF), which inhibits subsequent cytokine-triggered inflammatory processes.

Adalimumab is a recombinant monoclonal antibody that inhibits human TNF, which inhibits subsequent cytokine-triggered inflammatory processes.

Certolizumab pegol is a PEGylated (polyethylene glycolated) humanized antibody Fab fragment of TNF monoclonal antibody. It inhibits human TNF activity, which inhibits subsequent cytokine-triggered inflammatory processes. PEGylation delays elimination and prolongs the half-life of the drug.

Natalizumab is a monoclonal antibody against the alpha-4 subunit of integrin molecules. It blocks the association of integrin with vascular receptors, which limits adhesion and transmigration of leukocytes.

Golimumab is a monoclonal antibody that inhibits human TNF, which inhibits subsequent cytokine-triggered inflammatory processes.

Vedolizumab is a humanized monoclonal antibody that binds to the $\alpha4\beta7$ integrin and blocks its interaction with MAdCAM-1 (mucosal vascular addressin cell adhesion molecule-1) and inhibits the migration of memory T-lymphocytes across the endothelium into inflamed GI parenchymal tissue.

Ustekinumab is an anti-p40 monoclonal antibody that inhibits the cytokines interleukin-12 and -23, which are involved in the inflammatory process.

Tofacitinib inhibits Janus kinase (JAK) enzymes, which are intracellular enzymes involved in stimulating hematopoiesis and immune cell function through a signaling pathway. This prevents cytokine- or growth factor-mediated gene expression and intracellular activity of immune cells.

Common Adverse Effects

- Sulfasalazine may cause nausea, vomiting, anorexia, and headaches. The sulfapyridine moiety leads to hypersensitivity reactions (e.g., rash, fever, agranulocytosis, pancreatitis, nephritis, hepatitis) and altered spermatogenesis in males.
- Mesalamine is better tolerated than sulfasalazine. Olsalazine may cause self-limited watery diarrhea. Balsalazide causes abdominal pain in 10% of patients.
- Ciprofloxacin may cause nausea, diarrhea, headache, and vaginal candidiasis.
- Methotrexate frequently causes nausea and leukopenia. Asymptomatic elevations in liver function tests may occur.
- Infliximab may cause infusion-related reactions, upper respiratory infections, headache, rash, cough, and stomach pain. Allergic reactions have been reported. Infliximab increases the risk of serious infections (bacterial [including tuberculosis and those caused by *Legionella* and *Listeria*], viral, and fungal infections) and certain types of cancer. New onset or exacerbation of preexisting heart failure, hepatotoxicity, neuropathy, anemia, and lupus-like syndrome have also been reported.
- Adalimumab may cause injection-site reactions, upper respiratory infections, headaches, rash, and nausea. Allergic reactions have been reported. Adalimumab increases the risk of serious infections (bacterial [including tuberculosis and those caused by *Legionella* and *Listeria*], viral, and fungal infections) and certain types of cancer. New onset or exacerbation of preexisting heart failure, neuropathy, anemia, and lupus-like syndrome have also been reported.
- Certolizumab pegol may cause injection-site reactions, upper respiratory tract infections, rash, and urinary tract infections. Allergic reactions have been reported. Certolizumab pegol increases the risk of serious infections (bacterial [including tuberculosis and those caused by *Legionella* and *Listeria*], viral, and fungal infections) and certain types of cancer. New onset or exacerbation of preexisting heart failure, neuropathy, anemia, and lupus-like syndrome have also been reported.
- Natalizumab increases the risk of developing progressive multifocal leukoencephalopathy. Serious allergic reactions (usually within 2 hours of infusion) and hepatotoxicity have been reported. Natalizumab increases the risk of serious infections (bacterial [including tuberculosis], viral, and fungal infections). Natalizumab may cause headache, arthralgia, nasopharyngitis, fatigue, nausea, hypersensitivity reactions, and increased AST (aspartate aminotransferase) and ALT (alanine aminotransferase). It also increases the risk of serious infections and progressive multifocal leukoencephalopathy.
- Golimumab may lead to the formation of antibodies to the drug, cause a positive antinuclear antibody (ANA) titer, and causes upper respiratory tract infections. Serious bacterial, fungal, and viral infections have been reported. Patients taking golimumab have a higher risk of developing malignancies.
- Vedolizumab may cause headache, arthralgias and nasopharyngitis and elevated liver function tests. Vedolizumab increases the risk of serious infections and the risk of developing progressive multifocal leukoencephalopathy. It may also cause infusion and hypersensitivity reactions.
- Ustekinumab may cause nasopharyngitis and gastrointestinal upset. It increases the risk of serious infections and the development of reversible posterior leukoencephalopathy syndrome. Hypersensitivity reactions have also been reported.
- Tofacitinib may cause nasopharyngitis and serious bacterial, fungal, and viral infections. Deep vein thrombosis, pulmonary embolism, and arterial thrombosis have been reported. Patients taking tofacitinib have a higher risk of developing malignancies.

Monitoring parameters

Serum chemistries, complete blood counts, liver function tests, blood glucose concentrations, ESR, response to therapy, and the presence of adverse effects should be monitored. Tuberculosis skin testing should be performed before administering biologic agents. Patients should be monitored for the development of serious infections.

Drug interactions

Sulfasalazine may decrease the bioavailability of digoxin by inhibiting its absorption.

Azathioprine is converted into 6-mercaptopurine in vivo; 6-mercaptopurine then undergoes hepatic first-pass metabolism, which is catalyzed by xanthene oxidase. By inhibiting xanthene oxidase, **allopurinol** increases the bioavailability of azathioprine. The azathioprine dose should be lowered by 25% to 50% when the 2 agents are used concurrently.

Ciprofloxacin binds with antacids, zinc, and iron products. It also increases the therapeutic effects of **warfarin**, cyclosporine, and theophylline.

Corticosteroids should not be administered with natalizumab because of the increased risk of serious infections.

The use of methotrexate and concurrent NSAIDs has caused fatal interactions. Methotrexate may increase levels of 6-mercaptopurine.

Infliximab should not be administered with etanercept or anakinra because of the increased risk of serious infections. Live vaccines should not be administered to patients taking infliximab.

Adalimumab should not be administered with anakinra because of the increased risk of serious infections. Live vaccines should not be administered to patients taking adalimumab. Methotrexate may decrease the clearance of adalimumab; however, this effect has not been shown to be clinically significant.

Certolizumab pegol should not be administered with anakinra, abatacept, rituximab, or natalizumab because of the increased risk of serious infections. Live vaccines should not be administered to patients taking certolizumab pegol. Certolizumab pegol may falsely elevate the activated partial thromboplastin time and the lupus anticoagulant assays.

Natalizumab should not be administered with other immunosuppressants, such as 6-mercaptopurine, azathioprine, cyclosporine, and methotrexate, or with TNF inhibitors because of the increased risk of progressive multifocal leukoencephalopathy.

The dietary supplement echinacea may decrease the effectiveness of infliximab, adalimumab, certolizumab pegol, natalizumab, golimumab and ustekinumab.

Golimumab should not be administered with other biologic agents. Live vaccines should not be administered to patients taking golimumab.

Vedolizumab should not be administered with natalizumab or other TNF-alpha inhibitors.

Ustekinumab should not be administered with infliximab or natalizumab. The reader is directed to the prescribing information for an extensive list of significant drug interactions.

Tofacitinib is a substrate of the cytochrome P450 3A4 enzyme system of the liver. It should not be used with strong inducers of this system. Dose reductions are required if the drug must be combined with strong inhibitors of this system.

Patient counseling

Sulfasalazine should be taken after meals. Patients should avoid sun exposure while taking it. **Folic acid** supplementation should be given during sulfasalazine treatment to avoid anemia. Sulfasalazine may cause orange discoloration of urine and skin.

Mesalamine tablets should be swallowed whole. Suppositories should not be handled excessively, and foil wrappers should be removed before insertion. Suspension enemas should be shaken well before use.

Antacids and ciprofloxacin should be taken 4 to 6 hours apart. Iron- or zinc-containing products should be taken 4 hours before or 2 hours after taking ciprofloxacin. Patients should avoid excessive exposure to sunlight.

Patients taking methotrexate should avoid alcohol, salicylates, and prolonged exposure to sunlight. Female patients of childbearing age should be counseled on appropriate contraceptive measures during methotrexate therapy.

Patients receiving therapy with infliximab should be counseled on the possibility of infusion reactions, delayed hypersensitivity reactions, and increased risk of infections. Live vaccines should not be administered to patients taking infliximab.

Patients taking adalimumab and certolizumab pegol should be counseled on the increased risk of infections and be instructed to report any symptoms of infection to their health care provider immediately. They should also be counseled on the potential for injection site reactions and be taught proper injection technique and proper sharps disposal. Live vaccines should not be administered to patients taking adalimumab and certolizumab pegol.

Patients taking natalizumab and vedolizumab should be counseled on the risk of acute hypersensitivity infusion reactions. They should also be counseled on the increased risk of infections, particularly progressive multifocal leukoencephalopathy. Patients should report symptoms of infection to their health care provider immediately. Live vaccines should not be administered to patients taking vedolizumab unless benefits outweigh risks.

Patients taking ustekinumab should be counseled on the risk of acute hypersensitivity infusion reactions and the risk of serious infections. They should report severe headache and mental status or vision changes to their physician because of the risk of posterior reversible encephalopathy syndrome. Live vaccines should be avoided in patients taking ustekinumab.

Patients taking tofacitinib should report signs and symptoms of infections and venous or arterial thromboembolism. Live vaccines should be avoided in patients taking tofacitinib.

Nondrug Therapy

Individuals should eliminate foods that exacerbate symptoms. Patients with lactase deficiency should avoid dairy products or take lactase supplements to avoid symptoms.

Enteral or parenteral supplementation may be used in patients with severe ulcerative colitis or Crohn's disease to maintain adequate nutritional status.

Surgery may be necessary for patients with severe ulcerative colitis or Crohn's disease. Surgery involves removing diseased segments of bowel, repairing fistulas, and draining abscesses. Options are as follows:

In UC, surgery is indicated for patients with severe colitis with or without toxic megacolon refractory to maximal medical therapy, less severe but intractable symptoms or intolerable medication side effects, exsanguinating hemorrhage, perforation, and documented or strongly suspected carcinoma.

Surgery is required in Crohn's disease patients with intractable hemorrhage, perforation, persisting or recurrent obstruction, abscess, dysplasia or cancer, or medically refractory disease.

Cigarette smoking worsens Crohn's disease and accelerates its recurrence. All patients who smoke should be counseled on smoking cessation.

NSAIDs may exacerbate Crohn's disease and should be avoided whenever possible.

The presence of stress, depression, and anxiety in patients with Crohn's disease should be assessed and managed to improve health-related quality of life and adherence to treatment recommendations.

 **25-6** **Irritable Bowel Syndrome Disease Overview**

Pathophysiology

Irritable bowel syndrome (IBS) is defined as abdominal pain or discomfort that occurs in association with altered bowel habits over a period of 3 months.

The pathogenesis is multifactorial and includes abnormal gut sensorimotor activity, central nervous system (CNS) dysfunction, psychological disturbances, genetic predisposition, enteric infection, and other intestinal luminal factors:

- Colonic motor abnormalities commonly occur in IBS. Patients with IBS may exhibit an exaggerated gastrocolonic response lasting up to 3 hours.
- Small intestinal motor patterns are frequently disturbed in patients with IBS. Small intestinal transit is delayed in constipation-predominant IBS and is accelerated in diarrhea-predominant IBS.

- Bloating may be the result of abnormal retrograde reflux of intestinal gas, enhanced perception of the presence of intestinal gas, or obstructive intestinal motor patterns.
- Motor dysfunction of other smooth muscles may occur in IBS. The following abnormalities may also be found: decreased LES pressures, abnormal esophageal body peristalsis, gastric slow-wave dysrhythmias, delayed gastric and gallbladder emptying, and dysfunction of the sphincter of Oddi.
- Eighty percent of patients with IBS exhibit psychiatric disturbances. The onset of psychiatric disturbances usually predates or occurs concurrently with the onset of IBS. Psychological stress triggers symptoms in many patients. IBS is also associated with a history of sexual abuse.
- Other factors that may contribute to IBS are alterations in gut flora (controversial), antecedent GI infection, carbohydrate malabsorption, food allergies, neurohumoral disturbances, genetic factors, and abnormal stool characteristics (low concentrations of bile or short-chain fatty acids).
- Relief of pain with defecation, looser stool with pain onset, more frequent stools with pain onset, and abdominal distention are significantly more common in IBS than in organic disease.

Clinical Presentation

IBS is a heterogeneous disorder with various clinical presentations:

- Abdominal pain is generally described as crampy or achy, and the intensity and location are highly variable. Pain may be exacerbated by meals and may last from 1 to 3 hours. Stress and emotional turmoil can also exacerbate pain.
- Patients typically present with diarrhea, constipation, or alternating periods of both.
- Upper GI symptoms (heartburn, dyspepsia, early satiety, nausea) occur more frequently in patients with constipation. Women experience abdominal distention, bloating, and nausea more often than men.
- Extraintestinal symptoms are common. They include genitourinary symptoms (e.g., pelvic pain, dysmenorrhea, dyspareunia, urinary frequency, nocturia, sensation of incomplete bladder evacuation), impaired sexual function (e.g., decreased libido), and musculoskeletal complaints (e.g., lower back pain, headaches, chronic fatigue).
- Alarm features include rectal bleeding, weight loss, iron deficiency anemia, nocturnal symptoms, family history of colorectal cancer, IBD, or celiac sprue. These symptoms may indicate the presence of an organic disease.

Classification

No symptom-based diagnostic criteria have ideal accuracy for diagnosing IBS. For this reason, two different sets of criteria are often used in combination. Once the diagnosis is made, IBS may be classified according to its predominant symptom: diarrhea predominant, constipation predominant, or mixed (symptoms may alternate). Symptoms may also be further categorized as mild, moderate, or severe.

Drug Therapy

Treatment should be offered to patients seeking medical care if the patient and health care provider believe that the IBS symptoms decrease the patient's quality of life. Goals of therapy include improving IBS symptoms and improving quality of life. The American Gastroenterological Association (AGA) published guidelines on the pharmacological management of IBS. Table 25-4 shows selected medications used to treat IBS.

Antispasmodic agents (e.g., hyoscyamine) significantly improve IBS-related global symptoms and modestly improve abdominal pain. The AGA suggests their use (over no treatment), but the recommendation is weak because of low-quality evidence.

TABLE 25-4. Selected Medications Used in Treatment of Irritable Bowel Syndrome

Generic name	Trade name	Classification	Dosage range and frequency	Dosage forms
Dicyclomine	Bentyl	Antispasmodic, anticholinergic	10 to 20 mg 4 times daily as needed	T, C, L
Hyoscyamine	Various trade names	Anticholinergic	0.25 to 0.5 mg twice daily to 4 times daily	T, L
Amitriptyline ⚠	Elavil	Tricyclic antidepressant	10 to 50 mg nightly	T
Tegaserod	Zelnorm	Serotonin (5-HT4) receptor antagonist	6 mg twice daily	T
Polyethylene glycol	Various trade names	Osmotic laxative	250 mL every 10 minutes up to 4 L	L
Alosetron ⚠	Lotronex	Serotonin (5-HT3) receptor antagonist	1 mg daily to twice daily	T
Lubiprostone	Amitiza	C-2 chloride channel activator	8 mcg twice daily	C
Loperamide ⚠	Imodium	Antidiarrheal	2 mg after each loose stool; maximum 16 mg daily	T, C, L
Diphenoxylate/ atropine	Lomotil	Antidiarrheal	15 to 20 mg daily of diphenoxylate in 3 to 4 divided doses	T, L
Linaclotide ⚠	Linzess	Guanylate cyclase-C agonist	290 mcg once daily	C
Eluxadoline	Viberzi	Mixed opioid receptor agonist/antagonist	100 mg twice daily (gallbladder present), 75 mg twice daily (gallbladder absent)[a], 75 mg twice daily (OATP1B1 inhibitors)[b]	T

Boldface indicates one of top 100 drugs for 2020 by prescription volume.
C, capsule; DT, delayed-release tablet; L, liquid; T, tablet; OATP, organic anion transport polypeptide.
a. The FDA issued a warning that eluxadoline should not be used in patients who do not have a gallbladder. This is because of 120 case reports of serious pancreatitis and 2 deaths in these patients.
b. Some examples are cyclosporine, gemfibrozil, atazanavir, lopinavir, ritonavir, saquinavir, tipranavir, rifampin, and eltrombopag.

The AGA suggests that polyethylene glycol be used (weak recommendation) for specific symptom relief or as adjunctive therapy (over no therapy) in patients with constipation-predominant IBS. The quality of evidence for its use specifically for constipation-predominant IBS is low. However, it is well tolerated and inexpensive.

Loperamide significantly decreases stool frequency in patients with diarrhea and other diseases. It has no effect on global IBS symptoms in patients with diarrhea-predominant IBS, though the quality of this evidence is low. The AGA suggests using loperamide (over no treatment; weak recommendation) as an adjunct to other therapies because of its low cost, wide availability, and low incidence of side effects.

Tegaserod improves global IBS symptoms, bloating, abdominal pain, and altered bowel habits in patients with constipation-predominant IBS. It was withdrawn from the U.S. market in March 2007 because of an increased incidence (0.11%) of cardiovascular events in patients taking the drug. It is available only through the FDA under an emergency investigational drug protocol.

Tricyclic antidepressants (TCAs) modestly improve global symptoms and abdominal pain in patients with IBS, though the quality of the evidence is low. The AGA suggests using TCAs (over no treatment; weak recommendation) because of their low cost. They should not be used in patients at risk for QT interval prolongation.

Alosetron improves global IBS symptoms in women with diarrhea-predominant IBS. Because of the incidence of colon ischemia and complicated constipation, alosetron is available only through a prescribing program regulated by the FDA and administered by the drug's manufacturer. It is approved for use

FDA BOXED WARNINGS

Amitriptyline

Antidepressants increased the risk compared to placebo of suicidal thinking and behavior (suicidality) in children, adolescents, and young adults in short-term studies of major depressive disorder (MDD) and other psychiatric disorders. Anyone considering the use of **amitriptyline** hydrochloride tablets or any other antidepressant in a child, adolescent, or young adult must balance this risk with the clinical need.

Alosetron

Infrequent but serious gastrointestinal adverse reactions have been reported with the use of alosetron hydrochloride. These events, including ischemic colitis and serious complications of constipation, have resulted in hospitalization, and rarely, blood transfusion, surgery, and death.

Loperamide

Cases of Torsades de Pointes, cardiac arrest, and death have been reported with the use of a higher than recommended dosages of loperamide hydrochloride. Loperamide hydrochloride is contraindicated in pediatric patients less than 2 years of age. Avoid loperamide hydrochloride dosages higher than recommended in adults and pediatric patients 2 years of age and older due to the risk of serious cardiac adverse reactions.

Linaclotide

Contraindicated in pediatric patients up less than 6 years of age; in nonclinical studies in neonatal mice, administration of a single, clinically relevant adult oral dose of linaclotide caused deaths due to dehydration. Avoid use of linaclotide in pediatric patients 6 to less than 18 years of age. The safety and efficacy of linaclotide has not been established in pediatric patients under 18 years of age.

---

only in women with chronic, severe, diarrhea-predominant IBS who do not respond to other therapies. The AGA suggests using alosetron (over no treatment; weak recommendation) on the basis of moderate-quality evidence.

Lubiprostone has been shown to relieve global IBS symptoms in women with constipation-predominant IBS. The AGA suggests using lubiprostone (over no treatment; weak recommendation) on the basis of moderate-quality evidence.

Linaclotide improves global IBS symptoms, reduces abdominal pain, and increases the number of spontaneous bowel movements in patients with constipation-predominant IBS. The AGA suggests using linaclotide (over no treatment; strong recommendation) on the basis of high-quality evidence.

Eluxadoline reduces abdominal pain and improves stool consistency in diarrhea-predominant IBS.

The AGA suggests against (weak recommendation) using selective serotonin reuptake inhibitors (SSRIs) to treat IBS because of the lack of improvement in global IBS symptoms and abdominal pain, though the quality of the evidence is low.

Mechanism of action

The antispasmodic agent dicyclomine decreases GI motility by relaxing smooth muscle in the gut.

Hyoscyamine is an anticholinergic agent that decreases GI motility by decreasing smooth muscle tone through antimuscarinic activity in the gut.

Tricyclic antidepressants (TCAs), such as **amitriptyline**, delay intestinal transit and may blunt perception of visceral distention. The effect of TCAs on the cerebral processing of visceral pain is unknown.

Tegaserod maleate, a partial 5-hydroxytryptamine (HT)4 agonist that stimulates the peristaltic reflex and intestinal secretion, inhibits visceral sensitivity by binding to 5-HT4 receptors in the gut.

Polyethylene glycol solutions are osmotic laxatives that aid in the treatment of IBS patients with constipation.

Loperamide inhibits peristalsis by directly affecting the circular and longitudinal muscles of the intestinal wall.

Diphenoxylate is a meperidine congener that directly affects the circular smooth muscle in the gut, which slows GI transit time.

Alosetron is a selective 5-HT3 receptor antagonist that inhibits activation of nonselective cation channels in the gut, thereby modulating the enteric nervous system.

Lubiprostone is the only C-2 chloride channel activator available. By activating C-2 chloride channels in the gut, lubiprostone increases secretion of saltwater into the intestinal lumen. It is approved only for women with constipation-dependent IBS.

Linaclotide is a guanylate cyclase-C (GC-C) agonist. It binds to GC-C in the luminal surface of intestinal epithelium. This increases intra- and extracellular levels of cyclic guanosine monophosphate (cGMP). The increase in cGMP stimulates the secretion of chloride and bicarbonate in the intestinal lumen, causing an increase in intestinal fluid and faster transit time.

Eluxadoline is a mu-opioid receptor agonist and delta-opioid receptor antagonist. By stimulating mu-opioid receptors in the GI tract, eluxadoline leads to decreased muscle contractility, inhibition of water and electrolyte secretion, and increased rectal sphincter tone. Antagonism of delta-opioid receptors in the gut may reduce the risk of iatrogenic constipation and abdominal pain.

Common Adverse Effects

Dicyclomine, hyoscyamine, and TCAs may cause anticholinergic side effects (CNS depression, dry mouth, urinary retention, constipation, decreased sweating).

Tegaserod may cause diarrhea, nausea, headache, and abdominal pain. It was associated with an increased risk of cardiovascular events in clinical trials.

Osmotic laxatives may cause abdominal pain and cramping.

Alosetron may cause constipation, abdominal pain, and nausea. Intestinal obstruction, perforation, toxic megacolon, ischemic colitis, and death have occurred.

Lubiprostone's most common side effects are nausea, diarrhea, and headache. Allergic reactions and dyspnea within 1 hour of the first dose have also been reported. Though dyspnea may recur with repeated doses, it usually resolves within 3 hours.

Linaclotide causes diarrhea in 20% of patients. Loose stools may occur more frequently if the drug is given with a high-fat breakfast. Abdominal pain, flatulence, upper respiratory infection, abdominal distention, and sinusitis have also been reported.

Eluxadoline may cause dizziness, drowsiness, nausea, vomiting, abdominal pain, and upper respiratory symptoms. It may also cause mild elevations in ALT and AST.

Monitoring

Patients should monitor for the presence of IBS symptoms and for the side effects of medications, as discussed in the section on adverse drug effects.

Drug Interactions

Anticholinergics and antispasmodics may decrease the effectiveness of antipsychotic medications. Side effects from anticholinergics are increased when they are given concurrently with a TCA.

TCA concentrations may be increased or decreased by medications that induce or inhibit the activity of the CYP450 enzyme system in the liver. TCAs should not be given concurrently with monoamine oxidase inhibitors or sympathomimetic agents.

Other medications should not be taken within 1 hour of the start of therapy with osmotic laxatives.

The levels of alosetron may be decreased by concurrent administration of rifamycin derivatives. No significant drug interactions have been reported with tegaserod, lubiprostone, linaclotide, or eluxadoline.

Patient counseling

Antispasmodics and anticholinergic agents are best used on an as-needed basis up to 3 times per day during acute attacks or before meals when postprandial symptoms are present.

Patients taking a TCA should avoid prolonged exposure to sunlight and avoid concurrent use of CNS depressants.

Tegaserod should be taken 30 minutes before meals and should not be initiated during an acute exacerbation of IBS. It is available only through an emergency investigational drug protocol from the FDA.

Osmotic laxatives should be used on an as-needed basis. Patients should drink plenty of water.

Patients must be enrolled in the manufacturer's prescribing program to receive alosetron. Patients should not initiate therapy with alosetron if they are currently constipated. Alosetron should be discontinued if no improvement in symptoms is seen after 4 weeks of therapy.

Lubiprostone should be taken with food and water. Softgel capsules should be swallowed whole.

Linaclotide should be taken on an empty stomach at least 30 minutes before breakfast. Capsules should be swallowed whole. They should not be broken or chewed.

Eluxadoline should be taken with food. Patients should avoid chronic or acute excessive alcohol consumption to reduce the risk of pancreatitis.

Nondrug Therapy

An effective health care provider–patient relationship is necessary for successful treatment. Education should be provided regarding disease pathophysiology and treatment, and the patient should be reassured that the symptoms are real.

Although evidence supporting exclusion diets is lacking, patients may be counseled to avoid foods that exacerbate IBS symptoms. Foods commonly implicated are fatty foods, beans, gas-producing foods, alcohol, caffeine, lactose (in lactase-deficient individuals), and occasionally excess fiber.

Cognitive behavioral therapy, dynamic psychotherapy, and hypnotherapy are more effective than usual care in relieving global symptoms of IBS. Although the quality of the evidence regarding such therapy is low, the potential benefit outweighs the potential risks.

25-7   Pharmacist's Role

The pharmacist should use the Pharmacist Patient Care Process to aid in the selection, initiation, and monitoring of pharmacotherapy for gastrointestinal diseases. First, the pharmacist should collect all relevant information from the patient and any available medical records that pertain to gastrointestinal disease symptoms, medical history, and current medication use (including allergies). The pharmacist can then make an assessment and recommendation to the patient or another provider on the best course of treatment (e.g., nonprescription medications for GERD vs. referral to a physician) for the particular symptoms reported. The pharmacist should then collaborate with health care providers to develop a treatment plan and work with the patient and/or caregiver to implement the treatment plan. The pharmacist should then follow up with the patient to monitor and evaluate the plan and make recommendations for adjusting the treatment plan when necessary.

NAPLEX Competency Statements

The questions in this chapter cover the following 2021 NAPLEX Competency Statements: **AREA 1:** 1.1; 1.2; 1.4; 1.5; 1.6 **AREA 2:** 2.1; 2.2 **AREA 3:** 3.2; 3.4; 3.5; 3.6; 3.7; 3.8.

25-8   Questions

Use the following case to answer Questions 1 and 2.

A 59-year-old African American male was recently diagnosed with peptic ulcer disease on endoscopy. Tissue biopsy is positive for *H. pylori*. He has no known drug allergies and denies previous exposure to macrolide antibiotics.

1. Which of the following is the ideal therapeutic regimen for *H. pylori*–related PUD in this case?

   A. Proton pump inhibitor, clarithromycin, amoxicillin
   B. Proton pump inhibitor, bismuth, tetracycline
   C. Omeprazole, amoxicillin
   D. Omeprazole, bismuth, clarithromycin, furazolidone
   E. Omeprazole, sucralfate, clarithromycin, furazolidone

2. If the patient is allergic to penicillin, which of the following treatment recommendations would you choose?

   A. Proton pump inhibitor, clarithromycin, amoxicillin
   B. Proton pump inhibitor, bismuth, metronidazole, tetracycline
   C. Omeprazole, metronidazole
   D. Clarithromycin, metronidazole, tetracycline
   E. Clarithromycin, metronidazole, furazolidone

3. Which of the following is the leading cause of peptic ulcer disease in *H. pylori*–negative patients?

   A. Mineralocorticoids
   B. NSAIDs
   C. Disease-modifying antirheumatic drugs
   D. Antibiotics
   E. Corticosteroids

4. Which of the following are true of NSAIDs? (Mark all that apply.)

   A. They inhibit production of prostaglandins.
   B. They are directly toxic to gastroduodenal epithelium.
   C. They require dose adjustments in renal insufficiency.
   D. They cause only gastric ulcers.
   E. They allow healing of peptic ulcer during continued therapy.

5. Which of the following are goals of therapy for peptic ulcer disease? (Mark all that apply.)

   A. Reduce episodes of diarrhea
   B. Eliminate symptoms
   C. Reduce risk of gastric cancer
   D. Heal ulcerations
   E. Avoid spreading *H. pylori*

Use the following case to answer Questions 6 and 7.

A 45-year-old White female with a past medical history significant only for seizure disorder has experienced heartburn after meals intermittently for the past 2 weeks. It becomes worse when she is reclining at bedtime. Her medications include phenytoin 300 mg at bedtime. She says that her symptoms are not troublesome and that she is going to self-treat with OTC medications.

6. Which of the following should *not* be recommended for this patient?

   A. Aluminum hydroxide
   B. Cimetidine
   C. Famotidine
   D. Ranitidine
   E. Magnesium hydroxide

7. The patient's symptoms are not relieved after 2 weeks of OTC treatment with famotidine and lifestyle modifications. She states her symptoms are becoming "troublesome." Which of the following is the best choice?

   A. Add the prokinetic agent metoclopramide to famotidine.
   B. Endoscopy should be performed because she has symptoms suggestive of complications from GERD.
   C. Add alginic acid 2 tablets nightly to famotidine.
   D. Discontinue current therapy, and initiate therapy with omeprazole 20 mg daily.
   E. Continue famotidine for 1 more week to achieve maximum effectiveness.

8. Which of the following are the most common symptoms of the typical esophageal GERD syndrome? (Mark all that apply.)

   A. Heartburn
   B. Belching
   C. Regurgitation
   D. Hypersalivation
   E. Hoarseness

9. Which of the following diagnoses carries an increased risk for developing esophageal adenocarcinoma?

   A. Typical reflux syndrome
   B. Reflux cough syndrome
   C. Reflux laryngitis
   D. Nontroublesome symptoms of GERD
   E. Barrett's esophagus

10. Which of the following may exacerbate GERD symptoms by lowering the lower esophageal sphincter pressure?

    A. Quinidine
    B. Iron
    C. Potassium chloride
    D. Diltiazem
    E. Tetracycline

11. Which of the following is the best choice for the initial treatment of troublesome symptoms of the typical reflux syndrome?

    A. Nizatidine 75 mg daily
    B. Pantoprazole 40 mg daily
    C. Metoclopramide 10 mg 4 times daily
    D. A 3-month trial of lifestyle modifications
    E. Pantoprazole 40 mg daily with metoclopramide 10 mg 4 times daily

12. A 32-year-old White male is diagnosed with mildly active, left-sided ulcerative colitis. Which of the following is the best choice to induce remission in him?

    A. Azathioprine 1 to 2.5 mg/kg/d
    B. Tofacitinib 10 mg twice daily
    C. Mesalamine 1 g rectally nightly
    D. Infliximab 5 mg/kg I.V. at 0, 2, and 6 weeks
    E. Methylprednisolone 16 mg I.V. every 8 hours

13. A 41-year-old Black female is diagnosed with moderately-to-severely active ulcerative colitis. She is going to be treated with infliximab 5 mg/kg at 0, 2, and 6 weeks for induction. Which one of the following should be added to her infliximab therapy?

    A. Add methotrexate 25 mg SQ weekly
    B. Add azathioprine 1 to 2.5 mg/kg daily
    C. Add methylprednisolone 16 mg I.V. every 8 hours until remission is achieved
    D. Add ciprofloxacin 500 mg orally twice a day
    E. Add vedolizumab 300 mg at 0, 2, and 6 weeks

14. Which of the following are true for ulcerative colitis? (Mark all that apply.)

    A. Vedolizumab may be used to induce remission in moderately-to-severely active disease.
    B. Oral corticosteroids are the drugs of choice for maintenance therapy.
    C. Thiopurines should be used for maintenance of remission in patients who achieved remission with corticosteroids.
    D. Topical aminosalicylates are the drugs of choice for severe/fulminant disease.
    E. Metronidazole is alternative first-line therapy for moderately-to-severely active disease.

15. Which of the following is true for mild-to-moderately severe Crohn's disease? (Mark all that apply.)

    A. Some patients with only mild symptoms may not require drug therapy.
    B. Oral sulfasalazine may be used for the treatment of mildly-to-moderately severe colonic Crohn's disease.
    C. Ciprofloxacin may be used to induce remission.
    D. Topical mesalamine preparations are the mainstay of therapy.
    E. Vedolizumab is the drug of choice to induce remission.

16. Which of the following is associated with the development of progressive multifocal leukoencephalopathy?

    A. Prednisone
    B. Sulfasalazine
    C. Mesalamine
    D. Methotrexate
    E. Natalizumab

17. A 39-year-old female presents with mild abdominal pain and diarrhea for 12 weeks. She has no significant past medical history and occasionally takes days off from her full-time job. Her symptoms are worse after meals. Which of the following is the best choice for initial therapy?

    A. Paroxetine 10 mg daily
    B. Amitriptyline 10 mg at bedtime
    C. Tegaserod 6 mg twice daily
    D. Alosetron 1 mg daily
    E. Dicyclomine 10 mg 4 times daily after meals

18. A 39-year-old female presents with mild abdominal pain and diarrhea for 12 weeks. She has no significant past medical history and occasionally takes days off from her full-time job. Her symptoms are worse after meals. Her symptoms are controlled for several months until she loses her job. Her abdominal pain then returns. She has five episodes of diarrhea per day and complains of fatigue and insomnia. Which of the following are the most appropriate for this patient? (Mark all that apply.)

    A. Initiate psychological counseling.
    B. Prescribe amitriptyline 10 to 50 mg at bedtime.
    C. Add loperamide 2 mg after each loose stool (16 mg/d maximum).
    D. Add alosetron 1 mg daily.
    E. Start tegaserod 6 mg twice daily.

19. Which of the following is indicated for constipation-predominant IBS?

    A. Tegaserod 6 mg twice daily
    B. Alosetron 1 mg twice daily
    C. Loperamide 2 to 16 mg/d
    D. Paroxetine 10 to 40 mg daily
    E. Diphenoxylate + atropine 2 tabs 4 times daily

20. Which of the following is affected by medications that induce or inhibit the cytochrome P450 enzyme system?

    A. Tegaserod
    B. Alosetron
    C. Fibercon
    D. Polyethylene glycol
    E. Amitriptyline

21. Which life-threatening complication caused the restriction of alosetron?

    A. Stevens–Johnson syndrome
    B. Toxic epidermal necrolysis
    C. Aplastic anemia
    D. Ischemic colitis
    E. Chronic diarrhea

22. Alosetron is indicated for which group of IBS patients?

    A. Women with diarrhea-predominant IBS
    B. Men with diarrhea-predominant IBS
    C. Women with constipation-predominant IBS
    D. Men with constipation-predominant IBS
    E. Children with diarrhea-predominant IBS

 25-9   **Answers**

1. **A.** Clarithromycin-based, triple-drug regimen with a PPI, clarithromycin, and either amoxicillin or metronidazole is one of several first-line regimens recommended by the American Gastroenterological Association for the treatment of PUD caused by *H. pylori*. PPI, bismuth, and tetracycline is not a recommended treatment regimen. Two-drug regimens are less effective and are not recommended. Furazolidone is unavailable in the United States.

2. **B.** The patient is allergic to penicillin; therefore, amoxicillin cannot be used. Two-drug regimens are less effective and not recommended. Antisecretory therapy is an integral part of *H. pylori* regimens to promote ulcer healing. Furazolidone is unavailable in the United States.

3. **B.** NSAIDs are the leading cause of PUD in patients who are negative for *H. pylori* infection.

4. **A, B, C.** NSAIDs inhibit production of prostaglandins and are directly toxic to gastroduodenal epithelium. NSAIDs require dose adjustments in renal insufficiency. NSAIDs may cause gastric or duodenal ulcers and must be discontinued to allow for ulcer healing.

5. **B, D.** Elimination of symptoms and healing of ulcerations are goals of therapy for PUD.

6. **B.** Cimetidine is a potent inhibitor of the cytochrome P450 enzyme system and will increase serum concentrations of phenytoin in this patient.

7. **D.** Prokinetic agents are useful mainly in patients with concurrent gastric motility disorders and are not routinely recommended. She does not currently exhibit symptoms of GERD complications. Alginic acid is ineffective when the patient is lying in the supine position and should not be given at bedtime. Nonprescription medications for GERD should be discontinued if symptoms are not relieved after a 2-week trial.

8. **A, C.** Heartburn and regurgitation are the most common symptoms of the typical reflux syndrome.

9. **E.** Patients with Barrett's esophagus have an increased risk of developing esophageal adenocarcinoma.

10. **D.** Calcium channel blockers decrease LES pressure. Quinidine, iron, potassium chloride, and tetracycline have direct irritant effects on the esophageal mucosa.

11. **B.** The correct dose of nizatidine (prescription strength) would be 150 mg twice daily. Metoclopramide is not routinely recommended for the treatment of the typical reflux syndrome. When patients find their symptoms "troublesome," pharmacologic therapy should be initiated.

12. **C.** For left-sided UC, rectal 5-aminosalicylate enemas at a dose of 1 g/d may be used alone or in combination with oral 5-aminosalicylate at a dose of 2 g/d to induce remission. Azathioprine (A), tofacitinib (B), and infliximab are not indicated in mildly active UC. Methylprednisolone (E) is indicated for acute severe UC in hospitalized patients.

13. **B.** A thiopurine should be added to infliximab induction therapy because combination therapy is more effective than either agent alone for moderately-to-severely active ulcerative colitis. Methotrexate (A) is not effective for inducing remission in moderately-to-severely active ulcerative colitis. Methylprednisolone (C) is indicated for acute severe ulcerative colitis in hospitalized patients. Ciprofloxacin (D) has no role in the induction of remission in ulcerative colitis. Vedolizumab (E) should not be combined with other biologic agents.

14. **A and C.** Vedolizumab may be used to induce remission in moderately-to-severely active disease. Thiopurines may be used to maintain remission in patients who achieved remission with corticosteroids. Oral corticosteroids should not be used as maintenance therapy. Systemic drugs are required for severe/fulminant disease. Metronidazole has no role in the therapy of ulcerative colitis.

15. **A and B.** Ciprofloxacin (C) does not induce remission or heal mucosa in patients with active Crohn's disease. It may be used to treat abscesses and fistulas in patients with Crohn's disease. Topical mesalamine preparations (D) provide limited clinical benefit in Crohn's disease though they are commonly used. Vedolizumab (E) is indicated to induce and maintain remission in moderately-to-severely active Crohn's disease.

16. **E.** Natalizumab has been associated with the development of progressive multifocal leukoencephalopathy.

17. **E.** This patient has mild, diarrhea-predominant IBS. Symptomatic treatment with dicyclomine is appropriate initial therapy, especially because her symptoms are meal related. A TCA may be added to dicyclomine if needed. Tegaserod is indicated for constipation-predominant IBS. Alosetron is reserved for patients with severe, diarrhea-predominant disease that has not responded to other therapies. Paroxetine is an SSRI and is not recommended by the American Gastroenterological Association for treatment of IBS.

18. **A, B, C.** Alosetron is reserved for patients with severe, diarrhea-predominant disease that has not responded to other therapies. Several types of psychotherapy have been shown to be more effective than usual care in IBS. TCAs improve abdominal pain in IBS and may also help with insomnia. Loperamide may be used on an as-needed basis for diarrhea. Tegaserod is indicated for constipation-predominant IBS.

19. **A.** Alosetron is approved for restricted use in diarrhea-predominant IBS. Loperamide and diphenoxylate + atropine are antidiarrheal medications that will exacerbate constipation. Paroxetine is an SSRI and is not recommended by the American Gastroenterological Association for treatment of IBS.

20. **E.** Tricyclic antidepressant serum concentrations are affected by drugs that alter cytochrome P450 activity.

21. **D.** Severe constipation, ischemic colitis, and death have been reported with alosetron.

22. **A.** Alosetron is approved for women with diarrhea-predominant IBS. It was not found to be effective in men and is not approved for use in children.

  **25-10** **Additional Resources**

Peptic Ulcer Disease

Chey WD, Leontiadis GI, Howden CW, et al. American College of Gastroenterology guideline on the treatment of *Helicobacter pylori* infection. *Am J Gastroenterol.* 2017;112:212–238.

Del Valle, J. Peptic ulcer disease and related disorders. In: Jameson J, Fauci AS, Kasper DL, et al., eds. *Harrison's Principles of Internal Medicine.* 20th ed. McGraw-Hill; 2018. Accessed July 24, 2020.

Kavitt RT, Lipowska AM, Anyane-Yeboa A, et al. Diagnosis and treatment of peptic ulcer disease. *Am J Med.* 2019; 132:447–456.

Laine L, Jensen DM. American College of Gastroenterology Practice Guidelines: management of patients with ulcer bleeding. *Am J Gastroenterol.* 2012;107:345–360.

Love BL, Mohorn PL. Peptic ulcer disease. In: Dipiro JT, Talbert RL, Yee GC, et al., eds. *Pharmacotherapy: A Pathophysiologic Approach.* 11th ed. New York, NY: McGraw-Hill Education; 2020:483–506.

Gastroesophageal Reflux Disease

Gywali CP, Fass R. Management of gastroesophageal reflux disease. *Gastroenterology.* 2018;154:302–318.

Kahrilas PJ, Hirano I. Diseases of the esophagus. In: Jameson J, Fauci AS, Kasper DL, et al., eds. *Harrison's Principles of Internal Medicine.* 20th ed. McGraw-Hill; 2018. Accessed July 24, 2020.

Katz PO, Gerson LB, Vela MF. Guidelines for the diagnosis and management of gastroesophageal reflux disease. *Am J Gastroenterol.* 2013;108:308–328.

May DB, Thiman M, Rao SSC. Gastroesophageal reflux disease. In: Dipiro JT, Talbert RL, Yee GC, et al., eds. *Pharmacotherapy: A Pathophysiologic Approach.* 11th ed. New York, NY: McGraw-Hill Education; 2020:463–480.

Inflammatory Bowel Disease

Friedman S, Blumberg RS. Inflammatory bowel disease. In: Jameson J, Fauci AS, Kasper DL, et al., eds. *Harrison's Principles of Internal Medicine.* 20th ed. McGraw-Hill; 2018. Accessed July 24, 2020.

Hemstreet BA. Inflammatory bowel disease. In: Dipiro JT, Talbert RL, Yee GC, et al., eds. *Pharmacotherapy: A Pathophysiologic Approach.* 11th ed. New York, NY: McGraw-Hill Education; 2020:507–527.

Lichtenstein GR, Loftus EV, Isaacs KL, et al. ACG clinical guideline: management of Crohn's disease in adults. *Am J Gastroenterol.* 2018;113:481–517.

Rubin DT, Ananthakrishnan AN, Siegel CA, et al. ACG clinical guideline: ulcerative colitis in adults. 2019;114:384–413.

Ungaro R, Mehandru S, Allen PB, et al. Ulcerative colitis. *Lancet.* 2017;389(10080):1756–1770.

Irritable Bowel Syndrome

Chang L, Lembo A, Sultan S. American Gastroenterological Association technical review on the pharmacological management of irritable bowel syndrome. *Gastroenterology.* 2014;147:1149–1172.

Ford AC, Lacy BE, Talley NJ. Irritable bowel syndrome. *N Engl J Med.* 2017;376:2566–2578.

Owyang C. Irritable bowel syndrome. In: Jameson J, Fauci AS, Kasper DL, et al., eds. *Harrison's Principles of Internal Medicine.* 20th ed. McGraw-Hill; 2018. Accessed July 24, 2020.

Weinberg DS, Smalley W, Heidelbaugh JJ, et al. American Gastroenterological Association Institute guideline on the pharmacological management of irritable bowel syndrome. *Gastroenterology.* 2014;147:1146–1148.

Arthritis

MELANIE P. SWIMS

26-1 KEY POINTS

RHEUMATOID ARTHRITIS

- Rheumatoid arthritis (RA), a highly variable autoimmune disease characterized by symmetric, erosive synovitis, often affects extra-articular sites.
- RA usually affects diarthrodial joints, such as proximal interphalangeal joints, metacarpophalangeal joints, metatarsophalangeal joints, wrists, and ankles. Also commonly involved are the elbows, shoulders, sternoclavicular joints, temporomandibular joints, hips, and knees.
- Morning stiffness is the hallmark of RA.
- According to the American College of Rheumatology (ACR), the goals in managing RA are to prevent or control joint damage, prevent loss of function, and decrease pain.
- The ACR recommends the aggressive use of disease-modifying antirheumatic drugs (DMARDs).
- Unlike the nonsteroidal anti-inflammatory drugs (NSAIDs), DMARDs can reduce or prevent joint damage and preserve joint integrity and function. DMARDs carry the risk of various toxicities, and they must be monitored on a regular basis.

OSTEOARTHRITIS

- Osteoarthritis (OA) is the most common form of arthritis in the United States.
- Joint stiffness, a common complaint in osteoarthritis, differs from that in RA because it is relatively short in duration and resolves with movement.
- Unlike RA, pain relief is the primary treatment goal in OA.

GOUT

- Gout, a systemic disease caused by the buildup of uric acid in the joints, causes inflammation, swelling, and pain.
- Primary gout is a result of an innate defect in purine metabolism or uric acid excretion.
- Patients with gout are classified as overproducers or underexcreters on the basis of 24-hour uric acid concentration levels.
- Treatment of an acute gouty arthritis attack involves the use of colchicine, NSAIDs, or glucocorticoids.
- Uricosuric agents, xanthine oxidase inhibitors, and uricase agents may be used to prevent further gout attacks. These agents should not be started during an acute gouty arthritis attack.

SYSTEMIC LUPUS ERYTHEMATOSUS

- Systemic lupus erythematosus (SLE) is a chronic autoimmune inflammatory disorder that can affect any system in the body.
- Therapy for SLE is primarily driven by the clinical manifestations of the disease.

26-2 STUDY GUIDE CHECKLIST

The following topics may guide your study of this subject area:

- ☐ Autoimmune nature and pathophysiology of RA.
- ☐ Monitoring of RA.
- ☐ Mechanism of action of NSAIDs.
- ☐ Adverse effects of NSAIDs.
- ☐ Adverse effects and monitoring of DMARDs.
- ☐ Pathophysiology and diagnosis of OA.
- ☐ Drug therapy of OA.
- ☐ Pathophysiology and diagnosis of gout.
- ☐ Mechanism of action of gout drugs.
- ☐ Adverse effects and monitoring of gout drugs.
- ☐ Drugs for treatment of gout attacks versus prophylaxis.
- ☐ Pathophysiology and diagnostic criteria of lupus.
- ☐ Drugs used in lupus treatment.

26-3 Rheumatoid Arthritis

Rheumatoid arthritis (RA) is a highly variable, chronic autoimmune disorder of unknown etiology characterized by symmetric, erosive synovitis. Manifestations may extend to extra-articular sites.

Incidence

RA affects 1% of the population and is two to three times more common in women than in men. Certain families, monozygotic twins, and people with specific human leukocyte antigen (HLA) genetic markers have a greater incidence of RA, which suggests a genetic predisposition.

Clinical Presentation

The onset of RA is unpredictable and varies from rapid to insidious progression.

RA usually affects diarthrodial joints such as the proximal interphalangeal (PIP) joints, metacarpophalangeal (MCP) joints, metatarsophalangeal (MTP) joints, wrists, and ankles. Also commonly involved are the elbows, shoulders, sternoclavicular joints, temporomandibular joints, hips, and knees.

The initial complaints may include generalized fatigue and multiple joint pain.

Morning stiffness is a hallmark of RA.

Ulnar deviation, swan-neck deformities, boutonnière deformities, and hammertoe formation are common irreversible joint abnormalities that occur in RA.

The extra-articular features that occur in RA include rheumatoid nodules, vasculitis, anemia, thrombocytopenia, Felty's syndrome, and Sjögren's syndrome.

Etiology

The cause of RA remains a mystery. Factors that may be responsible are of environmental, genetic, endocrinologic, gastrointestinal, and infectious origin.

RA is widely held to have a strong genetic component. This assertion is supported by the fact that a greater prevalence of RA is found in patients with the major histocompatibility complex antigen HLA-DR4. In combination with environmental factors, an inappropriate immune response may occur, resulting in chronic inflammation.

Pathophysiology

For unknown reasons, the body's immune system (starting with macrophages) attacks the cells within the joint capsule, thereby causing synovitis (as indicated by the warmth, swelling, redness, and pain associated with RA). Specifically, helper T-lymphocytes stimulate B-cell lymphocytes to attack antigen (in this case, the body's own collagen). In addition, helper T-lymphocytes release cytokines (interleukins and tumor necrosis factor), which cause further inflammation and injury in the joints. During the inflammatory process, the cells of the synovium grow and divide abnormally, causing a normally thin synovium to become thick (pannus). These abnormal synovial cells begin to invade and destroy the cartilage and bone within the joint. These effects are responsible for the pain and deformities seen in patients with RA.

Treatment Goals

According to the American College of Rheumatology (ACR), the goals in managing RA are to prevent or control joint damage, prevent loss of function, and decrease pain.

Monitoring

At each visit, the patient should be evaluated for subjective evidence of active disease on the basis of the following criteria:

- Degree of joint pain
- Duration of morning stiffness
- Duration of fatigue
- Presence of actively inflamed joints on examination
- Limitation of function
- Evidence of disease progression on physical examination (loss of motion, instability, malalignment, deformity)
- Erythrocyte sedimentation rate or C-reactive protein elevation

Other parameters for assessing response to treatment (outcomes) include the following:

- Progression of radiographic damage of involved joints
- Health care provider's global assessment of disease activity
- Patient's global assessment of disease activity
- Functional status or quality-of-life assessment using standardized questionnaires

The majority of clinical studies use a benchmark of 20% improvement in the preceding criteria, also known as ACR 20.

Drug Therapy

Aggressive use of disease-modifying antirheumatic drugs (DMARDs) is suggested (Table 26-1).

The ACR recommendations focus on the use of biologic and nonbiologic therapies for the treatment of RA.

The 2015 ACR recommendations for the initiation or reinstitution of biologic and nonbiologic therapies depend on three factors:

- Disease duration:
  - Early (< 6 months)
  - Established RA (≥ 6 months)
- Disease activity:
  - Available indices:
    - Disease Activity Score in 28 joints
    - Simplified Disease Activity Index
    - Clinical Disease Activity Index
  - Mild disease: Typically fewer than six inflamed joints, no extra-articular disease, and no radiographic evidence of erosions
  - Severe disease: Typically more than 20 inflamed joints; elevation in C-reactive protein; and positive rheumatoid factor, extra-articular disease, or both
- Prognostic factors:
  - Physical examination, health questionnaire, and laboratory analysis
  - Poor prognosis: Functional limitation, extra-articular disease, rheumatoid factor or anti–cyclic citrullinated peptide (anti-CCP) antibodies (anti-CCP antibodies may be more specific than rheumatoid factor)

Nonsteroidal anti-inflammatory drugs

Salicylates, nonsteroidal anti-inflammatory drugs (NSAIDs ⚠), and selective cyclooxygenase-2 (COX-2) inhibitors are agents with analgesic and anti-inflammatory properties useful in the management of RA.

TABLE 26-1. Disease-Modifying Antirheumatic Drugs

Generic name	Trade name	Dosage range	Administration schedule	Dosage forms
Nonbiologic				
Hydroxychloroquine	Plaquenil	200 to 400 mg	1 to 2 doses per day	Oral
Sulfasalazine	Azulfidine	1000 to 3000 mg	2 to 3 doses per day	Oral
Methotrexate	Rheumatrex	7.5 to 25 mg	Once weekly	Oral, I.M., SQ
Auranofin	Ridaura	3 to 6 mg	1 to 2 doses per day	Oral
Azathioprine	Imuran	50 to 150 mg	1 to 2 doses per day	Oral, I.V.
Minocycline	Minocin	100 to 200 mg	2 doses per day	Oral
Leflunomide	Arava	10 to 20 mg	1 to 2 doses per day	Oral
Tofacitinib	Xeljanz	5 to 10 mg	Daily to twice daily	Oral
	Xeljanz XR	11 mg	Daily	Oral
Baricitinib	Olumiant	2 mg	daily	orally
Upadacitinib	Rinvoq	15 mg	daily	orally
Biologic				
Certolizumab pegol	Cimzia	200 to 400 mg	400 mg initially and at 2 weeks and 4 weeks, then 200 mg every other week or 400 mg every 4 weeks	SQ
Etanercept	Enbrel	50 mg	Once weekly	SQ
Golimumab	Simponi	50 mg	Once monthly	SQ
Infliximab	Remicade	3 mg/kg	Weeks 0, 2, and 6, then every 8 weeks	IV
Anakinra	Kineret	100 mg	1 dose per day	SQ
Adalimumab	Humira	40 mg	Every other week	SQ
Abatacept	Orencia	< 60 kg = 500 mg; 60 to 100 kg = 750 mg; > 100 kg = 1000 mg	Weeks 0, 2, and 4, then every 4 weeks	I.V.
		OR		
		125 mg	Weekly after I.V. dose × 1 as above	SQ
Rituximab	Rituxan	1000 mg	Every 2 weeks for 2 doses	I.V.
Tocilizumab	Actemra	4 mg/kg; may be increased to 8 mg/kg on the basis of clinical response	Every 4 weeks	I.V.
		OR		
		Patient < 100 kg = 162 mg	Every other week	SQ
		Patient > 100 kg = 162 mg	Every week	SQ
Sarilumab	Kevzara	200 mg		SQ

Boldface indicates one of top 100 drugs for 2020 by prescription volume.
I.M., intramuscular; I.V., intravenous; SQ, subcutaneous.

NSAIDs *FDA BOXED WARNING*

Increased risk of cardiovascular thrombotic events (e.g., MI, stroke). Increased risk of gastrointestinal (GI) adverse events (ex: bleeding, ulceration).

These agents reduce joint pain and swelling; however, they do not inhibit joint destruction or otherwise alter the course of the disease. For this reason, they should not be considered as a sole treatment option. These agents act by inhibiting prostaglandin synthesis and release. Cyclooxygenase is present in many cells, including platelets, endothelial cells, and cells of the gastric and intestinal mucosa. The initial choice of agent is based on the efficacy, safety, cost, and convenience for any given patient. A wide range of interpatient variability exists with regard to clinical effect; several NSAIDs may need to be tried before achieving patient satisfaction (Table 26-2).

TABLE 26-2. Drug Therapy with Nonsteroidal Anti-Inflammatory Drugs

Generic name	Trade name	Dosage range	Administration schedule (doses/day)	Available dosage forms
Acetic acids				
Diclofenac	**Voltaren**	150 to 200 mg/d	3 to 4	Oral, ophthalmic, I.V., topical gel (now OTC)
	Voltaren XR	100 to 200 mg/d	1 to 2	Oral
Etodolac	Lodine	600 to 1200 mg/d	2 to 4	Oral
	Lodine XL	400 to 1000 mg/d	1	Oral
Indomethacin	Indocin	100 to 200 mg/d	2 to 3	Oral, I.V., suppository
	Indocin SR	75 to 150 mg/d	1 to 2	Oral
Nabumetone	Relafen	1000 to 2000 mg/d	1 to 2	Oral
Tolmetin	Tolectin	600 to 1800 mg/d	3	Oral
Sulindac	Clinoril	300 to 400 mg/d	2	Oral
Propionic acids				
Fenoprofen	Nalfon	900 to 3200 mg/d	3 to 4	Oral
Flurbiprofen	Ansaid	200 to 300 mg/d	2 to 4	Oral
Ibuprofen	Motrin	1200 to 3200 mg/d	3 to 4	Oral, I.V.
Ketoprofen ⚠	Orudis	150 to 300 mg/d	3 to 4	Oral
Naproxen	Naprosyn	500 to 1500 mg/d	2 to 3	Oral
Oxaprozin	Daypro	1200 to 1800 mg/d	1	Oral
Fenamate				
Meclofenamate	Meclomen	200 to 400 mg/d	3 to 4	Oral
Oxicams				
Meloxicam	Mobic	7.5 to 15 mg/d	1	Oral
Piroxicam	Feldene	10 to 20 mg/d	1 to 2	Oral
COX-2 selective				
Celecoxib	Celebrex	200 to 400 mg/d	1 to 2	Oral

Boldface indicates one of top 100 drugs for 2020 by prescription volume.
I.V., intravenous.

Ketoprofen *FDA BOXED WARNING*

NSAIDs cause an increased risk of serious cardiovascular thrombotic events, including myocardial infarction and stroke, which can be fatal. Can cause peptic ulcers, gastrointestinal bleeding and/or perforation of the stomach or intestines, which can be fatal.

Contraindications

- treatment of perioperative pain in the setting of coronary artery bypass graft (CABG).
- patients with advanced renal impairment and in patients at risk for renal failure due to volume depletion.
- patients with suspected or confirmed cerebrovascular bleeding, patients with hemorrhagic diathesis, incomplete hemostasis and those at high risk of bleeding.
- prophylactic analgesic before any major surgery.
- for labor and delivery.
- nursing mothers.
- patients currently receiving **aspirin** or NSAIDs because of the cumulative risk of inducing serious NSAID-related side effects.

Special Populations

- Dosage should be adjusted for patients 65 years or older, for patients under 50 kilograms (110 pounds) of body weight and for patients with moderately elevated serum creatinine.

Boldface indicates one of top 100 drugs for 2020 by prescription volume.

NSAIDs

Mechanism of action

NSAIDs prevent prostaglandin formation by inhibiting the action of the enzyme cyclooxygenase. The antithrombotic effect of **aspirin** occurs by an irreversible inhibition of platelet cyclooxygenase. This irreversible inhibition is unique to **aspirin**, because the remaining NSAIDs do so in a reversible manner.

Patient instructions

NSAIDs should be taken with food or milk to decrease gastrointestinal (GI) intolerance. Patients should report any dark or black stools, abdominal pain, or swelling to their health care provider immediately. Patients with a hypersensitivity to **aspirin** should not take NSAIDs.

Adverse drug effects

Compared with patients with osteoarthritis, patients with RA on NSAID therapy are at increased risk for a serious complication.

As with **aspirin**, NSAIDs cause platelet dysfunction. Unlike **aspirin**, however, this effect is readily reversible with discontinuation of the medication.

All NSAIDs are capable of causing GI intolerance and peptic ulceration. Risk factors for the development of peptic ulcer disease include advanced age, history of previous ulcer, concomitant use of corticosteroids or anticoagulants, higher dosage of NSAID, use of multiple NSAIDs, or serious underlying disease. Options to decrease the risk of developing GI ulceration include using a selective COX-2 inhibitor or adding a proton pump inhibitor to the patient's regimen. Misoprostol ⚠, an oral prostaglandin analogue, may be added at a dose of 100 to 200 mcg four times daily to prevent ulceration but is not as well tolerated because of diarrhea. Misoprostol is available in combination with **diclofenac** and sold under the trade name Arthrotec. A 2008 joint consensus statement by the American College of Cardiology Foundation, the American Heart Association, and the American College of Gastroenterology recommends that patients with a history of ulcer disease or with risk factors for ulceration be treated with a proton pump inhibitor while on NSAID therapy. If the patient is taking low-dose **aspirin** for cardiovascular protection,

Misoprostol *FDA BOXED WARNING*

Avoid use in women of child-bearing age. Should not be used by pregnant women—increased risk of abortion, premature birth, and birth defects.

a nonselective NSAID may be used in combination. COX-2 inhibitors should not be used in patients with cardiovascular disease.

Hepatic failure has been reported with NSAID use.

Renal blood flow can be decreased by NSAIDs, which may lead to permanent renal damage. Prostaglandins are responsible for maintaining the patency of the afferent renal tubule. Inhibition by NSAIDs decreases glomerular filtration pressure, resulting in decreased blood flow. Because of this mechanism, patients with hypertension, severe vascular disease, and kidney or liver problems and those taking diuretics are not good candidates for NSAID therapy.

Central nervous system (CNS) side effects such as dizziness, drowsiness, and confusion may occur with all NSAIDs.

Within the class, some drug-specific adverse reactions occur. An example of this is indomethacin, which tends to have more severe CNS adverse effects, such as headache.

Concern exists about NSAIDs and their risk of cardiovascular events. The U.S. Food and Drug Administration (FDA) now requires that manufacturers include a boxed warning regarding the potentially serious cardiovascular and GI adverse events associated with these drugs. NSAIDs should not be used in patients with heart failure.

Drug–drug interactions

Interactions are the same as those associated with **aspirin**. **Ibuprofen** may diminish the antiplatelet mechanism of **aspirin** if it is taken before **aspirin** or taken daily on a scheduled basis. Taking **aspirin** 2 hours before taking **ibuprofen** is recommended.

COX-2 inhibitors

COX-1 is the isoenzyme constitutively found in most tissues that produce the prostaglandins PGI2 and PGE2, which protect the gastric barrier, and thromboxane A2, which is responsible for platelet function. COX-2 is the inducible isoenzyme present at sites of inflammation. Celecoxib (Celebrex) has been shown to have lower incidence of endoscopically demonstrated gastroduodenal lesions than **ibuprofen**, **naproxen**, and **diclofenac**. The lower risk for GI complications is apparently eliminated when patients take low-dose **aspirin** concomitantly.

Celecoxib

Mechanism of action

Celecoxib selectively inhibits prostaglandin synthesis by specifically targeting the COX-2 isoenzyme.

Patient instructions

Patients with a history of allergic reaction to sulfonamides should avoid the use of celecoxib.

Adverse drug effects

Although the rates of GI ulceration have been demonstrated to be lower with COX-2 inhibitors than with traditional NSAIDs, the risk is not completely eliminated. In addition, the risk of dyspepsia, abdominal pain, and nausea is not significantly less with COX-2 inhibitors than with traditional NSAIDs. Celecoxib now contains an FDA boxed warning regarding cardiovascular and GI risk associated with its use.

Drug–drug interactions

Interactions are the same as those associated with **aspirin.**

Parameters to monitor

Complete blood count (CBC) and creatinine should be monitored at least yearly.

Other aspects

Merck removed rofecoxib (Vioxx) from the market in September 2004 because its use was shown to be associated with an increased cardiovascular risk in the VIGOR (Vioxx Gastrointestinal Outcomes Research), APPROVE (Adenomatous Polyp Prevention on Vioxx), and VICTOR (Vioxx in Colorectal Therapy: Definition of Optimal Regimen) trials. The FDA has concluded that the benefits of celecoxib outweigh the risks in properly selected and informed patients. Celecoxib contains an FDA boxed warning about cardiovascular and GI risk. Patients with a high risk of cardiovascular events should not use celecoxib, including CABG patients. The PRECISION trial looked at the safety of celecoxib verses **ibuprofen** or **naproxen.** In this trial it was determined that celecoxib does not confer a greater risk of cardiovascular events than **naproxen** or **ibuprofen**, but patients at high risk of cardiovascular disease should not take any NSAID.

Disease-Modifying Antirheumatic Drugs

Unlike the NSAIDs, DMARDs have the ability to reduce or prevent joint damage and preserve joint integrity and function. The ACR recommends that patients with an established diagnosis of RA be offered treatment with DMARDs. Biologic DMARDs are reserved for use after failure of nonbiologic agents, unless the patient has early disease with high activity and poor prognosis risk factors. Methotrexate ⚠ is typically selected for initial therapy because of its track record to induce long-term response. Methotrexate or leflunomide may be used as monotherapy in patients with all disease durations and activity regardless of poor prognostic features. Unfortunately, all DMARDs tend to lose effectiveness over time.

 Methotrexate *FDA BOXED WARNING*

Can cause severe or fatal toxicities—closely monitor for infections and adverse reactions of bone marrow, kidneys, liver, nervous system, gastrointestinal tract, lungs, and skin. Contraindicated in pregnancy for non-neoplastic diseases due to embryo-fetal toxicity.

Nonbiologic DMARDs

Hydroxychloroquine

Mechanism of action

Hydroxychloroquine (Plaquenil) may inhibit interleukin-1 release by monocytes, thereby decreasing macrophage chemotaxis and phagocytosis. It also inhibits the function of toll-like receptors that contribute to autoimmune disease, limiting B-cell and dendritic cell activation.

Patient instructions

Beneficial effect may not be seen until 1 to 6 months of use. Patients should report any changes in vision to their health care provider immediately.

Adverse drug effects

The most serious potential adverse effect associated with hydroxychloroquine is retinal damage that can lead to vision loss. This damage is caused by the deposition of the drug in the melanin layer of the cones.

A cumulative dose of 800 g and age > 70 years increase the risk. Hydroxychloroquine may also cause rash, abdominal cramping, diarrhea, myopathy, skin pigment changes, and peripheral neuropathy.

Parameters to monitor

Ophthalmic evaluations should be performed at baseline. If the patient has no risk factors (liver disease, retinal disease, age > 60 years) and the baseline examination is normal, the 2016 American College of Ophthalmology Guidelines recommend no further testing for five years. High-risk patients should have annual exams.

Dose

The dose is 6 to 7.5 mg/kg of lean body weight daily or 200 mg twice daily (maximum dose).

Sulfasalazine

Mechanism of action

The intestinal flora breaks sulfasalazine (Azulfidine) down to 5-aminosalicylic acid and sulfapyridine, the active moiety in RA. Sulfapyridine likely inhibits endothelial cell proliferation, reactive oxygen species, and cytokines. In addition, it has been shown to slow radiographic progression of RA.

Patient instructions

A coated tablet form may help reduce adverse GI effects.

Adverse drug effects

The most common adverse reactions associated with sulfasalazine include headache, GI intolerance, dysgeusia, rash, leukopenia, and thrombocytopenia. A reversible oligozoospermia can occur in up to 33% of males and, thus, may impair fertility. The drug may cause a discoloration of tears, sweat, and urine.

Drug–drug interactions

Sulfasalazine may inhibit the absorption of **folic acid**.

Parameters to monitor

Patient tests should include baseline CBC and liver function tests (LFTs). Patients should then have a CBC every 2 to 4 weeks for the first 3 months and then once every 3 months thereafter. Patients with glucose-6-phosphate dehydrogenase (G6PD) deficiency should not receive sulfasalazine.

Dose

Begin with 500 mg daily and titrate up to 1 to 3 g/d divided twice daily.

Methotrexate

Mechanism of action

Methotrexate (Rheumatrex) inhibits dihydrofolate reductase, which reduces dihydrofolate to tetrahydrofolate. Tetrahydrofolate can be used as a carrier of single carbon units for the synthesis of nucleotides and thymidylate. Therefore, methotrexate interferes with deoxyribonucleic acid (DNA) synthesis, repair, and cellular replication.

Patient instructions

Patients should not take this medication more than once per week. Daily dosing would be disastrous. Patients should be instructed not to drink any alcohol. Methotrexate is a teratogen and is contraindicated in pregnancy. Pregnancy and lactation should be avoided. Females should wait 3 to 6 months after discontinuation before conception, and males should wait 3 months before fathering a child. Doses up to 30 mg weekly do not affect female fertility but can cause a reversible male sterility.

Adverse drug effects

- **Liver:** Methotrexate may cause liver damage. People with diabetes, liver problems, obesity, and psoriasis and those who are elderly or alcoholic are at higher risk. If LFTs are more than three times the upper limit of normal, methotrexate should be discontinued.
- **Bone marrow:** Leukopenia, thrombocytopenia, and pancytopenia are rare but serious adverse effects associated with methotrexate therapy.
- **Lung:** Pulmonary toxicity is thought to occur in 0.1% to 1.2% of people who take methotrexate. Risk factors for the development of pulmonary toxicity include age, diabetes, rheumatoid involvement of the lungs, protein in the urine, and previous use of sulfasalazine, oral gold, or penicillamine.
- **GI:** Nausea, vomiting, and stomatitis occur with an incidence of 5% to 30%.

Drug–drug interactions

Aspirin (especially high dose) and other NSAIDs may increase methotrexate concentrations by as much as 30% to 35%. Trimethoprim-sulfamethoxazole may cause additive hematologic abnormalities because of its similar affinity for dihydrofolate reductase. Any drug inhibiting tubular secretion, such as clavulanate, will increase methotrexate levels.

Parameters to monitor

CBC, LFTs, albumin, and creatinine should be monitored every 2 to 4 weeks for the first 3 months and every 8 to 12 weeks thereafter. Patients at risk for hepatitis B and C should be screened before initiation.

Dose

The dose is 7.5 to 25 mg once weekly.

Other aspects

Taking folate supplements may help minimize adverse effects such as liver toxicity and should be regularly prescribed with methotrexate. **Folic acid** in doses up to 3 mg/d has proved effective and does not diminish methotrexate activity.

Leflunomide

Mechanism of action

Leflunomide ⚠ (Arava) inhibits dihydroorotate dehydrogenase (an enzyme involved in de novo pyrimidine synthesis) and has antiproliferative activity. Several in vivo and in vitro experimental models have demonstrated its anti-inflammatory effect.

Patient instructions

Leflunomide is contraindicated in pregnancy. Women taking leflunomide who wish to become pregnant should follow the drug elimination procedure outlined below under "Other aspects." Patients on leflunomide should be instructed not to drink any alcohol.

 Leflunomide *FDA BOXED WARNING*

Contraindicated in pregnant women. Contraindicated in patients with hepatic impairment.

Adverse drug effects

Diarrhea, elevated LFTs, alopecia, hypertension, bone marrow suppression, and rash have been reported with leflunomide therapy.

Drug–drug interactions

An increased risk of liver toxicity exists when leflunomide is used in conjunction with methotrexate. Rifampin causes a 40% increase in levels of leflunomide's active metabolite, M1.

Parameters to monitor

CBC, LFTs, albumin, and creatinine should be monitored every 2 to 4 weeks for the first 3 months and every 8 to 12 weeks thereafter. If alanine aminotransferase exceeds two times the upper limit of normal, reduce the dose of leflunomide to 10 mg/d. Patients at risk for hepatitis B and C should be screened before initiation.

Kinetics

After absorption, 80% of the parent compound is converted to the active metabolite, M1, which is responsible for all of leflunomide's activity. Because the half-life is 2 weeks, a loading dose is often given. In addition, M1 undergoes extensive enterohepatic recirculation.

Dose

The dose is 100 mg daily for 3 days (loading dose) and then 20 mg daily.

Other aspects

Begin the following drug elimination procedure if a patient decides to become pregnant: 8 g of cholestyramine 3 times daily for 11 days; plasma levels of M1 < 0.02 mg/L must be verified on 2 separate occasions at least 14 days apart.

Many randomized controlled trials have established leflunomide as an alternative to methotrexate as monotherapy.

Gold compounds

The intramuscular (I.M.) gold compounds, although used for many years, are not currently available. Auranofin ⚠ (Ridaura) is given orally.

Mechanism of action

The mechanism of action of gold compounds is currently unknown; they appear to suppress the synovitis seen in RA. Current research indicates that they may stimulate specific protective factors, such as interleukin-6 and interleukin-10.

Patient instructions

Patients receiving gold therapy should avoid prolonged sun exposure, which may increase the risk of serious rash.

Adverse drug effects

Oral gold adverse reactions are rash, neutropenia, thrombocytopenia, and proteinuria. The oral formulation leads to GI complaints of nausea, diarrhea, emesis, and dysgeusia.

 Auranofin *FDA BOXED WARNING*

Contains gold—risk of gold toxicity.

Drug–drug interactions

Patients receiving concomitant penicillamine therapy may be subject to an increased risk of toxicity associated with gold therapy. The risk of rash is higher when gold therapy is used with hydroxychloroquine.

Parameters to monitor

At baseline, all patients should have a CBC, creatinine, and urinalysis for protein. Those on oral therapy should have a CBC, platelet count, and urinalysis for protein every 4 to 12 weeks.

Dose

For oral gold, the dose is 3 mg twice daily up to 3 mg 3 times daily.

Biologic DMARDs

Anti–tumor necrosis factor therapy

The drugs used in anti–tumor necrosis factor (anti-TNF) therapy are infliximab ⚠ (Remicade), etanercept ⚠ (Enbrel), adalimumab ⚠ (Humira), golimumab ⚠ (Simponi), and certolizumab pegol ⚠ (Cimzia).

Mechanism of action

Composed of human constant and murine variable regions, infliximab is an antibody that binds specifically to human tumor necrosis factor (TNF).

Similarly, by binding specifically to TNF, etanercept binds and blocks its interaction with the cell surface's TNF receptors. It is not an antibody.

Adalimumab, certolizumab pegol, and golimumab are recombinant human monoclonal antibodies that bind to TNF with high affinity. Certolizumab pegol is unique in that it is a PEGylated (polyethylene glycolated) antigen-binding fragment (Fab fragment) derived from a high-affinity humanized anti-TNF monoclonal antibody (Ab). The Fab fragments lack the fragment crystallizable (Fc) portion of immunoglobulin, so the Fc responses such as complement- or Ab-dependent cell-mediated cytotoxicity are not realized, which is distinct from the other anti-TNF Ab, but certolizumab pegol still neutralizes membrane anti-TNF.

Patient instructions

Patients should not receive live vaccines during treatment. Therapy should be temporarily discontinued in the event of an acute infection.

Adverse drug effects

Therapy has been associated with serious mycobacterial, fungal, and opportunistic infectious complications such as sepsis and tuberculosis, leading to the requirement of an FDA boxed warning. Other adverse reactions include rash, headache, nausea, and cough. Although rare, anti-TNF drugs have been associated with nerve damage that resembles the disease process in multiple sclerosis, congestive heart failure, skin cancers, and lupus-like syndromes. Lymphoma and other hematological malignancies have been reported with TNF antagonists, although risk of solid tumors appears neutral. These drugs should not be used in patients with active hepatitis B or C.

 Infliximab, Etanercept, Adalimumab, Golimumab, and Certolizumab Pegol *FDA BOXED WARNINGS*

Increased risk of serious infections (e.g., tuberculosis, invasive fungal infections, other opportunistic infections). Lymphoma and other malignancies have been reported in children and adolescent patients. Certolizumab pegol not indicated for use in pediatric patients.

Drug–drug interactions

Live vaccines may interact with these drugs. Biologic drugs should not be used in combination because that increases the risk of infection.

Parameters to monitor

Be clinically alert for tuberculosis, histoplasmosis, and other opportunistic infections.

Dose

The dose for infliximab is 3 mg/kg intravenous (I.V.) initially, at weeks 2 and 6, and then every 8 weeks in combination with methotrexate.

The dose for etanercept is 25 mg subcutaneous twice weekly or 50 mg subcutaneous once weekly.
The dose for adalimumab is 40 mg subcutaneous every second week.
The dose for golimumab is 50 mg subcutaneous every 4 weeks.
The dose for certolizumab pegol is 400 mg subcutaneous initially and at weeks 2 and 4, followed by a dose of 200 mg every other week. Maintenance dosing up to 400 mg every 4 weeks can be considered.

Other aspects

Patients should be tested for tuberculosis (skin testing, chest radiograph, or both) and hepatitis B (if risk factors are present) before initiating therapy with any biologic agent. Currently, infliximab is approved for therapy only in combination with methotrexate. Patients should receive appropriate vaccinations before initiation, such as pneumococcal, influenza, hepatitis B, and herpes zoster.

Anakinra

Mechanism of action

Anakinra (Kineret) blocks the biologic activity of interleukin-1 by competitively inhibiting interleukin-1 binding to the interleukin-1 type I receptor.

Patient instructions

Kineret is supplied in a single-use, prefilled syringe that should be stored in the refrigerator. Any syringe left unrefrigerated for more than 24 hours should be discarded.

Adverse drug effects

Like the anti-TNF agents, anakinra increases the risk of serious infections. Injection-site reactions are extremely common. Headache, nausea, diarrhea, sinusitis, flu-like symptoms, and abdominal pain have also been reported.

Drug–drug interactions

Live vaccines can interact with anakinra.

Parameters to monitor

Patients should have a CBC checked at baseline, then monthly for 3 months, and then once every 3 months for the first year of therapy.

Dose

The dose is 100 mg subcutaneous daily.

Abatacept

Mechanism of action

Abatacept (Orencia) selectively modulates T-cell activation causing downregulation and an anti-inflammatory effect.

Adverse drug effects

Like the other biologic DMARDs, abatacept increases the risk of infections, especially upper respiratory infections. Nausea and headache are also frequently reported. In addition, patients with chronic obstructive pulmonary disease developed adverse effects more frequently than with a placebo. More cases of lung cancer were observed in patients treated with abatacept than with a placebo. The lymphoma rate was higher as well.

Drug–drug interactions

Use of abatacept is contraindicated with other biologic DMARDs because of increased risk of infection. Live vaccines are contraindicated as well.

Dose

Dose is based on weight (< 60 kg = 500 mg; 60 to 100 kg = 750 mg; > 100 kg = 1000 mg). Infusions are given over 30 minutes. After the initial dose, give at 2 and 4 weeks, followed by every 4 weeks. Alternatively, 125 mg subcutaneous weekly may be prescribed after 1 weight-based loading dose.

Other aspects

Abatacept contains maltose and may falsely elevate blood glucose readings. Monitors that do not react to maltose are recommended.

Rituximab

Mechanism of action

Rituximab (Rituxan) causes a transient depletion of B-cell lymphocytes by binding to the CD20 surface antigens.

Dose

Administer 1000 mg every 2 weeks for 2 doses; patients should be premedicated with a glucocorticoid, diphenhydramine, and **acetaminophen** to decrease infusion-related reactions.

Other aspects

Rituximab should be used only in patients with moderate to severe RA who have had an inadequate response or a contraindication to anti-TNF products.

> ⚠ **Rituximab** *FDA BOXED WARNING*
>
> Risk of fatal infusion reactions, severe mucocutaneous reactions, reactivation of hepatitis B, and progressive multifocal leukoencephalopathy.

Inleukin 6 inhibitors Tocilizumab (Actemra), Sarilumab (Kevzara)

Mechanism of action

Tocilizumab ⚠ (Actemra) is an interleukin-6 receptor–inhibiting antibody. The FDA approved tocilizumab in 2010 for moderate to severe RA in adults who have not achieved an adequate response to 1 or more anti-TNF agents, with or without methotrexate. It can be used with other nonbiologic DMARDs.

Patient instructions

Side effects should be reported to the health care provider immediately.

Adverse drug effects

Like the anti-TNF agents, tocilizumab increases the risk of serious infections. It also has been reported to rarely cause generalized peritonitis, diverticulitis, lower GI perforation, fistulae, and intra-abdominal abscesses. Increased transaminases, especially with methotrexate, and decreased white blood cells and platelets have also been reported, as have increased total cholesterol, LDL (low-density lipoprotein), triglycerides, and HDL (high-density lipoprotein) levels. Multiple sclerosis and chronic inflammatory demyelinating polyneuropathy cases may occur, and tocilizumab may increase malignancy risk.

More common side effects include severe allergic reactions (0.2%), rash (2%), mouth ulcers (2%), abdominal pain (2%), dizziness (3%), hypertension (6%), infusion reactions (7%), headache (7%), upper respiratory infections (5% to 8%), and serious infections (18%).

Drug–drug interactions

In chronic inflammation, the formation of cytochrome P450 (CYP450) enzymes is suppressed by increased levels of cytokines such as interleukin-6. Tocilizumab could normalize the formation of CYP450 enzymes; thus, in hepatically metabolized narrow therapeutic index drugs, an increase in CYP450-mediated metabolism may lower the levels of these drugs (e.g., **warfarin**, theophylline, phenytoin, cyclosporine, carbamazepine, **simvastatin**, **omeprazole**).

Parameters to monitor

- Patients should have CBC and LFTs checked at baseline and then every 4 to 8 weeks.
- Assess lipid parameters at 4 to 8 weeks following initiation of therapy and every 6 months thereafter. The risk of tuberculosis is not known, but perform tuberculosis testing before starting therapy.

Dose

The dose is a 4 mg/kg I.V. infusion over 1 hour every 4 weeks. The dose may be increased to 8 mg/kg on the basis of clinical response. A new subcutaneous product is dosed for patients < 100 kg at 162 mg subcutaneous every other week. Patients > 100 kg should get 162 mg subcutaneous weekly. Sarilumab ⚠ is given 200 mg subcutaneously every 2 weeks.

⚠ **Tocilizumab and Sarilumab** *FDA BOXED WARNINGS*

Increased risk of serious infections (e.g., tuberculosis, invasive fungal infections, opportunistic infections).

Janus kinase inhibitors Tofacitinib (Xeljanz), Baricitinib (Olumiant), Upadacitinib (Rinvoq)

Mechanism of action

Tofacitinib ⚠ (Xeljanz) is a janus kinase (JAK) inhibitor. The JAK family (JAK1, JAK2, JAK3, tyrosine kinase 2 [TYK2]) comprises tyrosine kinase proteins that signal in pairs and facilitate the phosphorylation process of many proteins intracellularly. One such group of proteins is the signal transducers and activators of transcription (STAT). These proteins regulate the transcription of genes that control inflammatory responses. Tofacitinib affects the signaling pathway at the point of the JAK family by preventing phosphorylation and activation of STAT. Tofacitinib is approved for moderate-to-severe RA patients who have failed or cannot take methotrexate as monotherapy or take tofacitinib in combination with methotrexate or another nonbiologic DMARD. It cannot be combined with another biologic or immunosuppressing drug such as azathioprine or cyclosporine. It is called a *targeted synthetic DMARD* to differentiate it from traditional DMARDs (synthetics) and biologic DMARDs.

Tofacitinib *FDA BOXED WARNING*

Increased risk of serious infections (e.g., tuberculosis, invasive fungal infections, other opportunistic infections, other opportunistic infections), thrombosis, lymphoma and other malignancies. Increased risk of mortality in patients with rheumatoid arthritis taking 10 mg twice daily. Patients who have undergone a kidney transplant have an increased risk of Epstein-Barr virus-associated lymphoproliferative disorder.

Patient instructions

Patients should not receive live vaccines during treatment. Discontinue tofacitinib during infections.

Adverse drug effects

Serious infections, increased risk of malignancies, increased lipids, neutropenia, transaminase elevations, drops in hemoglobin, intestinal perforations, and increases in serum creatinine have been reported. Rheumatoid arthritis patient with at least 1 cardiovascular risk factor had a higher rate of mortality and thrombosis with the 10 mg twice-daily dose. This is a new black box warning for all 3 Janus kinase inhibitors approved for RA. A Risk Evaluation and Mitigation Strategy (REMS) medication safety guide is available for patients.

Drug–drug interactions

Tofacitinib is metabolized by CYP450 3A4; therefore, drugs that inhibit or induce CYP450 3A4 may affect its pharmacokinetics. Drugs that inhibit CYP450 2C19 alone or P-glycoprotein are unlikely to affect tofacitinib.

Parameters to monitor

Patients should have a baseline CBC, and then hemoglobin again at 4 to 8 weeks and every 3 months thereafter. Lymphocyte count should be done at baseline and every month. Lipids should be done at 4 to 8 weeks, and liver tests should be checked periodically. Patients should be vigilant to report any signs or symptoms of infection.

Dose

The dose is 5 mg twice daily of tofacitinib or 11 mg daily of tofacitinib sustained release or, in the following circumstances, 5 mg daily orally:

- Moderate or severe renal insufficiency
- Moderate hepatic impairment
- Concomitant therapy with potential inhibitors of CYP450 3A4 (e.g., ketoconazole)
- Concomitant therapy with 1 or more drugs causing moderate inhibition of CYP450 3A4 and potent inhibition of CYP450 2C19 (e.g., fluconazole)
- Baricitinib ⚠ dose is 2 mg orally daily
- Upadacitinib ⚠ dose is 15 mg orally daily

 Baricitinib *FDA BOXED WARNING*

Serious infections leading to hospitalization or death, including tuberculosis and bacterial, invasive fungal, viral, and other opportunistic infections have occurred.

Lymphoma and other malignancies have been observed. Thrombosis, including deep venous thrombosis, pulmonary embolism, and arterial thrombosis have occurred.

Upadacitinib *FDA BOXED WARNING*

Serious infections leading to hospitalization or death, including tuberculosis and bacterial, invasive fungal, viral, and other opportunistic infections have occurred.

Lymphoma and other malignancies have been observed. Thrombosis, including deep venous thrombosis, pulmonary embolism, and arterial thrombosis have occurred.

Other agents
Azathioprine

Azathioprine (Imuran) is a purine analogue immunosuppressive agent that is generally reserved for refractory RA. It is associated with dose-related bone marrow suppression, stomatitis, diarrhea, rash, pancreatitis, and liver failure. Patients must have a baseline CBC, creatinine, and liver profile. Patients should then have a CBC and platelet count every 1 to 2 weeks after any change in dosage and every 1 to 3 months thereafter. Azathioprine should not be administered with **allopurinol** because xanthine oxidase metabolizes 6-mercaptopurine.

 Azathioprine *FDA BOXED WARNING*

Increased risk of malignancy.

Cyclosporine A

By blocking T-cell activation, cyclosporine A (Sandimmune) produces powerful immunosuppressive effects and is beneficial as monotherapy in the treatment of RA. Serious adverse effects such as hypertension, nephrotoxicity, glucose intolerance, and hepatotoxicity have limited its use.

 Cyclosporine A *FDA BOXED WARNING*

Increased risk of malignancy. Must be prescribed by physicians experienced in immunosuppressive therapy. Sandimmune® and Neoral® are NOT interchangeable. Variable absorption—requires frequent monitoring.

Corticosteroids

Low-dose oral corticosteroids (< 10 mg/d of **prednisone** or the equivalent) and local injections of glucocorticoids are highly effective. Studies indicate that corticosteroids decrease the progression of RA. They may be useful for acute flare-ups and in patients with significant systemic manifestations of RA. RA is associated with an increased risk of osteoporosis (independent of steroid therapy), and the addition of steroidal anti-inflammatory agents increases the risk.

Nondrug Therapy

Joint surgery

Patients may have arthroscopy performed to clean out the bone and cartilage fragments that cause pain within the joint capsule. Patients may eventually require complete joint replacement surgery.

Lifestyle modifications

- A mild exercise regimen can be an effective therapy.
- Some evidence suggests a moderate increase in daily protein intake may be beneficial in RA.
- Patients with RA benefit from a formal support group.
- Rest is an important strategy as well.

26-4   Osteoarthritis

Osteoarthritis (OA), a disease that affects the weight-bearing joints of the peripheral and axial skeleton, is the most common form of arthritis in the United States. OA is also known as degenerative joint disease. Joints most commonly affected are the hands, hips, and knees. Osteoarthritis is a leading cause of disability among older adults.

Incidence

Approximately 50% of people over the age of 65 years have OA. Before the age of 50 years, men have a higher incidence primarily because of sports injuries; however, after the age of 50 years, women have a higher incidence.

Clinical Presentation

Pain is a common initial finding in patients with OA. This pain typically worsens with weight-bearing activity and improves with rest of the affected joint. Changes in weather and barometric pressure tend to influence the severity of pain.

Joint stiffness is another common complaint. This stiffness differs from that of RA. It is relatively short in duration, is related to periods of inactivity, and resolves with movement.

Crepitus is common, especially when the knee joint is involved.

Joint deformities also occur in OA. Heberden's nodes, Bouchard's nodes, and osteophytes on the distal interphalangeal and proximal interphalangeal joints are commonly seen.

Pathophysiology

Although the causes of OA are not completely understood, biomechanical stresses affecting the articular cartilage and subchondral bone are thought to be the primary factors in the development of OA. In addition, inflammatory, biochemical, and immunologic components play a role. The function of the normal cartilage—that is, to dissipate the force and stress caused by normal weight-bearing activity—is impaired in OA.

- Collagen fibers are destroyed and subsequently release proteoglycans. The hydration of the cartilage increases, and the cartilage becomes thick.
- Metalloproteinases, which degrade the proteoglycans, are released to initiate the reparation process. This degradation causes an increase in chondrocyte activity.
- The resulting cartilage is thin because the chondrocyte activity cannot match the rate at which proteoglycan degradation occurs. With this ever-thinning layer of cartilage now exposing bone, the grinding motion stimulates osteoclast and osteoblast activity, thereby causing bone resorption and vascular changes. Ultimately, these changes lead to the formation of osteophytes.

Treatment Principles

Treatment of patients with OA focuses on symptom control. Currently, no therapeutic options are known to change the course of the disease. The 2019 American College of Rheumatology/Arthritis Foundation

TABLE 26-3. Therapies for Hand, Knee, and Hip Arthritis

Strongly Recommended for all (in green): Exercise, Self Management Programs, Oral NSAIDs.

Conditionally Recommended for all (in bold): Heat or Therapeutic Cooling, Cognitive Behavioral Therapy, Acupuncture, **Acetaminophen, Tramadol, Duloxetine.**

Hand	Knee	Hip
First Carpometacarpal joint Orthosis	Weight Loss	Weight Loss
Kinesiotaping	Tai Chi	Tai Chi
Other Hand Orthoses	Cane	Cane
Paraffin	Tibiofemoral Brace	Balance Training
Topical NSAIDs	Topical NSAID	Intraarticular Steroids with Imaging Guidance
Intraarticular Steroids	Intraarticular Steroids	
Chondroitin	Kinesiotaping	
	Balance Training	
	Patellofemoral Brace	
	Yoga	
	Radiofrequency Ablation	
	Topical Capsaicin	

Guideline for Management of Osteoarthritis of the Hand, Hip, and Knee have now recommended against use of glucosamine, chondroitin, and hyaluronic acid intra-articular injections although these treatments are still often used (Table 26-3).

Drug Therapy

Pain relief is the primary treatment goal for patients with OA. The recommended initial drug of choice is usually an NSAID or **acetaminophen**. For those patients who do not respond fully to **acetaminophen**, an NSAID is added, but side effects preclude their use in many patients.

NSAIDs (see section 26-3 Rheumatoid Arthritis)

Acetaminophen

Mechanism of action

Acetaminophen centrally inhibits prostaglandin synthesis.

Patient instructions

Patients with hepatic disease or viral hepatitis are at risk of toxicity from chronic **acetaminophen** use.

Adverse drug effects

Hepatotoxicity is the most severe side effect associated with **acetaminophen** therapy. For this reason, patients should not ingest more than 4 g of **acetaminophen** per day. Long-term therapy has also been linked to renal failure.

Tramadol

Mechanism of action

Tramadol ⚠ is a central opioid agonist that binds to mu receptors and weakly inhibits norepinephrine and serotonin reuptake.

Tramadol *FDA BOXED WARNING*

Potential for addiction, abuse, and misuse. Potential for life-threatening respiratory depression, especially if used concomitantly with benzodiazepines or if ultra-rapid metabolizer. Monitor interactions with medications metabolized by CYP3A4 and CPY2D6. Avoid use in pregnant women due to risk of neonatal opioid withdrawal.

Adverse drug effects

Nausea, vomiting, constipation, and seizures are associated with **tramadol** use. Withdrawal symptoms may occur with abrupt discontinuation.

Drug interactions

Tramadol is contraindicated in patients taking monoamine oxidase inhibitors because of the risk of serotonin syndrome. It should be used with caution in combination with any other serotonergic drugs.

Other aspects

Tramadol is available as an immediate-release product (Ultram), as an extended-release product (Ultram ER), and in combination with **acetaminophen** 325 mg (Ultracet).

Duloxetine

Duloxetine ⚠ is a serotonin norepinephrine reuptake inhibitor that may help both pain and depression, which is common with chronic pain conditions like osteoarthritis.

Adverse drug effects

GI upset, anxiety, insomnia, and headache are associated with **duloxetine**. At higher doses blood pressure may go up.

Drug interactions

Serotonin syndrome may occur with other serotonergic drugs like **sumatriptan** (and other triptans), **tramadol**, and **trazodone**. A small risk of increased bleeding may occur when used in conjunction with anticoagulants. CYP450 1A2 inhibitors (e.g., cimetidine, quinolone antibiotics) and CYP450 2D6 inhibitors (e.g., **fluoxetine**, quinidine) increase **duloxetine** levels.

 Duloxetine *FDA BOXED WARNING*

Increased risk of suicidal thoughts and behavior in patients less than 24 years old.

Topical Agents

Capsaicin

Mechanism of action

Derived from the pepper plant, capsaicin works by inhibiting the release of substance P, which is responsible for transmitting pain from the peripheral to the central nervous system.

Patient instructions

Patients should avoid contact with eyes. It is important to wash hands thoroughly after use.

Adverse drug effects

Patients will experience mild burning and stinging at the site of application.

Other aspects

Patients usually derive benefit after several weeks of application. Capsaicin is often used in conjunction with oral agents.

Topical NSAIDs (*Diclofenac* gel)

Mechanism of action

NSAIDs prevent prostaglandin formation by inhibiting the action of the enzyme cyclooxygenase.

Patient instructions

For lower extremities, apply 4 g of the 1% topical gel to the affected foot, knee, or ankle 4 times daily. Do not apply more than 16 g of the 1% gel to any single joint of the lower extremities. For upper extremities, apply 2 g of the 1% topical gel to the affected hand, elbow, or wrist 4 times daily. Gently massage the gel into the skin to ensure application to the entire affected hand (palm, back of hands, fingers), elbow, or wrist. Do not apply more than 8 g of the 1% gel to any single joint of the upper extremities.

Adverse drug effects

Application site reactions may occur as well as the class effects of oral NSAIDs.

Other aspects

In persons 75 years and older, topical NSAIDs are preferred over oral NSAIDs.

Nondrug Therapy

Nondrug therapy for OA consists of the following:

- Patient education
- Self-management programs (e.g., Arthritis Foundation Self-Management Program)
- Psychosocial interventions
- Weight loss (if overweight)
- Aerobic exercise programs, tai chi
- Physical therapy
- Manual therapy, supervised exercise
- Assistive devices for ambulation
- Kinesiotaping, splint use, braces, hand orthoses
- Assistive devices for activities of daily living

26-5 Gout

Gout, a systemic disease caused by the buildup of uric acid in the joints, causes inflammation, swelling, and pain. Hyperuricemia is defined as a urate level > 7 mg/dL in men and > 6 mg/dL in women.

Incidence

Gout has been known as "the disease of kings and the king of diseases" and can be traced to the time of Hippocrates. Gout occurs in approximately 4% of the population. The vast majority of gout patients are men.

Clinical Presentation

Pain in one joint of the lower extremity is the most common first symptom of gout. The initial period of pain, usually monoarticular and self-limiting, is followed by a period in which the patient is completely asymptomatic.

Termed *intercritical periods,* the time between acute gouty arthritis attacks may be 3 months to 2 years. The length of time shortens as the disease progresses.

The first attack is typically at night or in the early morning.

Gout commonly affects the ankle, heel, knee, wrist, finger, elbow, and instep. The most common site of the initial attack is the first metatarsophalangeal (MTP) joint (big toe) and is known as podagra.

The patient may experience fever, chills, and malaise during an acute gouty arthritis attack. Left untreated, the attack may last 1 to 2 weeks.

The skin over the affected joint becomes red, hot, swollen, and tender. As the patient recovers from the attack, local desquamation may occur.

Pathophysiology

Uric acid is the end product of purine metabolism. Xanthine oxidase is the rate-limiting step in the formation of uric acid. Foods that are a source of purines (including organ meats and some seafood) and alcohol (especially beer) may need to be restricted. Intake of foods containing high fructose sweeteners should be reduced because these sweeteners increase uric acid levels.

Primary gout is a result of an innate defect in purine metabolism or uric acid excretion. In this case, hyperuricemia may result from uric acid overproduction (in "overproducers"), impaired renal clearance of uric acid (in "underexcreters"), or a combination of both.

Secondary gout is associated with increased nucleic acid turnover, decreased renal function, increased purine production, or drug-induced decreased elimination of uric acid. Hematologic disorders that are lymphoproliferative and myeloproliferative in nature are known causes of secondary hyperuricemia. Salicylates such as **aspirin** may inhibit tubular secretion of uric acid at low doses. Diuretics (loops and thiazides) may cause hyperuricemia. Ethambutol, pyrazinamide, nicotinic acid, ethanol, niacin, and cyclosporine are known to cause an increase in serum uric acid.

Acute gout attacks are caused by the deposition of monosodium urate in the synovium of the joint. This deposition results in the stimulation of the body's inflammatory cascade. The monosodium urate (MSU) crystals undergo phagocytosis by polymorphonuclear leukocytes. These leukocytes, damaged by the sharp crystals, burst and release their contents (interleukin-1, lysosomes, prostaglandins) into the synovium, resulting in the inflammatory reaction—that is, pain, swelling, and erythema.

If left untreated, deposits of MSU crystals, also known as tophi, lead to joint deformity and disability. Ultimately, patients may develop 1 of 2 types of renal disease: urate nephropathy or uric acid nephropathy. Urate nephropathy results from the deposition of MSU crystals in the renal interstitium. Uric acid nephropathy results from the deposition of uric acid in the collecting tubules.

Treatment Goals

- Relieve pain and inflammation
- Reduce serum uric acid concentration
- Prevent recurrent gout attacks

Drug Therapy

Drugs for the treatment of gout are outlined in Table 26-4.

TABLE 26-4. Drugs for the Treatment of Gout

Generic name	Trade name	Classification	Normal dose	Comments	Dosage forms
Colchicine		Anti-inflammatory	1.2 mg oral followed by 0.6 mg 1 hour later; maximum dose of 1.8 mg over 1 hour	Drug may be used for chronic suppressive therapy; dose must be adjusted for renal insufficiency.	Oral
Probenecid	Benemid	Uricosuric agent	250 to 500 mg twice daily	Avoid salicylates; take with plenty of water.	Oral
Allopurinol	Zyloprim	Xanthine oxidase inhibitor	100 to 300 mg daily or divided dose	Drug may cause rash; reduce dosage in renal failure.	Oral
Febuxostat	**Uloric**	Xanthine oxidase inhibitor	40 mg daily; if uric acid not less than 6 mg/dL, increase to 80 mg daily	Drug may be used in mild renal impairment.	Oral
Indomethacin	Indocin	NSAID	50 mg 3 times daily	Drug may cause fluid retention, GI bleeding.	Oral, I.V., suppository
Lesinurad	Zurampic	URAT1 Inhibitor	200 mg daily	Use in combination.	Oral

Boldface indicates one of top 100 drugs for 2020 by prescription volume.
URAT1, urate transporter 1.

Acute Gouty Arthritis Attack

Three treatments are available: colchicine, NSAIDs (indomethacin in particular), and corticosteroids. Avoiding initiation of treatments that affect serum uric acid concentration is best during an acute attack.

Colchicine

Mechanism of action

Colchicine inhibits the phagocytosis of urate crystals by leukocytes. Colchicine also inhibits the release of chemotactic factor, thus reducing the adhesion of polymorphonuclear leukocytes.

Patient instructions

Patients should immediately stop taking colchicine if abdominal cramping or diarrhea occurs. In the past, multiple doses were allowed and patients were told they should never exceed a total of 8 mg during an acute gouty arthritis attack. New recommendations state 3 tablets within the first day only to avoid toxicity.

Adverse drug effects

Nausea, bloating, emesis, and diarrhea occur in up to 80% of patients taking colchicine, especially at high doses. Rarely, it may cause bone marrow suppression. This effect occurs with a higher incidence in those patients with underlying renal or hepatic dysfunction.

Drug–drug and drug–disease interactions

Patients with active peptic ulcer disease should not take colchicine.

Inhibitors of the CYP450 enzyme 3A4 and P-glycoproteins such as (but not limited to) cyclosporine, ketoconazole, ritonavir, clarithromycin, **azithromycin**, verapamil, and **diltiazem** may markedly increase colchicine levels, leading to toxicity.

Parameters to monitor

With long-term therapy, patients should have a serum creatinine test, LFT, and complete white blood cell count periodically.

Dose

For the treatment of an acute gouty arthritis attack, patients should take 1.2 mg orally followed by 0.6 mg in 1 hour. Maximum dose is 1.8 mg.

Other aspects

Colchicine is most effective when initiated within 12 to 36 hours of the attack.

Indomethacin

Indomethacin is the most extensively studied NSAID in the treatment of an acute gouty arthritis attack. Unlike colchicine, indomethacin is effective at any point during the acute attack. For more information, see the review of NSAIDs in Section 26-3.

Corticosteroids

For the treatment of acute gout pain, corticosteroids are effective when given intra-articularly, intravenously, or orally. Their use is limited to treatment failures of colchicine and NSAIDs. The dose of **prednisone** for acute attacks usually is 30 to 60 mg **prednisone** equivalent once daily for 3 to 5 days; then taper in 5 mg decrements spread over 10 to 14 days until discontinuation.

Gout Prophylaxis (Intercritical Period)

Patients with asymptomatic hyperuricemia should not be routinely treated with pharmacologic agents. These patients should undergo a workup to determine the cause of hyperuricemia. The use of low-dose (0.6 to 1.2 mg/d) colchicine can prevent subsequent attacks of gout. Patients in the intercritical period (after an acute gouty arthritis attack) are candidates for long-term prophylactic therapy directed at affecting serum uric acid levels if they have at least 2 gout attacks per year or tophi. If the uric acid level is very high, then prophylactic therapy is often started early. Prophylactic treatment initiation should be held until at least 2 to 4 weeks after a flare's resolution. Choice of therapy is based on the patient's pathophysiologic cause of hyperuricemia. Patients are generally classified as overproducers or underexcreters. Placing the patient on a purine-restricted diet and performing a 24-hour urine collection to measure uric acid concentration may identify overproducers of uric acid. Those patients who excrete more than 600 mg of uric acid are considered overproducers. Once this diagnosis is made, patients are treated with 1 of 3 classes of agents: xanthine oxidase inhibitors, uricosurics, or uricase agents. Uricosurics can be used in underexcreters but are less commonly used and are contraindicated in nephrolithiasis. Xanthine oxidase inhibitors should be titrated to achieve a uric acid of less than 6 mg/dL. In late 2010, the FDA announced the approval of a uricase agent, pegloticase (Krystexxa), an I.V. treatment for chronic gout in adults whose conditions have been refractory to conventional therapy. Pegloticase is a PEGylated uric acid–specific enzyme that lowers serum uric acid levels by catalyzing the oxidation of uric acid to allantoin, an inert and water-soluble purine metabolite that is readily eliminated, primarily by renal excretion.

⚠ **Pegloticase** *FDA BOXED WARNING*

Risk of anaphylaxis and infusion reactions. Should be administered in health care setting and pretreated with anti-histamines and corticosteroids. Do not administer to patients with G6PD deficiency.

Probenecid

Mechanism of action

Probenecid (Benemid) is a uricosuric agent that promotes the excretion of uric acid by blocking its reuptake at the proximal convoluted tubule.

Patient instructions

Patients should drink at least 2 liters of water per day to decrease the risk of uric acid stone formation. Patients should take probenecid with food if GI intolerance occurs.

Adverse drug effects

Probenecid is generally well tolerated and is associated with very few adverse side effects. Up to 10% of patients receiving probenecid therapy develop uric acid stones. Probenecid may cause abdominal discomfort, but patients can often avoid it by taking probenecid with food.

Drug–drug interactions

Because probenecid prevents the tubular secretion of many weak organic acids, it has potential drug interactions — for example, with the penicillins, cephalosporins, nitrofurantoin, and rifampin. Although the interaction between probenecid, penicillins, and cephalosporins has been used therapeutically, the interaction with nitrofurantoin reduces nitrofurantoin's effectiveness. Using probenecid and **aspirin** together, even in low doses, is not advisable because **aspirin** blocks uric acid excretion. However, a crossover study in patients with gouty arthritis concluded that low-dose **aspirin** did not significantly interfere with the uricosuric effects of probenecid. Additionally, the diuretic effects of **furosemide** and **hydrochlorothiazide** are magnified when probenecid is taken concomitantly. Finally, patients receiving sulfonylureas should be monitored closely for hypoglycemia when started on probenecid.

Other aspects

Patients should never begin uricosuric therapy during an acute gouty arthritis attack because of the risk of exacerbating the attack. Probenecid should not be used in patients with a creatinine clearance < 50 mL/min.

Allopurinol

Mechanism of action

Allopurinol (Zyloprim) and its metabolite, oxypurinol, inhibit xanthine oxidase formation (the rate-limiting step in uric acid synthesis), thereby facilitating the clearance of the more water-soluble precursors of uric acid, oxypurines.

Patient instructions

Patients should immediately report any signs of rash to their health care providers. **Allopurinol** should be taken with food to minimize GI discomfort.

Adverse drug effects

Allopurinol is generally well tolerated; the overall occurrence of adverse effects is less than 1%. Patients should be advised that rash, the most common adverse effect, might occur at any time during therapy. The rash may be as simple as a maculopapular eruption or as serious as the life-threatening Stevens–Johnson syndrome (which is exfoliative and erythematous). Rarely, **allopurinol** may cause alopecia, neutropenia, and hepatitis.

Drug–drug interactions

The chemotherapeutic agents azathioprine and 6-mercaptopurine are metabolized via the xanthine oxidase pathway; therefore, **allopurinol** and its metabolite oxypurinol may increase serum levels of these agents. The concomitant administration of ampicillin or **amoxicillin** with **allopurinol** increases the risk of rash to approximately 20%.

Parameters to monitor

Patients should be encouraged to report the first signs of rash to their health care provider immediately. Patients should have serum creatinine and LFTs drawn periodically.

Kinetics

With a half-life of 30 hours, **allopurinol** is rapidly converted to its active metabolite (oxypurinol). This speed allows for once-daily dosing.

Other aspects

To reduce the risk of precipitating an acute gouty arthritis attack, **allopurinol** should be initiated at a dose of 100 mg/d and increased at 100 mg intervals weekly to an average dose of 300 mg/d. Doses of up to 800 mg daily may be prescribed. Patients with renal insufficiency require a dose adjustment. If the target dose is 300 mg/d, patients with a creatinine clearance of 10 to 20 mL/min should receive 200 mg/d. Those with a clearance of less than 10 mL/min should receive 100 mg/d. New data suggests that **allopurinol** has a beneficial effect on patients with coronary artery disease (CAD) although more studies are needed. Patients that are ethnically Han Chinese, Thai, and Korean have a higher risk of carrying the HLA-B*58:01 haplotype that may confer a greater risk of **allopurinol** toxicity. In these patients systematic screening may be cost effective.

Febuxostat (Uloric) was approved in February 2009 for the chronic management of hyperuricemia in patients with gout. It is also a xanthine oxidase inhibitor; however, unlike **allopurinol**, it is not a purine-based analog.

Febuxostat

Mechanism of action

Febuxostat ⚠ (Uloric) inhibits xanthine oxidase formation (the rate-limiting step in uric acid synthesis), thereby facilitating the clearance of the more water-soluble precursors of uric acid, oxypurines.

Adverse drug effects

Nausea, rash, elevated liver tests, and dizziness have been reported.

Drug–drug interactions

The chemotherapeutic agents azathioprine and 6-mercaptopurine are metabolized via the xanthine oxidase pathway; therefore, febuxostat may increase serum levels of these agents. The co-administration of theophylline and febuxostat results in higher levels of one of the metabolites of theophylline.

Parameters to monitor

Patients should have LFTs drawn at 2 to 4 months and then periodically thereafter.

Other aspects

Because of the risk of gout flare, prophylaxis with an NSAID medication or colchicine is recommended when febuxostat is started and may be continued for up to 6 months. Febuxostat may be used in patients with mild-to-moderate renal impairment.

 Febuxostat *FDA BOXED WARNING*

Increased risk of cardiovascular (CV) death in patients with established CV disease.

Secondary hyperuricemia

As discussed earlier, hyperuricemia may be caused by lymphoproliferative and myeloproliferative disorders, as well as by their chemotherapeutic treatments (e.g., tumor lysis syndrome). **Allopurinol** is commonly added to the prescribed chemotherapeutic regimen to prevent complications of hyperuricemia, for example, an acute gouty arthritis attack. Rasburicase ⚠ (Elitek) is an approved therapeutic agent that is used to prevent hyperuricemia in children and adults with leukemia, lymphoma, and solid-tumor malignancies. Rasburicase is a recombinant urate oxidase enzyme that converts uric acid to allantoin, thereby allowing it to be eliminated. Patients with G6PD deficiency should not use rasburicase.

> ⚠ **Rasburicase** *FDA BOXED WARNING*
>
> Risk of serious and fatal hypersensitivity reactions and methemoglobinemia. Contraindicated in patients with G6PD deficiency due to risk of hemolysis.

26-6   Systemic Lupus Erythematosus

Systemic lupus erythematosus (SLE) is a chronic autoimmune inflammatory disorder that can affect any system in the body, including the skin, joints, and internal organs. Women of childbearing age are primarily affected. Fifteen-year survival rates are now approximately 76%. Lupus nephritis and infectious complications are the primary cause of mortality.

Classification

The workup of SLE must include the consideration of an alternative diagnosis. Because other autoimmune diseases have similar characteristics and because the features of SLE, RA, and scleroderma overlap, a thorough assessment is warranted. Drug-induced lupus must be ruled out as well.

Clinical Presentation

Box 26-1 describes the signs and symptoms of SLE

Patients typically present with chronic fatigue and depression. Dermatitis and arthritis (in multiple joints) are the most common clinical manifestations. The arthritic pain patients describe is generally out of proportion to the amount of synovitis present. Although rare, serious renal abnormalities can occur in patients with SLE. CNS involvement, also rare, can be serious. Lupus-related encephalopathy may occur from scarring of arterioles in the subcortical white matter. In addition, patients with SLE are at risk of stroke because of the thromboembolic nature of the antiphospholipid antibody.

Pathophysiology

The exact pathophysiology of SLE remains unknown. It is an autoimmune disease (type III hypersensitivity) in which patients have an overactivity of B-cell lymphocytes. The result is hypergammaglobulinemia that ultimately precipitates immune complexes on the vascular membranes, thereby causing activation of complement. Drugs, procainamide ⚠ being the most predominant, may also cause SLE. Other such medications include phenytoin ⚠, chlorpromazine ⚠, hydralazine, quinidine ⚠, methyldopa, and isoniazid ⚠. Patients of the slow acetylator phenotype may have a greater risk for developing drug-induced lupus, particularly with procainamide and hydralazine. Musculoskeletal manifestations are the primary clinical manifestation of drug-induced lupus, but patients may also have fever, fatigue, pericarditis, pleurisy, and

BOX 26-1 Clinical Presentation of Systemic Lupus Erythematosus (SLE)

Signs and symptoms consistent with SLE include the following:

- Malar rash (a butterfly-shaped rash over the cheeks and across the bridge of the nose)
- Discoid rash (scaly, disk-shaped sores on the face, neck, or chest)
- Photosensitivity
- Oral ulcers
- Arthritis
- Serositis (inflammation of the lining around the heart, lungs, or abdomen that causes pain and shortness of breath)
- Proteinuria
- CNS problems
- Antinuclear antibodies (autoantibodies that react against the body's own cells)

- Anemia, leukopenia, lymphopenia, thrombocytopenia
- Fatigue
- Fever
- Skin rash
- Muscle aches
- Nausea
- Vomiting and diarrhea
- Anorexia
- Raynaud's phenomenon
- Weight loss

Procainamide *FDA BOXED WARNING*

Prolonged administration may lead to positive antinuclear antibody test. If this occurs weigh risks vs. benefits of therapy.

Phenytoin *FDA BOXED WARNING*

Cardiovascular risk associated with rapid infusion—cardiac monitoring required during and after intravenous administration.

Chlorpromazine *FDA BOXED WARNING*

Increased risk of mortality in elderly patients with dementia-related psychosis—not approved for use in patients with dementia-related psychosis.

Quinidine *FDA BOXED WARNING*

Increased risk of mortality when compared to other antiarrhythmics.

Isoniazid *FDA BOXED WARNING*

Increased risk of severe or fatal hepatitis. Close monitoring of liver function is required.

weight loss. These usually disappear with drug discontinuation. Antihistone antibodies are specific for drug-induced lupus occurring only in a small percentage of idiopathic lupus patients.

Drug Therapy

Therapy for each case of SLE is based on the particular symptoms of the patient. Arthritis is commonly treated with NSAIDs or glucocorticoids. Dermatologic complications can be treated with hydroxychloroquine (see Section 26-3). Patients should be told to avoid sun exposure as this may worsen the disease. Hydroxychloroquine may also be used for musculoskeletal manifestations that do not respond to NSAIDs. Thrombocytopenia generally responds to glucocorticoid therapy. Steroid dosing should remain as low as possible to minimize side effects. At times steroid sparing agents like methotrexate or azathioprine may be tried. Immunosuppressive agents are used in patients with lupus nephritis. Most commonly, cyclophosphamide ⚠ is used, sometimes in combination with glucocorticoids, especially I.V. for induction therapies. Azathioprine and mycophenolate ⚠ may be used as well. In early 2011, the FDA approved belimumab (Benlysta) for the treatment of adult patients with active, autoantibody-positive SLE who are receiving standard therapy. Belimumab is in the new class of drugs known as BLyS-specific inhibitors.

> **Cyclophosphamide and Mycophenolate** *FDA BOXED WARNINGS*
>
> Increased risk of first trimester pregnancy loss and congenital malformations. Increased risk of lymphomas and other malignancies. Increased risk of serious infections.

Belimumab

Mechanism of action

Belimumab is a monoclonal antibody that inhibits the binding of human B-cell lymphocyte stimulator protein (BLyS) to its receptors on the B-cells. Belimumab inhibits the survival of B-cells, including autoreactive B-cells, and reduces the differentiation of B-cells into immunoglobulin-producing plasma cells.

Adverse drug effects

Migraine (5%), depression (5%), pharyngitis (5%), pain in limb (6%), insomnia (7%), bronchitis (9%), nasopharyngitis (9%), fever (10%), diarrhea (12%), and nausea (15%) have been reported.

Drug–drug interactions

None have been noted.

Parameters to monitor

Monitor for infusion reactions.

Dose

The dose is 10 mg/kg I.V. every 2 weeks × 3 doses and then every 4 weeks.

Other aspects

Belimumab may be helpful in more severe disease.

26-7   Pharmacist's Role

Pharmacist can play an important role in patient education on the benefit, purpose, and use of the medications used to treatment arthritis. They can also teach patients what adverse effects may occur and how the monitoring should be done. Pharmacists are key to ensure patient safety with dosing and drug interactions and to alert prescribers if patients report side effects or inefficacy.

NAPLEX Competency Statements

The questions in this chapter cover the following 2021 NAPLEX Competency Statements: **AREA 1:** 1.1; 1.2; 1.3; 1.4; 1.5; 1.6 **AREA 2:** 2.1; 2.2; 2.3; 2.4 **AREA 3:** 3.2; 3.3; 3.4; 3.5; 3.6; 3.7; 3.8; 3.10; 3.11; 3.12 **AREA 4:** 4.1 **AREA 5:** 5.1.

 **26-8   Questions**

1. A 45-year-old man presents to his local health care provider with a complaint of extreme stiffness for the past 2 months that begins in the morning and lasts until noon on most days. He also states that he feels "drained" all the time and that both of his knees are swollen and painful. On examining the patient, the health care provider documents the presence of rheumatoid nodules. The patient's laboratory workup is significant for an elevated CRP (C-reactive protein) and ESR (erythrocyte sedimentation rate) and a positive rheumatoid factor. He states that he has been taking over-the-counter ibuprofen at a dose of 200 mg 2 or 3 times daily without relief. Which of the following represents the best drug therapy option for this patient?

   A. Increase the dose of ibuprofen to 800 mg 3 times daily.
   B. Increase the dose of ibuprofen, and add methotrexate 25 mg twice daily.
   C. Increase the dose of ibuprofen, and add celecoxib 100 mg twice daily.
   D. Increase the dose of ibuprofen, and add leflunomide at a dose of 100 mg daily for 3 days, followed by 20 mg daily.
   E. Increase the dose of ibuprofen and add omeprazole for GI prophylaxis.

2. Which of the following represents the best way to decrease potential toxicity with methotrexate while achieving optimal therapeutic benefit?

   A. Add 1 to 3 mg of folic acid per day to the patient's regimen.
   B. Decrease the dose of methotrexate to 25 mg once monthly.
   C. Add monthly injections of leucovorin to the patient's regimen.
   D. Change to subcutaneous administration of methotrexate.
   E. Add leflunomide to the patient's regimen.

3. Because combination DMARD therapy may be more efficacious in the refractory RA population, which of the following represents the best choice for combination therapy?

   A. Arava 20 mg once daily + Rheumatrex 5 mg once daily
   B. Remicade 3 mg/kg I.V. + Enbrel 50 mg once weekly
   C. Ridaura 3 mg 4 times daily + Plaquenil 200 mg twice daily
   D. Remicade 3 mg/kg I.V. every 2 months + Rheumatrex 25 mg once weekly
   E. Prednisone 5 mg daily + Omeprazole 20 mg daily

4. A young woman in the rheumatology clinic is diagnosed with systemic lupus. She is begun on daily hydroxychloroquine and daily prednisone. What important safety parameters should she follow?

   A. She should have weekly blood work because of the side effects of steroids.
   B. She should use 2 forms of birth control because of the hydroxychloroquine.
   C. She should self isolate as steroids are so immunosuppressive.
   D. She should only take the medicines as needed on days she feels the overwhelming fatigue.
   E. She should avoid sunlight and be sure to see an optometrist or ophthalmologist for drug-therapy monitoring.

5. Which of the following represents a method to decrease the GI toxicity associated with NSAIDs?

   A. Changing patients from a COX-2 inhibitor to nonspecific NSAID
   B. Adding a proton pump inhibitor such as Prevacid to the patient's NSAID
   C. Adding glucosamine to the patient's NSAID
   D. Instructing the patient to take the NSAID at night, when acid secretion is limited
   E. Using antacids to decrease dyspepsia

6. NSAID side effects about which a patient be counseled include _____.

   A. category X teratogenicity
   B. neurologic and immunologic effects
   C. gastrointestinal and dermatologic effects
   D. cardiovascular, renal, and gastrointestinal effects
   E. additive toxicity with biologic drugs

7. Which of the following would be a contraindication for the use of Enbrel?

   A. Renal insufficiency
   B. Active infection
   C. Patient over the age of 65 years
   D. Patient with class I or II congestive heart failure
   E. Use of methotrexate

8. Regarding the biologic DMARDs, which of the following statements is correct?

   A. Kineret is unique in that it is not immunosuppressive.
   B. Patients should have TB screening completed before initiation.
   C. Patients should take as needed for symptom control.
   D. FluMist is acceptable to use for influenza prevention.
   E. Patients receiving therapy are at increased risk for hepatitis.

9. The use of glucocorticoids is associated with numerous adverse effects and long-term consequences. Which of the following are initiatives to treat, prevent, or minimize these adverse effects?

   A. Instructing patients to take the glucocorticoid in divided daily doses.
   B. Instructing patients on long-term therapy to add elemental calcium and 400 to 800 IU of daily ergocalciferol to their regimen.
   C. Adding daily chondroitin for arthritis to help offset bone effects of steroids.
   D. Informing patients that stopping glucocorticoid abruptly is contraindicated.
   E. Not vaccinating as vaccines may cause a loss of effect of the steroid.

10. A young female enters your pharmacy and informs you that she plans on becoming pregnant and would like you to review her medication profile to see if any of her medications would be potentially harmful. On reviewing her profile, you notice that she is taking Arava for RA. Which of the following is the most appropriate response?

    A. Arava is a category C drug and could potentially harm the fetus. She should discuss the risks and benefits of becoming pregnant with her health care provider first.
    B. Arava is contraindicated drug in pregnancy, and she should undergo the drug elimination procedure with cholestyramine before trying to conceive.
    C. Arava is a category X drug with no active metabolites and a short half-life; therefore, she should discontinue the drug and wait 1 to 2 weeks before trying to become pregnant.
    D. Arava is a category C drug and should not be used in the first trimester.
    E. Arava is a category B drug, and the risk of toxicity to the fetus is extremely low.

11. A 67-year-old man has chief complaints of a swollen big left toe and extreme pain. The area is erythematous and tender. Laboratory analysis reveals a uric acid level of 10 mg/dL. Review of the patient's past medical history reveals hypertension and congestive heart failure. A diagnosis of gout is made. Which of the following is the best choice for the treatment of the patient's acute gouty arthritis attack?

    A. Probenecid 500 mg now, followed by 500 mg twice daily
    B. Indomethacin 50 mg now, followed by 50 mg 3 to 3 times daily
    C. Allopurinol 100 mg once daily
    D. Colchicine 1.2 mg followed by 0.6 mg in 1 hour if symptoms persist
    E. Prednisone 5 mg for 3 days

12. Which of the following are criteria to begin treating patients with gout prophylaxis?

    A. The presence of crystals in the affected synovial joint fluid
    B. Two gout attacks per year or tophi
    C. The presence of symmetrically swollen joints
    D. The presence of hyperuricemia
    E. The patient is over 70 years old

13. During a routine clinic appointment, you conduct a medication review with your patient, a 35-year-old-male with RA. He states he and his wife have been trying to conceive for 1 year with no results. After reviewing his medication list, which drug would you most suspect is contributing to this patient's infertility issues?

A. Methotrexate
B. Hydroxychloroquine
C. Leflunomide
D. Sulfasalazine
E. Etanercept

14. Drug-induced lupus usually manifests as
_____.

A. severe nephrotic syndrome
B. blood disorders including low red blood cell, white blood cell, and platelet counts
C. arthritis
D. severe neurologic disease
E. cardiac failure

15. Which of the following statements is true regarding Zyloprim?

A. It works to decrease the formation of uric acid by inhibiting xanthine kinase.
B. It does not require dosage adjustment in patients with renal insufficiency.
C. Skin reactions, including Stevens–Johnson syndrome, have been reported with its use.
D. It should be used for the treatment of an acute gouty arthritis attack.
E. Drugs interactions are not an issue.

16. Which of the following represent potentially dangerous drug interactions with Zyloprim?

A. Leflunomide and methotrexate
B. Amoxicillin and Imuran
C. Etanercept and infliximab
D. Hydroxychloroquine
E. Entanercept and adalimumab

17. Which of the following is consistent with the diagnosis of osteoarthritis?

A. It is normally associated with elevations in C-reactive protein and ESR.
B. A common initial finding of pain typically worsens with weight-bearing activity and subsides with rest.
C. It commonly occurs in the wrists or the elbows.
D. Crepitus is uncommon.
E. The joint is usually red and warm.

18. Which of the following medication combinations is contraindicated?

A. Tylenol and Ultram
B. Glucosamine sulfate and chondroitin
C. Ultram and Parnate
D. Tylenol and glucosamine sulfate
E. Adalimumab and methotrexate

19. Concerning treatment of osteoarthritis, which of the following statements is correct?

A. Tylenol is generally considered an initial drug of choice.
B. Tylenol should be given scheduled and not as needed, and it has minimal adverse effects, especially in doses greater than 4 g/d.
C. NSAIDs may be helpful, and they have minimal side effects to consider.
D. Hyaluronic acid derivatives have been approved by the FDA for the treatment of pain associated with osteoarthritis, and they are robustly effective.
E. DMARDs could be considered as second line therapy.

20. Which of the following medications is considered to be a DMARD?

A. Plaquenil
B. Allopurinol
C. Belimumab
D. Celecoxib
E. Omeprazole

 **26-9**   # Answers

1. **D.** Although the patient currently has room to increase his dose of the NSAID, he would benefit from the addition of a DMARD. This patient has disease duration of less than 6 months with moderate disease and poor prognostic factors. Methotrexate represents a viable option; however, the dose of 25 mg twice daily is excessive (it should be dosed once weekly). The addition of leflunomide is the best choice.

2. **A.** The addition of folic acid to the methotrexate regimen has been demonstrated to reduce the risk of liver toxicity. Lowering the dose of methotrexate is likely to decrease risk but is also likely to decrease its effectiveness. Leucovorin, an injectable formulation of folate, is normally used to reverse methotrexate toxicity.

3. **D.** Arava plus methotrexate (Rheumatrex) may be a very efficacious combination, but it increases the risk of liver toxicity significantly, and methotrexate should not be given daily. Gold therapy in combination with Plaquenil increases the risk of rash (although it may rarely be used together), and oral gold therapy should not be dosed 4 times daily. Remicade and Enbrel, 2 biologics, should not be used together. Prednisone should only be used as necessary, and a DMARD would be preferable. Remicade is approved for use in combination with Rheumatrex; this combination represents the best choice.

4. **E.** She should avoid sunlight as that can exacerbate SLE, and she should see an eye specialist to be sure the hydroxychloroquine is not toxic to the eye.

5. **B.** Use a proton pump inhibitor. Glucosamine offers no GI protection. Timing the dose of NSAIDs has never been shown to change their toxicity profile. COX-2 inhibitors are less likely to cause GI damage than are nonspecific NSAIDs.

6. **D.** Cardiovascular, renal, and gastrointestinal side effects are the primary counseling points to cover.

7. **B.** Because of its effects on tumor necrosis factor, Enbrel may decrease a patient's ability to fight infection. Enbrel is contraindicated in patients with an active infection. Its use should be temporarily discontinued until the acute process has resolved.

8. **B.** Do a TB screening test before initiation of biologic drugs because of their immune-suppressing properties, which could cause the reactivation of a disease such as tuberculosis.

9. **D.** Because of adrenal suppression that occurs with long-term glucocorticoid therapy, patients should taper off the agent.

10. **B.** Because Arava is a teratogenic agent with an active metabolite with a long half-life, a drug elimination procedure should be performed before becoming pregnant.

11. **D.** Both probenecid and allopurinol may exacerbate an acute gouty arthritis attack and should be reserved for the prevention of further attacks only. Indomethacin is an option for the treatment of an acute gouty arthritis attack; however, because of NSAIDs' tendency to cause fluid retention in the renal tubules, it would not be the ideal agent in a patient with congestive heart failure. Prednisone is given at a higher dosage than 5 mg daily when used acutely in gout. Colchicine represents the best option from this list.

12. **B.** Two gout attacks per year or tophi are criteria to begin treating patients with gout prophylaxis.

13. **D.** Sulfasalazine causes oligozoospermia.

14. **C.** Drug-induced lupus often manifests itself as arthritis, not the other, more severe manifestations.

15. **C.** Zyloprim's use has been associated with serious skin reactions that may occur at any point during therapy.

16. **B.** The co-administration of amoxicillin and allopurinol increases the risk of rash up to 20%. Imuran is metabolized via xanthine oxidase, whose activity is inhibited by allopurinol, thus increasing the risk of toxicity associated with Imuran.

17. **B.** RA usually exhibits elevations in ESR and C-reactive protein, unlike OA. OA typically affects the weight-bearing joints and is relieved with rest. The joints are usually cool and bony.

18. **C.** Tylenol and Ultram are marketed therapeutically as Ultracet. Glucosamine sulfate with or without chondroitin used to be recommended as an alternative therapy in the treatment of OA. The combination of Ultram and Parnate, a monoamine oxidase inhibitor, is contraindicated because of the risk of serotonin syndrome.

19. A. Tylenol is generally considered to be safe and effective, and it is considered the drug of choice initially. Doses greater than 4 g/d of Tylenol should never be used because of the risk of hepatic injury. Hyaluronidase derivatives are marginally effective. The adverse effects of NSAIDs are considerable and must always be taken into account when initiating therapy for OA. DMARDs are not used for osteoarthritis.

20. A. Allopurinol is a xanthine oxidase inhibitor used in the treatment of gout. Nalfon is an NSAID. Belimumab is a monoclonal antibody used in the treatment of SLE.

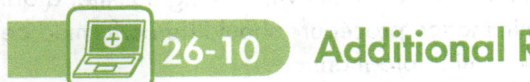 ## 26-10 Additional Resources

Rheumatoid Arthritis

Aletaha D, Neogi T, Silman AJ, et al. Rheumatoid arthritis classification criteria: an American College of Rheumatology/European League Against Rheumatism collaborative initiative. *Ann Rheum Dis.* 2010;69:1580–1588.

Bhatt DL, Scheiman J, Abraham NS, et al. ACCF/ACG/AHA 2008 expert consensus document on reducing the gastrointestinal risks of antiplatelet therapy and NSAID use. *Am J Gastroenterol.* 2008;103:2890–2907.

Furst DE, Keyston EC, Braun J, et al. Updated consensus statement on biological agents for the treatment of rheumatic diseases. *Ann Rheum Dis.* 2011;70(suppl 1):i2–i36.

Nissen SE, Yeomans ND, Solomon DH, et al. Cardiovascular Safely of Celecoxib, Naproxen, or Ibuprofen for Arthritis. *N Eng J Med* 2016;2519–2529.

Singh JA, Saag KG, Bridges SL Jr, et al. 2016 American College of Rheumatology Guideline for the Treatment of Rheumatoid Arthritis. *Arthritis Rheumatol.* 2016;68(1):1–26.

Smolen JS, Landewe RBM, Bijlsma JWJ, et al. EULAR recommendations for the management of rheumatoid arthritis with synthetic and biological disease-modifying antirheumatic drugs: 2019 update. *Ann Rheum Dis.* 2020;doi:10.1136/annrheumdis-2019-216655.

Osteoarthritis

Kolasinski SL, Neogi T, Hochberg MC, et al. American College of Rheumatology/Arthritis Foundation Guideline for the Management of Osteoarthritis of Hand, Hip, and Knee. *Arthritis Care Res.* 2020;72(2):149–162.

Gout

Khanna D, Fitzgerald JD, Khanna PP, et al. American College of Rheumatology guidelines for management of gout. Part 1: systemic pharmacologic and nonpharmacologic therapeutic approaches to hyperuricemia. *Arthritis Care Res.* 2012;64(10):1431–1446.

Khanna D, Khanna PP, Fitzgerald JD, et al. American College of Rheumatology guidelines for management of gout. Part 2: therapy and anti-inflammatory prophylaxis of acute gouty arthritis. *Arthritis Care Res.* 2012;64(10):1447–1461.

Richette P, Doherty M, Pascual E, et al. 2016 updated EULAR evidence-based recommendations for the management of gout. *Ann Rheum Dis* 2017;76:29–42.

Systemic Lupus Erythematosus

Fanouriakis A, Kostopoulou M, Alunno A, et al. 2019 update of the EULAR recommendations for the management of systemic lupus erythematosus. *Ann Rheum Dis* 2019;78:736–745.

Lupus Foundation of America. Web page: http://www.lupus.org.

Tsokos GC. Systemic lupus erythematosus. *N Engl J Med.* 2011;365(22):2110–2121.

Pain Management and Migraines

JAMES S. WHEELER

27-1 KEY POINTS

PAIN MANAGEMENT

- Opioids ⚠ relieve pain by mimicking the actions of endogenous opioid peptides at μ, δ, and κ receptors.
- Opioids fall into 3 categories: pure μ agonists, agonist–antagonists, and pure antagonists.
- With prolonged use, opioids produce tolerance to analgesia, euphoria, sedation, respiratory depression, and other adverse effects—but not to constipation.
- A growing body of evidence suggests the role of opioids in chronic, noncancer pain is limited.
- Opioid overdose induces coma, respiratory depression, and pinpoint pupils. Naloxone, a pure opioid antagonist, is used in cases of overdose to reverse most effects of opioids.
- Alcohol and other central nervous system (CNS) depressants can intensify opioid-induced sedation and respiratory depression. Tricyclic antidepressants and antihistamines may worsen opioid-induced constipation and urinary retention.
- Hydrocodone ⚠, codeine ⚠, fentanyl ⚠, methadone ⚠, and **oxycodone** ⚠ are metabolized by the cytochrome P450 (CYP450) system. Dose adjustments may be required in liver dysfunction. Fentanyl, morphine ⚠, and methadone require dosing adjustments in renal dysfunction.

MIGRAINE

- The pathogenesis of migraine is often multifactorial. Primary neuronal dysfunction originates in the CNS, leading to a sequence of changes that account for the different stages of migraine.
- The goal of abortive therapy is to eliminate headache pain and associated nausea and vomiting. The goal of preventive therapy is to reduce the incidence of migraine attacks.
- Triptans are drugs of choice for abortive therapy of migraines. They activate 5-hydroxytryptamine (HT)1B and 5-HT1D receptors, thereby causing constriction of cranial blood vessels and suppression of inflammatory neuropeptides.
- Triptans can cause coronary vasospasm and are contraindicated in patients with ischemic heart disease, prior myocardial infarction, and uncontrolled hypertension. If a triptan is combined with another triptan or with an ergot alkaloid, excessive prolonged vasospasms could result.
- Divalproex sodium ⚠, **topiramate**, **propranolol** ⚠, and timolol ⚠ are labeled by the U.S. Food and Drug Administration for use as first-line prophylaxis of migraine headaches. **Amitriptyline** ⚠, venlafaxine ⚠, **atenolol** ⚠, and nadolol ⚠ are among drugs used as second-line treatment.
- Nonopioid analgesics are effective for abortive therapy of mild to moderate pain.
- Opioid analgesics are reserved for a severe migraine that has not responded to other drugs.

27-2 STUDY GUIDE CHECKLIST

The following topics may guide your study of this subject area:

- ☐ Clinical presentation of various types of pain.
- ☐ Considerations for selection of pain management drugs based on patient's condition and prior drug experience.
- ☐ Trade names, available dosage forms, and dosing regimens of selected opioids.
- ☐ Major adverse drug effects of opioid drugs.
- ☐ Significant drug–disease and drug–drug interactions of opioid drugs.
- ☐ Ability to perform opioid dose conversions.
- ☐ Patient counseling points for specific pain management drugs.

Editor's Note: This chapter is based on the 11th edition chapter written by Elizabeth S. Miller and Sarah T. Stapleton.

Opioids *FDA BOXED WARNINGS*

Potential for addiction, abuse, and misuse. Potential for life-threatening respiratory depression, especially if used concomitantly with benzodiazepines. Monitor interactions with medications metabolized by CYP enzymes.

Avoid use in pregnant women due to risk of neonatal opioid withdrawal.

All immediate release (IR) and Extended-Release and Long-Acting (ER/LA) Opioid Analgesics are subject to the FDA's Risk Evaluation and Mitigation Strategy (REMS) to ensure that the benefits of opioid analgesics used in the outpatient setting outweigh the risks.

Butorphanol has an accidental exposure (intranasal) warning.

Fentanyl patches have warnings specific to exposure to heat (e.g., heating pads, electric blankets) may increase fentanyl levels. Risk of accidental exposure to children resulting in fatal overdose when using patch formulation.

Methadone has conditions for distribution and use of methadone products for the treatment of opioid addiction and Increased risk of QT prolongation.

Morphine's extended-release capsules have a warning with ethanol use, the oral solution has a risk of medication errors warning, and the brand names Infumorph, Duramorph, and Mitigo have risks with neuroaxial administration.

Meperidine should not be used concomitantly with MAOIs. The oral solution has a risk of medication errors.

Tapentadol's extended-release formulation has a warning for interaction with alcohol.

Tramadol has warnings of: accidental ingestion, ultra-rapid metabolism of **tramadol** and other risk factors for life threatening respiratory depression in children.

For further details on boxed warnings, refer to the product's package insert.

 ## Divalproex Sodium *FDA BOXED WARNING*

Valproic acid and its derivatives have FDA boxed warnings for hepatotoxicity, pancreatitis, fetal risk, and patients with mitochondrial disease. Children under 2 years of age are at a considerably increased risk of hepatotoxicity. Valproate is contraindicated in patients with known mitochondrial disorders and in children younger than two who are clinically suspected to have a mitochondrial disorder. In addition, valproate can cause neural tube defects, and is contraindicated in women of childbearing potential who are not using effective contraception.

Increased risk of hepatotoxicity. Increased risk of pancreatitis. Use in pregnant women is contraindicated due to increased risk of congenital malformations.

 ## Propranolol *FDA BOXED WARNING*

Cardiac ischemia after abrupt discontinuation with brand names Inderal LA, Inderal XL, and Innopral XL. Myocardial infarction and exacerbations of angina pectoris have occurred following abrupt discontinuation of therapy with beta-blockers.

Avoid abrupt discontinuation due to increased risk of cardiac adverse events.

Timolol *FDA BOXED WARNING*

Exacerbation of ischemic heart disease following abrupt withdrawal. Myocardial infarction and exacerbations of angina pectoris have occurred following abrupt discontinuation of therapy with beta-blockers. When discontinuing chronically administered timolol, gradually reduce the dose over 1 to 2 weeks.

Increased risk of ischemic heart disease exacerbation with abrupt withdrawal.

 Amitriptyline *FDA BOXED WARNING*

Suicidality and antidepressant drugs. Antidepressants increased the risk of suicidal thinking and behavior in children and young adults under age 24. Patients of all ages starting **Amitriptyline** should be monitored for suicidality and unusual changes in behavior.

Increased risk of suicidality.

 Venlafaxine *FDA BOXED WARNING*

Suicidality and antidepressant drugs. Antidepressants increased the risk of suicidal thinking and behavior in children and young adults under age 24. Patients of all ages starting **Venlafaxine** should be monitored for suicidality and unusual changes in behavior.

Increased risk of suicidality.

 Atenolol *FDA BOXED WARNING*

Cessation of therapy. Myocardial infarction and exacerbations of angina pectoris have occurred following abrupt discontinuation of therapy with beta-blockers.

Avoid abrupt discontinuation of therapy. Abrupt discontinuation increases risk of cardiac events.

 Nadolol *FDA BOXED WARNING*

Exacerbation of cardiac ischemia following abrupt withdrawal. Myocardial infarction and exacerbations of angina pectoris have occurred following abrupt discontinuation of therapy with beta-blockers. When discontinuing chronically administered nadolol, gradually reduce the dose over 1 to 2 weeks.

Avoid abrupt discontinuation of therapy. Abrupt discontinuation increases risk of cardiac events.

27-3   Pain Management

Pain is defined as real or potential tissue injury associated with any uncomfortable sensory or emotional experience, or both. Practitioners often define pain in terms of symptoms that the patient experiences or perceives.

Types and Clinical Presentation

Pain can be classified as acute, chronic, or cancer pain.

Acute pain is caused by an injury, illness, or surgery. It responds to medications and usually resolves when the underlying cause has been treated or healed. It is often associated with physiological symptoms such as tachycardia, hypertension, diaphoresis, and mydriasis.

Chronic pain exists beyond an expected time for healing, typically lasting months to years. It is often associated with psychological effects, including social isolation, depression, and anxiety.

Cancer pain may be acute, chronic, or intermittent and is often related to cancer progression or chemotherapy.

Pain is also defined by source. Such a classification divides pain into somatic, visceral, and neuropathic pain.

Somatic pain originates from the skin, muscles, tendons, ligaments, and bones. It is localized and described as sharp, stabbing, throbbing, or aching in nature. Although somatic pain can be severe, it tends to respond well to treatment with opioids.

The body's internal organs such as the liver, intestines, or stomach generate *visceral pain*. Visceral pain tends to be poorly localized and more likely to generate referred pain felt some distance away from the actual problem. Opioids are not as effective for visceral pain as they are for somatic pain.

Neuropathic pain results when the nerves themselves are damaged. It is typically burning in nature, although it may also cause numbness, aching, or a sensation like an electric shock. Opioid medications are not the most effective treatment for neuropathic pain and are recommended as second-line treatment. Specific tricyclic antidepressants, antiepileptics, and serotonin–norepinephrine reuptake inhibitors (SNRIs) are typically recommended as first-line treatment. Table 27-1 lists therapies for neuropathic pain.

Pathophysiology

Nociception, the pain sensation, begins when a sensory nerve ending is stimulated and sends repetitive signals to the spinal cord along ascending nerve fibers. Opioids chemically resemble neurotransmitters and modulate pain signal transmission.

Chronic pain is not a prolonged version of acute pain. As pain signals are repeatedly generated, neural pathways undergo changes that make them hypersensitive to pain signals and resistant to antinociceptive input.

Goals of Pain Management

Acute pain

The goal in acute pain management is to provide patients with pain relief that allows them to rest comfortably and allows postsurgery or postinjury rehabilitation. When opioids are used for acute pain, the lowest effective dose of immediate-release opioids should be used in no greater quantity than the expected duration of maximum pain (in many cases 3 days, rarely more than 7 days).

Chronic pain

In 2016, the U.S. Centers for Disease Control and Prevention published guidelines for prescribing opioids in chronic pain. Nonpharmacologic therapy and nonopioid pharmacologic therapy are preferred for

TABLE 27-1. Prescribing Recommendations for Neuropathic Pain

Medication class and generic name	Trade name	Available strengths	Starting dosage (maximum dose)	Major adverse effects
Antidepressants				
TCAs				
Nortriptyline ⚠	Pamelor	10, 25, 50, 75 mg	25 mg daily at bedtime (150 mg daily)	Cardiac toxicity, anticholinergic side effects (sedation, dry mouth, blurred vision, urinary retention)
Desipramine ⚠	Norpramin	10, 25, 50, 75, 100, 150 mg	25 mg daily at bedtime (150 mg daily)	
SNRIs				
Duloxetine ⚠	Cymbalta	20, 30, 60 mg	30 mg daily (60 mg daily)	Nausea
Venlafaxine	Effexor	25, 37.5, 50, 75, 100 mg	37.5 mg once or twice daily (225 mg daily)	Nausea, ↑ blood pressure
Calcium channel alpha 2–, delta ligands[a,b]				
Gabapentin	Neurontin	100, 300, 400 mg	100 to 300 mg bedtime or 3 times daily (3600 mg daily)	Dizziness, sedation, renal insufficiency
Pregabalin	Lyrica	25, 50, 75, 100, 150, 200, 225, 300 mg	50 mg 3 times daily or 75 mg twice daily (600 mg daily)	
Local anesthetic[a]				
Lidocaine patch	Lidoderm	5% patch	3 patches every 12 hours (starting and maximum)	Mild local reactions
Opioid agonists[c]				
Morphine, **oxycodone,** methadone, levorphanol ⚠	MSIR, Roxicodone, Dolophine, Levo-Dromoran[b]	Morphine 15, 30 mg; **oxycodone** 5, 15, 30 mg; methadone 5, 10 mg; levorphanol 2 mg	10 to 15 mg every 4 hours or as needed of morphine or equianalgesic dose of other opioid analgesic (no maximum dose)	Constipation, nausea, sedation
Tramadol ⚠	Ultram[b]	50 mg	50 to 100 mg daily or twice daily (400 mg daily)	Constipation, nausea, sedation, lowers the seizure threshold

Adapted from Dworkin RH, O'Connor AB, Audette J, et al., 2010; O'Connor AB, Dworkin RH, 2009.
Boldface indicates one of top 100 drugs for 2020 by prescription volume.
SNRI, serotonin–norepinephrine reuptake inhibitor; TCA, tricyclic antidepressant.
a. First-line treatment.
b. Consider lower starting doses and slower titration in the elderly.
c. Second-line treatment; may be appropriate as first-line treatment in certain circumstances.

FDA BOXED WARNINGS

Nortriptyline

Suicidality and antidepressants. Antidepressants including nortriptyline increased the risk of suicidal thinking and behaviors in children and young adults under the age of 24. Patients of all ages starting nortriptyline should be monitored for suicidality and unusual changes in behavior.

Increased risk of suicidality.

Desipramine

Suicidality and antidepressants. Antidepressants including desipramine increased the risk of suicidal thinking and behaviors in children and young adults under the age of 24. Patients of all ages starting desipramine should be monitored for suicidality and unusual changes in behavior.

Increased risk of suicidality.

Duloxetine

Suicidality and antidepressants. Antidepressants including **duloxetine** increased the risk of suicidal thinking and behaviors in children and young adults under the age of 24. Patients of all ages starting **duloxetine** should be monitored for suicidality and unusual changes in behavior.

Increased risk of suicidality.

Levorphanol

Levorphanol has FDA boxed warnings for addiction, abuse, and misuse, life-threatening respiratory depression, accidental ingestion, neonatal opioid withdrawal syndrome, and risks from concomitant use with benzodiazepines or other CNS depressants. Levorphanol also has an opioid analgesic risk evaluation and mitigation strategy (REMS) to ensure the benefits of therapy outweigh the risks.

Potential for addiction, abuse, and misuse. Potential for life-threatening respiratory depression, especially if used concomitantly with benzodiazepines. Avoid use in pregnant women due to risk of neonatal opioid withdrawal.

Tramadol

Potential for addiction, abuse, and misuse. Potential for life-threatening respiratory depression, especially if used concomitantly with benzodiazepines or if ultra-rapid metabolizer. Monitor interactions with medications metabolized by CYP3A4 and CPY2D6. Avoid use in pregnant women due to risk of neonatal opioid withdrawal.

chronic pain. If opioids are used, they should be combined with nonpharmacologic therapy and nonopioid pharmacologic therapy as appropriate. A growing body of evidence suggests the role of opioids in chronic, noncancer pain is limited. For patients initiated on opioids for chronic noncancer pain, these therapies should not be continued without evidence of a clear therapeutic benefit, given the risk of serious harm. The goal of chronic pain treatment is to restore the patient to the highest degree of function possible or a decrease in pain intensity of at least 30%, which can be measured by validated tools such as the "Pain average, interference with enjoyment of life, and interference with general activity" (PEG) assessment scale.

Multimodal therapy, the use of several different types of treatment, is usually required. Multimodal therapies include nerve blocks, rehabilitation, physical therapy, pharmacotherapy, acupuncture, and psychotherapy. Analgesics are categorized into nonopioid analgesics, opioid analgesics, and adjuvant analgesics. *Nonopioid analgesics,* such as **acetaminophen** and nonsteroidal anti-inflammatory drugs (NSAIDs), relieve all types of mild-to-moderate pain. Prescription products containing **acetaminophen** are limited to 325 mg per dosage unit because of the potential for severe liver failure. NSAIDs are commonly used as part of the treatment regimen for pain associated with inflammation and cancer-related bone pain. Unless contraindicated, all pain patients should first be given a trial of nonopioid analgesics. Nonopioids and opioids relieve pain via different mechanisms. Thus, combination therapy offers the potential for improved relief with decreased doses and fewer side effects. Nonopioids do not produce tolerance, physical dependence, or addiction Table 27-2 outlines available nonopioids.

Adjuvant analgesics are drugs with a primary indication other than pain. Commonly used adjuvant analgesics include antiepileptic drugs, tricyclic antidepressants, local anesthetics, and SNRIs. For further information on the antidepressants mentioned, refer to Chapters 28 (Seizure Disorders) and 29 (Psychiatric Diseases and Sleep Disorders).

TABLE 27-2. Common Nonopioid Analgesics

Generic name	Common trade name and strength	Dosing interval	I.V. starting dose	Oral daily starting dose (maximum dose)
Acetaminophen[a] ⚠				
Tablet	Tylenol	4 to 6 hours		325 to 600 mg (4000 mg daily)
Injection	Ofirmev		1000 mg	
Aspirin				
Tablet	Ecotrin			81 to 325 mg (4000 mg daily)
Diclofenac ⚠				
Tablet	Cataflam	8 to 12 hours		50 to 100 mg (150 mg daily)
Patch	Flector	Every 12 hours		
Ibuprofen ⚠				
Tablet	Motrin,	4 to 6 hours		200 to 400 mg (3200 mg daily)
Injection	Caldolor	6 hours	400 to 800 mg	
Ketoprofen ⚠				
Tablet		6 to 8 hours		25 to 50 mg (300 mg)
Naproxen ⚠				
Tablet	Naprosyn	12 hours		500 mg (1000 mg daily)
Naproxen sodium				
Tablet	Aleve, Anaprox	8 to 12 hours		440 mg (660 mg daily)
Ketorolac ⚠				
Tablet		4 to 6 hours oral		10 mg (40 mg daily, 5 days)
Injection		Single dose I.M., I.V., or every 6 hours I.V.	15 to 30 mg (maximum 5 days)	
Celecoxib ⚠				
Tablet	Celebrex	Every 12 hours		200 mg (400 mg daily)

Adapted from Herndon CM, Strickland JM, Ray JB, 2017.
Boldface indicates one of top 100 drugs for 2020 by prescription volume.
I.M., intramuscular; I.V., intravenous.
a. Rare but serious skin reactions have been reported.

FDA BOXED WARNINGS

Acetaminophen

Risk of medication errors and hepatotoxicity. **Acetaminophen** has been associated with cases of acute liver failure, at times resulting in liver transplant or death.

Increased risk of hepatotoxicity.

Diclofenac

Serious cardiovascular risk and serious gastrointestinal risk. Nonsteroidal anti-inflammatory drugs (NSAIDs) have an increased risk of serious cardiovascular events including myocardial infarction and stroke. NSAIDs also cause an increased risk of serious gastrointestinal adverse events including bleeding, ulceration, and perforation of the stomach or intestines.

Increased risk of cardiovascular thrombotic events. Increased risk of serious gastrointestinal adverse events (e.g., stomach bleed, ulcers).

Ibuprofen

Serious cardiovascular risk and serious gastrointestinal risk. Nonsteroidal anti-inflammatory drugs (NSAIDs) have an increased risk of serious cardiovascular events including myocardial infarction and stroke. NSAIDs also cause an increased risk of serious gastrointestinal adverse events including bleeding, ulceration, and perforation of the stomach or intestines.

Increased risk of cardiovascular thrombotic events. Increased risk of serious gastrointestinal adverse events (e.g., stomach bleed, ulcers).

Ketoprofen

Serious cardiovascular risk and serious gastrointestinal risk. Nonsteroidal anti-inflammatory drugs (NSAIDs) have an increased risk of serious cardiovascular events including myocardial infarction and stroke. NSAIDs also cause an increased risk of serious gastrointestinal adverse events including bleeding, ulceration, and perforation of the stomach or intestines.

Increased risk of cardiovascular thrombotic events. Increased risk of serious gastrointestinal adverse events (e.g., stomach bleed, ulcers).

Naproxen

Serious cardiovascular risk and serious gastrointestinal risk. Nonsteroidal anti-inflammatory drugs (NSAIDs) have an increased risk of serious cardiovascular events including myocardial infarction and stroke. NSAIDs also cause an increased risk of serious gastrointestinal adverse events including bleeding, ulceration, and perforation of the stomach or intestines.

Increased risk of cardiovascular thrombotic events. Increased risk of serious gastrointestinal adverse events (e.g., stomach bleed, ulcers).

Ketorolac

Serious cardiovascular risk and serious gastrointestinal risk. Nonsteroidal anti-inflammatory drugs (NSAIDs) have an increased risk of serious cardiovascular events including myocardial infarction and stroke. NSAIDs also cause an increased risk of serious gastrointestinal adverse events including bleeding, ulceration, and perforation of the stomach or intestines. Ketorolac has a warning for appropriate use as it is only indicated for the management of short term pain (up to 5 days in adults). It is not indicated for use in pediatric patients or for minor pain. It is contraindicated in intrathecal or epidural use due to its alcohol content. Hypersensitivity reactions ranging from bronchospasm to anaphylactic shock have occurred. Ketorolac is contraindicated in patients with advanced renal impairment and in patients at risk of renal failure due to volume depletion. It also has warnings to avoid use in patients with active bleeding or high risk of bleeds, concomitant use with other NSAIDs, and in labor and delivery. Dosage should be adjusted for patients over 65 years of age, patients under 50 kg, and for patients with moderately elevated serum creatinine.

Increased risk of cardiovascular thrombotic events. Increased risk of serious gastrointestinal adverse events (e.g., stomach bleed, ulcers). Maximum therapy duration is 5 days. Contraindicated in patients with advanced renal impairment, high bleed risk, or patients who are pregnant/delivering. Do NOT combine with other NSAIDs.

FDA BOXED WARNINGS (Continued)

Celecoxib

Serious cardiovascular risk and serious gastrointestinal risk. Nonsteroidal anti-inflammatory drugs (NSAIDs) have an increased risk of serious cardiovascular events including myocardial infarction and stroke. NSAIDs also cause an increased risk of serious gastrointestinal adverse events including bleeding, ulceration, and perforation of the stomach or intestines.

Increased risk of cardiovascular thrombotic events. Increased risk of serious gastrointestinal adverse events (e.g., stomach bleed, ulcers).

Cancer pain

A major goal of cancer pain management is to relieve the patient's pain without inducing disabling side effects. Cancer patients may suffer from constant pain that continues for months or years. For this reason, treatment with long-acting agents is more appropriate than treatment with short-acting medications. However, short-acting agents, referred to as "breakthrough" or "rescue" doses, are often available in addition to the long-acting medications.

Principles of opioid use

Opioids have no ceiling effect of analgesia.

Oral medications should be used whenever possible. Intramuscular injections are painful and should be avoided.

When patients have constant or near-constant pain, analgesics should be given around the clock. Long-acting opioid analgesics are often used for this purpose.

The use of short-acting opioids as rescue medication is controversial in chronic pain. If allowed, doses of rescue medications should range from 10% to 15% of the total daily long-acting opioid dose.

Mixed agonist–antagonist opioids are not used in chronic pain. They may induce a withdrawal syndrome in patients tolerant to opioids.

Drug Therapy

Mechanism of action

Morphine and other opioid agonists are thought to produce analgesia by mimicking the action of endogenous opioid peptides that bind at opioid receptors in the antinociceptive pathway.

Opioid receptors are located in the central nervous system (CNS), pituitary gland, and gastrointestinal (GI) tract. They are abundant in the periaqueductal gray matter of the brain and the dorsal horn of the spinal cord, 2 areas that are very active in pain reduction.

When a drug binds to 1 of these receptors as an agonist, it produces analgesia. When a drug binds to 1 of these receptors as an antagonist, analgesia and other effects are blocked.

The 3 major types of opioid receptor sites involved in analgesia are mu (μ), delta (δ), and kappa (κ):

- Binding to the μ receptor produces analgesia, sedation, euphoria, respiratory depression, physical dependence, constipation, and other effects.
- Activation of δ receptors produces analgesia without many adverse effects; however, there is no available δ-receptor agonist.
- Activation of the κ receptor produces analgesia and respiratory depression. In addition, psychotomimetic effects such as anxiety, strange thoughts, nightmares, and hallucinations are common.

Opioid analgesics

Opioids are classified by activity at the receptor site; that is, they are classified as pure opioid agonists, agonist–antagonists, or pure opioid antagonists.

Pure opioid agonists primarily activate μ receptors, although they may produce some κ-receptor activation. Pure opioid agonists are the most clinically useful opioid analgesics.

Morphine is the prototypical pure opioid agonist. Methadone is an opioid agonist with additional antagonist activity at the N-methyl-D-aspartate (NMDA) receptor. The NMDA receptor is believed to be active primarily in chronic pain.

Mixed agonist–antagonists bind as agonists at the κ receptor, producing weak analgesia. They bind as weak antagonists at the μ receptor (Table 27-3). The result is more dysphoria and psychotomimetic effects with a lower risk of respiratory depression.

Pentazocine ⚠ is the prototypical agonist–antagonist opioid. Buprenorphine ⚠ is actually a partial agonist at μ and κ receptors. This opioid has limited efficacy in pain management and is primarily used in detoxification programs.

Opioid antagonists such as naloxone and naltrexone block the μ and κ receptors (Table 27-4) and do not produce analgesia. Naloxone is used to reverse respiratory and CNS depression caused by overdose with opioid agonists. See Chapter 43 for more information. Tables 27-3 and 27-4 list starting opioid doses.

Box 27-1 lists the steps in the opioid conversion process.

TABLE 27-3. Opioid Dosing for Mild-to-Severe Pain in Adults

Generic name	Trade name and strength	Dosing interval	I.V. starting dose	Oral starting dose (maximum dose)
Moderate-to-severe pain: Moderate-severe opioid and opioid/antagonist				
Tapentadol (synthetic)				
Immediate-release tablet	Nucynta 50, 75, 100 mg	4 to 6 hours oral		50, 75, 100 mg (600 mg daily)
Extended-release tablet	Nucynta ER 50, 100, 150, 200, 250 mg	12 hours oral		50 mg (500 mg daily)
Liquid	20 mg/mL	4 to 6 hours oral		50, 75, 100 mg (600 mg daily)
Moderate-to-mild pain				
Codeine (natural)				
Tablet	Codeine sulfate 15, 30, 60 mg (CII)	4 hours	30 mg	15 to 60 mg (360 mg daily)
Liquid[a]	Codeine sulfate 6 mg/mL			
Tablet (codeine/acetaminophen)[a]	Tylenol with Codeine #3 (300/30 mg), #4 (300/60 mg)			
Liquid (codeine/acetaminophen)	Tylenol with Codeine Elixir 120/12 mg per 5 mL			
Hydrocodone (semisynthetic)				
Tablet (**hydrocodone/ acetaminophen**)	Vicodin 5/300 mg; Vicodin ES 7.5/300 mg; Vicodin HP 10/300 mg; Norco 5/325, 7.5/325, 10/325 mg	4 to 6 hours		2.5 to 10 mg

TABLE 27-3. Opioid Dosing for Mild-to-Severe Pain in Adults *(Continued)*

Generic name	Trade name and strength	Dosing interval	I.V. starting dose	Oral starting dose (maximum dose)
Liquid (**hydrocodone/ acetaminophen**)	Lortab Elixir 7.5/325 mg per 15 mL			
Tablet (hydrocodone/ ibuprofen)	Vicoprofen 7.5/200 mg; Reprexain 2.5/200, 5/200, 10/200 mg			
Moderate-to-severe pain: Agonists–antagonists				
Pentazocine ⚠				
Tablet (pentazocine/ naloxone)	50/0.5 mg	4 hours		50/0.5 to 100/1 mg (600 mg/d)
Butorphanol ⚠				
Injection	Butorphanol tartrate 1, 2 mg/mL	3 to 4 hours	0.5 to 2 mg	
Nasal spray	Butorphanol tartrate 1 mg/spray			1 spray in 1 nostril
Buprenorphine ⚠				
Injection	Buprenex 0.3 mg/mL	6 hours	0.3 to 0.6 mg	
Patch	Butrans 5, 10, 15, 20 mcg/h	7 days		5 mcg/h in opioid-naïve patients; 10 mg (opioid-tolerant patients) (20 mcg/h)
Miscellaneous				
Tramadol[b]				
Tablet	Ultram 50 mg	4 to 6 hours		50 to 100 mg (400 mg/d)
Controlled-release tablet	Ultram ER 100, 200, 300 mg	24 hours		100 mg (300 mg/d)
Tablet (tramadol/ acetaminophen)	Ultracet 325/37.5 mg	4 to 6 hours		2 tablets (650/75 mg) (8 tabs/d 2600/300 mg)

Boldface indicates one of top 100 drugs for 2020 by prescription volume.
I.M., intramuscular; I.V., intravenous.
a. Codeine contraindication effective April 2017: codeine should not be used to treat pain or cough in children younger than age 12 years.
b. Tramadol contraindication effective April 2017: tramadol should not be used in children younger than age 18 years to treat pain after surgery to remove the tonsils and/or adenoids, and it should not be used to treat pain in children younger than age 12 years.

 ### Pentazocine *FDA BOXED WARNING*

Pentazocine has FDA boxed warnings for addiction, abuse, misuse, life-threatening respiratory depression, neonatal opioid withdrawal syndrome, and risks from concomitant use with benzodiazepines and other CNS depressants.

Potential for addiction, abuse, and misuse. Potential for life-threatening respiratory depression, especially if used concomitantly with benzodiazepines. Avoid use in pregnant women due to risk of neonatal opioid withdrawal.

Buprenorphine *FDA BOXED WARNING*

Buprenorphine products have FDA boxed warnings for accidental exposure (buccal film, transdermal patch), addiction, abuse, and misuse (buccal film, immediate-release injection, transdermal patch), life-threatening respiratory depression (buccal film, immediate-release injection, transdermal patch), neonatal opioid withdrawal syndrome (buccal film, immediate-release injection, transdermal patch), risk associated with insertion and removal (subdermal implant), risks from concomitant use with benzodiazepines and other CNS depressants (buccal film, immediate-release injection, transdermal patch), risk of serious harm or death with IV administration (extended-release injection). Buprenorphine also has an opioid analgesic risk evaluation and mitigation strategy (REMS).

Potential for addiction, abuse, and misuse. Potential for life-threatening respiratory depression, especially if used concomitantly with benzodiazepines. Avoid use in pregnant women due to risk of neonatal opioid withdrawal. Accidental exposure to even one dose by children can result in a fatal overdose. Risk of serious harm or death with extended-release injection.

TABLE 27-4. Starting Doses for Strong Opioids for Severe and Moderate-to-Severe Pain in Adults: Mu Agonists

Generic name	Trade name and strength	Dosing interval	Equianalgesic dose I.V.	Equianalgesic dose Oral	Oral/ intranasal starting dose
Fentanyl (synthetic)					
Injection	Sublimaze 50 mcg/mL	0.5 to 2 hours I.M. or I.V.	0.1 mg	Not applicable	
Transdermal	Duragesic 12, 25, 50, 75, 100 mcg/h	Every 2 to 3 days			
Transmucosal lozenge[a]	Actiq 200, 400, 600, 800, 1200, 1600 mcg	4 hours			200 mcg
Disintegrating tablet[a]	Fentora 100, 200, 400, 600, 800 mcg	4 hours			100 mcg
	Abstral 100, 200, 300, 400, 600, 800 mcg	2 hours			100 mcg
Nasal spray[a]	Lazanda 100 mcg/100 mcL, 400 mcg/mcL	2 hours			100 mcg/mcL
Sublingual spray[a]	Subsys 100, 200, 400, 600, 800, 1200, 1600 mcg	4 hours			100 mcg
Hydrocodone (semisynthetic)					
Extended-release capsules	Zohydro ER 10, 15, 20, 30, 40, 50 mg	12 hours			10 mg
Extended-release tablets	Hysingla ER 20, 30, 40, 60, 80, 100, 120 mg				
Hydromorphone (semisynthetic)					
Immediate-release tablet	Dilaudid 2, 4, 8 mg	4 to 6 hours oral; 2 to 3 hours I.M., I.V., subcutaneous	1.3 to 2 mg	6.5 to 7.5 mg	2 to 4 mg
Liquid	Dilaudid 1 mg/mL	3 to 6 hours oral			2.5 to 10 mg
Injection	Dilaudid 1, 2, 4 mg/mL; Dilaudid HP 10 mg/mL				

Generic name	Trade name and strength	Dosing interval	Equianalgesic dose		Oral/intranasal starting dose
			I.V.	Oral	
Methadone (synthetic)					
Tablet	Dolophine 5, 10 mg; Methadose 5, 10 mg; Methadose dispersible 40 mg	8 to 12 hours oral; 4 to 12 hours I.M., I.V., or subcutaneous	Acute: 10 mg; chronic: 2 to 4 mg	Acute: 20 mg; chronic: 2 to 4 mg	2.5 to 10 mg
Liquid	Methadose 10 mg/mL; methadone HCl 1, 2, 10 mg/mL				
Injection	Methadone HCl 10 mg/mL				
Morphine (natural)					
Immediate-release tablet	MSIR 15, 30 mg	2 to 4 hours oral; 4 hours I.M., I.V., or subcutaneous; 4 hours per rectum	10 mg	30 mg	5 to 30 mg
Liquid	MSIR 2, 4, 20 mg/mL; morphine sulfate 2, 5 mg/mL; Roxanol 20 mg/mL				
Injection	Duramorph, Astramorph PF 0.5, 1 mg/mL; Infumorph 10, 25 mg/mL				
Controlled-release tablet	Kadian 10, 20, 30, 40, 50, 60, 70, 80, 100, 130, 150, 200 mg	12 to 24 hours oral	Not applicable		10 to 20 mg
	MS Contin 15, 30, 60, 100, 200 mg	8 to 12 hours oral			15 mg
Oxycodone (semisynthetic)					
Tablet	Roxicodone 5, 15, 30 mg	4 to 6 hours oral	Not applicable	20 mg	5 to 30 mg
	Oxecta 5, 7.5 mg	4 to 6 hours oral			5 to 15 mg
Capsule	Oxy IR 5 mg				
Liquid	Roxicodone 1, 20 mg/mL				
Tablet (**oxycodone/acetaminophen**)	Roxicet 5/325 mg; Percocet 2.5/325, 5/325, 7.5/325, 10/325 mg				
Liquid (**oxycodone/acetaminophen**)	Roxicet 5/325 mg per 5 mL				
Tablet (**oxycodone/ibuprofen**)	Combunox 5/400 mg	6 hours oral			
Controlled-release tablet	OxyContin 10, 15, 20, 30, 40, 60, 80 mg	12 hours oral		20 to 30 mg	10 mg
Oxymorphone (semisynthetic) ⚠					
Injection	Opana 1 mg/ml	4 to 6 hours oral; 4 hours I.M., I.V., or subcutaneous	1 to 1.5 mg	10 mg	5 to 20 mg
Immediate-release tablet	Opana 5, 10 mg	4 to 6 hours			10 to 20 mg

Boldface indicates one of top 100 drugs for 2020 by prescription volume.
I.M., intramuscular; I.V., intravenous.
a. For use in breakthrough cancer pain.

> **BOX 27-1. Steps in the Equianalgesic Conversion Process**

1. Total the 24-hour dose of current drug, including all breakthrough doses.
2. Convert 24-hour dose to new drug/route using an equianalgesic conversion table.
3. Divide the total dose of new drug by the dosing interval of the new drug.
4. In opioid-tolerant patients, consider reducing calculated dose of the new drug 25% to 50% to account for incomplete cross-tolerance.
5. Calculate a breakthrough dose—either 10% to 20% of the total daily opioid dose or 25% to 30% of the single standing dose.

Opioid analgesic adverse effects

Central nervous system

Opioids produce a number of CNS effects, including sedation, euphoria, dysphoria, changes in mood, and mental clouding. Confusion, disorientation, and cognitive impairment are also possible.

Mild-to-moderate muscle jerks, known as *myoclonus*, are common in patients on high doses of opioids. Myoclonus can be treated by changing the opioid dose, changing the opioid, or giving low doses of a benzodiazepine.

Neuroendocrine

Morphine acts in the hypothalamus to inhibit the release of gonadotropin-releasing hormone and corticotropin-releasing factor, thus decreasing levels of luteinizing hormone, follicle-stimulating hormone, adrenocorticotropic hormone, and beta endorphins.

Changes in hormone levels may cause decreased levels of testosterone and cortisol, disturbances in menstruation, and sexual dysfunction.

High doses of morphine and related opioids produce convulsions. Most convulsions occur at doses far in excess of those required to produce analgesia.

Respiratory

Respiratory depression is the most serious opioid-induced adverse effect. Opioids depress respiration by a direct effect on the brain-stem respiratory centers, making the brain stem less responsive to carbon dioxide.

The μ receptor is the primary receptor involved in respiratory depression, although activation of the κ receptor also contributes.

At equianalgesic doses, all pure opioid agonists depress respiration to the same degree. The agonist–antagonists have a ceiling effect (i.e., a dose beyond which no further respiratory depression or analgesia is produced), but this level is usually above recommended doses.

Opioids depress cough by inducing a direct effect on the cough reflex in the medulla.

Cardiovascular

Therapeutic doses of many opioids produce peripheral vasodilation, reduced peripheral resistance, and inhibition of the baroreceptor reflexes.

Peripheral vasodilation results primarily from opioid-induced release of histamine. Orthostatic hypotension and fainting can result. The naturally occurring and semisynthetic products are potent histamine releasers. Fentanyl has little propensity to release histamine.

Methadone has been associated with torsades de pointes, an atypical rapid ventricular tachycardia, at an average daily dose of 400 mg. Methadone should be used cautiously in patients on other QT-prolonging medications (see Chapter 14 on cardiac arrhythmias). Patients should receive an electrocardiogram before therapy, at day 30, and once yearly while receiving methadone.

Gastrointestinal

All clinically significant μ agonists produce some degree of nausea and vomiting by direct stimulation of the chemoreceptor trigger zone in the medulla, sensitization of the vestibular system, and slowing of GI motility.

Nausea and vomiting commonly occur in ambulatory patients (28% and 15%, respectively). Both can be pretreated with an antiemetic such as promethazine or prochlorperazine .

Opioids promote constipation by delaying gastric emptying, slowing bowel motility, and decreasing peristalsis. Opioids may also reduce secretions from the colonic mucosa. At its worst, GI dysfunction results in ileus, fecal impaction, and obstruction.

Because of the risk of developing opioid-induced constipation, patients exposed to around-the-clock opioid analgesics should be placed on prophylactic bowel regimens. Bowel regimens include increased fluid and fiber intake, daily stool softeners, and, if needed, stimulant laxatives. Severe constipation is managed with osmotic laxatives such as magnesium citrate and milk of magnesia.

Drugs specifically indicated for opioid-induced constipation include chloride channel activators: lubiprostone (Amitiza) and opioid receptor antagonists: naloxegol (Movantik), naldemedine (Symproic), and methylnaltrexone (Relistor).

⚠ Promethazine *FDA BOXED WARNING*

Respiratory depression in pediatrics. Promethazine should not be used in pediatric patients younger than 2 years. Promethazine also has a boxed warning for severe tissue injury including gangrene with the injection formulation, causing severe chemical irritation. The preferred route is deep intramuscular injection, subcutaneous injection is contraindicated.

Do not use in patients less than 2 years old—potential for fatal respiratory depression.

⚠ Prochlorperazine *FDA BOXED WARNING*

Dementia in elderly patients with dementia-related psychosis. These patients are at an increased risk of death when treated with an antipsychotic medication.

Increased risk of death in elderly patients with dementia-related psychosis.

Genitourinary

Opioids increase smooth muscle tone in the bladder and ureters and may cause bladder spasm and urgency.

An opioid-induced increase in urethral sphincter tone can make urination difficult. Urinary retention is most common in elderly men.

Biliary

Opioids increase smooth muscle tone in the biliary tract, especially in the sphincter of Oddi, which regulates the flow of bile and pancreatic fluids. This effect can result in a decrease in biliary and pancreatic secretions and a rise in the bile duct pressure. Patients may experience epigastric distress and, occasionally, biliary spasm.

All opioids are capable of causing constriction of the sphincter of Oddi and the biliary tract. Use caution when prescribing an opioid to a patient with biliary tract disease and pancreatitis.

Skin and eye

Therapeutic doses of morphine dilate cutaneous blood vessels, which causes flushing on the face, neck, and upper thorax. Sweating and pruritus may also occur. These changes may be caused in part by the release of histamine. Histamine release may induce or worsen asthmatic attacks in predisposed patients and can lead to wheezing, bronchoconstriction, and status asthmaticus.

Skin rash around the transdermal fentanyl patch is a common side effect caused by the patch adhesive.

Following a toxic dose of μ agonists, miosis is evident but insufficient alone to confirm a definitive diagnosis of opioid intoxication.

Overdose

Acute overdose with opioids is manifested by respiratory depression; somnolence progressing to stupor or coma; skeletal muscle flaccidity; cold, clammy skin; constricted pupils; and sometimes pulmonary edema, bradycardia, hypotension, and death.

An opioid antagonist such as naloxone is given to block opioid receptors and reverse the effects of overdose (see Chapter 43).

Antagonist administration may cause a complete reversal of opioid effects and precipitate an acute withdrawal syndrome in persons physically dependent on opioids.

Tolerance and physical dependence

The use of opioids is often limited by concerns regarding tolerance, physical dependence, and addiction.

Tolerance can be defined as a state in which a larger dose is required to produce the same response that could formerly be elicited by a smaller dose. Tolerance to analgesia is demonstrated by the need for an increased dosage of a drug to produce the same level of analgesia. Tolerance is sometimes mistaken for disease progression in cancer patients.

Tolerance to adverse effects of opioids occurs after weeks of continuous administration. Tolerance to the constipating and neuroendocrine effects of opioids does not occur.

Physical dependence is the occurrence of a withdrawal syndrome after an opioid is stopped or quickly decreased without titration. Warn patients to avoid abrupt discontinuation of such drugs.

Addiction is a behavior pattern involving the continued use of a substance for nonmedical reasons despite harm. It is characterized by impaired control over drug use, compulsive use, craving, and continued use despite harm.

Pharmacokinetics of Selected Opioids

Morphine

Compared with other opioids, morphine is relatively insoluble in lipids (e.g., in adults, only small amounts of the drug cross the blood–brain barrier).

Morphine does not accumulate in tissues when given in normal doses, allowing for frequent dosing. Morphine is primarily metabolized by glucuronidation during the first pass through the liver. Approximately 50% of morphine is converted by the liver to morphine-3-glucuronide and 15% to morphine-6-glucuronide (M6G). The pharmacologic effects of morphine (both analgesia and side effects) are in part caused by M6G.

Much of an oral dose is inactivated during this first pass through the liver; consequently, oral doses need to be much larger than parenteral doses to produce the same analgesic effects.

Fentanyl

Fentanyl is highly soluble in lipids. It accumulates in skeletal muscle and fat and is released slowly into the blood. Plasma half-life is 3 to 4 hours after parenteral administration.

Fentanyl is rapidly metabolized, primarily by dealkylation, to inactive metabolites in the liver. This process is mediated through the cytochrome P450 (CYP450) 3A4 hepatic enzyme system. The presence of inactive metabolites makes fentanyl a preferred drug in patients with liver dysfunction.

Transdermal fentanyl

The uptake of fentanyl through the skin is relatively slow and constant. The skin does not metabolize the drug, and 92% of the dose is delivered into the bloodstream as intact fentanyl.

Because of temperature-dependent increases in fentanyl release from the patch system as well as increased skin permeability, an increase in body temperature to 40°C (104°F) theoretically may increase serum fentanyl concentrations by approximately one-third.

Fentanyl is absorbed into the upper layers of the skin, forming a depot. Fentanyl then becomes available to systemic circulation. Serum fentanyl concentrations are measurable within 2 hours after application of the first patch, and analgesic effects can be observed 8 to 16 hours after application. Steady state is reached after several sequential patch applications.

Other fentanyl forms

Fentanyl is also available as a transmucosal fentanyl citrate lozenge, buccal tablet, soluble film, sublingual spray, or nasal spray. The transmucosal products are indicated only for those who are already receiving and exhibit tolerance to around-the-clock opioid therapy. Fentanyl soluble film is indicated for breakthrough pain in cancer patients 18 years of age and older who are opioid tolerant and are receiving around-the-clock opioid therapies.

Methadone

After therapeutic doses, about 90% of methadone is bound to plasma protein and is widely distributed in tissues. Methadone is found in low concentrations in the blood and the brain, with higher concentrations in the kidney, spleen, liver, and lung. Terminal half-life is extremely variable (15 to 55 hours); therefore, accumulation is possible, and dosing intervals need to be carefully monitored.

Methadone is extensively metabolized in the liver, mainly by N-demethylation. This process appears to be mediated primarily by CYP450 3A4 and to a lesser extent by CYP450 2D6. The major metabolites are excreted in the bile and urine.

Analgesic efficacy does not correspond to the half-life of the drug. Methadone may be dosed every 3 hours for pain control.

Oxycodone

Oxycodone is metabolized to noroxycodone, oxymorphone, and their glucuronides via the CYP450 enzyme system. The major circulating metabolite is noroxycodone. Noroxycodone is reported to be a weaker analgesic than **oxycodone**. Oxymorphone, although possessing good analgesic activity, is present in the plasma only in low concentrations. Its metabolism is mediated by CYP450 2D6.

Hydromorphone ⚠

Hydromorphone is metabolized to 3 major metabolites: hydromorphone 3-glucuronide, hydromorphone 3-glucoside, and dihydroisomorphine 6-glucoside. Whether hydromorphone is metabolized by the CYP450 system is not known. Hydromorphone is a poor inhibitor of CYP450 isoenzymes and is not expected to inhibit the metabolism of other drugs.

Meperidine ⚠

Normeperidine, a toxic metabolite of meperidine, produces anxiety, tremors, myoclonus, and generalized seizures when it accumulates with repetitive dosing. Patients with compromised renal function and concomitant use of benzodiazepines are particularly at risk. Naloxone does not reverse this hyperexcitability. For these reasons, meperidine should not be used for more than 48 hours in patients with renal or CNS disease or at doses greater than 600 mg every 24 hours.

Tapentadol ⚠

Tapentadol's dual mechanism activates the μ opioid receptor and inhibits reuptake of norepinephrine. It is metabolized to its major metabolite, tapentadol-O-glucuronide via glucuronidation and 2 minor metabolites, N-desmethyl tapentadol and hydroxy tapentadol, via the CYP450 enzyme system. The metabolism via CYP450 is not as significant as the phase 2 conjugation. Approximately 97% of the parent drug is metabolized. The major metabolic pathway is via conjugation with extensive metabolism through phase 2 pathways and minor metabolism by phase 1 oxidative pathways.

Tramadol ⚠

Tramadol is an analog of codeine, whose mechanism of action is not completely understood. Analgesia is apparently mediated by binding of the parent molecule and the O-desmethyltramadol (M1) active metabolite to μ opioid receptors, as well as by weak inhibition of neuronal uptake of norepinephrine and serotonin. In 2014, **tramadol** was listed as a DEA (U.S. Drug Enforcement Administration) schedule IV controlled substance.

The liver extensively metabolizes **tramadol**. The formation of the M1 active metabolite is dependent on CYP450 2D6. M1 appears to be up to 6 times more potent than **tramadol** in producing analgesia and 200 times more potent in binding to μ opioid receptors. CYP450 3A4 and CYP450 2B6 also play a role in **tramadol** metabolism. Caution should be exercised when administering **tramadol** to patients on CYP450 2D6 and CYP450 3A4 inhibitors.

The most common adverse effects are sedation, dizziness, headache, dry mouth, and constipation. Respiratory depression is minimal. Seizures have been reported; avoid use of **tramadol** in patients with seizure disorders or recognized risk for seizure (such as head trauma, metabolic disorders, alcohol and drug withdrawal, and CNS infections) and in patients taking antidepressants and neuroleptics.

Drug–Drug and Drug–Disease Interactions

Drug–drug interactions

All drugs with CNS-depressant actions (barbiturates, benzodiazepines, alcohol) can intensify sedation and respiratory depression caused by morphine and other opioids.

Antihistamines, tricyclic antidepressants, and atropine-like drugs can exacerbate morphine-induced constipation and urinary retention.

Antihypertensive drugs and others that lower blood pressure can exacerbate opioid-induced hypotension.

The combination of meperidine, hydromorphone, fentanyl sublingual tablets, or tapentadol with a monoamine oxidase inhibitor (MAOI) may produce a syndrome characterized by excitation, delirium, hyperpyrexia, convulsions, and severe respiratory depression. Death may also occur. Although this syndrome has not been reported with other opioids, combinations containing opioids and MAOIs should be avoided. Patients should not take an opioid medication within 14 days of taking an MAOI.

Agonist–antagonists can precipitate a withdrawal syndrome if administered to an individual who is physically dependent on a pure opioid agonist.

CYP450 enzymes metabolize codeine, hydrocodone, fentanyl, methadone, and **oxycodone**. Although not well documented, drug interactions through this system may exist. In particular, fentanyl and **oxycodone** should be used with caution in a patient on a CYP450 3A4 inhibitor. The patient should be monitored over an extended period and dose adjustments made as appropriate.

Codeine, hydrocodone, and **oxycodone** require metabolism through CYP450 2D6 to an active drug (Table 27-5). Approximately 7% of Whites, 3% of Blacks, and 1% of Asians are poor metabolizers of CYP450 2D6; they produce no CYP450 2D6 or produce undetectable levels of it. Poor metabolizers may experience little or no analgesia from drugs requiring CYP450 2D6 for conversion to active metabolites.

About 5% of patients have multiple copies of the CYP450 2D6 gene, making them ultrafast metabolizers. The clearance of some opioids may be increased, making more frequent dosing of the medications necessary.

TABLE 27-5. CYP450 2D6 Enzyme Activity

Substrates	Inhibitors	Inducers
Codeine	Celecoxib ⚠	Carbamazepine ⚠
Hydrocodone	Cimetidine	Ethanol
Meperidine	**Citalopram** ⚠	Phenobarbital
Methadone	**Fluoxetine** ⚠	Phenytoin ⚠
Oxycodone	Methadone	Rifampin
Tramadol	**Paroxetine** ⚠	
	Sertraline ⚠	

Boldface indicates one of top 100 drugs for 2020 by prescription volume.

FDA BOXED WARNINGS

Celecoxib

Serious cardiovascular risk and serious gastrointestinal risk. Nonsteroidal anti-inflammatory drugs (NSAIDs) have an increased risk of serious cardiovascular events including myocardial infarction and stroke. NSAIDs also cause an increased risk of serious gastrointestinal adverse events including bleeding, ulceration, and perforation of the stomach or intestines.

Increased risk of cardiovascular thrombotic events. Increased risk of serious gastrointestinal adverse events (e.g., stomach bleed, ulcers).

Carbamazepine

Serious dermatologic reaction and HLA-B*1502 allele and aplastic anemia and agranulocytosis. Serious and sometimes fatal dermatologic reactions including Stevens-Johnson syndrome have been reported in patients taking carbamazepine with HLA-B*1502. Aplastic anemia and agranulocytosis are rare, but patients should undergo a baseline blood count and be monitored for signs of bone marrow suppression.

Increased risk of serious dermatologic reactions (e.g., Stevens-Johnson syndrome), especially with HLA-B*1502 allele.

Citalopram

Suicidality and antidepressants. Antidepressants including **citalopram** increased the risk of suicidal thinking and behaviors in children and young adults under the age of 24. Patients of all ages starting **citalopram** should be monitored for suicidality and unusual changes in behavior.

Increased risk of suicidality.

Fluoxetine

Suicidality and antidepressants. Antidepressants including **fluoxetine** increased the risk of suicidal thinking and behaviors in children and young adults under the age of 24. Patients of all ages starting **fluoxetine** should be monitored for suicidality and unusual changes in behavior.

Increased risk of suicidality.

Phenytoin

Cardiovascular risk with rapid infusion (injection). The rate of phenytoin administration should not exceed 50 mg/minute due to the risk of severe hypotension and cardiac arrhythmias.

Cardiovascular risk with rapid infusion.

Paroxetine

Suicidality and antidepressants. Antidepressants including **paroxetine** increased the risk of suicidal thinking and behaviors in children and young adults under the age of 24. Patients of all ages starting **paroxetine** should be monitored for suicidality and unusual changes in behavior.

Increased risk of suicidality.

(continued)

FDA BOXED WARNINGS (Continued)

Sertraline

Suicidality and antidepressants. Antidepressants including **sertraline** increased the risk of suicidal thinking and behaviors in children and young adults under the age of 24. Patients of all ages starting **sertraline** should be monitored for suicidality and unusual changes in behavior.

Increased risk of suicidality.

Drug–disease interactions

In view of the extensive hepatic metabolism of opioids, their effects may be increased in patients with liver disease, particularly those with severe liver failure. Most opioids require dose reduction in patients with severe liver disease.

Fentanyl, morphine, and methadone require dosing adjustment in patients with renal impairment. Doses of fentanyl and morphine should be reduced 25% when creatinine clearance (CrCl) is 10 to 50 mL/min and by 50% when CrCl < 10 mL/min. The dosing interval of methadone should be increased to at least every 6 hours when CrCl is 10 to 50 mL/min and to every 8 hours when CrCl < 10 mL/min.

Renal impairment slows the clearance of morphine conjugates, resulting in accumulation of the active metabolite M6G. For this reason, dosage reduction may be advisable in the presence of clinically significant renal impairment.

Methadone appears to be firmly bound to protein in various tissues, including the brain. After repeated administrations, methadone gradually accumulates in tissues. The risk of accumulation is greater in patients with impaired renal or hepatic function because both organs are involved in the metabolism of methadone.

Patient Instructions and Counseling

Respiratory depression is increased by concurrent use of other drugs with CNS-depressant activity (e.g., alcohol, barbiturates, benzodiazepines). Outpatients should be warned against the use of alcohol with all other CNS depressants.

Constipation is commonly experienced with short- and long-term use of opioids. Suggest that patients take a stool softener and stimulant laxative if constipation occurs during the course of treatment. Inform patients about symptoms of hypotension (e.g., light-headedness, dizziness). Patients should minimize hypotension by moving slowly when changing from a supine to an upright position.

Advise patients that opioids are drugs of potential abuse and should never be taken by anyone other than the person for whom they are prescribed. Patients should never adjust the dose of their medication without first consulting their health care provider.

Liquid formulations should be measured with an appropriate dose-measuring cup or spoon and not a regular teaspoon or tablespoon.

Combinations should not exceed the maximum daily dose of **acetaminophen** (4 g/d, no liver damage present) to prevent liver toxicity.

Women who are pregnant or planning to become pregnant should consult their health care provider before starting therapy.

Fentanyl transdermal patch

The fentanyl transdermal patch must be applied to a clean, nonhairy site on the upper torso. Only water should be used to clean the area. Soap or alcohol can increase the effects of the medication and should not be used. The patch should not be applied to oily, broken, burned, cut, or irritated skin. It must be held in place for a minimum of 30 seconds to ensure adhesion.

Each new patch should be applied to a different area of skin to avoid irritation. If a patch comes off or causes irritation, it should be removed and a new patch applied to a different site.

To dispose of the patch, fold it in half and flush down the toilet.

Do not cut or damage the patch.

Temperature-dependent increases in fentanyl release from the patch could result in an overdose. Advise patients to avoid exposing the patch to direct external heat sources such as heating pads, electric blankets, heat lamps, saunas, hot tubs, and heated waterbeds. In addition, patients who develop a high fever while wearing the patch should contact their health care provider immediately.

For specific dosing, administration, and monitoring parameters for long acting formulations, refer to the product's package insert.

Parameters to monitor

Monitor the patient for respiratory depression. Higher risk for respiratory depression exists in patients who are not tolerant to opioid analgesics. Consider treatment when the respiratory rate is less than 8 to 12 respirations per minute for 30 minutes or longer despite stimulation or if oxygen saturation is less than 90%.

If a patient is easily arousable, he or she is unlikely to have respiratory depression.

The U.S. Food and Drug Administration (FDA) requires a Risk Evaluation and Mitigation Strategies (REMS) program for extended-release and long-acting opioids. A medication guide must be given with each prescription dispensed for a controlled substance in these classes. Pain medications with other REMS requirements are listed in Table 27-6.

TABLE 27-6. Risk and Evaluation Mitigation Strategies

Medication	REMS
Abstral (fentanyl sublingual tablet)	TIRF REMS Access program enrollment is required for prescribers (outpatient), pharmacies, and patients (outpatient).
Actiq (fentanyl citrate lozenge)	TIRF REMS Access program enrollment is required for prescribers (outpatient), pharmacies, and patients (outpatient).
Butrans (buprenorphine transdermal)	Prescribers must receive training.
Fentora (fentanyl citrate buccal tablet)	TIRF REMS Access program enrollment is required for prescribers (outpatient), pharmacies, and patients (outpatient).
Lazanda (fentanyl nasal spray)	TIRF REMS Access program enrollment is required for prescribers (outpatient), pharmacies, and patients (outpatient).
Methadone (40 mg tablet), indicated for detoxification and maintenance	Medication may be dispensed only in facilities that have been authorized for detoxification and maintenance treatment of patients with opioid addiction.
Opioids	Prescriber and patient education is required for all opioid analgesics intended for outpatient use.
Suboxone (sublingual buprenorphine/naloxone)	Drug Addiction Treatment Act waiver is required for prescribers. Prescribers will be issued a unique identification number (UIN) beginning with an "X," which is required to be present on the prescription.
Subsys (fentanyl sublingual spray)	TIRF REMS Access program enrollment is required for prescribers (outpatient), pharmacies, and patients (outpatient).
Subutex (sublingual buprenorphine)	Drug Addiction Treatment Act waiver is required for prescribers.
Vivitrol (naltrexone for extended-release injectable suspension)	Prescriber and patient education is required.

TIRF REMS, Transmucosal Immediate Release Fentanyl Risk Evaluation and Mitigation Strategy.

Nonpharmacologic Treatment of Pain

Nonpharmacologic strategies used in combination with appropriate drug regimens may improve pain relief by enhancing the therapeutic effects of medications and permitting use of lower doses.

Nonpharmacologic interventions should not be a substitute for analgesic use. Effective physical interventions include physical therapy, acupuncture, transcutaneous electrical nerve stimulation, yoga, and neurostimulation. Behavioral techniques, such as biofeedback or distraction and relaxation, have been found to improve pain control.

27-4   Migraine

Migraine is a chronic neurovascular disorder characterized by recurrent attacks of severe headache and autonomic nervous system dysfunction. Some patients also experience aura with neurologic symptoms (Figure 27-1).

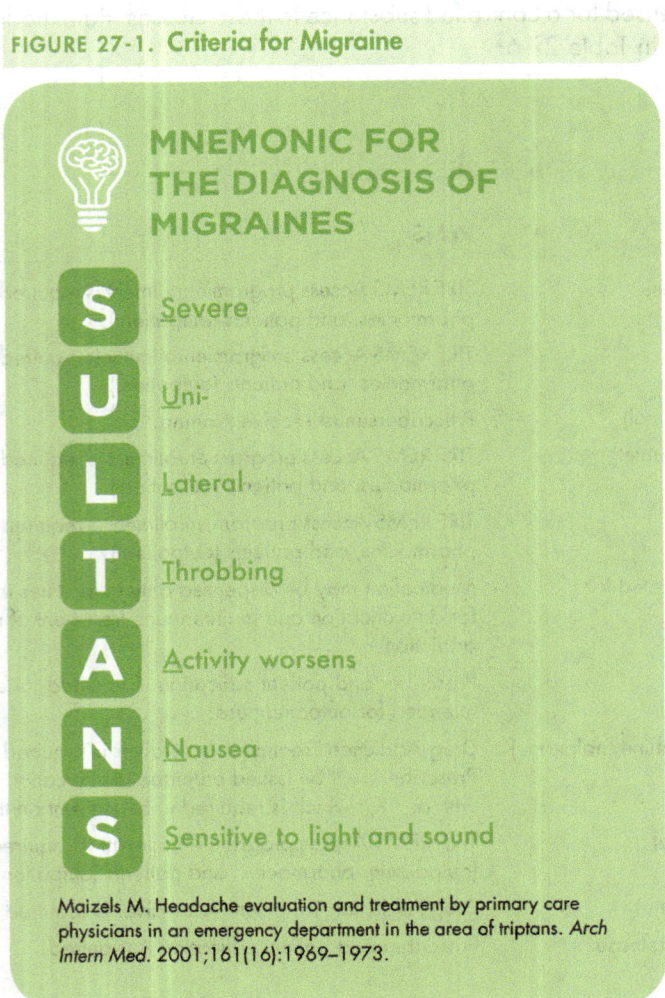

FIGURE 27-1. Criteria for Migraine

MNEMONIC FOR THE DIAGNOSIS OF MIGRAINES

S — Severe
U — Uni-
L — Lateral
T — Throbbing
A — Activity worsens
N — Nausea
S — Sensitive to light and sound

Maizels M. Headache evaluation and treatment by primary care physicians in an emergency department in the area of triptans. *Arch Intern Med.* 2001;161(16):1969–1973.

> **BOX 27-2. Criteria for Diagnosing Migraine Without Aura**

- The patient has at least 5 headaches lasting 4 to 72 hours each.
- The headaches have at least 2 of the following 4 characteristics:
  - Unilateral location
  - Pulsating quality
  - Moderate or severe intensity (inhibits or prohibits daily activities)
  - Aggravation with walking or similar routine physical activity

- During the headache, at least 1 of the following symptoms occurs:
  - Nausea or vomiting
  - Photophobia
  - Phonophobia
- Symptoms cannot be consistent with other headache types.

Clinical Presentation and Diagnostic Criteria

Migraine headaches usually occur in the frontotemporal region. Photophobia (increased sensitivity to light) and phonophobia (increased sensitivity to sound) also are frequent complaints. A *prodrome*, also referred to as a premonitory phase, of mood changes, stiff neck, fatigue, or other symptoms may occur hours or days before the onset of the headache. Migraine classification is based on whether an aura of visual or sensory symptoms is present. Migraine with aura is less common than migraine without aura (Box 27-2 and Box 27-3).

Pathophysiology

The pathogenesis of migraine is unclear and is thought to be multifactorial. A number of theories propose explanations of the vascular, electrophysical, and genetic mechanisms of migraines.

The most-agreed-upon theory is that of cortical-spreading depression. It suggests that a wave of depolarization spreads across the cerebral cortex from occipital to frontal regions, resulting in brain ion dysfunction and altered blood flow. These changes account for the progression and variety of symptoms that occur in patients with prodromal or aura phase.

The headache phase is probably related to inappropriate trigeminovascular activation with the release of inflammatory neuropeptides, such as substance P, neurokinin A, and calcitonin gene-related peptide.

Individuals prone to migraine may have inherited or environmentally acquired migraine thresholds that render them susceptible to a migraine attack on exposure to any of a range of patient-specific triggers. Once the threshold is exceeded, trigeminovascular activation is thought to be responsible for inducing a migraine.

> **BOX 27-3. Criteria for Diagnosis of Migraine With Aura**

- The patient has at least 2 attacks with the following criteria:
  - One or more completely reversible aura symptoms:
    - Visual
    - Sensory
    - Speech, language, or both
    - Motor
    - Brain stem
    - Retinal

- At least 2 of the following characteristics:
  - At least 1 aura symptom develops gradually (>5 minutes), 2 or more symptoms occur in succession, or both characteristics occur.
  - Each individual aura lasts 5 to 60 minutes.
  - At least 1 aura symptom is unilateral.
  - Headache follows or accompanies aura in <1 hour.
- Symptoms cannot be consistent with other headache types, and transient ischemic attack has been ruled out.

Treatment Principles

Abortive therapy

The U.S. Headache Consortium's 2015 guidelines identifies the following goals for successful treatment of acute attacks of migraine:

- Treat attacks rapidly and consistently, and prevent recurrence.
- Restore the patient's ability to function.
- Minimize the use of rescue medication.
- Optimize self-care, and reduce subsequent use of resources.
- Promote cost-effective therapies with minimal adverse effects.

Successful treatment of migraine depends on early intervention in relation to onset of headache and adequate dosing.

Preventive therapy (Box 27-4)

Two-thirds of patients taking preventive medication will have a 50% decrease in the frequency of attacks.

The minimum duration of trial for a daily preventive medication is 2 to 3 months. No consensus exists on the duration of the prophylaxis trial period; however, prophylaxis efficacy may continue to improve when a medication is taken continuously for months to years.

The goals of migraine preventive therapy are as follows:

- Reduce attack frequency, severity, and duration.
- Improve responsiveness to treatment of acute attacks.
- Improve function, and reduce disability.

Rebound headaches

Persons who take abortive medications daily can develop drug rebound headaches or headaches that begin upon discontinuation of a medication. Essentially all of the medications, such as analgesics, opioids, and triptans, can cause rebound headaches.

Abortive Drug Therapy

Nonprescription medications

Aspirin, acetaminophen, ibuprofen, and other aspirin-like analgesics provide adequate relief of mild to moderate migraines. Advil Migraine (**ibuprofen** 200 mg liquid-filled capsules) and Advil Migraine (**ibuprofen** 200 mg) is an example of a nonprescription medication indicated for migraine relief.

Combination products containing **aspirin, acetaminophen**, or both with caffeine are also available without a prescription. Caffeine has analgesic and possibly anti-inflammatory properties. It may also increase gastric acidity and perfusion, enhancing the absorption of **aspirin**. Excedrin Migraine (**acetaminophen** 250 mg, **aspirin** 250 mg, and caffeine 65 mg) is an example of an available combination nonprescription product.

BOX 27-4. Indications for Preventive Therapy in Migraine

Preventive therapy should be considered in the following situations:

- Attacks unresponsive to abortive medication
- Attacks causing substantial disability
- Attacks occurring twice or more monthly
- Patient at risk for rebound headache
- Trend in increasing frequency of attacks

Nonspecific prescription medications

Combination products containing an analgesic, caffeine, and butalbital or codeine are available. Butalbital may be useful for its sedative properties, but evidence is scant. Excessive use of these products can cause physical dependence and rebound headaches.

Opioids are well recognized as good analgesics, but strong evidence exists only for the efficacy of butorphanol nasal spray for migraine. Although opioids are commonly used, they should be a last resort after other therapies are not effective.

Given intravenously, the antiemetic metoclopramide may be appropriate as monotherapy for acute attacks, particularly in patients with significant nausea. Chlorpromazine and prochlorperazine may also be considered. Serotonin receptor antagonists (5-hydroxytryptamine [HT] 3) have not been shown to be useful migraine treatments.

⚠ Metoclopramide *FDA BOXED WARNING*

Tardive dyskinesia. Metoclopramide can cause tardive dyskinesia, a serious movement disorder. Avoid treatment with metoclopramide for over 12 weeks as this increases the risk of developing tardive dyskinesia.

Risk of tardive dyskinesia. Avoid treatment greater than 12 weeks.

⚠ Chlorpromazine *FDA BOXED WARNING*

Increased mortality in elderly patients with dementia-related psychosis. Elderly patients with dementia-related psychosis treated with antipsychotic drugs are at an increased risk of death.

Increased risk of death in elderly patients with dementia-related psychosis.

Ergotamine

Mechanism of action

In cranial arteries, ergotamine acts directly to promote constriction and reduce the amplitude of pulsations. In addition, the drug can affect blood flow by depressing the vasomotor center. Antimigraine effects are possibly due to agonist activity at serotonin receptor subtypes 5-HT1B and 5-HT1D.

Because of the risk of dependence, ergotamine should not be taken daily on a long-term basis.

Caffeine may be added to ergotamine to enhance vasoconstriction and ergotamine absorption

---

⚠ Ergotamine *FDA BOXED WARNING*

Co-administration of potent CYP3A4 inhibitors increases risk of severe peripheral ischemia.

Pharmacokinetics

Oral ergotamine has poor bioavailability because of extensive first-pass metabolism. Sublingual administration may not provide therapeutic blood levels.

Although the half-life of ergotamine is only 2 hours, pharmacologic effects can be seen for 24 hours after administration.

The drug is eliminated primarily by hepatic metabolism. Metabolites are excreted in the bile.

Adverse effects

Ergotamine is well tolerated at usual therapeutic doses.

The drug can stimulate the chemoreceptor trigger zone to cause nausea and vomiting in about 10% of patients. Concurrent treatment with metoclopramide or a phenothiazine antiemetic can help suppress this response.

Other common side effects include weakness in the legs, myalgia, numbness and tingling in the periphery, angina-like pain, tachycardia, and bradycardia.

Overdose

Acute or chronic overdose can cause serious toxicity (ergotism). Symptoms include ischemia, myalgia, and paresthesia. Ischemia can progress to gangrene.

The risk of ergotism is highest in patients with sepsis, peripheral vascular disease, and renal or hepatic impairment.

Drug–drug and drug–disease interactions

Ergotamines are contraindicated with potent inhibitors of CYP450 3A4 because of the risk of cerebral or peripheral ischemia. Concomitant use with selective serotonin receptor agonists should also be avoided because of the risk of a prolonged vasospastic reaction. Separate doses of ergotamine and other migraine medications by at least 24 hours.

Ergotamine is contraindicated for patients with hepatic or renal impairment, sepsis, coronary artery disease (CAD), and peripheral vascular disease.

Patient instructions and counseling

Monitor patients to avoid overuse of the medication.

Ergotamine and its derivatives are FDA pregnancy category X. They should not be taken during pregnancy because of their ability to promote uterine contractions and cause fetal harm or abortion.

Teach patients to recognize signs of ergotism. Muscle pain, paresthesia, and cold or pale extremities should be reported immediately.

Dihydroergotamine ⚠

Mechanism of action

The action of dihydroergotamine (DHE) is similar to that of ergotamine. Like ergotamine, DHE alters transmission at serotonergic, dopaminergic, and alpha-adrenergic junctions.

 Dihydroergotamine *FDA BOXED WARNING*

Co-administration of potent CYP3A4 inhibitors increases risk of severe peripheral ischemia.

In contrast to ergotamine, DHE causes minimal peripheral vasoconstriction, little nausea and vomiting, and no physical dependence. Diarrhea, however, is prominent.

Contraindications are the same as for ergotamine: CAD, peripheral vascular disease, sepsis, pregnancy, and hepatic or renal impairment.

As with ergotamine, do not administer DHE within 24 hours of a serotonin agonist.

Pharmacokinetics

DHE is not active orally because of extensive first-pass metabolism. An active metabolite, 8-hydroxy-dihydroergotamine, contributes to its therapeutic effects. The half-life of DHE plus its active metabolite is about 21 hours.

Concomitant administration of DHE with potent CYP450 3A4 inhibitors, including protease inhibitors and macrolide antibiotics, is contraindicated. Because CYP450 3A4 inhibition elevates the serum levels of DHE, the risk for vasospasm leading to cerebral ischemia or ischemia of the extremities is increased. Table 27-7 discusses the ergot alkaloids.

Selective serotonin receptor agonists

Mechanism of action

The selective serotonin receptor agonists, also known as *triptans*, are first-line drugs for terminating a migraine attack (Table 27-8). The triptans all activate 5-HT1B, 5-HT1D, and, to a lesser extent, 5-HT1A or 5-HT1F receptors. Triptans have no known affinity for 5-HT2 or 5-HT3 and other 5-HT receptor subclasses, nor do they bind to adrenergic, dopaminergic, muscarinergic, or histaminergic receptors.

Pharmacokinetics

The pharmacokinetics of the different triptans vary between agents.

Subcutaneous **sumatriptan** injection has the fastest onset of action when compared with other triptans. **Sumatriptan** nasal spray has a slightly slower onset than the injection.

The onset of the majority of oral triptans, including the disintegrating tablets, is similar among the available agents. Rizatriptan may have a slightly faster onset of action at 30 minutes; the disintegrating tablet does not offer a faster onset.

Migraine recurrence rates may be lower with long-half-life triptans such as naratriptan and frovatriptan. Triptans with longer half-lives, however, tend to have a slower onset of action.

TABLE 27-7. Ergot Alkaloids

Generic name	Trade name and strengths	Maximum daily dose (weekly maximum)	Dosing instructions
Ergotamine sublingual tablet	Ergomar 2 mg	6 mg oral (10 mg)	1 tablet at onset; then 1 every 30 min as needed
Ergotamine/caffeine tablet	Cafergot 1/100 mg	Ergotamine 6 mg oral (10 mg)	2 tablets at onset; then 1 every 30 min as needed
Ergotamine/caffeine suppository	Migergot 2/100 mg	Ergotamine 4 mg rectal suppository (10 mg)	Insert 1 at onset; repeat in 1 hour as needed
Dihydroergotamine (DHE)	Injection: DHE 45 1 mg/mL	DHE 3 mL I.M., 2 mL I.V. (6 mL I.V.)	0.5 to 1 mg I.V. or I.M. every hour as needed
	Nasal spray: Migranal 4 mg/mL	DHE 2 mg (6 mg)	Administer 1 spray (0.5 mg) in each nostril, followed in 15 minutes by an additional spray in each nostril

I.M., intramuscular; I.V., intravenous.

TABLE 27-8. Selective Serotonin Receptor Agonists (Triptans)

Generic name	Trade name	Available strengths	Dosage (maximum daily dose)	Half-life	Onset	Metabolism
Almotriptan	Axert	Tablet: 6.25, 12.5 mg	12.5 mg; repeat in 2 hours (25 mg)	3.5 hours	60 minutes	CYP450; MAO
Sumatriptan	Imitrex	Tablet: 25, 50, 100 mg	50 to 100 mg; repeat in 2 hours (200 mg)	2.5 hours	60 to 120 minutes	MAO
		Nasal: 5, 20 mg	5 or 20 mg; repeat in 2 hours (40 mg)		15 to 20 minutes	
	Imitrex STATdose, Sumavel DosePro	Subcutaneous injection: 4, 6 mg/0.5 mL	4 or 6 mg; repeat in 1 hour (12 mg)		10 to 15 minutes	
Eletriptan	Relpax	Tablet: 20, 40 mg	20 mg; repeat in 2 hours (80 mg)	4 hours	60 minutes	CYP450 3A4
Frovatriptan	Frova	Tablet: 2.5 mg	2.5 mg; repeat in 2 hours (7.5 mg)	26 hours	60 to 120 minutes	Renal 50%; CYP450 1A2
Rizatriptan	Maxalt	Tablet or wafer: 5, 10 mg	5 or 10 mg; repeat in 2 hours (30 mg)	2 to 3 hours	30 minutes	MAO
	Maxalt-MLT	Tablet[b]: 5, 10 mg	10 mg (30 mg)	2 to 3 hours	30 minutes	MAO
Zolmitriptan	Zomig	Tablet: 2.5, 5 mg	2.5 or 5 mg; repeat in 2 hours (10 mg)	2.5 to 4 hours	45 minutes	CYP450; MAO
		Nasal: 5 mg	5 mg; repeat in 2 hours (10 mg)	3 hours	10 to 15 minutes	CYP450; MAO
	Zomig-ZMT	Tablet[b]: 2.5, 5 mg	2.5 mg; repeat in 2 hours (10 mg)	3 hours	120 minutes	MAO-A
Naratriptan	Amerge	Tablet: 1, 2.5 mg	1 or 2.5 mg; repeat in 4 hours (5 mg)	6 hours	60 minutes	Renal 70%; CYP450
Miscellaneous agent						
Sumatriptan/ naproxen	Treximet	Tablet: 85/500 mg	1 tablet; may repeat in 2 hours (2 tablets) The safety of treating more than 5 migraines in a 30-day period has not been established.	**Sumatriptan** 2 hours/ naproxen 19 hours	60 to 120 minutes	**Sumatriptan:** MAO; naproxen: no significant CYP450 induction

Boldface indicates one of top 100 drugs for 2020 by prescription volume.
MAO, monoamine oxidase.
a. All triptans have a recommended total daily dose. The safety of treating an average of 4 or more headaches in a 30-day period with a triptan has not been established.
b. These dosage forms are orally disintegrating tablets placed on the tongue and are not intended for sublingual administration.

Adverse effects

Triptans are generally well tolerated with mild and transient side effects. The triptans differ slightly from one another in terms of tolerability but not safety.

The most frequent side effects are tingling and paresthesia and sensations of warmth in the head, neck, chest, and extremities. Dizziness, flushing, and neck pain or stiffness occur less frequently.

Chest symptoms

About 50% of patients on **sumatriptan** experience unpleasant chest symptoms, usually described as "heavy arms" or "chest pressure" rather than pain. These symptoms are transient and not related to ischemic heart disease. Possible causes are pulmonary vasoconstriction, esophageal spasm, intercostal muscle spasm, and bronchoconstriction.

Coronary vasospasm

Rarely, **sumatriptan** causes angina secondary to coronary vasospasm. Electrocardiographic changes have been observed in patients with CAD or Prinzmetal's (vasospastic) angina. To reduce the risk of angina, do not give **sumatriptan** to patients who have risk factors for CAD. These patients include postmenopausal women; men over age 40 years; smokers; and patients with hypertension, hypercholesterolemia, obesity, diabetes, or a family history of CAD.

Other adverse effects

Mild reactions include vertigo, malaise, fatigue, and tingling sensations. Transient pain and redness may occur at sites of subcutaneous injection. Intranasal administration may cause irritation in the nose and throat as well as an offensive or unusual taste.

Drug–drug and drug–disease interactions

The FDA issued a warning about the combination of triptans and serotonergic drugs such as selective serotonin reuptake inhibitors and serotonin–norepinephrine reuptake inhibitors, which can lead to the serotonin syndrome.

All triptans and ergot alkaloids cause vasoconstriction. Accordingly, if one triptan is combined with another or with an ergot alkaloid, excessive and prolonged vasospasm could result.

Do not use triptans within 24 hours of administering an ergot derivative or another triptan.

MAOIs can suppress degradation of triptans, which causes plasma levels to rise and results in toxicity. Furthermore, triptans should not be administered within 2 weeks of stopping an MAOI. Relpax is contraindicated with potent CYP450 3A4 inhibitors.

Triptans are contraindicated for patients with a history of ischemic heart disease, myocardial infarction, cerebrovascular events, uncontrolled hypertension, or other heart disease. Do not use triptans during pregnancy.

Patient instructions and counseling

Patients should be counseled to contact a health care provider if pain or tightness in the chest occurs.

Patients should not exceed daily maximum doses. If migraines occur more than 3 times a month, prophylactic treatment should be considered.

Calcitonin gene-related peptide (CGRP) receptor antagonists ("gepants")

Ubrogepant (Ubrelvy) and Rimegepant (Nurtec ODT) were approved in 2019 and 2020 for acute treatment of migraine with or without aura.

Mechanism of action

CGRP is a potent vasodilator and pain signaling neurotransmitter, which often increases during migraine attacks. By antagonizing the CGRP receptor, the migraine cascade is prevented.

Pharmacokinetics

The orally disintegrating tabs are rapidly absorbed. Rimegepant has a longer half-life than ubrogepant (~11 hours vs. 5 to 7 hours). Both are metabolized primarily by CYP3A4 and eliminated primarily in the feces.

Adverse effects

Both rimegepant and ubrogepant are well tolerated. Nausea is the most common adverse effect.

Drug–drug interactions

Concurrent use of rimegepant with strong inhibitors of CYP3A4, strong or moderate inducers of CYP3A, or inhibitors of P-gp or BCRP should be avoided. Ubrogepant is contraindicated for use with CYP3A4 inhibitors; use with strong CYP3A4 inducers should be avoided.

Serotonin 5-HT1F agonists (Ditans)

Lasmiditan (Reyvow) was approved by the FDA in 2020.

Mechanism of action

Lasmiditan selectively binds to 5-HT$_{1F}$ receptors preventing pain pathways in the trigeminal nerve system. Unlike triptans, lasmiditan has not been shown to have vasoconstrictive effects.

Pharmacokinetics

Rapid absorption with a Tmax = 1.8 hours, metabolized by hepatic and extra-hepatic, non-CYP enzymes. Elimination is primarily in the urine.

Adverse effects

The most commonly reported adverse effects include dizziness, paresthesia, and sedation.

Drug interactions

Lasmiditan inhibits P-glycoprotein (P-gp) and breast cancer resistance protein (BCRP); coadministration with P-gp or BCRP substrates should be avoided. Caution should be taken when using alcohol or other CNS depressants concomitantly. Coadministration of lasmiditan with serotonergic drugs might increase the risk of serotonin syndrome. Whether it is safe to use both lasmiditan and a triptan within a 24-hour period has not been determined.

Migraine Prophylactic Therapy

Table 27-9 summarizes selected migraine preventive treatments.

Beta-adrenergic blocking agents

Propranolol is one of the drugs of choice for migraine prophylaxis. This agent can reduce the number, duration, and intensity of migraine attacks. It and timolol are the only 2 beta blockers that have FDA approval for migraine prophylaxis.

Not all beta blockers are active against migraines. Recommended first-line agents include **metoprolol** ⚠, **propranolol**, and timolol. Additional agents with demonstrated efficacy include **atenolol** and nadolol. Adverse effects with these therapies include fatigue, dizziness, and hypotension. Because not all beta blockers are effective, a mechanism other than beta blockade is apparently responsible for the beneficial effects.

 Metoprolol *FDA BOXED WARNING*

Ischemic heart disease. Following abrupt cessation with certain beta blocking agents, exacerbations of angina pectoris and myocardial infarction have occurred.

Avoid abrupt discontinuation of therapy. Abrupt discontinuation increases risk of cardiac events.

TABLE 27-9. Selected Migraine Preventive Treatments

Drug	Recommended dose/day	Selected side effects
Beta-adrenergic receptor antagonists		
Propranolol	80 to 240 mg	Reduced energy, tiredness, postural symptoms
Metoprolol	100 to 200 mg	
Timolol	20 to 30 mg	
Atenolol	100 mg	
Antidepressants		
Amitriptyline	10 to 150 mg	Drowsiness
Fluoxetine	10 to 20 mg	Headache, nausea, nervousness, insomnia, drowsiness
Anticonvulsants		
Divalproex	400 to 600 mg	Drowsiness, weight gain, tremor, hair loss, hematologic and liver abnormalities, teratogenicity
Valproate	500 to 1500 mg	
Gabapentin	900 to 2400 mg	Somnolence, dizziness
Topiramate	100 mg	Confusion, paresthesias, weight loss
Dietary supplements		
Petasites (butterbur)	50 to 75 mg twice daily	
MIG-99 (feverfew)	50 to 300 mg twice daily; 2.08 to 18.75 mg 3 times daily for MIG-99 preparation	
Magnesium	400 to 600 mg	Diarrhea
Coenzyme Q10	300 mg	GI effects
Riboflavin	400 mg	Urine discoloration (yellow)

Adapted from Goadsby P, Lipton R, Ferrari M, 2002; D'Amico D, Tepper J, 2008; Fenstermacher N, Levin M, Ward T, 2011.
Boldface indicates one of top 100 drugs for 2020 by prescription volume.

Anticonvulsants

Good evidence supports the efficacy of divalproex sodium and sodium valproate. Both are considered first line for prevention. Divalproex sodium carries FDA approval for migraine prophylaxis. Adverse effects with these therapies include nausea, weight gain, hair loss, tremor, and teratogenic potential, such as neural tube defects. Both agents have boxed warnings for hepatotoxicity, pancreatitis, and teratogenicity. Valproate is contraindicated (pregnancy category X) for migraine prophylaxis in pregnant women because of decreased IQ (intelligence quotient) scores in exposed children.

Topiramate has evidence for clinical efficacy in reducing migraine frequency, duration, and intensity and is FDA approved for migraine prevention. **Topiramate** was the first medication approved for migraine prophylaxis in adolescents 12 to 17 years of age. Potential adverse effects include paresthesia, fatigue, nausea, dizziness, and difficulty concentrating. Anorexia and weight loss may also occur.

Antidepressants

Amitriptyline has efficacy for decreasing migraine frequency. In the past, it was considered first-line prophylaxis treatment. However, other agents moved to the forefront of migraine prophylactic therapy, and **amitriptyline** is considered second-line therapy. Somnolence, concentration difficulties, and anticholinergic symptoms are frequently reported with tricyclic antidepressants.

Venlafaxine effectively reduces migraine number and severity. It should be considered second-line therapy. Common side effects include nausea, vomiting, drowsiness, and tachycardia. SNRIs should not be used concomitantly with ergot derivatives or triptans because of increased risk of developing serotonin syndrome.

Calcium channel blockers

Calcium channel blockers were previously considered alternatives for migraine prevention. However, because there is inadequate data supporting their use in improving or preventing migraines, guidelines no longer recommend calcium channel blockers for migraine prevention.

Antispasmodics

OnabotulinumtoxinA (Botox) is the first and only FDA-approved agent for prevention of chronic migraine (defined as >15 migraine days per month with migraines lasting at least 4 hours).
    Calcitonin gene-related peptide (CGRP) antagonists:

Migraine patients have increased levels of the neuropeptide CGRP, which plays an important role in the migraine cascade. CGRP antagonists are humanized monoclonal antibodies that bind to the CGRP receptor or ligand, preventing the cascade of events triggering migraine. In 2018, the FDA approved 3 CGRP inhibitors for migraine prophylaxis: erenumab (Aimovig), fremanezumab (Ajovy), and galcanezumab (Emgality). As these agents lack hepatic and renal metabolism, drug interactions are uncommon. In 2020, an I.V. CGRP inhibitor was approved, eptinezumab (Vyepti). Table 27-10 provides an overview of these agents.

> ⚠️ **OnabotulinumtoxinA** *FDA BOXED WARNING*
>
> Spread of toxin effect. The effects of all onabotulinum toxin products may spread from the area of injection to product symptoms consistent with botulinum toxin effects. These can include asthenia, generalized muscle weakness, diplopia, ptosis, dysphagia, dysphonia, incontinence, and breathing difficulties.
>
> Risk of botulinum toxin spreading from injection area.

TABLE 27-10. Calcitonin Gene-Related Peptide (CGRP) Inhibitors for Migraine Prophylaxis

Generic name	Trade name	Available strengths	Dosage	Dosing instructions
Erenumab	Aimovig	70 mg/mL (1 mL), 140 mg/mL (1 mL)	Initial: 70 mg once a month; some patients may benefit from 140 mg once a month	Administer subcutaneously in abdomen (avoiding 2 inches around the navel), thigh, or upper arm, avoiding areas of skin that are tender, bruised, red, or hard.
Fremanezumab	Ajovy	225 mg/1.5 mL (1.5 mL)	225 mg once monthly or 675 mg (given as 3 consecutive injections of 225 mg each) every 3 months	Administer subcutaneously in the abdomen, thigh, or upper arm, avoiding areas that are tender, bruised, red, or indurated.
Galcanezumab	Emgality	100 mg/1 mL (1 mL), 120 mg/1 mL (1 mL)	Loading dose of 240 mg, given as 2 consecutive doses of 120 mg each, followed by monthly doses of 120 mg	Administer subcutaneously in the thigh, upper arm, or buttocks.

TABLE 27-10. Calcitonin Gene-Related Peptide (CGRP) Inhibitors for Migraine Prophylaxis *(Continued)*

Generic name	Trade name	Available strengths	Dosage	Dosing instructions
Eptinezumab	Vyepti	100 mg/mL (1 mL)	100 mg as an I.V. infusion over approximately 30 minutes every 3 months. Some patients may benefit from a dosage of 300 mg	Infuse over approximately 30 minutes. Use an I.V. infusion set with a 0.2 micron or 0.22 micron in-line or add-on sterile filter. After the infusion is complete, flush the line with 20 mL of 0.9% Sodium Chloride Injection, USP.

27-5 Nonpharmacologic Treatment of Migraines

General Principles of Nonpharmacologic Therapies

Nonpharmacologic approaches may be well-suited to patients who have exhibited a poor tolerance or poor response to drug therapy, who have a contraindication to drug therapy, or who have a history of long-term, frequent, or excessive use of analgesics or other acute medications. Nonpharmacologic interventions may also be useful in patients who are pregnant, are planning to become pregnant, or are nursing.

Treatment Recommendations

Patients with migraine pain may experience relief by resting or sleeping in a cool, quiet, dark environment. Half of migraine patients experience considerable relief by applying a cold compress to the head.

Trigger Management

Trigger management is important in preventing migraine attacks. Triggering factors can cause migraine. If recognized and avoided, they may impede an impending attack.

Triggers vary from person to person. Examples of triggers include changes in weather or air pressure; bright sunlight, glare, or fluorescent lights; chemical fumes; menstrual cycles; and certain foods such as processed meats, red wine, beer, dried fish, broad beans, fermented cheeses, aspartame, and monosodium glutamate.

27-6 Pharmacist's Role

Pharmacists have a vital role in ensuring safe and effective pain management. A comprehensive approach that includes medication reconciliation, designing multimodal pharmacotherapy regimens, collaborating with prescribers and interdisciplinary team members, monitoring pain regimens for safety and efficacy, and serving as patient educators are all critical components of the pharmacist's role in pain management. Treating and preventing migraines centers around appropriate pharmacotherapy. Pharmacists work close with patients and providers to plan treatments, assess their efficacy, and educate patients on these regimens.

NAPLEX Competency Statements

The questions in this chapter cover the following 2021 NAPLEX Competency Statements: **AREA 1:** 1.2; 1.4; 1.5 **AREA 2:** 2.1; 2.2; 2.3 **AREA 3:** 3.2; 3.4; 3.5; 3.6; 3.7; 3.8; 3.9; 3.10; 3.11; 3.12 **AREA 4:** 4.3; 4.4; 4.9 **AREA 5:** 5.1.

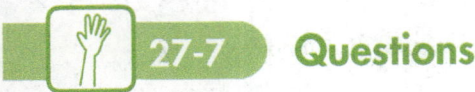

27-7   Questions

Use Patient Profile 27-1 to answer Question 1.

PATIENT PROFILE 27-1.

Patient name: Tyler George
Age: 37
Sex: Male
Diagnosis:
Chronic pain
Depression
Hypertension
Hyperlipidemia

Height: 5'11"
Weight: 189 lb
Allergies: NKDA

Laboratory and diagnostic tests

Vital signs:
BP: 134/80
Pulse: 80
RR: 20
Temp: 98.1
Lipid profile on 12/30/20
   Total cholesterol, 180 mg/dL
   LDL cholesterol, 105 mg/dL
   HDL cholesterol, 55 mg/dL
   Triglycerides, 120 mg/dL

Medication Record

Date	Rx #	Prescriber	Drug and Strength	Quantity	Sig	Refills
3/27	274789	Reed	Paroxetine 30 mg	90	Daily	3
3/20	273103	Reed	Simvastatin 40 mg	90	Daily	3
3/20	273004	Reed	Amlodipine 10 mg	90	Daily	3
10/18	268407	Owens	Quadrivalent inactivated influenza vaccine	1	0.5 mL I.M. in the deltoid muscle	0

1. T.G. is a 37-year-old male has chronic right hip pain following a work-related injury 6 months ago. His symptoms include a sharp, numb, and tingling pain that radiates from his hip to his knee. He currently uses ibuprofen 400 mg every 8 hours as needed for pain. He reports, however, worsening pain over the past month with little relief after taking ibuprofen. Which of the following agents would you recommend to treat his pain?

A. Carisoprodol
B. Fluoxetine
C. Hydrocodone/acetaminophen
D. Duloxetine
E. Acetaminophen

Use the following conversion table to answer Questions 2 to 4.

Equianalgesic Doses of Selected Opioids

Opioid	Parenteral	Oral
Morphine	10	30
Fentanyl[a]	0.1	n.a.
Hydromorphone	1.5	7.5
Methadone[b]	5	10
Oxycodone	n.a.	20
Oxymorphone	1	10

Adapted from McNicol 2008.
Boldface indicates one of top 100 drugs for 2020 by prescription volume.
n.a., not applicable.
a. Not for use to convert to transdermal products. Transdermal dose conversion in mcg/h is approximately 50% of the 24-hour *oral* morphine dose equivalent. This assumption can be used only when converting from an agent to the transdermal fentanyl product. The reverse conversion is *not* accurate!
b. Data suggest methadone may be more potent than originally thought. Consider reducing doses greater than the above conversion ratios, especially in patients receiving high doses of opioids chronically.

2. R.M. suffers from chronic pain that is aching and throbbing in nature. After failing numerous nonopioid therapies, his pain regimen consists of oxycodone 10/325 mg every 6 hours. His physician wishes to convert his regimen to a combination of long-acting and short-acting agents. Which of the following regimens is an accurate dose conversion for the long-acting opioid in this patient? Assume a 25% cross-tolerance reduction.

A. Morphine Sustained Release (SR) 20 mg twice daily
B. Morphine SR 40 mg twice daily
C. Oxymorphone Extended Release (ER) 20 mg twice daily
D. Fentanyl 50 mcg/h transdermal patch every 72 hours
E. Fentanyl 75 mcg/h transdermal patch every 72 hours

3. A patient is admitted to the hospital after developing an ileus. His total daily dose of oral morphine is 180 mg. Which of the following options is an appropriate hourly rate for this patient's morphine?

A. 2.5 mg/h infusion
B. 5 mg/h infusion
C. 7.5 mg/h infusion
D. 10 mg/h infusion
E. 12 mg/h infusion

4. L. R. is a 52-year-old male with a history of chronic back pain resulting from a work-related injury 3 years ago. His medications include pregabalin 75 mg twice daily, morphine SR 20 mg twice daily, morphine immediate release (IR) 5 mg 3 times daily as needed for breakthrough pain (he reports using all 3 doses of morphine IR daily). His pain is not well controlled and is affecting his personal relationships. His physician asks you to calculate an equianalgesic dose for a different long-acting opioid. Which of the following doses of long-acting opioids is the most appropriate for this patient? Do not use a cross-tolerance reduction in dosing.

A. Oxycodone controlled release (CR) 20 mg twice daily
B. Oxycodone CR 40 mg twice daily
C. Oxymorphone extended release (ER) 5 mg twice daily
D. Hydromorphone ER 4 mg daily
E. Hydromorphone ER 8 mg daily

5. Which of the following adverse effects are manifestations of μ opioid agonists? (Mark all that apply.)

A. Constipation
B. Respiratory depression
C. Nausea
D. Miosis
E. Pruritus

6. Addiction is defined by which of the following criteria? (Mark all that apply.)

A. Compulsive use of drugs
B. Physical dependence on a medication
C. Use of a substance for psychic effects
D. Impaired control of drug use and continued use despite harm
E. Natural tolerance developing after long-term drug use (typically 6 months or longer)

7. The preferred route of opioid administration is
_____.

A. oral
B. intravenous
C. subcutaneous
D. rectal
E. intramuscular

8. Which of the following opioids has the longest duration of analgesic effect?

A. Methadone
B. Controlled-release morphine
C. Hydromorphone
D. Transdermal fentanyl
E. Extended-release tapentadol

9. P. K. is a 67-year-old male with a past medical history including diabetes, stage II chronic kidney disease, and hypertension. He recently started hydrocodone and is complaining of constipation. His last bowel movement was 3 days ago. He usually has bowel movements once daily. Which of the following would you recommend to treat constipation?

A. Docusate sodium
B. Psyllium
C. Hydration and increased fiber intake
D. Docusate sodium + senna
E. Magnesium citrate

10. Which of the following statements regarding methadone pharmacokinetics is true?

A. The half-life corresponds to analgesic efficacy.
B. It is highly plasma protein bound and widely distributed in tissue.
C. The clearance of methadone is rapid, resulting in frequent dosing.
D. Methadone has low bioavailability from the GI tract and, therefore, is not useful when given orally.
E. Methadone is metabolized outside of the CYP450 system, therefore, making drug interactions uncommon.

11. Which of the following agents can be used to reverse respiratory effects caused by opioid overdose?

A. Naloxone
B. Pentazocine
C. Buprenorphine
D. Naltrexone
E. Methadone

12. Which of the following opioids has a toxic metabolite that can accumulate in renal dysfunction?

A. Hydromorphone
B. Fentanyl
C. Meperidine
D. Methadone
E. Buprenorphine

13. Which of the following medications is most likely to worsen opioid-induced constipation?

A. Paxil
B. Zocor
C. Premarin
D. Elavil
E. Glucophage

14. Which of the following medications is least likely to cause constipation?

A. Morphine IR
B. Morphine ER
C. Methadone
D. Oxycodone ER
E. Transdermal fentanyl patch

15. What is the rationale of adding caffeine to a simple analgesic for migraine treatment? (Mark all that apply.)

A. Decrease the required dose of acetaminophen and aspirin
B. Cause cerebral arterial vasoconstriction
C. Increase gastric acidity and perfusion, enhancing aspirin absorption
D. Prevent nausea during aura through phosphodiesterase induction
E. Decreasing heart rate and blood pressure

16. Which of the following agents is a selective serotonin receptor agonist?

A. Sumatriptan
B. Dihydroergotamine
C. Metoclopramide
D. Caffeine
E. Escitalopram

17. Which of the following statements is true regarding the adverse effects of ergotamine?

A. Ergotamine inhibits the chemoreceptor trigger zone to minimize nausea and vomiting.
B. Muscle weakness is an uncommon side effect of ergotamine.
C. Angina-like pain reported with the triptans is not seen with ergotamine use.
D. Overuse of ergotamine can result in ischemia.
E. Ergotamine is the drug of choice for migraine in pregnancy.

18. Which of the following statements about triptans is correct?

A. Triptans are contraindicated in ischemic cardiovascular disease.
B. Triptans are preferred for migraine treatment during pregnancy.
C. Patients taking ergot alkaloids can use triptans concomitantly.
D. Triptans are strictly contraindicated in patients with hypertension.
E. Newer triptans are indicated for both prophylaxis and abortive therapy.

19. Which of the following statements about Treximet is correct?

A. Treximet can be used concomitantly with over-the-counter products such as Aleve.
B. Treximet dose is limited to 3 capsules per 24 hours.
C. Treximet may cause dizziness.
D. Treximet is first-line therapy for migraine prophylaxis.
E. Treximet is safe for use in patients with cardiovascular disease.

20. Which of the following statements is true regarding initiation of prophylactic migraine therapy?

A. Patients requiring sumatriptan use 3 days per week or less are not candidates for prophylactic treatment.
B. Patients with migraines that occur with a frequency greater than twice monthly and an increasing frequency of attacks are candidates for prophylaxis.
C. Prophylactic therapy is required in patients with hypertension because hypertension is a contraindication to using abortive therapies.
D. Prophylactic treatment is contraindicated in migraines with aura.
E. Trigger avoidance is largely ineffective in preventing migraines.

21. Which of the following medications are appropriate for migraine prophylaxis? (Select all that apply.)

A. Divalproex
B. Propranolol
C. Dihydroergotamine
D. Hydrocodone
E. Erenumab

22. Rank the following triptans from fastest onset of action to slowest onset of action

Unordered response	Ordered response
Oral frovatriptan (Frova)	
Oral rizatriptan (Maxalt)	
Subcutaneous injection sumatriptan (Imitrex STAT dose)	

 **27-8** **Answers**

1. **D.** The patient is experiencing neuropathic pain. Specific tricyclic antidepressants, antiepileptics, and SNRIs are typically recommended as first-line treatment. Opioid medications are not the most effective treatment for neuropathic pain and are recommended as second-line treatment. Given the patient's blood pressure is well controlled, the slight risk of mild hypertension with duloxetine is outweighed by the benefit.

2. **A.** A total daily dose conversion of 40 mg of oxycodone/APAP IR (assuming a 25% cross-tolerance reduction) would result in a conversion to 45 mg of morphine total daily dose. The closest available product would be morphine SR 20 mg twice daily (40 mg total daily dose). An equivalent transdermal fentanyl patch dose would be 30 mcg/h (without a cross-tolerance reduction). An equivalent oxymorphone dose (assuming a 25% cross-tolerance reduction) would be 15 mg total daily dose.

3. **A.** A dose of 180 mg oral morphine converts to 60 mg of I.V. morphine, and 60 mg divided by 24 hours equals an infusion of 2.5 mg/h.

4. **A.** L. R.'s total daily dose (TDD) of morphine = 55 mg (40 mg + 15 mg of breakthrough). Converted to oxycodone, his TDD = 36.66 mg, which could be rounded up to 40 mg daily to allow for 20 mg twice daily dosing. A dose of 55 mg of morphine converted to oxymorphone = 18.3 mg daily. A daily dose of 55 mg of morphine converted to hydromorphone = 13.75 mg.

5. **A, B, C, D, E.** Other known adverse effects at therapeutic doses include peripheral vasodilation, reduced peripheral resistance, and inhibition of the baroreceptor reflexes.

6. **A, C, D.** Physical dependence is the occurrence of a withdrawal syndrome after an opioid is stopped or quickly decreased without titration. Addiction is the psychological dependence on the use of substances for psychical effects and is characterized by compulsive and continued use despite harm.

7. **A.** Oral medications should be used whenever possible because of convenience, flexibility, and steady serum levels.

8. **D.** Transdermal fentanyl provides analgesia for up to 72 hours. The analgesic effects of methadone do not correlate with its long half-life. Tapentadol ER is available as extended release tablet (nucynta ER) but must be dosed every 12 hours.

9. **D.** Patients on opiates do not develop tolerance to constipation. All patients taking around-the-clock opioid analgesics should be placed on prophylactic bowel regimens. Bulk laxatives are usually considered to be safe for chronic use; however, they are not recommended in opioid-induced constipation because these agents may increase the risk of bowel obstruction in patients with impaired GI motility. Stimulant laxatives are the most commonly used laxatives to treat opioid-induced constipation. Magnesium citrate should be avoided in patients with chronic kidney disease.

10. **B.** About 90% of methadone is bound to plasma protein and is widely distributed in tissues. Methadone has a long terminal half-life, resulting in slow clearance. This half-life does not correspond to analgesic dosing. It is metabolized via the CYP450 enzyme system.

11. **A.** Naloxone is a μ antagonist useful in opioid overdose. Naltrexone is also a μ antagonist, but it is reserved for use in alcoholism and opioid addiction.

12. **C.** Normeperidine, a metabolite of meperidine, can accumulate with chronic use, with renal impairment, and when the dose exceeds 600 mg every 24 hours.

13. **D.** The anticholinergic effects of tricyclic anti-depressants such as Elavil can exacerbate opioid-induced constipation and urinary retention.

14. **E.** Because transdermal delivery bypasses absorption from the GI tract, constipation has been reported to be less frequent with transdermal fentanyl than with other opioids.

15. **A, C.** Caffeine has analgesic and possibly anti-inflammatory properties. Therefore, reduced doses of acetaminophen and aspirin may be required. Caffeine may also increase gastric acidity and perfusion, enhancing the absorption of aspirin.

16. **A.** Sumatriptan is a selective serotonin receptor agonist.

17. **D.** Adverse effects of ergotamine include nausea and vomiting, physical dependence, muscle weakness, and angina-like pain. Overuse of ergotamine can result in ischemia that may progress to gangrene. Ergotamine is contraindicated for use during pregnancy.

18. **A.** Triptans are contraindicated in pregnancy and ischemic cardiovascular disease. They cannot be used within 24 hours of another triptan or ergot alkaloid.

19. **C.** Treximet is indicated for the acute treatment of migraine attacks with or without aura in adults. This medication may cause dizziness. The dose is limited to 2 tablets per 24 hours. Because of Treximet's naproxen content, other products containing naproxen should not be used concomitantly. Because of both Treximet's sumatriptan and naproxen components, it should be avoided in patients with cardiovascular disease.

20. **B.** Prophylactic therapy should be considered when migraines occur more than twice monthly and the frequency of attacks is increasing.

21. **A, B, E.** Propranolol has been shown to be effective for migraine prophylaxis. This agent can reduce the number and intensity of attacks in about 70% of patients. Erenumab (Aimovig) is a CGRP antagonist. Up to half of patients studied had fewer migraine days by at least 50%. Divalproex sodium carries FDA approval for migraine prophylaxis. Dihydroergotamine and hydrocodone are not approved for migraine prophylaxis.

22.

Drug	Onset of action
Sumatriptan subcutaneous injection (Imitrex STAT dose)	10 to 15 minutes
Rizatriptan (Maxalt)	30 to 60 minutes
Frovatriptan (Frova)	60 to 120 minutes

 **27-9** ## Additional Resources

Pain Management

American Society of Anesthesiologists Task Force on Pain Management. Practice guidelines for chronic pain management: an updated report by the American Society of Anesthesiologists Task Force on Chronic Pain Management and the American Society of Regional Anesthesia and Pain Medicine. *Anesthesiology.* 2010;112(4):810–833.

Approved risk evaluation and mitigation strategies (REMS). April 19, 2014. U.S. Food and Drug Administration website. https://www.accessdata.fda.gov/scripts/cder/rems. Accessed October 30, 2016.

Dowell D, Haegerich TM, Chou R. CDC Guideline for Prescribing Opioids for Chronic Pain—United States, 2016. *MMWR Recomm Rep.* 2016;65(RR-1):1–49. https://www.cdc.gov/mmwr/volumes/65/rr/pdfs/rr6501e1.pdf. Accessed June 12, 2020.

Dworkin RH, O'Connor AB, Audette J, et al. Recommendations for the pharmacological management of neuropathic pain: an overview and literature update. *Mayo Clinic Proc.* 2010;85:S3–S14.

Herndon CM, Strickland JM, Ray JB. Pain management. In: DiPiro JT, Talbert RL, Yee GC, et al., eds. *Pharmacotherapy: A Pathophysiologic Approach.* 10th ed. New York, NY: McGraw-Hill; 2017:909–926.

Krebs EE, Lorenz KA, Bair MJ, et al. Development and initial validation of the PEG, a three-item scale assessing pain intensity and interference. *J Gen Intern Med* 2009;24:733–738.

National Academies of Sciences, Engineering, and Medicine. 2020. *Framing opioid prescribing guidelines for acute pain: Developing the evidence.* Washington, DC: The National Academies Press. https://doi.org/10.17226/25555.

O'Connor AB, Dworkin RH. Treatment of neuropathic pain: an overview of recent guidelines. *Am J Med.* 2009;122 (10 suppl):S22–S32.

Migraines

D'Amico D, Tepper J. Prophylaxis of migraines: general principles and patient acceptance. *Neuropsychiatr Dis Treat.* 2008;4:1155–1167.

Fenstermacher N, Levin M, Ward T. Pharmacological prevention of migraine. *BMJ.* 2011;342:540–543.

Firnhaber J, Rickett K. What are the best prophylactic drugs for migraine? *J Fam Pract.* 2009;58(11):608–610.

Goadsby P, Lipton R, Ferrari M. Migraine: current understanding and treatment. *N Engl J Med.* 2002;346:257–270.

Holland S, Silberstein SD, Freitag F, et al. Evidence-based guideline update: NSAIDs and other complementary treatments for episodic migraine prevention in adults: Report of the Quality Standards Subcommittee of the American Academy of Neurology and the American Headache Society. *Neurology.* 2012;78:1346–1353.

Silberstein SD, Holland S, Freitag F, et al. Evidence-based guideline update: pharmacologic treatment for episodic migraine prevention in adults: Report of the Quality Standards Subcommittee of the American Academy of Neurology and the American Headache Society. *Neurology.* 2012;78:1337–1345.

Silberstein SD. Migraine. *Lancet.* 2004;363:381–391.

Silberstein SD. Topiramate in migraine prevention: evidence-based medicine from clinical trials. *Arch Neurol.* 2004;61:490–495.

Seizure Disorders

LESLIE A. HAMILTON

28-1 KEY POINTS

- Phenytoin injection should not be infused faster than 50 mg/min; fosphenytoin ⚠ can be administered at 150 mg phenytoin equivalents (PE)/min.
- **Gabapentin** and levetiracetam are not associated with any significant drug interactions.
- The following anticonvulsants (also known as antiepileptic drugs [AEDs]) carry a U.S. Food and Drug Administration (FDA) boxed warning: carbamazepine ⚠ (aplastic anemia, dermatologic reactions); valproic acid ⚠ (liver failure, teratogenicity, pancreatitis); felbamate ⚠ (aplastic anemia, hepatic failure); **lamotrigine** ⚠ (serious rash), and vigabatrin ⚠ (permanent vision loss). The FDA has also given a warning that AEDs may be associated with an increased risk of suicidal behavior or ideation.
- At high enough doses, all beta-lactam antibiotics, in addition to ciprofloxacin, and normeperidine (a metabolite of meperidine that accumulates in renal failure) may cause seizures.
- Carbamazepine undergoes autoinduction (i.e., it induces its own metabolism), and phenytoin has capacity-limited or saturable (i.e., Michaelis–Menten) pharmacokinetics.
- There may be an association between folic acid deficiency and spina bifida. All women of childbearing age should receive daily **folic acid** (0.4 mg/d); however, women with epilepsy should receive larger doses (1 mg/d). Doses of 4 mg/d may be required in women receiving phenytoin, carbamazepine, and/or phenobarbital.
- Unless a patient is experiencing a life-threatening adverse effect, an AED should not be abruptly discontinued.
- Patients with an allergy to sulfa medications should not be given zonisamide.

28-2 STUDY GUIDE CHECKLIST

The following topics may guide your study of this subject area:

- ☐ The various types of seizures, including generalized convulsive status epilepticus.
- ☐ Criteria for treatment, principles of treatment, and reasons for failure of an AED to adequately control epilepsy.
- ☐ Available formulations for the various anticonvulsants.
- ☐ FDA boxed warnings and the most prevalent and significant adverse effects for the various AEDs.
- ☐ Relevant pharmacokinetic characteristics and drug–drug or drug–nutrient interactions involving AEDs.
- ☐ Emergent treatment of status epilepticus.

Fosphenytoin *FDA BOXED WARNING*

Both fosphenytoin and phenytoin are associated with a boxed warning for the risk of severe hypotension and cardiac arrhythmias with rapid intravenous infusions.

 Carbamazepine *FDA BOXED WARNING*

Carbamazepine has been reported to be associated with aplastic anemia and agranulocytosis. In addition, Stevens-Johnson syndrome and toxic epidermal necrolysis have been reported.

 Valproic Acid *FDA BOXED WARNING*

Valproic acid has boxed warnings for serious hepatotoxicity, pancreatitis, and major congenital malformations.

 Felbamate *FDA BOXED WARNING*

Felbamate has been reported to be associated with aplastic anemia and acute liver failure.

 Lamotrigine *FDA BOXED WARNING*

Lamotrigine has been associated with Stevens-Johnson syndrome and toxic epidermal necrolysis.

 Vigabatrin *FDA BOXED WARNING*

Vigabatrin has been associated with permanent vision loss and is only available through a risk evaluation and mitigation strategy (REMS) program.

28-3 Epilepsy and Etiologies

Seizures occur when neurons become depolarized and repetitively fire action potentials. An individual who experiences a seizure may or may not have epilepsy. The term *epilepsy* is applied after 2 involuntary and unprovoked seizures. Many things, including drugs, can cause a person to seize (Table 28-1).

There are 3 main types of epilepsy: focal onset seizures, generalized onset seizures, and seizures of unknown onset. Figure 28-1 shows the classifications of epilepsy.

TABLE 28-1. Etiologies for Seizures

Category	Event
Genetic	Chromosomal abnormalities have been associated with some types of seizures
Mechanical	Birth injuries, head trauma, brain tumors, vascular abnormalities (stroke)
Metabolic	Electrolyte disturbances (sodium, elevated calcium), glucose abnormalities (low glucose), inborn errors of metabolism
Prescription medications	Antibiotics: All beta-lactam antibiotics and ciprofloxacin
	Anticonvulsants: May be proconvulsants and can exacerbate an existing seizure type or unmask a new seizure type in those with epilepsy when an AED is used for treatment of a nonindicated seizure type[a]
	Other: Local anesthetics (lidocaine), metoclopramide, theophylline, tricyclic antidepressants, **bupropion**, isoniazid, meperidine (normeperidine metabolite can cause seizures in patients with renal failure who receive normal doses), **tramadol**
Recreational drugs	Alcohol, amphetamines, cocaine and freebase cocaine, ephedra, **methylphenidate**, narcotics
Other	Fever, central nervous system infection, eclampsia, noncompliance

Boldface indicates one of top 100 drugs for 2020 by prescription volume.
a. Carbamazepine, phenytoin, or fosphenytoin may cause generalized nonmotor (absence) seizures. Carbamazepine may cause generalized motor seizures. **Lamotrigine** may cause myoclonic seizures. Ethosuximide may cause generalized motor seizures.

FIGURE 28-1. Classifications of Epilepsy

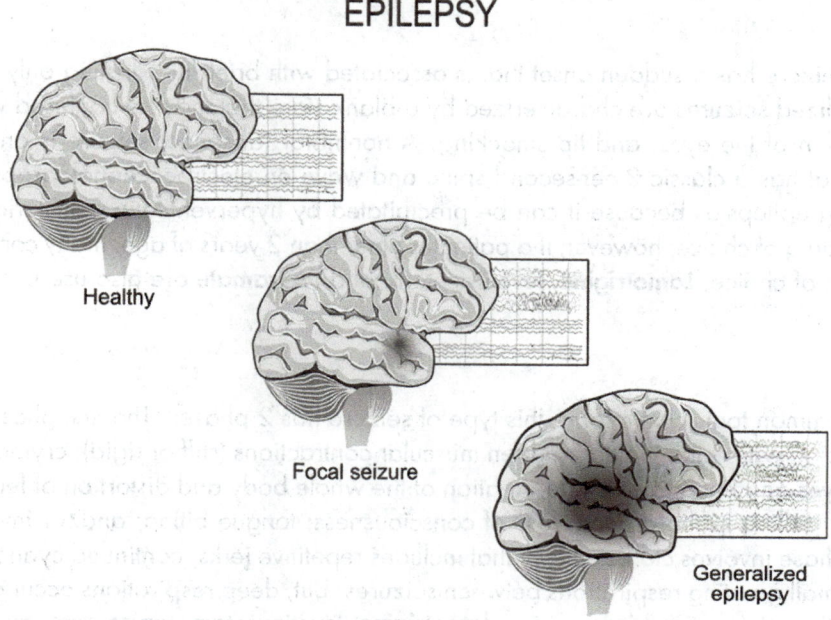

EPILEPSY

Healthy

Focal seizure

Generalized epilepsy

Focal Onset Seizures

Focal seizures begin in 1 hemisphere of the brain. They are unilateral, asymmetric movements, generally associated with an aura. An aura is a warning sensation experienced as a seizure begins. Focal seizures can be further divided into seizures with or without awareness and may have either a motor or nonmotor onset. When focal seizures are accompanied by altered consciousness, carbamazepine or oxcarbazepine are considered the drugs of choice. Other agents, such as lacosamide, **lamotrigine**, levetiracetam, and valproic acid are frequently used as first-line agents in treatment of new-onset focal seizures. Brivaracetam, cenobamate, eslicarbazepine, **gabapentin**, perampanel , phenobarbital, phenytoin, tiagabine, **topiramate**, and zonisamide are used less frequently because of concerns about adverse effects or less familiarity with newer agents. All agents are used in refractory disease.

> ⚠ **Perampanel** *FDA BOXED WARNING*
>
> Perampanel has a boxed warning for serious psychiatric and behavior reactions with its use.

Generalized Onset Seizures

Generalized onset seizures begin simultaneously in both brain hemispheres. They are characterized by bilateral movements and have no aura. Some are associated with altered consciousness or a total loss of consciousness. This chapter will focus on 2 types of generalized seizures: motor and nonmotor (absence) seizures. Juvenile myoclonic epilepsy, a generalized onset epilepsy syndrome, will also be discussed.

Nonmotor (absence) seizures

This type of seizure has a sudden onset that is associated with brief (i.e., lasting only seconds) seizures. These generalized seizures are characterized by a blank stare that may be confused with daydreaming, upward rotation of the eyes, and lip smacking. A nonmotor (absence) seizure is one of the few types of epilepsy that has a classic 3-per-second spike and wave on electroencephalography (EEG), and it is unique among epilepsies because it can be precipitated by hyperventilation. Historically, ethosuximide has been the drug of choice; however, if a patient is older than 2 years of age, many consider valproic acid to be the drug of choice. **Lamotrigine**, levetiracetam, and **topiramate** are also used.

Motor seizures

In the most common tonic-clonic form, this type of seizure has 2 phases. The first phase is a tonic activity that is associated with rigid, violent, sudden muscular contractions (stiff or rigid); crying or moaning; deviation of the eyes and head to one side; rotation of the whole body and distortion of features; suppression of respiration; falling to the ground; loss of consciousness; tongue biting; and/or involuntary urination. The second phase involves clonic activity that includes repetitive jerks, continued cyanosis, foaming at the mouth, and small grunting respirations between seizures; but, deep respirations occur as all muscles relax at the end of the seizure. Carbamazepine, **lamotrigine**, levetiracetam, **topiramate**, and valproic acid are frequently used as single agents or in adjunctive therapy. Although phenobarbital and phenytoin may be used, other AEDs are equally effective and are associated with fewer and more tolerable adverse effects and, in some instances, fewer drug–drug interactions.

Juvenile myoclonic epilepsy syndrome

Juvenile myoclonic epilepsy (JME) consists of generalized motor seizures (myoclonic and tonic-clonic) that generally occur on waking and may be provoked by sleep deprivation and alcohol. Because JME has a genetic basis, lifelong treatment with valproic acid, **lamotrigine**, levetiracetam, **topiramate**, or some combination of these agents is required.

Other Less Common Types of Epilepsy

Infantile spasms

These begin in the first 6 months of life, occur in clusters, may be associated with multiple seizures each day, and are associated with high mortality and morbidity. Before diagnosis, a parent may describe symptoms that resemble colic. These may be treated with adrenocorticotropic hormone (ACTH) or oral steroids, vigabatrin, or valproic acid (>2 years). **Topiramate** and zonisamide have also been used.

Lennox–Gastaut Syndrome

This syndrome accounts for 1% to 4% of childhood epilepsies and is characterized by a combination of various intractable seizures. It commonly appears between 2 and 6 years of age, is frequently accompanied by mental retardation and behavior problems, and carries a poor prognosis. This condition is treated with a combination of AEDs that include cannabidiol, clobazam, felbamate, **lamotrigine**, rufinamide, **topiramate**, and valproic acid (>2 years).

Posttraumatic epilepsy

Posttraumatic epilepsy presents following head trauma and may be treated prophylactically with phenytoin (or fosphenytoin) or levetiracetam. If no seizures occur within 7 days, medication should be discontinued. Valproic acid should not be used because it may cause central nervous system bleeding that may result in increased mortality.

Febrile seizure

While this is the most common seizure disorder in childhood, it should not be considered synonymous with epilepsy. Overall, the development of epilepsy in children who have experienced such seizures is rare (1% to 2%); however, about 15% of children who have complex febrile seizures will go on to develop epilepsy. Febrile seizures are generally benign and occur in a child with fever who does not have a central nervous system (CNS) infection. The age of onset is 4 months to 5 years (peaks at 14 to 18 months). Those at risk have at least 2 of the following risk factors: a first- or second-degree relative with a history of a febrile seizure; developmental delay; delayed discharge (>28 days) from a newborn center; or day care attendance. There are 2 types of febrile seizures: simple and complex. Simple febrile seizures are generalized seizures that last less than 15 minutes and do not recur within 24 hours. These are benign and are generally not treated. Complex febrile seizures are focal (i.e., involve an arm, leg, or face on 1 side only or eye deviation toward 1 side), prolonged (>15 minutes), or recur within 24 hours of the initial seizure. Drugs of choice for acute management of prolonged febrile seizures are rectal diazepam or intranasal midazolam. Daily AEDs are not indicated for the prevention of recurrent febrile seizures.

Generalized convulsive status epilepticus

Generalized convulsive status epilepticus (GCSE) is defined as a seizure that lasts longer than 5 minutes or 2 or more discrete seizures between which there is incomplete recovery of consciousness. It is a medical emergency. While GCSE is the most common type of status epilepticus, some patients may experience

FIGURE 28-2. American Epilepsy Society Proposed Treatment Algorithm for Status Epilepticus

Time Line	Interventions for emergency department, in-patient setting, or prehospital setting with trained paramedics

0-5 min Stabilization phase

1. Stabilize patient (airway, breathing, circulation, disability - neurologic exam)
2. Time seizure from its onset, monitor vital signs
3. Assess oxygenation, give oxygen via nasal cannula/mask, consider intubation if respiratory assistance needed
4. Initiate ECG monitoring
5. Collect finger stick blood glucose. If glucose < 60 mg/dl then
   Adults: 100 mg thiamine IV then 50 ml D50W IV
   Children ≥ 2 years: 2 ml/kg D25W IV   Children < 2 years: 4 ml/kg D12.5W
6. Attempt IV access and collect electrolytes, hematology, toxicology screen, (if appropriate) anticonvulsant drug levels

Yes ← **Does Seizure continue?** → No

No → If patient at baseline, then symptomatic medical care

5-20 min Initial therapy phase

A benzodiazepine is the initial therapy of choice (Level A):
Choose one of the following 3 equivalent first line options with dosing and frequency:
   Intramuscular midazolam (10 mg for > 40 kg, 5 mg for 13-40 kg, single dose, Level A) OR
   Intravenous lorazepam (0.1 mg/kg/dose, max: 4 mg/dose, may repeat dose once, Level A) OR
   Intravenous diazepam (0.15-0.2 mg/kg/dose, max: 10 mg/dose, may repeat dose once, Level A)
If none of the 3 options above are available, choose one of the following:
   Intravenous phenobarbital (15 mg/kg/dose, single dose, Level A) OR
   Rectal diazepam (0.2-0.5 mg/kg, max: 20 mg/dose, single dose, Level B) OR
   Intranasal midazolam (Level B), buccal midazolam (Level B)

Yes ← **Does seizure continue?** → No

No → If patient at baseline, then symptomatic medical care

20-40 min Second therapy phase

There is no evidence based preferred second therapy of choice (Level U):
Choose one of the following second line options and give as a single dose
   Intravenous fosphenytoin (20 mg PE/kg, max: 1500 mg PE/dose, single dose, Level U) OR
   Intravenous valproic acid (40 mg/kg, max: 3000 mg/dose, single dose, Level B) OR
   Intravenous levetiracetam (60 mg/kg, max: 4500 mg/dose, single dose, Level U)
If none of the options above are available, choose one of the following (if not given already)
   Intravenous phenobarbital (15 mg/kg, max dose, Level B)

Yes ← **Does seizure continue?** → No

No → If patient at baseline, then symptomatic medical care

40-60 min Third therapy phase

There is no clear evidence to guide therapy in this phase (Level U):
Choices include: repeat second line therapy or anesthetic doses of either thiopental, midazolam, pentobarbital, or propofol (all with continuous EEG monitoring).

Disclaimer: This clinical algorithm/guideline is designed to assist clinicians by providing an analytical framework for evaluating and treating patients with status epilepticus. It is not intended to establish a community standard of care, replace a clinician's medical judgment, or establish a protocol for all patients. The clinical conditions contemplated by this algorithm/guideline will not fit or work with all patients. Approaches not covered in this algorithm/guideline may be appropriate. Reprinted with permission from SAGE Publications.

nonconvulsive status epilepticus or repeated focal seizures. Figure 28-2 provides agents recommended for treatment. Therapy for GCSE consists of mainly intravenous (I.V.) formulations or continuous infusions. Many of the continuous infusions help to achieve burst suppression on EEG.

28-4   Treatment of Epilepsy

Almost no child should be treated after 1 seizure. Adults who have structural brain damage, a first seizure that is very severe, or an occupation that places them at risk of injury should a second seizure occur may be treated following 1 seizure. Monotherapy is always preferred. The addition of a second AED should not be considered until the serum concentrations or doses of the first AED have been maximized. Generally, the second AED should work through a different mechanism of action than the first. When the patient is at full doses of the second AED, the dose of the first drug should be slowly reduced and discontinued if possible. The use of 3 or more agents (i.e., polytherapy) is rarely needed. If a combination of 2 AEDs is tolerated and significantly reduces seizure frequency, polytherapy is indicated when greater control might be achieved or when doses of the 2 AEDs have been maximized, but enhanced efficacy is desired. Once a new AED has been added to the regimen, the response should be reassessed, and any unnecessary AED slowly discontinued.

Failure of an AED to manage seizures may be the result of a variety of factors. Approximately half of patients with epilepsy fail their first AED because of an incomplete response, intolerable adverse effects, or both. Despite further therapy, one-third will ultimately be refractory to anticonvulsant therapy.

Regardless of the reasons for failure, patient adherence to the prescribed regimen should be assessed in any patient with an inadequate response to AED therapy. This can be done using a combination of discussion with the patient, monitoring of AED serum concentrations, and review of medication refill record. Unanticipated or intolerable adverse effects can also contribute to poor adherence.

At times, a lack of response may be due to an incorrect diagnosis of the seizure type or use of an incorrect AED for a specific seizure type. For example, a patient with generalized nonmotor (absence) seizures who is incorrectly diagnosed with focal seizures and treated with carbamazepine will not respond to carbamazepine because it is not effective in generalized nonmotor (absence) seizures. At times the AED might be correct, but the dose, route, or formulation might be incorrect for a specific patient. The patient may also have altered pharmacokinetics that necessitate an alteration in dosage.

Research into factors that influence AED resistance has focused on genetic influences, in particular molecules that transport drugs out of target tissues using energy-dependent processes. One such molecule, P-glycoprotein (P-gp), is important in the transport of many AEDs. By promoting local efflux of a drug, P-gp can reduce the concentration of drug at sites of drug action. Because expression of multidrug resistance is under genetic control, research has focused on gene markers linked to polymorphisms of multidrug resistance among patients with refractory epilepsy. To date, these reports have generated conflicting results.

28-5 The Anticonvulsants

Regardless of official labeling, individual AEDs are used in virtually all seizure types. Several AEDs are high risk for medication errors and use bolded tall (uppercase) man lettering in their nomenclature to help draw attention to the dissimilarities in look-alike drug names (see Box 28-1).

Selection of an AED may be influenced by available dosage formulation, pharmacokinetic characteristics, the patient's pharmacogenomics profile, or the likelihood of anticipated or iatrogenic adverse effects, drug–drug, or drug–nutrient interactions. Although an agent may be an AED, some drugs have found greater utility outside of epilepsy in certain instances. For example, **gabapentin** is used for neuropathic pain, and **pregabalin** is used for fibromyalgia. The use of some AEDs has also been limited by concerns over serious adverse effects. For example, rufinamide is generally used only in Lennox–Gastaut syndrome, and vigabatrin is used in infantile spasms. Occasionally, non-AEDs such as acetazolamide, ACTH, oral steroids, and I.V. immune globulin are used to manage epilepsy.

> **BOX 28-1. Examples of Anticonvulsants with Tall Man Lettering**

carBAMazepine (TEGretol)	OXcarbazepine
cloBAZam	PENTobarbital
clonazePAM (KlonoPIN)	PHENobarbital
lamoTRIgine (LaMICtal)	tiaGABine
levETIRAacetam	

Dosage Formulation

Depending on the circumstance, an AED may be given by oral, I.V., intramuscular (I.M.), intranasal, buccal, or rectal routes. Oral administration of AEDs is the cornerstone of treatment and involves immediate release, including liquid formulations, or extended-release products (Table 28-2). Information regarding specific administration of the various AED oral products can be found in Table 28-3. As a general principle, slowly absorbed formulations are preferable for chronic therapy because they attenuate the fluctuations in drug concentrations between doses.

TABLE 28-2. Dosage Formulations for Antiepileptic Drugs[a]

Formulations	Dosing interval	Strength
Solutions		
Ethosuximide (Zarontin, generic)	bid to tid	250 mg/5 mL
Gabapentin (Neurontin, generic)	tid	250 mg/5 mL
Lacosamide (Vimpat)	bid	10 mg/mL
Levetiracetam (Keppra, generic)	bid	100 mg/mL
Phenobarbital (generic)	Daily to bid	20 mg/5 mL
Pregabalin (Lyrica)	tid to qid	20 mg/mL
Valproate sodium (Depakene, generic)	bid to qid	250 mg/5 mL
Suspensions		
Carbamazepine (Tegretol, generic)	tid to qid	100 mg/5 mL
Clobazam (Onfi)	bid	2.5 mg/mL
Felbamate (Felbatol, generic)	tid to qid	600 mg/5 mL
Gabapentin (Fanatrex FusePaq)	tid	25 mg/mL
Oxcarbazepine (Trileptal, generic)	bid	300 mg/5 mL
Perampanel (Fycompa)	Daily	0.5 mg/mL
Phenytoin (Dilantin, generic)	tid	125 mg/5 mL
Rufinamide (Banzel)	bid	40 mg/mL
Immediate release		
Carbamazepine (Tegretol, Epitol, generic)	bid	200 mg tablet
Clobazam (Onfi)	bid	5, 10, 20 mg tablets
Clonazepam (Klonopin)	Daily to bid	0.5, 1, 2 mg tablets
Eslicarbazepine acetate (Aptiom)	Daily	200, 400, 600, 800 mg tablets
Ethosuximide (Zarontin, generic)	bid to tid	250 mg capsule
Ezogabine (Potiga)	tid	50, 200, 300, 400 mg tablets
Felbamate (Felbatol, generic)	tid to qid	400, 600 mg tablets
Gabapentin (Neurontin, generic)	tid	100, 300, 400 mg capsules; 600, 800 mg tablets
Lacosamide (Vimpat)	bid	50, 100, 150, 200 mg tablets
Lamotrigine (Lamictal, generic)	bid	25, 100, 150, 200 mg tablets
Levetiracetam (Keppra, generic)	bid	250, 500, 750, 1000 mg tablets
Levetiracetam (Roweepra)	bid	500 mg tablet
Oxcarbazepine (Trileptal, generic)	bid	150, 300, 600 mg tablets
Perampanel (Fycompa)	Daily	2, 4, 6, 8, 10, 12 mg tablets

TABLE 28-2. Dosage Formulations for Antiepileptic Drugs[a] (Continued)

Formulations	Dosing interval	Strength
Phenobarbital (generic)	Daily to bid	15, 16.2, 30, 32.4, 60, 64.8, 97.2, 100 mg tablets
Pregabalin (Lyrica)	bid to tid	25, 50, 75, 100, 150, 200, 225, 300 mg tablets
Primidone (Mysoline, generic)	bid to tid	50, 250 mg tablets
Rufinamide (Banzel)	bid	200, 400 mg tablets
Tiagabine (Gabitril)	bid to qid	2, 4, 12, 16 mg tablets
Tiagabine (generic)	bid to qid	2, 4 mg tablets
Topiramate (Topamax, generic)	bid	15, 25 mg sprinkle capsules
Topiramate (Topamax, Topiragen, generic)	bid	25, 50, 100, 200 mg tablets
Valproic Acid (Depakene, generic)	bid to qid	250 mg capsule
Divalproex sodium (Depakote)	bid to qid	125, 250, 500 mg tablets
Vigabatrin (Sabril)	bid	500 mg tablet
Zonisamide (Zonegran, generic)	Daily to bid	25, 50, 100 mg capsules
Dispersible or chewable tablets		
Carbamazepine (generic)	bid	100 mg chewable tablet
Clonazepam (generic)	Daily to bid	0.125, 0.25, 0.5, 1, 2 mg dispersible tablets
Lamotrigine (Lamictal, generic)	bid	2, 5, 25 mg chewable tablets
Lamotrigine (Lamictal ODT, generic)	bid	25, 50, 100, 200 mg dispersible tablets
Levetiracetam (Spritam)	bid	250, 500, 750, 1000 mg dispersible tablets
Phenytoin (Infatabs, generic)	tid	50 mg chewable tablet
Powders		
Vigabatrin (Sabril)	bid	500 mg
Extended-release formulations		
Carbamazepine ER (Tegretol XR, generic)	bid	100, 200, 400 mg tablets
Carbamazepine ER (Carbatrol, Equetro)	bid	100, 200, 300 mg capsules
Gabapentin Enacarbil ER (Horizant ER, Gralise Starter)	Daily	300, 600 mg tablets
Lamotrigine ER (Lamictal XR)	Daily	25, 50, 100, 200, 250, 300 mg tablets
Lamotrigine ER (generic)	Daily	25, 50, 100, 200, 250, 300 mg tablets
Levetiracetam ER (Keppra XR, generic)	Daily	500, 750 mg tablets
Oxcarbazepine ER (Oxtellar XR)	Daily	150, 300, 600 mg tablets
Phenytoin Sodium (Dilantin, generic)	Daily	30, 100 mg capsules
Phenytoin Sodium (Phenytek, generic)	Daily	200, 300 mg capsules
Topiramate ER Capsule		
(Trokendi XR)	Daily	25, 50, 100, 200 mg capsules
(Qudexy XR)	Daily	25, 50, 100, 150, 200 mg sprinkle capsules
Valproic acid and derivatives		
Divalproex sodium (Depakote)	bid to qid	125 mg sprinkle capsule delayed release
Divalproex sodium (Depakote ER, generic)	Daily	250, 500 mg tablets
Divalproex sodium (generic)	Daily	125, 250, 500 mg capsules

Boldface indicates one of top 100 drugs for 2020 by prescription volume.
a. Available in the United States as of November 2016.

TABLE 28-3. Administration of Oral Antiepileptic Drugs

Anticonvulsant[a]	Effect of food	Administration
Brivaracetam	Take with or without food.	Solution: administer with an oral dosing syringe. Tablet: swallow whole with liquid, do not crush or chew.
Cannabidiol	Take consistently in fast or fed state.	Administer with an oral dosing syringe.
Carbamazepine	Suspension: Take with food. Extended-release capsule (Carbatrol, Equetro): Take with or without food. Extended-release tablet: Take with food.	Extended-release capsule (Carbatrol, Equetro): Capsule may be opened and contents sprinkled over food such as a teaspoon of applesauce. Extended-release tablet: Swallow whole; do not crush or chew.
Cenobamate	Take with or without food.	Swallow whole; do not crush or chew.
Clobazam	Take with or without food.	Suspension: Shake well, and administer with an oral dosing syringe. Tablet: Tablet may be crushed and mixed in applesauce.
Clonazepam	Tablet: Take with water. ODT: Take with or without water.	Tablet: Swallow whole. ODT: Open pouch, and peel back foil on the blister; do not push tablet through foil. Use dry hands to remove tablet and place in mouth.
Eslicarbazepine	Take with or without food.	Tablet: Swallow whole or crushed.
Ethosuximide	Take with or without food.	Solution: Administer with an oral dosing syringe.
Felbamate	Take with or without food.	Suspension: Shake well and administer with an oral dosing syringe.
Gabapentin	Capsule, tablet (excluding Gralise), solution: Take with or without food. Gralise: Take with evening meal.	Capsule: May be opened and sprinkled on food. Gralise: Swallow whole; do not break, split, crush, or chew. Solution: Administer with an oral dosing syringe.
Lacosamide	Take with or without food.	Solution: Administer with an oral dosing syringe. Tablet: Swallow whole; do not divide.
Lamotrigine	Take with or without food.	Chewable/dispersible tablets: Tablets may be chewed, dispersed in water or diluted fruit juice, or swallowed whole. Dispersible tablet: Add to enough liquid to cover tablet and let stand 1 minute until dispersed; swirl solution and consume immediately. ODT: Place on tongue and move around in the mouth. Tablets will dissolve rapidly and can be swallowed. Lamictal XR: Swallow whole; do not chew, crush, or cut.
Levetiracetam	Take with or without food.	Solution: Administer with an oral dosing syringe. Tablet (immediate and extended release): Swallow whole; do not chew or crush. Oral disintegrating tablet: Open pouch, and peel back foil on the blister; do not push tablet through foil. Use dry hands to remove tablet and place in mouth. Tablet disintegrates in <60 seconds; follow with sip of water. Do not swallow tablets intact. Add to enough liquid to cover tablet and let stand 1 minute until dispersed; swirl solution and consume immediately.

TABLE 28-3. Administration of Oral Antiepileptic Drugs *(Continued)*

Anticonvulsant[a]	Effect of food	Administration
Oxcarbazepine	Extended release: Administer on an empty stomach at least 1 hour before or 2 hours after food.	Extended release tablet: Swallow whole, do not cut, crush, or chew.
	Suspension and tablet: Take with or without food.	Suspension: Shake well and administer with an oral dosing syringe.
		Tablet: Swallow whole; do not cut, crush, or chew.
Perampanel	Take with or without food.	Suspension: Shake well and administer with an oral dosing syringe.
		Tablet: Swallow whole; do not cut, crush, or chew; take at bedtime.
Phenobarbital	Take with or without food.	Solution: Administer with an oral dosing syringe.
		Tablet: Swallow whole.
Phenytoin	Capsule: Take with or without food.	Chewable tablet: Chew thoroughly or swallow whole.
	Suspension: Absorption is impaired when given concurrently with continuous nasogastric feedings. Withhold nasogastric feedings for 1 to 2 hours before and after each dose.	Suspension: Shake well and administer with an oral dosing syringe.
		Extended release tablet: Swallow whole.
Pregabalin	Take with or without food.	Solution: Use an oral dosing syringe.
		Tablet: Swallow whole.
Primidone	Take with or without food.	Tablet: Swallow whole.
Rufinamide	Take with food.	Suspension: Shake well and administer with an oral dosing syringe.
		Tablet: Swallow whole or crushed.
Stiripentol	Take with food.	Capsule: swallow whole with water; do not crush, chew, or open capsule.
		Powder: Mix with water, consume immediately, and ensure entire contents taken.
Tiagabine	Take with food.	Tablet: Swallow whole or crushed.
Topiramate	Take with or without food.	Extended-release capsule: Swallow whole; do not break, crush, or chew.
		Sprinkle and Qudexy XR capsules: Swallow whole or open and sprinkle entire contents on a small amount of soft food; swallow immediately; and do not chew.
		Tablet: Do not crush, break, or chew because of bitter taste.
Valproic acid	Take with food.	Extended-release (Depakote), delayed release, or Depakene capsule: swallow whole; do not crush or chew.
		Solution: Administer with an oral dosing syringe.
		Sprinkle capsule: Swallow whole or open and sprinkle on small amount (1 teaspoonful) of soft food (e.g., pudding, applesauce); swallow immediately (do not store), and do not chew.
Vigabatrin	Take with or without food.	Solution: Administer with an oral dosing syringe; mix with water prior to administration.
Zonisamide	Take with or without food.	Capsule: Swallow whole.

Boldface indicates one of top 100 drugs for 2020 by prescription volume.
ODT, orally disintegrating tablet.
a. No medication names are in boldface in this table because the medication-prescribing patterns reflected in the prescription frequency of these medications address the medications' use in indications other than seizure disorders.

Extended-release products should be swallowed whole and should not be chewed, crushed, or cut. All suspensions should be shaken for at least 10 seconds before using and should only be administered using a dosing syringe. Likewise, solutions should be given with a dosing syringe. **Clonazepam, lamotrigine**, and levetiracetam are available as an orally disintegrating or dispersible tablet. The patient should be instructed to open the pouch and peel back the foil on the blister. The tablet should not be pushed through foil. Place the whole tablet on the tongue with a dry hand, follow with a sip of liquid, and swallow only after tablet disintegrates. Alternatively, the whole tablet can also be dispersed in enough liquid to cover the tablet and the entire contents consumed immediately. Any residue should be suspended by adding an additional small volume of liquid, and the full amount should be swallowed. Vigabatrin is available as a 500-mg powder packet, which should be dissolved in 10 mL of cold or room temperature water, fruit juice, milk, or infant formula to make a 50 mg/mL solution. When converting a patient from carbamazepine to oxcarbazepine, the dose of oxcarbazepine is 1.5 times the dose of carbamazepine in most patients and 1.2 times the dose of carbamazepine in patients receiving a slow-release formulation. Rectal administration is important for emergency situations when drugs cannot be administered either intravenously or orally (see Table 28-2). It is generally an at-home medication therapy for patients 2 years of age and older who are stable on AEDs but who require occasional use to control bouts of increased seizure activity or breakthrough seizures. Many AEDs have been given by this route, but rectal diazepam has an extensive history of successfully interrupting serial seizures and terminating status epilepticus. Diastat AcuDial is a commercially available gel of diazepam for rectal administration. The pharmacist should remove the 2 syringes from the case and confirm that the prescribed dose is visible in the display window. Both syringes should be locked (indicated by a green band) and returned to the case.

Midazolam can be given via intranasal and buccal routes and has been used successfully to control acute seizures in the home, in urgent situations by paramedics, and in hospital settings. This AED should be drawn up at the time it is needed and not stored in a plastic syringe because the plastic may leach into the drug. Effective intranasal delivery is best achieved by briskly compressing the syringe plunger to deliver a dose via a mucosal atomization device. This device enables the drug to be distributed as a mist rather than as larger droplets that may aggregate and run out of the nose or down the back of the throat, rendering it ineffective. In order to increase the surface area for absorption, half of the dose should be delivered into each nostril. I.M. delivery is often required when I.V. access is not available. Absorption is influenced by characteristics of the patient (e.g., blood flow to the site, muscle mass and activity, and quantity of adipose tissue) and the drug (e.g., pH). Among AEDs, phenobarbital, fosphenytoin, and midazolam are rapidly and reliably absorbed after I.M. administration. Hydrophobic medications such as diazepam and phenytoin have minimal systemic absorption when given by I.M. route. Phenytoin also may form insoluble crystals at the injection site that may be associated with local hemorrhage, tissue destruction, and muscle necrosis. Fosphenytoin should be used if I.M. administration of a hydantoin is needed.

I.V. administration is critical for the acute management of seizures or as replacement therapy in those temporarily unable to take oral medications. Unfortunately, not all AEDs have a parenteral dosage formulation (Table 28-4), and those that do may have limitations imposed by solubility, rate of administration, and adverse effects that may or may not be related to the AED. For example, phenytoin and fosphenytoin both carry a U.S. Food and Drug Administration (FDA) boxed warning for severe hypotension and cardiac arrhythmias that are related to the rate of administration. These adverse effects are most likely attributed to the propylene glycol solvent used to formulate parenteral phenytoin as well as diazepam, **lorazepam**, and phenobarbital. Large doses of propylene glycol have been associated with acute kidney injury, hyperosmolarity, and lactic acidosis. Although most patients respond to discontinuation of agents containing propylene glycol, those with multiorgan failure may require fomepizole or hemodialysis.

Other limitations of I.V. phenytoin include its lack of compatibility with I.V. solutions other than normal saline and its caustic pH (12). Fosphenytoin, a water-soluble phosphate ester, is a unique prodrug that is compatible with a variety of solutions and has a much lower pH (8.6 to 9). It has no known pharmacologic activity but is converted completely within minutes by blood and tissue phosphatases to phenytoin, the active metabolite. Fosphenytoin should be dosed using PE, thereby obviating the need for interconversion

TABLE 28-4. Adverse Drug Reactions and Monitoring of Patients Receiving Commonly Used Intravenous AEDs

Anticonvulsant	Adverse drug reaction	Monitoring parameter	Comments
Diazepam	Hypotension and cardiac arrhythmias	Vital signs and ECG during administration	Diazepam contains propylene glycol.ᵃ Administer at a rate not to exceed 5 mg/min.
Fosphenytoin	Hypotension and cardiac arrhythmias; paresthesia; pruritus; nystagmus	Vital signs and ECG during administration	Administer at a rate not to exceed 150 mg PE/min in adults and 2 mg PE/kg/min in pediatric patients. Doses should be given more slowly in elderly patients or in those with preexisting cardiac disease. Hypotension occurs less than that noted with phenytoin because this product does not contain propylene glycol; pruritus generally involves the groin, is dose- and rate-related, and subsides 10 minutes after infusion. Horizontal nystagmus suggests serum concentration above the reference range and toxicity; if a serum phenytoin concentration validates this, the dose should be decreased.
Lorazepam	Apnea, hypotension, bradycardia, cardiac arrest, respiratory depression, metabolic acidosis, renal toxicity	Vital signs and ECG during administration; HCO_3 and serum creatinine; cumulative dose of propylene glycol	**Lorazepam** contains propylene glycol.ᵃ Administer at a rate not to exceed 2 mg/min in adult and pediatric patients.
Midazolam	Apnea, hypotension, bradycardia, cardiac arrest, respiratory depression	Vital signs and ECG during administration	Tolerance may develop.
Pentobarbital	Hypotension, metabolic acidosis, respiratory depression, CNS depression, renal toxicity	Vital signs and ECG during administration; HCO_3 and serum creatinine; cumulative dose of propylene glycolᵃ, EEG if used in anesthesia doses	Rate of infusion should be decreased or vasopressors may be added if hypotension occurs.
Phenytoin	Hypotension and cardiac arrhythmias; paresthesia; nystagmus	Vital signs and ECG during administration	Phenytoin contains propylene glycol.ᵃ Administer at a rate not to exceed 50 mg/min in adults and 3 mg/kg/min (maximum 50 mg/min) in pediatric patients. Doses should be given more slowly in elderly patients or in those with preexisting cardiac disease. Horizontal nystagmus suggests serum concentration above the reference range and toxicity; if a serum phenytoin concentration validates this, the dose should be decreased.
Phenobarbital	Hypotension; respiratory and CNS depression	Vital signs and mental status; EEG if used in anesthesia doses	Phenobarbital contains propylene glycol.ᵃ Administer at a rate not to exceed 60 mg/min in adults and 30 mg/min in pediatric patients. Apnea and hypoventilation may occur.
Propofol	Progressive metabolic acidosis, hemodynamic instability, rhabdomyolysis, bradyarrhythmias	Vital signs, ECG, osmolar gap; triglycerides; EEG if used in anesthesia doses	Propofol infusion–related syndrome may occur with large doses or prolonged therapy and may prove fatal. Change I.V. tubing every 12 hours.

Boldface indicates one of top 100 drugs for 2020 by prescription volume.

CNS, central nervous system; ECG, electrocardiogram; EEG, electroencephalography; FDA, U.S. Food and Drug Administration; PE, phenytoin equivalent.

a. Propylene glycol causes hypotension and cardiac arrhythmias when administered too rapidly or when used in large doses. Accumulation may occur during prolonged continuous infusions and may cause acidosis.

between phenytoin and fosphenytoin. Accordingly, 1.5 mg of fosphenytoin sodium is equivalent to 1 mg phenytoin sodium and is referred to as 1 mg PE. The amount and concentration of fosphenytoin is always expressed in terms of mg PE. Serum phenytoin concentrations are used for therapeutic drug monitoring.

Pharmacokinetics

Absorption

When administered orally, most AEDs have good bioavailability. Exceptions are **gabapentin**, and vigabatrin whose bioavailabilities are <60% (Table 28-5). Gabapentin's absorption is regulated by the L-amino acid transporter system located in the proximal small bowel. Because absorption from the gastrointestinal system exhibits saturable capacity, gabapentin's absorption is dose dependent. As the dose of **gabapentin** is increased, the bioavailability disproportionately decreases. As noted above, following I.M. administration, the bioavailability of diazepam and phenytoin are erratic.

The majority of AEDs can be taken without regard to food (see Table 28-3). Carbamazepine, **gabapentin** (Gralise product), rufinamide, tiagabine, and valproic acid should be taken with food. Extended release oxcarbazepine tablets should be administered on an empty stomach at least 1 hour before or 2 hours after food. Phenytoin absorption is impaired when the suspension is given concurrently to patients who are receiving continuous nasogastric feedings; hence, nutritional supplements should be held for 1 to 2 hours before and after each phenytoin dose. Gabapentin's bioavailability is decreased 20% by concurrent administration of antacids; hence, the drug should be given 2 hours before or after antacids.

Protein binding

Various AEDs differ in the extent to which they are bound to serum proteins. The binding of ethosuximide, phenobarbital, and primidone is so low as to be clinically irrelevant. Those AEDs with significant binding are noted in Table 28-5. Carbamazepine (alpha-1-acid glycoprotein), phenytoin (albumin), and valproate (albumin) exhibit saturable protein binding at serum concentrations within their therapeutic serum concentration ranges. As the total serum concentration increases, the percentage of unbound drug disproportionately increases. Conditions that cause hypoalbuminemia, such as renal disease and hepatic disease, and certain drug interactions with acidic compounds such as fatty acids, **aspirin**, and valproate increase the unbound drug concentrations of phenytoin and carbamazepine. Phenytoin follows Michaelis–Menten pharmacokinetics.

TABLE 28-5. Pharmacokinetic Parameters That Are Clinically Significant

Poor or incomplete bioavailability	High protein binding	Predominant renal elimination unchanged
Gabapentin (<60%)	Cannabidiol (>94%)	Eslicarbazepine (>90%)
Vigabatrin (60 to 80%)	Carbamazepine (75%)	**Gabapentin** (100%)
	Clobazam (80 to 90%)	Oxcarbazepine (95%)
	Clonazepam (85%)	**Pregabalin** (90%)
	Lorazepam (91%)	Rufinamide (85%)
	Perampanel (95%)	**Topiramate** (70%)
	Phenytoin (95%)	Vigabatrin (80%)
	Stiripentol (99%)	
	Tiagabine (98%)	
	Valproate (80 to 90%)	

Boldface indicates one of top 100 drugs for 2020 by prescription volume.

Hepatic and renal elimination

AEDs are eliminated through either renal excretion of the unchanged parent drug, hepatic transformation to active or inactive metabolites, or a combination of both. The majority of AEDs undergo some degree of metabolism before renal elimination. Several AEDs are not significantly metabolized but are eliminated unchanged renally (see Table 28-5). Similarly, levetiracetam has minimal nonhepatic metabolism.

Drugs that are eliminated mainly by hepatic metabolism include carbamazepine, ethosuximide, phenytoin, **lamotrigine**, tiagabine, zonisamide, and various benzodiazepines. Several AEDs are eliminated both by hepatic biotransformation and by renal excretion of unmetabolized drug (i.e., phenobarbital, felbamate, oxcarbazepine, **topiramate**, and valproate). All of these are subject to considerable hepatic metabolism, which may alter hepatic processing and thereby substantially affect serum concentrations. Carbamazepine (10,11-epoxide), eslicarbazepine acetate (eslicarbazepine and oxcarbazepine), fosphenytoin (phenytoin), oxcarbazepine (licarbazepine), and primidone (phenylethylmalonamide [PEMA] and phenobarbital) have active metabolites.

Carbamazepine also induces its own metabolism (i.e., autoinduction or time-dependent metabolism) in a concentration- and time-dependent manner, which affects concentrations of both carbamazepine and the carbamazepine-10,11-epoxide. Autoinduction occurs during the first month of therapy, often at the point of dose titration. Because dosage increases may not result in linear increases in carbamazepine serum concentrations, low concentrations may be misconstrued as medication nonadherence. For phenytoin, the elimination mechanisms have a low capacity relative to the phenytoin serum concentrations that are usually present, so these mechanisms are partially saturated. This nonlinear elimination causes the relationship between the phenytoin dose and serum concentration to be extremely unpredictable. As the dose is increased, clearance decreases, resulting in a disproportionate increase in serum concentration.

There is a formula for correction of phenytoin that can approximate total serum phenytoin concentrations in patients with low albumin. In patients with normal renal function, phenytoin is corrected as follows:

$$\text{adjusted total concentration} = \text{measured concentration}/[(0.2 \times \text{albumin}) + 0.1]$$

In patients with renal dysfunction, the formula changes:

$$\text{adjusted total concentration} = \text{measured concentration}/[(0.1 \times \text{albumin}) + 0.1]$$

These formulas only approximate phenytoin total serum concentrations and may not be accurate in patients in intensive care units or in pediatric patients, for whom free serum phenytoin concentrations may be used.

Serum concentration monitoring

Following administration of an I.V. loading dose, assessment is generally indicated to confirm that a therapeutic concentration has been achieved or to calculate apparent volume of distribution. A serum concentration may also be obtained to establish the therapeutic concentration (effective dose) for an individual patient. Should a patient have a seizure, a concentration may be useful in assessing medication adherence or in determining the need for a loading dose. A concentration is also useful in the case of suspected AED toxicity. Finally, a serum concentration might prove beneficial in cases where a clinically significant change in physiologic function results in a change in the absorption, binding, metabolism, or elimination of an AED. The reference range for various AEDs is noted in Table 28-6. Because phenytoin is highly bound to albumin, both total and free serum concentrations can be measured. Although a free serum concentration provides a more accurate assessment, it may not be readily available in some clinical laboratories.

TABLE 28-6. Reference Range and Serum Concentration Monitoring

Anticonvulsant	Reference range (mg/L)	Time to steady state (days)
Brivaracetam	0.2 to 2	2
Cannabidiol	Not established	10
Carbamazepine	4 to 12	2 to 5 (may be longer with autoinduction)
Clobazam	0.03 to 0.3 (NDM: 0.3 to 3)	5 to 9
Eslicarbazepine acetate	3 to 35	4 to 5
Ethosuximide	50 to 100	7 to 10
Felbamate	30 to 60	3 to 4
Gabapentin	2 to 20	1 to 2
Lacosamide	10 to 20	3
Lamotrigine	3 to 15	Monotherapy: 3 to 6; VPA: 5 to 15
Levetiracetam	12 to 46[a]	1 to 2
Oxcarbazepine (MHD)	(MHD) 3 to 35[a]	2 to 3
Perampanel	0.1 to 1.2	14 to 21
Phenobarbital	10 to 40	11 to 30
Phenytoin, fosphenytoin	10 to 20 (free level: 1 to 2)	5 to 17
Pregabalin	2 to 8	2
Primidone	PRM: 5 to 12 (phenobarbital: 15 to 40)	2 to 4
Rufinamide	5 to 40	3
Stiripentol	4 to 22	1 to 3
Tiagabine	Not established	1 to 2
Topiramate	5 to 20	4 to 5
Valproate	50 to 100	2 to 4
Vigabatrin	0.8 to 36	1 to 2
Zonisamide	10 to 40	12 to 17

Boldface indicates one of top 100 drugs for 2020 by prescription volume.
MHD, monohydroxy derivative (active metabolite also known as licarbazepine); NDM, N-desmethylclobazam; PRM, primidone; VPA, valproic acid.
a. No clear correlation between efficacy and therapeutic levels.

Adverse Effects

Many of the AEDs are associated with adverse effects that occur during the initiation or dose-escalating phase of therapy. Some of the most frequently observed adverse reactions include dizziness, drowsiness, unsteadiness, headache, fatigue, insomnia, nausea, and vomiting. To minimize the possibility of such reactions, therapy should be initiated at the smallest recommended dosage and slowly titrated as appropriate. Many AEDs are associated with unique adverse effects (Table 28-7), and several carry similar warnings in their labeling and are noted below.

Suicidal ideation

All AEDs carry a warning for increased risk of suicidal behavior or ideation. The FDA has analyzed suicidality reports from placebo-controlled studies involving AEDs and found that patients receiving anticonvulsants had approximately twice the risk of suicidal behavior or ideation as did patients receiving a placebo.

TABLE 28-7. Common Adverse Effects

Adverse effect	Agent
Aplastic anemia	Carbamazepine[a], felbamate[a]
Behavioral changes	Clobazam, **clonazepam**, ethosuximide, **gabapentin**, levetiracetam, perampanel[a], phenobarbital (paradoxical hyperactivity)
Bone disorders (osteopenia, osteoporosis)	Oxcarbazepine, phenytoin
Cardiac changes	Barbiturates (hypotension), carbamazepine (conduction abnormalities), cenobamate (shortened QT interval), fosphenytoin (hypotension and arrhythmias)[a], lacosamide, phenytoin (hypotension and arrhythmias)[a], rufinamide (shortened QT interval)
Dermatologic reactions (SJS and TEN)	Carbamazepine[a], eslicarbazepine, ethosuximide, fosphenytoin, **lamotrigine**[a], oxcarbazepine, phenobarbital, phenytoin, rufinamide, tiagabine, zonisamide
Gingival hyperplasia	Phenytoin
Hair changes	Ethosuximide (hirsutism), phenytoin (hypertrichosis), **topiramate**, and valproic acid (alopecia)
Hepatotoxicity	Carbamazepine, cannabidiol, felbamate [a], fosphenytoin, phenobarbital, phenytoin, valproic acid[a]
Hyponatremia (SIADH)	Carbamazepine, eslicarbazepine, oxcarbazepine
Multiorgan hypersensitivity reaction or DRESS	Carbamazepine, cenobamate, eslicarbazepine, ethosuximide, **gabapentin**, lacosamide, **lamotrigine**, oxcarbazepine, phenobarbital, phenytoin, rufinamide, **topiramate**, valproic acid, zonisamide
Nephrolithiasis, oligohydrosis	**Topiramate**, zonisamide
Neuropsychiatric changes	Brivaracetam, **gabapentin**, **lamotrigine**, levetiracetam, perampanel[a], zonisamide
Ophthalmic changes	**topiramate** (glaucoma, visual field), vigabatrin[a]
Paresthesias	**Topiramate**, vigabatrin, zonisamide
Pancreatitis	Valproic acid[a]
Suicidal ideation	All AEDs
Teratogenicity	Benzodiazepines, carbamazepine, fosphenytoin, phenobarbital, phenytoin, **topiramate**, valproic acid[a]
Thrombocytopenia	Valproic acid, stiripentol
Weight change	Ethosuximide, felbamate, fosphenytoin, **topiramate**, and zonisamide (loss); **gabapentin**, perampanel, **pregabalin**, **topiramate**, valproic acid, vigabatrin (gain)

Boldface indicates one of top 100 drugs for 2020 by prescription volume.
DRESS, drug reaction with eosinophilia and systemic symptoms; SIADH, syndrome of inappropriate antidiuretic hormone; SJS, Stevens–Johnson syndrome; TEN, toxic epidermal necrolysis.
a. This drug has an FDA boxed warning for specific adverse effect.

Severe dermatologic reactions

Several AEDs (i.e., carbamazepine, eslicarbazepine, oxcarbazepine, fosphenytoin, phenytoin, phenobarbital, valproic acid, and **lamotrigine**) carry some form of labeling for Stevens–Johnson syndrome or toxic epidermal necrolysis (TEN). The labeling for both carbamazepine and **lamotrigine** carries an FDA boxed warning for this adverse effect. Recently, a relationship between the human leukocyte antigen (HLA) and these reactions has been identified in patients from Asia and of Asian descent. Specifically, in patients of Chinese descent, the HLA-B*1502 allele has been associated with a significantly higher risk of Stevens–Johnson syndrome. In fact, carbamazepine labeling includes the requirement to screen patients with Chinese ancestry for the presence of HLA-B*1502 before starting therapy and to avoid the use of carbamazepine in those who test positive for the allele. A cytochrome P450 (CYP) 2C variant that included CYP2C9*3, which is known to reduce drug clearance, was identified as an important genetic factor associated with phenytoin-related severe dermatologic reactions.

Most severe dermatologic reactions are associated with aromatic amine anticonvulsants (i.e., phenobarbital, phenytoin, **lamotrigine**, carbamazepine, oxcarbazepine). Because zonisamide contains a sulfonamide structure, it is contraindicated in patients with a prior allergy to sulfonamide antibiotics. When a reaction is severe (i.e., Stevens–Johnson syndrome or TEN) and the patient needs to continue on an AED, a nonaromatic amine (i.e., valproate, **gabapentin**, **topiramate**, or levetiracetam) should be used in order to avoid clinical cross-reactivity.

Anticonvulsant hypersensitivity syndrome

Also referred to as drug reaction with eosinophilia and systemic symptoms (DRESS), this syndrome is characterized by fever (90% to 100%), rash (90%), hepatitis (50%), and other multiorgan abnormalities (50%). Patients may or may not progress to develop severe dermatologic reactions (i.e., Stevens–Johnson syndrome or TEN). When signs or symptoms are present, the AED should be discontinued, and the patient converted to an AED that has a nonaromatic structure. The risk of developing a hypersensitivity reaction may be increased in patients with the variant HLA-A*3101 allele.

Withdrawal or abrupt discontinuation

A little over half of patients who remain seizure-free for 2 years can have their anticonvulsant successfully withdrawn. Most (90%) who are seizure-free for 4 years can be successfully withdrawn from anticonvulsants. Unless the patient is experiencing a severe or life-threatening adverse effect, never abruptly discontinue an anticonvulsant; taper slowly over 2 to 6 months.

Rebound or withdrawal seizures or symptoms may occur following abrupt discontinuation or large decreases in doses of a benzodiazepine. Use caution when reducing dose or withdrawing therapy; decrease slowly (e.g., decrease weekly) and monitor for withdrawal symptoms. Flumazenil (Romazicon) may cause withdrawal in patients receiving long-term benzodiazepine therapy.

Teratogenicity

In 1979, the FDA established 5 lettered risk categories—A, B, C, D, and X—to indicate the potential of a drug to cause birth defects if used during pregnancy; however, the Pregnancy and Lactation Labeling (Drugs) Final Rule letter categories have been phased out and replaced with pregnancy and lactation considerations for health care providers to discuss with patients. In addition, there is a North American AED Pregnancy Registry available that is studying the effects of AED in pregnant women.

Valproic acid is the only AED that carries an FDA boxed warning for teratogenicity. Exposure to this AED during pregnancy is associated with about a threefold increase in the rate of major anomalies, mainly spina bifida. It is also associated with a possible set of dysmorphic features, the valproate syndrome. A daily dose of > 1000 mg, polytherapy, or both are associated with a higher risk of teratogenicity. Thus, when valproate cannot be avoided in pregnancy, the lowest possible effective dose should be prescribed in 2 to 3 divided doses, preferably as monotherapy.

Certain AEDs, but not all agents, can potentially decrease folate levels, by either hepatic enzyme induction or decreased absorption. Consensus statements recommend 0.4 mg of **folic acid** per day in all women planning a pregnancy. Enzyme-inducing anticonvulsants, such as phenytoin, carbamazepine, primidone, and phenobarbital, are known to decrease folate levels, and valproic acid may interfere with folate metabolism. For these reasons, women with epilepsy who are of childbearing years should receive 0.8 to 1 mg/d of **folic acid**.

Medications

Many AEDs are associated with unique or significant adverse effects that are important to consider in drug selection and monitoring, many of which are listed below.

Carbamazepine

In addition to severe dermatologic reactions, carbamazepine has been given an FDA boxed warning for aplastic anemia and agranulocytosis. Baseline hematological testing should be performed before carbamazepine is begun. If on follow-up a patient exhibits low or decreased white blood cell or platelet counts, the patient should be monitored closely. If evidence of bone marrow suppression develops (e.g., fever, sore throat, mouth ulcers, easy bruising, and petechial or purpuric hemorrhage), the drug should be discontinued. Carbamazepine has a tricyclic structure that may cause cardiac conduction abnormalities; therefore, it should be used cautiously in patients with known electrocardiogram (ECG) abnormalities or preexisting cardiac damage.

Felbamate

This AED has an FDA boxed warning for both aplastic anemia and hepatotoxicity. Although the onset of aplastic anemia has ranged from 5 to 30 weeks, clinical manifestation may not be apparent for several months after discontinuation of the drug. Routine blood testing does not reduce the incidence of aplastic anemia but, in some cases, allows for early detection. Felbamate should be discontinued if any evidence of bone marrow suppression occurs.

Felbamate is also associated with hepatotoxicity that often occurs within 3 to 5 weeks of the onset of signs and symptoms of liver failure. Of the cases reported, approximately two-thirds resulted in death or required liver transplantation, usually within 5 weeks of the onset of liver failure. Although baseline and periodic monitoring of serum transaminase levels is recommended, there is no evidence that such testing will prevent serious injury. However, the general belief is that early detection of drug-induced hepatic injury along with immediate withdrawal of the suspect drug enhances the likelihood for recovery. Felbamate should be discontinued if liver enzymes increase to at least 2 times the upper limit of normal, or if clinical signs and symptoms are suggestive of liver failure. Felbamate is also associated with anorexia and may result in significant weight loss.

Gabapentin

Although not stated in an FDA boxed warning, **gabapentin** has been noted to cause neuropsychiatric symptoms including emotional lability, hostility (e.g., aggressive behaviors), changes in behavior and thinking (e.g., concentration problems and changes in school performance), and hyperkinesia (e.g., restlessness and hyperactivity). It may cause psychosis in patients with renal dysfunction who are given normal doses. The FDA has recently warned about the risk of breathing difficulties when **gabapentin** is used in patients with preexisting lung disease or concomitantly with opioids.

Lacosamide

Cardiovascular effects including prolonged PR interval and second-degree and complete atrioventricular (AV) block have been reported with lacosamide. Use cautiously in patients with preexisting cardiac conduction problems (e.g., first- or second-degree AV block and sick sinus syndrome without pacemaker), sodium channelopathies, myocardial ischemia, heart failure, or structural heart disease or those who are using another drug that prolongs the PR interval. An ECG is recommended before initiating therapy.

Levetiracetam

Although not stated in an FDA boxed warning, levetiracetam has been noted to cause neuropsychiatric symptoms including emotional lability, hostility, changes in behavior and thinking, and hyperkinesia.

Oxcarbazepine

Because Oxcarbazepine has a similar structure to carbamazepine, it may produce severe dermatologic reactions in those positive for the HLA-B*1502 allele. Although not specified by an FDA boxed warning, patients of Asian descent should be considered for screening for the HLA-B*1502 allele before initiation of therapy (see severe dermatological reactions earlier in this chapter). Oxcarbazepine also should be avoided in any patient who developed a dermatologic reaction to an AED with an aromatic amine structure.

Perampanel

Perampanel has been given an FDA boxed warning for dose-related, serious, or life-threatening neuropsychiatric events (e.g., aggression, anger, homicidal ideation and threats, hostility, and irritability). These often occur in the first 6 weeks of therapy even in patients without a psychiatric history, aggressive behavior, or use of concomitant medications associated with hostility and aggression. The patient should be monitored during dosage adjustments or when receiving large doses. The dose should be decreased or immediately discontinued if severe or worsening symptoms occur. It should be permanently discontinued if persistent severe or worsening psychiatric symptoms or behaviors are noted.

Phenobarbital

Phenobarbital may cause paradoxical responses, including agitation and hyperactivity, particularly in pediatric patients or those with acute or chronic pain.

Phenytoin

Chronic administration of oral phenytoin may cause significant gingival hyperplasia and hirsutism.

Pregabalin

The FDA has recently warned about the risk of breathing difficulties when **pregabalin** is used in patients with preexisting lung disease or concomitantly with opioids.

Topiramate

Although **topiramate** is not associated with any FDA boxed warnings, it is linked to numerous adverse effects that may affect therapy. It may cause cognitive dysfunction (e.g., confusion; psychomotor slowing; difficulty with concentration and attention; or difficulty with memory, speech, or language), psychiatric disturbances (e.g., depression or mood disorders), and sedation (e.g., somnolence or fatigue). Occurrence may be related to rapid titration and larger doses.

Because **topiramate** is a weak carbonic anhydrase inhibitor, it may cause paresthesias and kidney stones. The likelihood of kidney stones may be reduced by increasing fluid intake. **Topiramate** may also be associated with hyperchloremic nonanion gap metabolic acidosis as a result of inhibition of carbonic anhydrase and mild-to-moderate increased renal bicarbonate loss. The risk may be increased with a predisposing condition (e.g., renal, respiratory, or hepatic impairment), diarrhea, ketogenic diet, status epilepticus, or concurrent treatment with drugs known to cause acidosis. Serum bicarbonate and complications of chronic acidosis (e.g., nephrolithiasis, nephrocalcinosis, osteomalacia, or osteoporosis) should be monitored. Dose reduction or discontinuation (by tapering dose) should be considered in patients with persistent or severe metabolic acidosis.

Topiramate may also be associated with oligohydrosis and hyperthermia; hence, patients should be cautioned to monitor their ability to sweat during strenuous exercise, during exposure to high environmental temperature, or during administration of other carbonic anhydrase inhibitors and drugs with anticholinergic activity.

Valproic acid and derivatives

Valproic acid and derivatives contain FDA boxed warnings for hepatotoxicity, pancreatitis, and teratogenicity. Children <2 years of age, especially receiving multiple anticonvulsants, with congenital metabolic disorders, and with severe seizure disorders accompanied by mental retardation, have an increased risk of developing fatal hepatotoxicity. There is an increased risk of valproate-induced acute liver failure and resultant deaths in patients with hereditary neurometabolic mitochondrial disorders. Liver function tests should be performed before initiation of therapy and at frequent intervals thereafter, especially during the first 6 months. Valproic acid may also cause hyperammonemia. Pancreatitis, including hemorrhagic pancreatitis, has been reported and may prove fatal; thus, if diagnosed, valproate should be discontinued. Patients with abdominal pain, nausea, vomiting, or anorexia should seek medical attention. Valproic acid also is associated with weight gain and alopecia, as well as dose-related tremors and thrombocytopenia.

Vigabatrin

Vigabatrin may lead to permanent vision loss, including tunnel vision, and can result in disability. The risk of vision loss increases with increasing dose and cumulative exposure. Vision assessment is recommended at baseline, every 3 months during therapy, and about 3 to 6 months after discontinuation of therapy. Vigabatrin should be discontinued slowly in any patient who does not show clinical benefit within 3 months (refractory focal seizures) or 2 to 4 weeks (infantile spasms) of initiation, respectively. Because of the significance of this adverse effect, vigabatrin is available only through a special restricted program (i.e., specialty pharmacies) using a risk evaluation and mitigation strategy.

Zonisamide

Decreased sweating (oligohydrosis) and hyperthermia requiring hospitalization have been reported in children; hence, zonisamide should be used cautiously in those receiving other drugs that may predispose patients to heat-related disorders (e.g., anticholinergics). Severe metabolic acidosis may occur and is more likely in pediatric patients than in adults. Untreated metabolic acidosis may increase the risk of the development of nephrolithiasis or nephrocalcinosis, osteoporosis or osteomalacia (possibly resulting in rickets), and reduced growth rates.

Drug Interactions

A vast number of drug interactions among AEDs and between AEDs and other medications have been reported. An important difference between older and newer AEDs is the potential of older AEDs to cause clinically significant drug interactions. Many interactions involving older AEDs are reciprocal, meaning that each drug exerts an influence on the other. Conversely, newer AEDs have limited or no potential for drug interaction. The list of interactions is too numerous to note in this chapter; hence, the practitioner should rely on current medical information when combining medications with an AED.

The ability of an AED to cause a drug–drug interaction depends on a variety of factors that are related to the pharmacokinetic characteristics of the drug. Adopting a mechanistic approach in understanding how interactions occur may be helpful. The majority of clinically significant interactions can be attributed to effects on absorption, plasma protein binding, and elimination (see Table 28-5).

Absorption

Clinically significant interactions related to absorption are rare. Binding agents (e.g., cholestyramine and colestipol) can decrease bioavailability of a drug and thereby reduce its therapeutic effect. Some drugs are susceptible to chelation with cations such as aluminum, magnesium, and iron. The interaction between **gabapentin** and antacids is a perfect example of this because antacids decrease the bioavailability of **gabapentin** by 20%. Some drugs have pH-dependent absorption that is influenced by an increase or decrease in stomach pH. CYP3A4 is active in the stomach and may be responsible for metabolism of a drug before it can enter systemic circulation. Likewise, P-gp, located in intestinal mucosa, can actively pump drugs back into the intestinal lumen, which also results in metabolizing the drug before it reaches systemic circulation. An understanding of the activity of these gut enzymes has raised the possibility that some AED interactions attributed to enzyme induction may actually be due to reduced gastrointestinal absorption.

Protein binding

Drug interactions as a result of plasma protein binding generally involve either albumin or alpha-1-acid glycoprotein. These interactions occur when a drug with a greater affinity for binding displaces a drug with a lesser affinity for that protein. This leads to an increase in free concentration, which may cause toxicity. These types of interactions are clinically significant only when both drugs are highly bound (>90%) to the same protein. With the exception of carbamazepine, which is bound to alpha-1-acid glycoprotein, AEDs are bound to albumin (see Table 28-5). Most AEDs are monitored using total serum concentrations, which may not be as accurate in critically ill patients. In the face of a protein-binding interaction, this method of assessment may cause an unnecessary and incorrect dosage adjustment that could lead to toxicity.

Renal elimination

Although active secretion into the renal tubules is an important route of elimination for some drugs, this process does not affect AEDs.

Hepatic elimination

Newer AEDs are easier to use and perhaps safer, especially for patients taking multiple medications, than the first generation of AEDs. Important to hepatic clearance is the substrate responsible for an AED's individual elimination and the resultant capacity of that system given the relative amount of drug available (Table 28-8). Likewise, the ability of an AED to induce or inhibit an isoenzyme responsible for the elimination processes of another drug is critical (see Table 28-8). When depicting the potential for an interaction, one usually describes the likelihood as strong, moderate, or weak. Strongly and moderately inducing drugs decrease the area under the curve (AUC) of a sensitive substrate of a given metabolic pathway by ≥80% and between 50% to 80%, respectively. Strong, moderate, and weak inhibitors increase the AUC of sensitive substrates of a given metabolic pathway 5 times or more, 2 to 5 times more, and 1.25 to 2 times more, respectively.

Drugs that depend on hepatic biotransformation for elimination are most affected by pharmacokinetic interactions. Phenytoin is one of the most sensitive AEDs and is most likely to experience interactions, because its eliminating enzymes are partially saturated at usual doses and serum concentrations and because it is highly protein bound. Most older AEDs (e.g., phenytoin, carbamazepine, and phenobarbital) are inducers of various CYP450 isozymes. Carbamazepine is unique in that it induces its own metabolism, with peak effects generally noted by 21 days.

Major inducers of hepatic drug metabolism increase the activity of CYP2C9, CYP2C19, and CYP3A4 plus the activities of epoxide hydrolase and uridine diphosphate glucuronosyltransferase (UDPGT). UDPGT catalyzes the formation of glucuronide conjugates and plays a major role in the elimination of **lamotrigine**, oxcarbazepine, and valproate and a minor role for phenobarbital. Carbamazepine, felbamate, oxcarbazepine, phenobarbital, phenytoin, primidone, and **topiramate** induce the metabolism of the estrogen or progestogen components of oral contraceptives. Conversely, oral contraceptives may lower serum concentrations of **lamotrigine**.

Valproate and felbamate are inhibitors of hepatic drug metabolism. The addition of valproate substantially increases **lamotrigine** and phenobarbital concentrations because valproate inhibits and is a substrate of multiple CYP450 enzymes. Likewise, felbamate increases the concentrations of phenobarbital, phenytoin, and valproate. When valproate or felbamate is added to phenobarbital, phenytoin, or valproate, the doses of the preexistent drug should be reduced.

Several studies support the role of polymorphisms affecting the functioning of CYP2C9 and CYP2C19 in patients with epilepsy receiving phenytoin, phenobarbital, or diazepam. This is best exemplified in those with Asian ancestry who have adverse effects when given standard doses of diazepam. Additionally, the CYP2C variant CYP2C9*3 has recently been associated with delayed clearance of plasma phenytoin and severe cutaneous adverse reactions. Likewise, the HLA-B*1502 allele has been associated with a significantly higher risk of severe dermatologic reactions in those of Asian descent.

TABLE 28-8. Summary of AED Substrates and Isozymes Involved in Hepatic Elimination

AED	Substrate	Induces	Inhibits
Brivaracetam	CYP2C19	1	
Cannabidiol	CYP3A4, CYP2C19	CYP2C8, CYP2C9, CYP2C19, UGT1A9, UGT2B7	
Carbamazepine	CYP3A4ª, CYP2C8	CYP1A2, CYP3A4ª, P-gp, CYP2B6, CYP2C9, UGT1A1	
Cenobamate	CYP2E1, CYP2A6, CYP2B6, CYP2C19, CYP3A4, UGT2B7	CYP2B6, CYP3A4	CYP2C19
Clobazam	CYP2C19ª, CYP2B6, CYP3A4	CYP3A4	CYP2D6
Clonazepam	CYP3A4ª		
Eslicarbazepine	UGT2B4	CYP3A4	CYP2C19
Ethosuximide	CYP3A4ª		
Felbamate	CYP3A4,ª CYP2E1		CYP2C19
Lacosamide	CYP2C9, CYP2C19, CYP3A4		
Lamotrigine			OCT2
Oxcarbazepine		CYP3A4	
Perampanel	CYP3A4ª, CYP1A2, CYP2B6		
Phenobarbital	CYP2C19ª, CYP2C9, CYP2E1	CYP1A2, CYP2A6, CYP2C9, CYP3A4ª, CYP2B6, P-gp, UGT1A1	
Phenytoin	CYP2C9ª, CYP2C19ª, CYP3A4	CYP2C19, CYP2C8, CYP2C9, CYP3A4ª, CYP2B6, CYP1A2, P-gp, UGT1A1	
Primidone		CYP1A2, CYP2A6, CYP2C9, CYP3A4ª, CYP2B6, P-gp, UTG1A1	
Rufinamide		CYP3A4	CYP2E1
Stiripentol	CYP1A2, CYP2C19ª, CYP3A4ª		CYP1A2, CYP2C19
Tiagabine	CYP3A4ª		
Topiramate		CYP3A4	CYP2C19
Valproic acid	CYP2A6, CYP2B6, CYP2C9, CYP2C19, CPY2E1		CYP2C9
Vigabatrin		CYP2C9	
Zonisamide	CYP3A4,ª CYP2C19		

Boldface indicates one of top 100 drugs for 2020 by prescription volume.
OCT, organic cation transporter; UGT, UDP-glucuronosyltransferase.
a. Strong or major activity occurs.

Although most interactions are based on a drug's pharmacokinetic characteristics, some interactions are of a pharmacodynamic nature. An example of this is the FDA boxed warning for benzodiazepines. Concomitant use of benzodiazepines and opioids may result in profound sedation, respiratory depression, coma, and death. The combination of carbamazepine and **lamotrigine** may produce enhanced dizziness. Levetiracetam and **gabapentin** are minimally associated with drug interactions.

Patient Counseling Applicable to All AEDs

- The patient should keep a seizure diary and attend regular appointments with the health care provider to determine whether the medication is working properly and whether unwanted side effects occur.
- The full effects of this medication may not be seen for several weeks.

- Take with food or milk if upset stomach occurs.
- Do not drink alcohol or take CNS depressants or illegal drugs with this medication.
- If this medication causes blurred vision or drowsiness, the patient should not drive or operate heavy machinery while taking this medication until accustomed to its effects.
- Consult with a health care provider if anticipating pregnancy, becoming pregnant, or planning to breastfeed while taking this medication.
- Some medications decrease the effectiveness of birth control pills. The patient should discuss this with a health care provider or pharmacist, who may recommend a backup birth control method to prevent pregnancy.
- A woman capable of having children should take at least 1 mg of **folic acid** a day.
- Medication should not be stopped unless directed to do so by a health care provider; some medicines must be discontinued slowly. The patient should tell the health care provider or pharmacist if he or she plans to stop taking this medication.
- Check with a pharmacist or health care provider before taking or starting any new medication (prescription, over-the-counter, or herbal product).
- If a dose is missed, it should be taken as soon as it's remembered. If the time for the next dose is soon, skip the missed dose and resume the regular schedule. Do not take extra or double doses. If 2 or more doses are missed, contact the health care provider for further instructions.
- Contact a health care provider immediately if skin rash occurs.

28-6 Pharmacist's Role

Pharmacists can have an impact on the treatment of seizures in all patient care settings. Within the acute care setting, pharmacists can manage drug interactions with AEDs and other medications and monitor levels of these agents. In addition, pharmacists can assistant with the management of status epilepticus in the acute care setting. Pharmacists that practice in the community pharmacy setting can manage drug interactions with AEDs and other concomitant medications and counsel patients on compliance. Lastly, those pharmacists working in ambulatory care settings may work with providers and patients in the long-term monitoring of AEDs.

NAPLEX Competency Statements

The questions in this chapter cover the following 2021 NAPLEX Competency Statements: **AREA 1:** 1.1; 1.2; 1.3; 1.4; 1.5; 1.6 **AREA 2:** 2.1; 2.2; 2.3; 2.4 **AREA 3:** 3.1; 3.2; 3.3; 3.4; 3.5; 3.6; 3.7; 3.8; 3.9; 3.10; 3.11; 3.12 **AREA 4:** 4.3 **AREA 5:** 5.1.

28-7  Questions

1. Which of the following is true regarding phenytoin?

    A. The maximum rate of I.V. administration is 50 mg/min.
    B. If I.V. access cannot be established, phenytoin can be given I.M.
    C. Because phenytoin contains propylene glycol, it is soluble in any I.V. fluid.
    D. It is an inhibitor of the cytochrome P450 system.
    E. A major limitation to the use of the product in pediatric patients is the lack of a commercially available liquid formulation.

2. Which of the following is true regarding a patient with refractory status epilepticus who is placed in a medically induced coma with a barbiturate?

    A. If the patient is mechanically ventilated, the barbiturates will induce respiratory arrest.
    B. The goal of a coma that is medically induced with a barbiturate is to induce burst suppression (isoelectric) on electroencephalography.
    C. If hypotension develops, the patient should be given nitroprusside.
    D. The barbiturates are not associated with drug interactions.
    E. A major problem with this type of therapy is kidney failure.

3. Which of the following is associated with autoinduction?

   A. Phenobarbital
   B. Phenytoin
   C. Carbamazepine
   D. Gabapentin
   E. Levetiracetam

4. Which of the following agents reduces the likelihood of congenital malformations in epileptic women receiving valproate?

   A. Folic acid
   B. Vitamin B_{12}
   C. Ginkgo biloba
   D. Iron
   E. Selenium

5. Which of the following is true regarding anticonvulsants and their effect on weight?

   A. Valproic acid and phenytoin both decrease weight.
   B. Valproic acid increases weight, and topiramate decreases weight.
   C. Topiramate and phenytoin both increase weight.
   D. Topiramate, valproic acid, and phenytoin cause no change in weight.
   E. Phenytoin is the only anticonvulsant known to increase weight.

6. A 24-year-old woman has focal seizures that are currently controlled with valproic acid, gabapentin, and topiramate. She calls your pharmacy to ask if any of her medications can cause nosebleeds because she has had 1 or 2 in the past week. You refer her to her local health care provider, where her platelet count is reported to be $95,132/mm^3$. Which of the following is true?

   A. None of her anticonvulsants causes thrombocytopenia.
   B. Valproate can cause a dose-related thrombocytopenia.
   C. Gabapentin has inhibited the metabolism of topiramate, and the elevated concentration of topiramate is responsible for the thrombocytopenia.
   D. Gabapentin can cause idiosyncratic thrombocytopenia.
   E. Topiramate can cause thrombocytopenia.

7. A patient has hypertension, diabetes mellitus, and end-stage kidney disease (SCr = 6.8 mg/dL) and has developed seizures. Which of the following anticonvulsants would require dosage adjustment in this patient?

   A. Gabapentin and topiramate
   B. Lamotrigine and felbamate
   C. Phenobarbital and gabapentin
   D. Phenytoin and valproic acid
   E. Phenobarbital and levetiracetam

8. Which of the following anticonvulsants is metabolized to phenobarbital?

   A. Ethosuximide
   B. Primidone
   C. Zonisamide
   D. Levetiracetam
   E. Carbamazepine

9. A 7-year-old boy is receiving valproic acid for focal to bilateral tonic-clonic seizures that are refractory to phenobarbital, phenytoin, carbamazepine, and gabapentin. He has continued to have seizures and was started on lamotrigine 2 weeks ago. Today he presents with a diffuse maculopapular erythematous rash with lesions on his lips. Which of the following is correct?

   A. A rash associated with lamotrigine generally occurs within the first few days; hence, the rash is not associated with an anticonvulsant.
   B. The patient should be given diphenhydramine, and lamotrigine should be continued.
   C. Lamotrigine should be discontinued.
   D. The rash is secondary to a drug interaction between gabapentin and carbamazepine.
   E. All of the anticonvulsants are associated with a life-threatening rash. To prevent status epilepticus associated with abrupt discontinuation of the anticonvulsants, the medications should be slowly discontinued.

10. A new anticonvulsant has just been approved by the FDA. Its bioavailability is >95%, and it is highly protein bound to alpha-1-acid glycoprotein. It undergoes extensive hepatic metabolism by CYP2C9. Less than 5% is excreted unchanged in the urine. It is known to inhibit CYP3A4. A patient on this anticonvulsant has developed significant depression and is being started on an antidepressant that is 93% bound to albumin and is a potent inhibitor of CYP2C19. The antidepressant is a prodrug that is metabolized by CYP3A4 to an active metabolite that is hepatically cleared by CYP2C9. The neurologist wants to know if any drug interactions may occur that would necessitate a change in drug dosage. Which of the following is the appropriate response?

   A. No drug interactions should occur in this patient.
   B. The dose of the anticonvulsant should be reduced because of a potential protein-binding interaction that would increase the serum concentration of the anticonvulsant.
   C. The dose of the anticonvulsant should be increased.
   D. The patient may not benefit from the antidepressant, and another antidepressant that is not metabolized by CYP3A4 should be used.
   E. Because of an interaction in the gut that decreases bioavailability, the dose should be increased.

11. Which of the following AEDs is (are) not associated with any drug–drug interactions?

   A. Carbamazepine and gabapentin
   B. Carbamazepine and levetiracetam
   C. Gabapentin and levetiracetam
   D. Carbamazepine only
   E. Phenytoin and carbamazepine

12. A 42-year-old woman has been successfully treated with valproic acid for years, but she has experienced some undesirable side effects. She is slowly titrated onto a new anticonvulsant, and the valproic acid is gradually discontinued. She presents to the emergency department with severe flank pain and is diagnosed with a kidney stone. Which of the following may have precipitated her current situation?

   A. Gabapentin
   B. Lamotrigine
   C. Levetiracetam
   D. Topiramate
   E. Phenytoin

13. Which of the following drugs carry an FDA boxed warning?

   A. Carbamazepine and levetiracetam
   B. Felbamate and levetiracetam
   C. Lamotrigine and phenobarbital
   D. Carbamazepine and felbamate
   E. Phenobarbital and carbamazepine

14. Which of the following carries an FDA boxed warning for pancreatitis?

   A. Carbamazepine
   B. Felbamate
   C. Zonisamide
   D. Valproic acid
   E. Phenytoin

15. What is the drug of choice for generalized nonmotor (absence) seizures in a child <2 years of age?

   A. Phenytoin
   B. Phenobarbital
   C. Ethosuximide
   D. Valproic acid
   E. Primidone

16. Diastat is given by which of the following routes?

   A. Rectally
   B. Intramuscularly
   C. Intravenously
   D. Intranasally
   E. Subcutaneously

17. Which of the following is true?

   A. Febrile seizures must be accompanied by a CNS infection.
   B. Complex febrile seizures last >15 minutes.
   C. Most children who have a febrile seizure go on to develop epilepsy.
   D. The drug of choice for a simple febrile seizure is carbamazepine.
   E. Simple febrile seizures should never be treated.

18. Which of the following anticonvulsants is (are) available in a liquid, chewable tablet, and intravenous formulation?

   A. Phenytoin only
   B. Valproic acid and carbamazepine
   C. Oxcarbazepine and primidone
   D. Valproic acid only
   E. Primidone and valproic acid

19. Patients should be told to drink plenty of fluid when taking which of the following?

A. Carbamazepine
B. Topiramate
C. Levetiracetam
D. Gabapentin
E. Phenytoin

20. Which of the following medications may cause seizures in an adult patient with renal failure?

A. Meperidine
B. Phenobarbital
C. Carbamazepine
D. Lamotrigine
E. Theophylline

21. Which of the following is associated with Michaelis–Menten pharmacokinetics?

A. Carbamazepine
B. Valproic acid
C. Topiramate
D. Phenytoin
E. Phenobarbital

22. A patient on which of the following medications should be made aware of the importance of good oral hygiene?

A. Felbamate
B. Phenytoin
C. Zonisamide
D. Phenobarbital
E. Levetiracetam

 **28-8   Answers**

1. A. Because phenytoin contains propylene glycol and is itself cardiotoxic, the I.V. formulation should not be infused faster than 50 mg/min. Phenytoin is extremely alkaline (pH ~12). I.M. administration is not only associated with tissue damage but also erratically absorbed. Phenytoin can be admixed only with normal saline, is an inducer, and is also available as a suspension and a chewable tablet.

2. B. The goal is to produce a "flat" EEG, or burst suppression. If the patient is mechanically ventilated, the effect of a medication on respiration is not a factor in its administration. Although pentobarbital may cause hypotension if given too rapidly, nitroprusside is a vasodilator used to treat hypertension. The barbiturates are known inducers. A coma that is medically induced with a barbiturate does not cause kidney failure.

3. C. Carbamazepine induces its own metabolism, with peak effects seen about 21 days after beginning the medication or following an increase in dosage. Phenobarbital and phenytoin are inducers. Gabapentin and levetiracetam are not cleared hepatically.

4. A. Many of the anticonvulsants can cause folic acid deficiency. An association exists between folic acid deficiency and spina bifida; hence, all women with epilepsy who are of childbearing age should receive supplemental folic acid every day (1 mg).

5. B. Topiramate can cause significant weight loss, and valproate can cause significant weight gain. Phenytoin does not significantly affect weight.

6. B. Valproic acid can cause clinically significant thrombocytopenia. Gabapentin is not associated with any drug interaction that affects metabolism, and it does not cause a decrease in platelets. Topiramate does not cause thrombocytopenia.

7. A. Gabapentin and topiramate would require dosage adjustment because they are renally eliminated.

8. B. Primidone (Mysoline) is an active anticonvulsant, but it is also metabolized to phenobarbital.

9. C. Lamotrigine has an FDA boxed warning for severe rash. Because this patient has a diffuse rash and lesions on his lips, lamotrigine should be discontinued. Because the incidence of severe rash may be higher in children than in adults, current practice would be to discontinue lamotrigine and not "treat through" the rash with diphenhydramine. Gabapentin does not interact with lamotrigine. However, the combination of valproic acid and lamotrigine is associated with a higher incidence of rash. Although abrupt discontinuation of an anticonvulsant may induce status epilepticus, an anticonvulsant may be abruptly discontinued in the face of a life-threatening event.

10. D. Because the new anticonvulsant inhibits CYP3A4, D is the correct answer. Because the antidepressant is a prodrug, which must be metabolized by CYP3A4 to become active, it may not be effective. An alternative antidepressant should be considered.

11. C. At this time, neither gabapentin nor levetiracetam is associated with significant drug–drug interactions. The absorption of gabapentin may be reduced by concurrent administration of aluminum- or magnesium-containing antacids; hence, antacids should be given 2 hours before or after a dose of gabapentin. Carbamazepine is an inducer that is associated with numerous drug–drug interactions.

12. D. Both topiramate and zonisamide may cause kidney stones. Although neither agent is contraindicated in patients with a history of kidney stones, these drugs should be used cautiously in such patients. Patients should be counseled to remain adequately hydrated because doing so may decrease the risk of stone formation.

13. D. Both carbamazepine and felbamate are associated with aplastic anemia and hepatic failure. Levetiracetam has no FDA boxed warning.

14. D. Valproic acid may cause fatal hemorrhagic pancreatitis.

15. C. Although valproic acid is extremely effective and is frequently used as monotherapy for generalized

nonmotor (absence) seizures, it should not be given to a patient <2 years of age.

16. A. Diastat is a commercially available gel form of diazepam that is given rectally.

17. B. Unlike simple febrile seizures, which last for only a short period, complex febrile seizures are prolonged (>15 minutes) or recur within 24 hours of the initial seizure. Febrile seizures must occur in the absence of CNS infection in a child with fever. Most febrile seizures are benign, and children do not go on to develop epilepsy. Carbamazepine is ineffective in febrile seizures.

18. A. Only phenytoin is available as a liquid (125 mg/5 mL), as a chewable tablet (50 mg), and in an I.V. dosage form. Valproic acid is not available as a chewable tablet.

19. B. Because topiramate may cause kidney stones, patients should be encouraged to drink plenty of fluids. This would also be true for zonisamide.

20. A. Normeperidine, a metabolite of meperidine, can accumulate in patients with renal failure who receive normal doses and cause seizures. The other agents listed are not eliminated renally in adults.

21. D. Phenytoin has capacity-limited or saturable (i.e., Michaelis–Menten) pharmacokinetics.

22. B. Phenytoin may cause gingival hyperplasia (i.e., overgrowth of the gums). Hence, patients should be instructed to brush and floss daily and to have regular visits with the dentist.

28-9 Additional Resources

Baumann RJ, Duffner PK. Treatment of children with simple febrile seizures: the AAP practice parameter. *Pediatr Neurol.* 2000;23:11–17.

Brophy GM, Bell R, Claassen J, et al. Guidelines for the evaluation and management of status epilepticus. *Neurocrit Care.* 2012;17(1):3–23.

Brunbech L, Sabers A. Effect of antiepileptic drugs on cognitive function in individuals with epilepsy: a comparative review of newer versus older agents. *Drugs.* 2002;62:593–604.

Fisher RS, Cross JH, French JA, et al. Operational classification of seizure types by the International League Against Epilepsy: Position Paper of the ILAE Commission for Classification and Terminology. *Epilepsia.* 2017;58(4):522–530. doi: 10.1111/epi.13670.

Glauser T, Shinnar S, Glass D, et al. Evidence-based guideline: Treatment of convulsive status epilepticus in children and adults: Report of the Guideline Committee of the American Epilepsy Society. *Epilepsy Curr.* 2016;16 (1):48–61. doi: 10.5698 /1535-7597-16.1.48.

Italiano D, Perucca E. Clinical pharmacokinetics of new-generation antiepileptic drugs at the extremes of age: an update. *Clin Pharmacokinet.* 2013;52(8):627–645.

Krivoy N, Taer M, Neuman MG. Antiepileptic drug-induced hypersensitivity syndrome reactions. *Curr Drug Saf.* 2006;1(3):289–299.

Patsalos PN, Berry DJ, Bourgeois BFD, et al. Antiepileptic drugs—best practice guidelines for therapeutic drug monitoring: a position paper by the subcommission on therapeutic drug monitoring, ILAE Commission on Therapeutic Strategies. *Epilepsia.* 2008;49:1239–1276.

Perucca E. Clinically relevant drug interactions with antiepileptic drugs. *Br J Clin Pharmacol.* 2006;61(3):246–255.

Steering Committee on Quality Improvement and Management, Subcommittee on Febrile Seizures. Febrile seizures: clinical practice guideline for the long-term management of the child with simple febrile seizures. *Pediatrics.* 2008;121: 1281–1286.

Psychiatric Diseases and Sleep Disorders

29

WESLEY GEMINN   LANCE MORGAN

29-1 KEY POINTS

SCHIZOPHRENIA

- Antipsychotics are essential in the treatment of schizophrenia; atypical antipsychotics (i.e., risperidone, olanzapine, aripiprazole ⚠) are considered first line because they have lower risk of extrapyramidal symptoms and tardive dyskinesia compared to typical antipsychotics.
- Atypical antipsychotics are associated with development of metabolic syndrome.
- Clozapine ⚠ is the only agent proven effective for refractory schizophrenia but must be closely monitored for agranulocytosis.
- Long-acting injectable antipsychotics have been shown to increase medication adherence.

BIPOLAR DISORDER

- The acute treatment for bipolar disorder focuses on slowing down the patient and reducing harm to himself or herself and others.
- A mood stabilizer is an essential component in the treatment of bipolar disorder. First-line mood stabilizers include lithium ⚠, divalproex sodium (or valproic acid) ⚠, carbamazepine ⚠, **lamotrigine** ⚠, and atypical antipsychotics.
- Patients receiving lithium or divalproex should be closely monitored for signs and symptoms of toxicity and should have periodic serum drug concentration evaluations.

MAJOR DEPRESSION

- All antidepressants are equally effective, and drug choice should depend on patient-specific factors such as cost, drug–drug interactions, adverse effects, previous treatment, and patient choice.
- First-line antidepressants include selective serotonin reuptake inhibitors (SSRIs), serotonin norepinephrine reuptake inhibitors (SNRIs), and **bupropion** because of their more favorable adverse effect and drug–drug interaction profiles.

ANXIETY DISORDERS

- Anxiety disorders are serious, debilitating mental illnesses with extreme anxiety as the primary mood disturbance.
- Potential medications to treat anxiety include benzodiazepines, **buspirone**, antidepressants (especially SSRIs and certain SNRIs), beta blockers, and **hydroxyzine**.

EATING DISORDERS

- SSRIs may be helpful in treating eating disorders (especially bulimia). Optimal therapy should include psychotherapy in combination with drug therapy.

SLEEP DISORDERS

- Patients with insomnia have difficulty falling asleep, staying asleep, or both. Patients should be assessed for factors that may contribute to the insomnia before using drug therapy.
- Treatment with a nonbenzodiazepine receptor agonist (i.e., **zolpidem**, eszopiclone, zaleplon ⚠) should be limited to 2 to 4 weeks and continued only if no other options are viable because of the risk of developing dependence.
- Patients with excessive daytime somnolence may benefit from nonamphetamine stimulants (modafinil or armodafinil), which promote wakefulness.
- Sodium oxybate (Xyrem) ⚠ is indicated for patients with narcolepsy who have failed other therapies.

29-2 STUDY GUIDE CHECKLIST

The following topics may guide your study of this subject area:

- ☐ The *Diagnostic and Statistical Manual of Mental Disorders, Fifth Edition (DSM-5)*.
- ☐ General clinical presentation and symptoms of schizophrenia, bipolar disorder, major depressive disorder, anxiety disorders, eating disorders, and sleep disorders.
- ☐ General nonpharmacologic treatment options for psychiatric illness.
- ☐ Considerations for pharmacologic treatment based on a patient's clinical presentation and medication history.
- ☐ Mechanism of action of various classes of psychotropic drugs.
- ☐ Trade names and available dosage forms, particularly the "Top 100 Drugs".
- ☐ Frequency of dosing regimen, particularly long-acting injectable antipsychotics.
- ☐ Major adverse drug effects of psychotropic drugs.
- ☐ Significant drug–drug interactions of psychotropic drugs.
- ☐ Unique patient counseling points for specific psychotropic drugs.
- ☐ Monitoring of the safety and efficacy of psychotropic drugs.
- ☐ Guidelines for the pharmacological treatment of schizophrenia, bipolar disorder, major depressive disorder, anxiety disorders, eating disorders, and sleep disorders.

Editor's Note: This chapter is based on the 12th edition chapter written by Wesley Geminn and Lance Morgan.

Risperidone, Olanzapine, and Aripiprazole *FDA BOXED WARNINGS*

Increased mortality in elderly patients with dementia-related psychosis.

 Clozapine *FDA BOXED WARNING*

Risk of severe neutropenia, orthostatic hypotension, bradycardia, syncope, seizure, myocarditis, and cardiomyopathy. Increased mortality in elderly patients with dementia-related psychosis.

 Lithium *FDA BOXED WARNING*

Risk of lithium toxicity—monitor levels regularly.

 Divalproex Sodium (or valproic acid) *FDA BOXED WARNING*

Increased risk of hepatotoxicity. Increased risk of pancreatitis. Use in pregnant women is contraindicated due to increased risk of congenital malformations.

 Carbamazepine *FDA BOXED WARNING*

Increased risk of serious dermatologic reactions (e.g., Stevens-Johnson syndrome), especially with HLA-B*1502 allele.

 Lamotrigine *FDA BOXED WARNING*

Risk of serious skin rashes (e.g., Stevens-Johnson syndrome, toxic epidermal necrolysis).

Zolpidem, Eszopiclone, and Zaleplon *FDA BOXED WARNINGS*

Risk of complex sleep behaviors (e.g., sleep-walking, sleep-driving). Discontinue immediately if complex sleep behaviors occur.

 Sodium Oxybate (Xyrem) *FDA BOXED WARNING*

Risk of significant respiratory depression. Risk of respiratory depression, decreased consciousness, coma, and death when misused or abused. Required REMS program due to risks of CNS depression, abuse, and misuse.

29-3 Schizophrenia

Schizophrenia is a psychiatric disorder characterized by a profound disruption in perception, cognition, and emotion.

Epidemiology

Approximately 1% of the U.S. adult population has schizophrenia, with 200,000 new cases reported annually. Although the onset is earlier in males (average age 18 to 24 years) than in females (average age late 20s to early 40s), no gender or racial differences exist.

Clinical Presentation

The onset of schizophrenia is typically characterized by deterioration in occupational and social situations over a period of 6 months or more.

Symptoms

Symptoms are commonly referred to as *positive* (hallucinations or delusions), *negative* (flat affect, avolition, anhedonia, and poverty of thought), or *disorganized* (disorganized speech or behavior).

Most patients fluctuate between acute episodes and remission. Patients in remission may still exhibit residual symptoms.

Associated features

Morbidity

There are many comorbid disease states (mental and medical); for example, substance abuse is found in 60% to 70% of persons with schizophrenia.

Mortality

Shortened life expectancy is a feature of schizophrenia. Patients with schizophrenia are at an increased risk of suicide (10% commit suicide).

Etiology

The etiology is most likely multifactorial:

- Genetic
- Neurobiological
- Developmental (season of birth, viral illness, traumatic injury)

Treatment Principles and Goals

- All antipsychotics have been shown to be equally effective with the exception of clozapine, which is the only antipsychotic approved for treatment of refractory schizophrenia.
- The choice of antipsychotic medication is based on the following:
  - Past history of patient or family member response
  - Adverse effect profile of the antipsychotic
- Initiate therapy with a trial of an antipsychotic (at least 4 to 6 weeks at recommended doses).
- Nonadherence, adverse effects, complicated drug regimens, and lack of insight about the disease are common reasons for treatment failure.
- Consider long-acting injectable preparations in situations of poor adherence.

Drug Therapy

Typical (older) antipsychotics

Mechanism of action

These drugs block postsynaptic dopamine-2 (D2) receptors. They share anticholinergic, antihistaminic, and alpha-blocking properties.

Other conventional antipsychotics

Though not commonly used, perphenazine (Trilafon), thiothixene (Navane), trifluoperazine (Stelazine), and loxapine (Loxitane, Adasuve) are typical (also known as conventional or first generation) antipsychotics used to treat schizophrenia.

Adverse effects of typical antipsychotics

Typical antipsychotics are often described as high, medium, or low potency depending on their affinity for the D2 receptor. Low-potency typical antipsychotics also antagonize the histamine, alpha-adrenergic, and muscarinic receptors leading to more sedation, weight gain, orthostasis, and anticholinergic effects. High-potency typical antipsychotics are associated with higher rates of movement disorders related to extrapyramidal symptoms (EPSs). Symptoms of sedation and orthostasis may resolve or become more tolerant over time; however, EPS-related movement disorders may gradually worsen.

Extrapyramidal symptoms

EPSs are most likely attributed to an imbalance in dopamine and acetylcholine.

Dystonic reactions

Reactions usually occur within 24 to 96 hours of initiating or changing the dose. They present as painful, involuntary muscle spasms in skeletal muscles (most commonly in the facial or neck muscles but sometimes in the back, arm, and leg muscles).

Dystonic reactions are treated with benztropine (Cogentin) 1 to 2 mg intramuscular (I.M.) or diphenhydramine (Benadryl) 25 to 50 mg I.M. every 30 minutes until the reaction is relieved. Prophylaxis with oral therapy of these 2 agents is frequently used with high-dose, high-potency typical antipsychotics.

Akathisia

Akathisia usually occurs within a few weeks of initiating antipsychotic therapy. It is described as a subjective feeling of discomfort, usually seen as motor restlessness of the legs (inability to stand still or sit still). Akathisia may be treated by decreasing the dose, changing the drug, or adding lipophilic beta blockers (e.g., propranolol), benzodiazepines, **clonidine**, or anticholinergic agents.

Pseudoparkinsonism

Pseudoparkinsonism usually occurs after months or years of therapy. This condition resembles Parkinson's symptoms (e.g., cogwheel rigidity, bradykinesia, tremor, shuffling gait). It is treated with amantadine (Symmetrel) 100 mg twice daily or anticholinergics (including benztropine, diphenhydramine, and trihexyphenidyl [Artane]).

Other adverse effects

Tardive dyskinesia

Tardive dyskinesia (TD) is a medication-induced hyperkinetic movement disorder that can be irreversible and lifelong. TD typically occurs after years of antipsychotic therapy. It is caused by long-term suppression of dopamine.

A triad of symptoms characterize TD:

- Choreoathetosis (splayed, writhing fingers)
- Oral or buccal movements (grimacing, bruxism, lip smacking)
- Protrusion of the tongue

The best treatment is prevention (i.e., use the lowest effective dose of antipsychotic). Newer pharmacologic treatment that inhibits the vesicular monoamine transporter-2 (VMAT2 inhibitors), such as valbenazine, tetrabenazine, and duetetrabenazine, has shown to significantly reduce TD symptoms. Other various therapies (e.g., vitamin E, lecithin, vitamin B_6) may also help alleviate symptoms. Switching from the offending antipsychotic to clozapine may be helpful because it has not been reported to cause TD. Monitor for TD by administering the AIMS (Abnormal Involuntary Movement Scale) test to all patients initiating or increasing their dose of an antipsychotic and at least annually thereafter.

Neuroleptic malignant syndrome

Neuroleptic malignant syndrome (NMS) has a low incidence and high mortality. It is thought to be due to rapid dopamine blockade commonly associated with high-potency typical antipsychotics. Its clinical presentation can be found in Box 29-1.

NMS treatment is as follows:

- Transport the patient to an emergency room immediately.
- Discontinue antipsychotic medication.
- Administer supportive therapy (cooling blankets, hydration) or the dopamine agonist bromocriptine (Parlodel) or the smooth muscle relaxant dantrolene (Dantrium).

BOX 29-1. Clinical Presentation of Neuroleptic Malignant Syndrome

- Rapid progression (<24 hours)
- Body temperature >100.4°F
- Lead-pipe rigidity
- Hypertension
- Diaphoresis

- Increased heart rate
- Incontinence
- Increased liver function test (LFT), creatinine phosphokinase (CPK), and white blood count (WBC)

Cardiac effects

Because QT prolongation is possible, electrocardiogram (ECG) monitoring is recommended for all patients upon initiation of an antipsychotic and periodically thereafter.

Miscellaneous adverse effects

Miscellaneous adverse effects that may occur less frequently include hyperprolactinemia, temperature dysregulation, and ophthalmological and dermatological effects.

The U.S. Food and Drug Administration (FDA) has issued a boxed warning for increase in mortality with use of typical antipsychotics in elderly patients with dementia, and typical antipsychotics are not approved for the treatment of patients with dementia-related psychosis.

Atypical (newer) antipsychotics

These drugs are generally weak dopamine and D2 receptor blockers that also block serotonin, alpha-adrenergic, histaminic, and muscarinic receptors to varying degrees in the central nervous system (CNS).

No universally accepted definition of *atypical* exists, but these medications generally have the following features compared to typical (older) antipsychotics:

- Adverse effects are less severe (little or no EPS, minimal to no prolactin increase [except risperidone], less risk of TD).
- More weight gain, more lipid abnormalities, and a greater risk of diabetes are seen with these drugs (risk is lower with some agents, such as ziprasidone, aripiprazole, lurasidone, and iloperidone).
- A dose-dependent increased risk of ventricular arrhythmias and sudden cardiac death is seen, possibly because of prolongation of the QT interval similar to that with typical antipsychotics.
- Decreased affinity for the dopamine receptor results in less risk for EPS and decreased risk of developing drug-induced negative symptoms, such as avolition and cognitive impairment.
- Results from CATIE (Clinical Antipsychotic Trials in Intervention Effectiveness) showed high discontinuation rates for all antipsychotics secondary to inefficacy or intolerable adverse effects. No difference was seen between perphenazine and atypical antipsychotics (except olanzapine).
- The U.S. Food and Drug Administration (FDA) has issued a boxed warning for an increase in mortality with use of atypical antipsychotics in elderly patients with dementia, and atypical antipsychotics are not approved for the treatment of patients with dementia-related psychosis.

Treatment Strategies

Acute schizophrenia

- Goal is to decrease danger to self and others and reduce symptoms back to baseline.
- Increase dosage of the antipsychotic until symptoms improve or adverse effects limit the dose.
- Haloperidol or fluphenazine (immediate release) 5 to 10 mg I.M. and **lorazepam** 2 mg I.M. every 4 hours as needed may be used for psychosis or agitation. An anticholinergic may also be needed (e.g., benztropine or diphenhydramine for EPSs).
- Olanzapine 10 mg I.M. may be used and can be repeated in 2 hours and again 4 hours later, for a maximum of 30 mg/d for psychosis or agitation.
- Patients may use ziprasidone 10 mg I.M. administered every 2 hours or 20 mg I.M. administered every 4 hours, for a maximum of 40 mg/d for psychosis or agitation.

Maintenance

- Consider starting an atypical antipsychotic at a recommended dose or consider a typical antipsychotic if patient has had previous success with a typical agent or if other patient-

specific factors limit use of an atypical antipsychotic (e.g., cost, adverse effects, drug–drug interactions).
- Positive symptoms will often respond early in treatment, whereas negative symptoms often take longer to resolve.
- Monitor for adverse effects and emphasize medication adherence.
- Treatment is noncurative, and lifelong therapy is usually needed.
- Consider medications that are available in long-acting, injectable formulations.

Monitoring for patients on atypical antipsychotics

- Fasting glucose and lipids and blood pressure at baseline and at 12 weeks
- Weight (body mass index) at baseline, 4 weeks, 8 weeks, and 12 weeks, and then quarterly
- Waist circumference at baseline and then annually

Long-acting injectable dosage forms

Long-acting injectable dosage forms of antipsychotics are often used in patients who may be nonadherent to their medications or who prefer the convenience. Tolerability with oral dosage form should be assessed before switching to a long-acting injectable form. Some antipsychotics may require an overlap with the oral dosage forms during initiation of the long-acting injectable. See Tables 29-1 and 29-3 for more information.

TABLE 29-1. Typical (Conventional or Older) Antipsychotics

Drug and form	Trade name	Available dose forms	Potency	Daily dosage range	Equivalent oral dose	Clinical highlights
Chlorpromazine	Thorazine	Tablets, sustained-release capsules, oral liquid, injection, suppository	Low	50 to 2000 mg	100 mg	First antipsychotic used clinically; also drug of choice for intractable hiccups
Perphenazine	Trilafon	Tablets	Medium	4 to 64 mg in divided doses	10 mg	Moderate sedation, extrapyramidal symptoms; low anticholinergic effect, orthostasis
Fluphenazine	Prolixin, Prolixin Decanoate	Tablets, oral liquid, injection, long-acting injection	High	1 to 65 mg oral; 12.5 to 75 mg I.M. (decanoate) every 2 weeks	2 mg	Decanoate injection dosed at 1.25 times the total daily oral dose every 2 to 3 weeks; steady state reached within 6 weeks. Decanoate in thick sesame seed oil; monitor for allergies
Haloperidol	Haldol, Haldol-D	Tablets, oral liquid, injection, long-acting injection	High	1 to 100 mg oral; 50 to 300 mg I.M. (decanoate) every 4 weeks	2 mg	Decanoate injection dosed at 10 times the total daily oral dose every 4 weeks; steady state reached within 8 to 12 weeks. Decanoate in thick sesame seed oil; monitor for allergies

TABLE 29-2. Adverse Effects of Typical Antipsychotic Medications

Drug	Extrapyramidal symptoms	Sedation	Orthostasis	Weight gain	Anticholinergic effect
Chlorpromazine	+++	++++	++++	++	+++
Perphenazine	++++	++	+	+	++
Fluphenazine	++++	+	+	+	+
Haloperidol	++++	+	+	+	+

Typical antipsychotics are listed in increasing potency for dopamine receptor.

⚠ Chlorpromazine *FDA BOXED WARNING*

Increased risk of death in elderly patients with dementia-related psychosis.

⚠ Perphenazine *FDA BOXED WARNING*

Increased risk of death in elderly patients with dementia-related psychosis.

⚠ Fluphenazine *FDA BOXED WARNING*

Increased risk of death in elderly patients with dementia-related psychosis.

⚠ Haloperidol *FDA BOXED WARNING*

Increased risk of death in elderly patients with dementia-related psychosis.

TABLE 29-3. Atypical Antipsychotics

Drug	Trade name	Form	Usual dose	Adverse effects	Clinical highlights
Clozapine ⚠	Clozaril, FazaClo, Versacloz	Tablets, orally disintegrating tablets, oral suspension	12.5 mg titrated up to 300 to 900 mg/day	Sedation, weight gain, hypersalivation; boxed warning for seizure risk (> 600 mg/day), agranulocytosis, orthostasis, myocarditis, respiratory and cardiac arrest; no EPS or TD	Indicated for refractory schizophrenia only. Has REMS program for risk of agranulocytosis; ANC must be > 1500 to initiate and then monitor according to REMS schedule. Pregnancy category B.
Risperidone ⚠	Risperdal, Risperdal M-tabs, Risperdal Consta, Perseris	Tablets, oral liquid, orally disintegrating tablets, long-acting injection	1 mg bid up to 4 to 6 mg/day; maximum dose 16 mg/day; 25 to 50 mg IM every 2 weeks (Consta); 90 to 120 mg SQ every month (Perseris)	Dose-related EPS (> 8 mg/day), ± weight gain, ± sedation, prolactin elevation, orthostasis	Most "typical" acting of the atypical antipsychotics. Available in concentrate; do not mix with teas or colas. Commonly used in dementia (0.25 to 1 mg); patient must overlap long-acting injection, Consta, with oral risperidone for at least 3 weeks. No overlap needed with Perseris.
Olanzapine ⚠	Zyprexa, Zyprexa Zydis, Zyprexa Relprevv	Tablets, orally disintegrating tablets (Zydis), injection, long-acting injection (Relprevv)	10 to 20 mg/day; higher doses have been reported Long-acting injection maintenance dose: 150 mg q2wk, 300 mg q2wk, or 405 mg q4wk	Sedation, orthostasis, weight gain. Most likely to cause metabolic syndrome and induce diabetes. Long-acting injection, Relprevv, has REMS program owing to boxed warning for PIDSS, which can be fatal.	Also indicated for acute manic episodes of bipolar disorder. Zyprexa Zydis is useful for patients who are unable to swallow or are "cheeking" medications. Short-acting injections should not be used with injectable benzodiazepines. Relprevv must be administered in office and patient observed for at least 3 hours for PIDSS.
Quetiapine ⚠	Seroquel, Seroquel XR	Tablets, extended-release tablets	300 to 800 mg/day; higher doses have been reported	High sedation, dizziness, headache	Low EPS and prolactin elevation risk; do lens test at baseline and every 6 months owing to risk of forming cataracts. Boxed warning for suicidality in children, adolescents, and young adults. Dose at bedtime owing to sedation. Has potential for abuse.
Ziprasidone ⚠	Geodon	Capsules, injection	40 to 200 mg/day po; 20 mg IM × 1 dose (may repeat in 4h; maximum IM daily dose 40 mg)	Negligible weight gain or sedation, QT prolongation warning in package insert	Use caution with other medications that prolong QT interval. Dose with meals to increase absorption.
Aripiprazole ⚠	**Abilify,** Abilify Discmelt, Abilify Maintena, Aristada, Abilify Mycite	Tablets, oral liquid, orally disintegrating tablets, injection, long-acting injection, tablet with sensor	10 to 30 mg/day po; 5.25 to 15 mg/day IM; maximum IM daily dose 30 mg. Long-acting injection: 300 to 400 mg IM monthly (Maintena) or 441 to 662 mg monthly or 882 mg every 6 weeks (Aristada)	Possible insomnia, negligible weight gain or sedation, akathisia	Once-daily dosing benefit; partial agonist for D2 and 5-HT1A. Boxed warning for suicidality in children, adolescents, and young adults. Abilify Mycite uses a sensor in each tablet that is detected by a patch worn by the patient to track adherence using digital technology.

(continued)

TABLE 29-3. Atypical Antipsychotics (Continued)

Drug	Trade name	Form	Usual dose	Adverse effects	Clinical highlights
Paliperidone ⚠	Invega, Invega Sustenna, Invega Trinza	Extended-release tablets, long-acting injection	6 mg/day; maximum dose 12 mg/day. For Sustenna: 234 mg day 1, 156 mg 1 wk later, then 117 mg q month. Trinza (T) is given every 3 months, and dose is based off previous Sustenna (S) dose; 78 mg(S)→273 mg(T) 117 mg(S)→410 mg(T) 156 mg(S)→546 mg(T) 234 mg(S)→819 mg(T)	Headache, tachycardia, somnolence, anxiety, orthostasis, hyperprolactinemia (especially in geriatric patients)	Metabolite of risperidone. Sustained-release tablet: do not crush or chew; tablet shell may be seen in stool. Oral dose can be gradually stopped after initiating long-acting injection. May assess tolerability with risperidone. May switch to Trinza after receiving 4 months of Sustenna.
Iloperidone ⚠	Fanapt	Tablets	1 mg bid initial, 6 to 12 mg bid usual dose, maximum dose 12 mg bid; reduce dose by half with strong CYP450 2C9 and 3A4 inhibitors	Dizziness, nausea, somnolence, EPS, QT prolongation	Titrate dose to avoid significant orthostatic hypotension. If more than 3 days missed, retitrate dose.
Asenapine ⚠	Saphris, Secuado	Sublingual tablets, transdermal patch	5 mg bid can increase to 10 mg bid after 1 wk; 3.8 mg/24 hours daily for 1 week, then increase to 5.7 mg/24 hours or 7.6 mg/24 hours	EPS, insomnia, somnolence, dizziness, numbness of mouth and tongue; serious allergic reactions have been reported	For Saphris sublingual, do not crush, chew, or swallow and do not eat or drink for 10 minutes after dosing. Secuado daily patch avoids food and drink restrictions. Use dry hands when handling. May cause anaphylactic allergic reaction.
Lurasidone ⚠	**Latuda**	Tablets	40 mg initial dose, usual dose 40 to 160 mg/day, maximum 80 mg/day in moderate renal/hepatic dx or moderate CYP450 3A4 inhibitors	Somnolence, nausea and vomiting, EPS (dose related)	Take with food, at least 350 calories. Contraindicated with strong CYP450 3A4 inducers or inhibitors. Pregnancy category B.
Brexpiprazole ⚠	Rexulti	Tablets	1 mg/day on days 1 to 4, then 2 mg/day on days 5 to 7, then 4 mg/day thereafter	Akathisia, increased triglycerides and blood glucose, headache	Similar mechanism to aripiprazole with addition of 5-HT2A antagonism. Long half-life of 91 hours. Adjust dose for renal impairment (CrCl < 60) to 3 mg maximum for schizophrenia and 2 mg for MDD. Decrease dose by 50% for poor CYP2D6 metabolizers.
Cariprazine ⚠	Vraylar	Capsules	1.5 mg/day initially, then increase to 1.5 mg to 3 mg increments; maximum dose 6 mg/day	Akathisia, indigestion, vomiting, headache, insomnia	Concomitant use of CYP3A4 inducers is not recommended. Warn patients to avoid dehydration or overheating while using.
Lumateperone ⚠	Caplyta	Capsules	42 mg/day, no titration required	Somnolence, sedation, dry mouth	Warn patients to avoid dehydration or overheating while using.

Boldface indicates one of top 100 drugs for 2020 by prescription volume.

5-HT, 5-hydroxytryptamine; ANC, absolute neutrophil count; CrCl, creatinine clearance; dx, dysfunction; MDD, major depressive disorder; PIDSS, postinjection delirium/sedation syndrome; REMS, risk evaluation and mitigation strategy.

Clozapine *FDA BOXED WARNING*

Risk of severe neutropenia, orthostatic hypotension, bradycardia, syncope, seizure, myocarditis, and cardiomy-opathy. Increased mortality in elderly patients with dementia-related psychosis.

 Risperidone *FDA BOXED WARNING*

Increased risk of death in elderly patients with dementia-related psychosis.

 Olanzapine *FDA BOXED WARNING*

Increased risk of death in elderly patients with dementia-related psychosis.

 Quetiapine *FDA BOXED WARNING*

Increased risk of death in elderly patients with dementia-related psychosis.

 Ziprasidone *FDA BOXED WARNING*

Increased risk of death in elderly patients with dementia-related psychosis.

 Aripiprazole *FDA BOXED WARNING*

Increased risk of death in elderly patients with dementia-related psychosis.

 Paliperidone *FDA BOXED WARNING*

Increased risk of death in elderly patients with dementia-related psychosis.

Iloperidone *FDA BOXED WARNING*

Increased risk of death in elderly patients with dementia-related psychosis.

 Asenapine *FDA BOXED WARNING*

Increased risk of death in elderly patients with dementia-related psychosis.

 Lurasidone *FDA BOXED WARNING*

Increased risk of death in elderly patients with dementia-related psychosis.

 Brexpiprazole *FDA BOXED WARNING*

Increased risk of death in elderly patients with dementia-related psychosis.

 Cariprazine *FDA BOXED WARNING*

Increased risk of death in elderly patients with dementia-related psychosis.

 Lumateperone *FDA BOXED WARNING*

Increased risk of death in elderly patients with dementia-related psychosis.

29-4 Bipolar Disorder

Bipolar disorder is a recurrent mood disorder with a lifetime prevalence of 3.7% to 3.9%. This disorder is associated with significant morbidity and mortality. Incidence is equal in females and males. Onset is usually between ages 8 and 44 years with an average onset around age 25 years. The first episode for females is usually marked by a depressive episode. For males, it is usually marked by a manic episode.

Types and Classifications

- *Bipolar I:* This type is characterized by the occurrence of manic episodes plus or minus hypomanic or major depressive episodes.
- *Bipolar II:* This type is characterized by the occurrence of hypomanic episodes and major depressive episodes.
- *Cyclothymia:* This type is defined as numerous periods of hypomania and depressive symptoms that do not meet the criteria for a hypomanic or major depressive episode. Diagnosis requires that cyclothymia symptoms occur for at least a 2-year period in adults or 1-year period for children and adolescents.

Clinical Presentation

See the *Diagnostic and Statistical Manual of Mental Disorders Text Revision (DSM-5)* for complete diagnostic criteria.

Mania

Mania is characterized by heightened mood (euphoria), flight of ideas, rapid or pressured speech, grandiosity, increased energy, decreased need for sleep, irritability, and impulsivity. Judgment is significantly impaired (e.g., increased risk-taking behavior). Marked impairment also exists in social or occupational functioning.

Hypomania

Hypomania is a less severe form of mania. This disorder usually does not cause marked impairment in social or occupational functioning.

Mixed features

A specifier "with mixed features" may be applied to episodes of mania or hypomania when depressive features are also present.

Rapid cycling

In *rapid cycling,* the patient experiences more than 4 mood episodes in a year. Mood episodes may occur in any combination. Rapid cycling primarily occurs in women (70% to 90%). Rapid cycling typically occurs in more severe forms of the disease and is associated with poorer long-term outcomes such as hospitalizations and increased rates of suicide.

Treatment Principles and Goals

- Establish and maintain a therapeutic alliance.
- Monitor the patient's psychiatric status.
- Provide education regarding bipolar disorder.
- Enhance treatment adherence.
- Promote regular patterns of activity and sleep.
- Anticipate stressors.
- Identify new episodes early.
- Minimize functional impairments.

Drug Therapy

Mood stabilizers are first line for treatment of bipolar disorder. See Table 29-4 for current medications approved as mood stabilizers.

Lithium

Indications

Lithium is indicated for acute treatment and maintenance of manic episodes associated with bipolar disorders. It is effective for both the manic and depressive symptoms and may be beneficial in patients experiencing suicidal ideation.

TABLE 29-4. Mood Stabilizers

Drug	Trade name	Form	Usual dose	Adverse effects	Clinical highlights
Lithium	Lithobid, Eskalith, Eskalith CR	Capsules, extended-release tablets, oral liquid	Starting: 900 to 1200 mg in divided doses; titrate to desired response or level	Tremor, polydipsia or polyuria, nausea or diarrhea, weight gain, hypothyroidism, mental dulling	Many drug interactions; boxed warning for lithium toxicity. Teratogenicity is a concern (pregnancy category D); monitor blood levels—acute: 0.8 to 1.5 mEq/L, maintenance: 0.6 to 1.2 mEq/L.
Divalproex sodium	Depakote, Depakote ER	Tablets, delayed-release tablets, extended-release tablets	Starting: 500 mg 2 to 3 times daily or 15 mg/kg; maximum dose 60 mg/kg/d; ER dosed daily	GI upset, sedation, tremor, weight gain, alopecia, transient elevation in LFTs	Boxed warnings: hepatotoxicity, hemorrhagic pancreatitis, teratogenicity (pregnancy category D); monitor blood levels: 50 to 125 mcg/mL (85 to 125 mcg/mL for mania).
Carbamazepine	Tegretol	Tablets, chewable tablets, extended-release tablets, oral liquid	Starting: 200 mg twice daily; increase to 800 to 1200 mg/d (3 to 4 daily doses); usual range 400 to 1600 mg/d	Ataxia, dizziness, sedation, slurred speech, aplastic anemia	See text for contraindications; many drug interactions (pregnancy category C); monitor blood levels: 4 to 12 mcg/mL. Boxed warning for serious dermatological reactions and for agranulocytosis and aplastic anemia.
Lamotrigine	Lamictal	Tablets, chewable tablets	Starting: 25 mg/d weeks 1 and 2; 50 mg/d weeks 3 and 4; 100 mg/d week 5; 200 mg/d week 6; 200 mg/d usual dose	Dizziness, headache, ataxia, nausea, diplopia, rash	Boxed warning: severe rashes such as Stevens–Johnson syndrome; start at 25 mg and titrate to 200 mg over 6 weeks to help prevent rash.

Boldface indicates one of top 100 drugs for 2020 by prescription volume.

Mechanism of action

Lithium's mechanism of action is unknown. Various theories suggest that lithium facilitates gamma-aminobutyric acid (GABA) function, alters cation transport across cell membranes in nerve and muscle cells, or influences reuptake of 5-hydroxytryptamine (5-HT) or norepinephrine (NE).

Contraindications and precautions

Contraindications and precautions include renal disease, first trimester of pregnancy, unmasking of Brugada syndrome, encephalopathic syndrome with neuroleptic medications, previous lithium toxicity, or hypersensitivity to lithium.

Use with caution in patients who have thyroid disease or sodium depletion, patients who are receiving diuretics, or dehydrated patients.

Monitoring (baseline and follow-up)

- **Thyroid panel:** Lithium may cause hypothyroidism. Test baseline and thyroid-stimulating hormone (TSH) every 6 to 12 months or as clinically indicated.
- **Serum creatinine (SCr) and blood urea nitrogen (BUN):** Lithium is 100% renally eliminated. Test baseline and every 3 months for patients with renal dysfunction and every 6 to 12 months otherwise or as clinically indicated.
- **Electrolytes:** In the event of hyponatremia, lithium toxicity may occur. Test electrolytes every 6 to 12 months or as clinically indicated.
- **ECG:** Lithium causes flattened or inverted T-waves. This condition is reversible. Test baseline and every 6 to 12 months or as clinically indicated.
- **Urinalysis:** Lithium may decrease specific gravity. Perform urinalysis every 6 to 12 months.
- **Pregnancy test:** Lithium may cause cardiovascular defects (e.g., Ebstein's anomaly, floppy baby syndrome). Perform pregnancy test every 6 to 12 months or as clinically indicated.
- **Lithium level:** Lithium reaches steady-state levels in 3 to 5 half-lives (half-life = ~24 hours). Obtain the level in the morning immediately before next dose (acute: 0.8 to 1.5 mEq/L; maintenance: 0.6 to 1.2 mEq/L). Lithium levels should be checked after each dose increase and before the next dose increase. Periodic monitoring of lithium levels should occur every 6 months or more frequently if clinically indicated.

Drug–drug interactions

Table 29-5 summarizes the drug–drug interactions with lithium.

Concurrent use with calcium channel blockers increases the risks of neurotoxicity, and concurrent use with selective serotonin reuptake inhibitors (SSRIs) can result in diarrhea, confusion, tremor, dizziness, and agitation.

Adverse effects

Several concentration-related toxicity concerns are associated with the drug:

- **Mild toxicity (serum levels 1.5 to 2.5 mEq/L):** Gastrointestinal (GI) upset (nausea, vomiting, diarrhea), muscle weakness, fatigue, fine hand tremor, and difficulty with concentration and memory
- **Moderate toxicity (serum levels 2.5 to 3.5 mEq/L):** Ataxia, lethargy, nystagmus, worsening confusion, severe GI upset, coarse tremors, and increased deep tendon reflexes
- **Severe toxicity (serum levels > 3.5 mEq/L):** Severely impaired consciousness, coma, seizures, respiratory complications, and death

Toxicity is treated as follows:

- Discontinue lithium, and initiate gastric lavage, if indicated.
- Correct electrolyte and fluid imbalances.
- Monitor neurologic changes.

TABLE 29-5. Drug–Drug Interactions with Lithium

Increase level of lithium	Decrease level of lithium
Nonsteroidal anti-inflammatory drugs	Theophylline
Angiotensin-converting enzyme inhibitors	Caffeine
Angiotensin receptor blockers	Pregnancy
Fluoxetine	Osmotic diuretics (mannitol and urea)
Metronidazole	
Thiazide diuretics	
Sodium depletion:	
Low-sodium diet	
Excessive exercise or sweating	
Vomiting or diarrhea	
Salt deficiency	

Boldface indicates one of top 100 drugs for 2020 by prescription volume.

- Give supportive care.
- Give dialysis if indicated.

Patient information

- Routinely monitoring serum lithium levels is important.
- Maintain a steady salt and fluid intake.
- Do not crush or chew extended- or slow-release dosage forms.
- Common adverse effects of lithium include mild hand tremor, weakness, lack of coordination, dry mouth, altered taste perception, weight gain, increased thirst, increased frequency of urination, mild nausea, loss of appetite, stomach pain or upset stomach, loss of libido, impotence, diarrhea, thinning of the hair, itchy skin, and kidney abnormalities.

Divalproex sodium

Indications

Divalproex sodium is indicated for bipolar disorder. It is considered first-line treatment for acute manic episodes. It has unlabeled use for prophylaxis of manic episodes, is effective for rapid cyclers and patients with dysphoric mood, and is helpful in the management of agitation and aggression. Divalproex is rapidly metabolized to valproic acid (VPA) in the stomach.

Mechanism of action

Its mechanism of action is unknown, but divalproex sodium is thought to increase GABA or mimic its action at the postsynaptic receptor site.

Contraindications

Contraindications include the following:

- Hepatic dysfunction
- Hypersensitivity to divalproex sodium
- Patients <2 years old
- Pregnancy

With respect to pregnancy, VPA may cause neural tube defects and spina bifida. If the benefit outweighs the risk, consider supplementing with 4 to 5 mg/day of **folic acid** to decrease risk of fetal damage. Perform pregnancy test every 6 to 12 months.

Monitoring
Valproic acid (VPA)
- VPA level reaches steady state in 3 to 5 half-lives (half-life = 9 to 16 hours); serum drug concentration of 50 to 125 mcg/mL is optimal.
- Draw level periodically as clinically indicated.

Liver function test (LFT)
- Test baseline, every 6 to 12 months, with dose changes, or as clinically indicated.
- Divalproex/VPA is hepatically eliminated and carries an FDA boxed warning for hepatotoxicity.

Complete blood count with differential
- Test baseline complete blood count (CBC), every 6 to 12 months, with dose changes, or as clinically indicated.
- Divalproex/VPA may cause thrombocytopenia.
- Hematologic abnormalities may be seen with serum levels above 100 mcg/mL.

Serum ammonia
- Test at baseline with dose changes or as clinically indicated.
- Divalproex/VPA may cause hyperammonemia.

Drug–drug interactions
- Divalproex/VPA is a cytochrome P450 (CYP450) 2C19 enzyme substrate, a CYP450 2C9 and 2D6 inhibitor, and a weak CYP450 3A3/4 inhibitor.
- Interactions occur with carbamazepine, **lamotrigine**, and phenytoin. Increased sedative effects occur with phenobarbital and benzodiazepines.

Adverse effects
Common adverse effects include tremor, weight gain, alopecia, lack of coordination, nausea, abdominal pain, dyspepsia, vomiting, sleepiness, asthenia, and rash.

Patient information
- Take with food to avoid GI upset.
- Take a multivitamin with selenium and zinc if alopecia (hair loss) occurs.
- Monitoring VPA levels routinely is important.

Carbamazepine

Indications
Carbamazepine (CBZ) is considered a first-line therapy for acute and prophylactic treatment of bipolar disorder. It has limited utility, however, because of numerous clinically significant drug–drug interactions, especially with adjunctive antipsychotic treatment.

Mechanism of action
CBZ inhibits voltage-sensitive sodium channels.

Monitoring
Monitor CBC with differential, electrolytes, LFTs, SCr or BUN, pregnancy status, and ECG (if the patient > 40 years old or has a preexisting heart disease).

CBZ is an autoinducer. Monitor levels routinely, especially during first few months of therapy. The optimal serum drug concentration is 4 to 12 mcg/mL.

Contraindications
Contraindications include history of previous bone marrow depression and hypersensitivity to CBZ.

Drug–drug interactions

- CBZ is a CYP450 2C8 and 3A3/4 enzyme substrate.
- It is a CYP450 1A2, 2C, and 3A3/4 inducer.
- CBZ may induce the metabolism of benzodiazepines, clozapine, corticosteroids, oral contraceptives, VPA, **warfarin**, phenytoin, and tricyclic antidepressants (and others).
- CBZ may be inhibited by cimetidine, clarithromycin, **diltiazem**, verapamil, **metronidazole**, and **lamotrigine** (and others).

Adverse effects

Common adverse effects include nausea, vomiting, dizziness, lack of coordination, unsteadiness, drowsiness, dry mouth, and swollen tongue. Serious and sometimes fatal dermatologic reactions can occur, including toxic epidermal necrolysis (TEN) and Stevens–Johnson syndrome (SJS), have been reported during treatment with CBZ. Studies in patients of Chinese ancestry have found a strong association between the risk of developing SJS/TEN and the presence of HLA-B*1502. Patients with ancestry in genetically at-risk populations should be screened for the presence of HLA-B*1502 prior to initiating treatment with CBZ.

Lamotrigine (Lamictal)

Lamotrigine is approved for maintenance treatment of bipolar depression. Titration of the dose is required to monitor for signs and symptoms of severe and potentially life-threatening skin rashes, including SJS and TEN.

Drug–drug interactions

- CBZ, phenytoin, oral contraceptives, rifampin, and phenobarbital decrease **lamotrigine** concentrations.
- Divalproex/VPA doubles **lamotrigine** concentrations. **Lamotrigine** doses should be cut in half with coadministration of divalproex/VPA to decrease the risk of SJS.

Adverse effects

Common adverse effects include nausea, headache, tremor or anxiety, and sedation.

Atypical antipsychotics

Atypical antipsychotics have become a mainstay of treatment of bipolar disorder as monotherapy, as well as adjunctive therapy, with traditional mood-stabilizing agents. Some agents are approved for all phases of bipolar disorder, which include maintenance, acute mania, depression, and mixed/manic episodes. Although the FDA has not approved all atypical antipsychotics for treatment of bipolar disorder, most agents are considered to have mood-stabilizing abilities like those of traditional mood stabilizers.

Second-line therapies

Antidepressants

Antidepressants may be used adjunctively to treat bipolar depression. Current evidence suggests that treatment outcomes are not improved with antidepressant monotherapy for bipolar depression and that the risks of increased rates of switching to a manic or hypomanic episode may outweigh any benefits gained by the antidepressant. Concomitant use of antidepressant medication *with* a mood stabilizer is very important to lower the risks of switching to a hypomanic or manic episode when antidepressants are used.

Oxcarbazepine (Trileptal)

This agent is structurally similar to CBZ (a keto-analogue of CBZ). It is sometimes used as a mood stabilizer in patients with bipolar disorder, but further studies are needed. Recent guidelines suggest reserving oxcarbazepine as adjunctive treatment as an alternative to CBZ in the maintenance phase of treatment only.

No autoinduction problems exist, and there are no serum drug levels to monitor. Sodium levels must be monitored due to the risk of developing drug-induced hyponatremia. It appears to have fewer drug–drug interactions than CBZ.

29-5   Major Depressive Disorder

Major depressive disorder is treatable but often goes untreated or undertreated. Most cases go unrecognized, which may be due to the social stigma surrounding depression. Several myths contribute to the problem of undertreatment (e.g., major depression is caused by personal weakness or an inability to handle life's problems).

Epidemiology

The lifetime prevalence rate of depression is 20.6%. One in 4 females (26.14%) and 1 in 8 males (14.7%) are affected.

Major depression is most common between the ages of 25 and 44 years. Risk factors for major depression can be found in Box 29-2, and the clinical presentation for this condition can be found in Box 29-3. The proposed etiology is in Box 29-4.

BOX 29-2. Risk Factors for Major Depression

- Family history
- Female gender
- Previous depressive episode
- Previous suicide attempt
- Comorbid medical or substance abuse disorder

BOX 29-3. Clinical Presentation of Major Depression

Physical findings
- Fatigue
- Pain (i.e., headaches, back pain, GI upset)
- Sleep disturbances (usually insomnia)
- Appetite disturbances (usually decreased appetite)
- Psychomotor retardation or agitation

Emotional symptoms
- Anhedonia
- Depressed mood for most of the day
- Hopelessness or helplessness
- Inappropriate feelings of guilt and worthlessness
- Anxiety or worry
- Suicidal ideation

Cognitive symptoms
- Decreased ability to concentrate
- Indecisiveness

Laboratory studies

There are no diagnostic laboratory tests for depression, but the following lab work should be conducted to rule out other illnesses that may manifest as depressive symptoms or to test for medical conditions that may induce depression:
- CBC with differential
- Thyroid function tests
- Urine drug screen

> **BOX 29-4. Etiology of Major Depression**
>
> The etiology is unknown; however, there are many hypotheses, including the following:
>
> - Dysregulation of neurotransmitters
> - Decreased concentration of certain neurotransmitters
> - Genetic basis for the disorder
> - Certain medications
>   - Antihypertensives (e.g., reserpine, **propranolol**, **clonidine**, methyldopa)
>
> - Antiparkinsonian agents (e.g., levodopa, carbidopa, amantadine)
> - Hormonal agents (e.g., estrogens, progesterone)
> - Others, including corticosteroids, cycloserine, vinblastine, and vincristine
> - Certain medical conditions (e.g., recent myocardial infarction, chronic pain, cancer, multiple sclerosis) may also induce or worsen depression.
>
> **Boldface** indicates one of top 100 drugs for 2020 by prescription volume.

DSM-5 Diagnostic Criteria

At least 5 of the symptoms discussed earlier must be present nearly every day for a 2-week period and represent a change from previous functioning. At least 1 of the symptoms must be depressed mood or anhedonia.

Treatment Principles and Goals

Goals are as follows:

- Improve patient's quality of life and ability to function
- Reduce or eliminate target symptoms with an antidepressant
- Optimally, incorporate psychotherapy
- Prevent relapse

Although all antidepressants are equally effective in a given population, the following occurs:

- Response varies from person to person.
- Each differs in adverse effect and drug–drug interaction profiles.
- Drug selection should be based on patient-specific factors (e.g., accessibility, adverse effects, drug-interactions, previous treatment attempts).

Note: The FDA requires all antidepressant drugs to include boxed warnings about increased risk of suicidal ideation and behavior in children, adolescents, and young adults (up to age 24 years), and a medication guide highlighting these risks is to be distributed with each new or refilled prescription for antidepressants in this population.

Monitoring parameters

In the first week, the following should be noted:

- Trend toward normalization of appetite and sleep pattern

In the second to third week, the following should be noted:

- Increased energy
- Improved concentration and memory
- Improved somatic symptoms

Note: Risk for suicide increases at this time because the patient has the energy to carry out any ideations. This is often called the "danger period" when starting an antidepressant.

At 4 to 6 weeks, the following should be evident:

- Improved mood
- Decreased suicidal ideation
- Increased libido

Duration of therapy

Acute phase

The acute phase is usually 6 to 12 weeks or the length of time needed to stabilize depressive symptoms.

Maintenance phase

During this phase, maintain therapeutic doses of antidepressant. The duration is usually 1 year; antidepressant may be tapered for a period of time, but monitor for signs of relapse. The goal is to prevent relapse.

Prophylaxis

Chronic antidepressant therapy may be necessary for certain patients experiencing the following:

- A first-degree relative with bipolar disorder or recurrent depression
- Onset of depression before age 20 years or after age 60 years
- Recurrence of depression within 1 year after medication discontinuation
- Severe, sudden, or life-threatening depression requiring inpatient hospitalization

Drug Therapy

Tricyclic antidepressants

Mechanism of action

TCAs increase the synaptic concentration of 5-HT or NE in the CNS (i.e., TCAs inhibit the presynaptic neuronal membrane's reuptake of 5-HT or NE).

Adverse Effects (Box 29-5)

BOX 29-5. Adverse Effects of Tricyclic Antidepressants

Adverse effects include orthostatic hypotension, tachycardia, sedation, anticholinergic effects, arrhythmias (prolonged QT interval), weight gain, and sexual dysfunction.

Tertiary amines (e.g., **amitriptyline**, imipramine, doxepin, clomipramine) have more intense adverse effects compared to secondary amines (e.g., nortriptyline, desipramine).

Boldface indicates one of top 100 drugs for 2020 by prescription volume.

Contraindications

Concomitant use of a monoamine oxidase inhibitor (MAOI) within the past 14 days, during pregnancy or lactation, and with narrow-angle glaucoma is contraindicated.

Precautions

- Doses may be titrated to full dose range over 1 to 3 weeks.
- Many patients require half the usual dose because of sedative effects; however, for patients with insomnia, the sedating effects may be helpful.
- These agents can be lethal in overdose (block sinoatrial node in the heart).

- Use with caution in patients with cardiac conduction disturbances, seizure disorders, hyperthyroidism, and renal or hepatic impairment.
- Avoid abrupt withdrawal in patients with prolonged use.

Drug–drug interactions

- Co-administration of SSRIs, cimetidine, **diltiazem**, verapamil, labetalol, quinidine, haloperidol, or **methylphenidate** may increase serum drug concentration of TCAs through CYP450 inhibition, primarily 3A4 and 2D6.
- Co-administration of carbamazepine, phenytoin, or barbiturate may decrease serum drug concentration of TCAs by inducing CYP450 metabolism.
- Administration of MAOIs within 14 days may cause serotonin syndrome, a life-threatening syndrome similar to, and often misdiagnosed as, NMS characterized by neuromuscular hyperreactivity, hyperthermia, and altered mental status.
- Monitoring of blood pressure, pulse, ECG changes, and mental status changes is prudent. Drug serum monitoring are not commonly used in guiding therapy, but may be useful for **amitriptyline**, desipramine, imipramine, and nortriptyline.

TABLE 29-6. Selected Tricyclic Antidepressants

Drug	Trade name	Form	Indications	Initial dose	Dose range
Amitriptyline ⚠	Elavil	Tablets, injection (pregnancy category D)	Depression, chronic and neuropathic pain, migraine prophylaxis, peripheral neuropathy	50 to 75 mg/d	75 to 300 mg
Nortriptyline ⚠	Pamelor, Aventyl	Capsules, injection (pregnancy category D)	Depression, chronic pain	25 to 50 mg/d	40 to 200 mg
Doxepin ⚠	Sinequan, Silenor, Zonalon	Capsules, oral liquid, topical cream (pregnancy category C)	Depression; anxiety; insomnia; pruritis (cream); unlabeled: chronic and neuropathic pain	75 mg/d (in divided doses)	75 to 300 mg
Clomipramine ⚠	Anafranil	Capsules (pregnancy category C)	Obsessive-compulsive disorder, depression, panic attacks, chronic pain	25 to 100 mg daily, titrated up for 1 to 2 weeks	Usual effective dose 200 to 250 mg/d; maximum dose 250 mg because of dose-related increased risk of seizure

Boldface indicates one of top 100 drugs for 2020 by prescription volume.

 Amitriptyline *FDA BOXED WARNING*

Increased risk of suicidality, particularly in people under 24 years old. Not approved for pediatric use.

Nortriptyline *FDA BOXED WARNING*

Increased risk of suicidality, particularly in people under 24 years old. Not approved for pediatric use.

 Doxepin *FDA BOXED WARNING*

Increased risk of suicidality, particularly in people under 24 years old. Not approved for pediatric use.

 Clomipramine *FDA BOXED WARNING*

Increased risk of suicidality, particularly in people under 24 years old. Not approved for pediatric use.

Monoamine oxidase inhibitors

Table 29-7 summarizes information about MAOIs.

Mechanism of action

MAOIs increase the synaptic concentration of NE, 5-HT, and dopamine (DA) by inhibiting the breakdown enzyme monoamine oxidase.

Note: MAOIs may be useful for patients who do not respond to other antidepressants or for treatment of atypical depression, but they are rarely used because of the need for dietary restrictions, their adverse effect profile, and their potentially dangerous interactions with other medications.

TABLE 29-7. Monoamine Oxidase Inhibitors

Drug	Trade name	Form	Initial dose	Dose range
Phenelzine ⚠	Nardil	Tablets	15 mg 3 times daily (>16 years old); may increase as rapidly as tolerated to 90 mg/d	60 to 90 mg/d
Tranylcypromine ⚠	Parnate	Tablets	30 mg/d in divided doses; may increase by 10 mg/d every 1 to 3 weeks	30 to 60 mg/d
Selegiline ⚠	Emsam Patch	Transdermal patch	6 mg/24 h; may increase by 3 mg/24 h not less than every 2 weeks to maximum of 12 mg/24 h	6 mg/24 h to 12 mg/24 h

 Phenelzine *FDA BOXED WARNING*

Increased risk of suicidality, particularly in people under 24 years old. Not approved for pediatric use.

Tranylcypromine *FDA BOXED WARNING*

Increased risk of suicidality, particularly in people under 24 years old. Not approved for pediatric use. Avoid tyramine-containing foods due to risk of hypertensive crisis.

 Selegiline *FDA BOXED WARNING*

Increased risk of suicidality, particularly in people under 24 years old. Not approved for pediatric use.

Adverse effects (Box 29-6)

 BOX 29-6. Adverse Effects of MAOIs

Adverse effects include orthostatic hypotension, weight gain, sexual dysfunction, anticholinergic effects, and hypertensive crisis.

Contraindications

Be alert for renal or hepatic dysfunction, cardiovascular disease, and concomitant sympathomimetic therapy (e.g., pseudoephedrine, ephedra).

When a patient is switched from an MAOI to an SSRI, the MAOI must be discontinued 2 weeks before initiation of an SSRI to prevent serotonin syndrome. When a patient is switched from an SSRI to an MAOI, the SSRI must be discontinued 2 weeks before initiation of MAOI, with the exception of **fluoxetine**, which requires 5 weeks because of its long half-life.

Precautions

Be aware of drug–food interaction with tyramine-containing foods (e.g., red wine, aged cheeses, Marmite) for each MAOI with the exception of the low-dose (6 mg/24 h) selegiline patch. Excess tyramine can result in release of NE, leading to a hypertensive crisis.

Drug–drug interactions
- TCAs
- SSRIs
- Sympathomimetics
- Meperidine

Selective serotonin reuptake inhibitors

See Table 29-8 for information about SSRIs.

Mechanism of action

These agents selectively inhibit the reuptake of 5-HT.

All SSRIs should be tapered upon discontinuation of treatment (over 2 to 4 weeks). Adverse effects with abrupt withdrawal include flu-like symptoms, dizziness, nausea, tremor, anxiety, and palpitations. These withdrawal effects are less severe with **fluoxetine** because of its extended half-life. Other adverse effects of SSRIs can be found in Box 29-7.

TABLE 29-8. Selective Serotonin Reuptake Inhibitors

Drug	Trade name	Form	Initial dose	Usual dose	Clinical highlights
Citalopram ⚠	Celexa	Tablets, oral liquid	10 mg	20 to 40 mg/d; maximum dose 40 mg/d; >40 mg/d may cause QT prolongation. FDA issued revised recommendations for **citalopram** with maximum recommended dose of 20 mg for patients >60 years old.	Often preferred in geriatric patients; fewer drug interactions
Escitalopram ⚠	Lexapro	Tablets	10 mg	10 to 20 mg/d	S-isomer of **citalopram**; 20 mg Celexa = 10 mg Lexapro
Paroxetine ⚠	Paxil	Tablet, oral liquid	10 to 20 mg	10 to 40 mg; maximum dose 50 mg/d	Least-activating SSRI
	Paxil CR	Controlled-release tablets	12.5 to 25 mg	25 to 37.5 mg	CR formulation associated with fewer adverse effects; 10 mg Paxil = 12.5 mg Paxil CR
Fluoxetine ⚠	Prozac, Sarafem	Capsules, tablets, oral liquid	10 to 20 mg	20 to 80 mg/d	Longer half-life, so tapering unnecessary but must also wait longer before switching to MAOI (5 weeks); available in 90 mg capsule formulation given once weekly
Sertraline ⚠	Zoloft	Tablets, oral liquid	25 to 50 mg	50 to 100 mg/d; maximum dose 200 mg/d	Often used for geriatric patients; fewer drug interactions

Boldface indicates one of top 100 drugs for 2020 by prescription volume.

 Citalopram *FDA BOXED WARNING*

Increased risk of suicidality, particularly in people under 24 years old. Not approved for pediatric use.

 Escitalopram *FDA BOXED WARNING*

Increased risk of suicidality, particular in pediatric and young adult patients. Not approved for use under 12 years of age.

Paroxetine *FDA BOXED WARNING*

Increased risk of suicidality, particularly in pediatric and young adults.

 Fluoxetine *FDA BOXED WARNING*

Increased risk of suicidality, particularly in people under 24 years old. Not approved for use under 7 years of age.

 Sertraline *FDA BOXED WARNING*

Increased risk of suicidality, particularly in pediatric and young adults.

Adverse effects

 BOX 29-7. Adverse Effects of SSRIs

Effects include GI complaints, nervousness, insomnia, headache, fatigue, and sexual dysfunction, but SSRIs are safer in overdose than TCAs.

Drug–drug interactions

Drug–drug interactions exist with TCAs and MAOIs and among SSRIs. Interactions are variable depending on the SSRI. Reportedly, there are fewer drug–drug interactions with **escitalopram** and **citalopram**.

Serotonin–norepinephrine reuptake inhibitors

See Table 29-9 for information about serotonin–norepinephrine reuptake inhibitors (SNRIs).

Mechanism of action

These agents inhibit the reuptake of 5-HT and NE (and also DA at higher doses). Anticholinergic and antihistaminic effects are negligible. As the dose increases, NE and DA reuptake are more pronounced, which may lead to dose-dependent increase in heart rate and blood pressure.

Adverse effects (Box 29-8)

 BOX 29-8. Adverse Effects of SNRIs

Effects include GI upset, anxiety, insomnia, and headache. Elevation in blood pressure is possible; use with caution in patients with uncontrolled hypertension. Other adverse effects are similar to those of SSRIs. Withdrawal symptoms may occur if the medication is abruptly discontinued.

TABLE 29-9. Serotonin–Norepinephrine Reuptake Inhibitors

Drug	Trade name	Form	Initial dose	Maximum dose	Clinical highlights
Venlafaxine	Effexor	Capsules	37.5 mg twice daily	375 mg/d in divided doses	Take with food; monitor blood pressure.
	Effexor XR	Extended-release capsules	75 mg/d	225 mg/d	Extended-release formulation has less GI upset than immediate-release formulation; monitor blood pressure.
Desvenlafaxine	**Pristiq, Khedezla**	Extended-release tablets	50 mg/d	50 mg/d; CrCl < 30 mL/min every other day	Fewer drug interactions owing to conjugation; monitor blood pressure.
Duloxetine	Cymbalta	Capsules	30 mg/d	120 mg/d	Also used for diabetic peripheral neuropathy; monitor blood pressure.
Levomilnacipran	Fetzima	Extended-release capsules	20 mg/d	120 mg/d	Levomilnacipran is indicated for depression only. Counsel patient that alcohol may accelerate drug release from capsule.

Boldface indicates one of top 100 drugs for 2020 by prescription volume.
CrCl, creatinine clearance.

 Venlafaxine *FDA BOXED WARNING*

Increased risk of suicidality, particularly in people under 24 years old.

 Desvenlafaxine *FDA BOXED WARNING*

Increased risk of suicidality, particularly in people under 24 years old.

 Duloxetine *FDA BOXED WARNING*

Increased risk of suicidality, particularly in people under 24 years old.

 Levomilnacipran *FDA BOXED WARNING*

Increased risk of suicidality, particularly in people under 24 years old. Not approved for use in pediatric patients.

Drug–drug interactions

Serotonin syndrome may occur when SSRIs or SNRIs are used in combination with sibutramine, **sumatriptan**, **tramadol**, and **trazodone**. PT/INR (prothrombin time per international normalized ratio) elevations have been seen when **venlafaxine** is added to patients taking **warfarin**. All SSRIs and SNRIs may increase risk of abnormal bleeding when used with anticoagulants or nonsteroidal anti-inflammatory drugs. Desvenlafaxine is an active metabolite of **venlafaxine** and has fewer metabolic drug interactions. CYP450 1A2 inhibitors (e.g., cimetidine, quinolone antibiotics) and CYP450 2D6 inhibitors (e.g., **fluoxetine**, quinidine) increase **duloxetine** levels.

Bupropion (Wellbutrin, Wellbutrin SR, Wellbutrin XL, Forfivo XL, and Zyban)

Mechanism of action

Bupropion, an inhibitor of NE and DA reuptake (effects on 5-HT reuptake are minimal), is a norepinephrine–dopamine reuptake inhibitor.

Adverse effects (Box 29-9)

BOX 29-9. Adverse Effects of Bupropion	
GI upset	Headache
Insomnia	Psychosis (rare)
Anxiety	Lowering of seizure threshold

Drug–drug interactions

Cimetidine and ritonavir inhibit **bupropion** metabolism while CBZ induces **bupropion** metabolism.

Other aspects

There is an increased risk of seizure with **bupropion**, especially in patients with a seizure disorder, eating disorder, or electrolyte imbalance. The maximum daily dose is 450 mg (400 mg sustained release). Titrate the dose slowly to minimize seizure risk. **Bupropion** is marketed as Zyban for smoking cessation.

Trazodone (Desyrel) and trazodone extended release (Oleptro) ⚠

Mechanism of action

This agent inhibits 5-HT reuptake and blocks 5-HT2A receptors.

Adverse effects (Box 29-10)

BOX 29-10. Adverse Effects of Trazodone
Extreme sedation
Orthostatic hypotension
Priapism

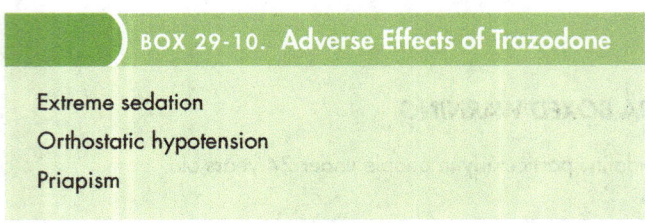

⚠ **Trazodone (Desyrel) and Trazodone Extended Release (Oleptro)**
FDA BOXED WARNINGS

Increased risk of suicidality. Not approved for use in pediatric patients.

Drug–drug interactions

Fluoxetine and ritonavir inhibit **trazodone** metabolism.

Other aspects

Because it causes excessive sedation, immediate-release **trazodone** is not often clinically used as an antidepressant; rather, it is commonly used to treat insomnia (usually dosed 25 to 150 mg at bedtime). Extended-release **trazodone** is dosed 150 to 375 mg daily at bedtime on an empty stomach.

Vilazodone (Viibryd) ⚠

Mechanism of action

Vilazodone's mechanism is similar to that of an SSRI and acts as a 5-HT1A partial agonist.

Adverse effects (Box 29-11)

BOX 29-11. Adverse Effects of Vilazodone	
Diarrhea	Insomnia
Nausea and vomiting	Decreased libido (less than with SSRIs and SNRIs)

Other aspects

Patient starter kit is used for dosing. Vilazodone should be dosed with food.

 Vilazodone (Viibryd) *FDA BOXED WARNING*

Increased risk of suicidality. Not approved for use in pediatric patients.

Mirtazapine (Remeron and Remeron SolTab) ⚠

Mirtazapine is also considered a first-line antidepressant in guidelines but is often used as second-line treatment because of adverse effects.

Mechanism of action

This agent antagonizes presynaptic alpha-2 autoreceptors and heteroreceptors that prevent the release of 5-HT and NE (resulting in increased 5-HT and NE in the synapses). It antagonizes 5-HT2A and 5-HT3 receptors, thereby resulting in less GI upset and less anxiety.

Adverse effects (Box 29-12)

BOX 29-12. Adverse Effects of Mirtazapine	
Sedation	Constipation
Increased appetite	Elevation in LFTs and increase in triglycerides may occur
Weight gain	Small risk of agranulocytosis or neutropenia

Mirtazapine (Remeron and Remeron SolTab) *FDA BOXED WARNING*

Increased risk of suicidality. Not approved for use in pediatric patients.

Vortioxetine (Trintellix)

Note: Name was changed to Trintellix from Brintellix because of name confusion with Brilinta (ticagrelor).

Mechanism of action

Vortioxetine inhibits reuptake of serotonin (5-HT); antagonizes 5-HT3, 5-HT1D, and 5-HT7 receptors; agonizes 5-HT1A receptors; and is a 5-HT1B receptor partial agonist.

Adverse effects (Box 29-13)

> **BOX 29-13. Adverse Effects of Vortioxetine**
>
> Nausea and vomiting
> Constipation

Other aspects

To avoid adverse effects, taper dose to 10 mg for 1 week before discontinuation.

 Vortioxetine (Trintellix) *FDA BOXED WARNING*

Increased risk of suicidality. Not approved for use in pediatric patients.

Aripiprazole (Abilify), quetiapine (Seroquel), brexpiprazole (Rexulti), and olanzapine/fluoxetine (Symbyax)

Aripiprazole, **quetiapine**, and brexpiprazole are approved for adjunct treatment of major depressive disorders. Olanzapine/**fluoxetine** is approved for treatment-resistant depression. Antipsychotic doses for the augmentation of antidepressant therapy are generally lower than doses used in the treatment of schizophrenia.

Adverse effects

See Section 29-3 on schizophrenia.

Esketamine (Spravato)

Nasal spray approved for the adjunct treatment of treatment-resistant major depressive disorder.

 Esketamine (Spravato) *FDA BOXED WARNING*

Risk of sedation, dissociation, abuse/misuse, and suicidality. Patients must be monitored in-clinic for at least 2 hours after administration.

Mechanism of action

Esketamine antagonizes the NMDA receptor.

Adverse effects (Box 29-14)

> **BOX 29-14. Adverse Effects of Esketamine**
>
> Nausea, dizziness, sedation, and dissociative disorder. Increased blood pressure has been reported, and caution is advised if systolic blood pressure is greater than 140 mmHg or diastolic greater than 90 mmHg before administration.

Other aspects

Esketamine is the s-enantiomer of ketamine, a known drug of abuse. Monitor for drug dependence, and use with caution in individuals with history of substance use disorder.

Nonpharmacologic Treatments

Psychotherapy

Psychotherapy is especially useful when combined with drug therapy.

Electroconvulsive therapy

Electroconvulsive therapy (ECT) is very safe and effective for treating depression. It is believed to physically "reset" receptors in the brain. ECT is usually reserved for refractory or psychotic patients. The procedure is administered every other day for 6 to 9 treatments. Maintenance treatment is variable for each patient, but ECT is usually administered monthly after acute treatment. Adverse effects include short-term memory loss and confusion on the day of treatment.

29-6 Anxiety Disorders

Anxiety disorders are serious, debilitating mental illnesses that include a group of conditions that share extreme anxiety as the primary mood disturbance.

Epidemiology

Anxiety disorders are the most common form of mental illness, affecting approximately 19.1% of adults in the United States. There is significant comorbidity with other psychiatric illnesses (e.g., substance abuse).

Types and Classifications

Generalized anxiety disorder

Generalized anxiety disorder (GAD) is characterized by unprovoked excessive worry and tension for more than 6 months and at least 3 of the following symptoms: restlessness, irritability, muscle tension, fatigue, sleep disturbances, and difficulty concentrating. GAD usually consumes the patient's day, affecting social and occupational functioning. Physical complaints (e.g., GI upset, headache, muscle tension, tremors, insomnia, fatigue) are common. Incidence of GAD is higher in females than in males.

Panic attacks and panic disorder

Panic attacks are characterized by feelings of terror that suddenly strike without warning and usually last for approximately 10 to 15 minutes.

Physical symptoms include increased heart rate, sweating, tremors, shortness of breath, chest pain, and dizziness. Patients feel a sense of dread or feel that they may die. Panic disorder is the resultant disorder after having more than 2 unexpected panic attacks and experiencing 1 of the following for more than 1 month: preoccupation with avoiding another attack, excessive worry about the consequences of another attack, or going to great lengths to avoid people, places, or things they associate with the panic attack.

Social anxiety disorder

Social anxiety disorder is characterized by feelings of anxiety in social situations (e.g., speaking in front of others, attending social gatherings). Patients feel as though everyone is staring at and judging them. People affected by social anxiety disorder usually do not seek treatment and may self-medicate with alcohol or other substances. There is equal male and female prevalence.

Substance-induced anxiety disorder

Anxiety symptoms are likely to be a direct result of use of an agent (e.g., amphetamines, toxin, medication). Symptoms may also occur with intoxication or withdrawal.

Associated features

High comorbidity exists with other psychiatric illnesses, especially depression. High comorbidity also exists with alcohol or substance abuse. This disorder is frequently associated with other chronic medical illnesses (e.g., chronic pain syndromes, long-term illnesses, GI distress, headaches).

Etiology

This disorder's etiology is presently unknown. Most current evidence suggests the cause is primarily biologic (imbalance of GABA, 5-HT, and NE) with genetic predisposition.

Drug Therapy

Benzodiazepines

Benzodiazepines (BZDs), the most commonly used anxiolytics, are described below. Additional dosing, pharmacokinetics, and metabolism information for commonly used benzodiazepines can be found in Table 29-10.

Mechanism of action

BZDs potentiate the actions of GABA by increasing the influx of chloride ions into neurons. One hypothesis is that, through their effects on neurons mediated by receptor complexes, BZDs reduce neuronal firing and, thus, the symptoms of anxiety.

TABLE 29-10. Benzodiazepines ⚠

Drug	Trade name	Time to peak plasma concentration (hours)	Half-life (hours)	Usual daily dose (mg/d)	Metabolic pathway
Alprazolam	Xanax, Xanax XR,	1 to 2	12 to 15	0.5 to 4	Oxidation
Chlordiazepoxide	Librium	2 to 4	5 to 30	5 to 200	Oxidation
Clonazepam	Klonopin	1 to 2	18 to 50	1 to 3	Nitro reduction
Diazepam	Valium	0.5 to 2	20 to 80	2 to 40	Oxidation
Lorazepam	Ativan	1 to 6	10 to 20	2 to 6	Conjugation
Oxazepam	Serax	2 to 4	5 to 20	30 to 120	Conjugation
Temazepam	Restoril	2 to 3	10 to 40	15 to 30	Conjugation

Boldface indicates one of top 100 drugs for 2020 by prescription volume.

Benzodiazepines *FDA BOXED WARNING*

Increased risk of profound sedation if use concomitantly with opioids. Risk of abuse, misuse, addiction, physical dependence, and withdrawal reactions.

Note: The rate of absorption varies with BZDs. The more lipophilic compounds (i.e., **alprazolam** , diazepam ⚠, clorazepate ⚠, flurazepam ⚠) are rapidly absorbed and result in quicker onset of action. The less lipophilic BZDs are chlordiazepoxide, **clonazepam**, and **lorazepam**.

Adverse effects (Box 29-15)

> **BOX 29-15. Adverse Effects of Benzodiazepines**
>
> Sedation, dizziness, confusion, blurred vision, diplopia, syncope, residual daytime sedation, and reduced psychomotor and cognitive dysfunction.

Metabolism

Lorazepam, oxazepam, and temazepam are metabolized through conjugation and are, therefore, preferred in patients with hepatic dysfunction and the elderly.

Drug–drug interactions

BZDs metabolized by CYP450 3A4 (e.g., **alprazolam**, diazepam, triazolam) have decreased clearance if taken concomitantly with CYP450 3A4 inhibitors (e.g., ketoconazole, erythromycin, nefazodone). BZDs are deadly in overdose or if taken concomitantly with alcohol.

Precautions

- BZDs may cause a paradoxical reaction in children, cognitively impaired elderly patients, developmentally or intellectually disabled patients, and post–head injury patients, leading to increased aggression or agitation.
- Never abruptly discontinue BZDs because doing so may precipitate status epilepticus. Always taper the dose to avoid seizure risk and withdrawal symptoms.
- In elderly patients, the BZDs of choice are those that are conjugated (**lorazepam**, oxazepam, and temazepam). There is an increased risk of falls in this population.
- Avoiding use of BZDs in pregnancy (especially first trimester) is best because of risk of cleft palate. BZDs are also present in breast milk and should be avoided in nursing females.
- The abuse potential is great; BZDs are not recommended for patients with a history of substance use disorders. BZDs should be used at the lowest effective dose and for the shortest amount of time necessary. BZDs are not recommended for long-term use.
- Tolerance is common, and increased doses are needed to control anxiety levels.

 Alprazolam, Diazepam, Clorazepate, and Flurazepam *FDA BOXED WARNINGS*

Increased risk of profound sedation if use concomitantly with opioids. Risk of abuse, misuse, addiction, physical dependence, and withdrawal reactions.

- Chlordiazepoxide and diazepam are also preferred for alcohol withdrawal treatment because of their long half-lives and self-tapering ability.
- **Alprazolam** extended release (Xanax XR) is dosed once daily; do not crush, chew, or break doses. It is also available as an orally disintegrating tablet.

Buspirone (BuSpar)

Mechanism of action

The mechanism of action is poorly understood; 5-HT1A is a partial agonist, and **buspirone** reportedly stimulates presynaptic 5-HT1A receptors. In addition, the agent has a moderate affinity for D2 receptors. **Buspirone** does not interact with the BZD-GABA receptor complex. Onset of anxiolytic effect is longer for **buspirone** than for BZD (2 to 3 weeks).

Adverse effects (Box 29-16)

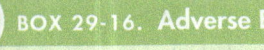

BOX 29-16. Adverse Effects of Buspirone

GI upset, headache, and nervousness.

Benefits

Possible benefits of **buspirone** over BZDs are as follows:

- Usually less sedating than BZDs
- Little to no psychomotor or cognitive impairment
- No association with withdrawal symptoms, abuse, or physical dependence
- Not cross-tolerant with BZDs or alcohol

Antidepressants as treatment for anxiety disorders

SSRIs and SNRIs are a first-line treatment for many anxiety disorders, especially in patients with comorbid depression and substance use disorders. Specific anxiety indication may vary by agent.

TCAs are usually a third-line treatment because of adverse effects and the danger of overdose.

MAOIs are usually a third-line treatment because of adverse effects and drug–food interactions.

Titrate doses of antidepressants slowly to decrease risk of initial anxiety symptoms. Often, maintenance doses of antidepressants are higher for anxiety than for depression.

Other classes of drugs used to treat anxiety disorders

Beta blockers (e.g., **propranolol**, **atenolol**) ease peripheral symptoms of anxiety and may be useful for panic disorders, social anxiety disorder, and performance anxiety.

Hydroxyzine reduces anxiety and is often used in patients with substance abuse issues. Nonpharmacological options for anxiety can be found in Box 29-17.

BOX 29-17. Nonpharmacologic Treatment of Anxiety Disorders

- Supportive psychotherapy (individual, group, family)
- Cognitive behavioral therapy
- Focus on coping with the fear of the symptoms of anxiety
- Relaxation techniques
- Exercise and lifestyle modifications (reduced caffeine and simple sugars)

29-7 Eating Disorders

Anorexia and Bulimia

Anorexia nervosa

Characteristics

Patients suffering from anorexia nervosa refuse to maintain body weight at or above a minimal, normal weight for their age and height (85% or less of expected body weight). They experience intense fear of gaining weight or becoming fat, although they are underweight. There is a disturbance in self-perception of body weight, size, proportion, and attractiveness.

Types

- Restricting
- Binge eating and purging

Bulimia nervosa

Characteristics

Recurrent episodes of binge eating occur (often followed by intense feelings of guilt). The patient may consume as much as 5000 to 20,000 calories over 2 to 8 hours. Recurrent and inappropriate compensatory behavior occurs to prevent weight gain.

A person binge eats at least once weekly for 3 months. Self-evaluation is primarily influenced by body shape and weight.

Types

- Purging (vomiting, abuse of laxatives or diuretics)
- Nonpurging (excessive exercise, fasting)

Prevalence

Eating disorders are most commonly seen in White, middle- to upper-class females.

The age of onset for anorexia nervosa is 13 to 20 years old. The male-to-female ratio is 1:10 to 20. For bulimia nervosa, the age of onset is 16 to 18 years old, and the male-to-female ratio is 1:10.

Medical Complications and Signs of Disease

- Eating disorders produce states of semistarvation and noticeable malnutrition, especially in anorexia.
- In bulimia, patients are more difficult to identify because they are commonly of normal body weight.
- Dehydration occurs.
- There is a high incidence of comorbid anxiety, depression, obsessive-compulsive disorder (OCD), and substance abuse.
- Dental caries and enamel erosion occur because of stomach acid exposure.
- Calluses on the dorsum of the hand or fingers develop because of induction of vomiting.
- Mortality rate is about 10% from starvation (primarily because of electrolyte imbalances), arrhythmia, or suicide.
- Long-term complications include endocrine or metabolic, cardiovascular, renal, gastroenterological, hematological, pulmonary, musculoskeletal, immunological, and dermatological issues.

Treatment

Psychotherapy is the mainstay of treatment. Therapy can be individual, group, family, supportive, cognitive behavioral, or insight oriented. Primary objectives are to define and examine the extent of the problem. The patient learns to accept the condition, and treatment results in a reconstruction of self-identity and self-confidence.

Dietary intake is slowly normalized with the goal of restoring normal body weight. Nutritional counseling is used. Distorted ideas about caloric intake and body shape are corrected.

Relapse prevention focuses on developing and using coping mechanisms and avoiding high-risk situations.

Drug Therapy

SSRIs are primarily used and may be more effective for patients with bulimia. Antidepressants do not appear to be beneficial in helping severely malnourished patients with anorexia nervosa gain weight, but they may help patients maintain weight after it has been gained. SSRIs may decrease binge–purge behavior, anxiety, obsessions, impulsivity, and depression symptoms. Low doses of olanzapine and **quetiapine** may improve weight gain and psychological symptoms in anorexia nervosa. Low-dose, short-acting BZDs have been shown to be beneficial in patients with severe anxiety associated with eating.

Fluoxetine (Prozac) is the only FDA-indicated medication for the treatment of bulimia nervosa. Higher doses are used; titrate to 60 to 80 mg/d every morning. **Bupropion** is contraindicated in bulimia nervosa because of seizure risk.

Lisdexamfetamine (Vyvanse) is FDA-approved for moderate to severe binge-eating disorder. Doses start at 30 mg once daily and can be titrated up at weekly intervals to a maximum dose of 70 mg/d. Counseling points for **lisdexamfetamine** are similar to other stimulants approved for attention-deficit/hyperactivity disorder.

Topiramate (Topamax) and zonisamide (Zonegran) may be beneficial in binge-eating disorder and bulimia nervosa, but evidence is limited and they are not FDA approved.

Ideally, treatment of eating disorders includes both psychotherapy and pharmacotherapy.

> ⚠ **Lisdexamfetamine (Vyvanse)** *FDA BOXED WARNING*
>
> High potential for abuse and dependence.

29-8 Sleep Disorders

Sleep disorders affect 70 million Americans and are the most frequent health care complaint. Failure to maintain a healthy sleep pattern contributes to poor health and possible development of chronic conditions such as depression and cardiovascular disease. The primary sleep disorders that prescription medications are used to treat are insomnia, narcolepsy, and restless leg syndrome.

Insomnia

Insomnia is characterized by the inability to initiate sleep, remain asleep, or return to sleep resulting in poor quality of sleep for at least 3 nights per week for at least 3 months. This contributes to daytime somnolence, fatigue, irritability, and decreased concentration.

Epidemiology

Insomnia is the most common sleep-wake disorder, affecting more than one-third of all adults. It is twice as likely to occur in women as in men. Concurrently, 40% of patients with insomnia are likely to have a psychiatric disorder. See Box 29-18 for substances that may induce or worsen insomnia, and Box 29-19 includes the clinical presentation of insomnia.

Treatment principles and goals

Patients must be assessed for underlying cause of insomnia such as a comorbid condition. Patients must also be assessed for any behaviors or substances that could be contributing. Therapy should be started with nonpharmacologic options before the use of medications is considered. Treatment goals can be found in Box 29-20.

Drug therapy

Antihistamines

Agents

- Doxylamine (Unisom, Nitetime Sleep Aid)
- Diphenhydramine (Benadryl, Nytol, Sominex, ZzzQuil)

Mechanism of action

Antihistamines block H1 receptors in the CNS. The over-the-counter, first-generation antihistamines diphenhydramine and doxylamine are used for insomnia but should be recommended for short-term use only.

BOX 29-18. Substances That May Induce or Worsen Insomnia

- Antidepressants
- Stimulants
- Decongestants
- Narcotic analgesics
- Cardiovascular medications
- Pulmonary medications
- Alcohol

BOX 29-19. Clinical Presentation of Insomnia

- Frequent or early morning awakening
- Disturbed quality of sleep with unusual or troublesome dreams
- Difficulty falling asleep
- Inability to fall back to sleep
- Impairment of daytime functioning
- Anxiety, fatigue, irritability, depression, memory impairment

---

BOX 29-20. Treatment Goals for Insomnia

- Improvement in sleep quality, duration, or both
- Improvement of daytime impairments
- Improvement in insomnia symptoms
- Formation of a positive and clear association between the bed and sleeping
- Improvement in sleep-related psychological distress
- Avoidance of adverse effects from selected therapies

Antihistamines can cause dry mouth, constipation, blurred vision, and other anticholinergic adverse effects. Maximum sedation occurs 3 to 6 hours after dosing. Tolerance to sedative effect occurs after 4 days of repeated use and may begin to have a paradoxical effect. Diphenhydramine has a greater pool of evidence supporting efficacy and is available in a variety of formulations leading it to be the more preferred agent.

Melatonin receptor agonists

See Table 29-11.

Agents

- Ramelteon (Rozerem)
- Tasimelteon (Hetlioz)
- Melatonin (OTC)

Mechanism of action

These agents regulate circadian rhythm through agonism of melatonin receptor subtypes MT1 and MT2. With either medication, onset of efficacy may take 3 to 5 weeks.

Tasimelteon is approved for non-24-hour sleep-wake disorder, which is caused by the patient's circadian rhythm differing from the normal day, common in people who are totally blind.

Sedating antidepressants

See Section 29-5 on major depressive disorder.

Agents

- Doxepin (Silenor)
- **Amitriptyline** (Elavil)
- **Trazodone** (Desyrel, Oleptro)
- Mirtazapine (Remeron)

Mechanism of action

These agents block H1 receptors within the CNS. Use of antidepressants for insomnia has not been well studied and should be used cautiously because of the risk of adverse effects. Dosing for these medications for insomnia is often lower than doses typically used for depression. The adverse effect profile for these medications is quite extensive and requires close monitoring.

Non-benzodiazepine receptor agonists

See Table 29-12.

Agents

- **Zolpidem** (Ambien, Ambien CR, Edluar, Intermezzo, Zolpimist)
- Zaleplon (Sonata)
- Eszopiclone (Lunesta)

TABLE 29-11. Melatonin Receptor Agonists

Drug	Trade name	Form	Usual dose	Adverse effects	Clinical highlights
Ramelteon	Rozerem	Tablets	8 mg nightly	Dizziness, somnolence, fatigue, worsened insomnia	Consider use when traditional hypnotics cannot be used.
Tasimelteon	Hetlioz	Capsules	5 to 10 mg nightly	Headache, abnormal dreams, urinary tract infection	Medication may take weeks or months to work owing to differences in circadian rhythms.

TABLE 29-12. Nonbenzodiazepine Receptor Agonists

Drug	Trade name	Form	Usual dose	Adverse effects	Clinical highlights
Zolpidem	Ambien	Tablets	5 to 10 mg nightly	Class effects: somnolence, dizziness, ataxia, parasomnias, dysgeusia	For sleep onset
	Ambien CR	Controlled-release tablets	6.25 to 12.5 nightly		For sleep onset
	Edluar SL tabs	Sublingual tabs	5 to 10 mg nightly		For sleep onset and awakenings
	Intermezzo SL	Sublingual tabs	1.75 mg for females, 3.5 mg for males		For sleep onset and awakenings
Zaleplon	Sonata	Capsules	5 to 10 mg nightly		Indicated for sleep onset and awakenings
Eszopiclone	Lunesta	Tablets	1 to 3 mg nightly		Indicated for sleep maintenance

Boldface indicates one of top 100 drugs for 2020 by prescription volume.

Mechanism of action

These agents selectively bind to GABA-A receptors to induce sleepiness. The nonbenzodiazepines are preferred over benzodiazepines because of lessened potential for abuse and dependency. Current guidelines recommend treatment for 2 to 4 weeks, then reevaluation. Chronic use of these medications is discouraged because of the lack of evidence of success and the potential for dependency. Discontinuation of therapy can result in rebound insomnia, typically lasting 1 to 3 days. Slowly tapering off the medication and initiating cognitive-behavioral therapy is the preferred method of discontinuation.

Benzodiazepines

Agents

- Estazolam (ProSom)
- Flurazepam (Dalmane)
- Quazepam (Doral)
- Temazepam (Restoril)
- Triazolam (Halcion)

Mechanism of action

These agents potentiate the GABA-A receptor and increase GABA levels. Because of the risk of abuse and dependence, BZDs are not recommended for patients unless other options have failed. Patients who are indicated for treatment are to take the lowest effective dose for the shortest duration. Elderly patients are particularly at risk for psychomotor and cognitive adverse effects, and their use should be closely monitored.

Orexin receptor antagonist

- Suvorexant (Belsomra)

Mechanism of action

Suvorexant antagonizes both orexin A and orexin B peptides that promote wakefulness and regulate the sleep-wake cycle. Adverse effects of headache, sleep paralysis, and next-day sleepiness have been reported. Avoid in hepatic impairment.

See Box 29-21 for some nonpharmacological options for insomnia.

Treatment strategies

- Identify and manage medical, psychiatric, and pharmacologic causes.
- Assess patient demographics, drug interactions, abuse potential, and comorbidities.

> ### BOX 29-21. Nonpharmacologic Therapy for Insomnia

- Cognitive behavioral therapy
- Stimulus control therapy
- Sleep hygiene
  - Exercise routinely but not within 4 hours of bedtime.

- Maintain a comfortable sleep environment.
- Avoid alcohol, caffeine, and nicotine.
- Find a relaxing and enjoyable activity before bedtime.

- Implement a trial of sleep hygiene.
- Determine the type of problem to be able to select the correct treatment approach:
  - *Onset:* Short-duration agent with a rapid onset
  - *Maintenance:* Intermediate-duration agent
  - *Awakenings:* Short duration with rapid onset or intermediate to long duration

Narcolepsy

Narcolepsy is characterized as excessive daytime somnolence with symptoms related to an intrusion of rapid eye movement (REM) sleep that causes sudden daytime bouts of sleep onset. The hallmarks of narcolepsy are cataplexy, hypnagogic hallucinations, and sleep paralysis. Genetic disorders, autoimmune disorders, brain lesions, and other disorders that result in orexin deficiency are thought to cause narcolepsy. HLA haplotype DQB1*0602 is found in approximately 90% of narcolepsy cases, and its presence increases the risk of narcolepsy 200-fold.

Epidemiology

Patients living with narcolepsy have difficulty managing work, school, and other activities of normal day-to-day life because of excessive daytime sleepiness. Narcolepsy affects 0.03% to 0.06% of adult Americans, is most commonly seen in men, and often increases in severity with age.

Clinical presentation

- Excessive daytime somnolence with sudden onset (i.e., sleep attacks)
- Cataplexy (emotionally triggered muscle weakness)
- Hypnagogic hallucinations (strong, vivid hallucinations that occur as the patient falls asleep)
- Sleep paralysis (complete inability to move for 1 to 2 minutes after waking)

Treatment principles or goals

Reduce symptoms that adversely affect quality of life. Use treatment to return normal function to the patient in all aspects of life.

Drug therapy

Nonamphetamine stimulants

Table 29-13 lists and describes nonamphetamine stimulants.

Agents

- Modafinil (Provigil)
- Armodafinil (Nuvigil)

TABLE 29-13. Nonamphetamine Stimulants

Drug	Trade name	Form	Usual dose	Adverse effects	Clinical highlights
Modafinil	Provigil	Tablets	200 to 400 mg/d	Headache, dizziness, anxiety, agitation, severe rash	Indicated for narcolepsy with excessive daytime somnolence C-IV
Armodafinil	Nuvigil	Tablets	150 to 250 mg/d	Similar adverse effects to modafinil, including severe rash	Indicated for narcolepsy with excessive daytime somnolence R-isomer of modafinil C-IV

C-IV, Schedule IV under the Controlled Substances Act.

Mechanism of action

These agents inhibit DA reuptake by binding to the DA transporter. They may also stimulate orexin-containing neurons in the hypothalamus and are considered first-line treatment for excessive daytime sleepiness.

CNS depressants

Agent

Sodium oxybate (Xyrem)

Mechanism of action

Although the exact mechanism is unknown, sodium oxybate is taken at night and is thought to allow restructuring of sleep architecture to resemble normal sleeping patterns. It is the only FDA-approved agent for cataplexy.

Patient takes first dose (2.25 g in ¼ cup of water) at bedtime at least 2 hours after a meal and then repeats the dose 2.5 to 4 hours later. The target dose range for Xyrem is 6 to 9 g per night. Dose adjustments are needed for patients with hepatic impairment and for patients currently taking divalproex sodium.

Instruct patients to take their doses while in bed and to lie down after taking their dose. Patients can fall asleep within 5 to 15 minutes and may not feel drowsy first.

Amphetamine stimulants

Agents

- **Dextroamphetamine** (Dexedrine)
- **Methylphenidate** (Methylin, Ritalin, Metadate ER, Ritalin SR)

Mechanism of action

These agents cause release of DA and NE to promote wakefulness.

Antidepressants

See Section–29-5 on major depressive disorder.

⚠ **Dextroamphetamine (Dexedrine)** *FDA BOXED WARNING*

High potential for abuse and dependence. Misuse may cause sudden death and serious cardiovascular events.

Agents

- **Venlafaxine** (Effexor)
- **Fluoxetine** (Prozac)
- Solriamfetol (Sunosi)

Mechanism of action

Antidepressants increase noradrenergic and serotonergic signaling that is thought to suppress REM sleep and reduce cataplexy. Solriamfetol is a selective NE-DA reuptake inhibitor approved for excessive sleepiness with narcolepsy and obstructive sleep apnea. Solriamfetol should be avoided in patients with uncontrolled hypertension or end-stage kidney disease.

Histamine Inverse Agonist

- Pitolisant (Wakix)

Mechanism of action

Pitolisant is a H3 receptor inverse agonist approved for daytime sleepiness with narcolepsy. It may also reduce cataplexy. Common adverse effects include nausea, headache, and anxiety and may also cause QT prolongation.

Treatment strategies

- Indication—excessive daytime somnolence
  - First line: Modafinil or armodafinil, solriamfetol
  - Second line: **Dextroamphetamine** or **methylphenidate**, pitolisant
  - Third line: Sodium oxybate
- Indication—cataplexy
  - First line: **Venlafaxine** or **fluoxetine**
  - Second line: Sodium oxybate

Restless Leg Syndrome

Restless leg syndrome (RLS) is the persistent urge to move the lower legs. RLS worsens at night and is relieved by movement. The clinical presentation can be found in Box 29-22. It is thought to be caused by dysregulation of DA in the basal ganglia. RLS occurs more frequently in the elderly (approximately 10% to 20% of adults over 60 years of age). It may be associated with chronic inflammatory disease, iron deficiency, or psychotropic medications such as SSRIs, SNRIs, lithium, and antidopaminergic medications such as antipsychotics.

Drug therapy

For RLS, DA agonists are the first-line therapy, but only the immediate release formulations of pramipexole and ropinirole and rotigotine transdermal patch are FDA approved (Table 29-14). These medications should be taken 1 to 3 hours before bedtime, and their dosing should be titrated up for maximum efficacy and tolerability. Adverse effects for DA agonists include orthostasis, somnolence, and nausea. **Gabapentin** is also approved for RLS.

> **BOX 29-22. Clinical Presentation of Restless Leg Syndrome**

- Urge to move the legs that is typically associated with paresthesia or dysesthesia
- Symptoms that start or become worse at rest
- Partial relief obtained from physical activity
- Worsening of symptoms at night

TABLE 29-14. Dopamine Agonists Used for Restless Leg Syndrome

Drug	Trade name	Form	Usual dose	Adverse effects	Clinical highlights
Ropinirole	Requip	Tablets	0.25 mg 1 to 3 hours before bedtime	Nausea, vomiting, confusion, dizziness, orthostatic hypotension, edema, decreased prolactin levels	Mainstay of restless leg syndrome
Pramipexole	Mirapex	Tablets	0.125 mg 2 to 3 hours before bedtime		Can be titrated up by 0.125 mg every 7 days to a maximum of 3 mg/d
Rotigotine	Neupro	Transdermal patch	1 mg/24 h initially, may increase by 1 mg/24 h weekly to max of 3 mg/24 h	Application site reactions, nausea, vomiting, dizziness, orthostasis	Approved for moderate-to-severe restless legs syndrome and Parkinson's disease. Higher doses are often used for Parkinson's disease (maximum is 8 mg/24 h).

29-9 Pharmacist's Role

Pharmacists can make a meaningful impact on mental health and sleep care in multiple treatment settings. Within the acute care setting, pharmacists can play a role in identifying and resolving psychotropic drug-related issues including, but not limited to, drug–drug interactions, drug–food interactions, ordering and interpreting pertinent laboratory data, and performing medication reconciliation. Pharmacists that practice in the community pharmacy setting play a crucial role in determining that psychotropic medications are being used for appropriate indications, that the medication regimens are being adhered to, and provide critical counseling to patients regarding their medications. Lastly, those pharmacists working in ambulatory care settings can identify if patients are experiencing drug-related adverse effects, access issues, or any other issues that may impact a patient's ability to meet their treatment goals.

NAPLEX Competency Statements

The questions in this chapter cover the following 2021 NAPLEX Competency Statements: **AREA 1:** 1.2; 1.3; 1.4; 1.5; 1.6; 1.7 **AREA 2:** 2.1; 2.2; 2.3; 2.4 **AREA 3:** 3.2; 3.3; 3.4; 3.5; 3.6; 3.7; 3.8; 3.9; 3.10; 3.11; 3.12.

29-10 Questions

1. S. J. is a 30-year-old White female with a 10-year history of schizophrenia. Her current therapy includes haloperidol 10 mg orally twice daily. Her psychiatrist wants to convert her to haloperidol decanoate. What would be the appropriate equivalent monthly dose of haloperidol decanoate?

   A. 100 mg
   B. 10 mg
   C. 500 mg
   D. 200 mg
   E. 12.5 mg

2. B. T. reports to the nursing station with his head pulled sharply to the side and rear. He complains of severe pain in his neck and back area. The most appropriate diagnosis and treatment would be which of the following?

   A. Akathisia; propranolol 20 mg I.M. until resolution
   B. Dystonic reaction; diphenhydramine 50 mg I.M. every 30 minutes until resolution
   C. Tardive dyskinesia; physical therapy
   D. Dystonic reaction; lorazepam 2 mg I.M. every 30 minutes until resolution
   E. None of the above

3. A 30-year-old patient with schizophrenia was receiving risperidone 3 mg twice daily for 12 weeks with very little response. She is currently taking quetiapine 400 mg twice daily for 12 weeks with little to no response. Which of the following recommendations is best for this patient?

A. Increase quetiapine dose to 600 mg twice daily.
B. Switch the patient to clozapine.
C. Add risperidone 3 mg twice daily to quetiapine.
D. Add fluoxetine and ECT.
E. Continue current therapy.

Use the following patient profile to answer Question 4.

4. Marvin presented to the emergency department complaining of stiffness and thinks he may have "the flu." After reviewing his profile, which recommendations should you make?

A. Discontinue oral fluphenazine and begin quetiapine.
B. Discontinue oral fluphenazine.
C. Continue oral fluphenazine and add bromocriptine.
D. Discontinue oral fluphenazine, and give fluphenazine decanoate 25 mg I.M. stat.
E. Do nothing; labs need to be evaluated first.

5. What class of medications has been shown to induce mania in patients with bipolar disorder?

A. Antidepressants
B. Antipsychotics
C. Mood stabilizers
D. Calcium channel blockers
E. Antibiotics

6. Which of the following is a common adverse effect of lithium?

A. Polyuria
B. Weight loss
C. Elevated hepatic enzymes
D. Akathisia
E. Euphoria

7. Which of the following statements is correct regarding the treatment of bipolar disorder?

A. Lithium and divalproex sodium are considered first-line therapy options for mood stabilization.
B. When treating a patient with lithium, one must monitor the WBC and ANC because of lithium's propensity to cause agranulocytosis.
C. Patients diagnosed with bipolar I disorder exhibit episodes of mania at all times.
D. Patients with bipolar I disorder can be successfully treated with antidepressants alone.
E. Symptoms associated with mild lithium toxicity are likely to occur when serum drug concentration is greater than 3 mEq/L.

PATIENT PROFILE

Patient name: Marvin Culpepper   **Height:** 5'6"

Age: 58   **Weight:** 190 lb

Sex: Male   **Allergies:** None

Diagnosis: Schizophrenia, hepatitis C

Current medications: Fluphenazine 10 mg orally 3 times daily

Laboratory and diagnostic tests

1/13/2020

BP: 176/110 mmHg

HR: 128 bpm

Temp: 102.1 degrees F

RR: 12 rpm

Sodium: 142 mEq/L   Calcium: 9.1 mg/dL

Potassium: 4.5 mEq/L   Glucose: 110 mg/dL

Chloride: 105 mEq/L   Creatinine: 2.12 mg/dL

Carbon Dioxide: 21 mEq/L   WBC: 19,000

8. Which of the following medications has a boxed warning for severe rashes, including Stevens–Johnson syndrome?

A. Olanzapine
B. Topiramate
C. Oxcarbazepine
D. Lamotrigine
E. Divalproex

Use the following patient profile to answer Questions 9 and 10.

9. Which additional laboratory tests should be completed before initiation of divalproex sodium for Mr. Jacob's bipolar disorder diagnosis? (Mark all that apply.)

A. Liver function tests
B. Thyroid panel
C. Electrocardiogram
D. CBC with differential
E. Ammonia level

10. Mr. Jacob's medication for hypertension, lisinopril, is likely to _____.

A. Decrease lithium levels
B. Increase lithium levels
C. Decrease valproic acid levels
D. Increase valproic acid levels
E. Have no effect on lithium or valproic acid levels

11. Which of the following antidepressants is well known for lowering the seizure threshold?

A. Fluoxetine
B. Bupropion
C. Venlafaxine
D. Mirtazapine
E. Selegiline

PATIENT PROFILE

Patient name: Henry Jacobs
Age: 34
Sex: Male
Diagnosis: Bipolar I disorder, most recent episode manic
Alcohol dependence
Hypertension
Current medications: Lisinopril 10 mg orally daily

Height: 6'0"
Weight: 205 lb
Allergies: Sulfa

Laboratory and diagnostic tests

1/13/2020

BP: 138/86 mmHg
HR: 87 bpm
Temp: 97.5 degrees F
RR: 12 rpm
Sodium: 142 mEq/L
Potassium: 4.7 mEq/L
Chloride: 106 mEq/L
Carbon dioxide: 21 mEq/L

Calcium: 9.0 mg/dL
Glucose (fasting): 70 mg/dL
Creatinine: 0.86 mg/dL

12. A 29-year-old depressed Black female has shown little improvement with fluoxetine treatment, so the psychiatrist decides to change her medication to tranylcypromine. What is your recommendation for the switch?

A. Gradually decrease fluoxetine dosage over a 4-week period, and then start tranylcypromine.
B. Wait 2 weeks after stopping fluoxetine, and then begin tranylcypromine.
C. Over 6 weeks, gradually decrease fluoxetine dosage as you gradually increase the tranylcypromine dosage.
D. Wait 5 weeks after stopping fluoxetine before initiating tranylcypromine.
E. Maintain fluoxetine dosage, and start tranylcypromine; stop the fluoxetine when the tranylcypromine has achieved a therapeutic level.

13. Which of the following has been shown to induce or worsen depression?

A. Propranolol
B. Amoxicillin
C. Thiamine
D. Methylphenidate
E. Phenelzine

Use the following case to answer the next 2 questions:

K. Y. is a 36-year-old female admitted to your mental health facility for the fifth time in the past 3 years for major depressive disorder. She presents with lack of appetite, avolition, anhedonia, and suicidal ideations with a plan. Vitals include BP 127/76 mmHg, P 82, R 18, T 98.6°F. Labs include TSH 4, FBG (fasting blood glucose) 135, (–) UDS (urine drug screen), and BAL (blood alcohol level) 0. Her current medications are fluoxetine 40 mg daily, metformin 1000 mg twice daily, and hydroxyzine 25 mg 3 times daily. K. Y. states compliance and denies adverse effects. Past medications include citalopram and venlafaxine.

14. What is the most likely indication for the use of hydroxyzine in this patient?

A. Pruritus
B. Anxiety
C. Hypertension
D. Appetite enhancement
E. Diabetes

15. The psychiatrist asks for your recommendation for K. Y.'s refractory depression. What is the best option?

A. Discontinue fluoxetine, and initiate desvenlafaxine.
B. Discontinue fluoxetine, wait 2 weeks, and start selegiline.
C. Add aripiprazole to current regimen.
D. Discontinue fluoxetine, and start escitalopram.
E. Add oxazepam to current regimen.

16. Which of the following classes of antidepressants is rarely used in routine treatment of depression because of strict dietary restrictions and dangerous drug interactions?

A. SSRIs
B. SNRIs
C. TCAs
D. MAOIs
E. Atypical antidepressants

17. Which of the following statements regarding the use of SSRIs in anxiety disorders is most accurate?

A. SSRIs are not usually effective in the treatment of anxiety.
B. Initial SSRI doses for anxiety should be lower than initial doses for depression.
C. SSRIs should be used only after a failed treatment trial with benzodiazepines.
D. SSRIs may be used on an as-needed basis when anxiety symptoms emerge.
E. SSRIs work very rapidly to resolve symptoms of anxiety.

18. Which of the following benzodiazepines is preferred in the elderly or patients with hepatic dysfunction? (Mark all that apply.)

A. Chlordiazepoxide
B. Clonazepam
C. Alprazolam
D. Lorazepam
E. Oxazepam

19. Which of the following is FDA approved for the treatment of moderate-to-severe binge-eating disorder?

A. Bupropion
B. Sertraline
C. Citalopram
D. Lisdexamfetamine
E. Fluoxetine

20. Which of the following is the most appropriate treatment for bulimia nervosa?

   A. Insight-oriented therapy
   B. Fluoxetine 20 mg daily
   C. Fluoxetine 60 mg every morning + cognitive behavioral therapy
   D. Olanzapine 10 mg at bedtime
   E. Olanzapine 20 mg at bedtime + family therapy

21. Which medication is most closely linked to insomnia?

   A. Nortriptyline
   B. Ethinyl/norgestimate
   C. Cetirizine
   D. Venlafaxine
   E. Paroxetine

22. Which of the following is true about Xyrem? (Mark all that apply.)

   A. Xyrem should be taken at bed and then again 2.5 to 4 hours later.
   B. Xyrem comes as a solution.
   C. Xyrem should be taken at least 2 hours after a meal.
   D. Xyrem requires dosage adjustment when taken with divalproex sodium.
   E. The usual effective dose of Xyrem is 6 to 9 g per night.

20-11 Answers

1. D. The patient is on haloperidol 10 mg twice daily. Therefore, to convert to the decanoate injection, the total oral daily dose is multiplied by 10. The dose would be Haldol-D 200 mg I.M. every 4 weeks.

2. B. The patient is experiencing a dystonic reaction, which can be treated with either benztropine 1 to 2 mg I.M. or diphenhydramine 25 to 50 mg I.M. every 30 minutes until resolved. The dystonic reaction is thought to occur because of an imbalance in dopamine and acetylcholine in the nigrostriatal region of the brain.

3. B. The only antipsychotic proven effective for refractory schizophrenia is clozapine. Because the patient has had little-to-no response to quetiapine,

raising her quetiapine dose is inappropriate. Little evidence supports the use of multiple antipsychotics in the treatment of schizophrenia. Augmenting quetiapine therapy with fluoxetine and ECT is inappropriate because the patient has had little response to quetiapine. Guidelines for the treatment of schizophrenia recommend 2 adequate trials of antipsychotic monotherapy before switching the patient to clozapine, unless clozapine use is contraindicated or inappropriate for the patient.

4. B. The symptoms that the patient is displaying appear to be the result of neuroleptic malignant syndrome. All neuroleptics have the propensity to cause this rare but deadly adverse effect. The first steps in treating NMS are to discontinue the offending agent, offer supportive therapy, and prescribe a dopamine agonist and (commonly) a skeletal muscle relaxant.

5. A. Antidepressants have been shown to increase the rates of hypomanic and manic episodes. Mood stabilizers and antipsychotics lower the rates of mania and hypomania. Antibiotics do not affect bipolar disorder to any known extent.

6. A. Common adverse effects that occur with lithium include polyuria, polydipsia, tremor, and GI upset. Common adverse effects that may occur later in therapy include weight gain and mental dulling. Elevated hepatic enzymes and alopecia are adverse effects that may occur with divalproex sodium. Akathisia is an extrapyramidal adverse effect induced by antipsychotics.

7. A. Lithium and divalproex are first-line therapy for bipolar disorder. Agranulocytosis is an adverse effect that is monitored with clozapine therapy. Bipolar I patients do not spend all of their time in mania. They also experience depression and normal mood at times. Antidepressants can increase the risks of experiencing a manic episode in patients with bipolar disorder, especially when used as monotherapy.

8. D. Lamotrigine has been associated with serious dermatological reactions, including Stevens–Johnson syndrome, in patients using the medication for epilepsy or bipolar/mood disorders. Risk factors for developing the serious reactions include increased age, concomitant use of valproate, or use of higher-than-recommended doses.

9. **A, D.** Liver function tests and a complete blood count with differential should be performed at baseline and periodically throughout divalproex treatment. Divalproex is not recommended for use in hepatic dysfunction and may cause thrombocytopenia during treatment. Thyroid levels and an ECG are recommended monitoring for lithium therapy. Ammonia levels are only recommended to be taken if patients are showing signs or symptoms of hyperammonemia.

10. **B.** Angiotensin-converting enzyme inhibitors such as lisinopril increase lithium levels when used in combination. These medications do not have a drug interaction with divalproex or valproic acid.

11. **B.** Bupropion is contraindicated in patients with seizure disorder because of its ability to lower the seizure threshold. The other antidepressants listed do not have this warning.

12. **D.** Because of fluoxetine's long half-life, 5 weeks should pass before initiating MAOI therapy. If fluoxetine is not cleared from the body by the time the MAOI is started, there is a risk of developing serotonin syndrome.

13. **A.** Many medications can cause or worsen depression, such as antihypertensives (reserpine, methyldopa, propranolol, clonidine), antiparkinsonian agents (levodopa, carbidopa, amantadine), hormonal agents (estrogens, progesterone), corticosteroids, cycloserine, and the anticancer agents vinblastine and vincristine.

14. **B.** Hydroxyzine reduces anxiety and is often used in patients with substance abuse issues. Hydroxyzine is indicated for pruritus but is likely being used for anxiety in this patient. Hydroxyzine may be confused with hydralazine, which is indicated for essential hypertension.

15. **C.** Abilify (aripiprazole) is approved as adjunctive treatment for refractory depression. The patient has already failed a trial with venlafaxine; therefore, initiating therapy with its isomer Pristiq (desvenlafaxine) may not be the best option. MAOIs are a viable fourth-line treatment option; however, you would wait 5 weeks after discontinuing fluoxetine before initiating an MAOI. Lexapro (escitalopram) is an isomer of citalopram, which had already failed to help the patient. Benzodiazepines are not recommended for treatment of depression.

16. **D.** MAOIs are rarely used because of numerous drug interactions, adverse effects, and the need for the strict dietary restrictions of tyramine-containing foods. MAOIs inhibit the metabolism of tyramine, an amino acid that helps regulate blood pressure, causing excessive catecholamine release and leading to hypertensive crisis.

17. **B.** Because SSRIs can be activating and may initially cause symptoms of anxiety, it is important to "start low and go slow" with these agents when used for anxiety disorders.

18. **D, E.** Lorazepam, oxazepam, and temazepam are preferred in the elderly or patients with hepatic dysfunction because they are metabolized by hepatic glucuronidation. The other benzodiazepines listed do not undergo glucuronidation and have active metabolites that may accumulate in the elderly or patients with liver dysfunction.

19. **D.** Lisdexamfetamine (Vyvanse) is FDA approved for moderate-to-severe binge-eating disorder.

20. **C.** Fluoxetine is approved for treating bulimia nervosa; 60 mg/d is the most common dose. A combination of psychotherapy and pharmacotherapy is preferred.

21. **D.** The norepinephrine effects of the SNRI, venlafaxine, have the potential to enhance wakefulness and cause or contribute to insomnia.

22. **A, B, C, D, E.** Xyrem is a CNS depressant that is indicated for excessive daytime somnolence, narcolepsy with cataplexy, sleep paralysis, and hypnagogic hallucinations. Dosing starts at 2.25 g at bedtime and an additional 2.25 g 2.5 to 4 hours later. The dose should be titrated to effect with a typical range of 6 to 9 g per night, the usual effective dose. Xyrem should be taken at least 2 hours after a meal. Xyrem has an additive effect with other CNS depressants and divalproex sodium and should be avoided.

29-12   Additional Resources

American Psychiatric Association. *Diagnostic and Statistical Manual of Mental Disorders,* Fifth Edition (DSM-5). Arlington, VA: American Psychiatric Association; 2013.

American Psychiatric Association. Practice Guidelines Web page: http://psychiatryonline.org/guidelines. Accessed April 25, 2017.

Connolly KR, Thase ME. The clinical management of bipolar disorder: a review of evidence-based guidelines. *Primy Care Companion for CNS Disord.* 2011;13(4):doi:10.4088/PCC.10r01097.

Leucht S, Corves C, Arbter D, et al. Second-generation versus first-generation antipsychotic drugs for schizophrenia: a meta-analysis. *Lancet.* 2009;373(9657):31–41.

National Institute of Mental Health. Clinical Antipsychotic Trials of Intervention Effectiveness (CATIE) Web page: https://www.nimh.nih.gov/funding/clinical-research/practical/catie/index.shtml. Accessed April 25, 2017.

National Institute of Mental Health. Sequenced Treatment Alternatives to Relieve Depression (STAR*D) Study Web page: https://www.nimh.nih.gov/funding/clinical-research/practical/stard/index.shtml. Accessed April 25, 2017.

Schutte-Rodin S, Broch L, Buysse D, et al. Clinical guideline for the evaluation and management of chronic insomnia in adults. *J Clin Sleep Med.* 2008;4(5):487–504.

Section 9: Psychiatric Disorders. In: DiPiro, JT., Nolin, TD, Yee, GC, et al., eds. *Pharmacotherapy: A Pathophysiologic Approach.* 11th ed. New York, NY: McGraw-Hill Education; 2020:1007–1228.

Wise MS, Arand DL, Auger RR, et al. Treatment of narcolepsy and other hypersomnias of central origin: an American Academy of Sleep Medicine Review. *Sleep.* 2007;30(12):1712–1727.

Thromboembolic Disease

30

GALE L. HAMANN

30-1 KEY POINTS

- Heparin, also known as unfractionated heparin, should be administered as a bolus of 80 IU/kg intravenous (I.V.), followed by a maintenance infusion of 18 IU/kg/h. Heparin is monitored by activated partial thromboplastin time (aPTT).
- Low molecular weight heparin (LMWH) offers a more predictable response at lower doses without the need to monitor levels, except in patients with severe renal impairment or in obesity.
- An acute venous thromboembolism (VTE) should be treated with I.V. heparin, LMWH, or fondaparinux to provide immediate anticoagulation, followed by the initiation of **warfarin** therapy. **Warfarin** should be initiated at 5 to 7.5 mg daily for most patients. Heparin, LMWH, or fondaparinux should be overlapped with **warfarin** for at least 4 to 5 days or until 2 consecutive international normalized ratios (INRs) are within the therapeutic range.
- **Apixaban** and rivaroxaban are oral factor Xa inhibitors used for the treatment of VTE. They provide immediate anticoagulation therapy without the need for parenteral anticoagulation. Rivaroxaban is dosed at 15 mg twice daily for 21 days, followed by 20 mg daily with the evening meal. **Apixaban** is dosed at 10 mg twice daily for 7 days followed by 5 mg twice daily. Edoxaban also is an oral factor Xa inhibitor used for the treatment of VTE after 5 to 10 days of parenteral anticoagulation. Edoxaban is dosed at 60 mg daily. Dose reductions of **apixaban**, rivaroxaban, and edoxaban are necessary with reduced renal function.
- **Apixaban** and rivaroxaban also are indicated for the prevention of VTE associated with hip and knee replacement surgery. **Apixaban** is dosed at 2.5 mg daily for 35 days after hip replacement and 12 days after knee replacement. Rivaroxaban is dosed at 10 mg daily for 35 days after hip replacement and for 12 to 14 days after knee replacement.
- Dabigatran is a direct thrombin inhibitor used to treat acute VTE. It is dosed at 150 mg twice daily after 5 to 10 days of parenteral anticoagulation. Dabigatran is contraindicated in creatinine clearance <30 mL/min.

30-2 STUDY GUIDE CHECKLIST

The following topics may guide your study of this subject area:

- ☐ Prophylactic therapies for the prevention of thromboembolic disease.
- ☐ Treatment of thromboembolic disease.
- ☐ Mechanisms of action and pharmacokinetic considerations of the various anticoagulants.
- ☐ Indications for the various anticoagulants.
- ☐ Trade names and available dosage forms of the various anticoagulants.
- ☐ Dosing regimens of the various anticoagulants.
- ☐ Major adverse drug reactions of the various anticoagulants.
- ☐ Significant drug interactions of the various anticoagulants.
- ☐ Patient counseling points for the various anticoagulants.

30-3   Venous Thromboembolic Disease

Definition

Venous thromboembolism (VTE) is a disease process that involves the development of a deep venous thrombosis, a pulmonary embolism, or both.

A *pulmonary embolism* (PE) is a thrombus or foreign substance from the systemic circulation that lodges in the pulmonary artery or its branches and causes a complete or partial occlusion of pulmonary blood flow. A PE is diagnosed based on a detailed history and clinical symptoms. A spiral computed tomography (CT) scan or a ventilation-perfusion scan confirms the diagnosis.

A *deep venous thrombosis* (DVT) is a thrombus that forms most commonly in the popliteal or femoral veins, the veins of the calf, or the iliac veins of the upper leg. A DVT is diagnosed based on a detailed history and clinical symptoms. A duplex ultrasound, which measures both blood flow and compressibility of the affected vessel, confirms the diagnosis.

VTE Treatment Options

- Heparin, also known as unfractionated heparin, low molecular weight heparin (LMWH), or fondaparinux overlapped with **warfarin** until 2 consecutive international normalized ratios (INRs) are within the therapeutic range
- **Apixaban**
- Dabigatran
- Edoxaban
- Rivaroxaban

Drug Therapy

Unfractionated heparin

Table 30-1 describes heparin in the treatment of VTE.

LMWHs and pentasaccharide

Table 30-2 describes LMWH and pentasaccharide.

Therapeutic use

- Prevention and treatment of VTE
- Prevention of VTE in patients with a previous VTE or a known hypercoagulability
- Prophylaxis for VTE in high-risk populations
- Arterial embolism prevention in patients with mechanical or tissue prosthetic heart valve replacement
- Arterial embolism prevention in patients with atrial fibrillation or atrial flutter
- Arterial embolism prevention in patients with an acute cardioembolic stroke

> ⚠️ **LMWHs** *FDA BOXED WARNING*
>
> Risk of life-threatening epidural or spinal hematoma if patient is receiving neuraxial anesthesia or undergoing a spinal puncture. Risk increases if patient has an indwelling epidural catheter, is taking other medications that affect hemostasis (e.g., NSAIDs, anticoagulants), has a history of traumatic or repeated epidural or spinal punctures, or has a history of spinal deformity or spinal surgery.

TABLE 30-1. Heparin in the Treatment of VTE

Characteristic	Comment
Indication	Prevention and treatment of VTE
	Prevention of VTE in patients with a previous VTE or a known hypercoagulability
	Prophylaxis for VTE in high-risk populations
Mechanism of action	Heparin binds to antithrombin and converts it from a slow progressive thrombin inhibitor to a rapid thrombin inhibitor. This catalyzes inactivation of factors XIIa, XIa, IXa, Xa, and IIa (thrombin).
Pharmacokinetics	Heparin is cleared by a rapid saturable mechanism that occurs at therapeutic doses.
	A slower, unsaturable first-order clearance (largely by renal means) occurs at high doses.
	The half-life of heparin varies from approximately 30 minutes (after an I.V. bolus of 25 IU/kg) to 60 minutes (after an I.V. bolus of 100 IU/kg).
Monitoring	Heparin is monitored by an aPTT, which is sensitive to the inhibitory effects of heparin on factors IIa (thrombin), IXa, and Xa.
	The therapeutic range for an aPTT is determined by an antifactor Xa chromogenic assay of 0.3 to 0.7 IU/mL.
	An aPTT should be measured 6 hours after a bolus dose of heparin or after any dosage change and then every 6 hours until a therapeutic aPTT is reached. Once a therapeutic aPTT is achieved, an aPTT may be evaluated every 24 hours.
	Platelet count and hematocrit should be evaluated at baseline and every 1 to 3 days.
	Signs and symptoms of bleeding or bruising, especially at surgical sites, should be monitored.
Dosing	Heparin should be dosed using a weight-based nomogram.
	Nomograms are specific only for the reagent and instrument used to validate that nomogram.
	Heparin is administered as an I.V. bolus of 80 IU/kg, followed by an infusion of 18 IU/kg/h. An aPTT is measured 6 hours after the infusion or after each dosage adjustment. The infusion is adjusted based on a dosing nomogram. An aPTT is measured every 24 hours once it is within therapeutic range.
	Heparin may be administered subcutaneously every 12 hours. The initial dose is 17,500 IU or 250 IU/kg subcutaneous every 12 hours. The dose should be adjusted to an aPTT within the therapeutic range, measured 6 hours after the injection.
	Heparin may be administered as a fixed dose that is unmonitored. An initial dose of 333 IU/kg is administered, followed by 250 IU/kg subcutaneous every 12 hours.
Adverse effects	The most common adverse effects are minor bleeding in the form of gingival bleeding, epistaxis, and ecchymosis.
	The most common serious adverse effects of heparin are gastrointestinal or urogenital bleeding.
	Fatal or life-threatening adverse effects often result from intracranial or retroperitoneal bleeding.
	Transient thrombocytopenia may occur within the first 2 to 4 days of therapy, which will resolve with continued therapy.
	Heparin-induced thrombocytopenia (defined as a reduction in platelets of 50% from baseline or <50,000) may occur in 1% to 2% of patients, which requires heparin discontinuation.
	Osteoporosis can occur with chronic use.
Contraindications	Active bleeding
	Severely uncontrolled hypertension
	History of heparin-induced thrombocytopenia

aPTT, activated partial thromboplastin time; I.V., intravenous.

TABLE 30-2. LMWH and Pentasaccharide

Characteristic	Enoxaparin	Dalteparin	Fondaparinux
Trade name	Lovenox	Fragmin	Arixtra
Dosage form	30, 40, 60, 80, 100, 120, 150 mg syringe	2500-, 5000-, 7500-, 10,000-, 12,500-, 15,000-, 18,000-IU syringe	2.5, 5, 7.5, and 10 mg syringe
Drug class	LMWH	LMWH	Pentasaccharide
Mechanism of action	Inhibits factor Xa and, to a much lesser extent, factor IIa	Inhibits factor Xa and, to a much lesser extent, factor IIa	Inhibits factor Xa
Bioavailability (%)	92	87	100
Half-life	3 to 6 hours	3 to 5 hours	17 to 21 hours
Anti Xa monitoring in obesity or significant renal impairment	Anti Xa levels drawn 4 hours after a dose Therapeutic levels: ■ 0.6 to 1 IU/mL for twice-daily dosing ■ 1 to 2 IU/mL for once-daily dosing	Anti Xa levels drawn 4 to 6 hours after a dose Therapeutic level: ■ 0.5 to 1.5 IU/mL	No monitoring
Monitoring	Platelet counts, hematocrit and hemoglobin, signs and symptoms of bleeding		
Adverse effects	Most common adverse effects are minor bleeding in the form of gingival bleeding, epistaxis, and ecchymosis. Most common serious adverse effects of heparin are gastrointestinal or urogenital bleeding. Fatal or life-threatening adverse effects often result from intracranial or retroperitoneal bleeding. Heparin-induced thrombocytopenia can occur with enoxaparin and dalteparin.		

Patient instructions and counseling

- Strict compliance is necessary to ensure a consistent level of anticoagulation.
- Notify a health care provider if bruising, hematuria, melena, hemoptysis, epistaxis, gingival bleeding, or any other abnormal bleeding occurs.
- Consult a health care provider or pharmacist before taking any over-the-counter medications.
- Avoid **aspirin** or nonsteroidal anti-inflammatory drugs (NSAIDs).
- The air bubble in the LMWH or fondaparinux syringe should be near the plunger before injection. This method ensures that all the drug is expelled from the syringe and helps minimize the amount of bleeding, bruising, and hematoma formation from the injection site.

Dosing LMWH and fondaparinux

See Tables 30-3 and 30-4 for indications and dosage regimens.

Direct thrombin inhibitor

Argatroban

See Table 30-5 for indication and dosing regimen.

Warfarin ⚠

See Table 30-6 for indications.

Warfarin *FDA BOXED WARNING*

Increased risk of bleeding—INR should be monitored regularly.

TABLE 30-3. Indications and Recommended Doses of LMWH and Fondaparinux

Indication	Enoxaparin	Dalteparin	Fondaparinux
Total hip replacement	30 mg subcutaneous every 12 hours *or* 40 mg subcutaneous every 24 hours	5000 IU subcutaneous 0 to 14 hours before surgery, then every 24 hours *or* 2500 IU subcutaneous 2 hours before surgery, then 5000 IU every 24 hours *or* 2500 IU subcutaneous 2 hours before surgery and 4 to 8 hours after, then 5000 IU every 24 hours	2.5 mg subcutaneous every 24 hours starting 6 to 8 hours after surgery
Total knee replacement	30 mg subcutaneous every 12 hours		2.5 mg subcutaneous every 24 hours starting 6 to 8 hours after surgery
Abdominal surgery	40 mg subcutaneous every 24 hours	2500 IU subcutaneous 1 to 2 hours before surgery, then 5000 IU every 24 hours	2.5 mg subcutaneous every 24 hours starting 6 to 8 hours after surgery
Hip fracture			2.5 mg subcutaneous every 24 hours starting 6 to 8 hours after surgery
Acute medical illness	40 mg subcutaneous every 24 hours	5000 IU subcutaneous every 24 hours	
Trauma	30 mg subcutaneous every 12 hours		
DVT treatment with or without PE	1 mg/kg subcutaneous every 12 hours *or* 1.5 mg/kg subcutaneous every 24 hours		5 mg for <50 kg; 7.5 mg for 50 to 100 kg; 10 mg for >100 kg subcutaneous every 24 hours
VTE in patients with cancer		200 IU/kg subcutaneous daily for 1 month, followed by 150 IU/kg subcutaneous daily for 5 months	

TABLE 30-4. Enoxaparin Dosage Regimens for Patients with Severe Renal Impairment (Creatinine Clearance < 30 mL/min)

Indication	Dosage regimen
Prophylaxis in abdominal surgery	30 mg subcutaneous once daily
Prophylaxis in hip or knee replacement surgery	30 mg subcutaneous once daily
Prophylaxis in medical patients during acute illness	30 mg subcutaneous once daily
Treatment of acute DVT with or without PE when administered in conjunction with **warfarin**	1 mg/kg subcutaneous once daily

Boldface indicates one of top 100 drugs for 2020 by prescription volume.

TABLE 30-5. Argatroban

Characteristic	Comment
Mechanism of action	Direct thrombin inhibitor
	Synthetic molecule that reversibly binds to thrombin
Pharmacokinetic	Metabolized in the liver to inactive metabolites
	Half-life of 0.5 to 1 hour
Indication	Prophylaxis and treatment of thrombosis associated with heparin-induced thrombocytopenia
Monitoring	Complete blood count (CBC) and signs and symptoms of bleeding should be monitored.
	The aPTT should be drawn 2 hours after an infusion is started and after each dosage change.
Dosing	Administer a continuous I.V. infusion at the rate of 2 mcg/kg/min.
	Adjust infusion rate to maintain an aPTT ratio of 1.5 to 2.5.
Adverse effects	Most common adverse effects are minor bleeding in the form of gingival bleeding, epistaxis, and ecchymosis.
	Most common serious adverse effects are gastrointestinal or urogenital bleeding.
	Fatal or life-threatening adverse effects from intracranial or retroperitoneal bleeding have been reported.
	No known antidote for argatroban exists, but the anticoagulant effect declines rapidly after discontinuation.

aPTT, activated partial thromboplastin time; I.V., intravenous.

TABLE 30-6. Warfarin

Characteristic	Comment
Trade name	Coumadin, Jantoven
Tablet size (color)	1 mg (pink), 2 mg (lavender), 2.5 mg (green), 3 mg (tan), 4 mg (blue), 5 mg (peach), 6 mg (teal), 7.5 mg (yellow), 10 mg (white)
Injectable	For I.V. use only: 5 mg powder for reconstitution (2 mg/mL)
Indication	Prevention and treatment of VTE
	Prevention of VTE in patients with a previous VTE or a known hypercoagulability
	Prophylaxis for VTE in high-risk populations
	Prevention of arterial embolism in patients with mechanical or tissue prosthetic heart valve replacement
	Prevention of arterial embolism in patients with atrial fibrillation or atrial flutter
	Prevention of arterial embolism in patients with a previous cardioembolic stroke
	Prevention of acute MI in patients with peripheral arterial disease
Mechanism of action	**Warfarin** is a vitamin-K antagonist interfering with the interconversion of vitamin K and its 2,3-epoxide.
	Warfarin reduces the activity of vitamin K–dependent coagulation factors II, VII, IX, X, and proteins C and S produced in the liver, which declines over 6 to 96 hours.
	At least 4 to 5 days of **warfarin** therapy are necessary before a patient is completely anticoagulated.
Pharmacokinetics	**Warfarin** is a racemic mixture of 2 active isomers (warfarin S and warfarin R) in roughly equal amounts.
	The S isomer is 3 to 4 times more potent than the R isomer.
	Warfarin is rapidly and completely absorbed from the gastrointestinal tract with peak concentration in approximately 90 minutes.
	Warfarin is 99% protein bound with a half-life of 36 to 42 hours.
	The S isomer of **warfarin** is metabolized by cytochrome P450 (CYP) 2C9 and, to a lesser extent, by CYP3A4.
	The R isomer is metabolized by CYP1A2 and CYP3A4 and, to a lesser extent, by CYP2C19.

TABLE 30-6. Warfarin (Continued)

Characteristic	Comment
Monitoring	**Warfarin** is monitored by use of the INR.
	The INR reflects the reduction in clotting factors II, VII, and X.
	A target INR of 2.5 and a therapeutic range of 2.0 to 3.0 are indicated for patients treated for VTE, atrial fibrillation, mechanical aortic valve, bioprosthetic valve, or antiphospholipid syndrome.
	A target INR of 3.0 and a therapeutic range of 2.5 to 3.5 are indicated for patients treated for a mechanical mitral valve or both mechanical aortic and mitral valves.
	Hematocrit and hemoglobin should be monitored.
	Signs and symptoms of bleeding should be monitored.

Boldface indicates one of top 100 drugs for 2020 by prescription volume.
INR, international normalized ratio; I.V., intravenous; MI, myocardial infarction.

Patient instructions and counseling

- **Warfarin** should be taken at the same time every day.
- Strict compliance is necessary to ensure a consistent level of anticoagulation.
- Strict compliance with a consistent vitamin K diet is necessary to ensure a consistent level of anticoagulation.
- Notify the health care provider in the event of hematuria, melena, epistaxis, hemoptysis, increased bruising, or any abnormal bleeding.
- Notify all health care providers, including dentists, of **warfarin** therapy.
- Blood monitoring to determine an adequate level of anticoagulation and compliance is necessary at regular intervals.
- Consult a health care provider or pharmacist before taking any new prescription or over-the-counter medications.
- Avoid **aspirin** or NSAIDs unless instructed otherwise by a health care provider.
- Women of childbearing age should use an effective form of birth control, because **warfarin** has teratogenic effects.

Dosing

Initiating **warfarin** at 5 mg daily should result in an INR around 2.0 in 4 to 5 days for most patients. **Warfarin** also may be administered between 7.5 and 10 mg for the first 1 to 2 days and then adjusted depending on the INR response.

Initiating **warfarin** at a dose of 7.5 to 10 mg daily may be appropriate for young, healthy, or obese patients.

Initiating **warfarin** at a dose of ≤5 mg daily may be appropriate in the elderly; in patients with liver disease, heart failure, or malnutrition; in patients taking drugs known to increase the responsiveness to warfarin; or in patients with a high risk of bleeding.

If a rapid anticoagulant effect is indicated, I.V. heparin, LMWH, or fondaparinux should be administered along with **warfarin** for at least 4 to 5 days until a therapeutic INR is reached. Heparin, LMWH, or fondaparinux may be discontinued when the INR is within the therapeutic range on 2 consecutive occasions. Dosage adjustments for patients already on **warfarin** therapy are made at 10% to 20% of the current dose.

Disease state interaction

Disease states that can increase the response to **warfarin** are hyperthyroidism, congestive heart failure, liver disease, fever, and genetic increased **warfarin** sensitivity.

Disease states that can decrease the response to **warfarin** are hypothyroidism and genetic warfarin resistance. Patient nonadherence also can result in a reduced warfarin response.

Drug–drug interactions

Warfarin is a drug with a narrow therapeutic index. Numerous drugs interact with **warfarin**. Drugs that either inhibit or induce cytochrome P450 (CYP) 2C9 or 3A4 (and, to a lesser extent, CYP1A2 or 2C19) potentiate or reduce the anticoagulant effect. The S isomer is more active than the R isomer; thus, drugs that inhibit or induce the S isomer will have a more significant effect on **warfarin** than drugs that inhibit or induce the R isomer (Table 30-7).

Drug–food interactions

Foods that contain high amounts of vitamin K can reduce the anticoagulant effect of **warfarin** (Table 30-7). Patients must be consistent in their consumption of these foods and should space their consumption evenly over a 7-day period. If a patient suddenly stops eating these foods, the INR may increase dramatically.

Adverse effects

The most common adverse effect is minor bleeding in the form of gingival bleeding, epistaxis, and ecchymosis. The most common serious adverse effects of **warfarin** are either gastrointestinal or urogenital bleeding.

Warfarin-induced skin necrosis is a rare but serious adverse effect. Skin necrosis begins within 10 days of **warfarin** initiation. It is characterized by painful, erythematous lesions on breasts, thighs, and buttocks, which may progress to hemorrhagic lesions. The concomitant use of heparin, LMWH, or fondaparinux with initiation of **warfarin** can prevent its occurrence.

Purple toe syndrome is a dark blue-tinged discoloration of the feet that occurs rarely 3 to 8 weeks after **warfarin** initiation.

Fatal or life-threatening adverse effects are related to intracranial or retroperitoneal bleeding.

Several treatment options are available for the reversal of anticoagulation. Treatment may be necessary for a supratherapeutic INR or before an invasive procedure. Withholding **warfarin** will reduce the level of anticoagulation. For an INR of 6 to 10, an estimated 2.5 days may be needed to reduce the INR to <4. Phytonadione (also referred to as vitamin K) will reverse the effects of **warfarin**. Phytonadione may be administered orally or intravenously. For intravenous (I.V.) administration, phytonadione should be diluted in at least 50 mL of I.V. fluid and administered over 20 minutes to minimize the risk of anaphylactic reactions. Administering oral phytonadione while also withholding **warfarin** therapy may reduce an INR of 6 to 10 to an INR of <4 in approximately 1.4 days. I.V. phytonadione begins reversing an INR within 2 hours. Other treatment options for reversing an INR include fresh frozen plasma, nonactivated prothrombin complex concentrate (PCC), or recombinant factor VII. PCC is available as a 3-factor or

TABLE 30-7. Drugs and Foods That Can Interact with Warfarin

Type of interaction	Interacting substance
Potentiation of anticoagulant effect	**Acetaminophen**, alcohol (acute use), anabolic steroids, cimetidine, clofibrate, disulfiram, piroxicam, **omeprazole**, **simvastatin**, sulfinpyrazone, cranberry juice
Highly significant potentiation of anticoagulant effect	Amiodarone, ciprofloxacin, erythromycin, fluconazole, isoniazid, itraconazole, ketoconazole, **levothyroxine**, **metronidazole**, phenytoin, trimethoprim-sulfamethoxazole, vitamin E (high doses)
Reduction of anticoagulation effect	Alcohol (chronic use), dicloxacillin, griseofulvin
Highly significant reduction of anticoagulation effect	Barbiturates, carbamazepine, cholestyramine, enteral feeding, nafcillin, rifampin, vitamin K–containing foods (broccoli, Brussels sprouts, cabbage, canola oil, cauliflower, coleslaw, collard greens, endive, green kale, lettuce, mayonnaise, mustard greens, soybean oil, spinach)

Boldface indicates one of top 100 drugs for 2020 by prescription volume.

> **BOX 30-1.** Recommendations for Managing Anticoagulation Therapy in Patients Requiring Invasive Procedures

Patients with Low Risk of Thromboembolism

- Discontinue **warfarin** 5 days before procedure.

Patients with Moderate Risk of Thromboembolism

- Discontinue **warfarin** 5 days before procedure.
- Consider bridging with prophylactic or therapeutic-dose subcutaneous LMWH or I.V. heparin during interruption of **warfarin** therapy depending on patient's thrombosis risk.

Patients with High Risk of Thromboembolism

- Discontinue **warfarin** 5 days before procedure.
- Bridge with therapeutic-dose subcutaneous LMWH or I.V. heparin during interruption of **warfarin** therapy.
- In patients whose INR is still elevated (>1.5) 1 to 2 days before surgery, administer 1 to 2 mg oral vitamin K to normalize INR.
- Discontinue therapeutic-dose LMWH 24 hours before procedure.
- Discontinue heparin approximately 4 to 6 hours before procedure.

- Restart **warfarin** 12 to 24 hours after procedure or when hemostasis is adequate.
- Resume therapeutic-dose LMWH approximately 24 hours after procedure or when hemostasis is adequate.
- In patients at high risk of bleeding, delay therapeutic-dose LMWH or heparin for 48 to 72 hours or administer low-dose LMWH or heparin when hemostasis is secured or completely avoid LMWH or heparin.
- Individualize treatment plans according to postoperative hemostasis and bleeding risk.

Patients Undergoing Minor Dental or Dermatologic Procedure or Cataract Removal

- Continue **warfarin** therapy around the time of the procedure.
- For dental procedures, co-administer an oral prohemostatic agent such as tranexamic acid or epsilon amino caproic acid mouthwash.

Boldface indicates one of top 100 drugs for 2020 by prescription volume.

4-factor concentrate; 3-factor PCC contains factors II, IX, and X, whereas 4-factor PCC contains factors II, VII, IX, and X.

Box 30-1 outlines the recommendations for managing anticoagulation in patients undergoing invasive procedures.

Direct-acting oral anticoagulants

Four direct-acting oral anticoagulants (DOACs) are available:

- **Apixaban (Eliquis)** ⚠
- Dabigatran (Pradaxa) ⚠
- Edoxaban (Savaysa) ⚠
- Rivaroxaban (Xarelto) ⚠

DOAC characteristics and dosing are outlined in Tables 30-8 and 30-9.

 Apixaban (Eliquis) *FDA BOXED WARNING*

Increased risk of thrombotic events when discontinued prematurely. Risk of epidural or spinal hematoma if receiving neuraxial anesthesia or undergoing spinal puncture.

Dabigatran (Pradaxa) *FDA BOXED WARNING*

Increased risk of thrombotic events when discontinued prematurely. Risk of epidural or spinal hematoma if receiving neuraxial anesthesia or undergoing spinal puncture.

 Edoxaban (Savaysa) *FDA BOXED WARNING*

Reduced efficacy in nonvalvular atrial fibrillation if creatinine clearance is greater than 95 ml/min. Increased risk of thrombotic events when discontinued prematurely. Risk of epidural or spinal hematoma if receiving neuraxial anesthesia or undergoing spinal puncture.

 Rivaroxaban (Xarelto) *FDA BOXED WARNING*

Increased risk of thrombotic events when discontinued prematurely. Risk of epidural or spinal hematoma if receiving neuraxial anesthesia or undergoing spinal puncture.

TABLE 30-8. Direct-Acting Oral Anticoagulants

Characteristic	Rivaroxaban	Apixaban	Edoxaban	Dabigatran
Trade name	**Xarelto**	**Eliquis**	Savaysa	Pradaxa
Mechanism of action	Inhibits factor Xa free and bound	Inhibits factor Xa free and bound	Inhibits factor Xa free and bound	Inhibits thrombin free and bound
Dosage form	10, 15, 20 mg	2.5, 5 mg	15, 30, 60 mg	75, 110, 150 mg
Prodrug	No	No	No	Yes
Bioavailability (%)	80	50	62	7
Time to peak	2 to 4 hours	1 to 3 hours	1 to 2 hours	1 to 3 hours
Half-life	5 to 9 hours	9 to 14 hours	10 to 14 hours	12 to 17 hours
Renal clearance (%)	33	25	35 to 50	80
Monitoring	Creatinine clearance should be calculated before beginning drug therapy and then used to determine the dosing regimen. No routine blood monitoring is necessary. Hematocrit and hemoglobin should be monitored. Signs and symptoms of bleeding should be monitored.			
Antidote	Andexanet Alfa[b]	Andexanet Alfa[b]	Andexanet Alfa[b]	Idarucizumab[a]
Drug interactions	CYP3A4 and P-gp	CYP3A4 and P-gp	P-gp	P-gp
Adverse effects	Most common adverse effects are related to bleeding. Minor bleeding includes gingival bleeding, epistaxis, or ecchymosis. Major bleeding most often involves gastrointestinal or urogenital system. Intracranial bleeding may be fatal or life threatening. Dabigatran may cause dyspepsia or gastritis.			
Pregnancy Category	C	B	C	C

Boldface indicates one of top 100 drugs for 2020 by prescription volume.
CYP, Cytochrome P450; P-gp, P-glycoprotein.
a. Praxbind (brand name).
b. Andexxa (brand name).

TABLE 30-9. Dosing for Direct-Acting Oral Anticoagulants

Indication	Rivaroxaban	Apixaban	Edoxaban	Dabigatran
Treatment of DVT and PE	15 mg twice daily with food for 21 days, then 20 mg daily with the evening meal CrCl < 30 mL/min: avoid use	10 mg twice daily for 7 days followed by 5 mg twice daily	60 mg after 5 to 10 days of initial parenteral anticoagulant Weight ≤ 60 kg: 30 mg daily after 5 to 10 days of initial parenteral anticoagulant CrCl 15 to 50 mL/min: 30 mg daily CrCl < 15 mL/min: not recommended	150 mg twice daily after 5 to 10 days or parenteral anticoagulation CrCl ≤ 30 mL/min: not recommended
Recurrent DVT/PE	20 mg daily with food CrCl < 30 mL/min: avoid use	2.5 mg twice daily after at least 6 months of treatment	Not indicated	150 mg twice daily CrCl ≤ 30 mL/min: not recommended
Total knee arthroplasty	10 mg daily without regard to meals for 12 days beginning at least 6 to 10 hours after surgery CrCl < 30 mL/min: avoid use	2.5 mg twice daily for 12 days beginning 12 to 24 hours postoperatively	Not indicated	Not indicated
Total hip arthroplasty	10 mg daily without regard to meals beginning at least 6 to 10 hours after surgery for 35 days CrCl < 30 mL/min: avoid use	2.5 mg twice daily for 35 days beginning 12 to 24 hours postoperatively	Not indicated	110 mg 1 to 4 hours after surgery, then 220 mg daily for 28 to 35 days CrCl ≤ 30 mL/min: not recommended
Heart valve replacement	Not indicated	Not indicated	Not indicated	Not indicated
Converting from **warfarin**	Stop **warfarin** and begin rivaroxaban when INR < 3.0.	Stop **warfarin** and begin **apixaban** when INR < 2.0.	Stop **warfarin** and begin edoxaban when INR < 2.0.	Stop **warfarin** and begin dabigatran when INR ≤ 2.5.
Contraindicated drugs	Strong inhibitors: ketoconazole, itraconazole, ritonavir, clarithromycin, erythromycin Strong inducers: rifampicin, carbamazepine, phenytoin, St. John's wort	Strong inducers: rifampicin, carbamazepine, phenytoin, St. John's wort	Strong inducer: rifampicin	Strong inducer: rifampicin

Boldface indicates one of top 100 drugs for 2020 by prescription volume.
CrCl, creatinine clearance.

Patient instructions and counseling

- DOACs are used for the treatment of a DVT or PE or to reduce the risk of the recurrence of a DVT or PE.
- **Apixaban** and rivaroxaban lower the risk of developing a blood clot after hip or knee replacement surgery.
- Rivaroxaban should be taken twice daily with food or once daily with the evening meal in patients with a DVT or PE. For prevention of a blood clot after hip or knee replacement surgery, rivaroxaban may be taken with or without food.
- Failure to take DOACs on a consistent basis greatly increases the chance of developing a blood clot.
- Strict compliance is necessary to ensure a consistent level of anticoagulation.
- If the patient forgets to take the rivaroxaban 20 mg daily, it should be taken as soon as remembered the same day. Do not take 2 doses to make up for the missed dose. If taking rivaroxaban 15 mg twice daily, take it as soon as remembered in order to get both doses within a 24-hour period.
- If the patient forgets to take the **apixaban** dose, it should be taken as soon as remembered the same day, then twice-daily dosing should be resumed. Do not take 2 doses to make up for the missed dose.
- If the patient forgets to take the dabigatran dose, it should be taken as soon as remembered the same day. The dose should be skipped if it cannot be taken at least 6 hours before the next dose. Do not take 2 doses to make up for the missed dose.
- Do not stop taking these medications without talking to a health care provider.
- Notify a health care provider in the event of hematuria, melena, epistaxis, hemoptysis, increased bruising, or any abnormal bleeding.
- Notify all health care providers, including dentists, of DOAC therapy.
- Avoid **aspirin** or NSAIDs unless instructed otherwise by a physician.

30-4 Pharmacist's Role

Pharmacist have long been involved in anticoagulation therapies both in the hospital and in ambulatory clinics. Pharmacists utilize collaborative practice agreements with physicians to manage anticoagulation therapy, traditionally with **warfarin** and now with the direct acting anticoagulants. Studies have demonstrated that a pharmacist-managed anticoagulation clinic improves the patient's time that their INRs are within the therapeutic range and reduces adverse effects.

NAPLEX Competency Statements

The questions in this chapter cover the following 2021 NAPLEX Competency Statements: **AREA 1:** 1.1; 1.2; 1.3; 1.4; 1.5; 1.6; 1.7 **AREA 2:** 2.1; 2.2; 2.3; 2.4 **AREA 3:** 3.1; 3.2; 3.3; 3.4; 3.5; 5.6; 3.7; 3.8; 3.9; 3.10; 3.11; 3.12 **AREA 5:** 5.1; 5.5 **AREA 6:** 6.1; 6.4.

30-5   Questions

Use the following case study to answer Questions 1 to 7.

A 24-year-old female presents to the emergency department with complaints of severe shortness of breath, dyspnea, and chest pain. She also is experiencing tachycardia and tachypnea. Two days earlier she noticed pain and swelling in her left lower extremity. Her medical history is negative for thrombosis. Her current medications include Tri-Levlen daily and ibuprofen 600 mg every 6 hours as needed for pain. A duplex ultrasound of the left lower extremity revealed a DVT. A CT scan of her chest reveals a pulmonary embolism. Her vital signs are T, 98.4°F; P, 124/min; R, 36/min; BP, 162/100 mmHg; Wt, 220 lb (100 kg); Ht, 5'4".

1. This patient is started on heparin therapy. Which dosage regimen is most appropriate?

   A. I.V. heparin 20,000 IU bolus, then 5000 IU/h
   B. I.V. heparin 8000 IU bolus, then 1800 IU/h
   C. I.V. heparin 5000 IU bolus, then 500 IU/h
   D. I.V. heparin 5000 IU every 12 hours
   E. Subcutaneous heparin 5000 IU every 12 hours

2. The physician would like to treat this patient with warfarin and enoxaparin. Which is the correct dose of enoxaparin if this patient's creatinine clearance is 80 mL/min?

   A. 30 mg subcutaneous every 12 hours
   B. 60 mg subcutaneous every 12 hours
   C. 80 mg subcutaneous every 12 hours
   D. 100 mg subcutaneous every 12 hours
   E. 120 mg subcutaneous every 12 hours

3. The physician would like to treat this patient with warfarin and enoxaparin. What is an appropriate starting dose of warfarin for this patient?

   A. 1 mg daily
   B. 7.5 mg daily
   C. 15 mg daily
   D. 20 mg daily
   E. 25 mg daily

4. Which laboratory test is used to monitor heparin therapy?

   A. aPTT
   B. No laboratory testing is needed.
   C. INR
   D. Clotting time
   E. Factor Xa

5. Which laboratory test is used to monitor warfarin therapy?

   A. aPTT
   B. No laboratory testing is needed.
   C. INR
   D. Clotting time
   E. Factor Xa

6. The physician has decided to use one of the direct-acting oral anticoagulants. Which of the following is the best answer?

   A. Rivaroxaban 150 mg twice daily
   B. Dabigatran 100 mg
   C. Apixaban 10 mg twice daily for 7 days, then 5 mg twice daily
   D. Pradaxa 60 mg daily after 3 days of a parenteral anticoagulant
   E. Edoxaban 20 mg twice daily for 21 days, then 10 mg daily

7. How long should enoxaparin be continued in a patient with an acute DVT or PE?

   A. At least 4 to 5 days, until the INR > 2.0 for 24 hours.
   B. At least 4 to 5 days, until the INR > 3.0 for 24 hours.
   C. At least 24 hours, until the INR > 4.0 for 24 hours.
   D. At least 48 hours, until the INR > 4.0 for 24 hours.
   E. At least 7 to 10 days, until the INR > 3.5 for 24 hours.

8. Which of the following statements is *false* regarding important information to communicate to a patient on warfarin therapy?

A. Take warfarin every day without missing any doses.

B. Eat a consistent amount of vitamin K–rich foods per week.

C. Report any symptoms of bleeding to your physician.

D. Warfarin is the preferred anticoagulant for use in women, because it is safe to take during pregnancy.

E. Do not take aspirin-containing products unless directed to do so by your physician.

9. Which of the following is an example of a vitamin K–rich food that can lower an INR?

A. Green beans

B. Spinach

C. Lima beans

D. Sweet peas

E. Green peppers

10. Which of the following cardiovascular drugs is most likely to affect an INR?

A. Sotalol

B. Eprosartan

C. Amiodarone

D. Disopyramide

E. Dofetilide

11. Which of the following drugs used to treat seizures is the most likely to interact with warfarin therapy?

A. Lamotrigine

B. Carbamazepine

C. Topiramate

D. Levetiracetam

E. Tiagabine

12. A 58-year-old male is scheduled for a total knee replacement the following day. He has a medical history of hypertension for which he is treated with amlodipine 5 mg daily. His height is 6'2", and his weight is 176 lb (80 kg). Which of the following is the best DVT prophylaxis therapy for this patient?

A. Fondaparinux 7.5 mg subcutaneous every 12 hours

B. Lovenox 80 mg subcutaneous every 12 hours

C. Rivaroxaban 10 mg daily

D. Xarelto 20 mg daily

E. Dabigatran 150 mg twice daily

13. A 58-year-old male is scheduled for a total knee replacement the following day. He has a medical history of hypertension for which he is treated with amlodipine 5 mg daily. His height is 6'2", and his weight is 176 lb (80 kg). Which of the following is the best answer for the duration of therapy for this patient?

A. 7 days

B. 12 days

C. 14 days

D. 17 days

E. 21 days

14. Fondaparinux is an anticoagulant that inhibits which of the following clotting factors?

A. IIa

B. IXa

C. Xa

D. XIa

E. VIIa

15. A 63-year-old patient is receiving warfarin 7.5 mg daily for a PE. What therapeutic INR range is indicated for this patient?

A. 1.0 to 2.0

B. 1.5 to 2.5

C. 2.0 to 3.0

D. 2.0 to 3.5

E. 2.5 to 3.5

16. A 56-year-old female presents to the emergency department with complaints of flank pain, dysuria, and increased urinary frequency. She is diagnosed with a urinary tract infection. Her past medical history includes type 2 diabetes, hypertension, and recurrent DVTs. Her medications include metformin 1 g twice daily, quinapril 40 mg daily, and warfarin 5 mg daily. What would be the most appropriate antibiotic to treat this patient's UTI?

A. Septra DS twice daily
B. Ciprofloxacin 500 mg twice daily
C. Rifampin 300 mg 4 times daily
D. Doxycycline 100 mg twice daily
E. Erythromycin 500 mg 4 times daily

17. A 45-year-old patient visits the pharmacy with a prescription for warfarin 7.5 mg daily that was written 5 months before. Which of the following is the best action to take?

A. Fill the prescription because it is valid.
B. Fill only half of the prescription and ask the patient to contact his or her physician.
C. Call the physician to verify that the warfarin dose is correct.
D. Ask the patient to return the following day to allow time to consult the managing pharmacist.
E. Refuse to fill the prescription because it is too old to process legally.

18. What color is warfarin 7.5 mg tablet?

A. White
B. Blue
C. Yellow
D. Pink
E. Green

19. Which of the following is *not* an advantage of using LMWH over heparin?

A. Subcutaneous administration
B. No dosage adjustment needed with renal insufficiency
C. Once- or twice-daily dosing
D. Predictable response at lower doses
E. Lower incidence of heparin-induced thrombocytopenia

20. Idarucizumab is a reversal agent for which of the following anticoagulants?

A. Rivaroxaban
B. Dabigatran
C. Edoxaban
D. Apixaban
E. Warfarin

21. Which of the following is an appropriate therapy for the prevention of a VTE after hip replacement surgery?

A. Enoxaparin 40 mg subcutaneous once daily
B. Enoxaparin 30 mg subcutaneous once daily
C. Rivaroxaban 20 mg daily
D. Apixaban 10 mg daily
E. Edoxaban 60 mg daily

 **30-6   Answers**

1. B. Several studies have indicated that weight-based dosing of heparin is more effective in obtaining therapeutic aPTT than standard heparin titration. A weight-based protocol with an 80 IU/kg I.V. bolus followed by an infusion of 18 IU/kg/h should produce an aPTT close to the therapeutic range. The other doses are not appropriate.

2. C. Enoxaparin provides rapid anticoagulation and is administered as a bridge with warfarin until an INR of 2.0 to 3.0 has been reached. The appropriate dose is 1 mg/kg subcutaneous every 12 hours, or 80 mg.

3. B. Warfarin 7.5 mg daily should result in an INR of about 2.0 within 4 to 5 days. The other doses are either extremely low or extremely high for the majority of patients. Higher doses of warfarin may elevate an INR, but this increase may not be associated with a level of anticoagulation. A rapid increase in INR is due to depletion of factor VII rather than the anticoagulant effect that is associated with depletion of factors II and X.

4. A. The aPTT is a laboratory test used to monitor heparin therapy. The aPTT should be checked 6 hours after a dosage change and every 24 hours if it is within the therapeutic range. An INR is used to monitor warfarin therapy.

5. **C.** An INR is used to monitor warfarin therapy. An aPTT, clotting time, and factor Xa are not useful for monitoring warfarin therapy.

6. **C.** For the treatment of a VTE, apixaban 10 mg twice daily for 7 days, then 5 mg twice daily is the appropriate dose. Rivaroxaban is dosed at 15 mg twice daily for 21 days, followed by 20 mg daily with the evening meal. Dabigatran (Pradaxa) is dosed at 150 mg twice daily after 5 to 10 days of a parenteral anticoagulant. Edoxaban is dosed at 60 mg daily after 5 to 10 days of a parenteral anticoagulant.

7. **A.** For the treatment of an acute DVT or PE, at least 4 to 5 days overlap of heparin or LMWH with warfarin is needed before an anticoagulant effect is produced by warfarin. Heparin or LMWH should be discontinued after an INR >2.0 for 24 hours.

8. **D.** Warfarin is a teratogen and should not be used during pregnancy. Statements A, B, C, and E are important to discuss with patients on warfarin. Patients should follow strict compliance with warfarin. They should eat vitamin K–rich foods consistently over the course of a week and report any symptoms of bleeding to their health care provider.

9. **B.** Green, leafy vegetables contain higher amounts of vitamin K; thus, spinach can reduce an INR. Although green beans, lima beans, sweet peas, and green peppers are green in color, they do not have a large amount of vitamin K.

10. **C.** Amiodarone can cause a dose-dependent increase in an INR by inhibiting CYP2C9. The warfarin dose may need to be reduced by 35% to 50% when amiodarone is added to warfarin therapy.

11. **B.** Carbamazepine induces the cytochrome P450 isozymes 1A2, 2C9, and 3A4; warfarin is a substrate for the isozymes 1A2, 2C9, and 3A4. Carbamazepine, therefore, induces the metabolism of warfarin. This results in the need for larger-than-normal doses of warfarin to achieve a therapeutic INR.

12. **C.** Rivaroxaban 10 mg daily is the correct dose for DVT prophylaxis associated with a knee replacement. Fondaparinux 7.5 mg subcutaneous daily, Lovenox 80 mg subcutaneous every 12 hours, and Xarelto 20 mg daily are all treatment doses rather than prophylactic doses, and dabigatran is not indicated for DVT prophylaxis associated with a knee replacement.

13. **B.** The recommended treatment duration for prophylaxis associated with a knee replacement is 12 days.

14. **C.** Fondaparinux inhibits factor Xa.

15. **C.** The therapeutic range for oral anticoagulation is an INR of 2.0 to 3.0, with a target of 2.5. Increased bleeding is associated with an INR >4.0, and embolic events are more common with an INR <1.5.

16. **D.** Doxycycline 100 mg twice daily would be the most appropriate therapy for a UTI. Septra DS, erythromycin, and ciprofloxacin will interact with warfarin to elevate the INR.

17. **C.** Warfarin is a drug that requires continuous blood monitoring to ensure that a therapeutic INR is maintained. Guidelines recommend that an INR be evaluated monthly. A prescription written for warfarin 5 months before may indicate that a patient is not being monitored appropriately. Therefore, the pharmacist should contact the prescriber to verify the warfarin prescription and to ensure the patient is being monitored.

18. **C.** Warfarin 7.5 mg is yellow, 1 mg is pink, 4 mg is blue, and 10 mg is white.

19. **B.** Because LMWHs are eliminated renally, their doses must be adjusted for patients with renal impairment (creatinine clearance < 30 mL/min). Guidelines recently have been released for enoxaparin dosing in patients with renal impairment. For DVT prophylaxis, enoxaparin should be administered 30 mg subcutaneous every 24 hours rather than every 12 hours. For DVT treatment, enoxaparin should be administered 1 mg/kg subcutaneous every 24 hours rather than every 12 hours.

20. **B.** Idarucizumab is the reversal agent for dabigatran. Vitamin K is the reversal agent for warfarin. As of July 2017, no reversal agent exists for rivaroxaban, edoxaban, or apixaban.

21. **A.** Enoxaparin 40 mg subcutaneous once daily or 30 mg subcutaneous twice daily are appropriate therapies for prevention of a VTE after hip replacement. Other therapies include rivaroxaban 10 mg daily or apixaban 2.5 mg twice daily. Edoxaban is not indicated for prevention of a VTE after hip replacement.

30-7 Additional Resources

Guyatt G, Akl E, Crowther D, et al. Executive summary: antithrombotic therapy and prevention of thrombosis panel, 9th ed.: American College of Chest Physicians Evidence-Based Clinical Practice Guidelines. *Chest.* 2012;141(suppl 2): e7S–e47S.

Kearon C, Akl E, Ornelas J, et al. Antithrombotic therapy for VTE disease: CHEST Guideline and Expert Panel Report. *Chest.* 2016;149(2):315–352.

Pediatrics

31

CATHERINE M. CRILL

31-1 KEY POINTS

- Counseling on appropriate medication administration in pediatric patients is vital to ensuring both safety and efficacy.
- Pharmacotherapy should be adjusted in pediatric patients according to developmental differences in absorption, distribution, metabolism, and elimination to optimize therapeutic efficacy while minimizing the risk of toxicity.
- Although spontaneous resolution does occur in many cases of acute otitis media, antibiotic therapy is initiated to prevent complications such as meningitis and mastoiditis. The observation option is an acceptable initial treatment for select patients.
- High-dose **amoxicillin** remains the drug of choice for uncomplicated acute otitis media because of its safety profile, cost, and excellent pharmacodynamic profile against sensitive and drug-resistant *S. pneumoniae*.
- An accurate diagnosis of attention-deficit/hyperactivity disorder (ADHD) should be obtained before initiating drug therapy.
- Pharmacotherapy for ADHD is stimulants (first line). Second-line agents are atomoxetine, guanfacine, and **clonidine**. Pharmacotherapy should be titrated to the desired functional effect without increasing the risk of side effects.
- ADHD therapy should include behavioral modification. Monitoring of drug and nondrug therapy should include input from different environments (e.g., parents, teachers).
- Bacterial and viral conjunctivitis may occur in the first month of life. Antimicrobial ointment administration should be instituted after delivery for prophylaxis.
- Bacterial, viral, and allergic conjunctivitis should be treated with antimicrobial therapy (bacterial), symptomatic therapy (bacterial, viral, allergic), and ocular antihistamines, decongestants, mast cell stabilizers, or combination products (allergic).

31-2 STUDY GUIDE CHECKLIST

The following topics may guide your study of this subject area:

- ☐ Medication administration recommendations specific to the pediatric population.
- ☐ Developmental considerations in pediatric patients with respect to drug absorption, distribution, metabolism, and excretion.
- ☐ Differentiation between acute otitis media, otitis media with effusion, and recurrent otitis media.
- ☐ Common bacterial organisms associated with acute otitis media and their resistance patterns.
- ☐ Recommended treatment regimens for an initial episode of acute otitis media and for patients unresponsive to initial therapy or observation therapy.
- ☐ Administration techniques for otic and ophthalmic medications.
- ☐ Recommended drug therapies for ADHD.
- ☐ Considerations for conjunctivitis management based on patient age and whether the cause is bacterial, viral, or allergic.

31-3   Special Drug Therapy Considerations in Pediatric Patients

Medication Administration Issues in Pediatric Patients

Medication administration issues extend across the pediatric age spectrum (see Box 31-1). Pediatric medication administration is complicated by many variables, including developmental alterations in the way drugs are absorbed, distributed, metabolized, and eliminated, as well as by medication adherence (palatability, administration routes) and accurate dosing and delivery. Medications are typically dosed in neonates, infants, and children as amount per kilogram (2.2 pounds = 1 kg) per day divided into doses per day compared to typical adult dosing of amount per day divided into doses per day. The transition to adult dosing generally begins in adolescence. Alternate routes of administration may be used in pediatric patients. For example, the dermal route is effective (and potentially excessive) for drug absorption in the neonate, particularly the premature neonate, because of an immature stratum corneum and increased skin hydration. The intraosseous and rectal routes are also effective for drug delivery in infants and children. Because small pediatric patients do not learn to swallow pills until later in childhood, liquid formulations are preferred. The use of inappropriate medication administration devices has resulted in toxicity and death in pediatric patients. See Box 31-2 that outlines appropriate and inappropriate medication administration devices.

Stickers demarcating the appropriate dose can also be applied to liquid measuring devices for further clarity when counseling caregivers. When liquid formulations are not commercially available, considerations include the medication's appropriateness for crushing and mixing with liquids or sprinkling capsules contents on food (and what type of food). See Table 31-5 later in the chapter for administration methods for otic and ophthalmic preparations. Development issues that impact pharmacotherapy in pediatric patients are described in Table 31-1.

Because of developmental immaturity in renal elimination as well as changes in muscle mass during pediatric development, a pediatric equation for estimation of creatine clearance (CrCl) is used in pediatric patients. Children do not reach adult CrCl until between 1 and 2 years of age. Average CrCl values (normal renal function) across the pediatric age spectrum and into adulthood are shown in Table 31-2.

BOX 31-1. Pediatric Age Definitions

- *Preterm:* <37 weeks gestation
- *Term:* ≥37 weeks gestation
- *Neonate:* <1 month

- *Infant:* 1 month to <1 year
- *Child:* 1 to 11 years
- *Adolescent:* 12 to 16 years

BOX 31-2. Inappropriate and Appropriate Medication Administration Methods in Pediatric Patients

Inappropriate	Appropriate
Different size table spoons (teaspoon, tablespoon, kids spoon, etc.)	Medicine dropper
Administration droppers and cups that do not go with the medicine to be given	Oral syringe
	Medicine cup
	Medicine spoon

TABLE 31-1. Pediatric Developmental Pharmacotherapy

Absorption	Distribution	Metabolism	Excretion

Compared to older children/adolescents/adults, neonates/infants and young children have:

Absorption	Distribution	Metabolism	Excretion
■ ↑ Relative increased gastric pH ■ Irregular and decreased motility ■ ↑ Longer GI transit time ■ ↓ Lower concentrativon of pancreatic enzymes and bile acids	■ ↓ Decreased plasma albumin and proteins ■ Competitive plasma protein binding by endogenous substances (unconjugated bilirubin) ■ Differences in body composition (neonates/infants: greater total body water, decreased adipose tissue) ■ Changes in muscle mass over time	■ ↓ Hepatic metabolism lower at birth ■ ↑ Longer half-life of drugs undergoing Phase I and Phase II reactions ■ Most developed/functional at birth: hydrolysis, methylation, oxidation, reduction, sulfation ■ Insufficiency of one pathway may lead to metabolism by another pathway	■ ↓ Decreased renal blood flow ■ ↓ Decreased GFR ■ ↓ Decreased tubular secretion ■ SCr in neonates may be falsely elevated due to presence of maternal SCr

Implications for drug therapy:

Absorption	Distribution	Metabolism	Excretion
■ ↑ Increased bioavailability of acid labile drugs and basic drugs ■ ↓ Decreased bioavailability of acidic drugs ■ Erratic absorption of sustained release products ■ ↓ Decreased absorption of lipid-soluble drugs and fat-soluble vitamins	Neonates/infants: ■ ↑ Increased free fraction of protein-bound drugs (e.g., phenytoin, sulfonamides) ■ ↑ Increased potential for drug displacement by endogenous substances (e.g., unconjugated bilirubin and kernicterus) ■ ↑ Greater Vd of hydrophilic drugs	■ **Acetaminophen** metabolized by sulfation in neonates/infants compared to glucuronidation (children/adults) ■ Infants convert theophylline to caffeine due to functional methylation that is not expressed in adults ■ Toxicity examples include gray baby syndrome with chloramphenicol (immature glucoronosyltransferase or UDPG activity responsible for glucuronidation) and gasping syndrome with benzyl alcohol accumulation (underdeveloped alcohol dehydrogenase)	■ GFR estimations during first week of life may be undervalued ■ Use Bedside Schwartz equation for GFR estimation (eGFR) in pediatric patients: eGFR (mL/min/1.73 m²) = 0.413 × (height in cm/SCr)

Boldface indicates one of top 100 drugs for 2020 by prescription volume.
GFR, glomerular filtration rate; GI, gastrointestinal; SCr, serum creatinine; UDPG, uridine diphosphate glucose; Vd, volume of distribution.

TABLE 31-2. Average Creatinine Clearance Values (Normal Renal Function)

Age (term)	Value (mL/min/1.73 m²)
5 to 7 days	50.6 ± 5.8
1 to 2 months	64.6 ± 5.8
5 to 8 months	87.7 ± 11.9
9 to 12 months	86.9 ± 8.4
>18 months (male)	124 ± 26
>8 months (female)	109 ± 13.5
Adult (male)	105 ± 14
Adult (female)	95 ± 18

31-4 Specific Infections and Disease States in the Pediatric Population

Otitis Media

Otitis media is an inflammatory process of the middle ear. It is classified as follows:

- *Acute otitis media* is the rapid onset of signs and symptoms of inflammation in the middle ear. Uncomplicated acute otitis media is not accompanied by otorrhea (discharge from the ear).
- *Nonsevere:* Mild otalgia (ear pain) for <48 hours and temperature <39°C or 102.2°F
- *Severe:* Moderate-to-severe otalgia, otalgia for at least 48 hours, or fever ≥39°C or 102.2°F
- *Recurrent otitis media* is the diagnosis of 3 or more separate episodes of acute otitis media within a 6-month period or 4 episodes within a year (with at least 1 episode in the past 6 months).
- *Otitis media with effusion* is inflammation of the middle ear with the presence of fluid in the middle ear (effusion) without the associated signs or symptoms of acute infection.

Clinical presentation

Signs and symptoms include fever, otalgia (often manifested as ear tugging or pulling), otorrhea, changes in balance or hearing, irritability, difficulty sleeping, lethargy, anorexia, vomiting, and diarrhea. Associated symptoms may be runny nose, congestion, or cough.

Pathophysiology

The infant's eustachian tube is shorter and more horizontal than that of the adult, thus preventing drainage of middle ear secretions into the nasopharynx and promoting pooling of secretions in the middle ear. Anatomic abnormalities increase risk (e.g., cleft palate, adenoid hypertrophy). An immature immune system or altered host defenses also increase risk, as do viral infections and allergies.

Risk factors include male gender; Native American, Canadian Eskimo, or Alaskan descent; family history of acute otitis media or respiratory tract infection; early age of first episode (earlier age is associated with greater severity and recurrence); day care environment; parental smoking; lack of breast-feeding in infancy; and pacifier use.

Microbial pathogens

Historically, up to 50% of cases of otitis media were thought to be viral in origin. However, with accurate diagnosis of acute otitis media (i.e., differentiating between acute disease and otitis media with effusion), the majority of cases are bacterial with or without a viral component. The primary bacteria responsible for acute otitis media are discussed below.

- *Streptococcus pneumoniae* has been responsible over time for the majority of bacterial otitis media cases. Bacterial resistance, which occurs primarily through alteration in penicillin-binding protein (decreased affinity for binding sites), is common.
- *Haemophilus influenzae* (primarily nonencapsulated or nontypeable strains) has been considered the second-most-common organism responsible for bacterial otitis media cases. Bacterial resistance occurs through beta-lactamase production.
- *Moraxella catarrhalis* is the third-most-common organism responsible for bacterial otitis media cases. Almost all strains are beta-lactamase producing.

With the advent of the pneumococcal 7-valent (PCV7) and 13-valent (PCV13) vaccines, the otopathogens responsible for acute otitis media are changing. The incidence of acute otitis media because of *S. pneumoniae* and *H. influenzae* strains is now approximately equal. With respect to *S. pneumoniae*, the majority of strains identified in acute otitis media cases are those that are not represented in the vaccine.

Diagnosis

The 2013 clinical practice guidelines by the American Academy of Pediatrics (AAP) and the American Academy of Family Physicians (AAFP) have established diagnostic criteria and recommend the use of pneumatic otoscopy or tympanometry to differentiate between episodes of acute otitis media and otitis media with effusion. The 2013 guidelines apply to the diagnosis and management of uncomplicated acute otitis media in infants and children 6 months to 12 years of age. For management in infants less than 6 months of age, the earlier 2004 guidelines may still be used.

Otoscopic examination determines color, translucency, and position of the tympanic membrane. Pneumatic otoscopic examination determines mobility of the tympanic membrane (i.e., presence or absence of effusion). The membrane will not move briskly with positive and negative pressure if effusion is present. Tympanometry may also be used to determine the presence of middle ear effusion. Tympanocentesis (i.e., a needle is inserted through the tympanic membrane to withdraw fluid) allows for culture and identification of the pathogen.

According to the 2013 guidelines, middle ear effusion on examination with pneumatic otoscope or with tympanometry must be present to diagnose acute otitis media. In addition, acute otitis media should be diagnosed with moderate to severe bulging of the tympanic membrane or new onset of otorrhea. Alternately, acute otitis media may be diagnosed with mild bulging of the tympanic membrane and recent onset (<48 hours) of ear pain or intense erythema of the tympanic membrane.

Treatment principles and goals

- Assess and control pain
- Eradicate infection
- Prevent complications
- Avoid unnecessary antibiotic therapy
- Improve compliance
- Eliminate presence of effusion
- Prevent recurrence

Drug therapy

Many episodes of otitis media will have spontaneous resolution; however, because of a risk of complications from untreated otitis media (e.g., mastoiditis, meningitis, subdural empyema), antimicrobials remain the mainstay of therapy. Observation therapy may be appropriate in select patients.

Antimicrobial treatment options are described in Table 31-3.

First-line therapy

High-dose **amoxicillin** (Amoxil) reaches good concentrations in the middle ear and has excellent in vitro activity against *S. pneumoniae* and most *H. influenzae*. **Amoxicillin** is palatable, inexpensive, and has an excellent safety and efficacy profile with a narrow spectrum of activity. While higher doses may overcome drug-resistant *S. pneumoniae*, **amoxicillin** does not eradicate beta-lactamase–producing organisms.

Amoxicillin-clavulanate (Augmentin) should be used as first-line therapy in patients who have received **amoxicillin** in the past 30 days, those with conjunctivitis, or those in whom beta-lactamase-positive *H. influenzae* or *M. catarrhalis* is suspected. It is recommended to keep the daily clavulanate dose <10 mg/kg to prevent diarrhea.

For penicillin-allergic patients, cefdinir, cefpodoxime, cefuroxime (Ceftin), or ceftriaxone may be used.

Duration of therapy

Two courses of therapy are possible:

- Standard course (10 days)
- Shorter course (1 to 7 days)

TABLE 31-3. Antimicrobial Therapy for Acute Otitis Media

Initial antibiotics or after treatment failure with observation		Treatment failure after 48 to 72 hours of antibiotics	
First line	**Alternative**	**First line**	**Alternative**
Amoxicillin (Amoxil) 80 to 90 mg/kg/d or Amoxicillin-clavulanate (Augmentin)ᵃ 90 mg/kg/d **amoxicillin** + 6.4 mg/kg/d clavulanate	Cefdinir 14 mg/kg/d in 1 or 2 doses or Cefuroxime (Ceftin) 30 mg/kg/d in 2 doses or Cefpodoxime 10 mg/kg/d in 2 doses or Ceftriaxone 50 mg/kg/d I.M. or IV for 1 to 3 daysᵇ	Amoxicillin-clavulanate (Augmentin) 90 mg/kg/d **amoxicillin** + 6.4 mg/kg/d clavulanate or Ceftriaxone 50 mg/kg/d I.M. or I.V. for 3 daysᵇ	Ceftriaxone 50 mg/kg/d for 3 daysᵇ or Clindamycinᶜ (Cleocin) 30 to 40 mg/kg/d in 3 doses ± 2nd- or 3rd-generation cephalosporin or Clindamycinᶜ (Cleocin) + 2nd- or 3rd-generation cephalosporin Tympanocentesis, consult specialist

Boldface indicates one of top 100 drugs for 2020 by prescription volume.

I.M., intramuscular; I.V., intravenous.

a. Amoxicillin-clavulanate is first-line therapy in patients who have received **amoxicillin** in the past 30 days, those with conjunctivitis, those with a history of recurrent otitis media unresponsive to **amoxicillin**, or those in whom beta-lactamase activity for *H. influenzae* or *M. catarrhalis* is indicated.

b. More than 1 ceftriaxone dose may be needed to prevent recurrence.

c. Clindamycin does not have activity against *H. influenzae*. It should be used when penicillin-resistant *S. pneumoniae* is suspected.

> ⚠ **Clindamycin (Cleocin)** *FDA BOXED WARNING*
>
> Clindamycin has been associated with severe *Clostridioides* (formerly *Clostridium*) *difficile*-associated diarrhea (CDAD) which may result in death. Do not use clindamycin for nonbacterial infections, such as most upper respiratory infections.

Advantages of the shorter course are improved compliance, decreased adverse effects of drug therapy, decreased risk of bacterial resistance, and lower costs. Disadvantages are delayed or no cure, increased risk of complications from untreated acute otitis media, and greater risk of recurrence.

The 2013 guidelines recommend the standard 10-day course in children <2 years of age or for severe symptoms at any age. A 7-day course may be used in children 2 to 5 years of age (and a 5 to 7 to day course in children age 6 years and older) with mild-to-moderate acute otitis media.

Other therapy

Antipyretics (**acetaminophen** [Tylenol] ⚠ and **ibuprofen** [Motrin]) ⚠ or analgesics may be used. Use **acetaminophen** with caution in high doses to avoid hepatotoxicity. Use **ibuprofen** only in patients >6 months of age and use with caution in patients with vomiting, diarrhea, and poor fluid intake, because dehydration predisposes them to **ibuprofen**-induced renal insufficiency. Avoid alternating antipyretic therapy. Encourage parents to choose 1 agent, inform them of any adverse effects, and educate them about symptoms of those effects (e.g., hepatotoxicity or renal insufficiency). The only topical analgesics available are naturopathic otic solutions.

Topical antimicrobials may have a place in therapy, particularly with ruptured tympanic membranes (fluoroquinolone or fluoroquinolone and steroid combination otic suspensions [ofloxacin otic, Cetraxal, Cipro HC, Ciprodex]).

⚠ Acetaminophen (Tylenol) *FDA BOXED WARNING*

Acetaminophen has been associated with cases of acute liver failure that may result in death or require liver transplant. The risk of liver injury is greater with doses that exceed the maximum daily limits as well as when taking more than one acetaminophen-containing product.

Acetaminophen injection carries to potential for dosing errors that could result in accidental overdose and death. Ensure the following: the dose in milligrams and milliliters is not confused; the dosing is based on weight for patients less than 50 kg; infusion pumps are properly programmed; and the total daily dose of **acetaminophen** from all sources does not exceed maximum daily limits.

⚠ Ibuprofen (Motrin) *FDA BOXED WARNING*

Ibuprofen use is associated with increased risk of serious cardiovascular thrombotic events including myocardial infarction and stroke. It is contraindicated in patients undergoing coronary artery bypass graft surgery. **Ibuprofen** is also associated with increased risk of gastrointestinal (GI) bleeding, ulcerations, and perforation during any time of use which may result in death. Elderly patients and those with a prior history of peptic ulcer disease or GI bleed are at greater risk for serious GI complications.

Patient instructions and counseling

- Complete the entire course of prescribed antibiotics.
- Shake bottle well before administering dose. Follow labeling regarding temperature for storage of medication.
- Contact the health care provider if patient develops a rash or has difficulty breathing, or if symptoms persist after 72 hours of initiating therapy.

Adverse drug effects

- *Gastrointestinal effects:* Nausea and diarrhea, discoloration of stools (with cefdinir)
- *Hypersensitivity:* Rash, anaphylaxis

Nondrug therapy

Local heat or cold therapy may be used (counsel the caregiver on appropriate use and technique to prevent burn injury).

Observation therapy

Observation therapy is appropriate only when follow-up at 48 to 72 hours can be ensured and antimicrobials initiated if symptoms persist or worsen. This therapy is *not* appropriate for the following patients:

- Infants <6 months of age
- Infants and children between 6 months and 2 years of age with otorrhea, severe symptoms (toxic-appearing child, otalgia >48 hours, or temperature ≥39°C or 102.2°F), or bilateral disease
- Children ≥2 years of age with otorrhea or severe symptoms as described above

Immunization and immunoprophylaxis

Pneumococcal conjugate vaccination should provide some protection against strains responsible for a majority of bacterial otitis media.

H. influenzae type B vaccination is of no benefit in otitis media. Most strains causing otitis media are non-typeable and not prevented by vaccination.

Killed and live-attenuated intranasal influenza vaccine may decrease episodes of acute otitis media during the respiratory illness season. Annual influenza vaccination is recommended for infants and children age 6 months and older as part of the childhood immunization schedule.

Risk reduction

- Encourage exclusive breast-feeding for 6 months.
- Eliminate passive exposure to tobacco smoke.
- Avoid supine bottle feeding.
- Reduce or eliminate pacifier use after 6 months of age.
- Reduce incidence of upper respiratory infections by altering day care attendance (when possible).

Recurrent otitis media

The use of antimicrobials for otitis media prophylaxis is not recommended. Risk factor reduction in this group of patients is important. Surgical placement of tympanostomy tubes may be recommended to decrease recurrent episodes, restore hearing, and relieve discomfort.

Otitis media with effusion

Effusion in the middle ear may persist for months after an episode of acute otitis media. Complications include hearing loss and delayed speech and language development. No role exists for antimicrobials, antihistamines, decongestants, or corticosteroids in otitis media with effusion. Thus, accurate diagnosis and distinguishing effusion from acute otitis media is important to avoid unnecessary antimicrobial use. The goal of management of otitis media with effusion is to prevent speech, language, and learning delays. Tympanostomy tube placement is indicated if any of these occur.

Otitis Externa

Otitis externa is an inflammation of the outer ear canal, also referred to as *swimmer's ear.*

Clinical presentation

Patients present with itching, pain, otic exudate, and hearing impairment.

Pathophysiology

With prolonged exposure to moisture, the ear canal is disrupted (e.g., loss of cerumen and altered pH) and susceptible to infection. The most common organisms are *Pseudomonas aeruginosa* and *Staphylococcus aureus.* Fungal pathogens account for a minority of cases.

Therapy consists of antibiotic or antibiotic/steroid otic preparations such as neomycin, polymyxin B, and hydrocortisone (generic), or neomycin, colistin, and hydrocortisone (Coly-Mycin S). Fluoroquinolone otic preparations such as ciprofloxacin (Cetraxal, generic) and ofloxacin (generic) and fluoroquinolone/steroid preparations (Ciprodex, Cipro HC) can also be used, as well as acetic acid (VoSol) and acetic acid/hydrocortisone (VoSol HC) otic preparations or oral analgesics. See Table 31-5 for administration of otic preparations in pediatric patients.

Preventive measures include drying ears after exposure to moisture; using drops containing isopropyl alcohol, with or without acetic acid to reduce pH; and avoiding cotton swabs.

Attention-Deficit/Hyperactivity Disorder

According to the American Psychiatric Association's *Diagnostic and Statistical Manual of Mental Disorders*, 5th edition (DSM-5), attention-deficit/hyperactivity disorder (ADHD) is a persistent pattern of inattention, hyperactivity/impulsivity, or both that interferes with development; has symptoms presenting in two or more settings; and has a direct, negative effect on social, academic, or occupational functioning. The DSM-5 defines the following ADHD classifications: predominantly inattentive presentation, predominantly hyperactive-impulsive presentation, combined presentation, and other specified and unspecified ADHD.

Pathophysiology

ADHD results from an imbalance in catecholamine neurotransmission (specifically between dopamine and norepinephrine). See Box 31-3 for diagnosis criteria of ADHD.

Treatment goals

- Educate the patient and family.
- Improve functioning and behavior.
- Achieve effective drug therapy with minimal side effects.

Drug therapy

Table 31-4 describes drug therapy for ADHD.

> ### BOX 31-3. Diagnosis of ADHD

Children must have 6 or more symptoms of inattention, hyperactivity/impulsivity, or both for at least 6 months.

- Symptoms must be present before 12 years of age.
- Impairment must present in 2 or more settings (e.g., home and school).

- Clinically significant impairment occurs in social, academic, or occupational environments.
- Symptoms do not occur exclusively during another psychotic or mental illness (e.g., schizophrenia, mood disorder).

TABLE 31-4. Drug Therapy for Attention-Deficit/Hyperactivity Disorder

Therapeutic category	Indication and mechanism of action	Comments
Stimulants (first-line therapy) *Mixed amphetamine salts* **(amphetamine/dextroamphetamine ⚠):** Short-acting (Adderall, Eveko, Eveko ODT) Long-acting (Adderall XR, Adzenys XR-ODT, Adzenys ER, Dyanavel XR, Mydayis)	Reuptake blockade of catecholamines (norepinephrine and dopamine) in presynaptic nerve endings	Products are classified as C-IIs with the potential for drug dependency. Doses given after 4 PM may cause insomnia. **Lisdexamfetamine ⚠** is the prodrug of **dextroamphetamine**; it was developed to discourage the potential for drug abuse. **Daytrana ⚠** is a transdermal patch and should be applied every morning to alternating hips and worn for 9 hours.

(continued)

TABLE 31-4. Drug Therapy for Attention-Deficit/Hyperactivity Disorder *(Continued)*

Therapeutic category	Indication and mechanism of action	Comments
Dextroamphetamine ⚠️ : Short-acting (ProCentra, Zenzedi) Long-acting (Dexedrine Spansule) **Lisdexamfetamine dimesylate** ⚠️ : Long-acting (Vyvanse) **Methylphenidate:** Short-acting (Methylin, **methylphenidate** (generic), Ritalin) Long-acting (Adhansia XR, Aptensio XR, Concerta, Cotempla XR-ODT, Daytrana, Jornay PM, Metadate CD, **methylphenidate** (generic), Ritalin LA ⚠️ , Quillivant XR ⚠️ , QuilliChew ER) Dexmethylphenidate ⚠️ : Short-acting (Focalin) Long-acting (Focalin XR)		Dexmethylphenidate ⚠️ , the d-threo-enantiomer of racemic **methylphenidate**, is thought to be the more active enantiomer. Methylin ⚠️ is available as an oral solution. Short-acting Adderall and Ritalin tablets may be crushed or chewed. The following long-acting products allow for opening the capsule and sprinkling contents on applesauce: Aptensio XR, Adderall XR, Focalin XR, Jornay PM, Metadate CD ⚠️ , Mydayis, Ritalin LA. Contents of Vyvanse capsules may be mixed with yogurt, orange juice, or water. Newly approved products offer additional options for pediatric dosing including liquid formulations (Adzenys ER, Dyanavel XR ⚠️ , ProCentra, Quillivant XR), chewable tablets (QuilliChew ER, Vyvanse chewables), and orally disintegrating tablets (Adzenys XR-ODT, Cotempla XR-ODT). Drug holidays may be recommended to determine if the need for stimulant is still present and to minimize side effects (e.g., summer is a good time to see if patient is outgrowing disease).
Second-line therapy		
Atomoxetine (Strattera)	Noradrenergic-specific reuptake inhibitor	Atomoxetine is a nonstimulant, noncontrolled agent. Maximum effects may take up to 4 to 6 weeks. Discontinue in patients who develop jaundice or laboratory evidence of liver injury. Capsule should not be opened.
Guanfacine (extended-release; Intuniv)	Alpha-2-receptor agonist	Guanfacine is FDA approved for use as monotherapy or as adjunctive therapy with stimulants. Maximum effects may take 2 to 4 weeks. Tablet must be swallowed whole; do not crush or chew. Label recommends taking with a high-fat meal.
Clonidine (extended-release; Kapvay)	Alpha-2-receptor agonist	**Clonidine** is FDA approved for use as monotherapy or as adjunctive therapy with stimulants. Maximum effects may take 2 to 4 weeks. **Clonidine** is a good option to use for ADHD and coexisting conditions such as sleep disturbances or tics. Tablet must be swallowed whole; do not crush or chew.

Boldface indicates one of top 100 drugs for 2020 by prescription volume.

Amphetamine/Dextroamphetamine *FDA BOXED WARNING*

CNS stimulants, including amphetamine-containing products and **methylphenidate**, have a high potential for abuse and dependence.

 Lisdexamfetamine Dimesylate *FDA BOXED WARNING*

CNS stimulants (amphetamines and **methylphenidate**-containing products), including **lisdexamfetamine**, have a high potential for abuse and dependence.

 Daytrana *FDA BOXED WARNING*

Daytrana should be given cautiously to patients with a history of drug dependence or alcoholism. Long term abusive use may lead to psychological dependence, abnormal behavior, and psychotic episodes. During withdrawal from abusive use, severe depression may occur.

 Dextroamphetamine *FDA BOXED WARNING*

Amphetamines have a high potential for abuse. Misuse of amphetamines may cause sudden death and serious cardiovascular adverse reactions.

 Dexmethylphenidate *FDA BOXED WARNING*

CNS stimulants, including dexmethylphenidate, **methylphenidate**-containing products, and amphetamines, have a high potential for abuse and dependence.

Methylin *FDA BOXED WARNING*

Methylin should be given cautiously to emotionally unstable patients, such as those with a history of drug dependence or alcoholism, because such patients may increase dosage on their own initiative. Long term abusive use may lead to psychological dependence, abnormal behavior, and psychotic episodes. During withdrawal from abusive use, severe depression as well as the effects of chronic overactivity may occur.

 Metadate CD *FDA BOXED WARNING*

Metadate CD should be given cautiously to patients with a history of drug dependence or alcoholism. Long term abusive use may lead to psychological dependence, abnormal behavior, and psychotic episodes. During withdrawal from abusive use, severe depression may occur.

 Dyanavel XR *FDA BOXED WARNING*

CNS stimulants, including DYANAVEL XR, other amphetamine-containing products, and **methylphenidate**, have a high potential for abuse and dependence.

 Ritalin LA *FDA BOXED WARNING*

CNS stimulants, including Ritalin LA, other **methylphenidate**-containing products, and amphetamines, have a high potential for abuse and dependence.

Quillivant XR *FDA BOXED WARNING*

CNS stimulants, including QUILLIVANT XR, other **methylphenidate**-containing products, and amphetamines, have a high potential for abuse and dependence.

The AAP released an updated clinical practice guideline for the diagnosis, evaluation, and treatment of ADHD in 2019. Recommendations for treatment vary on the basis of patient age as follows:

- *Preschool-age children (4 to 5 years of age):* First-line therapy is behavior therapy. **Methylphenidate** ⚠ (see Table 31-4 for brand names) may be added to behavior therapy with moderate-to-severe dysfunction if there is not significant improvement in the child's functioning with behavior therapy alone.
- *Elementary school–age children (6 to 11 years of age):* First-line therapy should be drug therapy in combination with behavior therapy.
- *Adolescents (12 to 18 years of age):* Drug therapy should be used with the assent of the patient and preferably in combination with behavior therapy.

Stimulants are recommended as first-line drug therapy. Second-line drugs include atomoxetine (Strattera) ⚠, extended-release guanfacine (Intuniv), and extended-release **clonidine** (Kapvay).

Patient counseling

Advise patients and caregivers of the need to store stimulants away from other children or siblings because of the potential for abuse.

 Methylphenidate *FDA BOXED WARNING*

CNS stimulants, including **methylphenidate**-containing products and amphetamines, have a high potential for abuse and dependence. Long term abusive use may lead to psychotic episodes.

 Atomoxetine (Strattera) *FDA BOXED WARNING*

Atomoxetine has been associated with increased risk of suicidal ideation in short-term studies in children or adolescents with attention deficit hyperactivity disorder (ADHD). Comorbidities may also increase the risk of suicidal ideation. The risk may be greater during early treatment. Closely monitor patients being started on atomoxetine for suicidal ideation or other changes in behavior.

Adverse drug effects

Stimulants may cause appetite suppression, abdominal pain, headache, insomnia, jitteriness, and weight loss (not height dependent). Stimulants may also lower the seizure threshold. **Methylphenidate** ⚠ is contra-indicated in patients with motor tics and Tourette syndrome.

Methylphenidate and atomoxetine ⚠ include warnings about the possibility of priapism.

Labeling for all the stimulants and for atomoxetine (Strattera) includes warnings for an increased risk of psychosis or mania, aggression or violent behavior, and anxiety or panic attacks.

In addition, atomoxetine (Strattera) labeling includes warnings for increased risk of suicidal ideation in children and adolescents and for the potential for severe liver injury. It is also contraindicated in patients with pheochromocytoma or a history of pheochromocytoma because of serious reactions (hypertension, tachyarrhythmia).

Warnings are included for stimulants (amphetamine ⚠ and **methylphenidate** ⚠ products) and atomoxetine (Strattera) regarding serious cardiovascular events, including sudden death, in children and adolescents. A large retrospective cohort study of over 1.2 million children and young adults (up to 24 years of age) has failed to demonstrate an association between the use of ADHD medications, including stimulants and atomoxetine (Strattera), and serious adverse cardiovascular events (myocardial infarction, stroke, sudden cardiac death). Atomoxetine labeling carried a contraindication in patients with severe cardiac or vascular disorders. The American Heart Association and American Academy of Pediatrics recommend a thorough cardiovascular assessment prior to initiation of therapy with stimulants or atomoxetine for ADHD.

Atomoxetine (Strattera) has been associated with gastrointestinal symptoms and sedation early in therapy; these side effects can be offset by starting with half the therapeutic dose for the first week of therapy. Appetite suppression can also occur.

Alpha-2 adrenergic agonists (guanfacine [Intuniv], **clonidine** [Kapvay]) may cause hypotension, bradycardia, syncope, and sedation, especially within the first month of therapy. Somnolence is a common effect with these agents. Rebound hypertension is also possible with abrupt withdrawal; thus, tapering is recommended when discontinuing these products.

 Amphetamine *FDA BOXED WARNING*

Amphetamines have a high potential for abuse and dependence. Access to drug supply should be limited as there is a potential for non-therapeutic use or distribution to others. Misuse of amphetamines may cause sudden death and serious cardiovascular adverse reactions.

Drug–drug interactions
Methylphenidate

- **Methylphenidate** should not be given with monoamine oxidase (MAO) inhibitors (severe hypertension has occurred).
- Caffeine may enhance stimulant effects.
- **Methylphenidate** may inhibit metabolism of phenytoin ⚠ (Dilantin), phenobarbital, **warfarin** ⚠ (Coumadin), and tricyclics.

Atomoxetine (Strattera)

- Atomoxetine should not be given with MAO inhibitors (serious, sometimes fatal reactions have occurred).
- Atomoxetine is a substrate for CYP2D6; dosing should be titrated more slowly with concomitant use of strong CYP2D6 inhibitors (e.g., **fluoxetine** ⚠ [Prozac], **paroxetine** ⚠ [Paxil], quinidine ⚠).

Phenytoin *FDA BOXED WARNING*

The rate of intravenous phenytoin administration should not exceed 50 mg/minute in adults and 1 to 3 mg/kg/minute (or 50 mg/minute, whichever is slower) in pediatric patients because of the risk of severe hypotension and cardiac arrhythmias. Careful cardiac monitoring is needed during and after administering intravenous phenytoin.

 Warfarin *FDA BOXED WARNING*

Warfarin is associated with major or fatal bleeding. Regular monitoring of international normalized ratio (INR) and patient education should be performed.

 Fluoxetine *FDA BOXED WARNING*

Antidepressants increased the risk of suicidal thinking and behavior in children, adolescents, and young adults with major depressive disorder (MDD) and other psychiatric disorders. Closely monitor patients being started on antidepressants for suicidal ideation or other changes in behavior.

 Fluoxetine is approved for use in children with MDD (aged 8 years and older) and obsessive-compulsive disorder (OCD; aged 7 years and older). Sarafem is not approved for use in children.

 Paroxetine *FDA BOXED WARNING*

Antidepressants increased the risk of suicidal thoughts and behaviors in pediatric and young adult patients. Closely monitor all antidepressant-treated patients for clinical worsening and for emergence of suicidal thoughts and behaviors. **Paroxetine** is not approved for use in pediatric patients.

Quinidine *FDA BOXED WARNING*

Active antiarrhythmic therapy has resulted in increased mortality; the risk of active therapy is probably greatest in patients with structural heart disease.

Guanfacine (Intuniv)

- Guanfacine is a substrate for CYP3A4; dosing should be adjusted accordingly when given concomitantly with strong CYP3A4 inhibitors (e.g., ketoconazole ⚠ [Nizoral]) or inducers (e.g., rifampin [Rifadin, Rimactane]).
- Co-administration with valproic acid ⚠ (generic) results in increased valproic acid concentrations; therapeutic drug monitoring of valproic acid should be conducted and dose adjustments made (if necessary) when using these agents together.

Recommendations for therapy and monitoring

The efficacy of therapy should be monitored. Assess behavior changes, and evaluate feedback from teachers and parents.

Monitor patients periodically for changes in blood pressure and heart rate. The American Heart Association also recommends that all children be screened for cardiovascular disease risk factors before initiating therapy. An electrocardiogram (ECG) is warranted only before initiation of stimulant or atomoxetine (Strattera) therapy in patients with risk factors for cardiovascular disease.

 Ketoconazole *FDA BOXED WARNING*

Ketoconazole is associate with serious hepatotoxicity that may result in liver transplantation or death. Due to serious adverse effects, ketoconazole tablets are not indicated for the treatment of onychomycosis, cutaneous dermatophyte infections, or Candida infections. Use ketoconazole only when other effective antifungal therapy is not available or tolerated and the potential benefits are considered to outweigh the potential risks.

Ketoconazole is contraindicated with the following drugs: dofetilide, quinidine, pimozide, cisapride, methadone, disopyramide, dronedarone, and ranolazine. Ketoconazole can cause elevated plasma concentrations of these drugs and may prolong QT intervals, sometimes resulting in life-threatening ventricular dysrhythmias, such as torsades de pointes.

 Valproic Acid *FDA BOXED WARNING*

Valproate is associated with liver failure resulting in death. Children <2 years of age are at increased risk of fatal hepatotoxicity and this risk is compounded in patients on multiple anticonvulsants, those with congenital metabolic disorders, severe seizures accompanied by mental retardation, and organic brain disease. There is an increased risk of liver failure and death in patients with mitochondrial disorders caused by POLG mutations and children <2 years of age suspected of having a mitochondrial disorder.

Valproate should not be used in pregnant women or women of child-bearing potential due to the risk of major congenital malformations, particularly neural tube defects and decreased IQ scores and neurodevelopmental disorders. If therapy is necessary, contraception should be used.

Cases of life-threatening pancreatitis have been reported in both children and adults receiving valproate.

Stimulants

Begin with a low dose, and titrate upward to optimal functioning ability. The patient may need a decreased dose if side effects occur or if no further improvement is seen with the larger dose. If 1 stimulant fails, try another stimulant for the patient. For children who fail 2 stimulants, second-line therapy includes atomoxetine (Strattera) or an alpha-2-adrenergic agonist.

Atomoxetine (Strattera)

Because of the boxed warning for suicidal ideation when initiating therapy, patients should be monitored for any changes in behavior that necessitate referral to a mental health clinician.

Pharmacokinetic considerations

Methylphenidate does not distribute well into adipose tissue (dose on milligram basis instead of milligrams per kilogram).

Nondrug therapy

- Behavioral techniques (e.g., positive reinforcement, time out, response cost, token economy)
- Environmental modifications
- Classroom management

Conjunctivitis

Conjunctivitis is an inflammation of the conjunctiva of the eye. Conjunctivitis may be bacterial, viral, or allergic.

Clinical presentation

Conjunctivitis is characterized by redness of the eye, itching, ocular discharge, foreign body sensation, and crusting of the eye and eyelid. The patient may have altered vision because of the presence of discharge.

Pathophysiology

Conjunctivitis of the newborn

Inflammation of the conjunctiva often occurs in the first month of life. Causative agents include topical antimicrobial agents, bacteria (primarily *N. gonorrhoeae*, *Chlamydia trachomatis*, *S. aureus*, *Staphylococcus epidermidis*, *S. pneumoniae*, *Escherichia coli*, and other gram-negative bacteria), and viruses (primarily herpes simplex).

Bacterial conjunctivitis (beyond first month of life)

The most common bacteria are *S. aureus*, *S. epidermidis*, *S. pneumoniae*, and *H. influenzae* (also gonococcal and chlamydial).

Viral conjunctivitis

Viral conjunctivitis, also known as pink eye, is contagious. Adenovirus is the most common causative agent. This condition is commonly preceded by a cold or sore throat or exposure to another person with viral conjunctivitis. Herpes simplex is another cause of viral conjunctivitis. Corneal involvement may lead to permanent visual damage.

Allergic conjunctivitis

Allergic conjunctivitis is caused by exposure to dander, pollen, or a topical eye preparation. Most patients exhibit itching of the eye.

Diagnosis

Diagnosis is based on patient age and the patient's symptoms.

Treatment goals

- Eliminate or avoid the allergen (allergic conjunctivitis).
- Treat the underlying infection (bacterial conjunctivitis).
- Decrease severity, and provide symptomatic relief (all forms).

Drug therapy

Neonatal

Preventive medicine includes prophylaxis after delivery with erythromycin ophthalmic ointment (generic):

- *Onset day 1:* No treatment (secondary to prophylaxis after delivery)
- *Onset days 2 to 4 (N. gonorrheae):* Penicillin G (Pfizerpen) or ceftriaxone for 7 days
- *Onset days 3 to 10 (C. trachomatis):* Oral erythromycin (Erythrocin) + erythromycin ointment (generic) for 14 days
- *Onset days 2 to 16 (herpes simplex):* Possibly I.V. acyclovir (generic)

Bacterial (beyond first month of life)

Ophthalmic antibiotic drops (trimethoprim-polymyxin B [generic] or fluoroquinolone [ciprofloxacin (Ciloxan), gentamicin, or tobramycin (Tobrex)]) should be used in combination with an ophthalmic antibiotic ointment (erythromycin [generic] or bacitracin [generic]) at bedtime for 5 to 7 days.

Gonococcal

Ceftriaxone should be used for 1 dose. With corneal ulceration, use systemic I.V. ceftriaxone therapy. Also treat for *Chlamydia* species.

Chlamydial

Administer a single dose of **azithromycin** (Zithromax) to children.

Viral

Ocular lubricant (e.g., artificial tears product) should be administered every 3 to 4 hours while the patient is awake.

Allergic

Remove allergen. Use ocular lubricant (e.g., artificial tears product), ocular decongestants (phenylephrine [generic], tetrahydrozoline [most Visine products], oxymetazoline: alpha-adrenergic agonist [Visine LR], ketotifen [Alaway, Zatidor]), antihistamines (olopatadine [Pataday]), antihistamine–decongestant combination products (pheniramine and naphazoline [Naphcon-A, Opcon-A]), topical mast cell stabilizer (cromolyn sodium [generic]), combination mast cell stabilizer and antihistamine, or oral antihistamine therapy.

Adverse drug effects

Ocular decongestants can cause rebound congestion of the conjunctiva. This reaction is less common with tetrahydrozoline (multiple products).

Patient instructions and counseling

- Wash hands before and after administration of ophthalmic preparations.
- Administration of ophthalmic preparations in pediatric patients is described in Table 31-5.
- Do not share towels or linens.
- Store products according to labeling instructions.

Nondrug therapy

Cold compresses are a helpful nondrug therapy.

Select Medication Issues, Drug Contraindications, Boxed Warnings, and Labeling Changes Specific to Pediatric Patients

- Sulfonamides should not be used in neonates and infants ≤2 months of age because of risk of kernicterus.
- Ceftriaxone should not be used in neonates ≤28 days of age because of the risk of kernicterus.
- Use of fluoroquinolones in patients ≤18 years of age may cause arthropathy and cartilage lesions while growth plate is open. They are used in a few conditions as second-line agents.
- Tetracyclines are contraindicated in children ≤8 years of age because of drug deposition into developing teeth and bone.
- **Aspirin** is contraindicated because of risk of Reye's syndrome. It is used in certain conditions (e.g., Kawasaki disease).
- Promethazine (Phenergan) is contraindicated for children ≤2 years of age because of risk of respiratory depression and death.
- All antidepressants carry a warning about the potential for increased suicidal behavior in children and adolescents.

TABLE 31-5. Counseling on Administration of Ophthalmic and Otic Products

Otic medication administration	Ophthalmic medication administration
1. Wash hands before and after administration.	*Instilling eye drops:*
2. Warm otic drops to room temperature by holding bottle in hands for several minutes. Avoid instilling cold or hot drops into the ear canal.	Wash hands before and after administration. Tilt head back, grasp lower eyelid and pull away from eye, place dropper over eye, and have the patient look up immediately before instilling the drop. Blot excess solution away from around the eye. Wait 5 minutes between drops for multiple drop therapy. For suspension, place that drop in the eye last.
3. Shake the bottle if indicated on the label.	
4. Tilt the child's head to the side, or have the child lie down.	
5. Pull the child's ear backward and upward (for children <3 years of age, pull ear backward and downward), and instill the drops in the ear canal. Do not put the dropper bottle inside the ear canal. To remain free from contamination, the dropper should not come into contact with the ear.	*Instilling ointment:* Tilt head back, grasp lower eyelid and pull away from eye. Use a sweeping motion to instill 0.25 to 0.5 inch of ointment inside eyelid. Close eye after instillation, and wait 1 to 2 minutes. Blot excess ointment away from around the eye. Vision may be temporarily blurred with ointment administration.
6. Press gently on the small flap over the ear to push the drops into the canal.	
7. Have the child remain in the same position for the period of time indicated in the labeling. If this is not possible, place a cotton ball gently into the ear to prevent the drops from draining out of the ear canal.	*Instilling both drops and ointment:* Instill drops first and wait 10 minutes before applying ointment.
8. Wipe excess medication from the outside of the ear.	

- Fentanyl (Duragesic) is contraindicated for children ≤2 years of age and should be used in children ≥2 years of age only if they are already using other opioid pain medications (i.e., they are opioid tolerant).
- The use of Elidel cream (pimecrolimus) and Protopic ointment (tacrolimus) in children ≤2 years of age is not recommended because of possible cancer risk.
- There is a risk of ceftriaxone and calcium precipitation with the concomitant use of ceftriaxone and I.V. calcium-containing products. Deaths attributable to intravascular and pulmonary precipitates have occurred in neonates. Ceftriaxone should not be used in neonates (≤28 days of age) if they are receiving or are expected to receive I.V. calcium-containing products. In all other patients, the lines may be flushed well with a compatible fluid between the use of ceftriaxone and an I.V. calcium-containing product.
- Over-the-counter cough and cold medicines are not to be used in infants and children ≤4 years of age because of the risk of serious and potentially life-threatening side effects. Combination products are not recommended in pediatric patients.
- Antiepileptic agents include a warning about the risk of suicidal thoughts or actions.

Heparin carries warnings for the potential for dosing errors and deaths in neonates.

- Tumor necrosis factor (TNF)–alpha blocking agents carry warnings for the risk of lymphoma and malignancy in children and adolescents with autoimmune disorders.
- Codeine-containing products carry warnings for the risk of respiratory depression and death in children who are cytochrome P450 (CYP) 2D6-ultrarapid metabolizers receiving codeine after tonsillectomy, adenoidectomy, or both. Codeine solutions are contraindicated in all children <12 years of age and in children <18 years following tonsillectomy and/or adenoidectomy.
- Morphine accumulation can occur in breastfed infants of mothers who are CYP 2D6-ultrarapid metabolizers and taking codeine for postpartum pain care. Patient counseling should include limiting codeine use to less than 2 to 3 days and advising on signs and symptoms of opioid toxicity.
- Kaletra (lopinavir/ritonavir) carries a warning for propylene glycol accumulation and toxicity (cardiac toxicity, lactic acidosis, acute renal failure, CNS depression, respiratory complications, death) in preterm neonates.

31-5   Pharmacist's Role

The pharmacist plays a key role in ensuring the safe and effective use of medications in pediatric patients. It is important that the pharmacist understand developmental issues related to how drugs are absorbed, distributed, metabolized, and eliminated across the pediatric age spectrum. In addition, pharmacists are important gatekeepers to ensure that medications are prescribed accurately. Pharmacists advise parents and caregivers on the appropriate use of prescription and nonprescription medications for common pediatric conditions, including the appropriate administration tools to safely give medications to pediatric patients.

NAPLEX Competency Statements

The questions in this chapter cover the following 2021 NAPLEX Competency Statements: **AREA 1**: 1.1; 1.2; 1.3; 1.4; 1.5; 1.6; 1.7 **AREA 2:** 2.1; 2.2; 2.3; 2.4 **AREA 3:** 3.2; 3.4; 3.5; 3.6; 3.7; 3.8; 3.9; 3.10; 3.11; 3.12 **AREA 4:** 4.1; 4.2; 4.5; 4.6; 4.9 **AREA 5:** 5.5 **AREA 6:** 6.3; 6.4.

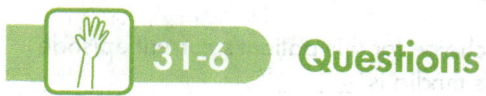

31-6   Questions

Use the following patient profile to answer Questions 1 and 2.

PATIENT PROFILE 31-1

Patient Name: Baby Boy Smith
Age: 4 days old
Sex: Male
Chief complaint:

Gestation: Term (37 weeks)
Birthweight: 3.2 kg
Length: 55 cm

Baby brought to emergency department by his parents due to fever and decreased oral intake and increased irritability since discharge from newborn nursery 2 days ago.

Emergency Department Medications

D5 1/2NS at 14 mL/h

Ampicillin 165 mg I.V. every 6 hours

Gentamicin 14 mg I.V. once daily

Laboratory and diagnostic tests

Cultures (blood, urine, and cerebrospinal fluid)—pending

Serum chemistries:

Sodium	142 mEq/L
Potassium	3.5 mEq/L
Chloride	108 mEq/L
Bicarbonate	22 mEq/L
Blood Urea Nitrogen	15 mg/dL
Serum Creatinine	0.9 mg/dL
Glucose	88 mg/dL

Bedside Schwartz equation is eGFR (mL/min/1.73 m²) = 0.413 × (height in cm/SCr)

---

1. What is the patient's estimated creatinine clearance (mL/min/1.73 m²)?

   A. 100
   B. 75
   C. 60
   D. 50
   E. 25

2. Which of the following is the most accurate reason for this patient's creatinine clearance estimate?

   A. Presence of maternal serum creatinine
   B. Increased water loss via postdelivery diuresis
   C. Increased glomerular filtration rate
   D. Increased tubular secretion rate
   E. Aminoglycoside-induced nephrotoxicity

3. Aminoglycosides are hydrophilic compounds. Which of the following is true regarding aminoglycoside pharmacokinetic parameters in neonates compared with those in adults?

   A. Decreased clearance
   B. Increased Vd
   C. Decreased half-life
   D. Unchanged elimination
   E. Increased liver metabolism

4. Which of the following is most likely to complicate phenytoin therapy in a 2-day-old breast-fed neonate with new-onset seizures?

A. Decreased renal elimination
B. Altered liver metabolism
C. Increased albumin stores
D. Decreased triglycerides
E. Physiological jaundice

5. A drug metabolized through which of the following reactions is a concern in the neonatal population?

A. Hydrolysis
B. Reduction
C. Sulfation
D. Glucuronidation
E. Methylation

Use the following patient profile to answer Questions 6 and 7.

6. Decisions for antimicrobial therapy in this patient should be based on coverage for which of the following bacterial pathogens? (Select all that apply.)

A. *Chlamydia trachomatis*
B. *Haemophilus influenzae*
C. *Moraxella catarrhalis*
D. *Pseudomonas aeruginosa*
E. *Streptococcus pneumoniae*

7. The drug of choice for this patient's current episode of acute otitis media is _____.

A. amoxicillin
B. amoxicillin-clavulanate
C. I.M. ceftriaxone
D. cefixime
E. trimethoprim-sulfamethoxazole

8. When a pharmacist is counseling an infant's caregiver about an antibiotic suspension prescribed for otitis media, which of the following is an appropriate recommendation?

A. Mix each dose with a full bottle of infant formula.
B. Keep suspension bottle at room temperature.
C. Administer dose with kitchen tablespoon.
D. Keep any remaining suspension for up to 1 year.
E. Use an oral syringe when delivering the suspension.

9. The pharmacy receives a prescription for amoxicillin-clavulanate 90 mg/kg/d for 10 days for a child weighing 30 pounds. Which of the following formulations and dosing regimens is the correct way to dispense this prescription?

A. Amoxicillin 125 mg/Clavulanate 31.25 mg per 5 mL; 1 tablespoon 3 times daily
B. Amoxicillin 250 mg/Clavulanate 62.5 mg per 5 mL; 2 teaspoons 3 times daily
C. Amoxicillin 600 mg/Clavulanate 42.9 mg per 5 mL; 1 teaspoon twice daily
D. Amoxicillin 400 mg/Clavulanate 57 mg per 5 mL; 1 teaspoon twice daily
E. Amoxicillin 200 mg/Clavulanate 28.5 mg per 5 mL; 2 teaspoons twice daily

---

PATIENT PROFILE

Patient Name: Baby Girl Jones	**Sex:** Female
Age: 7 months old	**Weight:** 8 kg
Chief complaint:	Baby brought to the pharmacy by her mother who describes new onset of fever (102.5°F) and increased irritability in the last 24 hours.
Past medical history:	formula-fed infant; acute otitis media episode at 3 months of age
Family history:	older sibling with recent upper respiratory tract infection
Social history:	infant attends daycare
Pneumatic otoscopic examination:	bulging, red tympanic membrane with no mobility on negative or positive pressure (right ear)

10. Which of the following is a common side effect of amoxicillin-clavulanate therapy?

A. Hemolytic anemia
B. Liver function test abnormalities
C. Pancreatitis
D. Diarrhea
E. Headache

11. Which of the following is a side effect that should be a concern in a child with acute otitis media, nausea, and vomiting who is receiving ibuprofen for fever?

A. Stevens–Johnson syndrome
B. Renal insufficiency
C. Hyponatremia
D. Oral candidiasis
E. Liver failure

12. How is otitis externa, or swimmer's ear, best treated?

A. Instill an antimicrobial and steroid solution into the ear canal.
B. Apply antimicrobial ointment into the ear canal with a cotton swab.
C. Instill an antihistamine solution into the ear canal.
D. Increase pH of the ear canal with administration of Burow's solution.
E. Decrease pH of ear canal with administration of dilute HCl solution.

13. An 8-year-old patient is newly diagnosed with attention-deficit/hyperactivity disorder. Which of the following is considered first-line therapy for this patient?

A. Intuniv
B. Kapvay
C. Strattera
D. Vyvanse
E. Wellbutrin

14. Atomoxetine is associated with which of the following serious adverse effects?

A. Hepatic injury
B. Renal failure
C. Cardiovascular collapse
D. Anaphylaxis
E. Toxic epidermal necrolysis

15. A 9-year-old male patient is being started on methylphenidate. This patient has 2 siblings, a 15-year-old brother and a 3-year-old sister. The pharmacist instructs the parents to keep the medication away from siblings and in a safe place. What is the most likely reason for the pharmacist's concern regarding methylphenidate?

A. Toxicity with overdose
B. Abuse potential
C. Stability of product
D. Increased suicide risk
E. Appetite suppression

16. A decrease in seizure threshold is a side effect of which of the following agents used for ADHD?

A. Atomoxetine
B. Clonidine
C. Guanfacine
D. Imipramine
E. Methylphenidate

17. A patient comes into your pharmacy and describes the development of itchy, red eyes, which are often swollen and draining. The patient says these symptoms occur every spring. Which of the following is the most likely cause of this patient's ocular disorder?

A. Viral conjunctivitis
B. Bacterial conjunctivitis
C. Allergic conjunctivitis
D. Blepharitis
E. Episcleritis

18. A patient comes into your pharmacy and describes the development of itchy, red eyes, which are often swollen and draining. The patient says these symptoms occur every spring. Which of the following therapies is the most appropriate recommendation for this patient's symptoms?

A. Intranasal steroid
B. Pseudoephedrine
C. Bacitracin ointment
D. Ocular phenylephrine
E. Ocular olopatadine

19. Which of the following is most commonly associated with bacterial conjunctivitis beyond the first month of life?

A. *Chlamydia*
B. *Clostridium*
C. *E. coli*
D. *Neisseria*
E. *Staphylococcus*

20. Which of the following is a side effect of the prolonged use of ocular decongestants?

A. Peripheral vasodilation
B. Rebound conjunctival congestion
C. Development of arrhythmias
D. Development of tolerance
E. Development of allergy to product

 **31-7** **Answers**

1. **E.** Using the Bedside Schwartz equation, this patient's estimated creatinine clearance is 25 mL/min/1.73 m² [0.413 × (50/0.9)].

2. **A.** The presence of maternal SCr that decreases in neonates over the first week of life may cause a false underestimate of calculated CrCl during this time. If one assumes that by the end of the first week of life, this patient's SCr has decreased to a more typical SCr of 0.4 mg/dL for a normal infant, the estimated CrCl would be 57 mL/min/1.73 m² [0.413 × 55/0.4). Although infants do experience postdelivery diuresis, it should not decrease creatinine clearance. Other factors that affect CrCl in the neonate and infant include a decreased glomerular filtration rate and a decreased tubular secretion rate. Finally, this infant has been started on a standard, once-daily aminoglycoside dose with no indications of renal insufficiency or drug-induced nephrotoxicity at this time.

3. **B.** Aminoglycosides are hydrophilic compounds; they will exhibit larger volumes of distribution in patients with greater total body water. Neonates and infants have greater total body water, greater extracellular fluid volume, and a relative lack of adipose tissue. With aminoglycosides, when the extracellular fluid volume decreases, the volume of distribution decreases, elimination rate increases, and the half-life decreases. In general, the elimination and clearance of aminoglycosides decreases with increasing age.

4. **E.** Phenytoin is a highly plasma protein–bound drug. The total and free concentrations of highly protein-bound drugs may be altered because of developmental differences in protein binding (decreased protein concentrations and altered binding capacity) and displacement by endogenous substances (e.g., free fatty acids and unconjugated bilirubin). Physiological jaundice, as exhibited by increasing total and unconjugated bilirubin concentrations, may occur in the neonatal period. Unconjugated bilirubin may displace drugs from albumin-binding sites. Additionally, 1 of the by-products of lipid metabolism, free fatty acids, may also displace drugs from albumin-binding sites (thereby increasing the free drug concentration). Kernicterus (also known as *yellow brain*) may occur when unconjugated bilirubin displaced by drugs or other endogenous substances (e.g., free fatty acids) crosses the blood–brain barrier, where it can deposit in the brain and cause neurologic complications. Because free fatty acids are not included in routine laboratory panels, serum triglycerides may serve as a surrogate marker of serum free fatty acid status.

5. **D.** UDPG (uridine diphosphate glucose glucuronyltransferase) is responsible for conjugation of endogenous substances (bilirubin) and medications (morphine and chloramphenicol). The capacity for glucuronidation metabolism does not begin until around 2 months of age and reaches adult capacity by 2 years of age. Medications metabolized through this system are potential toxins in the neonatal population. An example would be the use of chloramphenicol in neonates and the development of "gray-baby syndrome" because of drug accumulation. Hydrolysis, reduction, sulfation, and methylation are functional in the neonatal period and should not pose drug therapy complications in this population.

6. **B, C, E.** The most common bacterial pathogens in acute otitis media are *S. pneumoniae*, *H. influenzae*, and *M. catarrhalis*.

7. **A.** Despite the emergence of drug-resistant *S. pneumoniae*, high-dose amoxicillin (90 mg/kg/d)—because of its excellent pharmacodynamic profile, side-effect profile, and cost—remains the drug of choice in uncomplicated acute otitis media. Amoxicillin-clavulanate is considered first-line therapy in patients who have received amoxicillin in the past 30 days, those with conjunctivitis, those with recurrent otitis media unresponsive to amoxicillin, or those in whom beta-lactamase coverage for *H. influenzae* or *M. catarrhalis* is indicated. I.M. ceftriaxone is an acceptable alternative or second-line agent, whereas cefixime and trimethoprim-sulfamethoxazole are not recommended therapies for acute otitis media.

8. **E.** Counseling should include specific information about the antibiotic, its side-effect profile, storage information, information about administering the medicine, dosage instructions, the importance of taking the full course, and the need to shake the bottle before administering the dose. Liquid formulations should be given directly into the mouth using an approved pediatric dosage device (oral syringe or medicine spoon). Kitchen tablespoons are not approved pediatric dosage devices and can result in administration of greater than the desired dose of medication. While medicines can be mixed with a small amount of breastmilk or infant formula, a dose should never be mixed with an entire bottle feeding to ensure that the complete dose is given and it is administered all at one time. The recommended suspensions for acute otitis media should be refrigerated and the bottle discarded at the end of therapy (even if drug is remaining).

9. **C.** The amoxicillin 600 mg/clavulanate 42.9 mg per 5 mL formulation should be used when giving 90 mg/kg/d amoxicillin to keep the daily clavulanate dose < 10 mg/kg to prevent diarrhea. While answers D and E also provide < 10 mg/kg/d clavulanate, they result in a daily amoxicillin dose of 58 mg/kg.

10. **D.** The most common side effects with amoxicillin-clavulanate therapy include rash, urticaria, nausea, vomiting, and diarrhea. Although the other listed side effects may be seen with other antibiotic therapies, they do not typically occur with amoxicillin-clavulanate therapy.

11. **B.** Dehydration, which may develop in a child who is vomiting, is a risk factor for ibuprofen-induced renal insufficiency. If ibuprofen is used as an antipyretic or analgesic in pediatric patients, the parents or caregivers should be counseled regarding this risk and the need to follow intakes and outputs during the period of acute illness (i.e., gastroenteritis) when the child may be receiving ibuprofen therapy.

12. **A.** The treatment of otitis externa includes the instillation of an antimicrobial and steroid otic solution into the ear canal. Cotton swabs should be avoided to prevent otitis externa. Antihistamine solutions are not indicated in the treatment of otitis externa. Otic solutions containing acetic acid may also be of benefit in otitis externa by decreasing (not increasing) the pH of the ear canal and lowering its bacteria-harboring potential. Hydrochloric acid in any form should not be used in the ear canal.

13. **D.** Stimulants are considered first-line therapy for ADHD. Vyvanse (lisdexamfetamine dimesylate) is the only stimulant listed. Intuniv (guanfacine) and Kapvay (clonidine) are alpha-2-receptor agonists, and Strattera (atomoxetine) is a noradrenergic-specific reuptake inhibitor; both classes of drugs are considered second-line therapy for ADHD. Wellbutrin is an antidepressant and is not recommended for ADHD management.

14. **A.** Atomoxetine's labeling has a boxed warning about the potential for severe liver injury. Atomoxetine should be discontinued in any patient who develops jaundice or laboratory evidence of liver injury.

15. **B.** Because this patient has a younger sibling in the house, there is a potential for the child to get into her older brother's medicine. Stimulants may have the potential for abuse in patients who do not have ADHD (i.e., the 15-year-old brother). There are no stability issues with stimulants. Atomoxetine (Strattera) carries a warning for suicide risk. Appetite suppression can be seen with stimulants, but that would not be the reason for the pharmacist to keep the medicine away from other children.

16. **E.** Stimulants (methylphenidate) may lower the seizure threshold. The other agents listed are not associated with seizure occurrence.

17. **C.** Allergic conjunctivitis occurs after exposure to allergens, primarily dander or pollen. Patients suffering from allergic conjunctivitis will typically complain of eye itching.

18. E. Antimicrobial therapy (bacitracin ointment) has no place in therapy for allergic conjunctivitis. Ocular lubricants, decongestants, antihistamines (olopatadine), mast cell stabilizers, or combinations of these products are appropriate options for allergic conjunctivitis. Intranasal steroids may be used for allergic rhinitis, not conjunctivitis. Oral decongestants (pseudoephedrine) are not recommended for allergic conjunctivitis. Although ocular decongestants (phenylephrine) are recommended for allergic conjunctivitis, tetrahydrozoline products are preferred because of decreased rebound conjunctival congestion.

19. E. The most common pathogens in neonatal bacterial conjunctivitis are *N. gonorrhoeae, C. trachomatis, S. aureus, S. epidermidis, S. pneumoniae,* and *E. coli.* Bacterial conjunctivitis beyond the first month of life is most commonly caused by *S. aureus, S. epidermidis, S. pneumoniae,* and *H. influenzae. Clostridium,* an anaerobe, is not a common bacterial pathogen in conjunctivitis.

20. B. Not unlike reactions from prolonged use of nasal decongestants, prolonged use of ocular decongestants may cause rebound congestion of the conjunctiva. This effect is less pronounced with tetrahydrozoline.

 **31-8**   ## Additional Resources

American Psychiatric Association. *Diagnostic and Statistical Manual of Mental Disorders* (DSM-5). 5th ed. Washington, DC: American Psychiatric Association; 2013.

How to Give Ear Drops. Healthy Children. February 2013. Healthy Children.Org Website. https://www.healthychildren.org/English/safety-prevention/at-home/medication-safety/Pages/How-to-Give-Ear-Drops.aspx. Accessed June 28, 2021.

How to Give Eye Drops and Eye Ointment. Healthy Children. February 2013. Healthy Children.Org Website. https://www.healthychildren.org/English/safety-prevention/at-home/medication-safety/Pages/How-to-Give-Eye-Drops-and-Eye-Ointment.aspx. Accessed June 28, 2021.

Kearns GL, Abdel-Rahman SM, Alander SW, et al. Developmental pharmacology: drug disposition, action, and therapy in infants and children. *N Engl J Med.* 2003;349:1157–1167.

Lieberthal AS, Carroll AE, Chonmaitree T, et al. The diagnosis and management of acute otitis media. *Pediatrics.* 2013; 131:e964–e999.

Schwartz GJ, Work DF. Measurement and estimation of GFR in children and adolescents. *J Am Soc Nephrol.* 2009; 4(11):1832–1843.

Teoh DL, Reynold S. Diagnosis and management of pediatric conjunctivitis. *Pediatr Em Care.* 2003;19(1):48–55.

The ADHD Medication Guide. Northwell Health Inc. Copyright 2006, 2016, 2017, 2019, 2020 by Northwell Health, Inc., New Hyde Park, New York. http://www.adhdmedicationguide.com/. Accessed August 2, 2020.

Wolraich ML, Hagan JF, Allan C, et al. AAP Subcommittee on Children and Adolescents with Attention-Deficit/Hyperactivity Disorder. Clinical Practice Guideline for the Diagnosis, Evaluation, and Treatment of Attention-Deficit/Hyperactivity Disorder in Children and Adolescents. *Pediatrics.* 2019;144(4):e20192528.

Zeitlin D. Otic disorders. In: Krinsky DL, Ferreri SP, Hemstreet BA, et al., eds. *Handbook of Nonprescription Drugs: An Interactive Approach to Self-Care.* 20th ed. Washington, DC: American Pharmacists Association; 2020. https://pharmacylibrary.com/doi/10.21019/9781582123172.ch30.

Asthma and Chronic Obstructive Pulmonary Disease

32

CHRISTOPHER K. FINCH

32-1 KEY POINTS

ASTHMA

- Asthma is primarily an inflammatory airway disease.
- It is commonly undertreated, resulting in unnecessary suffering and economic loss.
- Managing patients via the principles of national and international guidelines has been shown to reduce emergency department visits and hospitalizations and to improve patient quality of life.
- Optimal long-term management includes objective assessment, environmental control, drug therapy, and patient education as a partnership.
- Patients with persistent asthma need daily controller therapy (anti-inflammatory agents).
- Inhaled corticosteroids (ICS) are the preferred first-step drug treatment for patients of all ages who have mild persistent asthma.
- Long-acting inhaled beta-2-agonists/ICS combinations are the preferred treatment for moderate or severe persistent asthma.
- Short-acting inhaled beta-2-agonists (SABA) do provide symptom relief but do not protect patients from severe exacerbations.
- Regular or frequent use of SABAs increases the risk for exacerbations.
- According to Global Initiative for Asthma (GINA) guidelines, SABAs should no longer be considered the agents of choice for quick relief.
- The preferred treatment for quick relief of symptoms and intermittent asthma is now as-needed, low-dose ICS-formoterol.
- Pharmacists should teach patients how to use all inhalers by demonstrations and *observation* of the patient.
- Patients must understand the purpose of daily controller medications versus quick-relief medications.
- Each patient should have a written action plan.

CHRONIC OBSTRUCTIVE PULMONARY DISEASE

- Chronic obstructive pulmonary disease (COPD) management should be a stepwise increase in treatment, tailored to reduce symptoms and enhance quality of life.
- Smoking cessation is highly important. None of the existing medications modify the long-term decline in pulmonary function. Drug treatment improves symptoms and decreases complications.
- Inhaled long-acting bronchodilators are central to management and preferred for reasons of efficacy and convenience.
- Combining bronchodilators improves efficacy and decreases the risk of side effects.
- ICS should be added to long-acting bronchodilators in patients with COPD at a high risk of exacerbations.
- The long-term administration of oxygen (>15 hours per day) to patients with COPD with chronic respiratory failure has been shown to increase survival.
- Influenza and pneumococcal vaccine(s) should be given based on current guidelines issued by the Centers for Disease Control and Prevention (CDC).

32-2 STUDY GUIDE CHECKLIST

The following topics may guide your study of this subject area:

- [ ] Risk factors and triggers for asthma and COPD.
- [ ] Importance of environmental control.
- [ ] Factors to consider when selecting drug therapy.
- [ ] Actions of different classes of drugs to treat asthma and COPD.
- [ ] Trade names and available dosage forms, particularly those in the "Top 100 Drugs."
- [ ] Major adverse effects and drug interactions.
- [ ] Proper peak expiratory flow measurement interpretation.
- [ ] Considerations when choosing doses and schedules for each drug.
- [ ] Importance of patient education, including correct inhaler technique.
- [ ] Management of acute exacerbations.
- [ ] Highly significant role of national and international evidence-based guidelines to manage asthma and COPD.

32-3   Asthma

Disease Overview

Asthma is a chronic inflammatory disorder of the airways in which many cells and cellular elements play a role, in particular mast cells, eosinophils, T-lymphocytes, neutrophils, and epithelial cells. In susceptible individuals, this inflammation causes recurrent episodes of wheezing, breathlessness, chest tightness, and cough, particularly at night and in the early morning. Asthma affects about 26 million Americans and is the most common cause of missed school days for children. Morbidity and mortality caused by asthma are unacceptably high; death rates are greatest among inner-city Blacks and Hispanics.

Types and Classifications

- *Childhood-onset (atopic):* Positive family history of asthma; allergy to tree or grass pollen, house dust mites, cockroaches, household pets, and molds
- *Adult-onset:* Frequently a negative family history and negative skin tests to common aeroallergens

Classification of severity criteria for children ≥ 12 years of age and for adults is shown in Tables 32-1 and 32-2. This classification is extremely important in defining treatment options (Table 32-3). See EPR-3 and GINA guidelines for ages 0 to 4 years and 5 to 11 years.

TABLE 32-1. Initiating Therapy in Adults and Adolescents ≥ 12 Years with Intermittent Asthma

Consideration	Initiating therapy in patients with intermittent asthma	
	Adults and adolescents ≥ 12 years	
Impairment Normal: FEV_1/FVC.	Symptom frequency	≤2 days/wk
	Number of nighttime awakenings	≤2 times per month
	Frequency of use of SABA to control symptoms	≤2 days/wk
	Extent of limitation of normal activity	No limitation
	Lung function	- Normal FEV_1 between exacerbations
	- Predicted FEV_1 or personal best peak flow	- FEV_1 >80% predicted
	- FEV_1/FVC	- FEV_1/FVC normal
Risk	Exacerbations that require oral systemic corticosteroids	0 to 1 times per year
	Considerations: severity and interval since last exacerbation	
Recommendation	Recommended step therapy	Step 1*
	- Should not replace clinical decision making and individual patient needs	
	- Re-evaluate level of asthma control in 2 to 6 weeks	

Impairment age/normal table:

Age	Normal
8 to 19	85%
20 to 39	80%
40 to 59	75%
60 to 80	70%

Adapted from NIH, National Heart, Lung, and Blood Institute. National guidelines for the diagnosis and management of asthma 2007 (EPR-3). Available at: https://www.nhlbi.nih.gov/guidelines/asthma/asthgdln.pdf, accessed May 26, 2020; and Global Initiative for Asthma. GINA 2020 guidelines. Available at: http://www.ginasthma.org. Accessed May 26, 2020.
SABA, short-acting beta-agonists; FEV_1, forced expiratory volume in 1 second; FVC, forced vital capacity.
GINA guideline preferred treatment recommendations:
* Step 1: as needed low dose ICS-formoterol
See Table 32-3 for preferred and alternative treatment options.

TABLE 32-2. Initiating Therapy in Adults and Adolescents ≥12 Years with Persistent Asthma

Consideration		Initiating therapy in patients with persistent asthma		
		Adults and adolescents ≥12 years		
		Mild	Moderate	Severe
Impairment Normal: FEV₁/FVC:	**Symptom frequency**	>2 days/wk, but not daily	Daily	Throughout the day
	Number of nighttime awakenings	3 to 4 times per month	>1 time per week, but not nightly	Often; 7 times per week
Age Normal 8 to 19 85% 20 to 39 80% 40 to 59 75% 60 to 80 70%	**Frequency of use of SABA to control symptoms**	>2 days/wk, but not daily and not more than once on any day	Daily	Several times/d
	Extent of limitation of normal activity	Minor limitation	Some limitation	Extreme limitation
	Lung function ▪ Predicted FEV₁ or personal best peak flow ▪ FEV₁/FVC	▪ FEV₁ >80% predicted ▪ FEV₁/FVC normal	▪ FEV₁ >60% but <80% predicted ▪ FEV₁/FVC reduced 5%	▪ FEV₁ <60% ▪ FEV₁/FVC reduced >5%
Risk	**Exacerbations that require oral systemic corticosteroids** Considerations: severity/interval since last exacerbation	≥2 times year		
Recommendation	**Recommended step therapy** Should not replace clinical decision making and individual patient needs Reevaluate in 2 to 6 weeks: level of asthma control	Step 2*	Step 3** Consider short course of oral systemic corticosteroids.	Steps 4 or 5***

Adapted from NIH, National Heart, Lung, and Blood Institute. National guidelines for the diagnosis and management of asthma 2007 (EPR-3). Available at: https://www.nhlbi.nih.gov/guidelines/asthma/asthgdln.pdf, accessed May 26, 2020; and Global Initiative for Asthma. GINA 2020 guidelines. Available at: http://www.ginasthma.org. Accessed May 26, 2020.
SABA, short-acting beta-agonists; FEV₁, forced expiratory volume in 1 second; FVC, forced vital capacity.
GINA guideline preferred treatment recommendations:
* Step 2 = daily low-dose inhaled corticosteroid (ICS)
** Step 3 = low-dose ICS-long-acting beta-agonist (LABA)
*** Step 4 = medium-dose ICS-LABA
*** Step 5 = high-dose ICS-LABA
See Table 32-3 for preferred and alternative treatment options.

Clinical Presentation

Presentation includes episodic wheezing, coughing, chest tightness, and shortness of breath that are worse at night, in the early morning, and with exercise.

Pathophysiology

▪ Asthma is an inflammatory airway disease often associated with bronchospasm.
▪ Common triggers of symptoms include aeroallergens, respiratory viral illness, exercise (especially in cold, dry air), environmental smoke, and fumes.

TABLE 32-3. Stepwise Approach for Managing Asthma in Adults and Adolescents ≥ 12 Years of Age

Asthma classification	Step	GINA recommendations			Notes
		Preferred controller therapy*	Alternative or addition	Quick relief	
Intermittent	1	As-needed, low-dose ICS-formoterol	As-needed SABA and low-dose ICS	As-needed, low-dose ICS-formoterol	■ This process should not replace clinical judgment.
Persistent	2	Daily low-dose ICS	As-needed, low dose ICS-formoterol or daily LTRA		■ At each step: evaluate patient education, environmental control, and comorbidity management.
	3	Low-dose ICS-LABA	Medium-dose ICS or low-dose ICS + LTRA	As-needed, low-dose ICS-formoterol or SABA**	
	4	Medium-dose ICS-LABA	High-dose ICS or add **tiotropium** or LTRA		■ After 3 months of asthma control, evaluate for step down in therapy.
	5	High-dose ICS-LABA	Consider **tiotropium**, immunotherapy, or low-dose OCS		■ Uncontrolled on Steps 4 to 5: consider immunotherapy.

Adapted from Global Initiative for Asthma. 2020 GINA Report, Global Strategy for Asthma Management and Prevention. Available at: http://www.ginasthma.org. Accessed June 4, 2020.
Boldface indicates one of top 100 drugs for 2020 by prescription volume.
ICS, inhaled corticosteroid; SABA, short-acting beta-agonist; LABA, long-acting beta-agonist; LTRA, leukotriene receptor antagonist; OCS, oral corticosteroids.
* Specific products can be found in Tables 32-4 and 32-5.
** ICS-formoterol should not be used as the reliever medication when maintenance therapy with a different LABA is used.

■ Drug-induced asthma includes asthma-like symptoms caused by **aspirin**, nonsteroidal anti-inflammatory drugs, and beta blockers. Low-to-moderate–dose beta-1-selective agents can be used if the patient has concurrent postmyocardial infarction (**atenolol** or **metoprolol** XL) or congestive heart failure (**metoprolol** XL) and does not have severe asthma. Cyclooxygenase-2 (COX-2) inhibitors can be used safely in many patients with aspirin-sensitive asthma.

■ There is a complex interaction among inflammatory cells (e.g., mast cells, eosinophils, Th2-type lymphocytes), mediators (e.g., leukotrienes), and cytokines (e.g., interleukin-4, interleukin-5). The result is airway inflammation (mucus and swelling in the lining of the airways) and airway hyperreactivity.

■ Early-phase response to inhaling an aeroallergen occurs immediately; late-phase response occurs 4 to 12 hours later.

■ Asthma is worsened by poorly controlled concurrent allergic rhinitis and sinusitis. Gastroesophageal reflux disease is common in asthma patients, but recent research revealed that although treatment with proton pump inhibitors may improve pulmonary function and asthma-related quality of life, the improvements are minor and of small clinical significance. Asthma may also worsen in the perimenstrual period.

Diagnostic Criteria

■ The main basis for diagnosis is a detailed history of episodic symptoms that are typically worse at night and in the early morning and that are associated with common triggers.

■ Reversible airway obstruction (improvement in pulmonary function tests [FEV_1, forced expiratory volume in 1st second] > 12% after inhaling a short-acting beta-2-agonist) is often detected.

■ Alternate diagnoses (e.g., chronic obstructive pulmonary disease [COPD] and vocal cord dysfunction) should be excluded.

Drug Therapy

Treatment Principles and Goals

- Optimal long-term management of asthma involves a continuous cycle of patient assessment, treatment adjustment (step-up or step-down), and review of the patient's response (Figure 32-1).
- Two primary treatment goals for asthma:
  - Reduce impairment by controlling symptoms.
  - Reduce risk of exacerbations and asthma deaths.
- Treatment goal to achieve asthma control by *reducing impairment*:
  - Prevent chronic and troublesome symptoms (e.g., coughing or breathlessness in the daytime, during the night, or after exercise).
  - Require infrequent use (<2 d/wk) of a rescue inhaler for quick relief of symptoms.
  - Maintain (near) "normal" pulmonary function.
  - Maintain normal activity levels (including exercise and other physical activity and attendance at work or at school).
  - Meet patients' and families' goals, expectations, and satisfaction with asthma care.
- Treatment goals are to achieve asthma control by *reducing risk*:
  - Prevent recurrent exacerbations and asthma deaths, and minimize the need for emergency department visits or hospitalization.
  - Prevent progressive loss of lung function; for children, prevent reduced lung growth.
  - Provide optimal pharmacotherapy with minimal or no adverse effects.
- A stepwise approach to managing asthma in adults and adolescents ≥12 years is shown in Table 32-3. These treatment guidelines are from EPR-3 and are consistent with 2020 guidelines from the Global Initiative for Asthma. Table 32-4 lists long-term control medications.
- Inhaled corticosteroids (ICS) are the most efficacious drugs for long-term management of persistent asthma. The addition of an inhaled, long-acting beta-2 agonist (LABA) ⚠ is recommended for patients with moderate or severe persistent asthma (always in combination products, e.g., Advair, Dulera, Symbicort). Recent trials have shown that **tiotropium** (Spiriva) therapy added to patients inadequately controlled with ICS or ICS/LABA combination provides additional benefit. In addition, Spiriva Respimat is FDA-approved for use in asthma for patients ≥12 years of age.

FIGURE 32-1. Asthma Management Cycle

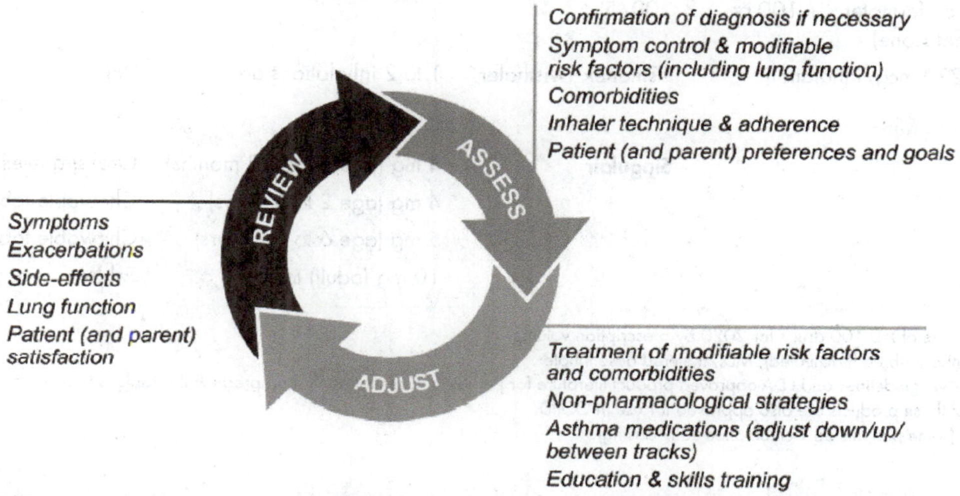

Confirmation of diagnosis if necessary
Symptom control & modifiable
risk factors (including lung function)
Comorbidities
Inhaler technique & adherence
Patient (and parent) preferences and goals

Symptoms
Exacerbations
Side-effects
Lung function
Patient (and parent)
satisfaction

Treatment of modifiable risk factors
and comorbidities
Non-pharmacological strategies
Asthma medications (adjust down/up/
between tracks)
Education & skills training

Adapted from Global Initiative for Asthma. 2020 GINA Report, Global Strategy for Asthma Management and Prevention. Available at: http://www.ginasthma.org. Accessed June 4, 2020.

Long-Acting Beta-2 Agonist (LABA) *FDA BOXED WARNING*

Long-acting beta-2 agonists (LABAs) increase the risk of asthma-related death when used as monotherapy.

TABLE 32-4. Examples of Long-term Asthma Control Medications[a]

Generic name	Trade name	Usual dosage range	Dosage form	Schedule[b]
Inhaled corticosteroids				
Beclomethasone HFA 40 mcg/puff; 80 mcg/puff	QVAR	80 to 480 mcg/d	MDI	Twice daily
Budesonide 200 mcg/inhalation	Pulmicort	1 to 3 inhalations/d	DPI (Flexhaler)	Twice daily
Budesonide–formoterol combination (each inhalation 4.5 mcg formoterol + budesonide 80 mcg or 160 mcg)	**Symbicort** (80/4.5, 160/4.5)	2 puffs	MDI	Twice daily
Budesonide 0.25 and 0.5 mg/dose	Respules	0.5 to 2 mg/d	Nebulized	Twice daily
Fluticasone 44, 110, 220 mcg/puff	**Flovent HFA**	88 to 660 mcg/d	MDI	Twice daily
Fluticasone 50, 100, 250 mcg/inhalation	**Flovent Diskus**	100 to 500 mcg/d	DPI	Twice daily
Fluticasone–salmeterol combination (each inhalation 50 mcg salmeterol + 100, 250, or 500 mcg fluticasone)	**Advair Diskus** (100/50, 250/50, 500/50)	1 inhalation	DPI (Diskus)	Twice daily
Fluticasone–salmeterol combination (each puff 21 mcg salmeterol + 45, 115, or 230 mcg fluticasone)	**Advair HFA** (45/21, 115/21, 230/21)	2 inhalations/dose	MDI	Twice daily
Fluticasone-vilanterol combination (each inhalation 25 mcg vilanterol + 100 or 200 mcg fluticasone)	Breo Ellipta (100/25, 200/25)	1 inhalation	DPI	Once daily
Mometasone-formoterol combination (each puff 5 mcg formoterol + 100 or 200 mcg mometasone)	Dulera (100/5, 200/5)	2 inhalations	MDI	Twice daily
Mometasone 220 mcg/inhalation	Asmanex Twisthaler	1 to 2 inhalations daily	DPI	At bedtime
Leukotriene modifier				
Montelukast	**Singulair**	4 mg (age 12 to 23 months)	Oral granules	Nightly
		4 mg (age 2 to 5 years)	Chewable tab	Nightly
		5 mg (age 6 to 14 years)	Chewable tab	Nightly
		10 mg (adult) tablet	Tablet	Nightly

Boldface indicates one of top 100 drugs for 2020 by prescription volume.
DPI, dry powder inhaler (breath activated); MDI, metered dose inhaler.
a. See EPR-3 or GINA guidelines and FDA-approved product literature for pediatric doses for each drug product; this table is NOT a comprehensive list; note that several of these products are also approved for use in COPD.
b. Usual schedule (some patients do well on once-daily dosing).

- For patients with evidence of elevated Type 2 inflammation biomarkers (eosinophils; interleukin-IL-4, -IL-5, and -IL-13; and exhaled nitric oxide) with exacerbations or poor symptom control despite high dose ICS, consider add-on biologic targeted treatments.

- Omalizumab (Xolair) ⚠: Anti-immunoglobulin E (anti-IgE) therapy is primarily indicated for severe, persistent, allergic asthma patients who have frequent emergency department visits and hospitalizations despite optimal therapy. It is given subcutaneously every 2 to 4 weeks. Similarly, anti-interleukin-5 therapy (mepolizumab [Nucala], benralizumab [Fasenra], and reslizumab [Cinqair]) ⚠ is indicated for the same populations. Most recently, add-on, anti-IL-4 receptor blocker therapy with dupilumab (Dupixent) has been approved for oral corticosteroid dependent, eosinophilic, severe asthma patients.

- For more information on the appropriate utility of these agents, see the section in the GINA guidelines—Difficult-to-Treat and Severe Asthma in Adults and Adolescents (https://ginasthma.org/wp-content/uploads/2018/11/GINA-SA-FINAL-wms.pdf).

- Drug therapy for acute exacerbations of asthma is shown in Table 32-5 (quick-relief medications). Refer to GINA guidelines for management of asthma exacerbations in the hospital and primary care office (https://ginasthma.org/wp-content/uploads/2020/04/Main-pocket-guide_2020_04_03-final-wms.pdf).

 Omalizumab (Xolair) *FDA BOXED WARNING*

Risk of anaphylaxis (e.g., bronchospasm, hypotension, syncope, urticaria, and/or angioedema of throat or tongue). Anaphylaxis may occur at first dose but has also occurred beyond 1 year after regularly administered doses. First dose should be given in a health care setting.

 Reslizumab (Cinqair) *FDA BOXED WARNING*

Risk of anaphylaxis. Patients should be observed after infusion.

TABLE 32-5. **Quick-Relief Asthma Medications**[a]

Generic name	Trade name	Usual dosage[b]	Dosage form	Schedule
Beta-2-agonists				
Albuterol HFA[c]	**Ventolin HFA, Proventil HFA**	2 puffs (90 mcg/puff)	MDI	Every 4 hours as needed
	ProAir HFA	2.5 mg	Nebulizer solution	Every 4 hours as needed
Levalbuterol[c]	Xopenex HFA	2 puffs (45 mcg/puff)	MDI	Every 4 hours as needed
	Xopenex	1.25 mg	Nebulizer solution	As needed
Budesonide/formoterol combination[d]	**Symbicort** (80/4.5, 160/4.5)	2 puffs	MDI	As needed

(continued)

TABLE 32-5. Quick-Relief Asthma Medications[a] *(Continued)*

Generic name	Trade name	Usual dosage[b]	Dosage form	Schedule
Anticholinergics				
Ipratropium	Atrovent HFA	2 puffs (17 mcg/puff)	MDI	Every 6 hours
		0.25 mg	Nebulizer solution	Every 6 hours
Ipratropium + **albuterol**	Combivent, Respimat	1 puff (20/100 mcg/puff)	Inhalation spray	Every 6 hours
	DuoNeb	0.5 mg ipratropium plus 2.5 mg albuterol	Nebulizer solution	Every 6 hours
Systemic corticosteroids[e]				
Methylprednisolone	Medrol	1 mg/kg/d	Tablets	Daily
Prednisone		1 mg/kg/d	Tablets or liquid	Daily
Prednisolone		1 mg/kg/d	Tablets	Daily

Boldface indicates one of top 100 drugs for 2020 by prescription volume.
MDI, metered dose inhaler.
a. See EPR-3 or GINA guidelines and FDA-approved product literature for more information, including pediatric doses for each drug product; this table is not a comprehensive list.
b. Usual dosage for routine home use. (Dose in emergency department is higher and more frequent.)
c. No longer the agent of choice for quick relief. For prevention of exercise-induced asthma, inhale 2 puffs 5 to 15 minutes before exercise. Increasing use indicates poor asthma control; increase anti-inflammatory therapy and reassess environmental control. (Good asthma control is indicated by infrequent need for quick-relief therapy.)
d. Considered the agent of choice for quick relief. Maximum dose is 72 mcg per day of formoterol.
e. Short courses are used for <2 weeks.

Monitoring

- Optimal management for the majority of patients will result in a dramatic reduction in symptoms (including nocturnal and early morning symptoms), as well as reduced acute care visits, fewer lost work or school days, and reduced need for quick-relief medications.
- Monitoring peak expiratory flow (PEF) using a peak flow meter at home is helpful in many patients (Box 32-1). *Green zone* is 80% to 100% of personal best value. *Yellow zone* is 50% to 79% of personal best and indicates that consultation with a health care professional is advisable. *Red zone*, or less than 50% of personal best, indicates that a written action plan should be implemented, and, if there is no quick response, immediate medical attention should be sought.
- Spirometry is usually performed in a health care provider's office.

BOX 32-1. Directions for Use of Peak Flow Meter

1. Stand while using the meter.
2. Position the indicator at the bottom of the scale.
3. Hold the peak flow meter so your fingers do not block the opening.
4. Inhale as deeply as possible, place the mouthpiece well into your mouth, and make sure your lips form a tight seal around it.
5. Blow out as fast and as hard as possible![a] BLAST! (Emphasize to the patient that the maneuver is highly effort dependent.)
6. Repeat steps 2 to 5 two more times, and record the highest of the 3 readings along with the date and time.[b]

a. Do not accelerate air with your tongue (i.e., use a spitting motion). This incorrect maneuver will give false elevation in PEF.
b. If a short-acting inhaled beta-2-agonist is required in the early morning, remember to check the peak expiratory flow before using the drug and record the value; then repeat PEF testing 15 minutes later.

Mechanism of Action

For more details, see the section on mechanism of action in EPR-3.

Long-term control medications

Corticosteroids

- Corticosteroids are anti-inflammatory. They block late reaction to an allergen and reduce airway hyperresponsiveness. They inhibit cytokine production, adhesion protein activation, and inflammatory cell migration and activation.
- Corticosteroids reverse beta-2-receptor downregulation and inhibit microvascular leakage.

Long-acting beta-2-agonists (LABA)

- With bronchodilation, smooth muscle relaxation follows adenylate cyclase activation and an increase in cyclic adenosine monophosphate (cAMP), producing functional antagonism of bronchoconstriction.
- In vitro, LABAs inhibit mast cell mediator release, decrease vascular permeability, and increase mucociliary clearance.
- Compared with a short-acting inhaled beta-2-agonist, salmeterol has a slower onset of action (15 to 30 minutes). Formoterol has an onset of action within 3 minutes. Both LABAs have a duration of action ≥12 hours.

Leukotriene modifiers

- Leukotriene receptor antagonist; selective competitive inhibitor of CysLT1 (cysteinyl leukotriene 1) receptors
- 5-Lipoxygenase inhibitor

> ⚠ **Leukotriene modifiers** *FDA BOXED WARNING*
>
> Risk of serious neuropsychiatric events (e.g., agitation, aggression, depression, sleep disturbances, suicidal thoughts). Risk versus benefit should be assessed prior to initiation of therapy.

Anti-IgE therapy

Omalizumab (Xolair) is a humanized monoclonal anti-IgE antibody that binds circulating IgE, thus inhibiting the allergic inflammatory cascade that results when aeroallergens bind to IgE on mast cells.

Anti-interleukin-5 therapy

Mepolizumab (Nucala) and reslizumab (Cinqair) are interleukin-5 (IL-5) antagonist monoclonal antibodies that bind to circulating IL-5, thus reducing the effects of eosinophils (e.g., IL-5 activates and prolongs the life of these inflammatory cells). Benralizumab (Fasenra) binds to the IL-5 receptor alpha subunit leading to apoptosis (cell death) of the eosinophils.

Anti-interleukin-4 therapy

Dupilumab (Dupixent) is a monoclonal antibody that binds to interleukin-4 (IL-4) receptor alpha and subsequently blocks both IL-4 and IL-13 signaling.

Quick-relief medications

Short-acting inhaled *beta-2-agonists*

With bronchodilation, smooth muscle relaxation follows adenylate cyclase activation and an increase in cAMP, producing functional antagonism of bronchoconstriction.

Anticholinergics

- With bronchodilation, there is competitive inhibition of muscarinic cholinergic receptors.
- Anticholinergics reduce intrinsic vagal tone to the airways. They may block reflex broncho-constriction secondary to irritants or to reflux esophagus.
- Anticholinergics may decrease mucus gland secretion.

Methylxanthines

Methylxanthines rarely are used for asthma; see EPR-3 for mechanisms.

Patient Instructions and Counseling

- Patient education is absolutely essential for optimal asthma management. Show patients or care-givers pictures or airway models of normal versus inflamed airways, and emphasize avoidance of (or minimizing exposure to) asthma triggers.
- Emphasize the need to take controller medications *every day*, even when the patient feels well and is having no breathing problems.
- Instruct patients regarding the dangers of overuse of short-acting inhaled beta-2-agonists. The patient should contact a health care provider if the usual dose does not give quick relief or start the written action plan given by the health care provider. Patients who purchase nonprescription racemic epinephrine (Asthmanefrin) may have persistent asthma and need daily controller medication. Even for intermittent asthma, patients need assessment by a health care provider, avoidance of asthma triggers, inhaler instruction, and written action plans. Recommendations now suggest the addition of low-dose ICS with as-needed SABA for intermittent asthma. Remember that if quick-relief medication is needed more than twice weekly, the patient has persistent asthma and needs daily controller treatment.
- Demonstrate the correct use of the metered dose inhaler (MDI), the MDI plus valved holding chamber (or other "spacer"), the soft mist inhaler, and the dry powder inhaler (DPI), and then observe the patient using the devices. Most patients do not perform well initially; the devices can be difficult to use at first (Figure 32-2 shows MDI or MDI spacer use). For the soft mist inhaler, the inhalation must be slow and deep to maximize lung deposition; however, for DPIs, remember to stress that inhalation must be rapid and deep.
- Demonstrate the correct use of peak flow meters, and observe patients using them (see Box 32-1). Explain about the green, yellow, and red zones (including the written action plan).
- Teach patients how to prevent exercise-induced asthma (e.g., ICS/formoterol combination or **albuterol** 15 minutes BEFORE exercise).
- Be sure patients receive an influenza vaccination every fall. For asthma patients 19 years of age and older, also administer the pneumococcal vaccine according to current recommendations from the Centers for Disease Control and Prevention.

Adverse Drug Effects

For more details, see the section on adverse drug effects in EPR-3.

Long-term control medications

Inhaled corticosteroids (ICS)

- ICS may cause coughing, dysphonia, and oral thrush. (Risk of candidiasis can be greatly minimized by using a valved holding chamber or "spacer.")
- In high doses, systemic effects may occur, although studies are not conclusive, and the clinical significance of these effects (e.g., adrenal suppression, osteoporosis, growth suppression, skin thinning, easy bruising) has not been established.

FIGURE 32-2. Steps for Using an Inhaler

Please demonstrate your inhaler technique at every visit.

1. Remove the cap and hold inhaler upright.
2. Shake the inhaler.
3. Tilt your head back slightly and breathe out slowly.
4. Position the inhaler in one of the following ways (A or B is optimal, but C is acceptable for those who have difficulty with A or B. C is required for breath-activated inhalers):

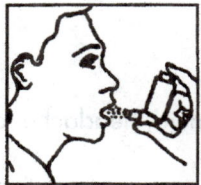 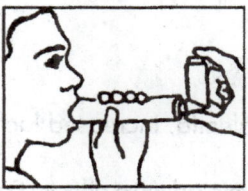 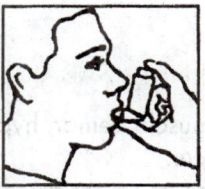 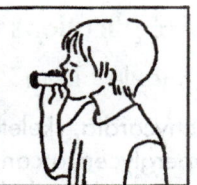

A. Open mouth with inhaler 1 to 2 inches away.

B. Use spacer/holding chamber (that is recommended especially for young children and for people using corticosteroids).

C. In the mouth. Do not use for corticosteroids.

D. NOTE: Inhaled dry powder capsules require a different inhalation technique. To use a dry powder inhaler, it is important to close the mouth tightly around the mouthpiece of the inhaler and to inhale rapidly.

5. Press down on the inhaler to release medication as you start to breathe in slowly.
6. Breathe in slowly (3 to 5 seconds).
7. Hold your breath for 10 seconds to allow the medicine to reach deeply into your lungs.
8. Repeat puff as directed. Waiting 1 minute between puffs may permit second puff to penetrate your lungs better.
9. Spacers/holding chambers are useful for all patients. They are particularly recommended for young children and older adults and for use with inhaled corticosteroids.

Avoid common inhaler mistakes. Follow these inhaler tips:

- Breathe out *before* pressing your inhaler.
- Inhale *slowly.*
- Breathe in through your mouth, not your nose.
- Press down on your inhaler at the *start* of inhalation (or within the first second of inhalation).
- Keep inhaling as you press down on inhaler.
- Press your inhaler only *once* while you are inhaling (one breath for each puff).
- Make sure you breathe in evenly and deeply.

NOTE: Other inhalers are becoming available in addition to those illustrated above. Different types of inhalers may require different techniques.

Source: *Expert Panel Report 2: Guidelines for the Diagnosis and Management of Asthma.* National Asthma Education and Prevention Program, National Heart, Lung, and Blood Institute, 1997.

Long-acting inhaled *beta-2*-agonists (LABA)

- Tachycardia, skeletal muscle tremor, and hypokalemia can occur.
- In asthma, LABA should always be in a combination product with inhaled corticosteroid (e.g., Advair, Dulera, Symbicort), whether used as a quick reliever for symptoms or in the long-term management of asthma. Use alone could mask inflammation and increase risk of severe exacerbations.

Leukotriene modifiers

- **Montelukast** and zafirlukast are usually well tolerated. **Montelukast** has a new boxed warning regarding the onset of neuropsychiatric events, including agitation, depression, sleeping problems, and suicidal thoughts.
- Zileuton can cause liver dysfunction.

Quick-relief medications

Short-acting inhaled *beta-2*-agonists (SABA)

- Tachycardia, skeletal muscle tremor, hypokalemia, increased lactic acid, headache, and, rarely, hyperglycemia can occur.
- In general, the inhaled route causes few systemic adverse effects. Patients with preexisting cardiovascular disease, especially the elderly, may have adverse cardiovascular reactions with inhaled therapy.
- Use of SABA alone for asthma management can lead to higher risk of asthma related death and urgent asthma related health care.

Anticholinergics

- Drying of mouth and respiratory secretions.
- Increased wheezing (rare).
- Blurred vision or acute angle-closure glaucoma can occur if aerosol inadvertently contacts eyes (e.g., ill-fitting nebulized facemask, touching of **tiotropium** dry powder capsule after inhalation followed by inadvertent touching of the eye).

Systemic corticosteroids

- With short-term use, reversible abnormalities in glucose metabolism, increased appetite, fluid retention, weight gain, mood alteration, hypertension, peptic ulcers, and, rarely, aseptic necrosis of the femur can occur.
- Consideration should be given to coexisting conditions that could be worsened by systemic corticosteroids, such as herpes virus infections, varicella, tuberculosis, hypertension, peptic ulcer disease, and strongyloidiasis.

Methylxanthines

- Dose-related acute toxicities include tachycardia, nausea and vomiting, tachyarrhythmias (supraventricular), central nervous system stimulation, headache, seizures, hematemesis, hyperglycemia, and hypokalemia.
- Adverse effects at usual therapeutic doses include insomnia, gastric upset, aggravation of ulcer or reflux, and an increase in hyperactivity in some children.

Drug–Drug and Drug–Disease Interactions

- For zafirlukast, administration with meals decreases bioavailability. Patients should take it at least 1 hour before or 2 hours after meals.
- Zileuton and zafirlukast may increase the effect of **warfarin** and increase theophylline levels.

- Well-known inducers of cytochrome P450 (carbamazepine, phenobarbital, phenytoin, and rifampin) are documented to decrease the effect of systemic corticosteroids.
- Examples of drugs that may increase the effect of systemic corticosteroids include erythromycin, clarithromycin, itraconazole, oral contraceptives, and conjugated estrogen.

Parameters to Monitor

- Refill record for daily controller medications (underuse) and quick-relief medications (overuse of **albuterol** [e.g., >1 canister/month]) is a sign of poorly controlled asthma.
- Reduction in symptoms (including nocturnal and early morning symptoms)
- Emergency department visits, hospitalizations, and unscheduled office visits
- Need for "bursts" of systemic corticosteroids
- Lost work or school days and the need for quick-relief medications
- PEF using a peak flow meter at home

In addition, if the patient also has rhinitis, monitor refills (e.g., intranasal corticosteroids) to ensure optimal control. If rhinitis is not well controlled, asthma control will likely suffer.

Kinetics

- Theophylline is no longer used extensively in asthma, but when it is used, knowledge of its kinetics is essential because of its high risk for adverse effects or suboptimal action. It may also be used for COPD.
- Other drugs, disease states, smoking, age, and diet can all affect theophylline kinetics and dose requirements (Table 32-6).
- Therapeutic serum theophylline concentrations are 5 to 15 mcg/mL. Elimination half-life in an otherwise healthy, nonsmoking adult is about 8 hours. In an adult who smokes, it is about 4 hours, and in a small child (1 year or older), it is about 4 hours.
- Neonates have greatly prolonged elimination half-life.
- Elimination half-life in patients with decompensated heart failure or cirrhosis is about 24 hours.
- High-fat meals may cause "dose dumping" for some products (check product literature).

Other

- MDIs should be stored at room temperature, between 59°F and 86°F. If left in a car during freezing or near-freezing temperatures, aerosol particles will be too large to inhale into the lungs.
- MDIs should be "primed" (number of doses to be released per each product's directions) only with first use or, in the case of a as-needed agent, only once every 2 weeks. (Frequent priming is unnecessary and wastes expensive medications.)
- Clean the actuator according to a manufacturer's instructions.
- The MDI dust cap should be kept on the inhaler when not in use.
- As with all inhalers, always check the mouthpiece for foreign objects before inhaling.
- For DPIs, don't exhale into the inhaler and make sure not to cover the vents located on the device. Rinse mouth after use.

Nondrug Therapy

- An essential component of optimal asthma management is environmental control.
- Without good control of the environment at home, school, and work, drug therapy will often be inadequate.
- Have the patient identify known asthma triggers, and help the patient identify potential triggers not yet realized. (Do not forget someone smoking at home or at work!)

TABLE 32-6. Examples of Factors Affecting Serum Theophylline Concentrations[a]

Factor	Decreases theophylline concentrations	Increases theophylline concentrations	Recommended action
Food	↓ or delays absorption of some sustained-release theophylline products	↑ rate of absorption (fatty foods) products	Select theophylline preparation that is not affected by food.
Diet	↑ metabolism (high protein)	↓ metabolism (high carbohydrate)	Inform patients that major changes in diet are not recommended while taking theophylline.
Systemic, febrile viral illness (e.g., influenza)		↓ metabolism	Decrease theophylline dose according to serum concentration level. Decrease dose by 50% if serum concentration measurement is not available.
Hypoxia, cor pulmonale, and decompensated congestive heart failure, cirrhosis		↓ metabolism	Decrease dose according to serum concentration level.
Age	↑ metabolism (1 to 9 years [of age])	↓ metabolism (<6 months [of age], elderly)	Adjust dose according to serum concentration level.
Phenobarbital, phenytoin, carbamazepine	↑ metabolism		Increase dose according to serum concentration level.
Cimetidine		↓ metabolism	Use alternative H2 blocker (e.g., famotidine or **ranitidine**).
Macrolides: TAO, erythromycin, clarithromycin		↓ metabolism	Use alternative antibiotic or adjust theophylline dose.
Quinolones: ciprofloxacin, enoxacin, pefloxacin		↓ metabolism	Use alternative antibiotic or adjust theophylline dose. Circumvent with ofloxacin if quinolone therapy is required.
Rifampin	↑ metabolism		Increase dose according to serum concentration level.
Smoking	↑ metabolism		Advise patient to stop smoking; increase dose according to serum concentration level.

Reproduced from NIH *Expert Panel Report 3*. (*Note:* Ticlopidine has been removed as it is rarely used.)
Boldface indicates one of top 100 drugs for 2020 by prescription volume.
↓, decreases; ↑, increases; TAO, triacetyloleandomycin.
a. This list is not all inclusive; for discussion of other factors, see package inserts.

32-4   Chronic Obstructive Pulmonary Disease

Disease Overview

COPD is characterized by airflow limitation that is not fully reversible. The airflow limitation is usually both progressive and associated with an abnormal inflammatory response of the lungs to noxious particles or gases. COPD is a major cause of death and suffering in the United States and around the world.

Types and Classifications

Some clinicians still refer to chronic bronchitis and emphysema in characterizing different levels of COPD (e.g., emphysema patients have destructive damage to the alveolar walls, whereas chronic bronchitis is associated with chronic productive cough). According to the Global Initiative for Chronic Obstructive Lung

Disease (GOLD), COPD severity classification of airflow limitation is as follows (in patients with FEV_1/FVC [forced vital capacity] <0.7):

- *GOLD 1. Mild:* FEV_1 ≥80% predicted
- *GOLD 2. Moderate:* 50% ≤FEV_1 <80% predicted
- *GOLD 3. Severe:* 30% ≤FEV_1 <50% predicted
- *GOLD 4. Very severe:* FEV_1 <30% predicted

In addition, examples of factors affecting the severity of COPD include frequency of exacerbations, presence of other disease states, overall health status, and severity of symptoms. The GOLD guidelines include a "Combined COPD Assessment," which includes symptomatic assessment with spirometric classification, exacerbation risk, or both. Using this assessment, 4 patient groups are summarized as follows: Group A (low risk, less symptoms), Group B (low risk, more symptoms), Group C (high risk, less symptoms), and Group D (high risk, more symptoms). These classifications are used in the initial choice for drug therapy of COPD (Figure 32-3).

Clinical Presentation

- Shortness of breath; dyspnea
- Cough and sputum production
- In the more severe form, respiratory failure and heart failure

Pathophysiology

- COPD is usually caused by long-term smoking; it may also be caused by exposure to other noxious particles and gases.
- Chronic inflammation is found throughout the airways but via different inflammatory cells and mediators than those that cause asthma. Thus, the response to inhaled corticosteroids is much less than that seen with asthma.
- An imbalance of proteinases and antiproteinases is found in the lung.

FIGURE 32-3. COPD Assessment and Primary Therapeutic Options
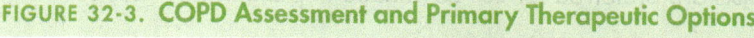
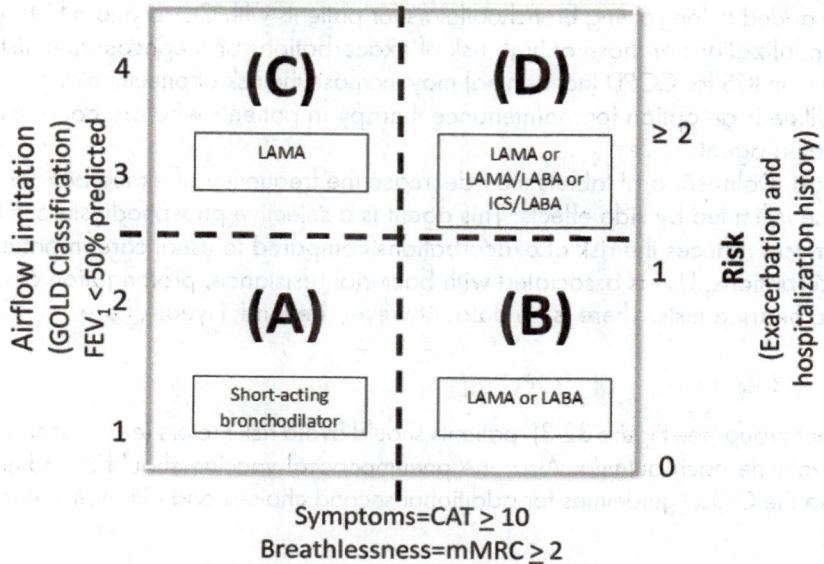

Adapted from Global Initiative for Chronic Obstructive Lung Disease 2020. Available at: http://www.goldcopd.com. Accessed May 20, 2020.
CAT, COPD assessment test; FEV_1, forced expiratory volume in 1 second; ICS, inhaled corticosteroid; LABA, long-acting beta agonist; LAMA, long-acting antimuscarinic agent; mMRC, modified Medical Research Council Dyspnea Scale.
See Table 32-7 for specific products.

- A rare hereditary cause of emphysema is alpha-1-antitrypsin deficiency.
- Pathologic changes are found in the central and peripheral airways as well as the alveoli and the pulmonary vasculature.
- The following pathological changes are also found:
  - Mucus hypersecretion
  - Ciliary dysfunction
  - Airflow limitation
  - Lung hyperinflation
  - Gas exchange abnormalities
  - Secondary pulmonary hypertension
  - Cor pulmonale

Diagnostic Criteria

- History of cigarette smoking or exposure to other noxious particles or fumes
- Chronic cough and sputum production
- Spirometry (e.g., reduced FEV_1)
- Ruling out of other lung diseases

Drug Therapy

Treatment Principles and Goals

- Management of COPD includes the following principles and goals: prevent progression of disease, relieve symptoms, enhance health status, increase exercise tolerance, prevent and treat exacerbations and complications, and decrease mortality.
- Bronchodilators are central to the symptomatic treatment of COPD. These agents will increase exercise capacity without necessarily improving FEV_1.
- Inhaled bronchodilators are preferred to oral bronchodilators for initial therapy; the specific choice of agent depends on patient response.
- Long-acting inhaled bronchodilators (Table 32-7) are more effective and convenient.
- Short-acting inhaled beta-2-agonists are preferred for use as needed in patients already receiving LABAs and antimuscarinics.
- ICSs are added to long-acting bronchodilators for patients with COPD and a history of exacerbations and hospitalizations or those at high risk of exacerbations or a concomitant history of asthma. Therapy with ICS for COPD (not asthma) may increase the risk of pneumonia.
- Theophylline is an option for maintenance therapy in patients who are not optimally controlled with inhaled agents.
- Roflumilast (Daliresp) oral tablets may decrease the frequency of exacerbations of severe COPD, but its use is limited by side effects. This agent is a selective phosphodiesterase type-4 inhibitor.
- **Azithromycin** reduces the risk of exacerbations compared to usual care in patients at high risk for exacerbations. Use is associated with bacterial resistance, prolongation of QT interval, and impaired hearing tests. There is no data, however, beyond 1 year of use.

Initial maintenance drug therapy of COPD (first choice and second choice)

For each patient group (see Figure 32-3), patients should avoid risk factors (e.g., cease smoking) and receive an influenza vaccine each autumn. Also, the pneumococcal vaccine should be administered per current guidelines. See the GOLD guidelines for additional second choices and alternative choice drug therapy.

- *Group A:*
  - Bronchodilator (short-acting) as needed (first choice)
  - Long-acting antimuscarinic agent (LAMA) *or* LABA *or* combination of short-acting anticholinergic and short-acting beta-2-agonist (second choice)

TABLE 32-7. Examples of Long-acting Bronchodilators for COPD[a,b]

Generic name	Trade name	Usual dose range	Dose form	Schedule
Aclidinium	Tudorza Pressair	One inhalation	DPI	Twice daily
Fluticasone + Umeclidinium + Vilanterol	Trelegy Ellipta	One inhalation	DPI	Once daily
Formoterol fumerate + glycopyrrolate	Bevespi Aerosphere	Two inhalations	MDI	Twice daily
Glycopyrrolate	Seebri Neohaler	One inhalation	DPI	Twice daily
Indacaterol	Arcapta Neohaler	One inhalation	DPI	Once daily
Indacaterol + glycopyrrolate	Utibron Neohaler	One inhalation	DPI	Twice daily
Olodaterol	Striverdi Respimat	One inhalation	Soft-mist inhaler	Once daily
Tiotropium	**Spiriva HandiHaler**[c]	One inhalation	DPI	Once daily
	Spiriva Respimat	One inhalation	Soft-mist inhaler	Once daily
Tiotropium + olodaterol	Stiolto Respimat	One inhalation	Soft-mist inhaler	Once daily
Umeclidinium	Incruse Ellipta	One inhalation	DPI	Once daily
Umeclidinium + vilanterol	Anoro Ellipta	One inhalation	DPI	Once daily

Boldface indicates one of top 100 drugs for 2020 by prescription volume.
MDI, metered dose inhaler; DPI, dry powder inhaler.
a. Including LAMA with or without LABA and ICS/LABA/LAMA combinations.
b. See Table 32-4 for ICS/LABA used in both asthma and COPD.
c. Make sure patient inhales at a rate to hear capsule rattle in HandiHaler.

- *Group B:*
  - LAMA *or* LABA (first choice)
  - Combination of long-acting inhaled bronchodilators (second choice)
- *Group C:*
  - LAMA alone (first choice)
  - Combination LABA/LAMA or LABA/ICS (second choice)
- *Group D:*
  - LAMA alone or LABA/LAMA combination if highly symptomatic (first choice)
  - Add ICS if exacerbation risk is high or history of asthma (second choice, one option)

Drug therapy for acute exacerbations of COPD

- Inhaled **albuterol** with or without ipratropium
- Systemic corticosteroids (e.g., **prednisone** 40 mg/d for 5 days)
- Oxygen

Antibiotics (usually oral) can be administered for patients experiencing the cardinal symptoms for a COPD exacerbation: purulent sputum in addition to increased sputum volume or increased dyspnea, or for patients who require mechanical ventilation. The choice of antibiotic depends on local patterns of bacterial resistance. Typical initial empiric therapy is **amoxicillin** with or without a beta-lactamase inhibitor, a macrolide, or doxycycline.

Monitoring

- Spirometry: FEV_1
- Symptoms of dyspnea, cough, sputum production, and change in sputum color and volume
- Exacerbation history

- PaO$_2$ (partial pressure of oxygen in the arterial blood)
- Exercise tolerance or fatigue
- Smoking status

Long-term drug therapy

See Tables 32-4 and 32-7 for specific drugs.

Nondrug therapy

- Smoking cessation—nicotine replacement therapy, **bupropion** (Zyban), varenicline (Chantix), support groups, and counseling
- Oxygen therapy
- Nutritional support
- Psychosocial support
- Pulmonary rehabilitation

Smoking cessation is the most important of these therapies.

NAPLEX Competency Statements

The questions in this chapter cover the following 2021 NAPLEX Competency Statements: **AREA 1:** 1.1; 1.2; 1.3; 1.4; 1.5; 1.6; 1.7 **AREA 2:** 2.1; 2.2; 2.3 **AREA 3:** 3.1; 3.2; 3.3; 3.4; 3.5; 3.7; 3.9; 3.11; 3.12 **AREA 5:** 5.5.

 **32-5   Questions**

1. In addition to airway inflammation, asthma is commonly associated with what problem?

A. Pulmonary fibrosis
B. Infection
C. Interstitial lung disease
D. Bronchospasm
E. Granulomas

2. Which objective measure is a component of the diagnosis of asthma?

A. PEF
B. FEV$_1$
C. FEF25-75
D. O$_2$ saturation
E. PD20

3. Which device requires slow inhalation?

A. Diskus
B. Flexhaler
C. Aerolizer
D. MDI plus spacer
E. Twisthaler

4. How many seconds is optimal for breath holding after inhaling from an MDI?

A. 4
B. 5
C. 15
D. 2
E. 10

5. Based on the GOLD guidelines, what would be the preferred initial therapy for a newly diagnosed COPD patient with an FEV$_1$ of 40%, minimal symptoms, and 2 exacerbations in the past year?

A. Methylprednisolone
B. LAMA
C. LABA
D. ICS/LABA
E. Theophylline

6. What is the trade name for mometasone + formoterol MDI?

A. Foradil
B. Pulmicort
C. Combivent
D. Symbicort
E. Dulera

7. Which of the following disease states decrease theophylline elimination and often result in reduced dosage requirements? (Mark all that apply.)

   A. Allergic rhinitis
   B. Heart failure (decompensated)
   C. Cirrhosis
   D. Hypertension
   E. Diabetes mellitus

8. Which of the following drugs are preferred for long-term treatment of moderate persistent asthma? (Mark all that apply.)

   A. Symbicort
   B. Breo Ellipta
   C. Anoro Ellipta
   D. Dulera
   E. Stiolto Respimat

9. Which of the following drugs is a once-daily antimuscarinic bronchodilator?

   A. Atrovent
   B. Serevent
   C. Foradil
   D. Spiriva
   E. Proventil

10. For patients with asthma or COPD exacerbations who are not responding adequately to inhaled short-acting bronchodilators, what is the agent of choice to add to manage the acute exacerbation?

   A. Fluticasone, high dose via spacer
   B. Budesonide, nebulized
   C. Montelukast, intravenously
   D. Theophylline, intravenously
   E. Prednisone, orally

11. Which drug may decrease serum theophylline concentrations?

   A. Clarithromycin
   B. Hydrochlorothiazide
   C. Cimetidine
   D. Rifampin
   E. Losartan

12. Which of the following side effects of inhaled corticosteroids is reduced by spacer devices?

   A. Hoarseness
   B. Decreased bone density
   C. Thinning of skin
   D. Oropharyngeal candidiasis
   E. Cataracts

13. What is the therapeutic range for theophylline for asthma management?

   A. 5 to 15 mcg/mL
   B. 8 to 12 mcg/mL
   C. 10 to 20 mcg/mL
   D. 15 to 25 mcg/mL
   E. 10 to 15 mcg/mL

14. Which asthma controller drug is preferred for mild persistent asthma in a 45-year-old woman?

   A. Accolate
   B. Singulair
   C. Xolair
   D. Pulmicort
   E. Medrol

15. Which of the following disease states may worsen asthma?

   A. Coronary artery disease
   B. Allergic rhinitis
   C. Diabetes
   D. Hypertension
   E. Arthritis

16. Which of the following classes of drugs is added to long-acting beta agonists (LABA) for long-term management of COPD in patients who have frequent exacerbations? (Mark all that apply.)

   A. Leukotriene receptor antagonists
   B. Long-acting antimuscarinic agents
   C. Anti-IgE agent
   D. Inhaled corticosteroids
   E. Methylxanthines

Use Patient Profile 32-1 to answer Questions 17 and 18.

17. Based on the GINA guidelines, which of the following classes of drugs is preferred for Mr. Johnson for optimal control of asthma?

A. Anticholinergics
B. Inhaled corticosteroids
C. Methylxanthines
D. Long-acting beta-2-agonists
E. Oral corticosteroids

18. What is an appropriate alternative to Lopressor for Mr. Johnson?

A. Lisinopril
B. Propranolol
C. Clonidine
D. Hydralazine
E. Carvedilol

Use Patient Profile 32-2 to answer Questions 19 and 20.

19. What concerns regarding theophylline should the pharmacist recognize for Mrs. Adams?

A. Cirrhosis is well documented to decrease elimination of theophylline.
B. The milligrams per kilogram dose is too low.
C. Mrs. Adams should be on a product administered every 12 hours.
D. Theophylline SR should be dosed in the morning, not evening.
E. Long-acting inhaled beta-2-agonists increase theophylline clearance.

20. Mrs. Adams has a friend who has COPD and has told her about Spiriva. Which of the following is the best response when she asks your opinion, as her pharmacist, about her taking Spiriva?

A. Spiriva is effective, but I am concerned about adverse effects.
B. Spiriva is a third-line drug for COPD; I would not use it now.
C. Spiriva is a good drug, but I want to talk to your doctor about starting a medicine called Flovent.
D. I will call your doctor and suggest adding Spiriva.
E. I think Symbicort would be better for you.

PATIENT PROFILE 32-1. Medication Profile

Patient Name: Thomas Johnson **Height:** 5'10"
Date of birth: 9-15-55 **Weight:** 75 kg
Drug allergies: Aspirin sensitivity
Allergies: NKA
Diagnosis:
(1) Asthma (childhood onset, mild persistent)
(2) Allergic rhinitis
(3) Hypertension

Medications

Date	Rx #	Physician	Drug and strength	Quantity	Sig	Refills
3/16	94385	Betts	Singulair 10 mg	30	1 at bedtime	3
3/16	94386	Betts	Albuterol MDI	1	2 puffs every 4 hours	6
3/16	94387	Betts	Fluticasone nasal spray	1	1 squirt both nostrils twice daily	3
3/25	95523	T. Jones	Lopressor 50 mg	60	1 twice daily	6
3/27	95734	Betts	Albuterol MDI	1	2 puffs every 4 hours	5

Pharmacist notes: 3/16—discussed proper use of MDI and observed patient use. Coached Mr. Johnson to inhale slowly (he was inhaling fast); he used the MDI correctly for the other steps.

PATIENT PROFILE 32-2. Medication Profile

Patient name: Mrs. S. T. Adams   **Height:** 5'5"

Date of birth: 1-16-37   **Weight:** 55 kg

Drug allergies: Sulfonamides

Diagnosis: (1) COPD—53 pack/year history of smoking (quit 2 years ago); no exacerbations in 10 years

           (2) Cirrhosis (diagnosed 3 months ago)

Medications

Date	Rx #	Physician	Drug and strength	Quantity	Sig	Refills
2/18	84389	Jones	Serevent Diskus	1	1 inhalation every 12 hours	6
2/18	84390	Jones	Albuterol MDI	1	2 puffs every 4 hours as needed	As needed
2/18	84392	Jones	Theophylline 600 mg	30	1 daily at 6 PM	2

Pharmacist notes: 2/18—discussed proper use of Diskus and observed patient use; taught Mrs. Adams to inhale deeply and rapidly (she was inhaling slowly for <2 seconds). Also observed use of MDI (she forgot to exhale gently before pressing down on MDI).

21. Based on the GINA guidelines, which of the following drugs is best for long-term management of intermittent asthma?

A. Low dose budesonide/formoterol, as needed
B. Montelukast daily
C. Albuterol, scheduled 4 times daily
D. Theophylline SR daily
E. Medium dose budesonide, scheduled

22. Which of the following is the best total daily dose of prednisone for home management of an acute exacerbation of asthma in an 82-kg male?

A. 40 mg
B. 20 mg
C. 80 mg
D. 60 mg
E. 120 mg

23. Which of the following drugs is most likely to cause an asthma exacerbation in a patient sensitive to aspirin? (Mark all that apply.)

A. Naproxen
B. Acetaminophen
C. Celecoxib
D. Salsalate
E. Ibuprofen

24. Which of the following types of inhalers does not work well in very cold temperatures?

A. Diskus
B. Flexhaler
C. Aerolizer
D. MDI
E. Twisthaler

25. Which of the following devices requires the patient to hear the capsule vibrating?

A. HandiHaler
B. Twisthaler
C. Flexhaler
D. Diskus
E. Respimat

 **32-6**   Answers

1. D. Asthma certainly has a bronchospastic component, yet it is primarily due to inflammation, so good control of inflammation dramatically reduces bronchospasm.

2. B. Spirometry, primarily the FEV_1, is part of the diagnosis of asthma.

3. D. Dry powder inhalers for asthma therapy that are currently available require rapid inhalation. MDIs require slow inhalation to minimize impaction of aerosol in the mouth and throat.

4. E. Ten seconds is best; there is no need to hold longer. If 10 seconds is uncomfortable, 4 to 5 seconds is acceptable.

5. B. A LAMA would be the preferred therapy for this patient as it has greater impact on exacerbations than LABA. ICS products are not beneficial to all COPD patients. Oral steroids and theophylline should not be used regularly.

6. E. Dulera is the combination of mometasone and formoterol.

7. B, C. Decompensated heart failure and cirrhosis can dramatically reduce theophylline clearance.

8. A, B, D. Combination products with ICS/LABA are correct. Items listed in answers C and E are COPD products.

9. D. Spiriva (tiotropium) is inhaled once daily.

10. E. Prednisone or other systemic corticosteroids (e.g., methylprednisolone) are well documented to be efficacious in asthma and acute exacerbations of COPD.

11. D. Rifampin is well documented to decrease serum theophylline concentrations. Clarithromycin and cimetidine are well documented to increase serum concentrations. Hydrochlorothiazide and losartan do not affect serum theophylline concentrations.

12. D. Oropharyngeal candidiasis or thrush is correct. The other side effects are not reduced by spacers.

13. A. The accepted range for asthma is 5 to 15 mcg/mL (*not* the old range of 10 to 20 mcg/mL). There is no benefit in exceeding 15 mcg/mL, and many patients receive benefit at lower doses.

14. D. Pulmicort or other inhaled corticosteroid is preferred (see GINA guidelines).

15. B. Allergic rhinitis that is not well controlled can worsen asthma control and outcomes.

16. B, D. Long-acting antimuscarinic agents and inhaled corticosteroids can be added to long-acting beta agonists in the treatment of COPD, especially if there are frequent exacerbations. Combination LABA/LAMA has greater impact on exacerbation reduction than monotherapy. The ICS class of drugs should *not* be used routinely in COPD patients with mild disease or without a significant history of exacerbations.

17. B. Inhaled corticosteroids are the preferred treatment (see Tables 32-2 and 32-3 for treatment choices). The pharmacist should share the asthma guidelines with Mr. Johnson's prescriber to help ensure optimal care. In addition, the pharmacist should educate the patient regarding the purpose of the medications and the proper use of inhalers. The pharmacist should observe the patient using the device.

18. A. An angiotensin-converting enzyme inhibitor, such as lisinopril, should be efficacious with few side effects (monitor for cough); beta blockers should be avoided in Mr. Johnson unless he is post–myocardial infarction or had congestive heart failure. In those situations, use a low dose of a beta-1-selective blocker and monitor carefully.

19. A. Cirrhosis is well documented to decrease elimination of theophylline. Given the recent diagnosis ensure a check of a steady-state theophylline level (peak), and anticipate dose reduction (usually 50% dose reduction in liver disease).

20. D. Because the patient has a prescription for Serevent, a logical change here would be to add the long-acting, once-daily anticholinergic tiotropium (Spiriva).

21. A. Per GINA guidelines, low-dose budesonide/formoterol combination, as needed, is the preferred treatment for intermittent asthma (remember, if it is needed more than twice per week during the day, the patient has persistent asthma, not intermittent asthma).

22. C. Eighty milligrams is an appropriate dose. If it is started as soon as the patient is in the red zone and not responding quickly to short-acting, inhaled beta-2-agonists, only a few days of treatment usually will be required (usually < 1 week).

23. A, D, E. Naproxen, ibuprofen, and salsalate have the same mechanism of action as aspirin and will predictably trigger symptoms in an aspirin-sensitive patient (i.e., increased production of leukotrienes). COX-2 inhibitors are usually safe (celecoxib). Acetaminophen is the choice agent for minor pain in these patients.

24. D. In cold temperatures, MDIs release large aerosol particles that do not penetrate deeply into the lungs. Dry powder inhalers are acceptable.

25. A. The HandiHaler requires that the patient hear the capsule vibrating (rattling) as the medication is being inhaled.

 ## 32-7 Additional Resources

Asthma

Beasley R, Holliday M, Reddel HK, et al. Controlled trial of budesonide-formoterol as needed for mild asthma. *N Engl J Med.* 2019;380:2020–30.

Global Initiative for Asthma. *Global Strategy for Asthma Management and Prevention, 2020.* Vancouver, WA: Global Initiative for Asthma; 2020.

Hardy J, Baggott C, Fingleton J, et al. Budesonide-formoterol reliever therapy versus maintenance budesonide plus terbutaline reliever therapy in adults with mild to moderate asthma (PRACTICAL): a 52-week, open-label, multicenter, superiority, randomized controlled trial. *Lancet.* 2019;394:919–928.

National Heart, Lung, and Blood Institute. *Expert Panel Report 3: Guidelines for the Diagnosis and Management of Asthma.* NIH Publication 07-4051. Bethesda, MD: U.S. Department of Health and Human Services, National Institutes of Health, National Heart, Lung, and Blood Institute; 2007. https://www.nhlbi.nih.gov/sites/default/files/media/docs/asthgdln_1.pdf. Accessed May 26, 2020.

Sanchis J, Gich I, Pedersen S. Systematic review of errors in inhaler use: has patient technique improved over time? *Chest.* 2016;150:394–406.

Stempel DA, Szefler SJ, Pedersen S, et al. Safety of adding salmeterol to fluticasone propionate in children with asthma. *N Engl J Med.* 2016;375:840–849.

Chronic Obstructive Pulmonary Disease

Global Initiative for Chronic Obstructive Lung Disease. *Global Strategy for the Diagnosis, Management, and Prevention of Chronic Obstructive Pulmonary Disease.* Updated 2021. http://www.goldcopd.org. Accessed September 10, 2021.

Leuppi JD, Schuetz P, Bingisser R, et al. Short-term vs. conventional glucocorticoid therapy in acute exacerbations of chronic obstructive pulmonary disease: the REDUCE randomized clinical trial. *JAMA.* 2013;309:2223–2231.

Lipson DA, Barnhart F, Brealey N, et al. Once-daily single-inhaler triple versus dual therapy in patients with COPD. *N Engl J Med.* 2018;378(18):1671–1680.

Infectious Diseases

33

MICHAEL P. VEVE

 ## 33-1 KEY POINTS

- Antimicrobial stewardship programs (ASPs) promote judicious antimicrobial use.
- Pharmacists are vital components of ASPs through communicating with and engaging stakeholders to improve prescribing practices.
- Empiric anti-infective therapy targets the most likely organism(s) associated with the infection type.
- After the identification of the organism causing the disease, anti-infective therapy should be narrowed to cover that specific organism (definitive therapy).
- Therapy should reflect the best medication for the organism while accounting for the patient's condition (renal function, concurrent disease states).
- Patient-specific factors (age, presence of prosthetic material, recent hospitalization, recent antibiotic use, chronic medical conditions, and receipt of certain types of medications) often infer risk of specific pathogens and are to guide empiric therapy for many infectious diseases.
- Many cases of bronchitis are viral in etiology, making routine antibiotic therapy controversial.
- The Centers for Disease Control and Prevention recommends direct observed therapy for treatment of active and latent tuberculosis.
- Treatment of diarrhea should be mainly supportive therapy, except in *Clostridioides difficile*–associated diarrhea for which oral vancomycin is the drug of choice.
- Fluoroquinolones are useful in the treatment of prostatitis.
- Patients testing positive for any sexually transmitted infection (STI) should be screened for the presence of other STIs.
- Penicillin is the drug of choice for the treatment of syphilis.
- Doxycycline is used in the treatment of tickborne infections.
- Antifungal agent selection is based on the suspected fungi and severity of illness.
- Amphotericin B products are reserved for severe fungal infections because of the high incidence of toxicity.
- Chronic hepatitis B is treated with nucleos(t)ide analogue therapies.
- Treatment for chronic hepatitis C virus is based on genotype. Patients are treated with a combination of 2 or 3 medications.
- Agents recommended for prophylaxis and treatment of influenza include oseltamivir and zanamivir.
- Acyclovir, valacyclovir, and famciclovir can be used to treat genital herpes simplex and varicella zoster infections.

 ## 33-2 STUDY GUIDE CHECKLIST

The following topics may guide your study of this subject area:

- ☐ Signs, symptoms, and laboratory findings of common infections.
- ☐ Culture and stain techniques used to identify infecting agent.
- ☐ Selection of empiric anti-infective therapy based on site of infection and risk factors.
- ☐ Spectrum of activity of individual anti-infective agents.
- ☐ De-escalation of therapy based on culture results.
- ☐ Frequency and duration of anti-infective therapy.

33-3   General Principles of Infectious Disease

Several infectious disease topics are addressed in other chapters of this review, including otitis media in Chapter 31, human immunodeficiency virus (HIV) and acquired immune deficiency syndrome (AIDS) in Chapter 35, and common colds in Chapter 39. For additional information about specific anti-infective agents, see Chapter 34.

Diagnosis

Diagnosis of most infectious diseases consists of isolation and identification of microorganisms, assessment of patient signs and symptoms for infection, and analysis of other laboratory data.

Isolation of organisms

For identification of the causative pathogen of a disease, samples should be taken from appropriate body sites before the initiation of anti-infective therapy to prevent the inhibition of organism growth. Organisms isolated from body sites that normally are sterile (blood, bone, spinal fluid) yield higher predictive value than do organisms isolated from body sites that are normally colonized with microorganisms (urine, skin, respiratory tract).

Identification of organisms

Once a specimen is obtained, a Gram stain is performed to determine the infectious organism's cell morphology and to guide empiric therapy (agents with either gram-positive or gram-negative coverage). After the species of organism has been determined, it is exposed to standardized concentrations of antibiotics to determine the concentrations that inhibit its growth. The lowest concentration that prevents microbial growth is called the minimum inhibitory concentration (MIC). The 3 breakpoint concentrations of antibiotics are susceptible, intermediate, and resistant. The breakpoint concentration determines whether the antibiotic can be used for therapy.

Physical signs and symptoms of infection (fever, redness, swelling, pain, and cough) must be considered both for initial diagnosis and for assessment of response to antibiotic therapy.

Laboratory tests

In the initial stage of infection, a patient's neutrophil count may increase above normal, and immature neutrophil forms (bands) may appear; therefore, a white blood cell (WBC) count should be taken. Laboratory tests may not be reliable in patients who are elderly, malnourished, neonatal, or severely infected.

Antimicrobial Stewardship and Treatment Strategies

Antimicrobial stewardship programs (ASPs) are multidisciplinary groups of pharmacists, physicians, nurses, and other health care professionals whose goal is to optimize clinical outcomes while minimizing unintended consequences of antimicrobial use, including toxicity, the selection of pathogenic organisms, and the emergence of resistance.

- ASPs are key components of hospitals and are active in outpatient, clinic settings. In short, they are responsible for developing antimicrobial use pathways, antimicrobial formulary management, and performing prospective audit and feedback to recommend appropriate antibiotic use.

Anti-infective agents should be used only when a significant infection has been diagnosed, when one is strongly suspected, or when prophylactic therapy is indicated.

Prophylactic anti-infective therapy is aimed at preventing infection and is commonly used after exposure to infection (tuberculosis) or before surgical intervention (bowel surgery).

Empiric therapy is directed toward all common pathogens associated with the suspected infection as well as local trends of susceptibility and prevalence.

Definitive therapy is guided by the isolated organisms. Antimicrobial therapy in this instance should be the narrowest spectrum agents that are active against the organism identified. Using appropriate definitive therapy (targeted and narrow in spectrum) can prevent the development of antimicrobial resistance as a result of unnecessary drug exposures, can avoid toxicities associated with broader-spectrum agents used empirically, and is generally more cost-effective.

Choice of Anti-infective Agents

The thought process of treating the infected patient is depicted in Figure 33-1.

To determine optimal anti-infective therapy or to review the appropriateness of other decisions, a clinician should consider the acronym DR. PLASMA:

DECISION MAKING FOR EMPIRIC ANTIMICROBIAL THERAPY

D — **Drug-drug interactions**
Are there potential serious drug-drug interactions that would prevent the use of certain antimicrobial classes?

R — **Renal and hepatic function**
What is the appropriate antimicrobial dose and interval? (Regimen design should consider patient size, renal or hepatic function, the disease state being treated, and pharmacodynamics of the agents used.)

P — **Primary source of infection**
What organisms are most likely to cause the suspected infection? Antibiotics should be tailored to these organisms.

L — **Location of acquisition**
Does the patient reside in a location at high-risk for drug-resistant pathogens (hospital-acquired infection, nursing home residents, international travelers)?

A — **Antimicrobial history**
Has the patient received previous antimicrobial therapy? Potential antibiotic failures could warrant use of alternative agents because of resistance and/or other factors.

S — **Severity of illness**
Is an antibiotic indicated on the basis of the clinical findings?

M — **Microbiological history**
Is there a recent infection history with a previously isolated organism? Empiric antimicrobial selection could include coverage for this organism.

A — **Allergy history**
Does the patient have a serious, true allergy to any antimicrobials that could be used to treat this infection?

"DR. PLASMA" concept developed by Dr. Julie Ann Justo, University of South Carolina College of Pharmacy

FIGURE 33-1. The Antibiotic Use Thought Process Front End and Back End

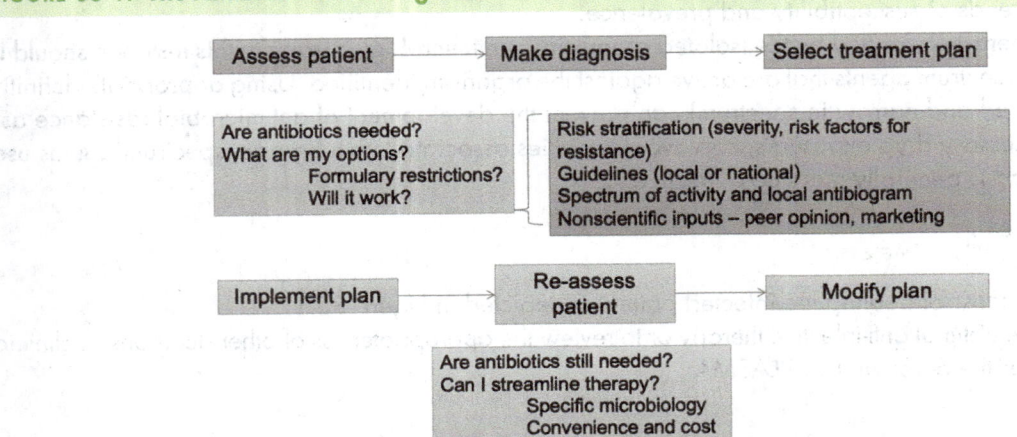

Lack of Therapeutic Effectiveness

When anti-infective therapy fails, careful analysis of possible causes should be made before changing the regimen. Factors associated with therapeutic failure include a lack of source control, infection misdiagnosis, inappropriate choice of antimicrobial agent, and the development of antimicrobial resistance.

33-4   Common Bacterial, Fungal, and Viral Infections

Meningitis

Meningitis is defined as inflammation of the meninges or the 3 outer protective layers of the brain (Figure 33-2). This section covers treatment of bacterial meningitis, which is most common. Risk factors for bacterial meningitis include age, head trauma, immunosuppression (e.g., steroids, organ transplant), alcoholism, diabetes mellitus, and crowding/dorm residential life.

Causative organisms

A variety of organisms are associated with bacterial meningitis, but *Streptococcus pneumonia* is predominate in adults. Patient age is one factor used to guide antibiotic selection, because age is associated with specific organisms (Table 33-1).

Clinical presentation

Patients may present with a fever, headache, photophobia, nuchal rigidity, seizures, vomiting, or altered mental status.

Diagnostic criteria

Blood and cerebrospinal fluid (CSF) samples should be obtained for culture and analysis if meningitis is suspected. In cases of bacterial meningitis, the following abnormalities occur in the CSF: increased WBCs and protein as well as decreased glucose.

FIGURE 33-2. Bacterial Meningitis

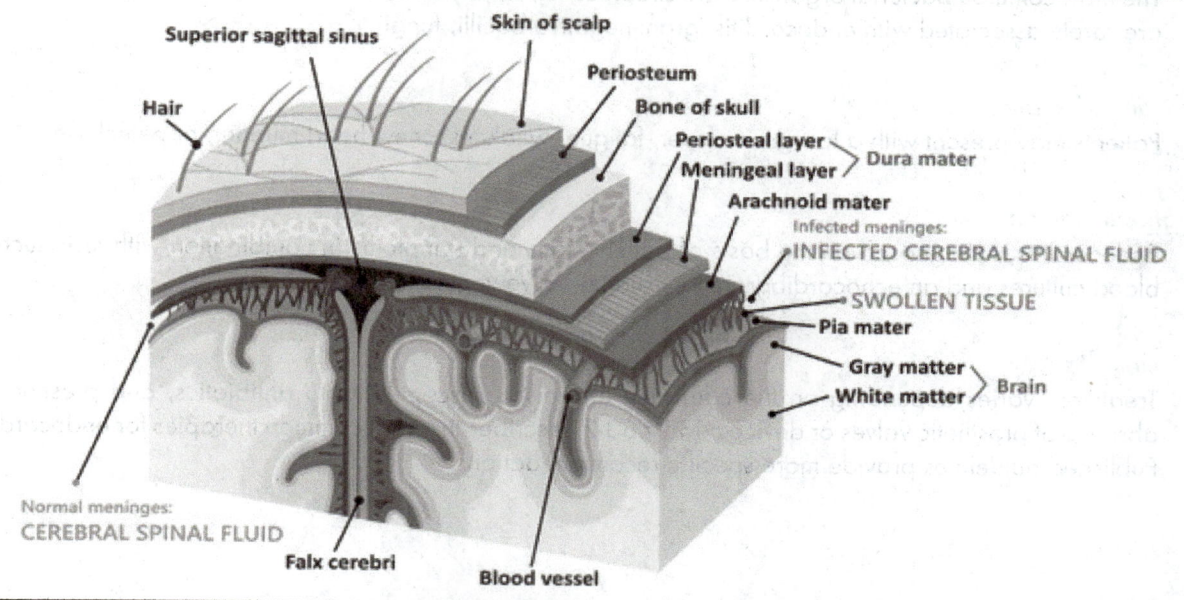

Figure comparing normal meninges to bacterial meningitis resulting in inflammation of the membranes that envelop the brain. Encephalitis is inflammation of the brain itself while meningoencephalitis is inflammation of both the meninges and the brain.

Treatment

Empiric treatment for bacterial meningitis is determined by patient age or comorbid conditions (see Table 33-1). Because of limited antibiotic penetration by many agents, the highest safe antibiotic doses are generally used. Adjunctive dexamethasone (Decadron) should be considered in select patient populations based on age and presumed causative bacteria (*S. pneumoniae*, *Haemophilus influenzae*). Once the pathogen has been identified, narrow spectrum, definitive therapy should be used based on susceptibility data and target site concentrations. Antibiotic characteristics associated with good CNS penetration are low molecular weight, low protein bound, and lipid soluble.

Endocarditis

Endocarditis is an infection of the endocardium, the membrane lining the heart chamber and valves. Injection drug use or heart abnormalities such as an artificial/prosthetic or damaged valve predispose patients to endocarditis.

TABLE 33-1. Empiric Therapy for Meningitis Based on Age

Age	Common organisms	Treatment
Newborn to 1 month	*Streptococcus agalactiae, Escherichia coli, Listeria monocytogenes, Klebsiella* spp.	Ampicillin plus either cefotaxime or an aminoglycoside
1 to 23 months	*Streptococcus pneumoniae, Neisseria meningitidis, S. agalactiae, Haemophilus influenzae, E. coli*	Vancomycin plus either ceftriaxone or cefotaxime
2 to 50 years	*N. meningitidis, S. pneumoniae*	Vancomycin plus either ceftriaxone or cefotaxime
50 years or older	*S. pneumoniae, N. meningitidis, L. monocytogenes, aerobic gram-negative bacilli*	Vancomycin plus ampicillin plus either ceftriaxone or cefotaxime

Tunkel AR, Hartman BJ, Kaplan SL, et al., 2004.

Causative organisms

The most common bacterial organisms are streptococci, staphylococci, and enterococci. Other organisms are rarely associated with endocarditis (gram-negative bacilli, fungi).

Clinical presentation

Patients may present with a low-grade fever, fatigue, weakness, new heart murmur, or petechiae.

Diagnostic criteria

Endocarditis is diagnosed on the basis of patient signs and symptoms in combination with tests such as blood cultures and an echocardiogram to visualize valve vegetations.

Treatment

Treatment varies depending on the causative organism, susceptibility to antibiotics, and presence or absence of prosthetic valves or devices. Table 33-2 describes the most common therapies for endocarditis. Published guidelines provide more specific recommendations.

TABLE 33-2. Treatment of Endocarditis

Organism or patient	Native valve (duration in weeks)	Prosthetic valve (duration in weeks)
Viridans group streptococci and *Streptococcus bovis:* MIC ≤ 0.12 mcg/mL	Penicillin G (4)	Penicillin G (6) ± gentamicin ⚠ (2)
	Ceftriaxone (4)	Ceftriaxone (6) ± gentamicin (2)
	Penicillin G (2) + gentamicin (2)	
	Ceftriaxone (2) + gentamicin (2)	
Viridans group streptococci and *S. bovis:* MIC 0.12 to 0.5 mcg/mL	Penicillin G (4) + gentamicin (2)	Penicillin (6) + gentamicin (6)
	Ceftriaxone (4)	Ceftriaxone (6) + gentamicin (6)
Oxacillin-susceptible staphylococci	Nafcillin or oxacillin (6)	Nafcillin (≥6) or oxacillin + rifampin (≥6) + gentamicin (2)
	Cefazolin[b] (6)	Cefazolin[b] (≥6) + rifampin (≥6) + gentamicin (2)
Oxacillin-resistant staphylococci	Vancomycin (6)	Vancomycin (≥6) + rifampin (≥6) + gentamicin (2)
	Daptomycin (6)	
Enterococci susceptible to penicillin and gentamicin in patients who can tolerate beta lactams	Ampicillin or penicillin G (4 to 6) + gentamicin (4 to 6)	Ampicillin or penicillin G (6) + gentamicin (6)
	Ampicillin (6) + ceftriaxone (6)	Ampicillin (6) + ceftriaxone (6)
Enterococci susceptible to aminoglycoside and vancomycin but resistant to penicillin or patients who cannot tolerate beta lactams	Vancomycin (6) + gentamicin (6)	Vancomycin (6) + gentamicin (6)
Enterococci resistant to penicillin, aminoglycosides, and vancomycin	Linezolid (>6)	Linezolid (>6)
	Daptomycin (>6)	Daptomycin (>6)

Baddour LM, Wilson WR, Bayer AS, et al., 2015.
a. Use vancomycin only if unable to use ampicillin or penicillin.
b. Cefazolin should be used for nonanaphylactoid, penicillin-allergic patients.

Gentamicin *FDA BOXED WARNING*

Close monitoring of serum concentrations and toxicities required due to risk of renal toxicity, neurotoxicity, and ototoxicity. Avoid concomitant use of other nephrotoxic and neurotoxic medications. Risk of fetal harm—avoid use in pregnancy.

Central Line–Associated Bloodstream Infections

Central line–associated bloodstream infections (CLABSIs) are common in hospital settings for patients with invasive central lines, such as in critically ill patients or those who require hemodialysis. CLABSIs result from introduction of microbes into the central line, usually by contamination.

Causative organisms

In general, coagulase-negative staphylococci and *Staphylococcus aureus* are the most common causes of intravascular device infections. Other pathogens including *Candida* spp., enterococci, *Pseudomonas aeruginosa,* and enteric gram-negative bacilli may be empirically covered on the basis of specific risk factors.

Clinical presentation

Intravascular catheter infection presentation is nonspecific, consisting of fever or hypothermia, chills, tachycardia, tachypnea, hypotension, and increased or decreased WBC count.

Diagnostic criteria

Blood cultures should be drawn from the catheter and from a peripheral site before initiating antibiotics. If possible, the catheter should be removed and cultured.

Treatment

The antibiotic selected and duration of treatment depend on the location and type of device, organism isolated, whether the device is removed, clinical response, and additional patient comorbidities. When possible, the infected device should be removed. If no specific risk factors are present, initial empiric treatment should include vancomycin to cover methicillin-resistant staphylococci. Selection of coverage for gram-negative organisms should be based on local susceptibility data and severity of disease. Empiric coverage of *Candida* spp. should be given to patients with a history of femoral catheter placement, use of total parenteral nutrition, prolonged use of antibiotics, hematologic malignancy, transplant, or colonization by *Candida* spp. at multiple sites.

Febrile Neutropenia

Patients with cancer often have marked decreases in WBCs caused by their chemotherapy regimen; this predisposes patients to infection. Neutropenia is defined as an absolute neutrophil count (ANC) below 500 cells/mL. When the ANC is less than 500 cells/mL, fever may be the only symptom of infection that the patient may display; therefore, fever in a neutropenic patient should prompt an investigation for an infection and the initiation of antibiotics.

Causative organisms

Because any infection can cause fever in neutropenic patients, a wide variety of bacterial, fungal, and viral pathogens may be implicated. The priority pathogen in neutropenic patients is *P. aeruginosa*, and empiric therapy should cover this organism in most cases. Other bacterial pathogens identified in neutropenic patients include coagulase-negative staphylococci, *S. aureus*, enterococci, and other enteric gram-negative bacilli (e.g., *E. coli*).

Clinical presentation

Patients with febrile neutropenia can present with a range of symptoms, from fever to severe pneumonia or septic shock.

Diagnostic criteria

An ANC of <500 cells/mL with either a single oral temperature of ≥38.3°C or a temperature of ≥38°C for over 1 hour is diagnostic of febrile neutropenia. An extensive clinical evaluation to determine the cause of infection is recommended.

Treatment

Treatment is based on a severity risk assessment such as the Multinational Association for Supportive Care in Cancer (MASCC) Risk-Index score. Empiric coverage should be based on suspected site of infection and risk factors for multidrug-resistant pathogens. When the site of infection is known (pneumonia, skin and soft tissue infection, catheter-related bloodstream infection), treatment should follow current guidelines. If the site of infection is not identifiable, coverage of gram-positive bacteria, enteric gram-negative bacilli, and *P. aeruginosa* should be provided with a single agent or combination of agents. Routine coverage for methicillin-resistant *S. aureus* (MRSA), other multidrug-resistant bacteria, and *Candida* spp. is not recommended. Double coverage of gram-negative bacteria is recommended for only select patients (critically ill) at risk of multidrug-resistant pathogens.

High-risk patients (MASCC score < 21) should be admitted and treated with intravenous antibiotics. Low-risk patients (MASCC score ≥ 21) may be candidates for oral antibiotic therapy or outpatient treatment. The site of infection and the organism identified determine the antibiotic treatment duration. If no infectious source is identified, antibiotic treatment should be continued until the ANC > 500 cells/mL. Table 33-3 lists treatment options.

TABLE 33-3. Initial Treatment of Febrile Neutropenia

Classification	Treatment
Infection site known	Treat as immunocompromised patient and health care–associated infection in accordance with national or institutional guidelines.
Infection site not known	

Risk severity	Treatment
Low risk	Oral ciprofloxacin ⚠ + amoxicillin/clavulanate
High risk	Cefepime, piperacillin/tazobactam, or an antipseudomonal carbapenem. The patient should be assessed for additional empiric anti-MRSA and/or antifungal therapy.

Ciprofloxacin *FDA BOXED WARNING*

Risk of serious adverse reactions including tendinitis, tendon rupture, peripheral neuropathy, central nervous effects, and exacerbation of myasthenia gravis.

Acute or Chronic Bronchitis

Acute bronchitis is a respiratory tract infection that typically presents with a cough as the predominant symptom with a clear chest radiograph. Chronic bronchitis is a disease of the bronchi that is manifested by cough and sputum expectoration occurring for at least 3 months per year for more than 2 consecutive years. Chronic bronchitis is most commonly caused by smoking or prolonged exposure to inhalation of noxious substances. When a person with chronic bronchitis experiences a worsening of symptoms, it is referred to as an acute exacerbation of chronic bronchitis.

Causative organisms

The majority of acute bronchitis infections are caused by respiratory viruses and predispose patients to develop secondary bacterial infections. Bacterial pathogens commonly implicated in acute bronchitis include *Mycoplasma pneumoniae*, *Chlamydophila pneumoniae*, *Bordetella pertussis*, and *Bordetella parapertussis*. Secondary bacterial infections are often caused by *S. pneumoniae*, *Moraxella catarrhalis*, or *H. influenzae*.

Clinical presentation

Acute bronchitis presents with cough as the predominant symptom, but fever, muscle aches, and fatigue can also be present.

Diagnostic criteria

There are no recommended diagnostic tests for acute bronchitis. Diagnosis is made by presentation with cough for less than 3 weeks with no radiological evidence of pneumonia. In addition, the common cold, asthma, and an exacerbation of chronic obstructive pulmonary disease should be ruled out.

Treatment

Acute bronchitis should not routinely be treated with antibiotics unless *B. pertussis* is suspected or known to be the cause. However, patients with acute exacerbations of chronic bronchitis should be treated with antibiotics because treatment of exacerbations with antibiotics has been shown to decrease the duration of illness (Table 33-4).

Pneumonia

Pneumonia is an inflammation of the lung tissue caused by bacterial, viral, or fungal infections. Pneumonia occurs in patients with underlying comorbid conditions (old age, smoking, diabetes, congestive heart failure) or structural lung disease, or in patients who are hospitalized and placed on mechanical ventilation.

TABLE 33-4. Treatment of Acute and Chronic Bronchitis

Illness	Treatment[a]
Acute bronchitis	Antibiotics are not to be offered or given.
Acute bronchitis caused by *Bordetella pertussis*	Erythromycin, clarithromycin, **azithromycin**
Exacerbation of chronic bronchitis	**Amoxicillin**, amoxicillin/clavulanate, erythromycin, clarithromycin, **azithromycin**, doxycycline, minocycline

Boldface indicates one of top 100 drugs for 2020 by prescription volume.
a. Usual duration is 7 to 10 days.

Causative organisms

Multiple viral or bacterial etiologies are possible, depending on age and predisposing conditions. Pneumonia is often classified as "community acquired" (CAP) or "hospital/ventilator associated" (HAP/VAP), and pathogen distribution varies based on pneumonia type (Table 33-5 and Table 33-6). In addition to those identified in CAP, organisms of greatest concern in HAP/VAP are *S. aureus,* including MRSA, and *P. aeruginosa.*

Clinical presentation

The onset of illness can be abrupt or subacute, with fever, chills, dyspnea, and productive cough predominating.

Diagnostic criteria

A diagnosis of pneumonia is based on patient signs and symptoms in combination with tests such as a chest x-ray or culture data. Blood and respiratory cultures (sputum, bronchoalveolar lavage) may be used to identify the causative pathogen.

TABLE 33-5. Empiric Treatment of Community-Acquired Pneumonia

Treatment location	Common organisms	Treatment
Outpatient treatment	*Streptococcus pneumoniae, Mycoplasma pneumoniae, Haemophilus influenzae, Chlamydophila pneumonia*	Previously health individuals: high-dose **amoxicillin**, doxycycline, or a macrolide
		Patients with comorbidities: respiratory fluoroquinolone or combination of beta lactam + macrolide
Inpatient treatment (non-ICU)	*S. pneumoniae, M. pneumoniae, C. pneumoniae, H influenzae, Legionella* spp.	Respiratory fluoroquinolone or combination of beta lactam + macrolide
Inpatient ICU treatment	*S. pneumoniae, Staphylococcus aureus, Legionella* spp., gram-negative bacilli, *H. influenzae*	Beta lactam (cefotaxime, ceftriaxone, or ampicillin/sulbactam) + either **azithromycin** or a respiratory fluoroquinolone
	Suspected multidrug resistant infection:	
	■ Recent hospitalization and receipt of I.V. antibiotics	Antipneumococcal antipseudomonal beta lactam + anti-MRSA antibiotic
	■ Prior isolation of MRSA or *P. aeruginosa*	
		Antipneumococcal antipseudomonal beta lactam + aminoglycoside + **azithromycin** or moxifloxacin ⚠

Mandell LA, Wunderink RG, Anzueto A, et al., 2007.
Boldface indicates one of top 100 drugs for 2020 by prescription volume.
ICU, intensive care unit; I.V., intravenous.

Moxifloxacin *FDA BOXED WARNING*

Risk of serious adverse reactions including tendinitis, tendon rupture, peripheral neuropathy, central nervous effects, and exacerbation of myasthenia gravis.

TABLE 33-6. Empiric Treatment of Hospital-acquired Pneumonia and Ventilator-associated Pneumonia

Patient risk	Treatment
Patient not at high risk of mortality without risk factors for MRSA	Monotherapy with antipseudomonal beta lactam Piperacillin/tazobactam Cefepime Imipenem/cilastatin Meropenem or Levofloxacin ⚠
Patient not at high risk of mortality with risk factors for MRSA	Add MRSA coverage Vancomycin Linezolid
Patient at high risk of mortality or received I.V. antibiotics in past 90 days	Add double gram-negative coverage to antipseudomonal beta lactam. Levofloxacin or Amikacin ⚠ Gentamicin Tobramycin ⚠

Metlay JP, Waterer GW, Long AC, et al. 2019.
I.V., intravenous.

 FDA BOXED WARNINGS

Levofloxacin
Risk of serious adverse reactions including tendinitis, tendon rupture, peripheral neuropathy, central nervous effects, and exacerbation of myasthenia gravis.

Amikacin
Close monitoring of serum concentrations, renal function, and toxicities required due to risk of renal toxicity, neurotoxicity, and ototoxicity. Avoid concomitant use of other nephrotoxic and neurotoxic medications.

Tobramycin
Close monitoring of serum concentrations, renal function, and toxicities required due to risk of renal toxicity, neurotoxicity, and ototoxicity. Avoid concomitant use of other nephrotoxic and neurotoxic medications. Risk of fetal harm—avoid use in pregnancy.

Treatment

CAP and HAP/VAP treatment is based on the pneumonia classification. In CAP, empiric antibiotic selection is determined by treatment location: outpatient, inpatient, or intensive care unit (Table 33-5).

HAP occurs when pneumonia develops 48 hours or more after a patient is admitted to the hospital. VAP occurs when pneumonia develops 48 hours after a patient is placed on a ventilator. Treatment for HAP or VAP is based on the onset of the infection and risk factors for multidrug-resistant organisms. Risk factors for multidrug-resistant organisms include treatment with antimicrobial agents within the past 90 days, septic shock, hospitalization for >5 days, immunosuppression, or a high rate of antibiotic resistance in the community or hospital unit. Table 33-6 outlines treatment for HAP and VAP.

Tuberculosis

Tuberculosis is a communicable infectious disease caused by *Mycobacterium tuberculosis*. It can produce a silent, latent infection as well as an active infection. This distinction is important because patients with active *M. tuberculosis* are considered infectious. Although infection of any tissue or organ with *M. tuberculosis* is possible, the usual site of infection is pulmonary.

Clinical presentation

The clinical presentation of tuberculosis is depicted in Figure 33-3

Diagnostic criteria

Diagnosis often is made by a combination of chest x-ray findings and a positive purified protein derivative (PPD) skin test or interferon-gamma release assay (IGRA).

Treatment

Tuberculosis is a very slow growing bacterium that requires prolonged treatment with multiple anti-infective agents to achieve a cure and to prevent development of resistance. To ensure compliance with therapy, the U.S. Centers for Disease Control and Prevention (CDC) recommends direct observed therapy for most treatment regimens for active and latent tuberculosis. See Table 33-7 for a summary of treatments.

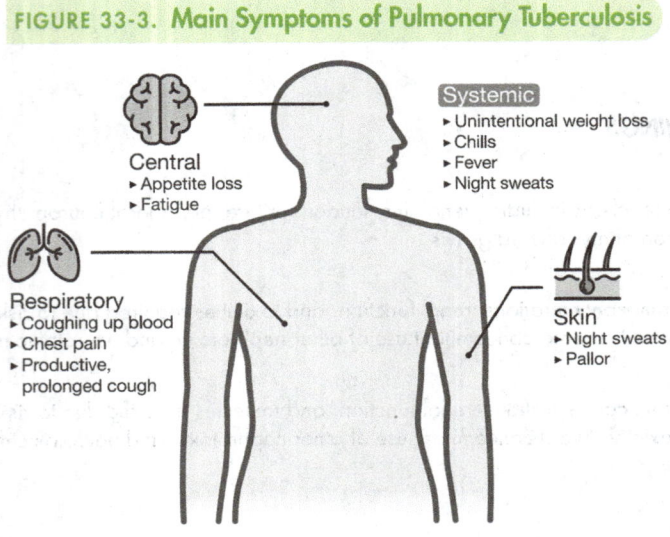

FIGURE 33-3. Main Symptoms of Pulmonary Tuberculosis

TABLE 33-7. Treatment of Tuberculosis

Disease stage	Treatment	Duration
Latent (preferred)	Isoniazid	9 months (for children and HIV-positive patients)
	Isoniazid	6 months
	Rifampin	4 months
Active disease (preferred)	Isoniazid + rifampin + pyrazinamide + ethambutol	2 months
	Followed by isoniazid + rifampin	4 months (6 months total)

⚠ **Isoniazid** *FDA BOXED WARNING*

Risk of severe or fatal hepatitis. Risk increases with age as well as alcohol consumption.

Intra-abdominal Infections

Intra-abdominal infections include infections of the retroperitoneal space or the peritoneal cavity.

Causative organisms

A variety of bacteria are associated with intra-abdominal infections including gram-negative and gram-positive aerobic bacteria but, importantly, anaerobic bacteria that live in the gut. Major causes of infection include *E. coli* and *Bacteroides* spp.

Clinical presentation

Patients may present with abdominal pain and fever. Systemic manifestation can occur in severe cases.

Diagnostic criteria

Generally, patient history and physical examination are sufficient to diagnose an intra-abdominal infection. Imaging studies or exploratory laparotomy may be necessary in select patients.

Treatment

In addition to antibiotics, fluid resuscitation may be required in cases of severe infections. Surgical procedures (source control) are essential to treatment in most patients, such as those with severe peritonitis or an abscess. Although cultures are not required in low-risk patients with a community-acquired infection, cultures of specimens obtained from the site of infection as well as susceptibility testing may prove beneficial to guiding therapy in hospital-acquired infections or higher-risk patients. Table 33-8 outlines the empiric treatment of adults with complicated intra-abdominal infections.

Infectious Diarrhea

Diarrhea is defined as an increase in frequency or liquidity of stool (or both), compared to a patient's normal stool. Infectious diarrhea is typically caused by uncooked food, fecal contamination, or antibiotic use in the case of *Clostridioides difficile*.

TABLE 33-8. Empiric Treatment of Adults with Complicated Intra-abdominal Infections

Type of infection	Treatment
Mild-to-moderately severe community-acquired extra-biliary infections	Single-agent treatment: cefoxitin, ertapenem, moxifloxacin, or tigecycline Combination treatment: **metronidazole** ⚠ plus 1 of the following: cefazolin, cefuroxime, ceftriaxone, cefotaxime, ciprofloxacin, or levofloxacin
High-risk or severe community-acquired extra-biliary infections	Single-agent treatment: imipenem, meropenem, or piperacillin/tazobactam Combination treatment: **metronidazole** plus 1 of the following: cefepime, ceftazidime, ciprofloxacin, or levofloxacin
High-risk community-acquired acute cholecystitis	**Metronidazole** plus 1 of the following: imipenem, meropenem, piperacillin/tazobactam, ciprofloxacin, levofloxacin, or cefepime
Health care–associated biliary infection	**Metronidazole** plus vancomycin plus 1 of the following: imipenem, meropenem, piperacillin/tazobactam, ciprofloxacin, levofloxacin, or cefepime

Solomkin JS, Mazuski JE, Bradley JS, et al., 2010.
Boldface indicates one of top 100 drugs for 2020 by prescription volume.

⚠ **FDA BOXED WARNINGS**

Tigecycline
Increase in all-cause mortality observed in a meta-analysis of phase 3 and 4 clinical trials-reserve for use in patients where alternative treatment is not suitable.

Metronidazole
Shown to be carcinogenic in mice and rats. Reserve use only for indicated conditions.

Causative organisms

Many disease states, drugs, and infectious organisms are associated with diarrhea. *C. difficile* is a common cause of infectious diarrhea and is associated with high mortality.

Clinical presentation

In addition to diarrhea, the patient may present with several of the following symptoms: fever, chills, nausea, vomiting, or abdominal cramping.

Diagnostic criteria

Etiology is usually determined by patient history and physical examination. Patient history should include factors such as immune status, recent travel, food exposure, or antibiotic use. Cultures and tests for toxins or parasites may be performed. Diagnosis of certain infectious organisms, such as those associated with foodborne illness, should be reported to appropriate agencies.

Treatment

Supportive care (hydration, electrolyte replacement, antipyretics, or antiemetics) is often the only treatment needed. Antimotility agents are discouraged because of the potential to cause toxic megacolon, especially in cases of bloody diarrhea, Shiga toxin–producing *E. coli* infections, or *C. difficile* infections. Antibacterial therapy is reserved for severe presentations, patients with risk factors, or patients diagnosed with specific pathogens. Table 33-9 provides an overview of treatments for immunocompetent patients.

TABLE 33-9. Treatment of Common Infectious Diarrhea for Immunocompetent Patients

Organism	Treatment
Clostridioides difficile	Initial episode or first recurrence
	Mild to severe: vancomycin (oral), fidaxomicin
	Severe, complicated: vancomycin (oral) with or without **metronidazole** (I.V.). Rectal vancomycin can be added if the patient has an ileus.
	Second recurrence: Tapered or pulsed vancomycin (oral) or fidaxomicin
Escherichia coli	
Enterotoxigenic, enteropathogenic, enteroinvasive	TMP-SMZ or fluoroquinolone
Enteroaggregative	Antimicrobial treatment not defined; can consider fluoroquinolone
Shiga toxin–producing *E. coli*	Generally supportive care only
Giardia	**Metronidazole**
Non-*typhi* species of *Salmonella*	Generally supportive care only
	Treatment if indicated: TMP-SMZ, fluoroquinolone, or ceftriaxone
Shigella spp.	TMP-SMZ, fluoroquinolone, ceftriaxone, or **azithromycin**
Vibrio cholera	Doxycycline, tetracycline, or fluoroquinolone
Yersinia spp.	Generally supportive care only

Cohen SH, Gerding DN, Johnson S, et al., 2010; Guerrant RL, Van Gilder T, Steiner TS, et al., 2001.
Boldface indicates one of top 100 drugs for 2020 by prescription volume.
I.V., intravenous; TMP-SMZ, trimethoprim-sulfamethoxazole.

Skin and Soft Tissue Infections

Bacterial infections of the skin and soft tissue can result in a variety of conditions. This chapter covers the following: impetigo, erysipelas, cellulitis, necrotizing infections, and infections caused by human or animal bites.

Causative organisms

Skin and soft tissue infections (SSTIs) are caused by a variety of organisms, but are mostly caused by streptococci and staphylococci. Staphylococcal skin infections, such as MRSA, are often characterized as abscess- or pus-forming, whereas streptococcal infections are nonpurulent. Necrotizing infections, such as gas gangrene, are often polymicrobial and include gram-positive, gram-negative, and anaerobic bacteria. Animal or human bites typically include mouth flora, such as *Eikenella* spp., *Pasturella* spp., and *Bartonella* spp., or other gram-positive organisms.

Clinical presentation

SSTIs are usually characterized by erythema and edema of the skin. More serious infections can result in systemic symptoms, such as fever, tachycardia, or hypotension. Table 33-10 describes signs and symptoms of selected SSTIs.

Diagnostic criteria

For mild infections, diagnosis is usually made by physical examination. Blood or biopsy cultures and surgical intervention may be necessary in patients with severe infections.

TABLE 33-10. Clinical Presentation of Selected Skin and Soft Tissue Infections

Infection	Signs and symptoms
Impetigo	Single or multiple localized, purulent lesions usually occurring on the head or extremities
Cellulitis	Progressive erythema and edema without raised demarcations; involvement extends into the deeper dermis and subcutaneous fat
Necrotizing infections	Rapidly progressive infection with systemic manifestations; skin necrosis and bullae may be present; involvement may extend into the fascia or muscle
Clostridial myonecrosis (gas gangrene)	Bronze or reddish-purple skin with systemic manifestations; crepitant tissue resulting from gas

Stevens DL, Bisno AL, Chambers HF, et al., 2014.

Treatment

Treatment is based on the type and severity of infection. Treatment is often empiric unless surgical cultures are obtained. Antistaphylococcal beta lactams, trimethoprim-sulfamethoxazole, clindamycin, or tetracyclines are typically used based on severity of illness. Because of the expanding incidence of MRSA, the need for empiric coverage of MRSA in SSTIs is increasing. MRSA should be considered in patients with purulent abscesses or who are unresponsive to initial therapies lacking MRSA coverage. In patients with a necrotizing infection, surgical intervention is often required in combination with antibiotic therapy that has gram-positive, gram-negative, and anaerobic activity. For human and animal bites, amoxicillin/clavulanate is often used.

Urinary Tract Infection

Urinary tract infections (UTIs) represent a wide variety of clinical syndromes, including urethritis, cystitis, prostatitis, and pyelonephritis. UTIs can result from urogenital abnormalities, lack of postcoital voiding, or improper catheter use, among others.

Causative organisms

The most common bacteria are enteric gram-negative bacilli (*E. coli*) and enterococci. Hospitalized, catheterized patients also may acquire *P. aeruginosa* or other resistant gram-negative bacilli.

Clinical presentation

Lower UTIs tend to present with dysuria, urinary urgency, polyuria, nocturia, and suprapubic heaviness or pain. Fever is rare in patients with lower UTIs. Upper UTIs, such as pyelonephritis, tend to present with flank pain and fever.

Diagnostic criteria

Diagnosis of UTIs is based on the presence of urinary or systemic symptoms, the presence of microorganisms in significant numbers, and the presence of WBCs in the urine sample. In general, higher numbers of organisms ($>10^5$ cells/mL) are needed to diagnose UTIs in females compared to males ($>10^3$ cells/mL) because more organisms can ascend the shorter female urethra.

Treatment

A variety of antibiotics may be useful for the treatment of UTIs (Table 33-11).

Fluoroquinolones are especially useful for the treatment of prostatitis resulting from high prostatic fluid concentrations. Length of therapy varies according to the severity of disease.

TABLE 33-11. Treatment of Urinary Tract Infections

Diagnosis	Organisms	Preferred treatments	Alternative treatment
Acute uncomplicated cystitis	Escherichia coli, Staphylococcus saprophyticus	TMP-SMZ × 3 days or nitrofurantoin × 5 days	Fluoroquinolone × 3 days or beta lactam × 3 to 7 days
Acute pyelonephritis	E. coli, Proteus mirabilis, Klebsiella pneumoniae, Enterococcus spp.	Fluoroquinolone × 7 days or TMP-SMZ × 14 days; if severe, can consider parenteral therapy with fluoroquinolone or broad-spectrum beta lactam or aminoglycoside	Broad-spectrum beta lactam plus aminoglycoside
Catheter-associated UTI	Coagulase-negative staphylococci, enteric gram-negative bacilli (E. coli), Pseudomonas aeruginosa	Broad-spectrum beta lactam or fluoroquinolone × 7 to 14 days based on resolution of symptoms Selection of regimen based on severity of infection and local bacterial susceptibility	Broad-spectrum beta lactam or fluoroquinolone plus additional gram-positive or gram-negative coverage if severe infection or suspicion of resistant pathogen
Prostatitis	E. coli, Proteus spp., K. pneumoniae	Quinolone × 4 to 6 weeks or TMP-SMZ × 4 to 6 weeks	

TMP-SMZ, trimethoprim-sulfamethoxazole; aminoglycoside: amikacin, tobramycin, or gentamicin; fluoroquinolone: ciprofloxacin, levofloxacin; carbapenem: ertapenem, imipenem/cilastatin, meropenem; beta lactam: amoxicillin/clavulanate, cefdinir, cefaclor, cefpodoxime; broad-spectrum beta lactam: piperacillin/tazobactam, cefepime, ceftazidime, aztreonam, or a carbapenem; gram-positive coverage: vancomycin, daptomycin, linezolid; gram-negative coverage: gentamicin, tobramycin, amikacin.

Bacterial Sexually Transmitted Infections (Chlamydia, Gonorrhea, and Syphilis)

Sexually transmitted diseases are diseases that can be transmitted via sexual intercourse. This section covers chlamydia, gonorrhea, and syphilis. Patients testing positive for any sexually transmitted disease should be screened for the presence of other venereal diseases. In addition, all sexual partners should be screened and treated if indicated.

Chlamydia

Chlamydia is caused by the bacterium *Chlamydia trachomatis*.

Clinical presentation

The majority of patients present asymptomatic, but men and women can present with discharge, dysuria, or abdominal pain. Chlamydia can result in serious complications in women if untreated, such as pelvic inflammatory disease, ectopic pregnancy, or infertility.

Diagnostic criteria

Chlamydia can be diagnosed by nucleic acid tests of a specimen swab obtained from the site of potential contact (endocervix, vagina, urethra, or rectum) or by testing urine.

Treatment

The recommended treatment of chlamydia is **azithromycin** 1 g orally for 1 dose. Alternatively, doxycycline 100 mg orally twice daily for 7 days is effective. Additional recommendations are available for pregnant women, infants, and children per CDC guidelines.

Gonorrhea

Gonorrhea is caused by the gram-negative cocci *Neisseria gonorrhoeae*.

Clinical presentation

Although patients with gonorrhea can be asymptomatic, gonorrheal infections may cause dysuria, penile discharge, or testicular pain in men. Women may experience dysuria, vaginal discharge, or vaginal bleeding. Women are also at risk of developing pelvic inflammatory disease, which can result in future infertility.

Diagnostic criteria

In symptomatic men, gonorrhea can be diagnosed by a Gram stain of a urethral swab; however, negative results in asymptomatic men are not sufficient to exclude an infection. In women and asymptomatic men, methods of diagnosis include cultures of specimen swabs and nucleic acid tests.

Treatment

N. gonorrhoeae has developed significant resistance to penicillins and fluoroquinolones; therefore, these agents are no longer recommended, leaving cephalosporins as the preferred treatment modality. Because of the high rate of comorbid chlamydia infections, patients diagnosed with gonorrhea should also receive therapy against chlamydia: **Zithromax (azithromycin)** 1 g orally once or doxycycline 100 mg orally twice daily for 7 days.

Syphilis

Syphilis is an infection caused by the spirochete *Treponema pallidum*.

Clinical presentation

Syphilis infections are classified into the following stages: primary, secondary, latent, and tertiary. Primary syphilis presents as a single lesion (chancre) or multiple lesions appearing at the site of infection. If not treated, primary syphilis progresses into secondary syphilis, characterized by a variety of rashes and flu-like symptoms. Untreated patients develop latent syphilis. Patients with latent syphilis lack signs or symptoms of syphilis, but the disease can progress further to tertiary syphilis. Symptoms of this stage include general paresis, deafness, progressive dementia, or aortic insufficiency.

Diagnostic criteria

Darkfield tests provide a definitive diagnosis of early syphilis. A variety of serologic tests are also available to aid diagnosis; however, more than 1 type of serologic test should be performed because of the limitations of these tests. Patients exhibiting any signs or symptoms of neurologic or ophthalmic involvement should have additional screening, including CSF analysis.

Treatment

Parenteral penicillin G is the treatment of choice for each stage of syphilis. Treatment guidelines describe the preparation, dosage, and duration of treatment based on the syphilis stage, as well as recommendations for children, patients with HIV, or pregnant patients.

Tickborne Systemic Febrile Syndromes

Tickborne illnesses are similar in transmission and natural history. The organisms responsible for these infections vary geographically, and serologic tests are used for diagnosis. The most common tick-borne illnesses are Lyme disease (caused by *Borrelia burgdorferi*), Rocky Mountain spotted fever (*Rickettsia rickettsia*), and ehrlichiosis (*Ehrlichia phagocytophila*). Patients present with a fever, specific rashes (bulls-eye or diffuse facial rash), and flu-like symptoms, as well as a history of tick exposure.

Treatment

The drug of choice in most tick-borne diseases is doxycycline. Additional considerations can be made for patients with tetracycline allergies or for pregnant patients.

Systemic Fungal Infections

Fungal infections fall into 2 categories: *primary* (able to cause infection in all patients) and *opportunistic* (able to cause infection only in immunocompromised patients). Fungal infections affect a variety of organ systems including the skin, central nervous system, pulmonary system, and gastrointestinal tract. The incidence of fungal infection is rising as a result of increased use of antibacterial agents and the increase in the number of immunocompromised patients.

Clinical presentation

Fungal infections can present in a variety of fashions but typically have a gradual onset with general malaise, fever, and weakness that are unrelieved by antibacterial therapy. Pulmonary infections can present with pneumonia-like symptoms or with asthma-like symptoms if bronchoallergic disease is present.

Diagnostic criteria

Diagnosis is made from patient history, cultures from infected fluids or tissues, and serologic tests.

Treatment

Treatment is based on the severity of the disease and often is empiric until the organism is isolated (Table 33-12). The duration of antifungal therapy is determined by the type of fungal infection, the site and severity of infection, and the immune status of the host. Because of the relatively slow growth of most fungi and the lack of commercial testing against antifungal agents, patient response is used to determine resistance to therapy.

TABLE 33-12. Treatment of Invasive Fungal Infections

Organism	Disease	Severity	Preferred treatment
Aspergillus spp.	Invasive pulmonary disease	Severe disease	Voriconazole
Blastomyces dermatitidis	Cutaneous, pulmonary, or extrapulmonary disease	Severe disease	L-AmB × 1 to 2 weeks, then itraconazole ⚠
		Mild disease	Itraconazole
Candida spp.	Bloodstream infection	Severe disease	Echinocandin, fluconazole, voriconazole
		Moderate disease	Fluconazole, echinocandin
Coccidioides immitis	Primary pulmonary disease	Severe disease	Fluconazole, itraconazole
Cryptococcus neoformans	Meningitis	Moderate disease	Fluconazole
		Immunocompromised	AmB ⚠ or L-AmB + flucytosine ⚠
		Immunocompetent	AmB or L-AmB + flucytosine
Histoplasma capsulatum	Pulmonary, disseminated, or localized	Severe disease	L-AmB × 2 weeks, then itraconazole
		Moderate disease	Itraconazole

AmB, amphotericin B; L-AmB, liposomal amphotericin B.

FDA BOXED WARNINGS

Itraconazole
May cause or exacerbate congestive heart failure (CHF). Do not administer for treatment of onychomycosis in patients with evidence of ventricular dysfunction. Significant number of drug–drug interactions and contraindications—see package insert for full list.

Amphotericin B
Only use in patients with progressive and potentially life-threatening fungal infections-should not be used to treat noninvasive fungal infections. Should not be given in doses greater than 1.5 mg/kg.

Flucytosine
Use with extreme caution in patients with renal impairment. Requires close monitoring of hematologic, renal, and hepatic status.

Viral Infections (Hepatitis, Influenza, and the Herpes Simplex Family)

Hepatitis

Hepatitis is a general term referring to a generalized inflammation of the liver. Five viruses (hepatitis types A-E) have been identified as causative agents for hepatitis and are commonly transmitted via injection drug use or fecal-oral contamination. Syndromes may be either acute or chronic.

Clinical presentation

Patients present with a history of anorexia, nausea, fatigue, and malaise that usually progresses to fever, right-upper-quadrant pain, dark urine, light-colored stools, and worsening of systemic symptoms. Some patients have no symptoms and little hepatic damage. In addition to physical signs, laboratory tests are remarkable for elevations in aspartate aminotransferase (AST), alanine aminotransferase (ALT), and serum bilirubin.

Diagnostic criteria

Additional laboratory antigen and antibody testing can be performed to diagnose and guide treatment of patients with hepatitis B and C. Genotyping is also required to guide treatment of hepatitis C. There are 6 major genotypes, which are identified as genotypes 1 to 6; hepatitis C genotype 1 is most common in the United States.

Treatment

Treatment of hepatitis depends on the viral strain and type of presentation. The decision to initiate treatment in patients with chronic hepatitis B depends on evaluation of factors such as hepatitis B surface antigen, hepatitis B e antigen, hepatitis B DNA levels, liver function tests, patient age, and liver biopsy results. In general, the first-line agents for chronic hepatitis B treatment are Baraclude (entecavir) ⚠ or Viread (tenofovir disoproxil fumarate) ⚠ or Temly (tenofovir alafenamide) ⚠. Other treatments include Epivir (lamivudine) ⚠, Hepsera (adefovir) ⚠, Tyzeka (telbivudine) ⚠, and Emtriva (emtricitabine) ⚠.

For patients with acute symptomatic hepatitis B, treatment is usually not indicated unless the patient has fulminant or prolonged, severe acute hepatitis. In these patients, treatment with peginterferon (Peg-IFN) ⚠, tenofovir, or entecavir is recommended.

Standard therapy and duration of treatment for chronic hepatitis C is based on genotype. Table 33-13 includes therapy for the most common hepatitis C genotype 1a and 1b. Treatment may require modifications in special patient populations, including patients with renal disease, HIV, or cirrhosis.

FDA BOXED WARNINGS

Baraclude (entencavir)
Risk of severe acute exacerbations of hepatitis B in patients who discontinue treatment-continue to monitor hepatic function for several months after treatment. Patients who have HIV/HBV coinfections should also be receiving anti-retroviral therapy for HIV (entecavir alone could promote resistance to nucleoside reverse transcriptase inhibitors). Risk of lactic acidosis and severe hepatomegaly with steatosis.

Viread (tenofovir disoproxil fumarate)
Risk of severe acute exacerbations of hepatitis B in patients who discontinue treatment-continue to monitor hepatic function for several months after treatment.

Temly (tenofovir alafenamide)
Risk of severe acute exacerbations of hepatitis B in patients who discontinue treatment-continue to monitor hepatic function for several months after treatment.

Epivir (lamivudine)
Risk of severe acute exacerbations of hepatitis B in patients who discontinue treatment-continue to monitor hepatic function for several months after treatment. Risk of HIV-1 resistance if used in patients with unrecognized or untreated HIV-1. Important to note that HIV-1 and HBV formulations have different doses and should not be interchanged.

Hepsera (adefovir)
Risk of severe acute exacerbations of hepatitis B in patients who discontinue treatment-continue to monitor hepatic function for several months after treatment. Risk of HIV-1 resistance if used in patients with unrecognized or untreated HIV-1. Risk of nephrotoxicity, lactic acidosis and severe hepatomegaly with steatosis.

Tyzeka (telbivudine)
Risk of severe acute exacerbations of hepatitis B in patients who discontinue treatment-continue to monitor hepatic function for several months after treatment.

Emtriva (emtricitabine)
Risk of severe acute exacerbations of hepatitis B in patients who discontinue treatment-continue to monitor hepatic function for several months after treatment.

Peginterferon (Peg-IFN)
May cause or aggravate fatal or life-threatening neuropsychiatric, autoimmune, ischemic, and infectious disorders.

TABLE 33-13. Treatment of Chronic Hepatitis C, Genotype 1a/b

Treatment	Standard duration
Zepatier (elbasvir 50 mg/grazoprevir 100 mg) ⚠ cannot have baseline NS5A RAVs for elbasvir	12 weeks (can be used in compensated cirrhosis)
Harvoni (ledipasvir 90 mg/sofosbuvir 400 mg)	12 weeks (can be used in compensated cirrhosis)
Viekira XR Viekira Pak (paritaprevir 150 mg/ritonavir 100 mg/ombitasvir 25 mg + dasabuvir 250 mg) ⚠ and weight-based Rebetol (ribavirin) ⚠	12 weeks
Epclusa (sofosbuvir 400 mg/velpatasvir 100 mg) ⚠	12 weeks (can be used in compensated cirrhosis)
Daklinza (daclatasvir 60 mg + sofosbuvir 400 mg) ⚠	12 weeks

American Association for the Study of Liver Diseases and Infectious Diseases Society of America, 2016.

FDA BOXED WARNINGS

Zepatier (elbasvir/grazoprevir)
Risk of reactivation of hepatitis B-patients should be tested for evidence of current or prior hepatitis B infection before initiation of treatment.

Viekira (paritaprevir/ritonavir/ombitasvir/dasabuvir)
Risk of reactivation of hepatitis B-patients should be tested for evidence of current or prior hepatitis B infection before initiation of treatment.

Rebetol (ribavirin)
Monotherapy is not effective for treatment of chronic hepatitis C virus. Risk of hemolytic anemia which may result in worsening of cardiac disease. Teratogenic and embryocidal effects have been demonstrated in animal species-contraindicated in pregnancy. Due to long half-life, pregnancy should be avoided for at least 6 months after completion of treatment.

Epclusa (sofosbuvir/velpatasvir)
Risk of reactivation of hepatitis B-patients should be tested for evidence of current or prior hepatitis B infection before initiation of treatment.

Daklinza (daclatasvir + sofosbuvir)
Risk of reactivation of hepatitis B-patients should be tested for evidence of current or prior hepatitis B infection before initiation of treatment.

Influenza

Influenza is a seasonal acute respiratory viral infection. Three viruses, influenza A, B, and C, are responsible for most infections.

Clinical presentation

Patients may present with a sudden onset of chills, fever, fatigue, headache, muscle aches, or cough. The primary viral infection may be followed by secondary bacterial infections.

Diagnostic criteria

Diagnosis is based on patient physical signs and symptoms. Rapid influenza diagnostic tests (RIDTs) are also available. RIDTs have a high specificity but low sensitivity; therefore, a negative result should not prevent treatment in patients with suspected influenza infection.

Treatment

Both prophylactic and treatment therapies are available and most commonly include oseltamivir. Exact therapies are determined by the viral strain present in the community. The CDC provides yearly recommendations concerning antiviral treatments based on current circulating strains. Recent circulating influenza A strains have demonstrated marked resistance to adamantanes; therefore, Symmetrel (amantadine) and Flumadine (rimantadine) are currently not recommended. Therapy should be initiated as soon as possible after symptoms develop, preferably within 48 hours of symptom onset.

Herpes family (herpes simplex and herpes zoster)

The herpes virus family is responsible for a variety of viral infections, including genital herpes simplex infections and varicella zoster infections (shingles).

Clinical presentation

Clinical presentation varies by disease.

- **Genital herpes simplex:** Patients with an initial genital herpes infection can present with flu-like symptoms including fever, headache, malaise, and myalgias in addition to development of painful lesions on the external genitalia. Recurrent infections may be preceded by a prodrome of tingling, dysesthesia, or numbness followed by the development of lesions. Infected patients may also be asymptomatic.
- **Varicella zoster:** Varicella zoster presents as a painful, pustular rash located on 1 or 2 dermatomes. The affected area may remain painful after the rash has resolved. Severe complications include ophthalmic manifestations and infections.

Diagnostic criteria

Diagnosis is based mostly on signs and symptoms, although additional testing may be performed.

- **Genital herpes simplex:** Virologic tests (cell culture and polymerase chain reaction [PCR]) and type-specific serologic tests for antibodies are available to diagnose genital herpes simplex and identify the type of infection. Two types of herpes simplex virus cause genital herpes: HSV-1 and HSV-2. HSV-1 also causes oral herpes infections.
- **Varicella zoster:** Diagnosis is typically based on patient signs and symptoms, but PCR, antibody staining, and serologic tests can also be used.

Treatment

Treatment depends on the type of herpes virus and disease state.

- **Genital herpes simplex:** Zovirax (acyclovir), Famvir (famciclovir), and Valtrex (valacyclovir) are approved for the treatment of genital herpes simplex viral infections; however, antiviral treatment does not eradicate the virus. Treatment can be prescribed for initial and recurrent episodes or for suppressive therapy.
- **Varicella zoster:** Acyclovir, valacyclovir, and famciclovir can be prescribed to decrease the duration and severity of varicella zoster infections.

33-5 Pharmacist's Role

Pharmacists are the key players of antimicrobial stewardship programs (ASPs) that help regulate antimicrobial use in the hospital and outpatient settings. Specifically, ASP pharmacists develop guidelines and pathways for appropriate antimicrobial selection given hospital or clinic susceptibility data (antibiogram) and drug formulary considerations. Ultimately, these documents are for end-users (physicians and other prescribers) to make smarter antimicrobial decisions.

NAPLEX Competency Statements

The questions in this chapter cover the following 2021 NAPLEX Competency Statements: **AREA 1:** 1.1; 1.2; 1.3; 1.4; 1.5; 1.6; 1.7 **AREA 2:** 2.1; 2.2; 2.4 **AREA 3:** 3.1; 3.2; 3.4; 3.5; 3.6; 3.7; 3.8; 3.9; 3.10; 3.11 **AREA 6:** 6.3.

33-6   Questions

1. The lowest concentration of anti-infective that prevents microbial growth is called the _____.

   A. minimum bactericidal concentration
   B. minimum bacteriostatic concentration
   C. minimum inhibitory concentration
   D. minimum inhibiting concentration
   E. minimum Schillings concentration

2. B. B. is a 52-year-old female with a past medical history of asthma. She presents to the walk-in clinic at a local pharmacy with complaints of cough, shortness of breath, fever, chills, and body aches for the past 24 hours. The local health department has reported a recent increase in influenza A in the region. What treatment should B. B. receive?

   A. Symptomatic management only with instructions to go to the emergency department if symptoms worsen.
   B. Symmetrel 100 mg twice daily for 5 days
   C. Tamiflu 75 mg twice daily for 5 days
   D. Flumadine 100 mg twice daily for 7 days
   E. Avelox 400 mg daily for 7 days

3. The hallmark of empiric therapy is _____.

   A. coverage of the most common pathogen associated with the infection
   B. coverage of the common pathogens associated with the infection
   C. coverage of all possible pathogens associated with the infection
   D. coverage of polymicrobial pathogens associated with the infection
   E. coverage of all viral organisms associated with the infection

4. Analysis of cerebrospinal fluid may give valuable clues to the identity of the pathogen in meningitis. Which of the following changes would be indicative of a bacterial infection?

   A. Increased WBCs, increased glucose, increased protein
   B. Increased WBCs, decreased glucose, increased protein
   C. Increased RBCs, decreased glucose, decreased protein
   D. Increased RBCs, increased glucose, increased protein
   E. A, B, and C

5. Empiric therapy for meningitis for patients up to 1 month of age includes _____.

   A. Vancomycin and ampicillin
   B. Aminoglycoside and ampicillin
   C. Ceftriaxone and vancomycin
   D. Vancomycin and aminoglycoside
   E. Ampicillin and ceftriaxone

6. C. F. is a 65-year-old male diagnosed with endocarditis. Blood cultures reveal a highly sensitive strain of *Streptococcus*. Which of the following is most appropriate if C. F. has an anaphylactoid penicillin allergy?

   A. Vancomycin
   B. Gentamicin
   C. Ceftriaxone and gentamicin
   D. Meropenem
   E. Rifampin and gentamicin

7. Which of following antibiotics should be used in a high-risk febrile neutropenia patient?

   A. Ceftriaxone
   B. Ertapenem
   C. Cefepime
   D. Vancomycin
   E. Moxifloxacin

8. Patients presenting with acute bronchitis without risk factors should be treated empirically with _____.

   A. Supportive care
   B. Clarithromycin
   C. Cefuroxime
   D. Ciprofloxacin
   E. Erythromycin

9. The most common organisms associated with CAP in adults treated as outpatients are _____.

   A. *Pseudomonas aeruginosa*, *Mycoplasma pneumoniae*, and *Haemophilus influenzae*
   B. *Streptococcus pneumoniae*, *Haemophilus influenzae*, and *Klebsiella pneumoniae*
   C. *Mycoplasma pneumoniae*, *Streptococcus pneumoniae*, *Haemophilus influenzae*, and *Klebsiella pneumoniae*
   D. *Mycoplasma pneumoniae*, *Streptococcus pneumoniae*, *Haemophilus influenzae*, and *Chlamydophila pneumoniae*
   E. *Mycoplasma pneumoniae*, *Streptococcus pneumoniae*, *Haemophilus influenzae*, and *Pseudomonas aeruginosa*

10. Which of the following is an appropriate regimen for a patient with HAP without risk factors for methicillin-resistant *Staphylococcus aureus*?

A. Doxycycline
B. Azithromycin
C. Piperacillin/tazobactam
D. Ciprofloxacin and vancomycin
E. Cefepime, ciprofloxacin, and vancomycin

11. Initial treatment of active tuberculosis infections in which no resistant strains of *Mycobacterium tuberculosis* are suspected should include _____.

A. Rifabutin and pyrazinamide
B. Rifampin and pyrazinamide
C. Ethambutol, rifampin, isoniazid, and pyrazinamide
D. Isoniazid, rifabutin, and pyrazinamide
E. Ethambutol and rifampin

12. The use of antimotility agents in a patient with suspected *Clostridium difficile* infection is _____.

A. Discouraged because of the potential to cause toxic megacolon
B. Encouraged because of increased cure rates
C. Discouraged because of increased reinfections
D. Encouraged because of decreased reinfections
E. Discouraged because of lack of efficacy

13. Which of the following is most likely to cause cellulitis?

A. *Candida albicans*
B. *Streptococcus* species
C. *Shigella boydii*
D. *Escherichia coli*
E. *Klebsiella pneumoniae*

14. The best empiric regimen to treat a prostate infection is _____.

A. Ciprofloxacin for 10 days
B. TMP-SMZ for 10 days
C. Ciprofloxacin and TMP-SMZ for 10 days
D. Ciprofloxacin for 4 to 6 weeks
E. Amoxicillin for 4 to 6 weeks

15. In adults, syphilis should be treated with _____.

A. Benzathine penicillin G
B. Azithromycin
C. Ceftriaxone
D. Ertapenem
E. Doxycycline

16. *Candida albicans* infections of mild-to-moderate severity may be treated with _____.

A. Fluconazole
B. Amphotericin B
C. Voriconazole
D. Caspofungin
E. Ketoconazole

17. The antiviral agent(s) with the best spectrum of activity against recent influenza A strains is _____.

A. Acyclovir
B. Rimantadine
C. Amantadine
D. Oseltamivir and zanamivir
E. Lamivudine and adefovir

18. Which of the following agents can be used to treat genital herpes simplex infections?

A. Valacyclovir
B. Rimantadine
C. Amantadine
D. Oseltamivir
E. Ritonavir

19. Which of the following is appropriate empiric treatment for a patient with a suspected tickborne illness?

A. Doxycycline
B. Azithromycin
C. Piperacillin/tazobactam
D. Ciprofloxacin and metronidazole
E. Chloramphenicol

20. Which of the following is the treatment of choice for an initial, mild *Clostridium difficile* infection?

A. Metronidazole I.V.
B. Metronidazole oral
C. Vancomycin I.V.
D. Vancomycin oral
E. Metronidazole I.V. and vancomycin oral

21. What is the recommended treatment for uncomplicated gonorrhea?

A. Ceftriaxone 125 mg I.M. once
B. Ceftriaxone 250 mg I.M. once plus azithromycin 1 g oral once
C. Gemifloxacin 320 mg oral once
D. Ceftriaxone 1 g I.M. or I.V. every 24 hours until improvement, then cefixime 400 mg oral twice daily to complete a total of at least 7 days of treatment
E. Treatment is not necessary in patients with uncomplicated gonorrhea.

22. Because J. B. has gonorrhea, she should also receive treatment for _____.

- **A.** Syphilis
- **B.** HIV
- **C.** Hepatitis
- **D.** Genital herpes
- **E.** Chlamydia

23. L. B. is a 45-year-old White female presenting to the emergency department with a fever of 103°F, flank pain, dysuria, urinary urgency, and frequency. Her laboratory tests are significant for an increased WBC count of 18,000 cells/mm³ and 3% immature forms (bands). Her urinalysis revealed >10⁵ cells/mL of gram-negative rods. What infection does L. B. have?

- **A.** Herpes simplex
- **B.** Gonorrhea
- **C.** Syphilis
- **D.** Urinary tract infection
- **E.** Food poisoning

24. What therapy is recommended for treatment of pyelonephritis severe enough to warrant hospitalization?

- **A.** Oral quinolone
- **B.** I.V. quinolone
- **C.** Oral penicillin
- **D.** I.V. carbapenem
- **E.** I.V. vancomycin

25. R. H. is a 45-year-old male recently diagnosed with hepatitis C. Genotyping reveals R. H. is infected with hepatitis C, genotype 1b. His health care provider decides to initiate treatment and asks you to select an appropriate treatment regimen. Which of the following could you recommend?

- **A.** Acyclovir 500 mg with lamivudine 150 mg daily for 10 weeks
- **B.** Ledipasvir 90 mg/sofosbuvir 400 mg for 12 weeks
- **C.** Entecavir 1 mg daily for 8 weeks
- **D.** Sofosbuvir 400 mg with ribavirin 600 mg daily for 10 weeks
- **E.** Tenofovir 300 mg daily with Peg-INF daily for 12 weeks

 **33-7**   **Answers**

1. C. The minimum inhibitory concentration determines the level of anti-infective to which dosing regimens may be set.

2. C. Tamiflu 75 mg twice daily started within 48 hours of symptom onset is recommended by current guidelines. Response A is incorrect because B. B. has a clinical diagnosis of influenza and symptoms began less than 48 hours ago. Responses B and D are both used to treat influenza; however, current guidelines recommend against use owing to increased resistance. Response E, Avelox, is an antibacterial antibiotic with no activity against the influenza virus.

3. B. Coverage of common pathogens associated with the infection increases the probability of curing the infection without increasing anti-infective exposure to other organisms, which increases the possibility of resistance.

4. B. Bacterial meningitis infections show an increase in WBCs and protein in the CSF, whereas CSF glucose is decreased.

5. B. This regimen covers the most likely organisms for meningitis in this age group: *S. agalactiae*, *E. coli*, and *L. monocytogenes* and *Klebsiella* species. Ampicillin and cefotaxime would be another appropriate choice for empiric therapy in patients up to 1 month of age.

6. A. Vancomycin is appropriate for penicillin-allergic patients with endocarditis caused by *Streptococcus* species. Other regimens for streptococci include penicillin or ceftriaxone (with or without gentamicin), which has a potential for cross-reactivity in patients with penicillin allergies.

7. C. High-risk patients with febrile neutropenia are at greatest risk for invasive *P. aeruginosa* infections. Cefepime is the only drug listed that has antipseudomonal activity. MRSA therapy should only be considered under certain circumstances (skin or line infections).

8. A. Because half of bronchitis infections have a viral etiology, antibacterial therapy for low-risk patients should not be attempted, with the exception of severe presentation.

9. D. *P. aeruginosa* is more likely in patients with risk factors for multidrug-resistant bacteria such as late-onset HAP or VAP. *K. pneumoniae* is also not commonly associated with CAP.

10. C. Empiric therapy for HAP without risk factors for methicillin-resistant *S. aureus* is as follows: piperacillin/tazobactam, cefepime, imipenem, meropenem, or levofloxacin. Doxycycline or azithromycin is appropriate for outpatient treatment of CAP. Cefepime, ciprofloxacin, and vancomycin in combination are appropriate for HAP in patients with risk factors for methicillin-resistant *S. aureus*.

11. C. The preferred treatment for active tuberculosis infections is a 4-drug regimen consisting of ethambutol, rifampin, isoniazid, and pyrazinamide for the initial 2 months, followed by rifampin with isoniazid for 4 additional months.

12. A. Use of antimotility agents in *C. difficile* infections increases the risk of toxic megacolon.

13. B. Most cellulitis infections are associated with *Streptococcus* species.

14. D. Prostate infections are difficult to treat, requiring 4 to 6 weeks of therapy. Although TMP-SMZ is a reasonable choice for treating most prostate infections, a duration of 10 days is not adequate; ciprofloxacin is preferred because of its ability to concentrate in prostate fluid.

15. D. Benzathine penicillin G is standard therapy for either late latent syphilis or tertiary syphilis. Single-dose benzathine penicillin (2.4 million units) is appropriate for primary, secondary, or early latent syphilis. Doxycycline should only be used in severe penicillin allergies and not in neurosyphilis.

16. A. Fluconazole is the preferred treatment for mild-to-moderate infections caused by *C. albicans*. Amphotericin B, voriconazole, and caspofungin are active against *Candida* but should be reserved for more severe infections or less susceptible *Candida* species. Ketoconazole is not a preferred treatment for *Candida* infections.

17. D. Recent influenza A strains have demonstrated marked resistance to amantadine and rimantadine; therefore, these agents are not currently recommended. Acyclovir, lamivudine, and adefovir are not active against influenza.

18. A. Acyclovir, famciclovir, and valacyclovir are approved for the treatment of genital herpes. All other answers are antiviral agents used in the treatment or prevention of viral infections other than herpes.

19. A. Doxycycline is recommended as primary treatment of almost all tickborne illnesses. Azithromycin and chloramphenicol are alternative treatments for specific tickborne diseases but are not first line.

20. D. Oral vancomycin is the treatment of choice for an initial, mild-to-moderate episode of *C. difficile*. An initial episode that is severe and complicated should be treated with oral vancomycin with or without metronidazole I.V. Vancomycin I.V. is inappropriate for a *C. difficile* infection.

21. B. Response A is not the appropriate dose of ceftriaxone in an adult. Response C is incorrect owing to increased resistance to fluoroquinolones. Response D is the treatment for disseminated gonococcal infections. Response E is incorrect because all cases of gonorrhea require treatment.

22. E. Because of the high rate of comorbid chlamydia infections, patients diagnosed with gonorrhea should also receive therapy against chlamydia: azithromycin 1 g orally once or doxycycline 100 mg orally twice daily for 7 days.

23. D. Given the clinical presentation and laboratory test results, L. B. has a severe UTI. The presence of systemic symptoms (fever and chills) suggests an upper UTI or pyelonephritis.

24. B. Given the severity of disease, parenteral therapy would be reasonable for initial therapy. Because the Gram stain of the urine revealed gram-negative rods, either a quinolone or an extended-spectrum beta lactam would be reasonable empiric therapy until the organism is identified and sensitivities obtained. A carbapenem would be adequate but should be reserved for infections when multidrug-resistant pathogens are suspected.

25. B. Response B is the recommended treatment for hepatitis C, genotype 1b. Responses A, C, D, and E are incorrect because they are either hepatitis B antivirals or are incorrect hepatitis C virus regimens.

33-8 Additional Resources

American Association for the Study of Liver Diseases and Infectious Diseases Society of America. Recommendations for testing, managing, and treating hepatitis C. http://www.hcvguidelines.org. Accessed June 2020.

Baddour LM, Wilson WR, Bayer AS, et al. Infective endocarditis in adults: diagnosis, antimicrobial therapy, and management of complications. A scientific statement for healthcare professionals from the American Heart Association. *Circulation.* 2015;132:1435–1486.

Centers for Disease Control and Prevention. Influenza Antiviral Medications: Summary for Clinicians. https://www.cdc.gov/flu/professionals/antivirals/summary-clinicians.htm. Accessed May 2021.

Centers for Disease Control and Prevention. Sexually transmitted diseases treatment guidelines 2015. *MMWR.* 2015;64(3):1–137.

Centers for Disease Control and Prevention. Shingles (herpes zoster) for healthcare professionals. https://www.cdc.gov/shingles/hcp/index.html. Accessed March 14, 2014.

Centers for Disease Control and Prevention. Treatment of tuberculosis, American Thoracic Society, CDC, and Infectious Diseases Society of America. *MMWR.* 2003;52(RR-11):1–74.

Chapman AS, Bakken JS, Folk SM, et al. Diagnosis and management of tickborne Rickettsial diseases: Rocky Mountain spotted fever, ehrlichiosis, and anaplasmosis—United States *MMWR.* 2006;55(RR-04):1–27.

Chapman SW, Dismukes WE, Proia LA, et al. Clinical practice guidelines for the management of blastomycosis: 2008 update by the Infectious Diseases Society of America. *Clin Infect Dis.* 2008;46:1801–1812.

Cohen SH, Gerding DN, Johnson S, et al. Clinical practice guidelines for *Clostridium difficile* infection in adults: 2010 update by the Society for Healthcare Epidemiology of America (SHEA) and the Infectious Diseases Society of America (IDSA). *Infect Control Hosp Epidemiol.* 2010;31(5):431–455.

Dellinger RP, Levy MM, Rhodes A, et al. Surviving Sepsis Campaign: international guidelines for management of severe sepsis and septic shock: 2012. *Crit Care Med.* 2013;41(2):580–637.

Dworkin RH, Johnson RW, Breuer J, et al. Recommendations for the management of herpes zoster. *Clin Infect Dis.* 2007;1(44):S1–S26.

Freifeld AG, Bow EJ, Sepkowitz KA, et al. Clinical practice guideline for the use of antimicrobial agents in neutropenic patients with cancer: 2010 update by the Infectious Diseases Society of America. *Clin Infect Dis.* 2011;52:e56–e93.

Galgiani JN, Ampel NM, Blair JE, et al. 2016 Infectious Diseases Society of America (IDSA) clinical practice guidelines for the treatment of Coccidioidomycosis. *Clin Infect Dis.* 2016;63(6):e112–e146.

Global Initiative for Chronic Obstructive Lung Disease. *Global Strategy for the Diagnosis, Management, and Prevention of Chronic Obstructive Pulmonary Disease.* Updated 2021. http://www.goldcopd.org. Accessed May 2021.

Guerrant RL, Van Gilder T, Steiner TS, et al. Practice guidelines for the management of infectious diarrhea. *Clin Infect Dis.* 2001;32:331–350.

Gupta K, Hooton TM, Naber KG, et al. International clinical practice guidelines for the treatment of acute uncomplicated cystitis and pyelonephritis in women: a 2010 update by the Infectious Diseases Society of America and the European Society for Microbiology and Infectious Diseases. *Clin Infect Dis.* 2011;52:e103–e120.

Hooton TM, Bradley SF, Cardenas DD, et al. Diagnosis, prevention, and treatment of catheter-associated urinary tract infection in adults: 2009 international clinical practice guidelines from the Infectious Diseases Society of America. *Clin Infect Dis.* 2010;50:625–663.

Kalil AC, Metersky ML, Klompas M, et al. Management of adults with hospital-acquired and ventilator-associated pneumonia: 2016 clinical practice guidelines by the Infectious Diseases Society of America and the American Thoracic Society. *Clin Infect Dis.* 2016;63:1–51.

Liu C, Bayer A, Cosgrove SE, et al. Clinical practice guidelines by the Infectious Diseases Society of America for the treatment of methicillin-resistant *Staphylococcus aureus* infections in adults and children. *Clin Infect Dis.* 2011;52:1–38.

Lok ASF, McMahon BJ. Chronic hepatitis B: update 2009. *Hepatology.* 2009;50(3):1–36.

Mandell LA, Wunderink RG, Anzueto A, et al. Infectious Diseases Society of America and the American Thoracic Society consensus guidelines on the management of community-acquired pneumonia in adults. *Clin Infect Dis.* 2007;44:27–72.

Mermel LA, Allon M, Bouza E, et al. Clinical practice guidelines for the diagnosis and management of intravascular catheter-related infection: 2009 update by the Infectious Diseases Society of America. *Clin Infect Dis.* 2009;49:1–45.

Pappas PG, Kauffman CA, Andes D, et al. Clinical practice guidelines for the management of candidiasis: 2016 update by the Infectious Diseases Society of America. *Clin Infect Dis.* 2016;62(4):e1–e50.

Patterson TF, Thompson GR, Denning DW, et al. Practice guidelines for the diagnosis and management of Aspergillosis: 2016 update by the Infectious Diseases Society of America. *Clin Infect Dis.* 2016;doi:10.1093/cid/ciw326.

Perfect JR, Dismukes WE, Dromer F, et al. Clinical practice guidelines for the management of cryptococcal disease: 2010 update by the Infectious Diseases Society of America. *Clin Infect Dis.* 2010;50:291–322.

Solomkin JS, Mazuski JE, Bradley JS, et al. Diagnosis and management of complicated intra-abdominal infection in adults and children: guidelines by the Surgical Infection Society and the Infectious Diseases Society of America. *Clin Infect Dis.* 2010;50:133–164.

Stevens DL, Bisno AL, Chambers HF, et al. Practice guidelines for the diagnosis and management of skin and soft tissue infections: 2014 update by the Infectious Diseases Society of America. *Clin Infect Dis.* 2014;59(2):e10–e52.

Tunkel AR, Hartman BJ, Kaplan SL, et al. Practice guidelines for the management of bacterial meningitis. *Clin Infect Dis.* 2004;39(9):1267–1284.

Wheat LJ, Freifels AG, Kleiman MB, et al. Clinical practice guidelines for the management of patients with histoplasmosis: 2007 update by the Infectious Diseases Society of America. *Clin Infect Dis.* 2007;45(7):807–825.

Anti-infective Agents

MICHAEL P. VEVE

 ## 34-1 KEY POINTS

AMINOGLYCOSIDES

- Aminoglycosides exhibit concentration-dependent bacterial killing, and dosing is tailored using pharmacokinetic drug monitoring.
- Primary uses include adjunct therapy for gram-positive synergy or severe infections with resistant gram-negative bacteria.

BETA-LACTAM ANTIBIOTICS

- Beta-lactam antibiotics exhibit time-dependent bacterial killing.
- First-generation cephalosporins display extensive gram-positive activity, whereas gram-negative activity is progressively enhanced with later generations (up to fourth generation).
- Ceftaroline displays activity against methicillin-resistant *Staphylococcus aureus* (MRSA).
- Beta-lactam/beta-lactamase inhibitors have extended coverage against some resistant gram-positive and gram-negative organisms, as well as anaerobes.
- Carbapenems possess very broad-spectrum activity, including gram-positive, gram-negative, and anaerobic coverage.
- Aztreonam, a monobactam, is active against only aerobic gram-negative bacteria.

GRAM-POSITIVE ANTIBIOTICS

- Vancomycin is primarily used in MRSA infections, and dosing is tailored using pharmacokinetic drug monitoring.
- Daptomycin and linezolid cover MRSA and vancomycin-resistant enterococci (VRE).

FLUOROQUINOLONES

- Fluoroquinolones have broad gram-positive and gram-negative coverage but are associated with several serious, albeit rare, adverse effects.

MACROLIDES

- Macrolides are often used for atypical pneumonia and chlamydial infections.

TETRACYCLINES AND GLYCYLCYCLINES

- Tetracyclines display activity against community-acquired MRSA strains and have reliable atypical coverage.

SULFONAMIDES

- Trimethoprim-sulfamethoxazole displays activity against community-acquired MRSA strains and is commonly used to treat urinary tract infections.

MISCELLANEOUS ANTIBIOTICS

- Clindamycin is an anaerobic antibiotic with activity against community-acquired MRSA.
- **Metronidazole** is active against only anaerobic bacteria, including *Bacteroides fragilis*.
- Fidaxomicin is an alternative to **metronidazole** or oral vancomycin for treatment of recurrent *Clostridium difficile* infection.
- The polymyxins treat severe infections caused by multidrug-resistant gram-negative pathogens but carry significant nephrotoxicity risk.

ANTIFUNGAL AGENTS

- Fluconazole is the drug of choice for *Candida albicans*, and echinocandins are drugs of choice for other resistant *Candida* spp.
- Voriconazole is the drug of choice for treatment of aspergillosis.
- Amphotericin B has activity against the majority of pertinent fungal pathogens, but is associated with several toxicities.
- Azole antifungals are potent inhibitors of hepatic metabolism.

ANTITUBERCULAR AGENTS

- Rifampin, isoniazid, pyrazinamide, and ethambutol (RIPE) are agents of first choice for active tuberculosis infection.
- Isoniazid monotherapy is the preferred treatment for latent tuberculosis infection.

 ## 34-2 STUDY GUIDE CHECKLIST

The following topics may guide your study of this subject area:

- ☐ General antimicrobial spectrum and mechanism of action of anti-infective agents.
- ☐ Agents that cover the bacterial pathogens MRSA and *Pseudomonas aeruginosa*, both of which are associated with antibiotic resistance and poor patient outcomes.
- ☐ Major toxicities associated with anti-infective agents.
- ☐ Antibiotic agents that require pharmacokinetic drug monitoring.
- ☐ Main indications for treatment with anti-infective agents.
- ☐ Drugs of choice for bacterial and fungal pathogens.
- ☐ Identification of major drug–drug interactions.
- ☐ Important patient counseling information for anti-infective agents.

34-3   Antibacterial Targets

There are several targets (Figure 34-1) for antibacterial agents, which can be summarized as the following: cell wall, cell membrane, ribosome, folic acid synthesis, and DNA/RNA inhibition. An understanding of antibacterial agent mechanisms can help clinicians select appropriate therapies.

FIGURE 34-1. Key Bacterial Cell Characteristics

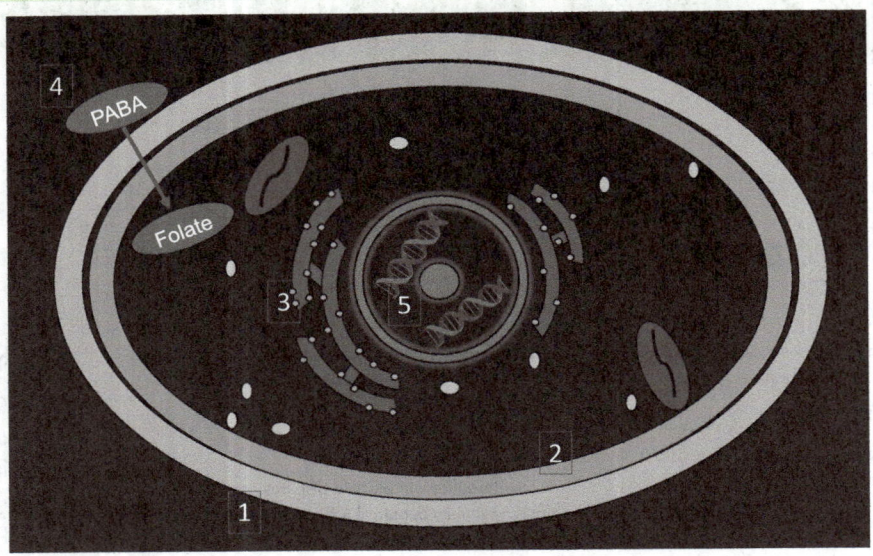

Cell Structure	Function	Antibacterial agent target
1. Cell wall	Provides shape and rigidity to the cell; made up of peptidoglycan	Glycopeptides, beta lactams
2. Cell membrane	Ion transport; cellular life activities	Daptomycin, polymyxins
3. Ribosome	Protein synthesis	Aminoglycosides, clindamycin, macrolides, oxazolidinones, tetracyclines, and glycylcyclines
4. Folic acid synthesis	Biosynthesis of nucleic acids and essential proteins	Trimethoprim-sulfamethoxazole
5. Cell DNA or RNA	Mechanisms for gene expression	Fluoroquinolones, **metronidazole** (anaerobes only), rifampin, fidaxomicin

⚠ **Metronidazole** *FDA BOXED WARNING*

Shown to be carcinogenic in mice and rats. Reserve use only for indicated conditions.

34-4   Aminoglycosides

Aminoglycosides are parental antibiotics that are active against most aerobic gram-negative bacteria, including *P. aeruginosa*, and display synergistic activity for select aerobic gram-positive bacteria such as MRSA and enterococci. They are not effective against anaerobic bacteria. Aminoglycosides are primarily used as adjunct treatment in serious infections due to their significant toxicity. The most commonly used aminoglycosides include amikacin, gentamicin, and tobramycin.

Mechanism of Action

Aminoglycosides inhibit bacterial protein synthesis through binding to the 30S ribosomal subunit, thereby irreversibly inhibiting bacterial ribonucleic acid (RNA) synthesis.

Spectrum of Activity

Amikacin, gentamicin, and tobramycin have a similar spectrum of activity that includes most gram-negative bacteria (Enterobacteriaceae, *P. aeruginosa*) and some gram-positives (not MRSA). They are generally active against more resistant gram-negative bacteria.

Adverse Drug Effects

Nephrotoxicity is demonstrated by an increase in blood urea nitrogen (BUN) and serum creatinine. Nephrotoxicity may occur in 10% to 25% of patients receiving aminoglycosides and is usually reversible on discontinuation of the agent if done promptly. Risk factors include a prolonged duration of therapy, concomitant use of other nephrotoxic agents, and elevated trough concentrations.

Neuromuscular blockade is an uncommon but potentially serious toxicity. Risk factors include the concomitant use of neuromuscular blocking agents and myasthenia gravis.

Ototoxicity includes both auditory and vestibular toxicity. Ototoxicity has been noted at all doses and durations of therapy; therefore, auditory and vestibular monitoring is necessary.

Dosing

Aminoglycosides are dosed on the basis of ideal body weight (IBW) unless the patient is obese. For obese patients, adjusted body weight is used. Traditional and extended interval dosing parameters for amino-glycosides are described in Table 34-1.

TABLE 34-1. Aminoglycosides[a] ⚠

Generic name	Trade name	Dosage forms	Normal dose	Elimination
Amikacin	Amikin	I.V., I.M.	Conventional dosing: 15 mg/kg daily divided every 8 to 12 hours	Renal
			Extended interval: 15 mg/kg every 24 to 72 hours	
Gentamicin	Garamycin	I.V., I.M.	Conventional dosing: 3 to 5 mg/kg daily divided every 8 hours	Renal
			Extended interval: 5 to 7 mg/kg every 24 to 72 hours	
Tobramycin	None	I.V., I.M., INHL	Conventional dosing: 3 to 5 mg/kg daily divided every 8 hours	Renal
			Extended interval: 5 to 7 mg/kg every 24 to 72 hours	
			Nebulized: 300 mg every 12 hours	

I.M., intramuscular; INHL, inhaled; I.V., intravenous.
a. Use ideal or adjusted body weight for all aminoglycoside dosing.

Aminoglycosides *FDA BOXED WARNING*

Close monitoring of serum concentrations, renal function, and toxicities required due to risk of renal toxicity, neurotoxicity, and ototoxicity. Avoid concomitant use of other nephrotoxic and neurotoxic medications. Risk of fetal harm—avoid use in pregnancy.

Extended interval dosing

Extended interval dosing is used to maximize efficacy and minimize nephrotoxicity of aminoglycosides. This strategy uses larger aminoglycoside doses that are typically given every 24, 48, or 72 hours. Use of a larger aminoglycoside dose yields a higher peak concentration than traditional dosing and is thought to maximize the concentration-dependent killing of bacteria, while allowing trough concentrations to fall below detectable levels to reduce toxicity. Aminoglycosides possess a significant postantibiotic effect and maintain efficacy even when concentrations fall below the minimum inhibitory concentration (MIC) of the causative pathogen. With extended interval dosing, peak and trough concentrations are typically obtained to calculate patient-specific pharmacokinetic parameters to assess with dosing frequency. Contraindications to extended interval aminoglycoside dosing include pregnancy, burns, ascites, and creatinine clearance <20 mL/min.

34-5 Penicillins

Mechanism of Action

Penicillins bind to penicillin-binding proteins in the bacterial cell wall, thereby inhibiting peptidoglycan cell wall synthesis and causing cell wall lysis and ultimately cell death.

Penicillins are classified as beta-lactam antibiotics because their chemical structure consists of a beta-lactam ring adjoined to a thiazolidine ring.

Spectrum of Activity and Dosing

The spectrum of activity and dosing for penicillins are listed in Tables 34-2 and 34-3.

Adverse Drug Effects

Penicillin allergies are the most commonly reported antibiotic allergy, but new data suggest that the majority of people with a history of a penicillin allergy can safely receive a beta-lactam antibiotic. True allergic or hypersensitivity reaction occurs in 1% to 10% of patients, and rash or anaphylaxis (0.01% to 0.05% of patients) can occur within 10 to 20 minutes. The potential for allergic reaction cross-reactivity with other beta lactams (cephalosporins, carbapenems, monobactams) is generally low.

Penicillinase-resistant penicillins can cause interstitial nephritis (nephrotoxicity) and increase transaminases.

Neurologic reactions (seizures) can be seen with high doses of penicillin given to patients with renal insufficiency.

Gastrointestinal (GI) effects, including nausea and vomiting, may occur with oral use.

Electrolyte abnormalities (hypo- or hyperkalemia, hypernatremia) may occur depending on the penicillin salt formulation.

Hematologic reactions (thrombocytopenia, neutropenia, hemolytic anemia) are possible.

TABLE 34-2. Spectrum of Activity of the Penicillins

Category	Agent	Spectrum
Natural penicillins	Penicillin G, Penicillin G benzathine, Penicillin G procaine, Penicillin VK	This group covers viridans group streptococci, *Streptococcus pyogenes, Clostridium perfringens* (gas gangrene), and *Treponema pallidum* (syphilis); some activity is found against enterococci, *Streptococcus pneumoniae*, and mouth anaerobes.
Penicillinase-resistant penicillins	Oxacillin, Nafcillin, Dicloxacillin	These are drugs of choice for MSSA; they cover some streptococci.
Aminopenicillins	Ampicillin, **Amoxicillin**	These are drugs of choice for enterococci and *Listeria monocytogenes*; they cover some *S. pneumoniae, Haemophilus influenzae, Escherichia coli, Klebsiella* spp., and *Proteus* spp.
Ureidopenicillin	Piperacillin; not commonly used as sole agent (see piperacillin/ tazobactam)	Enhanced gram-negative coverage is found compared with aminopenicillins, including *P. aeruginosa*.
Beta-lactamase inhibitors	Clavulanic acid, sulbactam, tazobactam (used only in combination)	Combinations of penicillin–beta-lactamase inhibitors improve gram-negative and anaerobic activity.
Aminopenicillins + beta-lactamase inhibitor	Ampicillin/sulbactam and **amoxicillin**/clavulanic acid	This combination is active against MSSA, *S. pneumoniae*, enterococci, *H. influenzae, Moraxella catarrhalis, Proteus* spp., *E. coli, Klebsiella pneumoniae*, and anaerobes.
Ureidopenicillin + beta-lactamase inhibitor	Piperacillin/tazobactam	This combination provides overall enhanced gram-positive, gram-negative (most notably *P. aeruginosa*), and anaerobic coverage.

Boldface indicates one of top 100 drugs for 2020 by prescription volume.
MSSA, methicillin-sensitive *Staphylococcus aureus*.

TABLE 34-3. Dosing of Penicillins

Type and generic name	Trade name	Elimination route	Administration route	Common doses
Natural penicillins				
Penicillin G	Pfizerpen	Renal	I.V., I.M., oral	2 million to 4 million units I.V. every 4 hours
Penicillin G benzathine	Bicillin L-A	Renal	I.M.	Strep throat: 1.2 million units; syphilis: 2.4 million units
Penicillin VK (phenoxymethylpenicillin potassium)	Pen-Vee-K, Veetids	Renal	Oral	250 to 500 mg oral 2 to 4 times daily (250 mg twice daily for prophylaxis)
Penicillinase-resistant penicillins				
Oxacillin	Prostaphlin, Bactocill	Hepatic	Oral, I.V., I.M.	1 to 2 g I.V. every 4 to 6 hours
Nafcillin	Nafcil, Unipen	Hepatic	I.V., I.M.	1 to 2 g I.V. every 4 to 6 hours
Dicloxacillin	Dynapen, Dycill	Renal	Oral	250 to 500 mg oral every 6 hours

(continued)

TABLE 34-3. Dosing of Penicillins *(Continued)*

Type and generic name	Trade name	Elimination route	Administration route	Common doses
Aminopenicillins				
Ampicillin	Omnipen, Principen	Renal	Oral, I.M., I.V.	1 to 2 g I.V. every 6 hours
Amoxicillin	**Amoxil, Trimox, Moxatag**	Renal	Oral	250 to 500 mg oral every 8 hours; 775 mg (ER) oral every 24 hours
Penicillin plus β-lactamase inhibitors				
Amoxicillin/clavulanic acid	Augmentin, Augmentin XR	Renal	Oral	250 to 500 mg oral 3 times daily, 500 to 875 mg oral twice daily; 2000 mg XR oral every 12 hours
Ampicillin/sulbactam	Unasyn	Renal	I.V., I.M.	1.5 g or 3 g I.V. every 6 to 8 hours
Piperacillin/tazobactam	Zosyn	Renal	I.V.	2.25 to 4.5 g I.V. every 6 hours; 3.375 g I.V. every 8 hours as 4-hour extended infusion

Boldface indicates one of top 100 drugs for 2020 by prescription volume.
I.M., intramuscular; I.V., intravenous.

Drug–Disease Interactions

Nafcillin and oxacillin are eliminated primarily by biliary excretion; therefore, there is no need to adjust dosage for patients with renal dysfunction. All other penicillins are renally eliminated and require dose adjustment with renal dysfunction.

34-6 Cephalosporins

Cephalosporins are beta-lactam antibiotics that are structurally and pharmacologically similar to penicillins but generally have a broader spectrum of activity against gram-positive and gram-negative organisms.

Mechanism of Action

Cephalosporins bind to penicillin-binding proteins in a manner similar to that of other beta lactams, thereby inhibiting peptidoglycan cell wall synthesis.

Spectrum of Activity

Cephalosporins are broad-spectrum antimicrobial agents; however, the spectrum of activity varies greatly among the individual agents. Thus, cephalosporins are grouped into 4 broad classes, or generations, according to their antimicrobial coverage (Table 34-4). Notably, no cephalosporin has clinically dependable coverage of enterococci.

Adverse Drug Effects

- Hypersensitivity, including fever, rash, pruritus, urticaria, anaphylaxis, and hemolytic anemia
- GI effects, such as nausea, vomiting, and diarrhea
- Seizures (potential risk with high doses in patients with renal impairment)
- *Clostridium difficile* colitis

TABLE 34-4. Cephalosporins

Generic name	Trade name	Dosage forms	Dose	Elimination	Notes
First generation					Gram-positive > gram-negative activity
Cefadroxil	Duricef, Ultracef	Oral	500 to 1000 mg every 12 hours	Renal	
Cefazolin	Ancef, Kefzol	I.V.	250 to 1000 mg every 8 hours	Renal	Drug of choice for MSSA infections
Cephalexin	Keflex	Oral	250 to 500 mg every 6 hours	Renal	Similar to cefazolin, just oral
Second generation					More gram-negative activity
Cefaclor	Ceclor	Oral	250 to 500 mg every 8 hours	Renal	
Cefotetan	Cefotan	I.V., I.M.	1 to 2 g every 12 hours	Renal	Anaerobic activity
Cefoxitin	Mefoxin	I.V.	1 to 2 g every 6 to 8 hours	Renal	Anaerobic activity
Cefprozil	Cefzil	Oral	250 to 500 mg every 12 to 24 hours	Renal	
Cefuroxime	Ceftin, Zinacef	I.V., I.M., Oral	750 to 1500 mg every 8 hours I.V. and I.M.; 250 to 500 mg oral every 12 hours	Renal	
Third generation					Gram-negative > gram-positive activity; CNS penetration
Cefdinir	Omnicef	Oral	300 mg every 12 hours	Renal	
Cefixime	Suprax	Oral	400 mg daily	Renal	
Cefotaxime	Claforan	I.V.	1 to 2 g every 6 to 8 hours	Renal	
Cefpodoxime	Vantin	Oral	100 to 400 mg every 12 hours	Renal	
Ceftazidime	Fortaz, Tazicef	I.V., I.M.	1 to 2 g every 8 to 12 hours	Renal	Antipseudomonal but no gram-positive activity
Ceftriaxone	Rocephin	I.V., I.M.	1 to 2 every 12 to 24 hours	Renal and biliary	No dosage adjustment in renal impairment
Fourth generation					Gram-positive and gram-negative activity
Cefepime	Maxipime	I.V., I.M.	1 to 2 g every 8 to 12 hours	Renal	Pseudomonas aeruginosa activity
Fifth generation					Enhanced gram-positive activity (MRSA); no P. aeruginosa activity
Ceftaroline	Teflaro	I.V.	600 mg every 12 hours	Renal	MRSA, drug-resistant Streptococcus pneumoniae activity
New generation: Cephalosporin plus beta-lactamase inhibitors					Enhanced gram-negative activity
Ceftazidime/ avibactam	Avycaz	I.V.	2500 mg every 8 hours	Renal	ESBL, CRE, P. aeruginosa activity
Ceftolozane/ tazobactam	Zerbaxa	I.V.	1500 mg every 8 hours	Renal	Multidrug-resistant P. aeruginosa activity

CRE, carbapenem-resistant Enterobacteriaceae; ESBL, extended-spectrum beta lactamase; I.M., intramuscular; I.V., intravenous; MRSA, methicillin-resistant Staphylococcus aureus.

Drug–Disease Interactions

All cephalosporins (except ceftriaxone) require dosage adjustments in patients with renal insufficiency.

Patient Instructions and Counseling

Cephalosporins should be avoided in patients with a severe hypersensitivity reaction (anaphylaxis) to penicillins.

34-7 Carbapenems

Carbapenems are beta-lactam-like antibiotics that are structurally and pharmacologically similar to penicillins and cephalosporins but are broader in spectrum (Table 34-5).

Mechanism of Action

Carbapenems bind to penicillin-binding proteins in a manner similar to that of other beta lactams, thereby inhibiting peptidoglycan cell wall synthesis.

Spectrum of Activity

Carbapenems are very broad-spectrum antibiotics with activity against most gram-positive and gram-negative aerobes and anaerobes. They are the drugs of choice for ESBL–producing Enterobacteriaceae. Carbapenems (other than ertapenem) cover *P. aeruginosa* and some *Acinetobacter* spp.

Adverse Drug Effects

Adverse GI effects include nausea, vomiting, diarrhea (including *Clostridium difficile* infection), gastroenteritis, and abdominal pain.

Neutropenia and thrombocytopenia have been reported.

TABLE 34-5. Carbapenems and Monobactam

Generic name	Trade name	Dosage forms	Dose	Elimination	Notes
Carbapenems					
Imipenem/cilastatin	Primaxin	I.V., I.M.	250 to 1000 mg every 6 to 12 hours, depending on the severity of infection	Renal	
Meropenem	Merrem	I.V.	500 to 2000 mg every 8 hours	Renal	
Ertapenem	Invanz	I.V., I.M.	1000 mg every 24 hours	Renal	Has no activity against *Acinetobacter* spp., *P. aeruginosa*, or enterococci (APE)
Monobactam					
Aztreonam	Azactam	I.V., I.M.	1 to 2 g every 6 to 12 hours, depending on the severity of infection	Renal	Useful in anaphylactic beta-lactam allergy; generally poor *P. aeruginosa* coverage

I.M., intramuscular; I.V., intravenous.

Carbapenems have the highest seizure-risk profile of the β-lactams, and imipenem likely poses the greatest risk of the carbapenem class, although seizures are rare (0.4% of patients). Risk factors include use in patients with previous seizures or head trauma and high doses in patients with renal dysfunction.

Drug–Drug Interactions

Carbapenems lower serum concentrations of valproic acid. When used concomitantly, they may put patients at risk for seizures.

Imipenem/Cilastatin

Imipenem is a semisynthetic carbapenem beta-lactam antibiotic. Cilastatin prevents renal metabolism of imipenem by dehydropeptidase, an enzyme present on the brush border of the proximal renal tubule, thereby increasing the concentrations of the active drug and preventing production of a nephrotoxic metabolite. Cilastatin has no antibacterial activity.

Meropenem

Meropenem is similar to imipenem but has a slightly lower seizure risk, is not hydrolyzed by dehydropeptidase, and has enhanced *P. aeruginosa* activity.

Ertapenem

Ertapenem is dosed once daily and does not cover *Acinetobacter* spp., *P. aeruginosa*, or enterococci (APE).

34-8　Monobactam

Monobactam antibiotics are cell wall–active antibiotics like the beta lactams, but structural differences make them weakly immunogenic, thereby decreasing allergic cross-reactivity with penicillins and cephalosporins.

Aztreonam

Aztreonam is the only monobactam antibiotic currently available (see Table 34-5).

Mechanism of action

Monobactams bind to penicillin-binding proteins in a manner similar to that of other beta lactams, thereby inhibiting peptidoglycan synthesis.

Spectrum of activity

Aztreonam is active only against some aerobic gram-negative bacteria. Though some strains of *P. aeruginosa* are susceptible, resistance is increasing.

Adverse drug effects

Similar to other beta-lactam agents, Aztreonam has a lower chance of allergic cross-reactivity with penicillin (<1%) except ceftazidime.

34-9   Gram-Positive Antibiotics

Linezolid

Linezolid is a synthetic oxazolidinone antibiotics (Table 34-6).

Mechanism of action

Oxazolidinones bind to the 23S site of the 50S ribosomal subunit that inhibits bacterial translation and, thus, protein synthesis.

Spectrum of activity

Linezolid is active against *Staphylococcus* spp., including MRSA; *Enterococcus faecalis* and *E. faecium* isolates, including VRE; and *Streptococcus* spp., including *S. pneumoniae*. Linezolid is also used for non-tuberculosis *Mycobacterium* spp.

Adverse drug effects

Reversible hematologic effects (most commonly thrombocytopenia) have been reported in prolonged durations. Neurotoxicity such as peripheral neuropathy and optic neuritis has been reported with prolonged use.

Linezolid is a weak monoamine oxidase inhibitor (MAOI), and caution should be exercised in patients receiving other serotonergic agents (MAOIs, selective serotonin reuptake inhibitors [SSRIs], tricyclic anti-depressants [TCAs], meperidine, triptans). Serotonin syndrome is rare but has been reported primarily in patients receiving multiple agents with serotonergic activity.

Daptomycin

Daptomycin is a cyclic lipopeptide antibiotic (see Table 34-6).

TABLE 34-6. Gram-Positive Antibiotics

Generic name	Trade name	Dosage forms	Dose	Elimination	Notes
Linezolid	Zyvox	I.V., oral	600 mg every 12 hours	Renal	Monoamine oxidase inhibitor; thrombocytopenia risk; no adjustment for renal dysfunction
Vancomycin	Vancocin	I.V., oral	15 to 20 mg/kg I.V.; 125 to 500 mg oral every 6 hours	Renal	Dose adjusted using trough concentrations; oral formulation used to treat *Clostridium difficile*
Daptomycin	Cubicin	I.V.	4 to 6 mg/kg every 24 hours	Renal	CPK to be monitored weekly
Telavancin ⚠	Vibativ	I.V.	10 mg/kg every 24 hours	Renal	Dose adjusted for renal function; interference with aPTT
Dalbavancin	Dalvance	I.V.	1500 mg once; 1000 mg then 500 mg a week later	Renal	
Oritavancin	Orbactiv	I.V.	1200 mg once	Hepatic	Interference with aPTT, PT, and INR testing

aPTT, activated partial thromboplastin; CPK, creatinine phosphokinase; INR, international normalized ratio; I.V., intravenous; PT, prothrombin time.

Telavancin *FDA BOXED WARNING*

Moderate to severe renal impairment, nephrotoxicity, and embryofetal toxicity. Avoid use in patients with CrCl less than 50 ml/min unless benefit outweighs risk. Monitor renal function in all patients.

Mechanism of action

Daptomycin binds to bacterial cell membranes, causing rapid depolarization, which results in loss of membrane potential, leading to cell death.

Spectrum of activity

Daptomycin has activity against gram-positive bacteria staphylococci (including MRSA), streptococci, and enterococci (including VRE).

Adverse drug effects

Musculoskeletal effects include increased creatinine phosphokinase (CPK), which can progress to rhabdomyolysis (baseline and weekly CPK monitoring recommended). Increased caution and CPK monitoring should be performed with concomitant daptomycin and statin therapy. Rarely, pulmonary eosinophilia manifesting as eosinophilic pneumonia has been reported.

Other

Daptomycin is inactivated by the surfactant in the lung and cannot be used to treat pneumonia.

Glycopeptide Antibiotics

Mechanism of action

The glycopeptides vancomycin, telavancin, dalbavancin, and oritavancin exhibit bactericidal killing through inhibition of peptidoglycan synthesis polymerization and cross-linking and, thus, cell wall synthesis. This binding occurs at a site different from that of the penicillins (see Table 34-6).

Vancomycin

Spectrum of activity

Vancomycin is active against most gram-positive bacteria, such as staphylococci (including MRSA), streptococci, and enterococci. Vancomycin is active against *C. difficile* and can be used to treat *C. difficile* infection when administered in oral dosage form.

Adverse drug effects

Vancomycin is associated with nephrotoxicity, which can occur with high trough concentrations, higher total daily doses, and when concomitant nephrotoxic agents are used.

Histamine release, or "red-man syndrome," is a reaction most commonly associated with rapid I.V. infusion. Histamine reactions can be minimized by slow I.V. infusion, not to exceed 500 mg/30 min and through the use of antihistamines such as diphenhydramine (Benadryl).

Monitoring parameters

Vancomycin is renally eliminated and renal function should be monitored via troughs. Typically, troughs of 10 to 20 mcg/mL are desired. For serious infections (bacteremia, endocarditis, osteomyelitis, meningitis, pneumonia) caused by MRSA, trough concentrations of 15 to 20 mcg/mL are recommended. However, troughs are considered a poor surrogate for vancomycin's pharmacodynamic target of an under-the-curve/minimum inhibitory concentration (AUC/MIC) of 400 to 600 mcg/hr/mL. Vancomycin dosing guidelines recommend more precise AUC/MIC dosing to prevent unnecessary nephrotoxicity. Lower trough concentrations of 10 to 15 mcg/mL are reserved for skin and soft tissue infections and non-MRSA infections.

Telavancin

Telavancin's mechanism of action and spectrum of activity are similar to those of vancomycin.

Telavancin is renally eliminated, and dose and interval must be adjusted for renal dysfunction. No drug monitoring is required for telavancin.

Adverse drug effects

Nephrotoxicity is reported more often with telavancin than with vancomycin.

Neurologic effects such as dizziness, headache, and insomnia are also common.

QT prolongation can occur. Telavancin can interfere with coagulation testing (activated partial thromboplastin time [aPTT]) for up to 18 hours.

Dalbavancin and Oritavancin

Dalbavancin's and oritavancin's mechanism of action and spectrum of activity are identical to those of vancomycin and telavancin. These single-dose agents are used for their long duration of action for skin and soft tissue infections.

Dalbavancin is renally eliminated, and dose must be adjusted for renal dysfunction. Oritavancin is hepatically eliminated without need for dose adjustment in renal dysfunction.

Adverse drug effects

Infusion site reactions are uncommonly observed. Oritavancin can interfere with coagulation testing (activated partial thromboplastin time [aPTT], prothrombin time [PT], and international normalized ratio [INR]) for 24 to 48 hours.

34-10   Fluoroquinolones ⚠

Quinolones are broad-spectrum antibacterial agents (Table 34-7).

Mechanism of Action

Fluoroquinolones are bactericidal agents. The mechanism of action of these agents is inhibition of topoisomerase II (deoxyribonucleic acid [DNA] gyrase) and topoisomerase I.V., resulting in disruption of bacterial DNA replication.

 Fluoroquinolones *FDA BOXED WARNING*

Risk of serious adverse reactions including tendinitis, tendon rupture, peripheral neuropathy, central nervous effects, and exacerbation of myasthenia gravis.

TABLE 34-7. Fluoroquinolones

Generic name	Trade name	Dosage forms	Normal dose	Elimination	Notes
Ciprofloxacin	Cipro	I.V.	400 mg every 8 to 12 hours	Renal	Marginally better *Pseudomonas aeruginosa* activity
		oral	250 to 750 mg every 12 hours		
Levofloxacin	Levaquin	I.V., oral	250 to 750 mg every 24 hours	Renal	Covers both *Streptococcus pneumoniae* and *P. aeruginosa*
Moxifloxacin	Avelox	I.V., oral	400 mg every 24 hours	Hepatic	Covers *S. pneumoniae*, but not *P. aeruginosa;* has some anaerobic activity

I.V., intravascular.

Spectrum of Activity

Gram-negative activity is extensive, including *Escherichia coli*, *Klebsiella* spp., *Proteus* spp., *Enterobacter* spp., *Citrobacter* spp., *Salmonella* spp., and *Shigella* spp., in addition to *Moraxella catarrhalis* and *H. influenzae*. Activity against *P. aeruginosa* varies among individual agents.

Newer fluoroquinolones (levofloxacin, moxifloxacin) demonstrate superior gram-positive coverage versus older agents (ciprofloxacin). Fluoroquinolones have limited enterococcal activity and are not recommended for the treatment of invasive staphylococcal infections. Moxifloxacin is unique in that is has some anaerobic coverage; it cannot be used for urinary tract infections because of limited urinary excretion.

All fluoroquinolones are highly active against *Legionella* spp. and display atypical coverage.

Adverse Drug Effects

- **CNS effects:** Peripheral neuropathy, headache, dizziness, mood swings, and insomnia have been reported.
- **Cardiovascular effects:** QT prolongation (moxifloxacin more than levofloxacin other flouroquinolones and ciprofloxacin)) and aortic aneurysm rupture can occur. Avoid use or closely monitor in patients with preexisting QT prolongation or multiple QT prolonging agents.
- **Endocrine effects:** Hypoglycemia or hyperglycemia (reason for FDA withdrawal of gatifloxacin) has been reported.
- **Other effects:** Tendinitis and tendon rupture might occur (highest-risk patients >60 years of age, concomitant use of corticosteroids, transplant patients).
- **Rare effects:** Rash, urticaria, leukopenia, and hepatotoxicity (reason for FDA withdrawal of trovafloxacin) have been reported.

Drug–Drug Interactions

Antacids, sucralfate, and divalent or trivalent cations (calcium, magnesium, iron) significantly decrease the absorption of fluoroquinolones.

Drug–Disease Interactions

Dosage adjustments should be made for renally cleared fluoroquinolones (ciprofloxacin, levofloxacin) based on specified creatinine clearance (CrCl). Avoid use in patients with myasthenia gravis.

Patient Instructions and Counseling

- Fluoroquinolones should be avoided in children or pregnant or nursing females.
- Do *not* take antacids, multivitamins, or other calcium, magnesium, or iron supplements for at least 2 hours after each dose.

34-11 Macrolides

Mechanism of Action

Macrolides are bacteriostatic against susceptible organisms (Table 34-8). The agents bind to the 50S ribosomal subunit, thereby inhibiting RNA synthesis.

Spectrum of Activity

Macrolides are active against some Gram-positive organisms, including penicillin-resistant streptococci. Macrolides are drugs of choice in atypical pneumonia (*Mycoplasma* spp., *Chlamydophila* spp., *Legionella* spp.) and *Chlamydia* sexually transmitted diseases. Erythromycin is now used more for its adverse effect to accelerate gastric motility than for its antibacterial activity.

Adverse Drug Effects

- **GI effects:** Erythromycin stimulates GI motility, leading to abdominal cramping and diarrhea.
- **Cardiac effects:** QT interval prolongation and arrhythmias have been reported. The risk of arrhythmia is highest in patients with known QT prolongation, hypokalemia, hypomagnesemia, bradycardia, and concomitant use of other antiarrhythmic agents.

Drug–Drug Interactions

Clarithromycin is a strong CYP3A4 inhibitor, but **azithromycin** is not.

TABLE 34-8. Macrolides

Generic name	Trade name	Dosage forms	Normal dose	Elimination	Notes
Azithromycin	**Zithromax**	Oral, I.V.	500 to 1000 mg once, then 250 mg every 24 hours, or 500 mg every 24 hours	Hepatic	Oral dose = I.V. dose; no adjustment for renal dysfunction
Clarithromycin	Biaxin, Biaxin XL	Oral	250 to 500 mg twice daily or 500 mg to 1 g XL every 24 hours	Renal	XL = daily dosing
Erythromycin	Various	Oral	250 to 500 mg every 6 hours	Hepatic	Erythromycin base, ethyl succinate, and stearate

Boldface indicates one of top 100 drugs for 2020 by prescription volume.
I.V., intravenous.

34-12   Tetracyclines and Glycylcyclines

Mechanism of Action

Tetracyclines and glycylcyclines inhibit bacterial protein synthesis by reversible binding on the 30S ribosomal subunit (Table 34-9).

Tigecycline, a glycylcycline, shares the same mechanism of action as tetracyclines but has a structural modification that increases affinity and binding to various bacterial ribosomes and decreases efflux from the cell.

Spectrum of Activity

Tetracyclines are used in a wide variety of disease states (respiratory tract, skin, genital infections, tick-borne disease). Doxycycline is used to treat infections caused by *Streptococcus pneumoniae* and community-acquired MRSA strains.

Tigecycline has enhanced broad-spectrum coverage including MRSA, VRE, and anaerobic coverage, including *B. fragilis*. It does not cover *Morganella* spp., *P. aeruginosa*, *Providencia* spp., and *Proteus* spp. (MP3).

Title	Explanation (MP3)	Reference
Holes in tigecycline coverage	**M**organella spp.	None
	Pseudomonas aeruginosa	
	Providencia spp.	
	Proteus spp.	

Patient Instructions and Counseling

Administering the drug with food can minimize GI distress.

Adverse Drug Effects

Photosensitivity reactions can occur. Tigecycline is associated with an abnormally high incidence of GI intolerance.

TABLE 34-9. Tetracyclines and Glycylcyclines

Generic name	Trade name	Dosage forms	Common doses	Primary mode of elimination
Tetracyclines				
Doxycycline	Vibramycin and others	Oral, I.V.	100 mg every 12 hours	Renal
Minocycline	Minocin	Oral, I.V.	100 to 200 mg every 12 hours	Hepatic
Tetracycline	Achromycin V, Sumycin, Tetracyn, and others	Oral, I.V., I.M.	1 to 2 g daily	Renal
Glycylcyclines				
Tigecycline ⚠	Tygacil	I.V.	100 mg once, then 50 mg I.V. every 12 hours	Hepatic

I.M., intramuscular; I.V., intravenous.

Tigecycline *FDA BOXED WARNING*

Increase in all-cause mortality observed in a meta-analysis of phase 3 and 4 clinical trials—reserve for use in patients where alternative treatment is not suitable.

Tetracyclines and glycylcyclines are generally contraindicated during pregnancy and breastfeeding and in children younger than age 8 years because of the association with tooth discoloration and interference with bone growth.

Drug–Drug and Drug–Disease Interactions

Similar to the fluoroquinolones, milk, antacids, iron supplements, and other substances with calcium, magnesium, aluminum, and iron decrease tetracycline GI absorption considerably and should be ingested at least 2 hours before or after administration of tetracycline.

Anticonvulsants (e.g., barbiturates, carbamazepine, phenytoin) induce hepatic microsomal metabolism of tetracyclines and, therefore, decrease tetracycline serum concentrations.

Tetracyclines and glycylcyclines may potentiate **warfarin**-induced anticoagulation; therefore, monitor PT and INR.

Tetracycline and glycylcycline doses do not have to be adjusted for renal dysfunction.

34-13 Sulfonamides

Sulfonamides are synthetic derivatives of sulfanilamide (Table 34-10).

Mechanism of Action

Sulfonamides interfere with bacterial folic acid synthesis by competitively inhibiting para aminobenzoic acid (PABA) utilization.

Spectrum of Activity

- **Gram-positive bacteria:** Staphylococci (MSSA, community-acquired MRSA strains), some streptococci (not enterococci)

TABLE 34-10. Sulfonamides

Generic name	Trade name	Dosage forms	Dose	Elimination	Notes
Sulfadiazine		I.V., Oral	2 to 4 g daily	Renal	Use to treat toxoplasmosis in combination with pyrimethamine.
Sulfamethoxazole (combined with trimethoprim)	Bactrim, Septra	I.V., Oral	1 to 3 g daily	Renal	Monitor for increases in K and SCr levels. Importantly, dosing is based on the trimethoprim component of this combination.

I.V., intravenous; K, potassium; SCr, serum creatinine.

- **Gram-negative bacteria:** *E. coli*, *Klebsiella* spp., *Proteus* spp., *Enterobacter* spp., *Salmonella* spp., *Shigella* spp.
- **Other organisms:** *Toxoplasma gondii*, *Plasmodium* spp., *Nocardia* spp.

Adverse Drug Effects

Hypersensitivity reactions appear to be cross-reactive with other sulfonamides, diuretics (including acetazolamide and thiazides), and sulfonylureas.

Dermatologic reactions include rash, urticaria, and Stevens–Johnson syndrome.

Increases in serum creatinine are common owing to inhibition of creatinine excretion (Bactrim, Septra).

Drug–Drug Interactions

Sulfamethoxazole is a CYP2C9 inhibitor and can significantly increase **warfarin** levels and INR.

34-14   Miscellaneous Antibiotics

A number of miscellaneous antibiotics are depicted in Table 34-11.

Clindamycin

Clindamycin is a semisynthetic antibiotic derived from lincomycin.

Mechanism of action

Clindamycin inhibits the 50S ribosomal subunit, thereby inhibiting RNA synthesis. Clindamycin is primarily bacteriostatic.

TABLE 34-11. Miscellaneous Antibiotics

Generic name	Trade name	Dosage forms	Dose	Elimination	Notes
Clindamycin	Cleocin	I.V., oral	600 to 900 mg I.V. every 8 hours; 300 to 600 mg every 6 hours oral	Hepatic	May predispose patient to *Clostridium difficile*; no renal dose adjustment
Metronidazole	**Flagyl**	I.V., oral	250 to 1000 mg 3 to 4 times daily	Hepatic	Disulfiram reaction; **warfarin** interaction; no renal dose adjustment
Colistimethate	Coly-Mycin M	I.M., I.V.	2.5 to 5 mg/kg daily divided every 8 to 12 hours	Renal	Dose based on IBW and adjusted for renal function
Polymyxin B ⚠		I.M., I.V.	15,000 to 25,000 units/kg daily divided every 12 hours for I.V.	Renal	1 mg = 10,000 units; dose adjusted for renal function
Fidaxomicin	Dificid	Oral	200 mg twice daily	Fecal	Nonabsorbable, for *C. difficile*

Boldface indicates one of top 100 drugs for 2020 by prescription volume.
IBW, ideal body weight; I.M., intramuscular; I.V., intravenous.

Polymyxin B *FDA BOXED WARNING*

Risk of nephrotoxicity and neurotoxicity—avoid concomitant use with other nephrotoxic or neurotoxic agents. Must be administered in a hospital setting for continuous monitoring. Do not use in pregnancy—safety has not been determined.

Spectrum of activity

Clindamycin is active against aerobic gram-positive, anaerobic gram-positive, and some anaerobic gram-negative bacteria. Clindamycin exhibits coverage against community-acquired MRSA strains. It has no activity against aerobic gram-negative bacteria.

Adverse drug effects

Enhanced adverse GI effects occur frequently with clindamycin. Clindamycin may induce *C. difficile* enterocolitis to a greater degree than many other antibiotics because it does not cover this organism.

Clindamycin can cause transient leukopenia, neutropenia, eosinophilia, thrombocytopenia, and agranulocytosis. These effects are usually reversible on discontinuation of the drug.

Metronidazole

Metronidazole is a nitroimidazole antibiotic that is active against anaerobic gram-negative and gram-positive bacteria as well as protozoa.

Mechanism of action

Metronidazole inhibits bacterial DNA synthesis.

Spectrum of activity

Metronidazole is active against anaerobic bacteria and is a drug of choice for *B. fragilis*. **Metronidazole** is effective for the treatment of *C. difficile* infection and other protozoa.

Adverse drug effects

- **GI effects:** Taste disturbance
- **Neurologic:** Dizziness, headache, paresthesia, peripheral neuropathy (particularly with longer courses of therapy)

Drug–drug interactions

Metronidazole inhibits drug metabolism through the cytochrome P450 (CYP450) system and increases the drug level or effect of **warfarin**, cyclosporine, carbamazepine, phenytoin, and tacrolimus. **Metronidazole** also produces a disulfiram-like reaction; therefore, alcohol should be avoided for at least 3 days before and after use.

Polymyxins

The polymyxins, polymyxin B and colistin, display broad gram-negative spectrum with dose-limiting side effects; therefore, they should be used only when no safe alternative exists. They have reemerged in clinical practice because of an increase in multidrug-resistant *Acinetobacter* spp. and *P. aeruginosa*.

Mechanism of action

The polymyxins act as anionic detergents that damage the external cell membrane of gram-negative bacteria and cause cell death.

Spectrum of activity

Polymyxins are active against most aerobic gram-negative bacilli, including multidrug resistant strains.

Adverse drug effects

- **Renal:** Electrolyte abnormalities (hypocalcemia, hyponatremia, hypokalemia) and significant incidence of renal failure (higher with colistin) limit use.
- **Neurologic:** Ataxia, dizziness, headache, myasthenia crisis, neuromuscular blockade, neurotoxicity, paresthesia, peripheral neuropathy, slurred speech, and vertigo have been reported.

Drug–drug interactions

The polymyxins have additive neurotoxic and nephrotoxic effects with neuromuscular blocking agents and aminoglycosides.

Fidaxomicin

Fidaxomicin is a nonabsorbable, oral macrolide antibiotic used in the treatment of recurrent *C. difficile* infection.

Mechanism of action

Fidaxomicin inhibits bacterial RNA polymerases.

Spectrum of activity

The most relevant activity of fidaxomicin is against *C. difficile*.

Adverse drug effects

GI adverse effects are the most commonly reported side effects.

Other

Some data suggest that *C. difficile* infection recurrence rates may be lower with fidaxomicin in comparison to oral vancomycin.

34-15   Antifungal Agents

Key antifungal targets are depicted in Figure 34-2. Specific antifungal agents are further described in Table 34-12.

Amphotericin B

Amphotericin B is a polyene antifungal agent used in the treatment of potentially life-threatening systemic fungal infections. There have been several lipid amphotericin B formulations developed in response to intolerances related to conventional amphotericin B use: Amphotericin B cholesterol sulfate complex (Amphotec), amphotericin B lipid complex (Abelcet), and amphotericin B liposomal (AmBisome).

FIGURE 34-2. Key Fungal Cell Characteristics

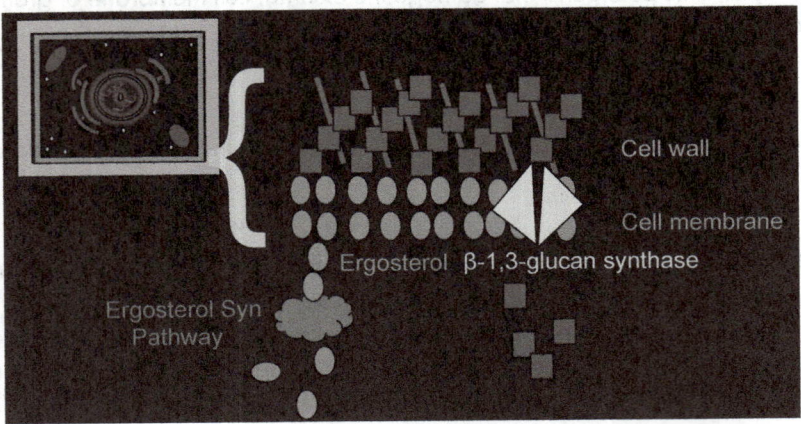

Cell structure	Function	Antibacterial agent target
1. Ergosterol	Make up fungal cell membrane	Amphotericin B
2. Ergosterol synthase	Enzyme that synthesizes ergosterol	Azoles
3. Beta-1,3 glucan synthase	Enzyme that creates beta-1,3 glucan that makes up the fungal cell-wall	Echinocandins
4. Cell DNA or RNA (not pictured)	Responsible for essential fungal cell operations	Flucytosine

Amphotericin B liposomal is used most commonly because of its similar efficacy and a 20% to 30% reduction in drug-related adverse effects compared with conventional formulations.

Mechanism of action

Amphotericin B is a broad-spectrum antifungal agent that binds to ergosterol in the fungal cell wall, leading to increased permeability and cell death.

Spectrum of activity

- *Aspergillus* spp., *Cryptococcus* spp., dimorphic fungi, and other molds such as mucorales.
- Most *Candida* spp.

Adverse drug effects

- **Infusion reactions:** Reactions can be severe to life threatening. Fever, chills, hypotension, rigors, pain, thrombophlebitis, and anaphylaxis can occur. Rates are lower with lipid formulations.
- **Renal and electrolyte effects:** Nephrotoxicity is the major dose-limiting toxicity, but significant hypokalemia, hypocalcemia, and hypomagnesemia can occur, and electrolytes should be supplemented and replaced. Lipid formulations decrease rates of nephrotoxicity.
- **FDA boxed warning:** Avoid use in patients with noninvasive fungal disease because of Amphotericin B's adverse effect profile. Use caution to verify dosing differences between drug formulations to avoid overdose.

TABLE 34-12. Antifungal Agents

Generic name	Trade name	Dosage forms	Dose	Elimination	Notes
Amphotericin B (liposomal, lipid complex, cholesterol complex)	AmBisome, Abelcet, Amphotec	I.V.	3 to 5 mg/kg every 24 hours	Unknown	Drug is 20% to 30% less nephrotoxic than conventional amphotericin B.
Caspofungin	Cancidas	I.V.	70 mg once and then 50 mg every 24 hours	Hepatic	Dose adjustment is made for patients with severe hepatic dysfunction.
Micafungin	Mycamine	I.V.	100 mg every 24 hours	Hepatic	
Anidulafungin	Eraxis	I.V.	200 mg once and then 100 mg every 24 hours	Chemical degradation	
Fluconazole	Diflucan	I.V., oral	100 to 800 mg every 24 hours	Renal	
Itraconazole	Sporanox	Oral	200 to 600 mg daily	Hepatic	Capsules require acidic environment; solution should be taken on an empty stomach.
Voriconazole	Vfend	I.V., oral	6 mg/kg every 12 hours × 2 doses then 4 mg/kg I.V. every 12 hours; 200 to 400 mg oral every 12 hours	Hepatic	Maximum oral dose is 800 mg per day to limit hepatotoxicity. Do *not* use I.V. formulation with CrCl <50 mL/min.
Isavuconazonium sulfate	Cresemba	I.V., oral	372 mg every 8 hours × 8 doses then 372 mg I.V. every 24 hours	Hepatic	I.V. must be administered with an in-line filter.
Posaconazole	Noxafil	I.V., oral (suspension and tablet)	200 to 400 mg 2 to 4 times daily	Hepatic	Suspension is best absorbed with high-calorie, high-fat meal or acidic environment.
Flucytosine	Ancobon	Oral	50 to 150 mg/kg daily	Renal	

CrCl, creatinine clearance; I.V., intravenous.

 Amphotericin B *FDA BOXED WARNING*

Only use in patients with progressive and potentially life-threatening fungal infections—should not be used to treat noninvasive fungal infections. Should not be given in doses greater than 1.5 mg/kg.

 Itraconazole *FDA BOXED WARNING*

May cause or exacerbate congestive heart failure (CHF). Do not administer for treatment of onychomycosis in patients with evidence of ventricular dysfunction. Significant number of drug–drug interactions and contraindications—see package insert for full list.

Flucytosine *FDA BOXED WARNING*

Use with extreme caution in patients with renal impairment. Requires close monitoring of hematologic, renal, and hepatic status.

Echinocandins

Echinocandins (caspofungin, micafungin, anidulafungin) are a class of I.V. antifungal agents with enhanced *Candida* spp. and *Aspergillus* spp. coverage. Echinocandins do not require dose adjustment for renal dysfunction; however, caspofungin should be dose adjusted in severe hepatic impairment. They are generally well-tolerated agents with a mild side effect profile.

Mechanism of action

Echinocandins inhibit beta-1,3 glucan synthase, thereby causing loss of cell wall integrity, resulting in cell lysis and death.

Spectrum of activity

Echinocandins are drugs of choice for resistant *Candida* spp. and *Aspergillus* spp., but they lack activity against other molds.

Adverse drug effects

Hepatic effects, including increased aspartate aminotransferase (AST) and alanine aminotransferase (ALT), have been reported.

Azole Antifungals

Mechanism of action

The azole antifungals inhibit fungal CYP450 14-alpha-demethylase, thereby decreasing ergosterol concentrations in susceptible fungi.

Drug–drug interactions

All azole antifungals are inhibitors of the CYP450 system and have many critical drug interactions attributable to decreased metabolism and, thus, toxicity.

The azole antifungals have also been shown to prolong the QT interval; thus, co-administration with other drugs that prolong the QT interval increases risk and should be monitored.

Fluconazole

Fluconazole is a synthetic triazole antifungal.

Spectrum of activity

Fluconazole is the drug of choice for *Candida albicans* infection. Fluconazole also displays good activity against *Cryptococcus* spp. and *Coccidioides* spp.

Adverse drug effects

Cholestasis and increased AST, ALT, and gamma-glutamyl transpeptidase (GGTP); hepatic necrosis; and, rarely, severe hepatic dysfunction have been reported.

Drug–drug interactions

Fluconazole is a significant inhibitor of CYP2C9, resulting in significant interactions with **warfarin** and phenytoin.

Itraconazole

Itraconazole is a synthetic triazole antifungal.

Spectrum of activity

Itraconazole is used mostly for the treatment of dimorphic fungi (*Histoplasma* spp., *Blastomyces* spp.).

Adverse drug effects

- ***Dermatologic and sensitivity reactions:*** Rash, pruritus, urticaria, angioedema, Stevens–Johnson syndrome
- ***Nervous system effects:*** Headache, dizziness, tremor, neuropathy
- ***FDA boxed warning:*** Congestive heart failure, peripheral edema, pulmonary edema, prolonged QT interval, ventricular dysrhythmias
- ***Hepatic effects:*** Increased AST and ALT
- ***Electrolyte and metabolic effects:*** Hypokalemia, adrenal insufficiency, gynecomastia

Patient instructions and counseling

- Capsules should be taken with food or acidic beverages to facilitate absorption.
- Oral solution should be taken on an empty stomach to help increase absorption.

Drug–drug interactions

Itraconazole is a significant inhibitor of CYP3A4 and is contraindicated when combined with various agents, including dofetilide, dronedarone, **lovastatin**, and **simvastatin**.

Voriconazole

Voriconazole is a synthetic triazole antifungal.

Spectrum of activity

Voriconazole is the drug of choice for *Aspergillosis* spp. It displays coverage of non–*Candida albicans* species as well as activity against *Histoplasma* and *Blastomyces* spp.

Adverse drug effects

- Hepatic effects such as hepatitis, cholestasis, and fulminant hepatic failure (mostly with the oral formulation at high doses)
- Visual disturbances and hallucinations
- Periostitis and squamous cell carcinoma reported rarely with prolonged use

Other

I.V. formulation should be avoided in patients with a CrCl <50 mL/min because of accumulation of the potentially nephrotoxic cyclodextrin vehicle component.

Isavuconazonium sulfate

Isavuconazonium sulfate is a triazole antifungal prodrug that is metabolized to isavuconazole.

Spectrum of activity

Isavuconazonium sulfate displays activity against *Aspergillus* spp. and has been effective for the treatment of mucormycosis.

Adverse drug effects

Elevations in liver enzymes have been reported and rarely hepatitis.

Drug–drug interactions

Coadministration of isavuconazonium sulfate with strong inhibitors or inducers of CYP3A4 is contraindicated.

Other

- I.V. formulation requires an inline filter.
- Isavuconazonium sulfate is potentially teratogenic, and pregnant women should avoid use.

Posaconazole

Posaconazole is a synthetic triazole antifungal.

Spectrum of activity

Posaconazole is primarily used for prophylaxis of invasive fungal infection in immunocompromised patients because of its coverage of *Aspergillus* and *Candida* spp. It can also be used for treatment of esophageal candidiasis. It has a broad in vitro spectrum of activity and has been effective as salvage treatment of mucormycosis.

Adverse drug effects

- **Nervous system effects:** Headache, dizziness, confusion
- **Cardiovascular effects:** Hypertension, hypotension, edema, prolonged QT interval, ventricular dysrhythmias
- **Hepatic effects:** Cholestasis, increased AST and ALT

Patient instructions and counseling

When administered as an oral suspension, posaconazole should be taken with food (ideally high fat and caloric content) or an acidic beverage to facilitate absorption. Proton pump inhibitors (PPIs) should be avoided because they can significantly reduce posaconazole absorption. Delayed-release tablet and I.V. formulations avoid absorption issues and can be administered without regard to food or PPI use.

Flucytosine

Mechanism of action

Flucytosine enters fungal cells and is converted to 5-fluorouracil, causing cell death.

Spectrum of activity

Flucytosine is active against most strains of *Cryptococcus* and *Candida* spp. It is commonly combined with amphotericin B for the treatment of cryptococcal meningitis.

Adverse drug effects

- **Renal effects:** Increased serum creatinine, BUN, and crystalluria have been reported. Use with caution in patients with renal impairment.

- **Nervous system effects:** Confusion, hallucinations, psychosis, headache, parkinsonism, paresthesias, peripheral neuropathy, hearing loss, and vertigo can occur.
- **FDA boxed warning:** Use with caution in patients with renal impairment, which can cause drug accumulation. Use requires frequent monitoring of kidney and liver function tests and hematology (WBC [white blood cell] and platelets).

34-16   Antitubercular Agents

First-Line Agents (RIPE Therapy)

For active tuberculosis (TB) infection, rifampin, isoniazid, pyrazinamide, and ethambutol (RIPE) are usually initiated for a 2-month period, and then rifampin and isoniazid are continued for an additional 4 months (Table 34-13). Various alternative regimens have been described.

Rifampin

Mechanism of action

Rifampin inhibits RNA synthesis in susceptible isolates.

Spectrum of activity

Rifampin is active against most *Mycobacterium* spp. and many gram-positive organisms such as MRSA.

Adverse drug effects

- **CNS effects:** Headache, dizziness, mental confusion, and psychosis have been reported.
- **Hepatic effects:** Increased bilirubin, AST, and ALT are common; fulminant hepatotoxicity has been reported.

TABLE 34-13. Antitubercular Agents

Generic name	Trade name	Dosage forms	Normal dose	Elimination	Notes
First-line agents					
Rifampin	Various	Oral, I.V.	10 to 20 mg/kg daily	Hepatic	Discoloration of body fluids, potent CYP3A4 inducer
Isoniazid ⚠	Various	Oral	5 to 10 mg/kg daily	Hepatic	Peripheral and optic neuropathy (use with pyridoxine)
Pyrazinamide	Various	Oral	15 to 30 mg/kg daily	Hepatic	Uric acid elevations, polyarthralgia
Ethambutol	Myambutol	Oral	15 to 25 mg/kg daily	Hepatic	Optic neuropathy

I.V., intravenous.

 Isoniazid *FDA BOXED WARNING*

Risk of severe or fatal hepatitis. Risk increases with age as well as alcohol consumption.

Patient instructions and counseling

Rifampin can cause an orange discoloration of body fluids such as tears, sweat, and saliva; patients should be counseled that this is expected. Rifampin may stain contact lenses.

Other

Rifampin is a potent inducer of CYP450 enzymes.

Isoniazid

Mechanism of action

Isoniazid appears to inhibit the bacterial cell wall of susceptible isolates and, therefore, is active only against actively dividing cells.

Spectrum of activity

Isoniazid is active against most *Mycobacterium* spp.

Adverse drug effects

- **CNS effects:** Peripheral neuropathy and, rarely, seizures, encephalopathy, and psychosis have been reported.
- **FDA boxed warning:** Increases in bilirubin, AST, and ALT are noted in up to 20% of patients receiving this agent. Isoniazid has led to fulminant hepatitis and death.
- **Hematologic effects:** Agranulocytosis, eosinophilia, thrombocytopenia, and hemolytic anemia have been reported.

Other

- Isoniazid is the drug of choice for latent TB infection (monotherapy treatment for 9 months).
- Supplementing with pyridoxine (25 mg daily) will decrease chances of neuropathy.
- Concomitant use with alcohol will increase risk of liver damage.

Pyrazinamide

Mechanism of action

Mycobacterium tuberculosis converts pyrazinamide to pyrazinoic acid, which possesses antitubercular activity.

Spectrum of activity

Pyrazinamide is active against *M. tuberculosis* only.

Adverse drug effects

- **Hepatic effects:** Increased liver enzymes are common, and fulminant hepatitis has been reported.
- **Pain and gout:** Pyrazinamide inhibits renal excretion of uric acid and may induce or worsen gout. Pyrazinamide can cause polyarthralgia.

Ethambutol

Mechanism of action

Ethambutol appears to inhibit bacterial cellular metabolism.

Spectrum of activity

Ethambutol is active against most *Mycobacterium* spp.

Adverse drug effects

Ocular effects may occur. Optic neuritis with decreased visual acuity, central and peripheral scotomas, and loss of red–green color discrimination have been noted. Peripheral neuropathy is also a common adverse effect.

34-17 Pharmacist's Role

Pharmacists can improve patient outcomes by providing appropriate antimicrobial therapy recommendations given a specific infectious disease state and/or identification of an organism. This concept is referred to as antimicrobial stewardship. Inpatient pharmacists play a pivotal role in pharmacokinetic dosing of vancomycin and aminoglycosides to ensure the safety and efficacy of these antibiotics with narrow therapeutic indexes. Antimicrobial monitoring is routinely performed by inpatient pharmacists, particularly regarding nephrotoxic agents or with antimicrobials associated with drug–drug or drug–disease interactions. In community settings, pharmacists provide important counseling to patients receiving antimicrobials and can identify serious drug–drug interactions.

NAPLEX Competency Statements

The questions in this chapter cover the following 2021 NAPLEX Competency Statements: **AREA 2:** 2.1; 2.2; 2.4 **AREA 3:** 3.1; 3.2; 3.3; 3.4; 3.5; 3.6; 3.7; 3.8; 3.9; 3.10; 3.11 **AREA 5:** 5.1; 5.5.

34-18 Questions

1. Which of the following is an antibiotic that exhibits concentration-dependent bacterial killing?

   A. Penicillin G
   B. Ceftriaxone
   C. Gentamicin
   D. Aztreonam
   E. Linezolid

2. Which of the following most accurately characterizes aminoglycoside toxicity?

   A. Thrombocytopenia and neutropenia
   B. CPK elevations and myalgias
   C. QT prolongation and risk of arrhythmia
   D. Nephrotoxicity and ototoxicity
   E. Serotonin syndrome

3. Which of the following beta-lactam antibiotics displays the best activity against enterococci?

   A. Ampicillin
   B. Cefepime
   C. Meropenem
   D. Aztreonam
   E. Ceftriaxone

4. Which of the following beta-lactam antibiotics displays activity against MRSA?

   A. Piperacillin/tazobactam
   B. Imipenem/cilastatin
   C. Aztreonam
   D. Cefazolin
   E. Ceftaroline

5. Which of the following penicillins does not have to be dose adjusted for renal insufficiency yet can cause interstitial nephritis?

   A. Nafcillin
   B. Amoxicillin
   C. Ampicillin/sulbactam
   D. Penicillin G
   E. Piperacillin/tazobactam

6. Which of the following cephalosporins is classified as a first-generation agent with enhanced gram-positive activity against MSSA?

   A. Cefuroxime
   B. Ceftazidime
   C. Cefepime
   D. Cefazolin
   E. Cefpodoxime

7. Which antibiotic displays broad-spectrum antibiotic activity yet does not cover *P. aeruginosa*?

   A. Amikacin
   B. Ciprofloxacin
   C. Colistin
   D. Ertapenem
   E. Ceftolozane/tazobactam

8. Which beta-lactam antibiotic would be most appropriate to treat gram-negative pathogens in a patient with a serious anaphylactic penicillin allergy?

   A. Oxacillin
   B. Aztreonam
   C. Cephalexin
   D. Penicillin V
   E. Imipenem/cilastatin

9. Which of the following reversible adverse effects is associated with rapid infusion time of vancomycin?

   A. Nephrotoxicity
   B. Ototoxicity
   C. Red-man syndrome
   D. Neurologic toxicity
   E. Neutropenia

10. Which of the following can be used as an oral formulation to treat infections caused by MRSA?

    A. Linezolid
    B. Daptomycin
    C. Vancomycin
    D. Ceftaroline
    E. Ciprofloxacin

11. For which of the following antibiotics should weekly CPK levels be drawn?

    A. Vancomycin
    B. Linezolid
    C. Levofloxacin
    D. Daptomycin
    E. Trimethoprim-sulfamethoxazole

12. Which of the following should be targeted for a patient receiving vancomycin for the treatment of MRSA pneumonia?

    A. Trough of 5 to 10 mcg/mL
    B. Peak of 10 to 15 mcg/mL
    C. Trough of 15 to 20 mcg/mL
    D. Trough monitoring is not necessary
    E. AUC/MIC of 800 mcg*h/mL

13. Which of the following antibiotics covers both *S. pneumoniae* and *P. aeruginosa*?

    A. Moxifloxacin
    B. Ciprofloxacin
    C. Trimethoprim-sulfamethoxazole
    D. Daptomycin
    E. Levofloxacin

14. Which of the following is an important patient counseling point for a patient receiving a fluoroquinolone antibiotic?

    A. Avoid antacids or calcium-containing substances within 2 hours of administration.
    B. Take only on an empty stomach.
    C. Take only with a high fat meal or an acidic beverage.
    D. Avoid proton pump inhibitors with use.
    E. Take with probiotic to prevent *C. difficile* infection.

15. Which of the following drugs displays the most significant drug–drug interaction with warfarin?

    A. Amoxicillin
    B. Cefdinir
    C. Fluconazole
    D. Azithromycin
    E. Anidulafungin

16. Which of the following drugs has the best activity to target a bloodstream infection resulting from an ESBL-producing *E. coli*?

    A. Ceftriaxone
    B. Amoxicillin/clavulanate
    C. Ertapenem
    D. Rifampin
    E. Daptomycin

17. Which of the following drugs could adequately treat a skin and soft tissue infection caused by community-acquired MRSA?

    A. Metronidazole
    B. Fidaxomicin
    C. Colistimethate
    D. Moxifloxacin
    E. Sulfamethoxazole-trimethoprim

18. Which of the following antibiotics may have a higher incidence of predisposing a patient for a *Clostridium difficile* infection?

- **A.** Clindamycin
- **B.** Fidaxomicin
- **C.** Metronidazole
- **D.** Oral vancomycin
- **E.** Amoxicillin

19. Which of the following agents has the best activity against the gram-negative anaerobe *Bacteroides fragilis*?

- **A.** Clindamycin
- **B.** Colistin
- **C.** Fidaxomicin
- **D.** Metronidazole
- **E.** Ciprofloxacin

20. Which of the following drugs is used only for severe infections caused by multidrug-resistant gram-negative pathogens because of a significant risk of nephrotoxicity?

- **A.** Rifaximin
- **B.** Colistin
- **C.** Clindamycin
- **D.** Fidaxomicin
- **E.** Vancomycin

21. Which of the following antifungal agents is the drug of choice for infection caused by *Candida albicans*?

- **A.** Amphoteracin B
- **B.** Fluconazole
- **C.** Flucytosine
- **D.** Posaconazole
- **E.** Voriconazole

22. Which of the following well-tolerated antifungal agents is commonly used to treat disseminated candidiasis caused by *Candida krusei*?

- **A.** Caspofungin
- **B.** Amphotericin B
- **C.** Posaconazole
- **D.** Fluconazole
- **E.** Flucytosine

23. Which of the following oral antifungal medications is the drug of choice in treating *Aspergillus* spp.?

- **A.** Amphotericin B
- **B.** Caspofungin
- **C.** Posaconazole
- **D.** Fluconazole
- **E.** Voriconazole

24. Which of the following antitubercular agents is the drug of choice for latent TB infection?

- **A.** Isoniazid
- **B.** Rifampin
- **C.** Ethambutol
- **D.** Linezolid
- **E.** Pyrazinamide

25. Which of the following agents can cause red-colored staining of body fluids?

- **A.** Rifampin
- **B.** Isoniazid
- **C.** Pyrazinamide
- **D.** Ethambutol
- **E.** Tigecycline

 **34-19   Answers**

1. **C.** Aminoglycoside antibiotics exhibit concentration-dependent bacterial killing, whereas beta-lactam antibiotics display time-dependent bacterial killing.

2. **D.** Aminoglycosides cause both nephrotoxicity and ototoxicity. Nephrotoxicity is usually reversible and seldom requires dialysis. Ototoxicity can be auditory and vestibular and sometimes is irreversible.

3. **A.** Ampicillin is a drug of choice for enterococci that are susceptible. No cephalosporins display reliable activity against enterococci.

4. **E.** Ceftaroline is currently the only beta-lactam antibiotic that displays activity against MRSA.

5. **A.** Nafcillin and oxacillin are penicillinase-resistant penicillins that do not have to be dose adjusted for renal insufficiency. This class of medications, however, can cause interstitial nephritis. The first medication in this class, methicillin, was removed from the market because of high incidence of interstitial nephritis.

6. **D.** Cefazolin is an intravenous, first-generation cephalosporin considered an agent of choice for MSSA, along with the penicillinase-resistant penicillins.

7. **D.** Ertapenem is a carbapenem that does not exhibit coverage against *P. aeruginosa*. It is also the only carbapenem that is administered once daily.

8. **B.** Aztreonam displays a purely gram-negative spectrum of activity and tends to have the lowest allergic cross-reactivity in patients with anaphylactic penicillin allergies. Carbapenems do have lower risks for cross-reactivity in most cases but should still be avoided in serious IgE-mediated allergies.

9. **C.** Red-man syndrome is a histamine-related adverse reaction that occurs when vancomycin is administered rapidly. Notably, this is not a true drug allergy and can be minimized by slowing the infusion time and pre-medicating with antihistamines such as diphenhydramine before infusion.

10. **A.** Linezolid is the only gram-positive antibiotic agent (covering MRSA) listed with an oral formulation. This can be helpful in the outpatient setting. Monitoring for thrombocytopenia should occur, particularly with longer courses of therapy (greater than 14 days). Ciprofloxacin does have an oral formulation but does not have reliable activity against MRSA. All other agents are I.V. only.

11. **D.** Baseline and weekly CPK levels should be drawn when patients are initiated on daptomycin therapy. Daptomycin therapy should be discontinued when CPK levels reach 5 times the upper limit of normal when patients are symptomatic (myalgias) or 10 times the upper limit of normal when patients are asymptomatic. Close monitoring should be performed when patients are on concomitant statin therapy.

12. **C.** Vancomycin trough concentration targets of 15 to 20 mcg/mL are now recommended for the majority of vancomycin treatment indications for MRSA with the exception of skin and soft tissue infections, which require lower targets (10 to 15 mcg/mL). The AUC/MIC target for vancomycin is 400 to 600 mcg*h/mL, higher exposures are associated with nephrotoxicity.

13. **E.** Levofloxacin displays broad-spectrum activity against both pneumococci and *P. aeruginosa*. In contrast, ciprofloxacin does not display reliable activity against pneumococci, and moxifloxacin does not display reliable activity against *P. aeruginosa*. Trimethoprim-sulfamethoxazole and daptomycin do not cover *P. aeruginosa*.

14. **A.** Absorption and drug concentrations can be greatly reduced by the concomitant administration of divalent and trivalent cations that bind fluoroquinolone (and tetracycline) antibiotics. Administration of these cations should be separated from fluoroquinolone and tetracycline dosing by at least 2 hours (some sources suggest 2 hours before and 4 hours after antibiotic dose). This patient counseling point can reduce the chances of treatment failure.

15. **C.** Fluconazole (and also trimethoprim/sulfamethoxazole) is a significant CYP2C9 inhibitor and can considerably increase INR levels when given concomitantly with warfarin. Other drugs listed display only minor risk of INR elevations.

16. **C.** Carbapenems such as meropenem are drugs of choice for systemic ESBL infections. Newer cephalosporin agents such as ceftazidime/avibactam and ceftolozane/tazobactam also display activity against ESBL isolates.

17. **E.** The 3 oral antibiotics commonly used to treat community-acquired MRSA skin and soft tissue infections include doxycycline, clindamycin, and sulfamethoxazole-trimethoprim.

18. **A.** Although all antibiotics can cause *C. difficile* infection, clindamycin's spectrum of activity covers many anaerobes except those for *C. difficile*. For this reason, it is commonly implicated as a predisposing factor for *C. difficile* infection.

19. **D.** Metronidazole displays a purely anaerobic spectrum of activity and is a drug of choice for one of the main gram-negative anaerobes, *B. fragilis*, which is typically located in the lower gastrointestinal tract.

20. **B.** Colistin is a polymyxin antibiotic that can be used for multidrug resistant gram-negative pathogens such as *P. aeruginosa* and *Acinetobacter* spp. Its main limiting side effect is significant nephrotoxicity, and it should be reserved for severe or multidrug-resistant infections.

21. **B.** Fluconazole is a drug of choice for *C. albicans*, yet it does not effectively cover some non–*Candida albicans* species, including *C. glabrata* or *C. krusei*. Although fluconazole can display dose-dependent

susceptibility for some *C. glabrata,* it is inherently resistant to *C. krusei.*

22. A. Echinocandins are drugs of choice for disseminated candidiasis caused by non–*C. albicans* or fluconazole-resistant *Candida* spp. Echinocandins are often initiated as empiric therapy for disseminated candidiasis until the fungal species is known by culture.

23. E. Voriconazole is an I.V. and oral antifungal agent that is commonly used to treat *Aspergillus* spp.

24. A. Isoniazid daily therapy is the preferred regimen for latent TB infection. Patients should be supplemented with pyridoxine and should avoid alcoholic beverages while taking isoniazid.

25. A. An important patient counseling point for patients being administered rifampin is to be aware of discoloration of body fluids such as tears, sweat, and saliva. Patients who wear contact lenses, for example, should be notified that the lenses may be permanently discolored.

34-20 Additional Resources

Bennett, J, Dolin R, Blaser MJ, eds. *Mandell, Douglas, and Bennett's Principles and Practice of Infectious Diseases.* 9th ed. New York, NY: Elsevier; 2019.

Lewis RE. Current concepts in antifungal pharmacology. *Mayo Clin Proc.* 2011;86(8):805–817.

Liu C, Bayer A, Cosgrove SE, et al. Clinical practice guidelines by the Infectious Diseases Society of America for the treatment of methicillin-resistant *Staphylococcus aureus* infection in adults and children. *Clin Infect Dis.* 2011;52:285–292.

Payam N, Dorman SE, Alipanah N, et al. Official American Thoracic Society/Centers for Disease Control and Prevention/Infectious Diseases Society of America Clinical Practice Guidelines: treatment of drug-susceptible tuberculosis. *Clin Infect Dis.* 2016;63(7):e147–e195.

Human Immunodeficiency Virus and the Acquired Immune Deficiency Syndrome

35

DREW L. ARMSTRONG

 35-1 KEY POINTS

- Human immunodeficiency virus (HIV) is a virus that destroys the immune system.
- Acquired immune deficiency syndrome (AIDS) is caused by HIV and is defined as a CD4 cell count less than 200/mm³ or the presence of an opportunistic infection.
- Acute HIV infection occurs within the first 2 to 4 weeks of infection with HIV and presents as nonspecific flu-like symptoms.
- The viral load indicates the amount of virus in the body and is an indication of how well antiretroviral medications are working.
- The CD4 cell count refers to the status of the immune system and a patient's degree of risk for developing an opportunistic infection.
- Nucleoside reverse transcriptase inhibitors (NRTIs), nonnucleoside reverse transcriptase inhibitors (NNRTIs), protease inhibitors (PIs), entry inhibitors (fusion inhibitors, chemokine [C-C motif] receptor 5 [CCR5] antagonists), postattachment inhibitors, and integrase strand transfer inhibitors (INSTIs) are the currently available classes of medications used to treat HIV.
- First-line regimens for HIV contain 1 or 2 NRTIs and an INSTI
- Vertical transmission is prevented by treating the mother with combination antiretroviral regimens.
- *Pneumocystis jiroveci* pneumonia requires primary prophylaxis at a CD4 cell count <200/mm³. Trimethoprim-sulfamethoxazole is the preferred treatment.
- *Mycobacterium avium* complex no longer requires primary prophylaxis in those that immediately initiate antiretroviral therapy (ART).
- All other opportunistic infections require treatment followed by secondary prophylaxis.

 35-2 STUDY GUIDE CHECKLIST

The following topics may guide your study of this subject area:

- ☐ Class side effects of NRTIs, NNRTIs, PIs, INSTIs.
- ☐ Medications that contain sulfa.
- ☐ Medications that need normal gastric pH for absorption.
- ☐ Medications that are contraindicated with PIs and NNRTIs.
- ☐ Medications that inhibit CYP3A.
- ☐ When HIV medication should be started.
- ☐ Preferred treatment regimens for HIV-naïve patients.
- ☐ Opportunistic infections that require primary prophylaxis.
- ☐ Preferred treatments for most common opportunistic infections.
- ☐ When to start postexposure prophylaxis (PEP) for occupational and nonoccupational exposures.
- ☐ Preferred regimen for PEP for occupational and nonoccupational exposures.
- ☐ Pre-exposure prophylaxis (PrEP) regimens.
- ☐ Preferred regimens to prevent mother-to-child transmission.

Editor's Note: This chapter is based on the 11th edition chapter written by Camille W. Thornton.

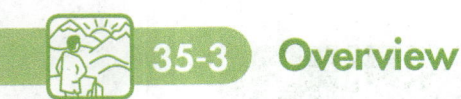

35-3 Overview

Human immunodeficiency virus (HIV) is a retrovirus that depletes the helper T-lymphocytes (CD4 cells), resulting in continued destruction of the immune system and subsequent gradual development of opportunistic infections and malignancies. See Box 35-1 for clinical presentation of HIV and Box 35-2 for testing recommendations. Box 35-3 lists common transmission methods.

Acquired immune deficiency syndrome (AIDS) is HIV with a CD4 cell count lower than 200 cells/mm³ or a history of opportunistic infection (e.g., *Pneumocystis jiroveci* pneumonia, toxoplasmosis, cryptococcal meningitis, histoplasmosis, *Mycobacterium avium*).

Monitoring Tools

Viral load

Viral load testing measures the amount of virus in blood. It can assess disease progression and evaluate the efficacy of antiretroviral therapy (ART). The goal of HIV treatment is to achieve and maintain an undetectable viral load. This is considered to be a viral load <200 copies/mL, although some ultrasensitive assays have a lower limit of detection of <20 copies/mL.

Acute illness and immunizations can cause increases in viral load for 2 to 4 weeks. Testing should not be performed during this time.

BOX 35-1. HIV Clinical Presentation

- Patient has an opportunistic infection and subsequently tests positive for HIV.
- Patient is not ill but has tested positive for HIV.
- Patient has acute retroviral syndrome:
  - Of patients acutely infected with HIV, 50% to 90% experience some of the symptoms.
  - Symptoms generally appear 2 to 4 weeks after virus exposure.
  - Duration of the clinical syndrome is about 14 days (the range is a few days to >10 weeks).
  - The disease is not readily recognized in the primary care setting because its symptoms are similar to those of the flu, mononucleosis, and other common illnesses.

BOX 35-2. Testing Recommendations from U.S. Centers for Disease Control and Prevention

- Perform routine, voluntary, opt-out HIV screening for all persons 13 to 64 years of age in health care settings. Testing is not based on risk factors.
- Perform HIV screening of pregnant women as part of the routine panel of prenatal screening tests. Testing is not based on risk factors.
- Repeat HIV screening of persons with known risk at least annually
  - Injection drug users and their sex partners
  - Persons who exchange sex for money or drugs
  - Sex partners of HIV-infected persons
  - Men who have sex with men
  - Heterosexual persons who themselves or whose sex partners have had more than 1 sex partner since their most recent HIV test

> ### BOX 35-3. Common Routes of HIV Transmission
>
> Transmission is through infected blood or hazardous body fluids, which can occur during the following activities:
>
> - Unprotected sexual contact with an infected person
>   - Multiple partners increase risk.
>   - Ongoing or past medical history of sexually transmitted disease increases risk.
> - Sharing of needles or syringes with an infected person
> - Transfusions of infected blood or blood clotting factors (the United States began screening the blood supply in 1985)
> - Vertical transmission (infected mother to infant)
> - Breast-feeding
>
> Occupational exposure and household contact are rare.

Monitoring of viral load in patients not on ART should occur every 3 to 4 months. Monitoring of viral load in patients starting a new regimen should occur 2 to 8 weeks after treatment initiation and then every 3 to 4 months.

CD4 cell count

CD4 cell count indicates the extent of immune system damage and the risk of developing opportunistic infections. Normal CD4 cell count is 800 to 1200 cells/mm^3.

CD4 cell count should be measured every 3 to 6 months in patients on or off ART. In clinically stable patients with suppressed viral load, CD4 cell count can be monitored every 6 to 12 months.

Resistance testing

Genotypes should be performed to determine if resistance to medications is present. Testing should be done on all patients before starting the first treatment regimen and whenever viral loads are persistently >500 to 1000 copies/mL and the patient is currently on medications for HIV or has taken them in the past 4 weeks before testing.

Treatment Principles and Goals

Goals of therapy

Therapy has the following goals:

- Maximal and durable suppression of viral load
- Restoration or preservation of immunologic function
- Improvement in quality of life
- Reduction of HIV-related morbidity and mortality
- Prevention of HIV transmission

Factors involved in achieving goals of therapy are as follows:

- Adherence to the antiretroviral regimen
- Performance of pretreatment drug resistance testing
- Selection of individualized initial combination regimen

Guidelines for prevention and treatment and medications used for the treatment of HIV can be located as a living document at https://clinicalinfo.hiv.gov/en/guidelines, which is updated regularly.

35-4   Drug Therapy

Tables 35-1 and 35-2 list antiretroviral agents recommended by the U.S. Department of Health and Human Services for initial treatment of established HIV infection.

Nucleoside Reverse Transcriptase Inhibitors ⚠

Commonly used nucleoside reverse transcriptase inhibitors (NRTIs) are described in Table 35-3 (not all inclusive). The mechanism of action of NRTIs is to interfere with HIV viral ribonucleic acid (RNA)–dependent deoxyribonucleic acid (DNA) polymerase, resulting in chain termination and inhibition of viral replication.

Didanosine (ddI), stavudine (d4T), and lamivudine (3TC) are dosed on the basis of weight. Most NRTIs are not affected by food (except didanosine). NRTIs have a low pill burden as a class and few drug interactions. All are prodrugs requiring 2 or 3 phosphorylations for activation. See Box 35-4 for five common NRTIs.

TABLE 35-1. Recommended First-Line Regimens for Initiation of Antiretrovirals

Regimen	Brand	Comments
Bictegravir/TAF/emtrictabine	Biktarvy	
Dolutegravir/abacavir/lamivudine	Triumeq	Only in patients who are HLA-B*5701 negative
Dolutegravir + TAF/emtricitabine or TDF/emtricitabine		
Raltegravir + TAF/emtricitabine or TDF/emtricitabine		
Dolutegravir/lamivudine	Dovato	Not for patients with VL >500,000 copies/mL, HBV co-infection

HBV, hepatitis B virus; TAF, tenofovir alafenamide; TDF, tenofovir disoproxil fumarate; VL, viral load.

TABLE 35-2. Alternative Regimens for Initiation of Antiretrovirals

Regimen	Brand	Comments
Elvitegravir/cobicistat/TAF/emtricitabine or TDF/emtricitabine	Stribild (TDF) Genvoya (TAF)	Stribild only in patients with pretreatment CrCl of >70 mL/min
Darunavir/cobicistat or ritonavir + TAF/emtricitabine or TDF/emtricitabine		
Atazanavir/cobicistat or ritonavir + TAF/emtricitabine or TDF/emtricitabine		
Darunavir/cobicistat or ritonavir + abacavir/lamivudine		Only in patients who are HLA-B*5701 negative
Doravirine/TDF/lamivudine	Delstrigo	
Efavirenz/TDF or TAF/emtricitabine or lamivudine	Atripla Symfi Symfi Lo	
Rilpivirine/TDF or TAF/emtricitabine	Complera (TDF) Odefsey (TAF)	Only in patients with pretreatment VL <100,000 and CD4 >200

CrCl, creatinine clearance; TAF, tenofovir alafenamide; TDF, tenofovir disoproxil fumarate; VL, viral load.

TABLE 35-3. Commonly Used Nucleoside Reverse Transcriptase Inhibitors

Characteristic	Lamivudine (3TC)[a]	Abacavir (ABC)[a]	Tenofovir (TDF)[a]	Tenofovir alafenamide (TAF)[a]	Emtricitabine (FTC)[a]
Trade name	Epivir	Ziagen	Viread	(currently not available)	Emtriva
Form	Capsule, tablet, oral solution Combination: Delstrigo (Doravirine/TDF/emtricitabine); Symfi/Symfi Lo (efavirenz/TDF/lamivudine); Epzicom (abacavir/lamivudine); Combivir (lamivudine/zidovudine); Trizivir (abacavir/lamivudine/zidovudine)	Tablet, oral solution Combination: Epzicom (abacavir/lamivudine); Trizivir (abacavir/lamivudine/zidovudine); Triumeq (abacavir/lamivudine/dolutegravir)	Tablet, oral powder Combination: Truvada (tenofovir/emtricitabine); Atripla (tenofovir/emtricitabine/efavirenz); Stribild (tenofovir/emtricitabine/elvitegravir/cobicistat); Complera (tenofovir/emtricitabine/rilpivirine); Delstrigo (Doravirine/TDF/emtricitabine); Symfi/Symfi Lo (efavirenz/TDF/lamivudine)	— Combination: Descovy (TAF/emtricitabine); Genvoya (TAF/emtricitabine/elvitegravir/cobicistat); Odefsey (TAF/emtricitabine/rilpivirine); Biktarvy (TAF/emtricitabine/bictegravir); Symtuza (darunavir/cobicistat/TAF/emtricitabine)	Tablet, oral solution Combination: Truvada (tenofovir/emtricitabine); Atripla (tenofovir/emtricitabine/efavirenz); Stribild (tenofovir/emtricitabine/elvitegravir/cobicistat); Complera (tenofovir/emtricitabine/rilpivirine); Biktarvy (TAF/emtricitabine/bictegravir); Symtuza (darunavir/cobicistat/TAF/emtricitabine)
Dosing	150 mg twice daily or 300 mg daily; Epzicom: daily; Combivir: twice daily; Trizivir: twice daily; Delstrigo: once daily; Symfi/Symfi Lo: once daily on empty stomach	300 mg twice daily or 600 mg daily; Epzicom: daily; Trizivir: twice daily; Triumeq: daily	300 mg daily; Truvada: daily; Atripla: daily on an empty stomach; Stribild: daily with food; Complera: daily with largest meal; Delstrigo: once daily; Symfi/Symfi Lo: once daily on empty stomach	Descovy: daily; Genvoya: daily with food; Odefsey: daily with largest meal; Biktarvy: daily; Symtuza: daily with food	Tablet: 200 mg daily; oral solution: 240 mg daily; Truvada: daily; Atripla: daily on empty stomach; Stribild: daily with food; Complera: daily with largest meal; Biktarvy: daily; Symtuza: daily with food
Food	Take without regard to meals.	Take without regard to meals.	Take without regard to meals except where noted above.	Take without regard to meals except where noted above.	Take without regard to meals except where noted above.
Adverse effects	Exacerbation of HBV in co-infected patients who discontinue lamivudine	Hypersensitivity reaction (test for HLA-B*5701 before initiation); some cohort studies suggest increased risk of myocardial infarction, but this has not been substantiated in other studies.	Renal insufficiency; Fanconi syndrome, osteomalacia, potential decrease in bone mineral density; exacerbation of HBV in co-infected patients who discontinue tenofovir	Renal insufficiency, Fanconi syndrome, osteomalacia, potential decrease in bone mineral density	Hyperpigmentation or skin discoloration; exacerbation of HBV in co-infected patients who discontinue emtricitabine
Drug interactions	No clinically significant drug interactions	Alcohol increases abacavir levels by 41%.	Didanosine, atazanavir, cidofovir, ganciclovir, valganciclovir, telaprevir	Not yet evaluated	No clinically significant drug interactions
Monitoring	None necessary.	Signs and symptoms of hypersensitivity reaction	Renal function	Renal function	None necessary

HBV, hepatitis B virus.
a. Monitor for signs and symptoms of NRTI class toxicities, lactic acidosis, and hepatic steatosis.

Nucleoside Reverse Transcriptase Inhibitors (NRTIs) *FDA BOXED WARNING*

NRTIs have increased risk of lactic acidosis and severe hepatomegaly with steatosis.

> **BOX 35-4. Five NRTI Combination Products**

- Combivir (zidovudine 300 mg + lamivudine 150 mg) every 12 hours
- Trizivir (zidovudine 300 mg + lamivudine 150 mg + abacavir 300 mg) every 12 hours
- Truvada (tenofovir disoproxil fumarate 300 mg + emtricitabine 200 mg) every 24 hours
- Descovy (tenofovir alafenamide [TAF] 25 mg + emtricitabine 200 mg) every 24 hours
- Epzicom (lamivudine 300 mg + abacavir 600 mg) every 24 hours

No special storage requirements are necessary for drugs in this class.

Usually, 2 NRTIs are used in combination with 1 nonnucleoside reverse transcriptase inhibitor (NNRTI), 1 protease inhibitor (PI), or 1 integrase strand transfer inhibitor (INSTI).

All NRTIs have a boxed warning concerning the following class toxicities:

- Lactic acidosis
- Severe hepatomegaly with steatosis

The following precautions should be kept in mind regarding NRTIs:

- Most patients should be dose adjusted for renal impairment (exception: abacavir).
- Lamivudine and emtricitabine are chemically similar and should not be used in the same regimen.
- Do not use zidovudine with stavudine because of antagonism (both require thymidine for activation).
- Do not use didanosine with stavudine during pregnancy because of increased risk of lactic acidosis and liver damage.
- Tenofovir increases didanosine levels and decreases atazanavir levels. Dosage adjustments are required.
- Patients should be tested for HLA-B*5701 to determine risk for hypersensitivity reaction to abacavir. Only patients testing negative should start abacavir.
- The "D" drugs (ddI and d4T) can cause pancreatitis and peripheral neuropathy; when used together, this effect can be additive. These drugs are more closely associated with lactic acidosis.

Non-nucleoside Reverse Transcriptase Inhibitors

NNRTIs are described in Table 35-4. Their mechanism of action is to competitively inhibit reverse transcriptase, thereby resulting in inhibition of HIV replication.

All should be dose adjusted for hepatic impairment.

Efavirenz should be taken on an empty stomach. Rilpivirine should be taken with the largest meal of the day. Efavirenz should be avoided in the first trimester of pregnancy but can be continued if adequate viral suppression is already achieved (increased risk of neural tube defects). Usually, 1 NNRTI is used in combination with 2 NRTIs.

No special storage requirements are necessary for drugs in this class. Class toxicities include rash and hepatic toxicity. See Box 35-5 for single-tablet regimens with NNRTI included.

TABLE 35-4. Commonly Used Nonnucleoside Reverse Transcriptase Inhibitors

Characteristic	Efavirenz (EFV)[a]	Nevirapine (NVP)[a]	Rilpivirine (RPV)[a]	Etravirine (ETR)[a]
Trade name	Sustiva	Viramune	Edurant	Intelence
Form	Capsule, tablet	Tablet, XR tablet, oral suspension	Tablet	Tablet
	Combination: Atripla (tenofovir/emtricitabine/efavirenz)		Combination: Complera (tenofovir/emtricitabine/rilpivirine); Odefsey (TAF/emtricitabine/rilpivirine)	
	Symfi/Symfi Lo (TDF/lamivudine/efavirenz)			
Dosing	600 mg daily on empty stomach; Atripla, Symfi, Symfi Lo: daily on empty stomach	200 mg daily × 14 days, then 200 mg twice daily or 400 mg XR daily	25 mg daily with largest meal; Complera: daily with largest meal; Odefsey: daily with largest meal	200 mg twice daily
Food	Take on empty stomach to reduce side effects.	Take without regard to meals.	Take with largest meal.	Take following a meal.
Adverse effects	CNS side effects, rash, increase in LFTs	Rash (including SJS) hepatotoxicity	Rash, depression, insomnia, prolonged QT interval	Rash (including SJS)
Drug interactions	CYP2B6 and 3A4 substrate	CYP450 substrate	CYP3A4 substrate	CYP3A4, 2C9, and 2C19 substrate
	CYP3A4 mixed inducer/inhibitor	CYP3A4 and 2B6 inducer	Requires acidic environment; contraindicated with PPIs: space administration from H2RAs and antacids.	CYP3A4 inducer; CYP2C9 and 2C19 inhibitor
	Avoid use with carbamazepine, itraconazole, ketoconazole, posaconazole, simeprevir, St. John's wort (not inclusive list).	Avoid use with atazanavir, carbamazepine, dolutegravir, itraconazole, ketoconazole, rifampin, St. John's wort (list is not inclusive).	CI with strong CYP3A4 inducers and PPIs	Avoid use with **clopidogrel**, carbamazepine, phenobarbital, phenytoin, rifampin, St. John's wort (list is not inclusive)
Monitoring	CNS side effects,[b] LFTs, rash	LFTs	LFTs, rash, QT interval	LFTs, rash

Boldface indicates one of top 100 drugs for 2020 by prescription volume.
CI, contraindication; CNS, central nervous system; H2RA, histamine 2–receptor antagonist; LFT, liver function test; PPI, proton pump inhibitor; SJS, Stevens–Johnson syndrome; XR, extended release.
a. Monitor for signs and symptoms of NNRTI class toxicities, rash, and hepatic toxicity.
b. CNS side effects include dizziness, somnolence, insomnia, abnormal dreams, confusion, abnormal thinking, impaired concentration, amnesia, agitation, depersonalization, hallucinations, and euphoria. Use caution in patients with a psychiatric history or previous addictions.

> ### BOX 35-5. Single-Tablet Regimens with NNRTI Included
>
> - Atripla (tenofovir 300 mg + emtricitabine 200 mg + efavirenz 600 mg) every 24 hours
> - Complera (tenofovir 300 mg + emtricitabine 200 mg + rilpivirine 25 mg) every 24 hours
> - Odefsey (tenofovir alafenamide 25 mg + emtricitabine 200 mg + rilpivirine 25 mg) every 24 hours
> - Delstrigo (tenofovir 300 mg + lamivudine 300 mg + doravirine 100 mg) every 24 hours
> - Symfi (tenofovir 300 mg + lamivudine 300 mg + efavirenz 600 mg) every 24 hours
> - Symfi Lo (tenofovir 300 mg + lamivudine 300 mg + efavirenz 400 mg) every 24 hours
> - Juluca (rilpivirine 25 mg + dolutegravir 50 mg) every 24 hours

Drug interactions can occur. All are cytochrome P450 (CYP) 3A4 inducers or inhibitors. Many are also inducers or inhibitors or are metabolized via other CYP pathways. Rilpivirine requires normal acid levels in the stomach for absorption. Class side effects include rash and elevations in liver enzymes.

Protease Inhibitors

Commonly used PIs are described in Table 35-5 (not all inclusive). Their mechanism of action is to inhibit protease, which then prevents the cleavage of HIV polyproteins and subsequently induces the formation of immature noninfectious viral particles.

All PIs should be dose adjusted for hepatic impairment. Most should be taken with food (except fosamprenavir, tipranavir, lopinavir/ritonavir tablets, and indinavir). Atazanavir and indinavir require normal acid levels in the stomach for absorption and are associated with kidney stone formation and increases in indirect bilirubin. Darunavir, fosamprenavir, and tipranavir contain sulfa. Caution is warranted for patients with a history of severe sulfa allergies.

Most PIs are CYP3A4 inhibitors. Ritonavir is the most potent inhibitor in the class and is primarily used for intensification "boosting" of other PIs. The following medications are contraindicated to be given with PIs: alfuzosin, ergot derivatives, flecainide, **lovastatin**, rifampin, sildenafil (when given for pulmonary hypertension), **simvastatin**, St. John's wort, and propafenone. Use caution with other medications that are metabolized via the CYP pathways (e.g., phosphodiesterase-5 inhibitors, statins, azole antibiotics, methadone, hormonal contraceptives), and always use drug interaction tools with regard to patients receiving PIs.

Lopinavir/ritonavir solution and tipranavir should be refrigerated.

Goals of boosting are as follows:

- Decrease pill burden.
- Decrease frequency of doses (i.e., decrease from every 8 to 12 hours).
- Increase drug levels, resulting in decreased resistance.

Baseline PI monitoring is done 4 to 6 weeks after starting the PI. Monitoring should then occur every 3 to 6 months thereafter. See Box 35-6 for PI toxicities and Box 35-7 for required lab monitoring.

Usually, 1 PI (boosted PIs preferred) is used in combination with 2 NRTIs. There is 1 STR with a medication from this class

- Symtuza (tenofovir alafenamide 10 mg + emtricitabine 200 mg + darunavir 800 mg + cobicistat 150 mg) every 24 hours

Entry Inhibitors

Entry inhibitors include enfuvirtide (T20) and maraviroc. Enfuvirtide is a fusion inhibitor, whereas maraviroc is a CCR5 (chemokine [C-C motif] receptor 5) antagonist. See Table 35-6 for information.

TABLE 35-5. Commonly Used Protease Inhibitors

Characteristic	Atazanavir[a]	Darunavir[a]	Ritonavir[a]	Fosamprenavir[a]	Lopinavir/Ritonavir[a]
Trade name	Reyataz	Prezista	Norvir	Lexiva	Kaletra
Form	Capsules	Tablets, liquid	Tablets, liquid	Tablets	Tablets
Dosing	300 mg orally once daily (with booster), or two 200 mg orally once daily (without booster)	600 mg orally twice daily (with booster) or 800 mg orally once daily (with booster)	Only used as a booster with other PIs	Two 700 mg tablets orally twice daily (without booster), or two 700 mg tablets orally once daily (with booster), or 700 mg tablets orally twice daily (with booster)	4 tablets (200 mg/50 g) once daily or 2 tablets twice daily (dependent on lopinavir resistance)
	Combination: with 150 mg cobicistat (Evotaz) once daily	Combination: with 150 mg cobicistat (Prezcobix) once daily; Symtuza (darunavir/cobicistat/TAF/emtricitabine)			
Food	Take with food.	Take with food.	Take with food.	Take with or without food.	Take with or without food.
Adverse effects	Skin rash, indirect hyperbilirubinemia, prolonged PR interval, increased LFTs	Skin rash, Stevens–Johnson syndrome (contains sulfa moiety), increased LFTs	GI intolerance, paresthesias, increased LFTs	GI intolerance, skin rash (contains sulfa moiety), increased LFTs, nephrolithiasis	GI intolerance, increased LFTs, prolonged QT, pancreatitis
Drug interactions	Requires normal stomach acidity (PPI, H2RA, antacids), metabolized by CYP3A	CYP3A4 substrate and inhibitor	CYP3A4 and 2D6 substrate and inhibitor	CYP3A4 substrate, inhibitor, and inducer	CYP3A4 and 2D6 (ritonavir portion) substrate and inhibitor
Monitoring	LFTs, glucose	LFTs, glucose, skin rash	LFTs, glucose	LFTs, glucose	LFTs, glucose

GI, gastrointestinal; H2RA, histamine 2–receptor antagonist; LFT, liver function test; PPI, proton pump inhibitor.

a. Class side effects of all PIs: hyperlipidemia, particularly hypertriglyceridemia, hyperglycemia, fat maldistribution, possible increased bleeding episodes in patients with hemophilia.

> **BOX 35-6. Protease Inhibitor Class Toxicities**

- Fat maldistribution
- Hyperglycemia
- Hyperlipidemia
- Possible increased bleeding episodes in patients with hemophilia

> **BOX 35-7. Protease Inhibitor Required Lab Monitoring**

- Glucose test
- Liver function tests (LFTs)
- Total cholesterol panel (particularly triglycerides)
- Signs and symptoms of gastrointestinal (GI) side effects
- Signs and symptoms of fat redistribution

Enfuvirtide (T20) (Fuzeon)

Enfuvirtide's mechanism of action is to bind to glycoprotein 41 on the HIV surface, thus inhibiting HIV binding to the CD4 cell. Side effects include injection-site reactions, an increased rate of bacterial pneumonia, and hypersensitivity.

Enfuvirtide is generally reserved for deep salvage regimens. Preferably, it should be used with at least 2 other active drugs. Resistance develops quickly with less potent regimens and in cases of poor adherence.

No known significant drug interactions have been seen to date. Enfuvirtide can be taken without regard to meals. It should be stored at room temperature; the reconstituted form should be stored in the refrigerator, where it will be stable for 24 hours.

TABLE 35-6. Entry Inhibitors

Characteristic	Maraviroc	Enfuvirtide
Trade name	Selzentry	Fuzeon
Form	Tablets	Injection
Dosing	150 mg orally twice daily (if given with certain strong CYP inhibitors)	90 mg injection twice daily
	300 mg orally twice daily (without strong CYP inhibitors or inducers)	
	600 mg orally twice daily (if given with certain strong CYP inducers)	
Food	Take with or without food.	Take with or without food.
Adverse effects	Hepatotoxicity, rash, fever, cough, abdominal pain	Local injection site reactions
Drug interactions	Avoid use with St. John's wort. Dose is adjusted dependent on CYP inducers and inhibitors.	None currently identified
Monitoring	Tropism test, rash	Injection site reactions

CYP, cytochrome P.

Maraviroc (Selzentry)

Maraviroc's mechanism of action is to bind to CCR5 receptors on the CD4 cell surface, which inhibits HIV binding and entry into the CD4 cell.

Perform Trofile testing before using maraviroc to determine the patient's tropism. The patient must be CCR5 tropic only.

Maraviroc is a CYP3A4 substrate. The dose depends on drug reactions

- Use 150 mg orally every 12 hours when giving maraviroc with strong CYP3A4 inhibitors (most PIs).
- Use 300 mg orally every 12 hours when giving maraviroc with enfuvirtide, tipranavir/ritonavir, nevirapine, or weak CYP3A4 inhibitors.
- Use 600 mg orally every 12 hours when giving with CYP3A4 inducers (efavirenz, rifampin, etc.).

Side effects include abdominal pain, cough, dizziness, musculoskeletal symptoms, pyrexia, rash, upper respiratory tract infections, hepatotoxicity, and orthostatic hypotension.

Preferably, use maraviroc with at least 2 other active drugs. Take it without regard to meals.

Postattachment Inhibitor

Ibalizumab-uiyk (Trogarzo) is a monoclonal antibody that blocks HIV from infecting CD4 cells by inhibiting the interaction of gp120 and HIV coreceptors. It is active against CCR5 and CXCR4 isolates.

Ibalizumab-uiyk is an intravenous (I.V.) infusion that consists of a 2000 mg loading dose followed by 800 mg maintenance doses every 2 weeks.

Side effects include primarily infusion site reactions. The infusion rate can be slowed to prevent these from occurring during subsequent administrations.

Integrase Strand Transfer Inhibitors

INSTIs include raltegravir (Isentress), dolutegravir (Tivicay), elvitegravir, and bictegravir. (Table 35-7). INSTIs block activity of the integrase enzyme, thereby preventing HIV DNA from meshing with the CD4 cell DNA. INSTIs chelate with polyvalent cations and should be separated from medications that contain them.

Raltegravir is metabolized through UDP-glucuronosyltransferase 1A1 (UGT1A1)-mediated glucuronidation. Drug interactions occur with rifampin and other drugs that affect UGT1A1. There are 2 dosing

TABLE 35-7. Integrase Strand Transfer Inhibitors

Characteristic	Raltegravir	Elvitegravir	Dolutegravir
Trade name	Isentress		Tivicay
Form	Tablet, oral liquid		Tablet
Dosing	400 mg orally twice daily or two 600 mg tablets once daily (Isentress HD)		50 mg orally once daily
Food	Take with or without food.		Take with or without food.
Adverse effects	Headache, insomnia, increase in CPK		Headache; insomnia; possible increase in SCr (no change to GFR), increase in CPK, increase in LFTs
Drug interactions	Give 2 hours before or 6 hours after polyvalent cations. Drug is metabolized by UGT1A1. Avoid giving with rifampin.		Give 2 hours before or 6 hours after polyvalent cations.
Monitoring	CPK, LFTs	CPK, LFTs	CPK, LFTs

CPK, creatinine phosphokinase; GFR, glomerular filtration rate; SCr, serum creatinine; UGT1A1, UDP-glucuronosyltransferase 1A1.

strategies: 400 mg orally every 12 hours or two 600 mg tablets once daily (Isentress HD). Side effects include nausea, headache, diarrhea, pyrexia, and creatinine phosphokinase (CPK) elevation. Take it without regard to meals.

Dolutegravir is metabolized through UGT1A1 and, to a minor extent, CYP3A. It inhibits the organic cation transporter 2 (OCT2) renal transporter; therefore, mild elevations in serum creatinine may be seen. Drug interactions occur with **metformin** and other drugs that are eliminated through the OCT2 renal transporter and with medications that are strong inhibitors or inducers of UGT1A1 (rifampin) or CYP3A (nevirapine, fosamprenavir/ritonavir, tipranavir/ritonavir, anticonvulsants). Data exist potentially linking neural tube defects with dolutegravir initiation in the first trimester of pregnancy. Discussion with the patient is recommended before any attempt to conceive.

Elvitegravir is metabolized through UGT1A1/3 and CYP3A enzymes. It is only commercially available as part of the single tablet regimes (STRs) Stribild and Genvoya.

Bictegravir is metabolized through UGT1A1 and CYP3A enzymes. Drug interactions occur with medications that are strong inhibitors or inducers of UGT1A1 (rifampin) or CYP3A (nevirapine, fosamprenavir/ritonavir, tipranavir/ritonavir, anticonvulsants). It is only commercially available as part of the STR Biktarvy.

When to Start Antiretrovirals

Current recommendations are for all persons with HIV to start antiretrovirals regardless of CD4 count. The Strategic Timing of Antiretroviral Treatment (START) study reported overwhelming mortality and morbidity benefits for both HIV and non-HIV associated diseases with earlier initiation of antiretrovirals. Emerging evidence supports "rapid initiation" of ART, which could even be as soon as the same day as diagnosis.

Counseling

All patients should be counseled on the importance of adherence. Greater than 95% adherence is necessary to decrease the incidence of resistance. Patients should be given tools to facilitate adherence to complicated regimens (e.g., pillboxes, calendars, pagers).

Patients should be counseled on class side effects especially any that are unique or potentially serious. Patients should also be counseled concerning important drug interactions (prescription, over-the-counter, herbal, vitamin, natural remedies) that could affect their regimen (e.g., proton pump inhibitors, H2 blockers, antacids with atazanavir and rilpivirine, polyvalent cations with integrase inhibitors) and any food requirements or restrictions.

Antiretroviral Therapy in the HIV-Infected Pregnant Woman

All pregnant HIV-infected women should receive combination antiretroviral regimens to prevent perinatal transmission regardless of viral load or CD4 cell count. Preferred regimens include 2 nucleosides (abacavir/lamivudine, tenofovir and emtricitabine or lamivudine, or zidovudine/lamivudine) combined with a boosted PI (atazanavir/ritonavir or lopinavir/ritonavir) or NNRTI (efavirenz, which may be initiated after 8 weeks of pregnancy). Transmission rates can be reduced to less than 1% in women treated with combination therapy, and undetectable viral loads can be maintained for the majority of the pregnancy. If possible, regimens should given during labor and delivery. Intravenous zidovudine during labor is now recommended only if the viral load of the woman is above 1000 copies/mL at delivery time. The 6-week neonatal component of the zidovudine chemoprophylaxis regimen is generally recommended for all HIV-exposed neonates to reduce perinatal transmission of HIV.

Guidelines for prevention of vertical transmission can be located as a living document at https://clinicalinfo.hiv.gov/en/guidelines, which is updated regularly.

Post- and Preexposure Prophylaxis

Postexposure prophylaxis

Universal precautions should be taken. The most common infectious exposure is through needlesticks or cuts (1 in 300 risk). The risk with mucous membrane exposure is much lower (1 in 1000 risk).

Postexposure prophylaxis (PEP) can reduce HIV infection by about 80%. Start therapy within 72 hours of exposure. The length of therapy is 4 weeks. The preferred treatment regimen is with tenofovir/emtricitabine and raltegravir. Guidelines for PEP can be located as a living document at https://hivinfo.nih.gov/, which is updated regularly.

Patients with exposure to HIV through a known positive source, such as sexual exposure or injection drug use, should receive nonoccupational PEP (nPEP) within 72 hours of the exposure. The length of therapy is 28 days.

Preexposure Prophylaxis (PrEP)

After exposure to HIV through sex or injection drug use, Truvada (tenofovir and emtricitabine) and Descovy (TAF and emtricitabine) can reduce the risk of permanent infection by 92% when taken daily and consistently. Descovy is the only currently FDA-approved medication for PrEP in cisgender males and transgender females (assigned male sex at birth). There is no data for PrEP use in cisgender females with Descovy. Additional information is available at https://www.cdc.gov/hiv/risk/prep/.

Opportunistic Infections

Only 2 opportunistic infections require primary prophylaxis:

- **Pneumocystis jiroveci *pneumonia (PCP):*** Treatment is required when CD4 cell count falls below 200/mm^3. The treatment of choice is trimethoprim-sulfamethoxazole (TMP-SMX) DS oral daily (see Table 35-8 for alternatives).
- **Mycobacterium avium *complex (MAC) bacteremia:*** Treatment is only required in those not immediately starting ART when CD4 cell count falls below 50/mm^3. **Azithromycin** 1200 mg oral every week is the treatment of choice.

All other primary prophylaxis occurs only if the patient is antigen positive or at high risk of exposure to the causative factor. All other opportunistic infections are treated when the patient is diagnosed. After treatment, patients receive suppressive therapy.

Some primary and secondary prophylaxis could possibly be discontinued with immune reconstitution (undetectable viral load and an increase in CD4 cells in response to ART; see Table 35-8).

Guidelines for prophylaxis and treatment of opportunistic infections can be located as a living document at https://hivinfo.nih.gov, which is updated regularly.

35-5   Pharmacist's Role

Pharmacists can impact the management of persons living with HIV in all settings. In the acute care setting, pharmacists are easily positioned to assess appropriateness of an ART regimen for completeness and for pertinent drug–drug interactions (for example, acid suppression in a ventilated patient). Pharmacists in the ambulatory setting can assist in regimen selection and can counsel patients on their medicine as well as on the importance of medication adherence at each office visit. Finally, pharmacists in the community setting can help ensure ART regimens are complete and can assess for drug–drug interactions prior to dispensing. They are also easily positioned to counsel patients on over-the-counter/herbal medications to avoid with their ART (for example, Tums with an integrase inhibitor).

TABLE 35-8. Opportunistic Infections

Pathogen	Indication	First choice	Alternative regimens	Comments
Pneumocystis jiroveci pneumonia	Prophylaxis: CD4 cell count <200/mm³; thrush; unexplained fever ≥2 weeks; history of PCP	TMP-SMX	Dapsone, atovaquone, or aerosolized pentamidine	Primary and secondary prophylaxis can be stopped for PCP on immune reconstitution (patients on HAART with CD4 cell count >200/mm³ for >3 months).
	Acute infection	TMP 15 to 20 mg/kg/d + SMX 75 to 100 mg/kg/d orally or I.V. × 21 days in 3 to 4 divided doses	Pentamidine I.V., primaquine + clindamycin, dapsone + TMP, or atovaquone	Patients with PO_2 <70 mmHg or A–a gradient >35 mmHg should receive a corticosteroid taper; treatment is for 21 days.
Candida	Treatment	Fluconazole, clotrimazole troches, nystatin suspension, itraconazole, posaconazole, amphotericin B, anidulafungin, caspofungin, micafungin, or voriconazole	Any of the preferred regimens	*Thrush:* treat for 10 to 14 days; CD4 cell count. *Esophagitis:* treat for 2 to 3 weeks. Chronic use of azoles might promote development of resistance.
Cryptococcal meningitis	Induction therapy (for at least 2 weeks)	Amphotericin B or lipid formulation amphotericin + flucytosine	Amphotericin B + fluconazole, amphotericin B alone, or fluconazole	Condition is spread through inhalation of soil contaminated with bird droppings.
	Consolidation therapy (for at least 8 weeks)	Fluconazole	Itraconazole	Managing increased intracranial pressures is critical.
	Maintenance therapy	Fluconazole	Itraconazole	Maintenance therapy is lifelong or until CD4 cell count ≥200/mm³ for >6 months as a result of ART.
Toxoplasmosis	Treatment (for at least 6 weeks)	Pyrimethamine + leucovorin + sulfadiazine	Pyrimethamine + leucovorin + clindamycin or atovaquone or **azithromycin**, TMP-SMX, atovaquone alone, or atovaquone + sulfadiazine	Condition is spread through raw or undercooked meat (lamb, beef, pork) and by contact with infected cat feces. Dexamethasone may be required if significant cerebral edema is present.
	Chronic maintenance therapy	Pyrimethamine + leucovorin + sulfadiazine	Pyrimethamine + leucovorin + clindamycin or atovaquone	Maintenance therapy is lifelong or until CD4 cell count ≥200/mm³ for >6 months as a result of ART and patient is free of signs and symptoms.

Disease	Therapy	Drug	Alternative	Comments
Histoplasmosis	Induction therapy (treat for at least 2 weeks)	Liposomal amphotericin B or itraconazole	Amphotericin B, amphotericin B lipid complex, or posaconazole	Condition is spread through inhalation of dust particles. Histoplasmosis is found in soils heavily contaminated by avian or bat feces. The Ohio and Mississippi River valleys are endemic areas in the United States.
	Maintenance therapy (for at least 12 months)	Itraconazole	Posaconazole	Maintenance therapy can be stopped after 12 months of treatment, CD4 cell count ≥ 150/mm³, ART for >6 months, and urine and serum antigen < 4.1 units.
Mycobacterium avium complex	Treatment and maintenance therapy	Clarithromycin + ethambutol ± rifabutin	**Azithromycin** + ethambutol Alternative third drugs: amikacin, streptomycin, ciprofloxacin, levofloxacin, **moxifloxacin**	Maintenance therapy may be discontinued after 12 months of treatment, CD4 cell count > 100/mm³ for 6 months on ART after treatment and patient is asymptomatic.
	Primary prophylaxis: recommended at CD4 cell count < 50/mm³ in those not immediately starting ART	**Azithromycin** or clarithromycin	Rifabutin or **azithromycin** + rifabutin	Treatment may possibly be discontinued when CD4 cell count > 100/mm³ for > 6 months in patients on ART.
Cytomegalovirus retinitis	Treatment (for 21 days)	Intraocular ganciclovir, valganciclovir, foscarnet, or ganciclovir	Cidofovir	Oral ganciclovir should not be used as sole induction therapy. Optimization of ART is an important part of initial therapy.
	Maintenance	Valganciclovir or intraocular ganciclovir	Ganciclovir, foscarnet, or cidofovir	Maintenance therapy can be stopped with inactive disease, CD4 cell count > 100 to 150/mm³ for 3 to 6 months in patients on ART.

Boldface indicates one of top 100 drugs for 2020 by prescription volume.
ART, antiretroviral therapy; HAART, highly active antiretroviral therapy; PCP, pneumocystis jiroveci pneumonia; TMP-SMZ, trimethoprim-sulfamethoxazole.

NAPLEX Competency Statements

The questions in this chapter cover the following 2021 NAPLEX Competency Statements: **AREA 1:** 1.1; 1.2; 1.3; 1.4; 1.5; 1.6; 1.7 **AREA 2:** 2.1; 2.2; 2.3; 2.4 **AREA 3:** 3.1; 3.2; 3.3; 3.4; 3.5; 3.6; 3.7; 3.8; 3.9; 3.10; 3.11; 3.12 **AREA 6:** 6.4.

35-6   Questions

Use the following case study to answer Questions 1 to 4.

C. T. is a 23-year-old, HIV-positive female who presents to the emergency department with shortness of breath and a fever. A physical exam reveals a temperature of 102°F, heart rate of 100 bpm, and decreased breath sounds in the left lower lobe of lungs. Her chest x-ray is positive for infiltrates in the left lung. She is diagnosed with *Pneumocystis jiroveci* pneumonia (PCP). She has no previous history of opportunistic infections and is not on any medications at this time (she has not been seen by a health care provider in over a year). Her CD4 cell count is 13 cells/mm^3, and her viral load is 170,198 copies/mL.

1. What is the treatment of choice for C. T.'s PCP?

   A. TMP-SMX DS 2 tabs orally every 8 hours for 21 days, then 1 tab orally daily
   B. Azithromycin 500 mg orally on day 1, then 250 mg orally daily indefinitely
   C. Doxycycline 100 mg orally twice daily for 7 days, then 100 mg orally daily
   D. Clarithromycin 500 mg orally twice daily for 10 days, then 250 mg orally daily
   E. Vancomycin 1 g I.V. every 12 hours for 10 days, then TMP-SMX DS orally daily

2. With a CD4 of 13 cells/mm^3, should C. T. receive any other prophylaxis against opportunistic infections in addition to PCP?

   A. Yes, against *Mycobacterium avium* complex: Zithromax 1200 mg orally weekly
   B. Yes, against thrush: Diflucan 100 mg orally daily
   C. Yes, against toxoplasmosis: Bactrim DS 1 tab orally every Monday, Wednesday, and Friday
   D. Yes, against cytomegalovirus: Valcyte 450 mg orally every Monday, Wednesday, and Friday
   E. No

3. Six weeks later, C. T. presents to the HIV clinic for follow-up. Her CD4 cell count is 12 cells/mm^3, and her viral load is 140,202 copies/mL. Should C. T. be started on HIV therapy?

   A. Yes, because her CD4 cell count is <200 cells/mm^3 and she has had an opportunistic infection.
   B. Yes, because her viral load is >100,000 copies/mL.
   C. Yes, because her Western blot was positive for HIV.
   D. Yes, because all patients with HIV should be treated regardless of CD4 count.
   E. No.

4. C. T. wishes to be started on HIV therapy. Which of the following would be an appropriate first-line regimen? (Mark all that apply.)

   A. TAF/emtriticitabine/bictegravir
   B. TAF/emtricitabine + dolutegravir
   C. Stavudine + didanosine + fosamprenavir
   D. Tenofovir/emtricitabine + atazanavir + ritonavir
   E. Dolutegravir/lamivudine

5. HIV can be transmitted by _____. (mark all that apply.)

   A. unprotected sexual contact with an infected person
   B. sharing of needles or syringes with an infected person
   C. infected mother to infant (vertical transmission)
   D. transfusion of blood (before 1985)
   E. breast-feeding

6. M. J. is 13-weeks pregnant and just tested positive for HIV. Her viral load is 22,434 copies/mL, and her CD4 cell count is 425 cells/mm^3. M. J. wishes to receive treatment for her HIV. Which of the following would be an appropriate regimen for M. J.?

   A. Zidovudine + stavudine + indinavir
   B. Tenofovir/emtricitabine + atazanavir + ritonavir
   C. Zidovudine/lamivudine + nelfinavir
   D. Stavudine + didanosine + nevirapine
   E. No treatment is necessary

7. Which of the following would be an important drug interaction with Isentress?

A. Metoprolol
B. Tums
C. Citalopram
D. Sulfamethoxazole/trimethoprim
E. Truvada

8. R. C. is a nurse in the emergency department. She has just been stuck with a needle that was used for an HIV-positive patient with a known high viral load. Which of the following is true concerning postexposure prophylaxis? (Mark all that apply.)

A. The regimen should be started within 72 hours of exposure.
B. R. C. will need to be treated only with zidovudine.
C. R. C. will need to be treated with a combination of tenofovir/emtricitabine and raltegravir.
D. Treatment will continue for 4 weeks.
E. Treatment will continue for 2 weeks.

9. The CD4 cell count relates to _____. (mark all that apply.)

A. the activity of the virus
B. the status of the immune system
C. how much a patient is at risk for acquiring an opportunistic infection
D. when the patient was infected
E. the last dose of antiretrovirals taken by the patient

10. The viral load relates to _____.

A. the activity of the virus and efficacy of antiretroviral therapy
B. the status of the immune system
C. when the patient was infected
D. how much a patient is at risk for acquiring an opportunistic infection
E. the last dose of antiretrovirals taken by the patient

11. S. J. presents to the emergency department with extreme flank pain with nausea and vomiting. He is diagnosed with a kidney stone. His past medical history is positive for HIV and diabetes. His medications include indinavir, lamivudine, didanosine, metformin, and dapsone. Which of his medications might have caused his kidney stone?

A. Indinavir
B. Lamivudine
C. Didanosine
D. Metformin
E. Dapsone

12. L. L. comes to the clinic with a chief complaint of burning and tingling in his feet that started about 1 month ago. His current medications include nelfinavir, stavudine, lamivudine, sertraline, and gemfibrozil. Which medication might be causing this problem?

A. Nelfinavir
B. Stavudine
C. Lamivudine
D. Sertraline
E. Gemfibrozil

13. S. E. presents to the emergency department with a 2-day history of extreme nausea, vomiting, and abdominal pain. Labs reveal elevations in amylase and lipase, and a diagnosis of pancreatitis is made. His medications include nevirapine, tenofovir, didanosine, and amitriptyline. Which of his medications could have caused his pancreatitis?

A. Nevirapine
B. Tenofovir
C. Didanosine
D. Amitriptyline
E. Dolutegravir

14. Which HIV medication should not be used until HLA-B*5701 testing has been performed to assess risk for hypersensitivity?

A. Efavirenz
B. Ritonavir
C. Zidovudine
D. Abacavir
E. Lamivudine

15. C. J. is starting efavirenz, tenofovir, lamivudine, and TMP-SMX. What should C. J. be counseled about concerning efavirenz?

   A. Anemia
   B. CNS side effects
   C. Neutropenia
   D. Renal toxicity
   E. Kidney stones

16. Which of the following would be a pertinent drug–drug interaction with Biktarvy (TAF/emtricitabine/bictegravir)? (Mark all that apply.)

   A. Ferrous sulfate
   B. Amlodipine
   C. Carbamazepine
   D. Rifampin
   E. Acetaminophen

17. Which of the following can cause hyperglycemia, hyperlipidemia (particularly elevations in triglycerides), and lipodystrophy?

   A. Lopinavir/ritonavir
   B. Delavirdine
   C. Didanosine
   D. Abacavir
   E. Lamivudine

18. Lactic acidosis and hepatic steatosis have been reported with which of these antiretroviral medications?

   A. Nevirapine
   B. Efavirenz
   C. Stavudine
   D. Saquinavir
   E. Nelfinavir

19. The mechanism of action of nucleoside reverse transcriptase inhibitors is to _____.

   A. directly inhibit reverse transcriptase
   B. prevent entry of the proviral DNA into the nucleus of the CD4 cell
   C. cause chain termination, resulting in a defective copy of proviral DNA
   D. prevent entry of HIV into the CD4 cell
   E. prevent cleavage of the newly formed polypeptide chains into viable HIV

20. The mechanism of action of nonnucleoside reverse transcriptase inhibitors is to _____.

   A. prevent cleavage of the newly formed polypeptide chains into viable HIV
   B. prevent entry of HIV into the CD4 cell
   C. prevent entry of the proviral DNA into the nucleus of the CD4 cell
   D. directly inhibit reverse transcriptase
   E. cause chain termination, resulting in a defective copy of proviral DNA

21. The mechanism of action of protease inhibitors is to _____.

   A. cause a defective copy of proviral DNA to be made
   B. prevent entry of the proviral DNA into the nucleus of the CD4 cell
   C. prevent cleavage of the newly formed polypeptide chains into viable HIV
   D. prevent entry of HIV into the CD4 cell
   E. directly inhibit reverse transcriptase

22. Which of the following medications if used with atazanavir can result in decreased levels and effectiveness of atazanavir?

   A. Loratadine
   B. Tenofovir
   C. Esomeprazole
   D. Metoclopramide
   E. Glipizide

23. Which of the following opportunistic infections require primary prophylaxis?

   A. *Pneumocystis jiroveci* pneumonia (PCP)
   B. Toxoplasmosis
   C. *Mycobacterium avium* complex (MAC)
   D. Cytomegalovirus (CMV)
   E. Thrush

24. The antifungal of first choice for maintenance therapy after treatment of cryptococcal meningitis is _____.

   A. itraconazole
   B. fluconazole
   C. ketoconazole
   D. amphotericin B
   E. terbinafine

25. The first-choice antifungal for treatment of histoplasmosis is _____.

A. itraconazole
B. fluconazole
C. ketoconazole
D. caspofungin
E. terbinafine

 **35-7** **Answers**

1. **A.** The treatment of choice for PCP is TMP-SMX in patients who are not allergic to sulfa medications. Duration of treatment is 21 days. Because this patient's CD4 cell count is <200 cells/mm^3 and she has had PCP, she will require secondary prophylaxis once treatment is completed. Preferred prophylaxis is once-daily TMP-SMX DS.

2. **A.** This patient's CD4 cell count is <50 cells/mm^3; therefore, she requires primary prophylaxis against MAC. Zithromax is the drug of choice. Prophylaxis against other opportunistic infections is generally not required.

3. **D.** Current guidelines state that all patients with HIV should receive antiretrovirals regardless of CD4 count.

4. **A, B, E.** Most regimens contain 2 NRTIs and either 1 INSTI, PI or 1 NNRTI (answer D contains 2 NRTIs and a boosted PI). All first-line regimens contain an INSTI (answer A and B). While answer D does contain 2 NRTIs and a PI, INSTIs are recommended first line. Didanosine and stavudine should not be used together because of increased toxicity (which makes Answer C incorrect). Dolutegravir/lamividuine is a new 2-drug STR that is indicated in treatment-naïve individuals with viral loads <500,000 copies/mL

5. **All apply.** All items are important risk factors for transmission of HIV. History of sexually transmitted diseases, occupational exposure to HIV-infected fluids (rare), and household exposure to HIV-infected fluids (rare) are also risk factors.

6. **B.** All HIV-positive pregnant women should receive treatment for HIV to decrease the risk of transmission to their offspring. Zidovudine and stavudine competitively inhibit each other and should not be used together. Nelfinavir is an unboosted PI and is not recommended in pregnancy. Stavudine and didanosine together are contraindicated in pregnancy because of increased risk of lactic acidosis and liver damage.

7. **B.** Integrase inhibitors chelate with cations and should be separated from medications that contain them.

8. **A, C, D.** The approved regimen for postexposure prophylaxis is tenofovir/emtricitabine and raltegravir. Treatment should continue for 4 weeks and should start within 72 hours of exposure.

9. **B, C.** CD4 cell count describes the status of the immune system (i.e., how much a patient is at risk for acquiring an opportunistic infection).

10. **A.** Viral load relates to the activity of the virus and efficacy of antiretroviral therapy.

11. **A.** Indinavir can cause kidney stones. Patients should drink at least 48 oz of water a day to decrease the risk of developing a kidney stone.

12. **B.** The "D" drugs, d4T (stavudine) and ddI (didanosine), can cause peripheral neuropathy and pancreatitis.

13. **C.** The "D" drugs, d4T (stavudine) and ddI (didanosine), can cause peripheral neuropathy and pancreatitis.

14. **D.** HLA-B*5701 testing should be performed prior to use of abacavir to assess risk of hypersensitivity.

15. **B.** Efavirenz can cause CNS side effects such as dizziness, trouble sleeping, drowsiness, trouble concentrating, and unusual dreams during the first 2 to 4 weeks of treatment.

16. **A, C, D.** Bictegravir chelates with polyvalent cations and is metabolized by CYP3A enzymes as well as UGT1A1. Rifampin and carbamazepine are potent inducers of these pathways.

17. **A.** Class side effects of PIs include hyperglycemia, hyperlipidemia, fat maldistribution, and increased bleeding in hemophiliacs.

18. **C.** Class side effects of NRTIs include lactic acidosis and hepatic steatosis.

19. **C.** NRTIs affect reverse transcriptase by causing chain termination, resulting in a defective copy of proviral DNA.

20. **D.** NNRTIs affect reverse transcriptase by directly inhibiting reverse transcriptase, resulting in less proviral DNA being made.

21. C. PIs prevent cleavage of the newly formed polypeptide chains into viable HIV, resulting in an immature virus that is unable to infect other CD4 cells.

22. C. Atazanavir levels are decreased by proton pump inhibitors, H_2 blockers, and antacids.

23. A. PCP requires primary prophylaxis when the CD4 cell count falls below 200 cells/mm^3. The preferred medication is TMP-SMX. MAC requires primary prophylaxis when the CD4 cell count falls below 50 cells/mm^3 only in those not starting ART

immediately. More information would be needed to determine if toxoplasmosis prophylaxis is indicated.

24. B. Generally, cryptococcal meningitis is initially treated with amphotericin B during the induction phase and then fluconazole for the consolidation phase and maintenance therapy.

25. A. Histoplasmosis is generally initially treated with amphotericin B and itraconazole for induction therapy and then itraconazole for maintenance therapy.

 ## 35-8 Additional Resources

Bartlett JG, Gallant JE. *Medical Management of HIV Infection.* Baltimore, MD: Johns Hopkins University Press; 2012:357–360.

Carr A, Miller J, Law M, et al. A syndrome of lipoatrophy, lactic acidaemia, and liver dysfunction associated with HIV nucleoside analog therapy: contribution to protease inhibitor-related lipodystrophy syndrome. *AIDS.* 2000;14:F25–F32.

Carr A, Samars K, Thorisdottir A, et al. Diagnosis, prediction, and natural course of HIV-1 protease-inhibitor-associated lipodystrophy, hyperlipidaemia, and diabetes mellitus: A cohort study. *Lancet.* 1999;353:2093–2099.

Centers for Disease Control and Prevention. 1993 revised classification system for HIV infection and expanded surveillance case definition for AIDS among adolescents and adults. *MMWR.* 1992;41:1–19.

Centers for Disease Control and Prevention, Perinatal HIV Guidelines Working Group. Public Health Service Task Force recommendations for the use of antiretroviral drugs in pregnant women infected with HIV-1 for maternal health and for reducing perinatal HIV-1 transmission in the United States. *MMWR.* 1998;47:1–30.

Chaisson RE, Keruly JC, Moore RD. Association of initial CD4 cell count and viral load with response to highly active anti-retroviral therapy. *JAMA.* 2000;284:3128–3129.

Chesney MA. Factors affecting adherence to antiretroviral therapy. *Clin Infect Dis.* 2000;30(suppl 2):S171–S176.

Finzi D, Hermankova M, Pierson T, et al. Identification of a reservoir for HIV-1 in patients on highly active antiretroviral therapy. *Science.* 1997;278:1295–1300.

Furrer H, Egger M, Opravil M, et al. Discontinuation of primary prophylaxis against *Pneumocystis carinii* pneumonia in HIV-1 infected adults treated with combination antiretroviral therapy: Swiss HIV Cohort Study. *N Engl J Med.* 1999;340:1301–1306.

Hoen B, Dumon B, Harzic M, et al. Highly active antiretroviral treatment initiated early in the course of symptomatic primary HIV-1 infections: Results of the ANRS 053 trial. *J Infect Dis.* 1999;180:1342–1346.

INSIGHT START Study Group. Initiation of antiretroviral therapy in early asymptomatic HIV infection. *N Engl J Med.* 2015;373:795–807.

Mellors JW, Munoz A, Giorgi JV, et al. Plasma viral load and CD4 lymphocytes as prognostic markers of HIV-1 infections. *Ann Intern Med.* 1997;126:946–954.

National Institutes of Health. Report of the NIH panel to define principles of therapy of HIV infection. *MMWR.* 1998;47(RR-5):1–41.

Sperling RS, Shapiro DE, Coombs RW, et al. Maternal viral load, zidovudine treatment, and the risk of transmission of human immunodeficiency virus type 1 from mother to infant: Pediatric AIDS Clinical Trials Group Protocol 076 Study Group. *N Engl J Med.* 1996;335:1621–1629.

U.S. Food and Drug Administration; Health Resources and Services Administration; National Institutes of Health; National Center for HIV, STD, and TB Prevention; National Institute for Occupational Safety and Health; and National Center for Infectious Diseases. Notice to readers update: Provisional Public Health Service recommendations for chemoprophylaxis after occupational exposure to HIV. *MMWR.* 1996;45:468–472.

U.S. Public Health Service and Infectious Diseases Society of America. 1999 USPHS/IDSA guidelines for the prevention of opportunistic infections in persons infected with human immunodeficiency virus. *MMWR.* 1999;48(RR-10):1–67.

Vittinghoff E, Scheer S, O'Malley P, et al. Combination antiretroviral therapy and recent declines in AIDS incidence and mortality. *J Infect Dis.* 1999;179:717–720.

Yeni PG, Hammer SM, Hirsch MS, et al. Treatment for adult HIV infection: 2004 recommendations of the International AIDS Society–USA Panel. *JAMA.* 2004;292:250–265.

Immunization

36

CHASITY M. SHELTON

 36-1 KEY POINTS

- The 2 types of vaccine antigens are (1) live viruses and (2) inactivated viruses or bacterial components.
- There are 2 types of immunity: active and passive.
- Adverse effects of inactivated vaccines include pain at the injection site and mild systemic symptoms (mild fever). Adverse effects of live vaccines include local injection site reactions and may mimic a mild case of the disease.
- Live vaccines should be avoided during pregnancy and in immunosuppressed persons.
- Influenza viruses undergo shifts and drifts, which account for the need for yearly vaccine changes.
- Diphtheria toxoid and tetanus toxoid should always be given together, unless a contraindication to 1 of the components exists. If there is a need for 1, then there is a need for both.
- A combination vaccine of tetanus, diphtheria, and pertussis (Tdap) is available for use in children over 7 years of age, adolescents, and adults. Children under the age of 7 years receive the pediatric version of the diphtheria, tetanus, and pertussis (DTaP) or diphtheria and tetanus toxoid (DT) vaccine (if they are unable to tolerate the pertussis vaccine). Revaccination with either tetanus and diphtheria (Td) or Tdap vaccine following the receipt of the first dose of Tdap should occur every 10 years.
- The hepatitis B vaccine is recommended for all infants, starting at birth, as well as all adolescents. Other indications include adults with diabetes, high-risk occupations, or high-risk behaviors.
- The hepatitis A vaccine is recommended for all children over the age of 1 year and for persons traveling to most parts of the world.
- Inactivated polio vaccine is the only polio vaccine recommended for use in the United States. Oral polio vaccine is not recommended because of the high incidence of vaccine-associated paralytic poliomyelitis.
- A second dose of the measles, mumps, and rubella vaccine and the varicella vaccine is recommended at 4 to 6 years of age.
- Combination vaccines are available to decrease the number of injections.

 36-2 STUDY GUIDE CHECKLIST

The following topics may guide your study of this subject area:

- ☐ Understanding of the immune system.
- ☐ Type of vaccines.
- ☐ Interpreting a vaccine schedule.
- ☐ Timing and spacing issues.
- ☐ Contraindications and precautions.
- ☐ Storage and handling of vaccines.
- ☐ Knowledge of vaccine-preventable diseases.
- ☐ Vaccine indications by age and comorbid conditions and dosages.

36-3 **Introduction**

Definitions

- *Immunity:* A naturally or artificially acquired state resulting in an individual's resistance or relative resistance to the occurrence or effects of a foreign substance. Immunity is the mechanism the body develops for protection from infectious disease. It is usually very specific to a single organism or to a group of closely related organisms.
- *Antigen:* A live or inactivated substance capable of evoking antibody production. An antigen can be a live organism, such as bacteria or a virus, or an inactivated or killed organism or portion of an organism. A live organism generally evokes the most effective immune response.
- *Antibody:* A protein evoked by an antigen that acts to eliminate that antigen.

Mechanisms for Acquiring Immunity

Active immunity

Active immunity is produced by an individual's own immune system. Immunity acquired in this manner has a delayed onset and is usually permanent. Active immunity may be acquired by having an active disease or by vaccination. B lymphocytes (B cells) circulate in the blood and bone marrow for many years. Re-exposure to the antigen causes the cells to replicate and to produce antibodies. These cells are also called *memory B cells* (Figure 36-1).

Passive immunity

Passive immunity is produced by an animal or human and transferred to another. Immunity acquired in this manner has a rapid onset and usually has a brief duration. An infant receives this type of immunity from

FIGURE 36-1. Acquisition of Active Immunity Through B Cell (Memory Cells) Production

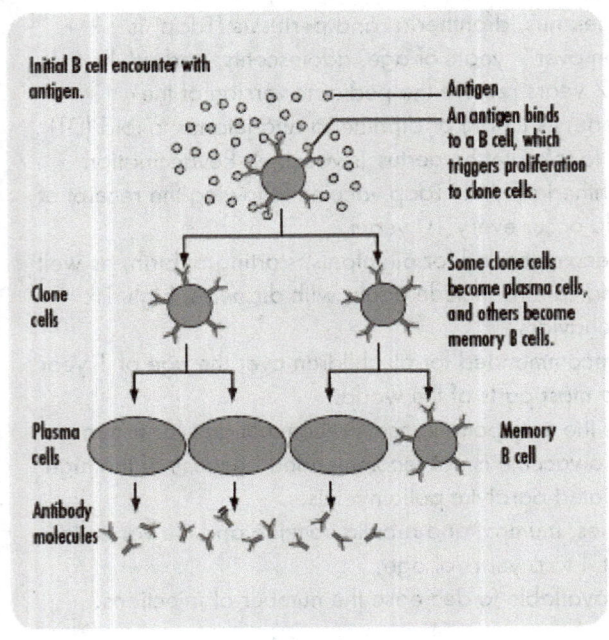

his or her mother. All types of blood products contain varying amounts of antibodies. Immune globulins and hyperimmune globulins are also used to induce passive immunity. One source of passive immunity is antitoxins, which contain antibodies against a known toxin.

36-4 Vaccines

Classification of Vaccines

Live attenuated vaccines

Live vaccines are produced by modifying a virus or bacteria to produce immunity. These vaccines usually do not produce disease-like symptoms, but when those occur they usually are much milder than the natural disease. These vaccines must replicate to be effective. They require special handling, such as protection from heat and light, to keep them alive. Circulating antibodies from another source may destroy the vaccine virus and cause vaccine failure.

The live vaccines available in the United State are listed in Box 36-1, and a memory aid for remembering these vaccines is in the mnemonic below.

BOX 36-1. Live Vaccines Available in the United States

- Adenovirus oral
- Cholera oral
- Dengue
- Ebola Zaire
- Influenza (live attenuated)
- Measles
- Mumps

- Rotavirus
- Rubella
- Typhoid oral
- Varicella
- Vaccinia (smallpox) ⚠
- Yellow fever

⚠ **Vaccinia (smallpox)** *FDA BOXED WARNING*

Injection (Powder for Solution)

Suspected cases of myocarditis and/or pericarditis have been observed in healthy adult primary vaccinees (at an approximate rate of 5.7 per 1000, 95% confidence interval (CI): 1.9 to 13.3) receiving ACAM2000™ (smallpox (vaccina) vaccine, live).

Encephalitis, encephalomyelitis, encephalopathy, progressive vaccinia, generalized vaccinia, severe vaccinial skin infections, and erythema multiforme major (including Stevens-Johnson Syndrome) and eczema vaccinatum resulting in permanent sequelae or death, ocular complications, blindness, and fetal death have occurred following either primary vaccination or revaccination with smallpox vaccines.

Risk of encephalitis, encephalomyelitis, encephalopathy, progressive vaccinia, generalized vaccinia, and severe skin infections or reactions. Suspected cases of myocarditis and/or pericarditis have been observed in healthy adults. Risk of smallpox transmission to people with close contact with vaccinated individual.

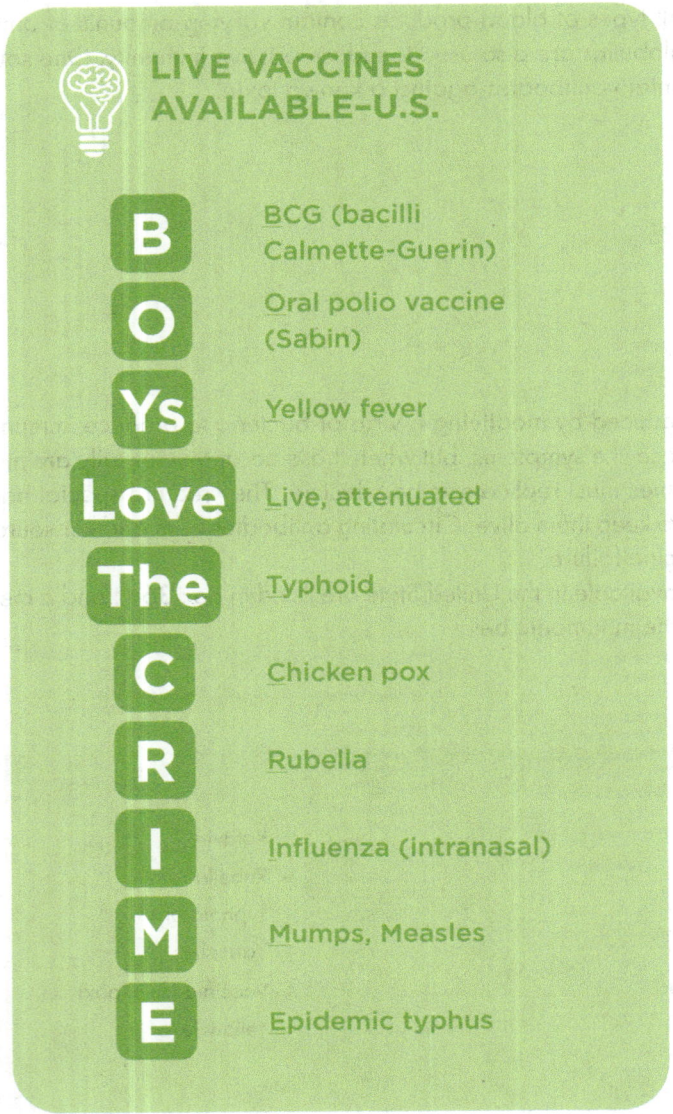

LIVE VACCINES AVAILABLE–U.S.

B — BCG (bacilli Calmette-Guerin)

O — Oral polio vaccine (Sabin)

Ys — Yellow fever

Love — Live, attenuated

The — Typhoid

C — Chicken pox

R — Rubella

I — Influenza (intranasal)

M — Mumps, Measles

E — Epidemic typhus

Inactivated vaccines

Inactivated vaccines are composed of all or a fraction of a virus or bacteria. These fractions include subunits (subvirions), bacterial cell wall polysaccharides, conjugated (attached to a protein carrier) bacteria cell wall polysaccharides, or inactivated toxins (toxoids). The bacteria or virus is inactivated using heat, chemicals, or both. Inactivated vaccines are not alive and cannot replicate; therefore, they are unable to induce disease.

The inactivated vaccines available in the United States are listed in Box 36-2, and a memory aid for remembering these vaccines is in the mnemonic below.

Vaccination Schedules

Vaccination schedules are available for children, adolescents, and adults from the U.S. Centers for Disease Control and Prevention (CDC). These schedules are updated yearly by the Advisory Committee on

---

BOX 36-2. Inactivated Vaccines Available in United States

- Anthrax
- Diphtheria
- *Haemophilus influenzae* type B
- Hepatitis A
- Hepatitis B
- Herpes zoster recombinant, adjuvanted
- Human papillomavirus
- Influenza (inactivated)
- Japanese encephalitis

- Meningococcal A, C, Y, W-135 polysaccharide and conjugate
- Meningococcal B
- Pertussis, acellular
- Pneumococcal polysaccharide and conjugate
- Polio
- Rabies
- Tetanus toxoid
- Typhoid injectable

Immunization Practices (ACIP) and can be found at https://www.cdc.gov/vaccines/schedules/index.html. The schedules indicate the best times to administer vaccines. Additional catch-up schedules are available for children and adolescents who are behind in their vaccinations.

The CDC schedules describe intervals between doses of the same vaccine in a series. The minimum interval in a series for most vaccines is 4 weeks. Decreasing the interval may interfere with antibody response and protection. Increasing the interval does not affect vaccine effectiveness. Restarting a series is never necessary except for the oral typhoid vaccine. Minimal intervals must be observed if repeating a dose.

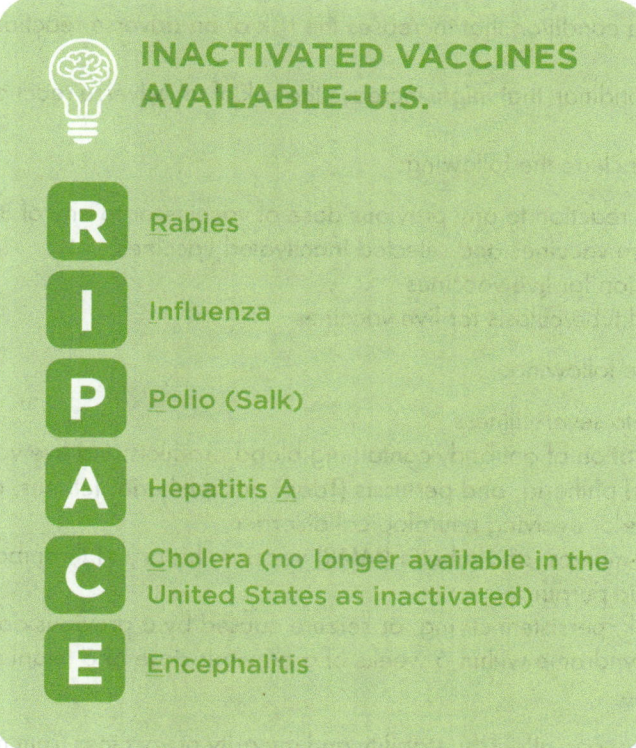

INACTIVATED VACCINES AVAILABLE–U.S.

R Rabies

I Influenza

P Polio (Salk)

A Hepatitis A

C Cholera (no longer available in the United States as inactivated)

E Encephalitis

Administration of Multiple Vaccines

There are no contraindications to the simultaneous administration of any vaccines. Inactivated and live vaccines may be given in any combination at the same time.

Most live vaccines must be separated from the administration of antibodies, such as blood products and immune globulins. Inactivated vaccines are not affected by a circulating antibody.

If 2 live vaccines are not given at the same time, a 4-week minimum interval must be observed. The exception to this is oral live vaccines (oral cholera, typhoid, and rotavirus vaccines), which can be administered simultaneously or at any interval with other live vaccines. One exception is that oral cholera vaccine should be administered before oral typhoid, and 8 hours should separate the cholera vaccine and the first dose of oral typhoid. No specific time interval is necessary between 2 inactivated vaccines or an inactivated plus a live vaccine.

Adverse Vaccine Reactions

Local reactions are the most common type of adverse reaction. They include pain, swelling, and redness at the site of injection. They usually occur within minutes to hours of the injection and are usually mild and self-limiting. Systemic adverse reactions include fever, malaise, myalgias, and headache. Systemic adverse reactions are more common following live vaccines and are similar to a mild case of the disease.

Allergic reactions are reactions to the vaccine antigens or to some component of the vaccine. Although rare, these reactions may be life threatening.

Another potential problem is syncope; therefore, monitoring patients for at least 15 minutes following vaccination is important.

The Vaccine Adverse Events Reporting System (VAERS) is a surveillance system monitored by the CDC that should be notified within 30 days of an adverse event that requires medical attention.

Contraindications and Precautions

A *contraindication* is a condition that increases the risk of an adverse reaction or decreases the effect of a vaccine.

A *precaution* is a condition that *might* increase the risk of an adverse reaction or decrease the effectiveness of a vaccine.

Contraindications include the following:

- An anaphylactic reaction to any previous dose of vaccine or to any of its components
- Pregnancy for live vaccines and selected inactivated vaccines
- Immunosuppression for live vaccines
- Active, untreated tuberculosis for live vaccines

Precautions include the following:

- Acute moderate to severe illness
- Recent administration of antibody-containing blood products and live vaccines
- For the tetanus, diphtheria, and pertussis (Tdap) or diphtheria, tetanus, and pertussis (DTaP) vaccine, unstable or evolving neurological disorder
- For the measles, mumps, and rubella (MMR) vaccine, history of thrombocytopenia or thrombocytopenic purpura
- High fever, shock, persistent crying, or seizure caused by a previous dose of DTaP or Tdap
- Guillain–Barré syndrome within 6 weeks of a previous dose of a tetanus-containing vaccine or influenza vaccine

Due to many factors that can affect the stability and integrity of vaccines from manufacturers to administration, employing appropriate management of vaccines (see Box 36-3) is important.

> ### BOX 36-3. Vaccine Management
>
> - Maintain cold chain from manufacturer until vaccine is administered.
> - Follow manufacturers' recommendation for shipping.
> - Keep nonfrozen vaccines from freezing during transport.
> - Refrigerate or freeze vaccines—depending on the specific vaccine—immediately on arrival.
> - Use stand-alone refrigerators and freezers
>   - Monitor temperatures daily.
>   - Do not store vaccines in refrigerator door.
>   - Store vaccines in the middle of the refrigerator.
>   - Stabilize temperature with water bottles in the refrigerator and frozen coolant packs in the freezer.
>   - Use a calibrated thermometer in each storage unit and monitor at least twice a day.
>   - Keep a temperature log.
> - Perform proper inventory management
>   - Maintain inventory log.
>   - Rotate stock.
>   - Follow manufacturer's guidelines for shelf life.
>   - Check expiration dates.
>   - Designate a person to be responsible for vaccines.
>   - Train all staff members to recognize vaccine shipment arrivals.
> - Follow manufacturers' directions for reconstitution.

36-5   Diseases and Vaccines

Pneumococcal Disease

There are over 90 known serotypes of gram-positive *Streptococcal pneumoniae* bacteria with a polysaccharide capsule. Serious primary diseases associated with *S. pneumoniae* include pneumonia, sepsis, and meningitis.

Rates of disease

Highest rates are seen in children less than 2 years of age. Patients over the age of 50 years have fatality rates of 30% to 60%. Pneumococcal disease is one of the leading causes of vaccine-preventable diseases. Pneumococcal bacteria are common respiratory tract inhabitants. Transmission is through direct person-to-person droplet contamination or auto-inoculation by carriers.

23-valent polysaccharide vaccine (Pneumovax-23 by Merck)

The vaccine is ineffective in children less than 2 years old.

Recommendations

- Adults 65 years and older
- Everyone over 2 years of age with certain chronic diseases
- Smokers 19 to 64 years of age

Dose

The dosage is 0.5 mL intramuscular (I.M.) or subcutaneous (SQ).
Revaccination is recommended in the following cases:

- Patients at high risk of selected diseases if more than 5 years have passed since the previous dose
- Everyone age 65 years and older who received an initial dose under the age of 65 years and if more than 5 years have passed since the previous dose

Adverse reactions

Adverse reactions include pain, swelling, and redness at the injection site and slight to moderate systemic reactions such as fever and myalgias.

13-valent conjugated polysaccharide vaccine (Prevnar by Pfizer)

Indications

- All children less than 2 years of age
- Children 24 to 59 months of age with high-risk medical conditions
- One dose for all adults who are immunocompromised (e.g., asplenia, cerebrospinal fluid leaks, cochlear implants)
- One dose for all immunocompetent adults age 65 years and older based on shared clinical decision-making

Dose

The usual dose is 0.5 mL administered I.M.
Revaccination is not routinely recommended, but if warranted high-risk persons 2 years of age and older should receive the 23-valent polysaccharide vaccine.

Adverse reactions

Adverse reactions include pain, swelling, and redness at the injection site and slight to moderate systemic reactions such as fever and myalgias.

Influenza

Influenza is an RNA (ribonucleic acid) virus of the orthomyxovirus family. There are 3 types of influenza viruses that cause illness in humans: A, B, and C. The etiology of these types are included in Table 36-1.
Antigenic drift, which is frequent minor changes in the antigenic structure of the virus, is the reason for yearly adjustments in vaccine formulations. *Antigenic shift,* which is major changes in 1 or both of the major antigens in influenza A, resulting in a different subtype, can cause major pandemics.

TABLE 36-1. Etiology of Influenza

	Influenza A	Influenza B	Influenza C
Natural host	Humans, swine, equine, birds, marine mammals, bats, canines	Humans	Humans, swine
Epidemiology	Antigenic shift or drift	Antigenic drift	Antigenic drift
Disease burden	Large pandemics with significant mortality in young patients possible	Severe disease usually confined to elderly or high-risk patients	Mild disease Not seasonal

Subtypes of influenza A are based on 2 surface antigens: hemagglutinin and neuraminidase. Six types of hemagglutinin (H1, H2, H3, H5, H7, H9) cause disease in humans. Two types of neuraminidase cause disease in humans (N1, N2). Influenza B has no subgroups but has 2 distinct genetic lineages (Victoria and Yamagata).

Influenza disease

Serious complications in all types include pneumonia, Reye's syndrome (progressive neurological symptoms associated with **aspirin** use in children), myocarditis, worsening of chronic bronchitis, and death.

Influenza can cause 20,000 to 40,000 deaths during epidemics. Pandemics could result in the deaths of millions of people. Rates of disease are highest in the elderly (≥65 years of age), children less than 2 years of age, and persons of any age with medical conditions.

The virus is shed in respiratory secretions for 5 to 10 days, and transmission is through direct person-to-person droplet contamination or contact. The incubation period is approximately 2 days (range, 1 to 4 days).

Clinical features include abrupt onset of fever, myalgia, sore throat, nonproductive cough, and headache.

Disease peaks between December and March in the Northern Hemisphere but may occur earlier or later. Year-round cases may be seen in tropical climates.

Influenza vaccines contain 3 antigens (2 type A viruses and 1 type B virus—trivalent) or 4 antigens (2 type A viruses and 2 type B viruses—quadrivalent). Vaccines are effective in up to 90% of healthy adults, 50% to 60% of the elderly, and 30% to 40% of the frail elderly.

Influenza vaccines

Influenza vaccines available in the United States are listed in Table 36-2.

Indications

Vaccination is indicated for all persons over 6 months of age unless contraindications exist. The ACIP recommendation for FluMist was renewed beginning with the 2018 to 2019 influenza season after preliminary studies showed improved protection after strain modification in the vaccine. During the 2018 to 2019 influenza season, the American Academy of Pediatrics (AAP) issued a preference for inactivated influenza vaccines over the intranasal live, attenuated influenza vaccine over concerns for a decrease in efficacy; however, beginning with the 2019 to 2020 influenza season, the AAP recommended any indicated influenza vaccine with no preference for the formulation administered.

Contraindications

Contraindications include severe allergic reactions to previous dose. FluMist should not be given to children 2 to 4 years of age with a history of wheezing or asthma, persons with chronic medical diseases, close contacts of severely immunocompromised persons who require a protective environment, pregnant women, or children receiving **aspirin** therapy.

Precautions

Use precaution with moderate-to-severe illness or a history of Guillain–Barré syndrome within 6 weeks of receipt of a previous dose of influenza vaccine.

Dose

Injectable vaccine normal doses are age 6 to 35 months: 0.25 mL I.M.; 3 to 8 years: 0.5 mL; >8 years: 0.5 mL. The dose of FluMist is 0.1 mL sprayed in each nostril (0.2 mL total). Children age 6 months to 8 years who have received fewer than 2 doses of influenza vaccine need 2 doses separated by at least 4 weeks.

All influenza vaccines must be shaken before use.

Revaccination yearly is needed.

TABLE 36-2. Influenza Vaccines

Trade name	Manufacturer	Age indications	Trivalent (IIV3) or quadrivalent (IIV4) Live, attenuated quadrivalent (LAIV4)
Fluzone	Sanofi Pasteur	≥6 months	IIV4
Fluzone Intradermal	Sanofi Pasteur	18 to 64 years	IIV4
Fluzone High-Dose	Sanofi Pasteur	≥65 years	IIV3
Fluzone High-Dose Quadrivalent	Sanofi Pasteur	≥65 years	IIV4
Fluarix	GlaxoSmithKline	≥3 years	IIV3
Fluarix Quadrivalent	GlaxoSmithKline	≥6 months	IIV4
FluLaval	GlaxoSmithKline	≥6 months	IIV3
FluLaval Quadrivalent	GlaxoSmithKline	≥6 months	IIV4
Afluria	Seqirus	≥5 years, needle 18 to 64 years, jet injector	IIV3
Afluria Quadrivalent	Seqirus	≥6 months, needle	IIV4
Agriflu	Seqirus	≥18 years	IIV3
Flucelvax	Seqirus	≥4 years	IIV3
Flucelvax Quadrivalent	Seqirus	≥4 years	IIV4
Fluvirin	Seqirus	≥4 years	IIV3
Fluad	Seqirus	≥65 years	IIV3
Fluad	Seqirus	≥65 years	IIV4
Flublok	Protein Sciences	≥18 years	IIV3
Flublok	Protein Sciences	≥18 years	IIV4
FluMist (intranasal live virus vaccine)	MedImmune	2 to 49 years	LAIV4

Adverse reactions

Adverse reactions include pain, swelling, and redness at the injection site and slight to moderate systemic reactions such as fever, myalgias, chills, and malaise. Severe neurologic reactions are rare.

Tetanus

Tetanus is caused by an exotoxin produced by *Clostridium tetani* and is characterized by generalized rigidity and convulsive spasms of skeletal muscles.

Complications include laryngospasm, fractures, hypertension, nosocomial infections, pulmonary embolism, aspiration, and death.

Tetanus toxoid vaccine

Tetanus toxoid is usually combined with diphtheria toxoid and pertussis vaccine.

Diphtheria

Diphtheria toxin is produced by *Corynebacterium diphtheriae* and presents with nonspecific upper respiratory infection symptoms that develop into pharyngitis. Two to 3 days later, a bluish-white membrane starts to form that can cover the entire soft palate. Airway obstruction may occur.

Other complications may include myocarditis, neuritis with paralysis, respiratory failure, and death.

Diphtheria toxoid vaccine

Diphtheria toxoid vaccine is combined with tetanus toxoid and pertussis vaccine. A single-toxoid antigen is not available.

Pertussis

Pertussis, or whooping cough, is caused by *Bordetella pertussis,* which produces a toxin that paralyzes the respiratory cilia and causes inflammation of the respiratory tract.

Pertussis complications may include pneumonia, encephalopathy, seizures, and death. Pertussis is highly contagious and is commonly spread by teens and adults to infants and small children.

Pertussis vaccine

Pertussis vaccine is combined with tetanus toxoid and diphtheria toxoid for children. A whole-cell vaccine was developed in the 1930s but is no longer available in the United States. Acellular pertussis vaccine was first licensed in 1991 and has fewer side effects than the whole-cell vaccine. However, it appears to have a shorter duration of protection than the whole-cell vaccine.

Available vaccines

- DTaP (Daptacel by Sanofi Pasteur and Infanrix by GlaxoSmithKline) is indicated for children age 2 months to 7 years.
- Diphtheria and tetanus toxoid (DT) is available for pediatric patients with a contraindication to pertussis vaccine.
- Tdap (Adacel by Sanofi Pasteur, approved by the U.S. Food and Drug Administration [FDA] for ages 10 to 64 years, and Boostrix by GlaxoSmithKline, approved for >10 years of age) is indicated for everyone over the age of 10 years.
- A tetanus and diphtheria (Td) vaccine (various manufacturers) or a tetanus, diphtheria, and acellular pertussis (Tdap) vaccine is recommended every 10 years for everyone over the age of 7 years following 1 dose of Tdap.
- The ACIP recommends a single dose of Tdap in all children 7 years of age and older and all adults who have not received pertussis vaccination regardless of the interval since their last Td vaccination. Additional recommendations include vaccination of pregnant women during every pregnancy at 27 to 36 weeks gestation.
- Recommendations for wound management may or may not include Tdap, Td, or tetanus immune globulin (Table 36-3).

Dose

- **Pediatric dose:** A 0.5 mL I.M. dose of DTaP vaccine is given at 2, 4, 6, and 15 to 18 months of age. A booster dose should be given at 4 to 6 years.

TABLE 36-3. Guidelines for Tetanus Wound Management

Vaccination history	Clean, minor wounds		All other wounds	
	Td or Tdap[a]	TIG	Td or Tdap[a]	TIG
Unknown or <3 doses	Yes	No	Yes	Yes
Three or more doses	No[b]	No	No[c]	No

TIG, tetanus immune globulin.
a. Tdap should be used if the patient has not previously received Tdap and ≥10 years of age.
b. Yes, if >10 years since last dose.
c. Yes, if >5 years since last dose.

- **Adolescent dose:** A 0.5 mL I.M. dose of Tdap vaccine is given at 11 to 12 years.
- **Adult dose:** A 0.5 mL I.M. dose of Tdap is given at least once. It is to be administered regardless of the interval since a previous Td was administered. A booster dose of Td or Tdap is recommended every 10 years following the initial dose of Tdap.

Adverse reactions

Adverse reactions include pain, swelling, and redness at the injection site; systemic reactions are uncommon. An exaggerated (Arthus-type) reaction with extensive, painful swelling from shoulder to elbow can occur at the injection site and is thought to be caused by too-frequent injections of the tetanus antigen component of the combination vaccines.

Hepatitis A

Hepatitis A is the most common hepatitis infection in the United States. Transmission is human to human by the fecal–oral route of exposure. Recent exposure (within 2 weeks) of an unimmunized person to hepatitis A requires administering hepatitis A vaccine alone for persons ages 1 to 40 years and immune globulin intramuscular (IGIM), as well as beginning the hepatitis A vaccine series for persons under the age of 1 year, over the age of 40 years, or if vaccination is contraindicated. The efficacy of IGIM if administered more than 2 weeks following exposure has not been established.

Hepatitis A vaccine

The available vaccines are Havrix by GlaxoSmithKline and VAQTA by Merck. These are inactivated whole-virus vaccines. Both vaccines are available in pediatric and adult formulations.

Hepatitis A vaccine is indicated for all high-risk patients and routinely for all children 1 to 2 years of age. Catch-up immunization should be given to all children up to 18 years of age. The 2 vaccines use different potency measurements, but the volume and schedule of the dose are the same.

Dose

Children and adolescents over 1 year of age are given 0.5 mL, repeated in 6 to 12 months (Havrix) or 6 to 18 months (VAQTA) for two doses total.

Adults over 18 years of age are given 1 mL, repeated in 6 to 12 months (Havrix) or 6 to 18 months (VAQTA) for two doses total.

Adverse reactions

Adverse reactions include pain, swelling, and redness at the injection site; systemic reactions are uncommon.

Combination vaccine

Twinrix, by GlaxoSmithKline, is a combination product with hepatitis B (adult dose) and hepatitis A (pediatric dose) indicated for persons 18 years of age and older.

Dose

The usual dose is 1 mL, given at 0, 1, and 6 to 12 months. An accelerated schedule can be given at 0, 7 days, and 21 to 30 days, followed by a booster at 1 year, if protection is needed earlier.

Hepatitis B

Hepatitis B is one of the most common infections worldwide.

Complications are usually related to chronic infections with hepatitis B virus and include chronic hepatitis, cirrhosis, liver failure, hepatocellular carcinoma, and death. Twenty-five percent of all carriers develop chronic, active hepatitis. The risk of becoming a carrier following infection ranges from 6% to 50%.

Hepatitis B vaccine

Three products are currently marketed: Heplisav-B (Dynavax), Recombivax HB (Merck) and Engerix-B (GlaxoSmithKline). Heplisav-B is a recombinant, adjuvanted hepatitis B vaccine currently approved for use in adults 18 years and older. Recombinvax HB and Engerix-B are recombinant vaccines. Although the antigen contents are different, these 2 vaccines are interchangeable.

Combination vaccines are available.

Dose
Recombivax HB or Engerix-B (3-dose series)

The usual pediatric dose is 0.5 mL I.M. given at birth, 2 months, and 6 months. The usual adult dose is 1 mL given at 0, 2, and 6 months. Adolescents 11 to 15 years of age may be given a 2-dose series separated by 4 months. This dose is approved for only Recombivax HB.

Heplisav-B (2-dose series)

The usual adult dose is 0.5 mL given at 0 and 1 month.

Indications for hepatitis B vaccination include all infants, all adolescents, and high-risk adults (e.g., those with multiple sex partners or sexually transmitted diseases, injection drug abusers, patients on dialysis, patients with hemophilia, and patients with diabetes).

Serological testing may not reflect immune status after 2 years following vaccination, but immunity continues. Booster doses should not be given.

Adverse reactions

Adverse reactions include pain, swelling (nodule may form), and redness at the injection site; systemic reactions are uncommon.

Haemophilus Influenzae Type B

Haemophilus influenzae type B (Hib) is a gram-negative coccobacillus, whose outer shell consists of a polyribosyl-ribitol-phosphate (PRP) polysaccharide capsule.

The organism enters through the nasopharynx and may cause disease or may colonize the nasopharynx, creating an asymptomatic carrier.

The most common clinical infections caused by Hib are meningitis, epiglottitis, pneumonia, arthritis, and cellulitis. Hib is primarily a disease of children, with a peak at age 6 to 7 months. It rarely attacks after the age of 5 years. Transmission is human to human by respiratory droplet spread to susceptible individuals.

Haemophilus influenzae type B vaccine

Current vaccines are polysaccharide vaccines conjugated to protein carriers. The specific carriers vary by manufacturer.

PRP-T (polyribosyl-ribitol phosphate–tetanus) (ActHIB by Sanofi Pasteur) and PRP-OMB (polyribosyl-ribitol phosphate–outer membrane protein) (PedvaxHIB by Merck) are indicated for infants ≥6 weeks of age. PRP-T (Hiberix by GSK) is approved as a booster dose only among children ≥12 months.

Combination products include DTaP-Hib-IPV (inactivated polio vaccine) (Pentacel by Sanofi Pasteur) and meningococcal C, Y, and Hib (MenHibrix by GlaxoSmithKline).

Dose

The usual dose for infants is 0.5 mL I.M. given at 2, 4, 6, and 12 to 15 months of age. If PRP-OMB (PedvaxHIB) is used for the pediatric series, the 6-month dose should be omitted.

Vaccination of children over 59 months of age is not indicated unless certain medical indications exist. These include persons with asplenia, those with immunodeficiency conditions, and those undergoing immunosuppressive therapy.

Adverse reactions

Adverse reactions include pain, swelling, and redness at the injection site; systemic reactions are uncommon.

Meningococcal Disease

Meningococcal disease is caused by *Neisseria meningitidis,* a gram-negative bacterium with a polysaccharide capsule. The clinical diseases caused by *N. meningitidis* include meningitis, sepsis, pneumonia, myocarditis, and urethritis. The types of *N. meningitidis* that cause over 95% of disease are serogroups A, B, C, W-135, and Y.

Approximately 800 to 1200 cases occur per year, with a fatality rate of approximately 10%. Conjugated polysaccharide meningococcal vaccines (Menactra and MenQuadfi by Sanofi Pasteur and Menveo by GlaxoSmithKline) are polysaccharide vaccines that are conjugated to a protein to increase efficacy. They are effective against serogroups A, C, W-135, and Y.

Indications

Menactra is approved for persons 2 to 55 years of age as a single dose and from 9 to 23 months as a 2-dose series. An additional dose may be needed in immunocompromised persons age 24 months and older (e.g., asplenia, sickle cell disease, or human immunodeficiency virus [HIV] infection). MenQuadfi is approved for individuals 2 years of age and older as a single dose, and a booster dose is approved for individuals 15 years of age and older at continued risk for meningococcal disease if at least 4 years have lapsed since a prior dose of quadrivalent meningococcal conjugate vaccine. Menveo is FDA approved starting at age 2 months as a 4-dose series. The number of doses and the interval vary if the series is started at a later age. It is given as a single dose and may be repeated after 2 or 3 months (depending on initial age for dose 1) for select high-risk conditions. The ACIP does not recommend these vaccines for routine use in infants and children. The ACIP recommends routine vaccination with conjugated vaccine for persons ages 11 to 12 years with a booster dose at age 16 years (5 years after previous dose), and 2 doses given 2 or 3 months apart for persons ages 2 months through 54 years for certain chronic diseases (see ACIP recommendation). Revaccination with conjugated vaccine is recommended every 5 years for persons who were previously vaccinated and who remain at high risk for the disease.

High-risk conditions include those with anatomic or functional asplenia, patients with HIV, anyone with potential exposure (such as laboratory workers), and travelers to the "meningitis belt" of Sub-Saharan Africa. Vaccine may also be useful during an outbreak.

Dose

The dose is 0.5 mL given intramuscularly.

Adverse reactions

Adverse reactions include pain, swelling, and redness at the injection site, as well as mild systemic reactions, such as fever, headaches, and malaise.

Meningococcal B vaccine (Bexsero by GlaxoSmithKline and Trumenba by Pfizer)

Indications

Both vaccines are FDA approved for patients age 10 to 25 years. They are recommended for patients with complement deficiencies, those with asplenia, microbiologists with risk of exposure, and those exposed during outbreaks. They may be given to adolescents to provide short-term protection based on shared clinical decision-making.

Dose

The dose is 0.5 mL given intramuscularly. Bexsero is given as a 2-dose series (0, 1 to 6 months), and Trumenba is given as a 2-dose series (0, 6 months) or a 3-dose series (0, 1 to 2 months, 6 months) depending on risk factors. Products are not interchangeable, and the same product should be used for all doses in a series.

Adverse reactions

Adverse reactions include pain, swelling, and redness at the injection site, as well as mild systemic reactions, such as fever, headaches, and malaise.

Polio

The 3 poliovirus types are identified as P1, P2, and P3.

Up to 95% of all infections are asymptomatic; however, infected persons may transmit the infection to others. One percent to 2% of infections present as nonparalytic aseptic meningitis, which typically resolves in 2 to 10 days. Flaccid paralysis occurs in less than 1% of those infected.

Polio vaccine (IPOL by Sanofi Pasteur)

The current vaccine available in the United States is an inactivated, trivalent injectable vaccine (IPV, or inactivated polio vaccine). Use of oral polio vaccine (OPV) was discontinued in the United States because of the elimination of wild-type polio disease and because yearly cases of vaccine-associated paralytic poliomyelitis were reported.

Dose

The pediatric dose is 0.5 mL I.M. given at 2, 4, 6 to 18 months, and 4 to 6 years of age. Routine vaccine or booster doses for adults are not recommended unless traveling to an endemic area.

Adverse reactions

Adverse reactions include minor pain, swelling, and redness at the injection site; systemic reactions are uncommon.

Measles, Mumps, and Rubella

Measles

Measles is a viral infection. The main presentation is a maculopapular rash. The virus is shed through the nasopharynx.

The incubation period is 10 to 12 days. Transmission is person to person through large respiratory droplets. Measles is highly contagious. Complications may include pneumonia, otitis, encephalitis, and death.

Mumps

Mumps is a viral infection with a presentation of parotitis in 30% to 40% of cases. The virus is shed through the nasopharynx.

The incubation period is 14 to 18 days (range, 14 to 25 days). Transmission is person to person through large respiratory droplets.

Complications can include orchitis, oophoritis, pancreatitis, and deafness.

Rubella

Rubella is a viral infection with up to 20% to 50% of cases subclinical and inapparent. The virus is shed through the nasopharynx. Fourteen to 17 days after exposure, a maculopapular rash appears, first on the face and then descending to cover the rest of the body. The rash disappears after about 3 days.

The incubation period is 14 days (range, 12 to 23 days). Transmission is person to person through large respiratory droplets.

Complications may include arthritis, arthralgias, encephalitis, and hemorrhaging. The major complication is congenital rubella syndrome (CRS), which occurs in the offspring of a woman who had rubella during pregnancy. Babies born with CRS have major birth defects that can affect many organs.

Measles–mumps–rubella vaccine (M-M-R II by Merck)

The current vaccine available in the United States is a live attenuated vaccine against all 3 diseases.

Contraindications

This vaccine is contraindicated in pregnancy. Pregnancy should be avoided for 4 weeks following vaccination. Other contraindications include immunosuppressive disease or patients receiving immunosuppressive therapy, as well as those receiving antibody-containing blood products.

Dose

The usual pediatric dose is 0.5 mL I.M. given at 12 months of age. A second dose is recommended at 4 to 6 years of age to produce immunity in those who did not respond to the first dose.

Serologic testing may be necessary to document immunity.

Adverse reactions

Adverse reactions include minor pain, swelling, and redness at the injection site and systemic reactions that mimic a mild case of the diseases.

Varicella (Chickenpox)

Varicella is a viral infection caused by the herpes zoster virus. The primary infection is called *chicken pox,* and the recurrent disease is herpes zoster (called *shingles*).

The virus enters through the respiratory tract and replicates in the nasopharynx and regional lymph glands. The incubation period is 14 to 16 days (range, 10 to 21 days).

The rash progresses from a macule to a papule to a vesicle before it crusts over. The rash first appears on the face and then the trunk (where most of the rash occurs) and the extremities.

Recurrent disease (herpes zoster) appears to be related to aging and immunosuppression. Recurrent disease usually presents as an outbreak of lesions along a dermatome and is usually unilateral. Neuralgia and intense pain may be present.

Transmission of varicella is person to person by infected respiratory secretions. Transmission by patients with herpes zoster is by direct contact with a nonimmune person.

Complications may include pneumonia, secondary bacterial infections, central nervous system infections, and sepsis.

Varicella vaccine (Varivax by Merck)

The current vaccine is a live attenuated vaccine.

Contraindications

This vaccine is contraindicated in pregnancy, and pregnancy should be avoided for 4 weeks following vaccination. Other contraindications include severe allergic reaction to neomycin or gelatin, immunosuppressive disease or patients receiving immunosuppressive therapy, as well as those receiving antibody-containing blood products.

Dose

The pediatric dose is 0.5 mL I.M., given at 12 to 18 months of age. A second dose is recommended at 4 to 6 years of age.

The adult dose (age > 13 years) is 2 doses of 0.5 mL, each separated by 4 to 8 weeks.

Refrigerator-stable and freezer-stable formulations of the vaccine are available. The freezer-stable vaccine must be stored frozen at 5°F (−15°C) or colder. Before reconstitution, the refrigerator-stable vaccine has a shelf-life of 2 years when stored at 2°C to 8 °C (36°F to 46°F) or colder, but it can also be frozen. Once the refrigerator-stable formulation is transferred to a refrigerator, the vaccine should not be refrozen. The diluent used to reconstitute either formulation of the vaccine should be stored at room temperature or refrigerated.

Adverse reactions

Adverse reactions include minor pain, swelling, and redness at the injection site and systemic reactions that mimic a mild case of the disease, including a mild generalized rash.

Combination Vaccine

There are 3 ProQuad formulations (refrigerator-stable, frozen recombinant human albumin [RHA], and frozen human serum albumin [HSA]) available that contain a combination of measles, mumps, rubella, and varicella (MMRV) vaccine indicated for prevention of measles, mumps, rubella, and varicella in children 12 months through 12 years of age. Routine dosing is 0.5 mL subcutaneous at 12 to 15 months followed by a booster dose at 4 to 6 years of age.

Herpes zoster vaccine (Shingrix by GlaxoSmithKline)

Shingrix (GSK) is a recombinant, adjuvanted zoster vaccine (lyophilized gE antigen component requiring reconstitution with an adjuvant suspension) shown to reduce the risk of developing herpes zoster by 97% and 91% in patients ≥50 years and ≥70 years, respectively. The ACIP prefers Shingrix (GSK) over Zostavax (Merck), a live, attenuated herpes zoster vaccine that is no longer available, for the prevention of herpes zoster and related post-herpetic complications.

Indication

Shingrix (GSK) is indicated for all adults over the age of 50 years, regardless of previous zoster disease or previous receipt of Zostavax (Merck).

Dose

Shingrix (GSK) is a 2-dose series of 0.5 mL I.M. (must be reconstituted) separated by 2 to 6 months. Wait at least 2 months after the last dose of live attenuated zoster vaccine to administer recombinant zoster vaccine when indicated. The recombinant, adjuvanted vaccine and the adjuvant suspension must both be refrigerated at 2°C to 8°C (36°F to 46°F) and discarded if frozen.

Adverse reactions

Adverse reactions include pain, redness, and swelling at the injection site and an increased incidence of headache.

Rotavirus

Rotavirus is the most common cause of severe gastroenteritis in infants and small children. Symptoms range from mild, watery diarrhea of limited duration to severe diarrhea with vomiting and fever that can result in dehydration.

A significant reduction in clinical disease and hospitalization rates has occurred since the introduction of the vaccine.

Rotavirus is transmitted by the fecal–oral route by close person-to-person contact through contaminated objects, food, and water.

Rotavirus vaccines

Two rotavirus vaccines are available:

- Pentavalent human–bovine reassortant rotavirus vaccine (RotaTeq [RV5] by Merck)
- Monovalent human rotavirus vaccine (Rotarix [RV1] by GlaxoSmithKline)

RV5 is a live oral vaccine that contains 5 reassortant rotaviruses and is available as a liquid that requires no reconstitution. RV1 is a live oral vaccine that contains 1 human rotavirus strain and is a lyophilized powder that must be reconstituted before administration.

Indications

The rotavirus vaccine can be administered simultaneously with all other pediatric vaccines indicated at the same age. It should not be given to infants who had a severe reaction to a previous dose.

Contraindications

Contraindications include altered immunocompetence, acute gastroenteritis, moderate or severe acute illness, preexisting chronic gastrointestinal disease, and a previous history of intussusception.

Dose

Both vaccines are administered orally. RV5 contains 2 mL per dose, and RV1 contains 1 mL per dose.

RV5 is a 3-dose series given at 2, 4, and 6 months of age. RV1 is a 2-dose series given at 2 and 4 months of age. The rotavirus series should be started no sooner than 6 weeks of age and must be completed by 8 months, 0 days of age.

Adverse reactions

Adverse reactions may include diarrhea and vomiting.

Human Papillomavirus

Human papillomavirus (HPV) is the most common sexually transmitted disease in the United States. Although most HPV infections are asymptomatic and self-limiting, persistent infection can cause cervical cancer and genital warts.

Approximately 100 HPV types exist, with 40 types affecting the genital area and the remainder associated with skin warts. High-risk viruses can cause low- and high-grade cervical cell abnormalities and anogenital cancers. The HPV types in the vaccine cause approximately 90% of cervical cancers. HPV types 6 and 11 cause 90% of all genital warts.

HPV vaccine

One HPV vaccine is now available in the United States:

- Human papillomavirus vaccine (Gardasil by Merck) protects against HPV types 6, 11, 16, 18, 31, 33, 45, 52, and 58 (HPV9).

Indications

HPV9 is indicated for the prevention of disease caused by the types of HPV in the specific vaccine; it is not used for the treatment of HPV infection.

The HPV vaccine is indicated for all 9 to 45 years of age and should be given routinely to all children aged 11 to 12 years.

Contraindications

HPV vaccine is contraindicated in persons who had a reaction to a previous dose.

Dose

The HPV vaccine is inactivated and administered as a 2-dose series given at 0 and 6 to 12 months if administered between 9 and 14 years of age, or a 3-dose series given at 0, 1 to 2, and 6 months if administered between 15 and 45 years of age. Persons with immunocompromising conditions (e.g.,

HIV infection) should receive the 3-dose series regardless of age at administration. The vaccine must be shaken, and 0.5 mL is administered intramuscularly in the deltoid area.

The HPV vaccine may be given simultaneously with other recommended vaccines.

Adverse reactions

Adverse reactions are primarily local and include pain, redness, and swelling at the injection site. A systemic reaction of fever may occur.

Combination Vaccines

As mentioned in previous sections, several vaccination combinations are on the market (Box 36-4).

Always review manufacturer and/or ACIP recommendations when using various combination products along with other individual products to complete a dosing series as some products are not interchangeable.

BOX 36-4. Combination Vaccines Available in the United States

- Tetanus, diphtheria, and pertussis combinations (various manufacturers): DTaP, DT, Td, Tdap
- Twinrix by GlaxoSmithKline: a combination product with hepatitis B (adult dose) and hepatitis A (pediatric dose) approved for those ≥18 years of age
- Pediarix (GlaxoSmithKline)
  - DTaP + hepatitis B + inactivated polio
  - Indicated when all vaccine components indicated
  - Not approved for patients <6 weeks or >7 years of age
  - Efficacy, contraindications, and adverse reactions similar to those of the vaccine components given separately
  - Dose: 0.5 mL I.M. given at 2, 4, and 6 months of age
  - Must be shaken vigorously before drawn up in syringe
  - Can be given even if infant receives birth dose of hepatitis B vaccine
- Pentacel (Sanofi Pasteur)
  - DTaP + Hib + inactivated polio
  - Indicated when all vaccine components indicated
  - Not approved for patients <6 weeks or >4 years of age
  - Efficacy, contraindications, and adverse reactions similar to those of the vaccine components given separately
  - Dose: 0.5 mL I.M. given at 2, 4, and 6 months of age
  - Must be shaken vigorously before drawn up in syringe
- ProQuad by Merck: a combination of measles, mumps, rubella, and varicella vaccines
- Kinrix by GlaxoSmithKline and Quadracel by Sanofi Pasteur: a combination of DTaP and IPV to be given at 4 to 6 years of age
- Vaxelis (MSP Vaccine Company)
  - DTaP + inactivated polio + Hib + HepB
  - Indicated when all vaccine components indicated
  - Not approved for patients <6 weeks or >4 years of age
  - Efficacy, contraindications, and adverse reactions similar to those of the vaccine components given separately
  - Dose: 0.5 mL I.M. given at 2, 4, and 6 months of age
  - Must be shaken vigorously before drawn up in syringe

36-6   Pharmacist's Role

Pharmacists play an important role in combating infectious diseases that are preventable with vaccines. With a growing number able to vaccinate, pharmacists can not only help immunize but also educate the community and dispel misconceptions surrounding vaccines.

NAPLEX Competency Statements

The questions in this chapter cover the following 2021 NAPLEX Competency Statements: **AREA 1:** 1.1; 1.6 **AREA 2:** 2.2; 2.4 **AREA 3:** 3.4; 3.5; 3.6; 3.7.

36-7   Questions

1. A 67-year-old patient presents to your pharmacy for a refill of his blood pressure medication. It is June, and he asks you to review his immunization status with him. About which adult vaccine(s) do you need to ask his status? (Mark all that apply.)

   A. Influenza
   B. Pneumococcal
   C. Meningococcal
   D. Tetanus, diphtheria, and acellular pertussis (Tdap)
   E. Hepatitis B

2. An immunocompetent 70-year-old patient states that he received a pneumococcal vaccine 4 years ago (PPSV23-Pneumovax 23). When should he receive another?

   A. He never needs another dose.
   B. He should receive a dose every year.
   C. He should receive another dose in 1 year.
   D. He should receive a PCV13 (Prevnar) vaccine if indicated based on shared clinical decision-making.
   E. Every 5 years

3. Which of the following describes the current injectable influenza vaccine used in the United States?

   A. Inactivated virus
   B. Live attenuated virus
   C. Conjugated vaccine
   D. Toxoid
   E. Toxin

4. Which one of the following is an indication for meningococcal conjugate vaccine?

   A. All adolescents 11 to 12 years of age, with a booster at age 16 years or 5 years after last dose
   B. All infants
   C. Patients with liver disease
   D. An adult backpacking in Europe
   E. College graduate students

5. At what age does one switch from DTaP to Tdap?

   A. 2 years
   B. 5 years
   C. 7 years
   D. 10 years
   E. DTaP can be used in all age groups.

6. Which of the following vaccines has *both* a polysaccharide and a conjugated vaccine on the U.S. market?

   A. Influenza
   B. Hepatitis A vaccine
   C. *Haemophilus influenzae* type B vaccine
   D. Pneumococcal vaccine
   E. MMR vaccine

7. Which polio vaccine schedule is recommended in the United States?

   A. Four doses of IPV
   B. Four doses of OPV
   C. Four doses of IPV plus a booster at 18 years of age
   D. Three doses of IPV
   E. Polio vaccine is no longer recommended in the United States.

8. Hepatitis B vaccine is _____.

A. a polysaccharide vaccine
B. an inactivated vaccine
C. a live vaccine
D. a conjugate vaccine
E. a toxoid

Use Patient Profile 36-1 to answer Questions 9 and 10.

PATIENT PROFILE 36-1

Patient Name: Sarah Jones   **Height:** 5'4"

Age: 18 yo   **Weight:** 140 lb

Sex: Female   **Allergies:** Penicillin

Current Medical History: No chronic medical conditions

Immunization History: Up to date on all childhood vaccines through age 5 years

9. Which of the following vaccine is indicated for Ms. Jones for routine vaccination before starting college?

A. Hepatitis B vaccine
B. Hepatitis A vaccine
C. Meningococcal A, C, W-135, Y vaccine
D. Pneumococcal vaccine
E. Herpes zoster vaccine

10. Ms. Jones is notified by the health department that she was exposed to a patient with hepatitis A yesterday. She should receive which of the following?

A. Hepatitis A vaccine series only
B. Hepatitis B vaccine series only
C. Hepatitis A vaccine series plus IGIM
D. Hepatitis A vaccine plus hepatitis B vaccine series
E. IGIM only

11. Which of the following is a high-risk group that should be targeted for pneumococcal vaccination? (Mark all that apply.)

A. Persons over 65 years of age
B. Persons with diabetes
C. Patients 21 to 49 years of age with hypertension
D. 35-year-old who smokes cigarettes
E. 40-year-old health care worker

12. Which complication of rubella infection is the most significant health problem?

A. Congenital rubella syndrome
B. Secondary infection
C. Patent ductus arteriosus
D. Diarrhea
E. Arthritis

13. Which of the following is a valid contraindication to the receipt of an injectable live-virus vaccine?

A. Current administration of antibiotics
B. Recent administration of antibody-containing blood products
C. Age over 12 months
D. Allergies to penicillin
E. A parent or sibling with a cold who is living in the same household

14. The most common adverse reaction to an inactivated vaccine is _____.

A. rash
B. severe headache
C. injection-site reaction
D. rhinorrhea
E. stomach pain

15. The only vaccine recommended at birth is _____.

A. DTaP
B. IPV
C. Hib
D. pneumococcal conjugate vaccine
E. hepatitis B

16. A 32-year-old female is injured in an automobile accident, and her spleen is removed. Which of the following vaccines are recommended for asplenic adult patients? (Mark all that apply.)

A. Pneumococcal vaccine
B. Meningococcal vaccine
C. IPV
D. *Haemophilus influenzae* type B vaccine
E. Influenza vaccine

17. If a second dose of a vaccine were given too soon (before the minimal interval time has passed), the correct course of action would be _____.

    A. restarting the entire series
    B. not counting that dose and repeating it after the minimal time has passed since the incorrect dose
    C. not worrying about it and continuing with the next dose as scheduled
    D. drawing antibody titers to confirm immunity
    E. doubling the next dose

18. Which of the following high-risk groups are at increased risk for pneumococcal disease and should be vaccinated? (Mark all that apply.)

    A. All adolescents at age 11 to 12 years
    B. Adults 65 years or older
    C. Black teenagers
    D. Adults with diabetes
    E. Children infected with HIV

19. Which of the following statements is true concerning Hib vaccine?

    A. One dose of Hib is recommended for all children over the age of 5 years if they have not received a previous dose.
    B. Standard dosing for Hib vaccine is 2, 4, 6, and 12 to 15 months of age.
    C. The 6-month dose is omitted if ActHIB is used for the first 2 doses.
    D. Hib vaccine is not routinely recommended for children 12 to 15 months of age.
    E. Hib vaccine is given only to high-risk infants.

20. Which of the following vaccines available in the United States is a live, attenuated virus vaccine?

    A. Polio (IPV)
    B. *Haemophilus influenzae* type B vaccine (Hib)
    C. DTaP
    D. Varicella vaccine
    E. Pneumococcal vaccine

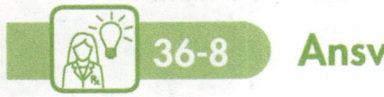 **36-8   Answers**

1. **B, D.** Routine vaccinations in an adult are a yearly influenza vaccine (if in season), Tdap vaccine if not previously vaccinated, and a single pneumococcal vaccine for patients over the age of 65 years or younger with select chronic illnesses (such as diabetes). June is too early in the season to indicate the influenza vaccine. Meningococcal and hepatitis vaccines are recommended only for certain indications.

2. **D.** Routine revaccination with pneumococcal polysaccharide vaccine (PPSV23) is not recommended. Revaccination is recommended for select high-risk groups and everyone age 65 years and older who received an initial dose under the age of 65 and if more than 5 years have elapsed since the previous dose. Immunocompetent individuals can receive a single dose of conjugated pneumococcal vaccine (PCV13) at 65 years or older if they have not received one before the age of 65 years based on shared clinical decision-making.

3. **A.** Injected influenza vaccine is an inactivated, split-virus vaccine. The live attenuated influenza vaccine is administered intranasally.

4. **A.** The ACIP recommends including all adolescents age 11 to 12 years with a booster at age 16 years (or 5 years since last dose) among the other high-risk recommendations (asplenia, travel to endemic areas, meningococcal outbreaks).

5. **C.** DTaP is indicated for children under the age of 7 years. Because of adverse effects of DTaP in children 7 years of age and older, Tdap is used.

6. **D.** Polysaccharide pneumococcal vaccine (23-valent) is indicated for those over the age of 2 years, and conjugated polysaccharide vaccine (13-valent) is approved for ages 2 months to 7 years (FDA approved but not ACIP recommended).

7. **A.** OPV is no longer recommended in the United States, and vaccination with 4 doses of IPV will continue until poliovirus is eradicated worldwide.

8. **B.** Hepatitis B vaccine is an inactivated vaccine.

9. **C.** Meningococcal A, C, W-135, Y vaccine is routine for adolescents, and catch-up is recommended if they missed it at a younger age.

10. **A.** The hepatitis A vaccine alone will protect a healthy individual between 1 and 40 years of age who has previously been exposed to the virus.

11. **A, B, D.** All persons over the age of 65 years, patients between 2 and 64 years of age with certain medical conditions, and adult smokers age 19 to 64 years are in need of pneumococcal vaccination.

12. **A.** Complications of rubella may include arthritis, arthralgias, encephalitis, and hemorrhaging; however, the major complication is congenital rubella syndrome, which occurs in the offspring of a woman who had rubella during pregnancy. Babies born with CRS have major birth defects that can affect many organs.

13. **B.** Live-virus vaccines will be killed if antibodies have been administered recently. The length of time that must separate these 2 products depends on the dose and type of antibody-containing blood product being used.

14. **C.** Local reactions are the most common type of adverse reaction and include pain, swelling, and redness at the site of injection. These reactions usually occur within minutes to hours of the injection and are usually mild and self-limiting. Systemic adverse reactions include fever, malaise, myalgias, and headache and are more common following live vaccines.

15. **E.** All the other listed vaccines are first given at 2 months of age. Hepatitis B vaccine is recommended at birth to decrease the incidence of hepatitis B in infants of hepatitis B–infected mothers.

16. **A, B, D, E.** Asplenic patients require protection against the encapsulated bacteria (pneumococcus, meningococcus, and *Haemophilus*), as well as common viral infections. The meningococcal vaccine is to be repeated every 5 years. Completion of previous series of routine vaccines, such as measles, varicella, and polio, are adequate for protection. Td vaccines should be repeated every 10 years following a single dose of Tdap, and influenza vaccine should be administered yearly.

17. **B.** The minimal interval in a series for most vaccines is 4 weeks. Decreasing the interval may interfere with antibody response and protection. Usually, the last dose in a series is separated from the previous dose by 4 to 6 months. Increasing the interval does not affect vaccine effectiveness. You never need to restart a series except for oral typhoid vaccine.

18. **B, D, E.** Rates of pneumococcal disease are highest in children <2 years of age (vaccination is routine in all infants); those with asplenia; patients with HIV; and patients with certain chronic conditions, such as diabetes. Those with the highest risk are indicated to receive both polysaccharide and conjugate vaccines. Obesity is not considered a high-risk disease for pneumococcal infection.

19. **B.** Hib vaccine is routinely administered to all infants and may be indicated for children over the age of 5 years with certain chronic conditions. This vaccine is relatively complicated to use because recommendations vary among manufacturers (PedvaxHIB does not require the 6-month dose). Please consult package inserts before administering.

20. **D.** Varicella vaccine, live attenuated influenza vaccine, measles–mumps–rubella vaccine, and rotavirus vaccine are the only live vaccines routinely administered in the United States. Other nonroutinely administered live vaccines include oral typhoid vaccine, vaccinia (smallpox) vaccine, and yellow fever vaccine. The majority of vaccines are inactivated or killed vaccines.

 **36-9** **Additional Resources**

Centers for Disease Control and Prevention. *Epidemiology and Prevention of Vaccine-Preventable Diseases* (Pink Book). 13th ed. Washington, DC: Public Health Foundation; 2015. Available at: https://www.cdc.gov/vaccines/pubs/pinkbook/index.html. Accessed June 1, 2020.

Centers for Disease Control and Prevention. Vaccine and Immunizations. Available at: https://www.cdc.gov/vaccines/index.html. Accessed June 1, 2020.

Centers for Disease Control and Prevention. Vaccine Recommendations of the ACIP. Available at: https://www.cdc.gov/vaccines/hcp/acip-recs/index.html. Accessed June 1, 2020.

Immunization Action Coalition. Available at: https://immunize.org/. Accessed June 1, 2020.

Osteoporosis

ANDREA S. FRANKS

 ## 37-1 KEY POINTS

- Patients should be counseled about the preventive measures to increase and maintain bone mineral density throughout the lifespan. Key measures include adequate calcium and vitamin D intake, moderation in alcohol use, and smoking avoidance. Regular weight-bearing and strengthening exercises that help reduce falls, build bone density, and prevent fractures should be encouraged.
- Medications that most commonly cause osteoporosis include some chemotherapy agents and long-term corticosteroids.
- Medication therapy should be considered for postmenopausal women and men over the age 50 who have a history of hip or vertebral fracture, T-score of −2.5 or less, or osteopenia (T-score between −1.0 and −2.5) with a FRAX indicating high fracture risk.
- Osteoporosis therapy should be tailored to each patient considering risks and benefits, concomitant diseases, and medications.
- Denosumab and some bisphosphonates (**alendronate**, risedronate, zoledronic acid) are first-line treatments for osteoporosis. They have been shown to decrease hip, vertebral, and nonvertebral fractures.
- Other medications have been shown to decrease some types of fractures, but do not have hip fracture data. These include ibandronate, raloxifene, abaloparatide, teriparatide, and romosozumab.
- Most oral bisphosphonate formulations must be taken with a full glass of plain water, 30 to 60 minutes before the first meal of the day or any other medications. The patient must remain upright for at least 30 minutes after taking an oral dosage. Bisphosphonates are contraindicated in patients with significant kidney disease.

 ## 37-2 STUDY GUIDE CHECKLIST

The following topics may guide your study of this subject area:

- ☐ Recommended intake of calcium for older adults.
- ☐ Recommended intake of vitamin D for older adults.
- ☐ Medications that may increase risk of osteoporosis.
- ☐ Contraindications and potential adverse effects of osteoporosis agents, including bisphosphonates, denosumab, calcitonin, estrogen therapy, estrogen agonist/antagonists or selective estrogen receptor modulators, teriparatide, abaloparatide, and romosozumab.

 **37-3** **Osteoporosis Disease Overview**

Osteoporosis is characterized by low bone mineral density and poor bone strength/quality that increases the risk of fractures. Osteoporosis increases the fragility of bone with a subsequent risk of fracture. The most common sites of osteoporosis-related fractures are the hip and vertebra.

Diagnostic Criteria

Dual-energy x-ray absorptiometry (DXA) scans are used to diagnose osteoporosis. The WHO classifications of bone mineral density (BMD) uses T-scores to guide osteoporosis diagnosis and treatment (see Figure 37-1).

Osteopenia (low bone density): T-score 1 to 2.5 standard deviations below the young adult mean (−1 to −2.5)
Osteoporosis: T-score *below* 2.5 standard deviations below the young adult mean (−2.5 or greater)

Risk for osteoporosis and fracture is determined by modifiable and unmodifiable factors. Key risk factors are included in a mnemonic in Figure 37-2.

Box 37-1 lists medical conditions associated with risk of osteoporosis.

Box 37-2 lists medications associated with an increased risk of osteoporosis.

Screening for Osteoporosis

The FRAX tool is useful for screening and making treatment decisions for osteoporosis. It calculates the percent probability of hip fracture and any major osteoporotic fracture in the subsequent 10 years for postmenopausal women and men 50 years of age or older. The FRAX tool can be accessed at https://www.sheffield.ac.uk/FRAX/ and is available through cell phone apps. BMD is measured by central DXA scan. DXA scan results provide T-scores used to diagnose, classify, and monitor osteoporosis and low bone mass (osteopenia).

Clinical Presentation

- Loss of height
- Vertebra, hip, or forearm fracture
- Kyphosis
- Bone pain (especially back pain, which could indicate vertebral compression fracture)

FIGURE 37-1.

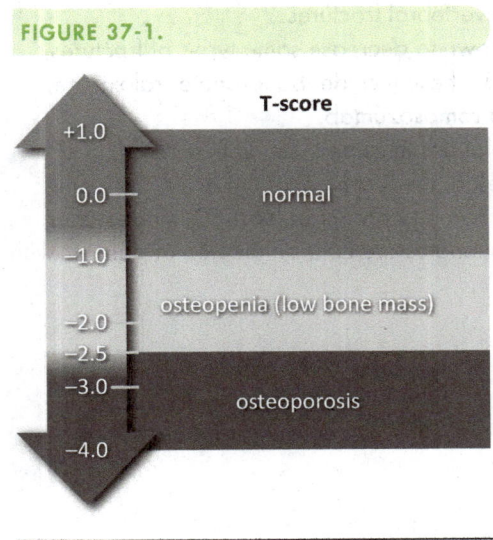

FIGURE 37-2. Risk Factors for Osteoporosis

MNEMONIC FOR OSTEOPOROSIS RISK FACTORS

O   LOw calcium intake

S   Seizure meds (anticonvulsants)

T   Thin build

E   Ethanol intake

O   HypOgonadism

P   Previous fracture

O   ThyrOid excess

R   Race (Asian, white)

O   Other relatives with osteoporosis

S   Steroids

I   Inactivity

S   Smoking

Source: Bethel M. Osteoporosis. https://emedicine.medscape.com/article/330598-overview#a4. Accessed March 31, 2019.

> ### BOX 37-1. Medical Conditions Associated with Increased Risk of Osteoporosis
>
> - Acquired immune deficiency syndrome (AIDS)
> - Cushing's disease
> - Diabetes, type 1 and type 2
> - Eating disorders
> - Hyperthyroidism
> - Hyperparathyroidism
> - Inflammatory bowel disease
>
> - Malabsorption syndromes (bariatric surgery, gastrectomy, Crohn's disease)
> - Rheumatoid arthritis
> - Chronic kidney disease
> - Chronic obstructive pulmonary disease
> - Low testosterone levels in men (hypogonadism)

Pathophysiology

Osteoblasts (formation) and osteoclasts (resorption) create a constant state of bone remodeling. During childhood and adolescence, bone formation exceeds resorption until peak bone mass is reached around age 25 to 35 years. Bone density then begins to decline. In women, bone loss accelerates after menopause.

General Treatment Principles

Adequate calcium and vitamin D intake through diet or supplementation is recommended throughout the lifespan (calcium 1000 to 1200 mg daily plus 600 to 1000 IU vitamin D daily).

Recommended lifestyle modifications include weight-bearing and muscle-strengthening exercise, exercises to help with balance, smoking cessation, and limited alcohol intake.

Medication for osteoporosis should be initiated on the basis of individual risk factors, bone mineral density, fracture history, and concomitant diseases and medications

> ### BOX 37-2. Medications Associated with an Increased Risk of Osteoporosis
>
> Antiretroviral therapy
> - Nucleoside/nucleotide reverse transcriptase inhibitors (NRTI)
> - Protease inhibitors
> - Nonnucleoside reverse transcriptase inhibitors (NNRTI)
>
> Antiseizure medications
> - Carbamazepine
> - Phenobarbital
> - Phenytoin
> - Valproic acid
>
> Aromatase inhibitors
> - Anastrozole
> - Letrozole
>
> Glucocorticoids (≥ 5 mg prednisone equivalent daily for ≥ 3 months)
>
> Heparin or low molecular weight heparin (≥ 6 months)
>
> Immunosuppressants
>
> Medroxyprogesterone acetate depot (DMPA)
>
> Proton pump inhibitors (long-term)
>
> Selective serotonin reuptake inhibitors (SSRI)
>
> Sodium glucose cotransporter 2 (SGLT2) inhibitors
>
> Tamoxifen (premenopausal)
>
> Thiazolidinediones
> - Pioglitazone
> - Rosiglitazone

Initiation of Treatment

The National Osteoporosis Foundation recommends initiation of medication in postmenopausal women and men ≥50 years of age who meet at least 1 of the following criteria:

1. Low bone mass (T-score between −1.0 and −2.5 at the femoral neck or spine) and A and/or B below:
   A. ≥3% FRAX-calculated 10-year probability of hip fracture and/or
   B. ≥20% FRAX-calculated 10-year probability of major osteoporosis-related fracture (defined as fractures resulting from low-impact trauma, excluding fractures of face, fingers, and toes)
2. A hip fracture or vertebral fracture regardless of T-score
3. T-score more than 2.5 SD below normal at the femoral neck or spine after appropriate evaluation to exclude secondary causes

Drug Therapy

Calcium and vitamin D

Mechanism of action

Calcium is necessary to maintain and improve bone mass. It is absorbed through the gastrointestinal (GI) tract, stored in the bone, and made available when calcium levels become low. Vitamin D facilitates absorption and regulation of calcium levels. In addition to facilitating calcium absorption, vitamin D may play a role in fall prevention.

Recommended requirements

Calcium

Both the Institute of Medicine (IOM) and National Osteoporosis Foundation (NOF) recommend calcium 1000 mg per day for men age 50 to 70 and 1200 mg per day for women age 51 and older and men age 71 and older (Table 37-1).

Vitamin D

The NOF recommends 800 to 1000 units of vitamin D/daily for adults age 50 years and older. The IOM recommends vitamin D intake of 600 units daily until age 70 years and 800 units for patients 70 and over. Because higher serum 25(OH)D levels (>30 to 32 ng/mL) are associated with optimal calcium absorption, the NOF and some other societies recommend daily vitamin D intake of 800 to 1000 units (Table 37-1).

TABLE 37-1. Recommended Daily Intake of Calcium and Vitamin D for Older Adults

Population	Calcium	Vitamin D (IOM)	Vitamin D (NOF)
Women			
51 to 70 years old	1200 mg	600 units	800 to 1000 units
Men			
51 to 70 years old	1000 mg	600 units	800 to 1000 units
Women and Men			
≥71 years old	1200 mg	800 units	800 to 1000 units

Adapted from NOF Healthcare Professionals Toolkit.
NOF, National Osteoporosis Foundation; IOM, Institute of Medicine.

Product selection

Calcium carbonate contains the highest level of elemental calcium. Because it requires acid to be absorbed, it should be taken with food. Absorption is decreased in patients taking proton pump inhibitors.

Calcium citrate products may be administered without regard to meals as they do not require acid to be absorbed. Calcium citrate is the best choice for patients taking proton pump inhibitors. Approximately 500 mg of calcium can be absorbed from the gastrointestinal tract at a time. To enhance absorption and minimize adverse effects, separate doses appropriately to achieve a total daily dose of 1000 to 1200 mg.

Patient instructions and counseling

- Only take 500 mg of calcium at a time so it can be absorbed.
- If the patient takes take calcium carbonate, it should be taken with meals.
- Calcium citrate can be taken with or without meals, and is the best choice if you take a medication to decrease acid secretion in your stomach.

Adverse drug effects

- **GI:** Nausea, vomiting, cramping, flatulence, especially with carbonate
- **Electrolytes:** Hypophosphatemia and hypercalcemia
- **Renal:** Nephrolithiasis (especially with higher doses and in patients predisposed to calcium oxalate kidney stones)

Drug–drug and drug–disease interactions

Concomitant administration with calcium may decrease the bioavailability of fluoroquinolones, tetracyclines, and **levothyroxine**. Calcium supplements should be used with caution in patients with a history of nephrolithiasis.

Bisphosphonates

Table 37-2 provides summary information about bisphosphonates and other antiresorptive medications.

Mechanism of action

Bisphosphonates are incorporated into the hydroxyapatite of the bone to increase and stabilize bone mass. They inhibit osteoclasts and have a very long half-life in the bone.

Bisphosphonates are considered first-line therapy for osteoporosis treatment, and several randomized, controlled clinical trials demonstrate reduction in fractures of the hips and vertebrae in addition to beneficial effects on BMD. Adherence may be increased with extended dosing intervals (weekly, monthly, quarterly); however, the studies that demonstrated fracture risk reduction used daily dosing.

Appropriate calcium and vitamin D intake must be assured when taking bisphosphonates. Bisphosphonates have very poor oral bioavailability and cannot be taken with any other food, beverage, or medication. Due to the risk of esophageal ulceration/irritation, they must be taking with 8 ounces of plain water and the patient must remain standing or sitting up for at least 30 minutes afterward.

Patient instructions and counseling

- Bisphosphonates must be taken with a full glass of water (8 oz) 30 to 60 minutes before the first meal of the day and any other medications, vitamins, or supplements.
- Atelvia, delayed-release risedronate, should be taken immediately after breakfast.
- Binosto, effervescent tablet of **alendronate**, should be dissolved in 4 oz of plain water. After bubbling stops, wait at least 5 minutes, then stir for 10 seconds and drink.
- Remain in an upright position for at least 30 minutes following ingestion, and do not lie down until after eating the first meal of the day.
- The patient should notify a health care provider if experiencing any pain in the chest or stomach while taking this medication.

TABLE 37-2. Antiresorptive Agents

Medication	Dosing
Bisphosphonates	
Alendronate (Fosamax)	Prevention: 5 mg orally daily or 35 mg orally weekly
(Binosto—effervescent tablet)	Treatment: 10 mg daily or 70 mg weekly
Risedronate (Actonel) (Atelvia—35 mg delayed release)	5 mg orally daily or
	35 mg orally weekly or
	150 mg orally monthly
Ibandronate (Boniva)	150 mg orally monthly, 3 mg I.V. every 3 months
Zoledronic acid (Reclast)	Prevention: 5 mg I.V. every 2 years
	Treatment: 5 mg I.V. once yearly
Estrogen Agonist/Antagonists or Selective estrogen receptor modulators	
Raloxifene (Evista)	60 mg orally daily
Conjugated equine estrogens (CEE)/bazedoxifene (Duavee)	0.45 CEE/20 bazedoxifene mg orally daily
Other antiresorptive agents	
Denosumab (Prolia)	60 mg subcutaneously every 6 months
Calcitonin (Miacalcin)	Intranasal: 200 IU daily, alternating nostrils
	Intramuscular or subcutaneous: 100 IU every other day

Boldface indicates one of top 100 drugs for 2020 by prescription volume.

- Be sure to get adequate calcium and vitamin D through diet and supplements.
- Major dental work should be completed before starting this medication to avoid rare but serious dental problems.

Adverse drug effects

- **GI:** Abdominal pain, dyspepsia, constipation, diarrhea, flatulence, nausea, gastritis, and esophageal ulceration
- **Dental:** Osteonecrosis of the jaw (rare, mostly in cancer patients on intravenous bisphosphonates)
- **Neuromuscular:** Myalgia, arthralgia, or flu-like symptoms (especially with intravenous zoledronic acid)
- **Orthopedic:** Low-trauma atypical femur fractures (rare, more common in patients taking for 3 to 5 years)

Drug–drug and drug–disease interactions

Concomitant administration with any other medications or supplements will significantly reduce the absorption of oral bisphosphonates. Bisphosphonates are contraindicated for patients with creatinine clearance <30 to 35 mL/min. Oral bisphosphonates are contraindicated in patients with abnormalities of the esophagus (stricture, achalasia).

Monitoring for safety and efficacy

- Monitoring for safety includes appropriate calcium and vitamin D intake and, in some cases, serum calcium and vitamin D levels.
- Monitor for signs/symptoms of esophageal or gastric irritation.
- Efficacy monitoring includes incidence of fractures and DXA scan.

Denosumab (Prolia)

Mechanism of action

Denosumab is a monoclonal antibody that binds to RANKL (receptor activator of nuclear factor kappa-B ligand), preventing osteoclast formation and decreasing bone resorption. It is considered first-line therapy in high-risk patients. Unlike bisphosphonates, it can be used in patients with decreased creatinine clearance/chronic kidney disease. Denosumab is FDA approved to treat osteoporosis in postmenopausal women and men at high risk for fracture due to multiple risk factors, including prior fractures and treatment with medications that decrease BMD (long-term systemic glucocorticoids, androgen deprivation, or aromatase inhibitors). When denosumab treatment is discontinued, bone loss can be rapid and may result in multiple vertebral fractures, especially in patients with a prior vertebral fracture. A bisphosphonate or other antiresorptive therapy is recommended after discontinuing denosumab therapy.

Patient instructions and counseling

- Prolia is administered by a health care professional every 6 months as an injection under the skin.
- Treatment should also include supplemental calcium (at least 1000 mg/d) and vitamin D (at least 400 IU/d).
- Major dental work should be completed before starting Prolia.

Adverse drug effects

- **Central nervous system (CNS):** Fatigue, headache
- **GI:** Nausea, diarrhea
- **Dermatologic:** Rash, dermatitis, eczema
- **Electrolytes:** Hypocalcemia
- **Neuromuscular:** Weakness, arthralgia
- **Dental:** Osteonecrosis of the jaw (rare)
- **Orthopedic:** Atypical femur fracture (rare)
- **Infectious:** Endocarditis, upper respiratory infection

Drug–drug and drug–disease interactions

Patients who are immunocompromised or who are taking immunosuppressants may have an increased risk of infection. Hypocalcemia should be resolved before initiating therapy.

Monitoring for safety and efficacy

- Monitor serum calcium, creatinine, phosphorus, and magnesium.
- To assess efficacy, monitor for fractures and bone mineral density with DXA scan. DXA scans are generally recommended after 2 years of treatment, but monitoring is individualized for each patient.

Estrogen therapy

Estrogen therapy (ET) has a beneficial effect on bone mineral density and hip and vertebral fracture risk, but the risks of long-term therapy appear to outweigh that benefit. Although ET should not be used specifically for osteoporosis, it will provide bone benefit in women who are prescribed ET for vasomotor symptoms and/or vulvovaginal atrophy. Bone loss can increase when ET is discontinued, so alternative medications should be considered to maintain BMD.

See Chapter 38 for adverse effects, drug–drug and drug–disease interactions, warnings, and monitoring of hormone therapies.

Estrogen agonist–antagonist or selective estrogen receptor modulator (SERM): Raloxifene (Evista)

Mechanism of action

Raloxifene ⚠ is an estrogen receptor agonist (EAA) in the bone where it decreases bone resorption and bone turnover. It acts as an antagonist in breast tissue. Raloxifene is indicated for both prevention and

Raloxifene *FDA BOXED WARNING*

Increased risk of deep vein thrombosis (DVT) and pulmonary embolism (PE). Avoid use in patients with current or history of venous thromboembolic disorders. Increased risk of stroke in postmenopausal women with history of coronary heart disease.

treatment of osteoporosis in postmenopausal women. While raloxifene has been shown to decrease vertebral fracture risk, reduction in hip and other nonvertebral fractures has not been documented. Raloxifene is also indicated for reduction in risk of invasive breast cancer in postmenopausal women with osteoporosis.

Patient instructions and counseling

This medication will not treat symptoms of menopause such as hot flashes and may aggravate them.

In the event of prolonged immobilization (surgery, hospitalization), discontinue raloxifene 3 days before and during the period of immobility due to the risk of thrombosis.

Adverse drug effects

- **Thrombotic:** DVT, PE
- **Cardiovascular:** Hot flashes, chest pain, syncope
- **GI:** Nausea, diarrhea, vomiting
- **Musculoskeletal:** Arthralgia, myalgia, nocturnal leg cramps

Tissue-selective estrogen complex (conjugated estrogens/bazedoxifene, Duavee)

Mechanism of action

Bazedoxifene is an EAA or SERM that reduces the risk of endometrial hyperplasia that can occur from taking estrogen alone. Conjugated estrogens/bazedoxifene (Duavee) is indicated for women experiencing moderate-to-severe vasomotor symptoms associated with menopause and to prevent postmenopausal osteoporosis.

Patient instructions and counseling

In the event of prolonged immobilization (surgery, hospitalization), when possible discontinue Duavee 3 days before and during the period of immobility.

Adverse drug effects

The most common adverse drug effects are similar to those of other estrogen and EAA/SERM agents. Duavee does not cause hot flashes like raloxifene, but it does have increased risks of thrombotic complications and has the same contraindications and precautions as other estrogens (see Chapter 38).

Calcitonin (Miacalcin, Fortical)

Mechanism of action

Calcitonin is involved in the regulation of calcium and bone metabolism and inhibits bone resorption by binding to osteoclast receptors. Salmon calcitonin is FDA-approved for the treatment of osteoporosis in women who are at least 5 years postmenopausal when other treatments are not suitable. Data show a decrease in vertebral fractures in patients who had a previous fracture. Calcitonin is available as nasal spray and injectable formulations and is considered last-line therapy. It may provide pain relief in some patients with acute vertebral fractures.

Patient instructions and counseling

- Patients should be counseled regarding administration techniques for the injection or nasal spray dosage forms.
- Store the nasal spray in the refrigerator until time for use. Warm the spray to room temperature before first use and then store at room temperature. Prime the pump before first use, and alternate nostrils each day.

Adverse drug effects

- **Skin:** Flushing
- **GI:** Nausea, diarrhea, vomiting, abdominal pain
- **Nasal (with nasal spray):** Rhinitis, nasal dryness, irritation, itching, congestion
- **Ophthalmic:** Blurred vision, abnormal lacrimation

Drug–drug and drug–disease interactions

Salmon calcitonin should be avoided in patients with a true allergy to seafood.

Anabolic/Formation Agents

While the medications above increase bone mass by decreasing bone resorption, 3 agents have anabolic effects in the bone, increasing bone formation. These anabolic agents are FDA approved to treat osteoporosis in postmenopausal women and men at high risk for fracture with multiple risk factors, including glucocorticoid therapy, and those who failed or cannot tolerate treatment with other antifracture medications. The dosages for the parathyroid hormone analogs, teriparatide and abaloparatide, and the humanized monoclonal antibody, romosozumab, are described in Table 37-3.

Parathyroid hormone: Teriparatide (Forteo)

Mechanism of action

The recombinant human product representing the first 34 amino acids in human PTH, teriparatide ⚠, stimulates osteoblasts to increase bone density and decrease fracture risk. Because of limited long-term

TABLE 37-3. Medications That Increase Bone Formation

Formation/Anabolic	Administration
Recombinant human parathyroid hormone [PTH (1-34)]	
Teriparatide (Forteo)	20 mcg subcutaneously daily for up to 2 years
Human parathyroid hormone-related peptide [PTHrP (1-34)] analog	
Abaloparatide (Tymlos)	80 mcg subcutaneously daily for up to 2 years
Antiresorptive and Formation	
Romosozumab (Evenity)	210 mg subcutaneously every month for 1 year (followed by antiresorptive therapy)

Adapted from McConnell et al.

 Teriparatide *FDA BOXED WARNING*

In rats, teriparatide caused an increase in the incidence of osteosarcoma. Teriparatide should be used only for patients for whom potential benefits outweigh potential risk. It should not be prescribed for patients at increased baseline risk for osteosarcoma.

safety data (<2 years) and risks of dose- and duration-dependent osteosarcoma in animal models, this medication is recommended for use only in patients at high risk of fracture and <2 years of therapy cumulatively across the lifetime.

Patient instructions and counseling

Patients should be educated regarding appropriate use of the prefilled pen delivery device, storage (refrigeration), and adverse effects (orthostasis, especially with first dose).

Adverse drug effects

- **Electrolytes:** Hypercalcemia (transient), hypercalciuria, increased uric acid
- **Musculoskeletal:** Pain, arthralgia, leg cramps
- **Cardiovascular:** Orthostasis, syncope
- **CNS:** Dizziness
- **GI:** Nausea, diarrhea, abdominal cramps
- **Skin:** Injection pain, urticaria

Drug–drug and drug–disease interactions

Teriparatide is contraindicated for patients with hypercalcemia or hyperparathyroidism or at an increased risk of osteosarcoma (history of bone cancer or radiation therapy to the bone) and other metabolic bone disease, such as Paget's disease, or children and adolescents whose bones are still growing.

Monitoring for safety and efficacy

- DXA scan for BMD 1 to 2 years after initiating therapy
- Serum calcium, urine calcium, if appropriate (history of hypercalciuria, active nephrolithiasis)

Abaloparatide (Tymlos)

Mechanism of action

Abaloparatide is an analog of human parathyroid hormone related peptide [PTHrP (1-34)], which stimulates osteoblast function by acting as an agonist at the PTH1 receptor. Abaloparatide therapy should not exceed 24 months and must be followed by antiresorptive therapy to retain the beneficial effects on bone.

> ⚠ **Abaloparatide** *FDA BOXED WARNING*
>
> Dose-dependent increase in incidence of osteosarcoma observed in rats. Use is not recommended in patients at increased risk of osteosarcoma. Cumulative use of this medication should not exceed 2 years.

Patient counseling

- Abaloparatide should be injected in the periumbilical area once daily, at approximately the same time each day.
- The injection site should be rotated daily.
- Because of the risk of dizziness/orthostasis, the first few doses should be given when the patient is able to sit or lie down.

Adverse drug effects

- **Electrolytes:** Hypercalcemia (transient), hypercalciuria, increased uric acid
- **Cardiovascular:** Orthostasis, palpitations

- **CNS:** Dizziness, headache
- **GI:** Nausea, abdominal pain
- **Skin:** Injection site pain and swelling

Drug–drug and drug–disease interactions

Like teriparatide, abaloparatide is contraindicated in patients with hypercalcemia or hyperparathyroidism or at an increased risk of osteosarcoma (history of bone cancer or radiation therapy to the bone) and other metabolic bone disease, such as Paget's disease, or children and adolescents whose bones are still growing.

Abaloparatide should be used with caution in patients with a history of urolithiasis due to the risk of hypercalciuria.

Monitoring for safety and efficacy

- Serum calcium, urine calcium, if appropriate (history of hypercalciuria, active nephrolithiasis)
- DXA scan for BMD 1 to 2 years after initiating therapy

Romosozumab-aqqg (Evenity)

Mechanism of action

Romosozumab-aqqg is unique in that it both increases bone formation and decreases bone resorption. This humanized monoclonal antibody inhibits sclerostin, a regulatory factor in bone metabolism. It improves bone structure and strength primarily by stimulating osteoblastic activity to increase new bone formation.

> ⚠ **Romosozumab-aqqg** *FDA BOXED WARNING*
>
> May increase risk of MI, stroke, and cardiovascular death. Do not initiate therapy for patients who have had a MI or stroke within the preceding year.

Patient counseling

- Evenity is administered by a health care professional once monthly for 12 doses. The patient receives 2 injections under the skin for each dose. After a year, the health care provider will most likely change to a different osteoporosis medication.
- Calcium and vitamin D should be adequately supplemented during treatment.

Adverse drug effects

- **Cardiovascular:** myocardial infarction, stroke
- **Musculoskeletal:** arthralgia
- **CNS:** headache
- **Hypersensitivity:** angioedema, dermatitis, rash, urticaria
- **Electrolytes:** hypocalcemia
- **Dental:** osteonecrosis of the jaw
- **Orthopedic:** atypical femoral fracture

Drug–drug and drug–disease interactions

Romosozumab-aqqg should not be initiated in patients who have had a myocardial infarction or stroke within the preceding year because of an increased risk of major adverse cardiac events in a study in postmenopausal women. For patients with cardiovascular disease risk factors, a decision regarding risk versus benefit should be made.

Hypocalcemia should be corrected before initiation treatment with romosozumab-aqqg.

Patients with severe renal impairment or receiving dialysis have an increased risk of hypocalcemia.

Monitoring for safety and efficacy

- Monitor serum calcium and supplement with calcium and vitamin D as needed. (especially with severe renal impairment or dialysis).
- Monitor for signs and symptoms of myocardial infarction or stroke, and advise patients to seek medical attention immediately if they develop symptoms.

37-4   Pharmacist's Role

Pharmacists play an important role in osteoporosis prevention and treatment. Pharmacists can prevent osteoporosis by assuring that patients have adequate calcium and vitamin D intake throughout the lifespan. This can be achieved through individual patient consultation or by participating in public health initiatives and community programs.

Pharmacists can recommend bone mineral density testing, provide screening, and help patients assess their fracture risk. They can collaborate to develop a treatment plan that includes calcium, vitamin D, and prescription medication. Pharmacists can help by promoting adherence, counseling patients about the medications, and monitoring for adverse effects and persistence with the prescribed regimen. Pharmacists can assist prescribers in determining the best initial treatment plan or adjusting therapy based on patient response or tolerance.

NAPLEX Competency Statements

The questions in this chapter cover the following 2021 NAPLEX Competency Statements: **AREA 1:** 1.1; 1.2; 1.4; 1.6; 1.7 **AREA 2:** 2.1 **AREA 3:** 3.2; 3.4; 3.5; 3.6; 3.8; 3.9; 3.11; 3.12: **AREA 5:** 5.5 **AREA 6:** 6.3; 6.4.

37-5   Questions

1. A. J. is a 35-year-old premenopausal woman who is concerned about her family history of osteoporosis. She does not eat dairy products because she is lactose intolerant. Her recent bone mineral density screening revealed a T-score of – 1 in the hip and vertebrae. Select the appropriate therapy recommendation from the following choices:

A. Daily estrogen therapy
B. Daily calcium and vitamin D supplementation
C. Weekly alendronate
D. Daily teriparatide injections
E. Daily calcitonin nasal spray

2. The pharmacist receives a prescription for Fosamax 70 mg daily for prevention of osteoporosis with instructions to the patient to take with food and remain upright for at least 30 minutes following ingestion. Identify the errors in this prescription. (Mark all that apply.)

A. The dose of Fosamax should be 35 mg weekly for prevention.
B. Fosamax should be taken at least 30 minutes before a meal.
C. Fosamax should not be taken with food.
D. Patients should lie down for 1 hour following administration of Fosamax.
E. Fosamax is used only for the treatment of osteoporosis.

3. What is the recommended daily dosage of calcium intake for a 53-year-old woman?

A. 250 mg
B. 500 mg
C. 750 mg
D. 1000 mg
E. 1200 mg

4. Which of the following agents is considered first-line therapy for postmenopausal osteoporosis? (Mark all that apply.)

A. Risedronate
B. Calcitonin
C. Prempro
D. Denosumab
E. Teriparatide

5. Which of the following products is available in both injectable and nasal spray dosage forms?

A. Raloxifene
B. Alendronate
C. Teriparatide
D. Calcitonin
E. Prempro

6. Which of the following drugs may increase the risk of osteoporosis? (Mark all that apply.)

A. Hydrochlorothiazide
B. Warfarin
C. Lisinopril
D. Enoxaparin
E. Depo-Provera

7. What is the recommended dose of raloxifene in the prevention and treatment of postmenopausal osteoporosis?

A. 10 mg daily
B. 15 mg daily
C. 40 mg daily
D. 60 mg daily
E. 120 mg daily

Use Patient Profile 37-1 to answer Questions 8 to 10

PATIENT PROFILE 37-1

Patient name: Elizabeth McLerran
Age: 62
Sex: Female
Diagnosis:

Height: 5'11"
Weight: 145 pounds
Allergies: NKDA, allergic to dairy and seafood

Hypertension
Postmenopausal osteoporosis
Gastroesophageal reflux disease/esophageal stricture

Laboratory and diagnostic tests

DXA scan: T-score hip −2.8; lumbar spine −2.6.
Creatinine Clearance (Cockroft-Gault): 60 mL/min

Medication Record

Date	Rx #	Physician	Drug and Strength	Quantity	Sig	Refills
9/1	4242	Gonzales	Pantoprazole 40 mg	90	1 tab daily	3
9/15	5555	Gonzales	Lisinopril 20 mg	30	1 tab daily	11
9/15	5556	Gonzales	HCTZ 25 mg	30	1 tab daily	11

8. Ms. McLerran seeks the pharmacist's advice about calcium supplementation. What do you recommend?

   A. Calcium carbonate 500 mg elemental calcium once daily on an empty stomach
   B. Calcium citrate 325 mg elemental calcium 2 tablets twice daily with or without food
   C. Calcium carbonate 500 mg elemental calcium twice daily with meals
   D. Calcium citrate 200 mg elemental calcium 3 times daily with meals
   E. Calcium carbonate 1000 mg once daily with breakfast

9. The pharmacist also recommends over-the-counter vitamin D supplementation for Ms. McLerran. What regimen(s) of vitamin D_3 (cholecalciferol) would be appropriate for this patient? (Mark all that apply.)

   A. 400 international units once daily
   B. 400 international units twice daily
   C. 1000 international units once daily
   D. 1000 international units twice daily
   E. 5000 international units once daily

10. In addition to assuring adequate calcium and vitamin D intake above, what treatment plan is most appropriate for Ms. McLerran's osteoporosis?

    A. Fosamax 10 mg orally daily
    B. Prolia 60 mg subcutaneously every 6 months
    C. Miacalcin 200 IU intranasally daily
    D. Forteo 20 mcg subcutaneously daily
    E. Actonel 5 mg orally daily

11. Which of the following may contribute to the development of osteoporosis? (Mark all that apply.)

    A. Nucleoside/nucleotide reverse transcriptase inhibitors (NRTI)
    B. Carbamazepine
    C. Phenobarbital
    D. Phenytoin
    E. Anastrozole

12. Which agent below is contraindicated in a patient with a history of radiation therapy to the bone?

    A. Ibandronate
    B. Calcitonin
    C. Teriparatide
    D. Raloxifene
    E. Denosumab

Use Patient Profile 37-2 to answer questions 13 to 14.

PATIENT PROFILE 37-2

Patient name: Nisha Patel
Age: 68
Sex: Female

Height: 5′3″
Weight: 140 pounds
Allergies: NKDA

Diagnosis:
Hypertension
Chronic kidney disease
Generalized anxiety disorder
Postmenopausal osteoporosis
Gastroesophageal reflux disease (mild)

Diet: Eats 1 cup of yogurt daily

Laboratory and diagnostic tests

DXA scan: T-score hip −3.2; lumbar spine −3.6.
Creatinine Clearance (Cockroft-Gault): 30 mL/min

PATIENT PROFILE 37-2. (Continued)

Medication Record

Date	Rx #	Physician	Drug and Strength	Quantity	Sig	Refills
10/1	5252	Smith	Prednisone 20 mg	10	2 tab daily	0
6/15	5555	Smith	Lisinopril 20 mg	30	1 tab daily	11
6/15	5556	Smith	Amlodipine 10 mg	30	1 tab daily	11
6/15	5557	Smith	Famotidine 20 mg	60	1 tab twice daily	11
6/15	5558	Smith	Sertraline 50 mg	30	1 tab daily	11
6/15	OTC	—	OsCal + D 500/200	—	1 tab twice daily with meals	

13. Which of Ms. Patel's medications is expected to increase her risk of osteoporosis and fracture?

   A. Prednisone
   B. Lisinopril
   C. Amlodipine
   D. Famotidine
   E. Sertraline

14. What treatment plan is most appropriate for Ms. Patel's osteoporosis?

   A. Fosamax 70 mg orally weekly
   B. Prolia 60 mg subcutaneous every 6 months
   C. Raloxifene 60 mg orally daily
   D. Risedronate 35 mg orally weekly
   E. Abaloparatide 80 mcg subcutaneously daily for up to 2 years

15. Which of the following may have a drug–drug or drug–disease interaction with calcium supplements? (Mark all that apply.)

   A. Levofloxacin
   B. Kidney stones
   C. Hypertension
   D. Cholelithiasis
   E. Levothyroxine

16. Osteonecrosis of the jaw is a rare but serious adverse effect of which of the following? (Mark all that apply.)

   A. Actonel
   B. Miacalcin
   C. Prolia
   D. Forteo
   E. Evenity

17. Which of the following are potential adverse effects of raloxifene? (Mark all that apply.)

   A. Deep vein thrombosis
   B. Myocardial infarction
   C. Hot flashes
   D. Leg cramps
   E. Atypical femur fracture

18. Which of the following are indicated for women experiencing moderate-to-severe vasomotor symptoms associated with menopause and to prevent postmenopausal osteoporosis and increases the risk of thrombotic events?

   A. Evista
   B. Prolia
   C. Duavee
   D. Forteo
   E. Miacalcin

19. Which of the following is/are adverse effect(s) of Evenity? (Mark all that apply.)

   A. Myocardial infarction
   B. Stroke
   C. Hypersensitivity reaction
   D. Osteonecrosis of the jaw
   E. Atypical femoral fracture

20. Which medication is FDA approved for the treatment of osteoporosis in women who are at least 5 years postmenopausal when other treatments are not suitable and may have analgesic effects in patients with painful, new vertebral fractures?

   A. Ibandronate
   B. Zoledronic acid
   C. Teriparatide
   D. Calcitonin
   E. Denosumab

 **37-6**   **Answers**

1. **B.** A. J. has neither osteopenia nor osteoporosis with a T-score of 1. At this point, preventive therapy is appropriate, with adequate calcium and vitamin D intake. Prescription therapy is not indicated at this time. Patient should also be counseled on lifestyle factors that can maintain bone mineral density and decrease fracture risk.

2. **A, B, C.** Fosamax (alendronate) is used for the prevention and treatment of osteoporosis. The appropriate dosage of alendronate sodium for prevention of osteoporosis includes a 35 mg weekly or 5 mg daily dose. The 70 mg weekly dose is for osteoporosis treatment. Oral bisphosphonates should be taken with a full glass of water at least 30 minutes before ingesting food or other beverages to optimize absorption. Patients should remain in the upright position for at least 30 minutes following ingestion of bisphosphonates to avoid esophageal irritation or ulceration.

3. **E.** According to the National Osteoporosis Foundation (NOF) and Institute of Medicine (IOM), daily calcium intake should be 1000 mg per day for men age 51 to 70 years and 1200 mg per day for women age 51 years and older and men age 71 years and older.

4. **A, D.** Bisphosphonates (e.g., risedronate) and denosumab are considered first-line therapy for osteoporosis because data demonstrate that they reduce the risk of hip fracture in addition to increasing bone mineral density.

5. **D.** Injectable and nasal spray dosage forms of calcitonin are available. Teriparatide is available as an injection only. Prempro, raloxifene, and alendronate are available only in oral dosage forms.

6. **D, E.** Depo-Provera may have a negative effect on bone mineral density. Long-term use of heparin and low molecular weight heparins, like enoxaparin, can increase risk of osteoporosis.

7. **D.** The FDA-approved dose of raloxifene is 60 mg once daily.

8. **B.** Calcium carbonate is not an appropriate salt form for this patient because she is taking pantoprazole chronically. Calcium carbonate requires acid to be absorbed, and absorption is decreased in patients taking proton pump inhibitors. According to NOF and IOM, women 51 and older should get at least 1200 mg of elemental calcium per day. The dosage in answer choice B, 650 mg twice daily, would provide 1300 mg daily. Products containing calcium citrate may be administered without regard to meals or proton pump inhibitors as they do not require acid to be absorbed.

9. **B, C.** For women age 51 to 70, the NOF recommends 800 to 1000 international units of vitamin D daily, while the IOM recommends 600 international units. Vitamin D can be administered once daily or in smaller doses throughout the day. Some patients prefer to take combination calcium + vitamin D supplements to minimize pill burden and enhance adherence.

10. **B.** Because of her esophageal stricture, this patient is at increased risk of esophageal ulceration from oral bisphosphonates, so oral bisphosphonates (Fosamax, Actonel) should be avoided. Raloxifene is not first-line therapy because it does not have hip fracture data. Forteo (Teriparatide) is reserved for patients who are at significant risk of fracture or who have failed first-line therapies. Reclast (zoledronic acid) has hip fracture and mortality data. This patient's creatinine clearance is 60 mL/min, well above zoledronic acid's contraindication of <35 ml/min. Prolia (denosumab) is also considered first-line therapy but specifically for patients at high risk. This patient has postmenopausal osteoporosis with T-scores and medical history that do not indicate that she is at very high fracture risk. Micacalcin (calcitonin) lacks efficacy with no data demonstrating a decrease in hip fractures.

11. **A, B, C, D, E.** All of these agents may contribute to the development of osteoporosis.

12. **C.** Because of increased risk of osteosarcoma in animal models, teriparatide and abaloparatide are both contraindicated in patients an increased risk of osteosarcoma. They are also contraindicated in patients with hypercalcemia or hyperparathyroidism.

13. **E.** Serotonin reuptake inhibitors (SSRIs), like sertraline, have been associated with decreased bone mineral density (BMD) and fracture risk,

especially in patients over 65. While longer courses of prednisone (>3 months) can decrease BMD, a short course for an acute problem like this patient had should not be problematic. While proton pump inhibitors contribute to osteoporosis, H2 antagonists like famotidine have not been shown to have a negative effect on bone.

14. **B.** While generally first-line therapy, the bisphosphonates, alendronate, and risedronate, should not be used with CrCl <35 and <30, respectively. Raloxifene (Evista) has only shown benefit in reducing vertebral fractures. Abaloparatide (Tymlos) is indicated for the treatment of postmenopausal women with osteoporosis at high risk for fracture (history of osteoporotic fracture, multiple risk factors for fracture, or failed or are intolerant to other available osteoporosis therapy). Denosumab (Prolia) is recommended as first-line therapy for patients at high risk of fracture with T-score exceeding 2.5 SD below normal. Denosumab is especially appropriate for those who cannot take oral agents or who have renal insufficiency as it is not renally excreted.

15. **A, B, E.** Calcium can decrease the absorption of oral quinolones, tetracyclines, and levothyroxine if administered concomitantly. Calcium supplements may increase the risk of calcium oxalate nephrolithiasis by increasing calcium in the urine.

16. **A, C, E.** Osteonecrosis of the jaw is a rare side effect of bisphosphonates, denosumab, and Romosozumab-aqqg. It most commonly occurs in patients with cancer receiving I.V. bisphosphonates and has been reported with oral bisphosphonates.

17. **A, C, D.** Raloxifene increases the risk of DVT and PE, similar to other hormone therapies (estrogen therapy, contraceptives). It can also cause hot flashes, which may be problematic in perimenopausal females already experiencing vasomotor symptoms. Raloxifene can also cause nocturnal leg cramps.

18. **C.** Duavee (conjugated equine estrogens/bazedoxifene) is indicated for women experiencing moderate-to-severe vasomotor symptoms associated with menopause and to prevent postmenopausal osteoporosis. Like other estrogenic products, it increases the risk of thrombotic events including DVT and PE.

19. **A, B, C, D, E.** Cardiovascular events including myocardial infarction and stroke; hypersensitivity reactions including rash, urticaria, and angioedema; osteonecrosis of the jaw; and atypical femoral fracture are all potential adverse effects of Romosozumab-aqqg (Evenity).

20. **D.** Calcitonin is FDA approved for the treatment of osteoporosis in women who are at least 5 years postmenopausal when other treatments are not suitable. While it has some data showing it decreases subsequent vertebral fractures in patients with a history of vertebral fractures, it does not have data showing hip fracture risk reduction. It may have analgesic effects that may benefit patients with painful, new vertebral fractures.

37-7 Additional Resources

Black DM, Rosen CJ. Postmenopausal Osteoporosis. *N Engl J Med.* 2016;374:254–262.

Cosman F, deBeur SJ, Lewiecki EM, et al. Clinician's guide to prevention and treatment of osteoporosis. *Osteoporosis Int.* 2014;25:2359–2381.

FRAX. Fracture Risk Assessment Tool. Available at: https://www.sheffield.ac.uk/FRAX/index.aspx?lang=En. Accessed July 10, 2020.

National Osteoporosis Foundation. Available at: https://www.nof.org/professionals/. Accessed February 12, 2021.

O'Connell MB, Borchert JS, Slazak EM, et al. Osteoporosis. In: DiPiro JT, Yee GC, Posey LM, et al., eds. *Pharmacotherapy: A Pathophysiologic Approach*, 11th ed. New York, NY: McGraw-Hill; 2020:1537–1566.

Shoback D, Rosen CJ, Black DM, et al. Pharmacological management of osteoporosis in postmenopausal women: an Endocrine Society Guideline Update. *J Clin Endocrinol Metab.* 2020;105(3):587–594.

Women's Health: Menopause and Contraception

38

TRACY M. HAGEMANN

38-1 KEY POINTS

POSTMENOPAUSAL THERAPY

- Postmenopausal hormone therapy (HT) must be individualized on the basis of patient-specific risks and benefits, medical/surgical history, and medications.
- The primary indication for initiating HT is to relieve vasomotor and genitourinary symptoms of menopause.
- HT should be used at the lowest effective dose and for the shortest duration for symptom relief.
- Combined estrogen–progestin therapy may be indicated in a woman with a uterus to protect from endometrial hyperplasia/cancer. Estrogen alone is indicated in women who have had hysterectomies.
- HT should not be prescribed for chronic disease prevention.
- Systemic HT and low-dose vaginal estrogen therapy are very effective treatments for moderate-to-severe symptoms of vulvar and vaginal atrophy.
- Nonhormonal therapy is an option for women with contraindications to HT.

CONTRACEPTION

- Oral contraceptives are safe and effective when used according to the manufacturer's recommended dose and administration. Selection of prescription contraceptives requires careful consideration of patient medical history, lifestyle, adherence, and preference.
- In addition to the contraceptive benefit of these products, other menstrual-related health problems may be resolved or lessened (e.g., menstrual pain, irregular menses).
- Changes in dose or product are often necessary to achieve an appropriate balance of estrogen and progestin while minimizing adverse effects.
- Patients should be advised to seek immediate medical care if they experience severe abdominal pain, severe chest pain, shortness of breath, severe headache, visual disturbances, or severe pain and swelling in the leg.

38-2 STUDY GUIDE CHECKLIST

The following topics may guide your study of this subject area:

- ☐ Indications for HT.
- ☐ Contraindications to HT.
- ☐ Commonly prescribed dosage forms and regimens of HT.
- ☐ Common adverse effects with oral contraceptives.
- ☐ Medical conditions that determine which type of contraceptive, if any, is appropriate.
- ☐ Commonly prescribed contraceptive dosage forms and regimens.

 **38-3** ## Menopause Overview

Definitions

Menopause, defined as 12 consecutive months of amenorrhea, is the permanent cessation of menses. The median age of onset in the United States is 51 years of age (range 40 to 55 years). Perimenopausal symptoms may begin up to 8 years before the cessation of menses (Box 38-1).

Perimenopause is the time before menopause and the first year following menopause. Ovarian function and production of estrogen decline during this time, menstrual cycles may be irregular, and women may experience vasomotor symptoms (see Box 38-1). Consideration of contraception during the perimenopausal period is important.

Pathophysiology

■ Ovarian production of **estradiol** and progesterone diminishes.
■ Follicle-stimulating hormone and luteinizing hormone concentrations increase.
■ Primary estrogen available is estrone (which is converted peripherally from androstenedione and is less potent), not **estradiol**.

Risk factors for menopause include age, surgery (removal of ovaries, total abdominal hysterectomy), history of pelvic irradiation, and certain medications (chemotherapy).

Treatment Principles

■ Hormone therapy (HT) should be initiated on an individual basis with careful consideration of the individual woman's risks and benefits. Box 38-2 lists the contraindications to estrogen therapy (ET).

BOX 38-1. Clinical Presentation of Menopause

- Cessation of menses for at least 12 consecutive months
- Symptoms of perimenopause related to declining estrogen:
  - Anovulation
  - Irregular menstrual cycles
- Symptoms of menopause directly related to lack of estrogen:
  - Vaginal dryness and vulvar or vaginal atrophy
  - Vasomotor symptoms (night sweats, hot flashes)

- Symptoms associated with menopause but without a proven link to estrogen deficiency:
  - Arthralgia/myalgia
  - Depression
  - Insomnia
  - Mood swings
  - Cognitive changes (memory, concentration)
  - Migraines
  - Urinary frequency

BOX 38-2. Contraindications to Estrogen Therapy

- Abnormal, undiagnosed genital bleeding
- Known, suspected, or history of breast cancer
- Active or history of deep vein thrombosis (DVT) or pulmonary embolism (PE)
- Estrogen-dependent neoplasia
- Pregnancy

- Active or history of arterial thromboembolic disease (stroke or myocardial infarction [MI])
- Liver dysfunction or disease
- Known protein C, protein S, or antithrombin deficiency, or other known thrombophilic disorders

- A woman with an intact uterus must be treated with estrogen plus progestin to reduce the risk of endometrial hyperplasia and endometrial cancer.
- A female who has had a hysterectomy may safely take unopposed estrogen.

Drug Therapy

Table 38-1 provides an overview of selected HT products.

TABLE 38-1. Selected Hormone Therapy Products

Medication	Dose frequency	Product names
Oral products ⚠		
Conjugated equine estrogens	Daily oral tablet	Premarin
Esterified estrogens	Daily oral tablet	Menest
17beta-estradiol	Daily oral tablet	**Estrace**
Conjugated equine estrogens and medroxyprogesterone acetate	Daily oral tablet	Prempro
Ethinyl estradiol and **norethindrone**	Daily oral tablet	Femhrt
Estradiol and **drospirenone**	Daily oral tablet	Angeliq
Estradiol and norethindrone	Daily oral tablet	Activella
Conjugated equine estrogens and bazedoxifene	Daily oral tablet	Duavee
Transdermal products ⚠		
Estradiol patch	Apply 1 patch twice weekly to lower abdomen, buttocks, or outer hip	**Alora**
		Minivelle
		Vivelle
		Vivelle Dot
Estradiol patch	Apply 1 patch once weekly to lower abdomen	**Menostar**
	Apply 1 patch once weekly to lower abdomen or upper buttocks	**Climara**
Estradiol and levonorgestrel	Apply 1 patch weekly to lower abdomen	Climara-Pro
Estradiol and Norethindrone	Apply 1 patch twice weekly to lower abdomen	Combipatch
Estradiol gel	Apply 1 pumpful 1 to 2 times daily to entire upper arm and shoulder	**Elestrin**
	1 packet applied once daily to upper thigh, alternating legs	**Divigel**
17beta-estradiol micronized gel	Apply 1 pumpful to inside and outside arm from wrist to shoulder once daily	**Estrogel**
Estradiol transdermal spray	1 spray daily to forearm; may be increased to 2 to 3 sprays daily	**Evamist**
Vaginal products ⚠		
17beta-estradiol cream	2 to 4 g daily for 1 to 2 weeks, then 50% of dose for 1 to 2 weeks, then 1 g 1 to 3 times daily	**Estrace**
17beta-estradiol ring	1 ring inserted vaginally every 3 months	**Estring**
Conjugated equine estrogens cream	0.5 to 2 g intravaginally for 21 days, then 1 week off OR 0.5 g intravaginally twice weekly continuously	Premarin
Estradiol acetate ring	1 ring inserted vaginally every 3 months	**Femring**
Estradiol hemihydrate tablet	1 tablet intravaginally once daily for 2 weeks, then 1 tablet twice weekly	**Vagifem**
Estradiol capsule	1 capsule intravaginally daily for 2 weeks, then insert 1 capsule twice weekly	Imvexxy

Boldface indicates one of top 100 drugs for 2020 by prescription volume.

FDA BOXED WARNINGS

Oral products

Estrogen-Alone Therapy: Increased risk of endometrial cancer if woman still has a uterus. Do not use for the prevention of cardiovascular disease or dementia. Should be used at lowest dose possible for the least amount of time that is necessary.

Estrogen plus Progestin Therapy: Do not use for the prevention of cardiovascular disease or dementia. Increased risk of DVT, PE, and MI in postmenopausal women. Increased risk of invasive breast cancer. Should be used at lowest dose possible for the least amount of time that is necessary.

Transdermal products

Estrogen-Alone Therapy: Increased risk of endometrial cancer if woman still has a uterus. Do not use for the prevention of cardiovascular disease or dementia. Should be used at lowest dose possible for the least amount of time that is necessary.

Estrogen plus Progestin Therapy: Do not use for the prevention of cardiovascular disease or dementia. Increased risk of DVT, PE, and MI in postmenopausal women. Increased risk of invasive breast cancer. Should be used at lowest dose possible for the least amount of time that is necessary.

Evamist: Breast budding and breast masses in prepubertal females and gynecomastia and breast masses in prepubertal males have been reported following unintentional secondary exposure. Ensure that children do not come into contact with application sites.

Vaginal products

Estrogen-Alone Therapy: Increased risk of endometrial cancer if woman still has a uterus. Do not use for the prevention of cardiovascular disease or dementia. Use should be limited to lowest dose and least amount of time necessary.

Estrogen plus Progestin Therapy: Do not use for the prevention of cardiovascular disease or dementia. Increased risk of DVT, PE, and MI in postmenopausal women. Increased risk of invasive breast cancer. Use should be limited to lowest dose and least amount of time necessary.

Estrogen and progestin

Mechanism of action

ET is used alone (if no uterus) or in combination with progestin to replace diminished levels of endogenous hormones.

Combined estrogen–progestin therapy (EPT) includes progestin to prevent endometrial hyperplasia and cancer.

Adverse drug effects

- Increased risks for venous thromboembolism (DVT, PE), stroke, coronary heart disease, and breast cancer were identified in the Women's Health Initiative (WHI) with postmenopausal women receiving HT. The beneficial effects may include reductions in fractures and colorectal cancer.
- Both ET and EPT should be used at the lowest doses and for the shortest possible time period for women who are experiencing moderate-to-severe vasomotor symptoms or vulvovaginal atrophy. Consider topical estrogen, particularly if the primary complaint is vulvovaginal atrophy.
- U.S. Food and Drug Administration (FDA) boxed warnings for ET and EPT include breast cancer, endometrial cancer, and dementia for women >65 years of age. An additional boxed warning states that ET and/or EPT should not be used to prevent cardiovascular disease. Data from the WHI studies show an increased risk of DVT and stroke with conjugated estrogen (CE) and an increased

risk of DVT, stroke, PE, and MI with CE and medroxyprogesterone acetate in postmenopausal women 50 to 79 years of age.

Common adverse effects with estrogen include breast tenderness, heavy or irregular menstrual bleeding, headache, and nausea. The most common adverse effects attributed to progestin are depression, headache, and irritability.

Drug–drug and drug–disease interactions

Estrogen may exacerbate illness in the following diseases:

- Depression
- Hypertriglyceridemia (minimize by using transdermal product)
- Thyroid disorder (patients may require an increased dose of thyroid supplement)
- Cholelithiasis
- Gastroesophageal reflux disease

Interaction with the following may result in decreased pharmacologic effect of estrogens:

- Cytochrome P450 (CYP450) 3A4 inducers:
  - Barbiturates
  - Carbamazepine
  - Rifampin
  - St. John's wort
  - Phenytoin

Interaction with the following may result in increased pharmacologic effect of estrogens:

- CYP450 3A4 inhibitors:
  - Azole antifungals
  - Macrolide antibiotics
  - Ritonavir

Parameters to monitor

Patients should be monitored for symptom improvement, adverse effects, and appropriate health maintenance (e.g., annual mammograms). Because the risk of breast cancer increased after 4 years of treatment with combined HT in the WHI, this is a target time frame for discontinuation. Patients with continued abnormal bleeding should have an ultrasound. Women over 65 years of age or those less than 65 years with risk factors for osteoporosis should have a bone mineral density test.

- If the patient has persistent vasomotor symptoms, estrogen dose should be increased.
- If the patient has breast tenderness, the estrogen dose should be decreased, or she may be switched to a transdermal estrogen product.
- If bloating or other premenstrual-like symptoms occur, consider changing to a different progestogen product.
- Using continuous estrogen/progesterone regimens may reduce or prevent monthly withdrawal bleeding and may be preferred by some women.

Patient instructions and counseling

- Adverse effects of estrogen may be diminished by starting with a low dose and may be alleviated by changing products. Most adverse effects improve with time.
- Adverse effects of progestin may be alleviated or diminished by changing products or changing from a continuous to a cyclic regimen.
- Patients should be instructed to immediately report any unusual vaginal bleeding or any signs or symptoms of stroke, MI, DVT, or PE.

Androgens (testosterone)

Mechanism of action

Androgens are the precursor hormones to estrogen production by the ovaries and peripheral sites. Ovarian testosterone production declines with menopause. Androgens act at androgen receptor sites or exhibit action following conversion to estrogen. Androgen replacement improves deficiency-related symptoms (i.e., decreased sexual desire, decreased energy, diminished well-being).

Adverse drug effects

- Fluid retention
- Lipid effects (increased triglycerides)
- Hepatic dysfunction
- Hepatocellular carcinoma (prolonged use of high doses)
- Facial hair growth, acne, and voice deepening

Patient instructions and counseling

- Testosterone therapy should be administered only to postmenopausal women who are receiving concurrent estrogen therapy.
- Relative contraindications to testosterone therapy include androgenic alopecia, hirsutism, and moderate-to-severe acne.
- Use of testosterone in postmenopausal women is controversial and not routinely recommended.

Other Medications

- Several other medications have FDA indications for use in the treatment of menopausal symptoms and are an option for women who do not want to take HT and those with contraindications to HT.
- Ospemifene ⚠, a selective estrogen receptor modulator (SERM), can be used for the treatment of moderate-to-severe dyspareunia and vaginal dryness associated with menopause. Use with opposing progesterone is required, and the most common adverse effect is hot flashes. Ospemifene is associated with an increased risk for stroke and VTE.
- Duavee ⚠ (conjugated estrogens and basedoxifene) is approved for the treatment of moderate to severe vasomotor symptoms associated with menopause and the prevention of postmenopausal osteoporosis. Duavee has a boxed warning for endometrial cancer, cardiovascular disease, and dementia. Adverse reactions include dizziness, abdominal pain, and nausea.

 Ospemifene *FDA BOXED WARNING*

Increased risk of endometrial cancer if used concurrently with unopposed estrogens by a woman with a uterus. Increased risk of thromboembolic and hemorrhagic stroke. Use should be limited to lowest dose and least amount of time necessary.

 Duavee *FDA BOXED WARNING*

Increased risk of endometrial cancer in a woman with a uterus who uses unopposed estrogens. Do not use for the prevention of cardiovascular disease or dementia. Do not use concurrently with any other estrogen therapy. Use should be limited to lowest dose and least amount of time necessary.

- The SSRIs and SNRIs have been used as alternatives to estrogen for the treatment of vasomotor symptoms associated with menopause. **Paroxetine** (Brisdelle) is the only agent in this drug class FDA approved for this indication. **Citalopram** (Celexa) and **Escitalopram** (Lexapro) have been used off-label, however, **fluoxetine** (Prozac) and **sertraline** (Zoloft) have not been shown to have significant reductions in hot flashes in placebo-controlled studies. Both **venlafaxine** (Effexor) and desvenlafaxine (Pristiq) are also alternatives to estrogen therapy for vasomotor symptoms; however, these are also used off-label. See Chapter 29 for mechanism of action and adverse effect information.
- Both **gabapentin** (Neurotin) and **pregabalin** (Lyrica) have been used off-label for treatment on vasomotor symptoms and have been shown to be superior to placebo for relief of hot flashes. (See Chapter 27 for mechanism of action and adverse effect information.)

Nondrug Therapy

- Most women with mild symptoms that do not affect daily activities will not require medication therapy.
- For mild hot flashes, lowering room temperature, the use of fans, avoiding triggers such as stressful situations and spicy foods, weight loss, as well as dressing in light layers of clothing that can be easily removed, can help.
- Water-based vaginal lubricants and moisturizers can mitigate vaginal dryness and help relieve pain associated with sexual intercourse.
- For urinary stress incontinence, Kegel exercises, which strengthen the pelvic floor muscles, can help keep the urinary sphincter from relaxing inappropriately during coughing, sneezing, laughing or when lifting objects.

38-4 Pharmacist's Role

- Pharmacists have a role in the team approach to treatment and management of menopausal symptoms. In the ambulatory and community setting, pharmacists can assist with screening for contraindications to HT and monitor patients for symptom relief and adverse effects due to HT. In the acute care setting, pharmacists may identify patients who may no longer have an indication for HT, or who may have developed a contraindication (MI, stroke) while on HT.
- Pharmacists can educate women on their HT, monitor for potential drug interactions, and assist the patient with adherence strategies.
- In the clinic setting, pharmacists can assist the prescriber with determination of optimal therapy as well as the most appropriate dosage form of HT for the patient.

38-5 Contraception

Contraception is the prevention of pregnancy by 1 of 3 methods.

- Preventing ovulation
- Preventing implantation of the fertilized ovum in the endometrium
- Inhibiting contact of sperm with mature ovum

Box 38-3 lists the estrogens and progestins used in prescription contraceptives. Table 38-2 lists estrogen-containing contraceptive products.

BOX 38-3. Estrogens and Progestins in Prescription Contraceptives

- Estrogens
- **Ethinyl estradiol**
- Estradiol valerate (metabolized to estradiol)
- Progestins
- *First generation:* norethindrone, norethindrone acetate, ethynodiol diacetate

- *Second generation:* norgestrel, levonorgestrel (more potent than first generation)
- *Third generation:* desogestrel, norgestimate
- *Other:* **drospirenone** (progestogenic, antiandrogenic, and antimineralocorticoid activity)

Boldface indicates one of top 100 drugs for 2020 by prescription volume.

TABLE 38-2. Estrogen-Containing Contraceptive Products ⚠

Estrogen dose	Progestin dose	Selected products
Monophasic products		
EE 20 mcg	Norethindrone acetate 1 mg	Loestrin 21 1/20, Loestrin 24 Fe, Junel 1/20, Larin 1/20, Microgestin 1/20, Microgestin Fe 1/20
EE 20 mcg	Levonorgestrel 0.1 mg	Aviane, Falmina, Lessina, Vienva
EE 20 mcg	**Drospirenone 3 mg**	Beyaz, Loryna, Vestura, Yaz
EE 30 mcg	Drosporenone 3 mg	Ocella, Safyral, Yasmin, Zarah
EE 30 mcg	Levonorgestrel 0.15 mg	Altavera, Levora, Marlissa, Portia
EE 30 mcg	Norgestrel 0.3 mg	Cryselle, Lo/Ovral-28, Low-Ogestrel
EE 30 mcg	Desogestrel 0.15 mg	Apri, Desogen
EE 35 mcg	Norethindrone 0.4 mg	Briellyn, Ovcon-35, Zeosa
EE 35 mcg	Norgestimate 0.25 mg	MonoNessa, Ortho-Cyclen, Sprintec
EE 35 mcg	Norethindrone 1 mg	Neocon 1/35, Norinyl 1/35, Ortho-Novum 1/35
EE 50 mcg	Norethindrone 1 mg	Necon 1/50, Ovcon 50
Biphasic products		
EE 10 mcg days 1 to 26	Norethindrone acetate 1 mg days 1 to 24	Lo Loestrin Fe
EE 20/10 mcg	Desogestrel 0.15 mg × 21 days	Mircette, Kariva, Viroele
EE 35 mcg	Norethindrone 0.5/1 mg	Necon 10/11
Triphasic products		
EE 20/30/35 mcg	Norethindrone acetate 1 mg	Estrostep Fe
EE 25 mcg	Desogestrel 0.1/0.125/0.15 mg	Cyclessa, Velivet
EE 35 mcg	Norethindrone 0.5/1/0.5 mg	Aranelle, Leena, Tri-Norinyl
EE 35 mcg	Norethindrone 0.5/0.75/1 mg	Necon 7/7/7, Ortho-Novum 7/7/7
EE 35 mcg	Norgestimate 0.18/0.215/0.25 mg	Ortho Tri-Cyclen
Quadriphasic products		
Estradiol valerate 3/2/2/1 mg	Dienogest 0/2/3/0 mg	Natazia
Extended-cycle products		
EE 20 mcg × 24 days	Norethindrone 1 mg × 24 days	Minastrin 24 Fe Chewable
EE 20/25/30/10 mcg	Levonorgestrel 0.15 mg	Quartette
EE 30 mcg × 84 days	Levonorgestrel 0.15 mg × 84 days	Jolessa, Quasense
EE 30/10 mcg	Levonorgestrel 0.15 mg	Seasonique

TABLE 38-2. Estrogen-Containing Contraceptive Products ⚠ *(Continued)*

Estrogen dose	Progestin dose	Selected products
Continuous-cycle product		
EE 20 mcg	Levonorgestrel 90 mcg	Amethyst
Transdermal product		
EE 35 mcg/24 hours	Norelgestromin 0.15 mg/24 hours	Xulane ⚠
Vaginal ring product		
EE 15 mcg/24 hours	Etonogestrel 0.12 mg/24 hours	NuvaRing ⚠

Boldface indicates one of top 100 drugs for 2020 by prescription volume.

 FDA BOXED WARNINGS

Estrogen-Containing Contraceptive Products
Cigarette smoking increases risk of serious cardiovascular effects including myocardial infarction, thromboembolism, and stroke. Avoid use in women over 35 years old who smoke.

Xulane
Cigarette smoking increases risk of serious cardiovascular effects including myocardial infarction, thromboembolism, and stroke. Avoid use in women over 35 years old who smoke. Contraindicated in women with a BMI greater than or equal to 30 due to increased risk of VTE.

NuvaRing
Cigarette smoking increases risk of serious cardiovascular effects including myocardial infarction, thrombo-embolism, and stroke. Avoid use in women over 35 years old who smoke.

Prescription Contraception Options

Combined hormonal contraception

- Combined oral contraceptive (COC)
- COCs contain estrogen plus progestin.
- They may be mono-, bi-, tri-, or quadriphasic.
- Extended cycle and continuous regimens are also available.
- Transdermal contraceptive patch (Xulane)
- Applied to skin once weekly, followed by patch-free week
- Higher adherence than oral agents
- May be less effective in women whose weight exceeds 198 pounds (88 kg)
- Contraceptive vaginal ring (NuvaRing)
- Inserted once monthly, left in for 3 weeks, and then removed for 1 week
- Lowest estrogen exposure of combined hormonal products

Progestin-only hormonal contraception

- Progestin-only oral contraceptive (norethindrone, **drospirenone**) (Table 38-3)
- Appropriate for breast-feeding women
- Less efficacious than combined oral contraceptives with shorter half-life, so must be taken at the same time daily
- May cause weight gain

TABLE 38-3. Progestin-only Contraceptive Products

Oral products	Instructions	Selected products
Norethindrone 0.35 mg	Take at the same time every day Start without regard to cycle Use backup method for 1 week after initiating No placebo pills	Aygestin, Camila, Heather, Jencycla, Lyza, Micronor, Sharobel, Tulana
Drospirenone 4 mg	Take at the same time every day Start on the first day of menses Use backup method for 7 days after a missed dose	Slynd
Injectable progestins		
Medroxyprogesterone acetate 150 mg/mL	I.M. dose every 3 months (13 weeks) Use deltoid or gluteal muscle	Depo-Provera ⚠
Medroxyprogesterone acetate 104 mg	Subcutaneous injection ever 3 months (12 to 14 weeks) Inject in thigh or abdomen	Depo-SubQ Provera 104 ⚠
Implant progestins		
Etonorgestrel 68 mg	Insert 1 implant subdermally in the inner side of the upper, nondominant arm Must be placed by a trained professional Removed no later than 3 years after insertion	Nexplanon
Intrauterine device progestins		
Levonorgestrel 19.5 mg	Must be placed by a trained professional Insert within the first 7 days of menstrual cycle Effective for up to 5 years	Kyleena
Levonorgestrel 13.5 mg	Must be placed by a trained professional Insert within the first 7 days of menstrual cycle Effective up to 3 years	Skyla
Levonorgestrel 52 mg	Must be placed by a trained professional Insert within the first 7 days of menstrual cycle Effective up to 4 years (Liletta) or 5 years (Mirena)	Liletta, Mirena

Boldface indicates one of top 100 drugs for 2020 by prescription volume.

 FDA BOXED WARNINGS

Depo-Provera
Risk of significant bone mineral density loss which may not be completely reversible. Unknown if use in adolescence or early adulthood increases risk of osteoporotic fracture later in life. Avoid use for longer than 2 years.

Depo-SubQ Provera 104
Risk of significant bone mineral density loss which may not be completely reversible. Unknown if use in adolescence or early adulthood increases risk of osteoporotic fracture later in life. Avoid use for longer than 2 years.

- May not be as effective in women whose weight exceeds 154 pounds (70 kg)
- Injectable depot medroxyprogesterone acetate (DMPA)
- Intramuscular (Depo-Provera) or subcutaneous (Depo-SubQ Provera 104) every 3 months
- May take longer to conceive after discontinuing than other contraceptives
- Has adverse effects including weight gain, menstrual irregularity, and decreased bone density
- Safe to use in breast-feeding because it contains progestin only

Intrauterine device (IUD)

- One of the most effective forms of reversible contraception
- May contain copper (Paragard), effective for 10 years, or levonorgestrel (Mirena, Skyla, Liletta, Kyleena), effective for 3 to 5 years
- Contraindicated in women who have an active pelvic infection, are pregnant, or have significantly distorted uterine anatomy
- Has adverse effects including irregular menstrual spotting the first few months and hormone-related symptoms (headache, nausea, breast tenderness, depression)
- Subdermal progestin-releasing implant (etonogestrel, Nexplanon)
- Effective up to 3 years
- Resumption of fertility within 1 week after removal
- Possible decrease in efficacy in women over 130% of ideal body weight
- May cause menstrual irregularity

Drug Therapy

Mechanism of action

Estrogens prevent development of a dominant follicle by suppression of follicle-stimulating hormone. They do not block ovulation.

Progestin inhibits ovulation. It contributes to the production of thick and impermeable cervical mucus. It also contributes to involution and atrophy of the endometrium.

Adverse drug effects (Box 38-4)

For medical conditions listed in Box 38-4, use of progestin-only oral contraceptives (OCs), DMPA, or an IUD may be an appropriate contraceptive choice.

> **BOX 38-4. The World Health Organization (WHO) Suggests Refraining from Prescribing COCs to Women with Certain Diagnoses**

- Breast cancer
- DVT or PE
- Cerebrovascular disease or coronary artery disease
- Diabetes with nephropathy, neuropathy, retinopathy, or other vascular disease
- Migraine headache, especially with aura
- Uncontrolled hypertension (≥160/90 mmHg)
- Breast-feeding women (<6 weeks postpartum)
- Liver disease
- Pregnancy

- Surgery with prolonged immobilization or any surgery on the legs
- Age >35 years and currently smoking
- Hypercoagulable states (e.g., factor V Leiden, protein C or S deficiency)
- Complicated valvular heart disease (pulmonary hypertension, risk of atrial fibrillation, history of endocarditis)
- Peripartum cardiomyopathy
- Systemic lupus erythematosus

The most common adverse drug effects with COCs include the following:

- Nausea and vomiting (usually resolves within 3 months)
- Breakthrough bleeding, spotting, amenorrhea, altered menstrual flow
- Melasma (hyperpigmentation of the skin, usually on the face)
- Headache or migraine
- Weight change or edema

Serious but less common effects are venous thrombosis, PE, MI, coronary thrombosis, arterial thrombo-embolism, and cerebral thrombosis. Patients should be advised to immediately discontinue taking their contraceptive and seek medical attention. A mnemonic to remember is ACHES.

Potential hormonal effects are associated with an imbalance in estrogen and progestin (Table 38-4).

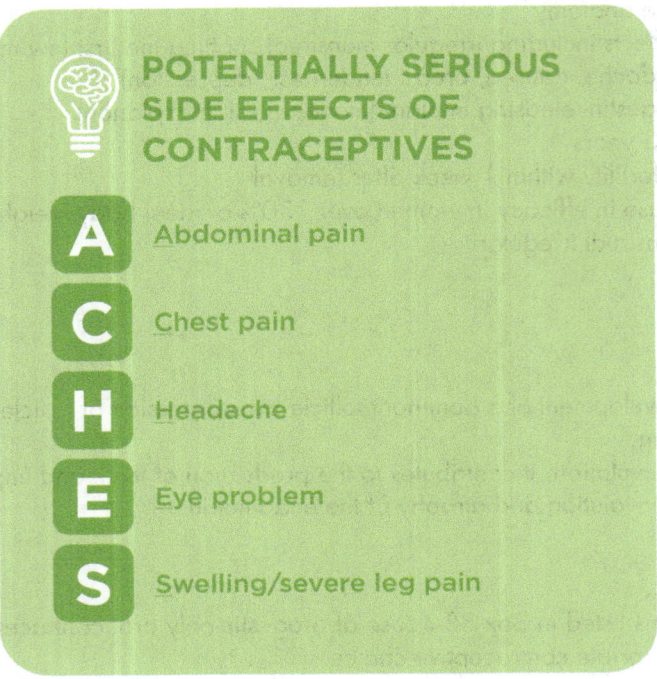

POTENTIALLY SERIOUS SIDE EFFECTS OF CONTRACEPTIVES

A — Abdominal pain

C — Chest pain

H — Headache

E — Eye problem

S — Swelling/severe leg pain

Drug–drug and drug–disease interactions

Interaction with some drugs (Table 38-5) may result in alterations in effectiveness of oral contraceptives or decreased effectiveness of the medication.

Patient instructions and counseling

- Efficacy is high (99%) with perfect adherence but averages 92% with typical use.
- Oral contraceptives do not prevent the transmission of sexually transmitted infections.
- Patients should be educated on warning signs of serious complications including DVT, PE, MI, or stroke. Remember ACHES.
- Patients should be advised to expect changes in characteristics of the menstrual cycle.
- Hormonal contraceptives can be started at any time in a women's cycle but should be used with a backup method for the first 7 days after initiation. Conversely, start first dose on the first day of the menstrual cycle or within the first 2 to 5 days of the menstrual cycle or the first Sunday after the start of the menstrual cycle then no backup method is required.
- Advice for the patient on what to do in case of missed doses (Table 38-6).

Table 38-7 lists drugs and instructions for emergency contraception.

TABLE 38-4. Hormonal Effects Resulting from Estrogen–Progestin Imbalance

Type of imbalance	Effect	Management
Too much estrogen	Breast tenderness/fullness	Decrease estrogen dose
	Nausea	Consider progestin-only contraceptive or IUD
	Edema and bloating	Consider extended cycle or continuous regimen
	Melasma	
	Headache	
	Mood changes	
Too much progestin	Acne or oily scalp	Decrease progestin dose
	Breast tenderness	Choose a less androgenic progestin such as
	Depression or irritability	ethynodiol, desogestrel, or **drospirenone**
	Hypomenorrhea	
	Increased appetite and weight gain	
	Fatigue	
	Constipation	
Too little estrogen	Breakthrough bleeding (early, days 1 to 9 of cycle)	Increase estrogen dose
	Hypomenorrhea	Rule out pregnancy
	Vasomotor symptoms	
Too little progestin	Amenorrhea	Increase progestin dose
	Breakthrough bleeding (late, days 14 to 21 of cycle)	Consider extended cycle or continuous regimen
	Hypermenorrhea	Consider progestin only product or IUD

Boldface indicates one of top 100 drugs for 2020 by prescription volume.

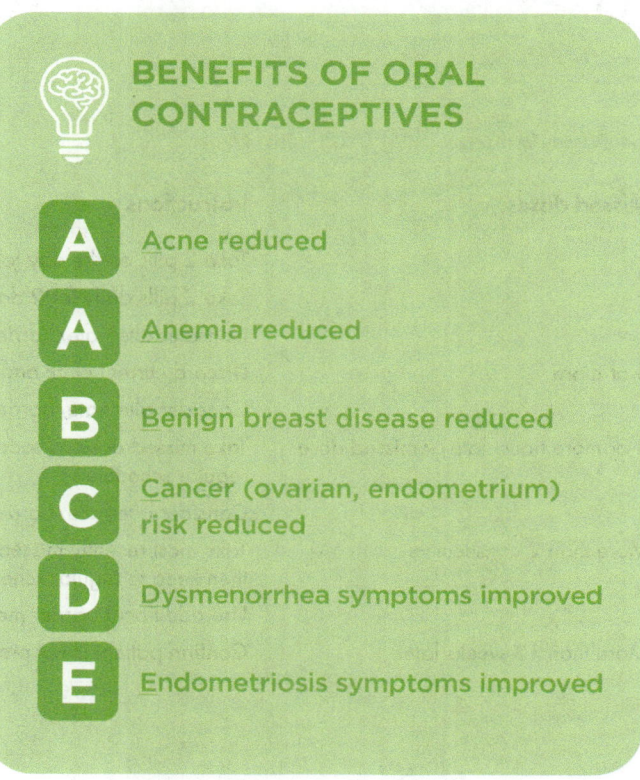

BENEFITS OF ORAL CONTRACEPTIVES

A Acne reduced

A Anemia reduced

B Benign breast disease reduced

C Cancer (ovarian, endometrium) risk reduced

D Dysmenorrhea symptoms improved

E Endometriosis symptoms improved

TABLE 38-5. Selected Drug Interactions with Oral Contraceptives

Drugs that increase OC effects	Drugs that decrease OC effects	Drugs that have altered metabolism or clearance with OCs
Atorvastatin	Antimicrobials*	**Acetaminophen**
Atazanavir	Barbiturates	Tricyclic antidepressants
Indinavir	Carbamazepine	**Aspirin**
	Griseofulvin	Benzodiazepines
	Lopinavir	Beta Blockers
	Nelfinavir	Caffeine
	Oxcarbazepine	Corticosteroids
	Phenobarbital	Cyclosporine
	Phenytoin	**Lamotrigine**
	Rifamycins	Theophyllines
	Ritonivir	
	St. John's Wort	
	Tipranavir	

Boldface indicates one of top 100 drugs for 2020 by prescription volume.
*Antimicrobials that do not decrease the effectiveness of oral contraceptives according to American College of Obstetrics and Gynecology (ACOG):

- Ampicillin
- Doxycycline
- Fluconazole
- **Metronidazole**
- Miconazole
- Fluoroquinolones
- Tetracyclines

TABLE 38-6. Instructions for When Contraceptive Doses Are Missed

Type of contraceptive	Missed doses	Instructions
COC	1	Take 2 pills on the day following the missed dose
COC	2	Take 2 pills daily for 2 days following the missed doses
		Consider alternate/barrier method for next 7 days
COC	3 or more	Discard current pack and start new packet
		Consider alternate/barrier method for next 7 days
Progestin only pill	3 or more hours late or missed dose	Take missed dose as soon as remembered, then keep to regular schedule
		Consider alternate/barrier method for next 2 days
Progestin only pill	More than 2 consecutive	Take most recently missed tablet as soon as remembered, then keep to regular schedule
		Use additional barrier method for next 7 days
Injectable progestin	More than 13 weeks late	Confirm patient is not pregnant before next dose

TABLE 38-7. Emergency Contraception

Type	Drug	Instructions	Note
Progestin*	Levonorgestrel 0.75 mg (Plan B)	2 tablets orally 12 hours apart within 72 hours after unprotected sex	Nonprescription for age >17
Progestin*	Levonorgestrel 1.5 mg (Plan B One-Step, My Way, others)	1 tablet orally once within 72 hours after unprotected sex	Nonprescription for age >17. Obese patients may need 3 mg dose
Selective progesterone receptor modulator	Ulipristal 30 mg (Ella)	1 tablet orally once within 120 hours of unprotected sex	Prescription only
Intrauterine device	Copper IUD (Paragard T 380A)	Placed by clinician within 120 hours of unprotected sex	Nonhormonal

*Prevents 95% of pregnancies if taken within 24 hours; 50% if taken within 72 hours.

Nondrug Contraception

- Condoms (see Chapter 39)
  Male: 17% failure rate; prevent sexually transmitted infections; recommend latex
  Female: More expensive and higher failure rate; can be inserted up to 8 hours before intercourse.
- Diaphragms (should be used with spermicide)
- Spermicides (ineffective when used alone; 29% failure rate)

38-6 Pharmacist's Role

- Pharmacists play an integral role on the health care team for the provision of preconception care for women of childbearing potential including education on family planning options, medication use and selection, disease state management (pregestational diabetes), weight loss, smoking cessation, alcohol and recreational drug use, and provision of indicated immunizations.
- Some states allow pharmacists to provide hormonal contraception to their patients.
- Pharmacists in the ambulatory and community setting may be the best resource for provision of emergency contraception.
- Pharmacists should educate women on the correct use of their choice of contraception, monitor for potential drug interactions, and assist the patient with adherence strategies including when to use a backup method in case of a missed dose.
- In the clinic setting, pharmacists can assist the prescriber with determination of optimal therapy as well as the most appropriate dosage adjustment for the patient.

NAPLEX Competency Statements

The questions in this chapter cover the following 2021 NAPLEX Competency Statements: **AREA 1:** 1.1; 1.2; 1.4; 1.5; 1.6; 1.7 **AREA 3:** 3.1; 3.2; 3.4; 3.5; 3.6; 3.7; 3.8; 3.12.

38-7   Questions

1. S. T. is a 32-year-old woman who wants to begin using a prescription contraceptive product. She is a new mother and would like to know if any products are safe for use during breast-feeding. S. T. states that she is not interested in using a device intravaginally and experiences irritation and inflammation with condom use. Which of the following product(s) would be an appropriate choice for S. T.? (Mark all that apply.)

A. Ortho Tri-Cyclen
B. Micronor
C. Depo-Provera
D. Seasonale
E. Premarin

2. Which of the following oral contraceptives is a biphasic product?

A. Ortho Tri-Cyclen
B. Necon 10/11
C. Ortho-Novum 1/35
D. Yasmin
E. Amethyst

3. A 20-year-old female comes to the pharmacy counter and asks how to prevent pregnancy after unprotected sex. She is currently on birth control pills, and her boyfriend typically wears a condom, but last night he forgot. What do you recommend?

A. Schedule an appointment with her OB-GYN immediately.
B. Take 2 birth control pills today instead of just 1, and then continue her normal regimen.
C. Sell her Ella from behind the counter.
D. Instruct her to purchase Plan B One-Step over the counter and take immediately.
E. It is too late to prevent pregnancy. She will have to wait and take a pregnancy test.

4. A 26-year-old female who is recently initiated on a combination hormonal oral contraceptive complains of late-cycle breakthrough bleeding. Which of the following is she most likely experiencing?

A. Too much estrogen
B. Too little estrogen
C. Too much progestin
D. Too little progestin
E. Too much androgen

5. What is the highest dose of estrogen (ethinyl estradiol) offered in an oral contraceptive?

A. 25 mcg
B. 30 mcg
C. 35 mcg
D. 40 mcg
E. 50 mcg

6. A combination oral contraceptive would be the preferred contraception in which of the following cases? (Mark all that apply.)

A. A 24-year-old graduate student who is in a monogamous relationship
B. A 28-year-old woman who is breast-feeding her infant
C. A 38-year-old obese woman who smokes 1 pack of cigarettes daily
D. A 48-year-old perimenopausal female with irregular menstrual cycles
E. A 28-year-old woman with migraine with aura taking warfarin for hypercoagulable state

Use Patient Profile 38-1 to answer Questions 7 and 8.

7. N. G. usually takes her pill at 9 PM every night, but last night she fell asleep early and didn't take her usual dose. It is now 10 AM, and she calls your pharmacy to ask what she should do. What do you tell her?

A. Take the missed dose as soon as possible, continue taking the remaining pills at the usual time. No additional contraceptive protection needed.
B. Take the missed dose as soon as possible, continue taking the remaining pills at the usual time. Use an additional barrier contraceptive product for the next 7 days if having intercourse.
C. Take the missed dose with your usual dose at 9 PM, effectively taking 2 pills tonight, then continue taking the remaining pills at the usual time. Use an additional barrier contraceptive product for the next 2 days if having intercourse.
D. Skip the missed dose, continue taking remaining pills at the usual time. No additional contraception protection needed.
E. Skip the missed dose, continue taking the remaining pills at the usual time. Use emergency contraception within the next 24 hours.

PATIENT PROFILE 38-1.

Patient Name: Nancy Greene   **Height:** 5'4"

Age: 24 years   **Weight:** 130 lb

Sex: Female   **Allergies:** Tetracyclines (rash)

Occupation: Case worker at area homeless shelter

Past Medical History: Acne

Tonsillectomy/Adenoidectomy (age 8 years)

Hyperlipidemia

Laboratory tests

Blood pressure: 130/70 mmHg

Heart Rate: 80 bpm

Positive TB Skin Test (Mantoux technique)

Negative sputum culture

Medication Record

Date	Rx #	Physician	Drug and strength	Quantity	Sig	Refills
2/9	11342	Patel	Adapalene gel 3%	45 g	Apply to affected areas once daily at bedtime	6
7/10	12650	Patel	Yasmin 28	1 pack	Take 1 tablet daily	12
10/19	14222	Farmer	Rifampin 300 mg	240	Take 2 daily for 4 months	0

---

8. Two weeks later, N.G. comes to refill her Yasmin and has a new prescription that she has to take for a few months to treat tuberculosis. Which of the following choices describes appropriate action taken by the pharmacist?

A. Call the prescriber, and request a change to other medications to avoid a drug interaction between Yasmin and rifampin.

B. Dispense the rifampin, and counsel her on the appropriate administration and duration of therapy for the antibiotic.

C. Dispense the rifampin, and counsel her regarding the potential for rifampin to interfere with the efficacy of Yasmin. Instruct her to use a backup method of contraception throughout her course of rifampin therapy.

D. Refuse to fill the rifampin prescription, and counsel her that she should not take antibiotics while she is on oral contraceptives.

E. Dispense the rifampin, and stop the patient's Yasmin prescription. Counsel her on nonhormonal methods of contraception.

9. NuvaRing would be the most appropriate contraceptive for which of the following women?

A. 25-year old woman with a history of DVT

B. 31-year old woman who smokes 2-packs a day

C. 37-year old woman with seasonal allergies and controlled asthma

D. 24-year old woman who is breastfeeding

E. 17-year old woman with lupus

10. Upon discontinuation, which of the following contraceptives has been shown to have the greatest effect on return to fertility status?

A. Nexplanon

B. Ortho Tri-Cyclen

C. Depo-Provera

D. Kyleena

E. Xulane

11. O. H. is a 17-year-old woman who has come to your pharmacy to pick up her new prescription of Loestrin. This is her first time starting oral contraceptives, and she indicates that she just finished her menses last week. How will you tell her to start the packet? (Mark all that apply)

A. She can start today but will need to use a backup barrier method for the next 7 days if having intercourse.
B. She can start today, and there is no need to use a backup barrier method.
C. She can take the first dose on the first day of her next menstrual cycle. She will not need to use a backup barrier method in this instance.
D. She can take the first dose on the first day of her next menstrual cycle. She will need to use a backup barrier method for the first 7 days after initiation.
E. She can start on the first Sunday after the start of her next menstrual cycle. She will not need to use a backup barrier method in this instance.

12. R. J. is a 55-year-old woman who presents to your pharmacy with a prescription for Premarin 0.625 mg daily. She has an intact uterus and has been recently diagnosed with menopause. Which of the following statements describes the appropriate action to be taken by the pharmacist?

A. Refuse to fill the prescription, and recommend a phytoestrogen supplement.
B. Call the physician to confirm that the patient has an intact uterus, and recommend a product containing estrogen plus progestin.
C. Fill the prescription, and counsel the patient regarding administration instructions and potential adverse effects.
D. Call the physician to confirm that the patient has an intact uterus, and suggest a transdermal estrogen product.
E. Call the physician, recommend cancelling the Premarin prescription, and recommend starting a Provera prescription.

13. Which of the following factors is a contraindication to the use of hormone replacement therapy in postmenopausal women?

A. Diabetes
B. Basal cell skin cancer
C. Thromboembolic disease
D. Depression
E. Obesity

14. From the following choices, select the most common side effect associated with estrogen therapy. (Mark all that apply.)

A. Breast tenderness
B. Depression
C. Nausea
D. Brittle fingernails
E. Hair loss

15. The Women's Health Initiative study found an association between combination (estrogen + progesterone) hormone therapy and which of the following conditions? (Mark all that apply.)

A. Breast cancer
B. Stroke
C. Cardiovascular disease
D. Colon cancer
E. Deep-vein thrombosis

16. Which of the following product dosing regimens is correct?

A. Climara Transdermal: Apply to skin once daily.
B. Vagifem: 1 tablet vaginally once daily for 2 weeks, then 1 tablet vaginally twice weekly.
C. Estring: Insert ring intravaginally once daily at bedtime.
D. Premarin tablets: 0.625 to 2.5 mg 3 times daily.
E. Premarin vaginal cream: 20 to 40 g vaginally once daily.

17. Which of the following drug interactions may result in increased pharmacologic effect of estrogen? (Mark all that apply.)

A. Macrolide antibiotics
B. Phenytoin
C. Fluconazole
D. Itraconazole
E. Carbamazepine

18. S. M. is a 51-year-old female with a past medical history that includes hypothyroidism and invasive ductal carcinoma of the left breast. She is at your clinic today to discuss options for controlling her moderate vasomotor symptoms associated with menopause. Which of the following medications are options for her? (Mark all that apply)

A. Effexor
B. Duavee
C. Brisdelle
D. Celexa
E. Vagifem

19. J. H. is a 56-year-old female who has recently noticed that sex has become quite painful, and she also describes vaginal dryness and itching. She has never had this problem before. She denies any hot flashes, irritability or night sweats. When you ask her about when her last menstrual period was, she informs you that she had a partial hysterectomy (uterus only) at age 36 due to severe uterine fibroids. Her medications include loratadine 10 mg daily for allergies and occasional ibuprofen for sinus headaches. What is the best option for her symptoms?

A. Prempro oral tablet daily
B. Ortho-Cyclen oral tablet daily
C. Depo-Provera I.M. injection
D. Premarin vaginal cream twice weekly
E. Premarin oral tablet daily

20. K. G. is a 51-year-old postmenopausal woman with a history of hysterectomy. She was initiated on 0.3 mg oral conjugated equine estrogens 3 months ago for treatment of severe vasomotor symptoms. Today she says that while her symptoms are somewhat improved, she still has daily hot flashes and experiences night sweats about 3 to 4 times a week. What is the best option for managing her symptoms?

A. Increase her daily estrogen dose
B. Decrease her daily estrogen dose
C. Do not change her current treatment
D. Change to ospemifene
E. Change to paroxetine

 **38-8** **Answers**

1. **B, C.** Micronor is a progestin-only oral contraceptive and is considered compatible with breast-feeding. Depo-Provera is an injectable progestin-only contraceptive option that is considered safe for women who desire to breast-feed because it does not affect milk production or adversely affect infant development. Ortho Tri-Cyclen and Seasonale are combined oral contraceptives that may decrease the quantity of breast milk available and may adversely affect the infant. Premarin is indicated for hormone replacement therapy, not contraception.

2. **B.** Necon 10/11 is a biphasic oral contraceptive.

3. **D.** Plan B (levonorgestrel) and generic products are over-the-counter emergency contraceptives that reduce the risk of pregnancy when started within 72 hours after unprotected sex. The medication is more effective the sooner it is initiated. The patient has no need to see her OB-GYN for emergency contraception alone. Ella (ulipristal acetate) is also an emergency contraceptive that can be used for up to 5 days after unprotected sex; however, it requires a prescription. Taking multiple oral contraceptive pills is no longer recommended because it is less effective and has greater side effects than the emergency contraceptives. Because the patient is well within the 72-hour window, she is still eligible for emergency contraception.

4. **D.** Too little progestin may result in breakthrough bleeding late in the menstrual cycle. She should be changed to a product with a higher progestin content.

5. **E.** The highest dose of estrogen (ethinyl estradiol) offered in an oral contraceptive is 50 mcg.

6. **A, D.** Progestin-only oral contraceptives are preferred in breast-feeding women because they do not negatively affect milk supply. Women who are over age 35 years and smoke should not use combined oral contraceptives. Perimenopausal females may take combined oral contraceptives to regulate their menstrual cycle. Oral contraceptives may increase the risk of ischemic stroke in patients with migraine with aura and may increase the risk of thrombosis in patients with a history of hypercoagulability and those on warfarin or other anticoagulants.

7. A. Since Yasmin is a combination oral contraceptive and she has only missed 1 dose, she should not need any back up method and should only take the next dose as soon as possible. Missing more than 1 dose of a combination contraceptive would require use of a backup method for a week afterward.

8. C. Rifampin has a pharmacokinetic interaction with combined hormonal contraceptives. Women taking rifampin should be educated about the possibility of oral contraceptive failure and should be encouraged to use nonhormonal contraception throughout the course of therapy. There is no need to stop the oral contraceptive while concomitantly taking rifampin, but a backup method should be used consistently during treatment.

9. C. NuvaRing is an estrogen-containing contraceptive and is not recommended in women who smoke, have lupus, are breastfeeding, or have a history of clotting disorders.

10. C. It may take up to 3 to 6 months for regular ovulation to occur once Depo-Provera is discontinued. All other types of contraception products are immediately or almost-immediately reversible.

11. A, C, E. Because she is not at the start of her menses right now, if she takes her first pill today, she will need to use backup barrier contraception for the first week after starting. If she waits, then she can start on the first day of her next cycle, 2 to 5 days after her cycle starts, or the first Sunday after her cycle begins and will not need to use a backup barrier method.

12. B. Unopposed estrogen is not recommended in women with an intact uterus because of an increased risk of endometrial hyperplasia and endometrial cancer. Women with an intact uterus should receive a product containing estrogen plus progestin.

13. C. Thromboembolic disease is a definite contra-indication to the use of HT in postmenopausal women.

14. A, C. Breast tenderness and nausea are the most common side effects associated with estrogen therapy.

15. A, B, C, E. The WHI study demonstrated a decreased risk of colon cancer with HT.

16. B. Vagifem dosage is 1 tablet vaginally once daily for 2 weeks; then 1 tablet vaginally twice weekly.

17. A, C, D. Macrolide antibiotics, fluconazole, and itraconazole may result in increased pharmacologic effect of estrogen by inhibiting CYP450 3A4. Phenytoin and carbamazepine may result in decreased pharmacologic effects of estrogen by CYP450 3A4 induction.

18. A, C, D. Estrogen containing products are contraindicated in patients with a history of breast cancer, so options B and E not be appropriate choices. Brisdelle has an FDA indication for treatment of postmenopausal vasomotor symptoms, and Effexor and Celexa, while off-label, have been successfully used to treat these symptoms in women who have a contraindication to estrogen.

19. D. Because her symptoms are primarily related to vulvar atrophy and she has no other menopausal symptoms, a topical vaginal cream is the best option at this time. Premarin oral tablets may be an option if she was experiencing other menopausal symptoms such as moderate-to-severe hot flashes and night sweats. Prempro is a combination estrogen/progestin product, and because she does not have a uterus, she would not require a progestin. Both Depo-Provera and Ortho-Cyclen are contraceptive products and are not used for menopausal symptoms.

20. A. She is currently taking a low dose of estrogen that may not be sufficient to manage her vasomotor symptoms. Increasing her dose to 0.625 mg will provide additional symptom relief.

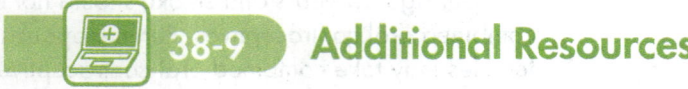

38-9   Additional Resources

Postmenopausal Hormone Therapy

Dang DK, Wheeler KE, Chen JT. Hormone therapy in women. In: DiPiro JT, Yee GC, Posey ML, et al., eds. *Pharmacotherapy: A Pathophysiologic Approach*. 11th ed. New York, NY: McGraw-Hill; 2019:1e–47e.

North American Menopause Society. Clinical Care Recommendations. Available at: http://www.menopause.org/publications /clinical-care-recommendations. Accessed May 27, 2020.

Torkelson C, Westberg SM, Drake D, et al. Menopause. In: O'Connell M, Smith JA, eds. *Women's Health Across the Lifespan,* 2nd ed. New York, NY: McGraw-Hill; 2019:1e–28e.

Contraception

El-Ibiary SY, Shrader SP, Ragucci KR. Contraception. Hormone therapy in women. In: DiPiro JT, Yee GC, Posey ML, et al., eds. *Pharmacotherapy: A Pathophysiologic Approach.* 11th ed. New York, NY: McGraw-Hill; 2019.

Mitchell JS, El-Ibiary SY, Downing D. Hormonal and Emergency Contraception. In: O'Connell MB, Smith JA, eds. *Women's Health Across the Lifespan,* 2nd ed. New York, NY: McGraw-Hill; 2019.

Use of hormonal contraception in women with coexisting medical conditions. ACOG Practice Bulletin No. 206. American College of Obstetricians and Gynecologists. *Obstet Gynecol.* 2019;133:396–399.

Men's Health

MICHELLE MOSELEY

39-1 KEY POINTS

ERECTILE DYSFUNCTION

- While the incidence of erectile dysfunction (ED) is more common in men of advanced age, the majority of ED cases result from physical and emotional issues. Risk factors to consider include obesity, diabetes, smoking, and depression.
- Management of underlying causes, including elimination of exacerbating medications, should be addressed.
- ED is a warning sign of underlying cardiovascular disease.
- Oral phosphodiesterase-5 inhibitors are first line unless the patient is taking a nitrate.

BENIGN PROSTATIC HYPERPLASIA

- Benign prostatic hyperplasia (BPH) is characterized by lower urinary tract symptoms as a result of androgen-driven prostatic growth. Medications also may cause or exacerbate symptoms.
- Based on the severity of symptoms and the size of the prostate, treatment options include watchful waiting, alpha-1-receptor blockers with or without 5-alpha-reductase inhibitors (5-ARIs), tadalafil, or surgery.
- Alpha blockers are considered first-line therapy and do not affect prostate size. Third-generation alpha blockers are more selective and are associated with fewer adverse cardiovascular effects than are the second generation.
- 5-ARIs are preferred for men with enlarged prostates to prevent disease progression. 5-ARIs decrease prostate size and reduce prostate-specific antigen levels, but they have a slow onset of action.

HYPOGONADISM

- Signs and symptoms of hypogonadism are nonspecific. Before a diagnosis is made, laboratory testing should be conducted to confirm testosterone deficiency.
- Testosterone replacement therapy (TRT) is available in several dosage formulations. Patients should be educated on proper administration.
- TRT requires careful monitoring to balance effectiveness with adverse effects such as erythrocytosis.

CONTRACEPTION

- Male contraception methods generally are less efficacious than hormonal contraception for women. Exceptions include abstinence and vasectomy.
- Male condoms and spermicide (nonoxynol-9) are widely available barrier methods that prevent sperm from reaching the ovum.
- Latex and polyurethane condoms prevent transmission of human immunodeficiency virus (HIV) and other sexually transmitted infections (STIs). Men allergic to latex may use lamb cecum condoms, but they do not prevent HIV or STIs.
- Men should use water-based lubricant with condoms. Oil-based lubricants can cause latex to breakdown.

39-2 STUDY GUIDE CHECKLIST

The following topics may guide your study of this subject area:

- ☐ Pathophysiology of ED, BPH, and hypogonadism.
- ☐ Risk factors for ED, BPH, and hypogonadism.
- ☐ First-line therapy for ED and BPH.
- ☐ Testosterone dosage formulations and application sites.
- ☐ Contraindications and potential adverse effects of the various pharmacotherapy options for ED, BPH, and hypogonadism.
- ☐ Medications that cause or worsen ED, BPH, and hypogonadism.
- ☐ Male contraceptive methods stratified by the ability to prevent unintended pregnancies or transmission of HIV and STIs.

39-3   Erectile Dysfunction

Disease Overview

Erectile dysfunction (ED) is defined as the persistent failure to achieve or maintain an erection to allow for satisfactory sexual performance. ED is one of the most common types of sexual dysfunction reported in men.

Pathophysiology and etiology

The incidence of ED increases with age, affecting up to one-third of men in their lifetime. After adjusting for age, the risk of ED is higher in men with heart disease, diabetes, and hypertension. Additional risk factors include obesity, cigarette smoking, hyperlipidemia, neurological and psychological conditions, and hypogonadism. ED may occur because of compromised organic factors (vascular, neurological, or hormonal), psychogenic factors, a combination of both organic and psychogenic factors, or medication side effects (Table 39-1). Organic ED is more common than psychogenic ED.

Normal erectile response results from the complex interaction of vascular, neurological, hormonal, and psychosocial factors. Sexual stimulation triggers the sympathetic and parasympathetic nervous system to release nitric oxide from penile epithelial cells. Nitric oxide promotes intracavernosal production of cyclic guanosine monophosphate (cGMP), which causes arterial dilation. Attaining and maintaining an erection requires optimum arterial influx of blood to the corpora cavernosa as well as efficient reduction in venous outflow. Catabolism of cGMP by the phosphodiesterase type 5 (PDE-5) enzyme results in detumescence, or loss of an erection.

Older adult males with complaints of ED should undergo screening for cardiovascular disease (CVD), because the symptoms of ED typically present on average 3 years before the onset of cardiovascular symptoms. Treatment of ED in patients with CVD is complicated by the concern that increased sexual activity might result in a small increase in myocardial infarction. Patients with ED and CVD are stratified on the basis of risk factors to determine if they should receive treatment.

Treatment principles

Shared decision-making is the cornerstone of treatment and management of ED. Initial treatment involves identifying and optimally managing or reversing potentially contributing factors. Underlying diseases such as hypertension, diabetes, and hypogonadism should be treated. Men should be instructed on lifestyle modifications including smoking cessation, consuming a diet low in cholesterol, engaging in routine physical

TABLE 39-1. Causes of Erectile Dysfunction

Dysfunction	Cause
Vasculogenic	Cardiovascular disease, hypertension, hyperlipidemia, diabetes, smoking
Neurogenic	Stroke, polyneuropathy, degenerative diseases, spinal cord trauma, surgery
Hormonal	Hypogonadism, hypo- or hyperthyroidism, hyperprolactinemia
Psychogenic	Performance-related anxiety, traumatic experience, relationship problems, anxiety, depression, stress, mental illness
Drug-induced	Diuretics, beta blockers, **clonidine**, antidepressants (serotonin reuptake inhibitors, tricyclics), antipsychotics, antihistamines, opioids, benzodiazepines, **spironolactone**, alpha blockers, 5-alpha-reductase inhibitors, antiandrogens, estrogens, antiparkinsonian agents, recreational drugs (alcohol, cocaine, marijuana, heroin)

Boldface indicates one of top 100 drugs for 2020 by prescription volume.

activity, maintaining ideal body weight, and eliminating excessive alcohol consumption. If possible, contributing medications should be discontinued.

If ED does not improve with initial management methods, specific treatment often is necessary (Figure 39-1). Treatment is guided by affordability, availability, ease of use, onset of action, concomitant medications, and risk for adverse effects. Generally, the least invasive treatment approaches are implemented first, but any treatment option is a valid choice.

Pharmacotherapy options for ED target smooth muscle relaxation to allow for corpora cavernosa filling. The 2 primary drug classes used for ED are PDE-5 inhibitors (sildenafil, vardenafil, tadalafil, avanafil) and prostaglandins (alprostadil). Doses may be titrated to produce a suitable erection not exceeding 1 hour. PDE-5 inhibitors are orally administered and considered first-line pharmacologic treatment for ED. Prostaglandins are second-line agents, because they require more invasive administration. Prostaglandins often are used when patients do not respond or exhibit intolerance or contraindications to PDE-5 inhibitors.

Penile devices are used in men who fail to respond or have contraindications to pharmacologic therapy. Psychotherapy, such as counseling, can be used alone or as adjunct therapy for psychogenic ED.

Drug Therapy

Phosphodiesterase-5 inhibitors

Phosphodiesterase-5 inhibitors (Table 39-2) are similar in effectiveness with differences in onset of action, duration of therapeutic effect, and dosing. All PDE-5 inhibitors require sexual stimulation for response to treatment and are limited to 1 dose per day. Tadalafil has the longest duration of action (approximately 36 hours). Men who have renal or hepatic dysfunction, are older than 65 years of age, or are taking a potent cytochrome P450 (CYP450) 3A4 inhibitor may require a lower dose of the PDE-5 inhibitor or may need to avoid it altogether.

Mechanism of action

PDE-5 inhibitors block the breakdown of cGMP, resulting in increased nitric oxide production that leads to arterial dilation and allows the corpora cavernosa to engorge with blood.

Patient instructions and counseling

- Food can impair absorption of sildenafil and vardenafil for up to 1 hour.
- The patient should inform his health care provider if he is taking nitrates for chest pain.
- The patient should talk to his health care provider before drinking alcohol with this medication.
- Reduce the chance of dizziness or passing out by rising slowly after sitting or lying down.
- PDE-5 inhibitors do not protect against the spread of human immunodeficiency virus (HIV) and other sexually transmitted infections (STIs).
- The patient should contact his health care provider immediately if any of the following effects occur:
  - Allergic reaction
  - Chest pain, sudden or severe headache, trouble breathing, or abnormal heartbeat
  - Sudden loss of vision
  - Sudden decrease or loss of hearing, ringing in the ears, or dizziness
  - Painful erection or an erection lasting longer than 4 hours

FIGURE 39-1. Treatment Approach for Erectile Dysfunction

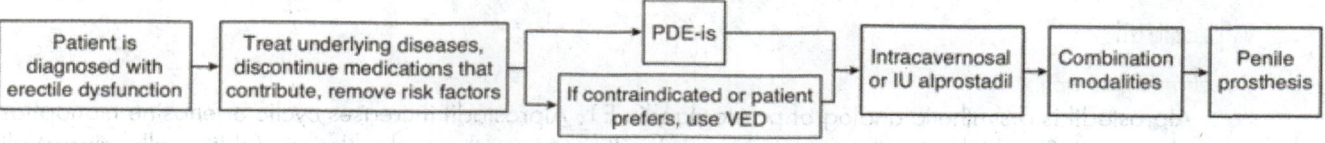

TABLE 39-2. Dosing Regimens for Selected Treatment Options for Erectile Dysfunction

Generic name	Trade name	Dosing	Comments
Phosphodiesterase-5 inhibitors			
Sildenafil	**Viagra** (ED), Revatio (PAH)	25 to 100 mg orally 1 hour before intercourse	Fatty meals can impair absorption.
Vardenafil	Levitra	5 to 20 mg orally 1 hour before intercourse	Fatty meals can impair absorption, but patient can take regardless of meals.
	Staxyn ODT	10 mg to dissolve on the tongue 1 hour before intercourse	Do not take with food or liquid.
Tadalafil	**Cialis** (ED, BPH), Adcirca (PAH)	10 to 20 mg orally 1 hour before intercourse for ED; 2.5 to 5 mg once daily for BPH with or without ED	Extended duration of action occurs. Drug may be taken with or without food.
Avanafil	Stendra	50 to 200 mg orally 30 minutes before intercourse	Drug may be taken with or without food.
Prostaglandin E1 Analog			
Alprostadil intracavernosal injection	Caverject, Edex	2.5 to 20 mcg intracavernosally 5 to 10 minutes before intercourse	Inject laterally into the proximal ⅓ of one corpus cavernosum. Limit to 1 dose per day and not more than 3 doses per week.
Alprostadil intraurethral suppository	MUSE	125 to 1000 mcg intraurethrally 5 to 10 minutes before intercourse	Urinate before use. Prefilled applicator is included. Limit to 2 doses per day.

Boldface indicates one of top 100 drugs for 2020 by prescription volume.
ED, erectile dysfunction; PAH, pulmonary arterial hypertension; ODT, orally disintegrating tablet; BPH, benign prostatic hyperplasia.

Adverse drug effects

The following adverse effects may occur: headache, dizziness, facial flushing, nasal congestion, nose bleed, dyspepsia, back and/or muscle pain (tadalafil), priapism, loss of vision, difficulty with blue-green color discrimination or halos (sildenafil), loss of hearing, tinnitus, vertigo, and cardiovascular events.

Drug interactions

Administration of the following with PDE-5 inhibitors may result in severe hypotension:

- Nitrates (contraindicated)
- Riociguat (Adempas)
- Alpha blockers
- Alcohol

Enhanced adverse effects may result from interaction with CYP450 3A4 inhibitors: azole antifungals, macrolides (erythromycin, clarithromycin), and ritonavir.

Decreased efficacy of the PDE-5 inhibitor may result from interaction with CYP450 3A4 inducers: rifampin, carbamazepine, phenobarbital, phenytoin, and St. John's wort.

Monitoring parameters

Monitor hepatic and renal function. Patients should be monitored for improvement of symptoms, adverse effects, and drug interactions.

Alprostadil

Mechanism of action

Alprostadil is a synthetic analog of prostaglandin E1. Alprostadil increases cyclic adenosine monophosphate (cAMP), which activates protein kinase, leading to smooth muscle dilation. Additionally, alprostadil may block norepinephrine, thus preventing vasoconstriction and detumescence. Alprostadil is available as an intraurethral suppository and an intracavernosal injection. Avoid using the injection in patients with sickle cell anemia, multiple myeloma, leukemia, or severe coagulopathy. See Table 39-2 for general information about prostaglandin E1 analogs.

Patient instructions and counseling
- The first dose can be administered under medical supervision to monitor for efficacy and the presence of hypotension.
- Intraurethral suppository (MUSE)
  - Urinate before use. Approximately 5 to 10 minutes before sexual activity, insert the prefilled applicator into the urethra, press the button on the top of the plunger, wait at least 5 seconds, remove the applicator, and then massage the penis to promote absorption.
  - A condom should be used with pregnant women or women of childbearing age to avoid alprostadil exposure.
- Intracavernosal injection (Caverject, Edex): The injection should occur 5 to 10 minutes before sexual activity in the upper one-third of the spongy tissue (corpus cavernosum) on 1 side of the penis only.
- Alprostadil does not protect against the spread of HIV and other STIs.

Adverse drug effects
The following adverse effects may occur:

- Intraurethral suppository: penile pain, burning or bleeding, urethral stricture, headache, dizziness, hypotension, and priapism. As a result of transfer during sexual activity, exposed females may experience vaginal burning, irritation, or stinging. Animal studies have reported embryotoxicity with MUSE; therefore, a condom barrier must be used during sexual intercourse with pregnant women.
- Intracavernosal injection: penile pain, plaque, corporal fibrosis, dizziness, hypotension, and priapism.

Drug interactions
PDE-5 inhibitors may enhance adverse effects.

Monitoring parameters
Patients should be monitored for improvement of symptoms and adverse effects.

Testosterone

Testosterone supplementation in men with ED resulting from hypogonadism can improve erections, sexual function, and desire. Treatment of testosterone deficiency will be addressed later in this chapter in section 39-5, Hypogonadism.

Miscellaneous Agents

Phentolamine (a nonselective alpha agonist) and papaverine (a nonselective PDE inhibitor) are intracavernosal injections that have been used in men with ED. No injectable nonprostaglandin agents are FDA approved for this indication.

Yohimbine is a centrally acting alpha-2-adrenergic antagonist that is used as an aphrodisiac. Use of yohimbine is not recommended because of the lack of efficacy data and the potential for adverse effects including anxiety, tachycardia, hypertension, and insomnia.

Nondrug therapy

- Mental health referral to promote treatment adherence and reduce performance anxiety
- Vacuum erection devices
- Penile prosthesis surgery

39-4 ▸ Benign Prostatic Hyperplasia

Disease Overview

Benign prostatic hyperplasia (BPH) is the noncancerous enlargement of the prostate gland stemming from an increase in the number of smooth muscle and epithelial cells. BPH affects more than half of men over the age of 60 and nearly 90% of men by age 80. Risk factors include increasing age, family history of BPH, obesity, ethnicity (Black or Latino), current or former smoker, and heavy alcohol consumption.

Pathophysiology and Etiology

The prostate is a walnut-sized reproductive organ found deep in the pelvis, surrounding the urethra at the bladder neck. BPH is a progressive condition that develops as a result of aging and androgen hormones. Testosterone is converted by 5-alpha-reductase to dihydrotestosterone (DHT), a primary stimulator of prostate cell proliferation. There are 2 types of 5-alpha-reductase. Type I has predominant expression in the liver and skin, with minor activity in the prostate, whereas Type II has predominant expression and activity in the prostate. The outer layer of prostatic tissue (the capsule) restricts overgrowth of the prostate, which compresses the urethra and leads to bladder outlet obstruction (BOO). Prostatic smooth muscle found in the bladder neck and capsule contains alpha-1 receptors that cause constriction when activated.

Prostate size does not always correlate with symptom burden or degree of obstruction. Lower urinary tract symptoms (LUTS) (Table 39-3) develop from increased smooth muscle tone and decreased size and force of the urinary system, resulting in incomplete emptying of the bladder, rapid refilling of the bladder, and thickening and irritation of the bladder wall. Untreated BPH can lead to the development of urinary tract infections, overflow incontinence, hematuria, bladder diverticula, stones, and renal failure. Suppression of androgens reduces prostate size, which may slow disease progression and decrease the risk of complications. Inhibition of alpha-1 receptors leads to improved symptoms, urine flow, and reduced residual urine volume.

Diagnosis Principles

Diagnosis is based on medical history (comorbid conditions, medications, surgery or trauma, lifestyle habits, emotional and psychological factors) and focused physical exam (digital rectal exam, urinalysis, prostate-specific antigen). Health care providers should rule out whether symptoms are secondary to BPH or another cause, such as diabetes, bladder or prostate cancer, prostatitis, or medications (diuretics, anticholinergics, antihistamines, alpha agonists, or antidepressants). Symptoms can be quantified using validated questionnaires such as the American Urological Association Symptom Index or International Prostate Symptoms Score.

Treatment Principles

Treatment options are guided by the patient's perception of the severity of his BPH symptoms and the patient's education regarding the benefits and harms of each treatment modality. Goals of therapy are to

TABLE 39-3. Lower Urinary Tract Symptoms Attributable to Benign Prostatic Hyperplasia

Type	Symptom
Obstructive (static)	Straining to void, interruption of voiding, weak stream, terminal dribbling, urinary hesitancy, feeling of incomplete voiding
Irritative (dynamic)	Urinary frequency, urgency, nocturia, enuresis

decrease LUTS, improve urine flow rate, reduce postvoid residual (PVR), slow the rate of progression of the disease, decrease complications, and avoid adverse effects of treatment.

Treatment options include lifestyle changes, watchful waiting, pharmacologic therapy, and surgical intervention:

- Lifestyle modifications alone or in combination with other treatment modalities may reduce symptoms or progression of LUTS. Changes include avoiding medications that can exacerbate symptoms, minimizing caffeine and alcohol intake, restricting fluids close to bedtime, and frequently emptying the bladder during the day.
- Watchful waiting is appropriate for patients with mild LUTS who are not bothered by the symptoms or who do not want to start treatment. Patients may return for annual reassessments.
- Patients with bothersome moderate-to-severe symptoms are treated with medications, minimally invasive surgery, or prostatectomy.
  - The mainstays of pharmacotherapy include alpha-receptor blockers, 5-alpha-reductase inhibitors (5-ARIs), or both. 5-ARIs are reserved for men with a significantly enlarged prostate and predominantly obstructive symptoms. A PDE-5 inhibitor (tadalafil) may be selected as an alternative agent for patients with BPH with or without ED. Muscarinic receptor antagonists for overactive bladder may be used as add-on therapy in men with bladder storage symptoms and a PVR <250 to 300 mL to avoid urinary retention (see Chapter 19 for more information on urinary incontinence).
  - Most of the surgical options are transurethral, accessing the prostate through the urethra. The gold standard intervention is the transurethral resection of the prostate (TURP). Complications that arise include urinary incontinence and sexual dysfunction, both of which resolve for most patients after a few months or a year, respectively.

Drug Therapy

Table 39-4 provides summary information about pharmacotherapy options for BPH. Figure 39-2 depicts receptor targets for BPH medications.

Alpha blockers

Mechanism of action

Inhibition of alpha-1 receptors found in prostatic smooth muscle alleviates LUTS by relaxing the tissue surrounding the bladder neck and allowing urine to expel more easily from the bladder. There are 3 types of alpha-1 receptors: 1A (bladder, prostate), 1B (vascular smooth muscle), and 1D (bladder, spinal cord). Compared to selective alpha-1A blockers, nonselective alpha-1 blockers are more likely to cause side effects such as orthostatic hypotension and dizziness as a result of their effect on alpha-1B receptors. Alpha blockers work within days to weeks, but they may require up to 4 to 6 weeks to reach maximal effectiveness. This medication class does not affect prostate volume, PSA levels, or progression of BPH.

Patient instructions and counseling

- Use caution when taking other medications that lower blood pressure, including PDE-5 inhibitors.
- To reduce the chance of dizziness or passing out, rise slowly after sitting or lying down (this adverse effect is more likely to occur after the first few doses or after a dose increase but could occur at any time).
- Do not crush, chew, or break **tamsulosin** or alfuzosin. Swallow the medication whole.
- Take **tamsulosin** 30 minutes to 1 hour after a meal to increase absorption.
- Consult an ophthalmologist if taking an alpha blocker and planning to undergo cataract surgery.

Adverse drug effects

The following adverse effects may occur: first dose syncope, orthostatic hypotension, dizziness, fatigue, headache, nasal congestion, ejaculatory disorders, intraoperative floppy iris syndrome, and priapism.

TABLE 39-4. Dosing Regimens for Selected Treatment Options for Benign Prostatic Hyperplasia

Generic name	Trade name	Dosing	Comments
Nonselective alph-a-1 receptor blockers			
Prazosin	Minipress		Not recommended because of cardiovascular effects.
Terazosin	Hytrin	1 to 20 mg orally at bedtime	Start at a low dose, and titrate slowly to avoid adverse effects. Take at bedtime to avoid first-dose syncope.
Doxazosin	Cardura	1 to 8 mg orally at bedtime	
	Cardura XL	4 to 8 mg orally at bedtime	
Alfuzosin	Uroxatral	10 mg orally once daily with food	Extended-release formulation; do not crush. Drug may cause QT prolongation. Avoid use in patients who have severe renal dysfunction or moderate to severe hepatic dysfunction, or who take potent CYP450 3A4 inhibitors.
Selective alpha-1A receptor blockers			
Tamsulosin	Flomax	0.4 mg orally daily 30 minutes following the same meal	Extended-release formulation; do not crush. Avoid use with potent CYP450 3A4 inhibitors.
Tamsulosin/ dutasteride	Jalyn	0.5/0.4 mg orally daily 30 minutes following the same meal	
Silodosin	Rapaflo	8 mg orally once daily following the same meal	Adjust dose for renal dysfunction. Avoid use in patients who have severe hepatic dysfunction or who take potent CYP450 3A4 or P-gp inhibitors.
5-Alpha-reductase inhibitors			
Finasteride	Proscar	5 mg orally once daily	Drug is pregnancy category X.
Dutasteride	Avodart	0.5 mg orally once daily	Drug is pregnancy category X.
Phosphodiesterase-5 inhibitor			
Tadalafil	Cialis	5 mg orally once daily	Adjust for renal dysfunction and CYP450 3A4 inhibitors.

Boldface indicates one of the top 100 drugs for 2020 by prescription volume.
P-gp, P-glycoprotein.

Drug interactions

Interaction with antihypertensives or PDE-5 inhibitors may result in severe hypotension. Alfuzosin may prolong the QT interval, especially when taken with other QT-prolonging agents. CYP450 3A4 inhibitors may enhance the adverse effects of alfuzosin, **tamsulosin**, and silodosin.

Monitoring parameters

Monitor blood pressure and urinary symptoms.

5-Alpha-reductase inhibitors

Clinical benefits of 5-ARIs include the reduction of prostate volume, decrease in circulating PSA levels, increase in peak urine flow rate, and improvement in voiding symptoms. This class also reduces urinary retention, risk of renal insufficiency, and need for surgical intervention resulting from disease progression. Results may be observed after 3 to 6 months; however, for maximal benefit, up to 12 months may be necessary. Generally, this class of drugs is reserved for men with an enlarged prostate.

FIGURE 39-2. Receptor Targets for Benign Prostatic Hyperplasia Medications

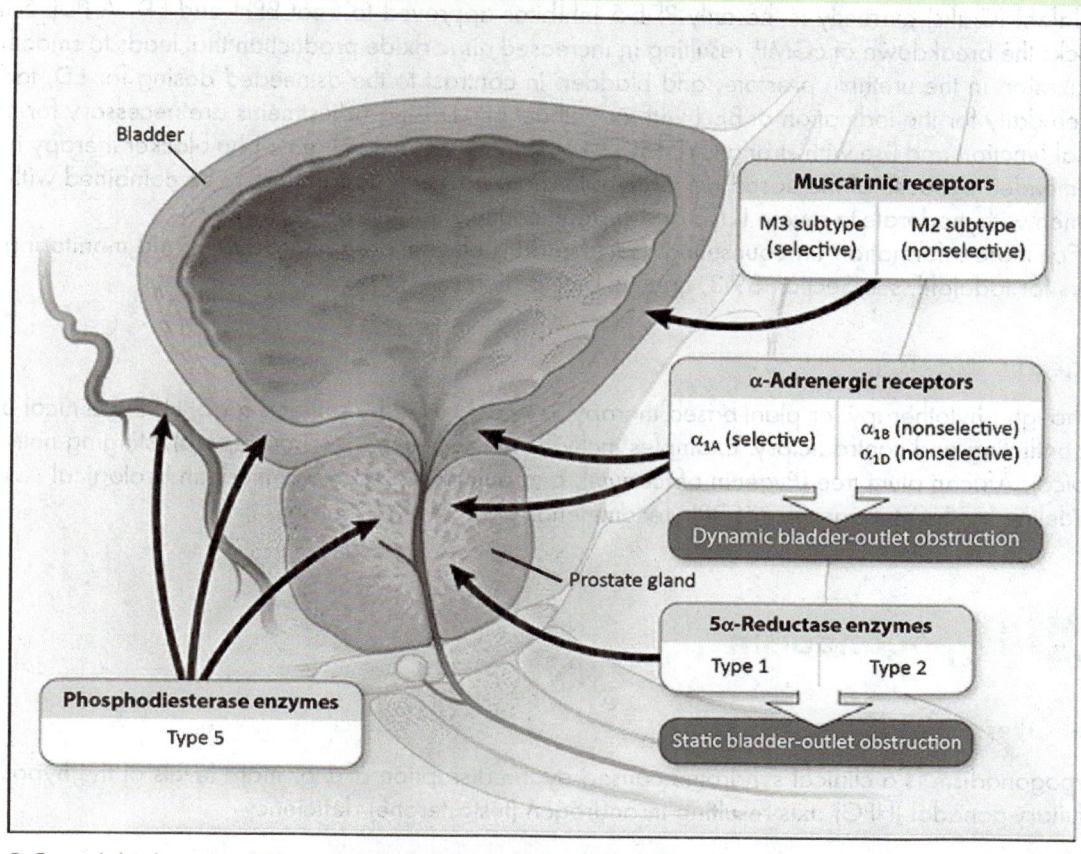

© Copyright American Pharmacists Association PharmacyLibrary.
All rights reserved. Any use is subject to the Terms of Use.

This figure depicts the bladder and prostate with receptor types as related to where the medications work. Selective agents target receptors that are located in these areas, whereas nonselective agents are less targeted and have more systemic side effects. Adapted from: Sarma AV and Wei JT. Benign prostatic hyperplasia and lower urinary tract symptoms. *N Engl J Med* 2012;367:248–57.

Mechanism of action

Inhibition of 5-alpha-reductase prevents the conversion of testosterone to DHT resulting in apoptosis of prostate epithelial cells. No particular 5-ARI has a pharmacodynamic advantage over another.

Patient instructions and counseling

- Pregnant women and women of childbearing age should not take or handle 5-ARIs because they pose a risk to unborn male fetuses.
- Talk to a health care provider if sexual dysfunction or decreased libido is experienced.
- Rarely, breast enlargement with tenderness may develop in men.

Adverse drug effects

The following adverse effects may occur: gynecomastia, ED, decreased libido, and ejaculatory disorders.

Monitoring parameters

Monitor PSA and urinary symptoms.

Phosphodiesterase-5 inhibitor

Tadalafil (Cialis) currently is the only PDE-5 inhibitor approved to treat BPH and ED. A PDE-5 inhibitor blocks the breakdown of cGMP, resulting in increased nitric oxide production that leads to smooth muscle relaxation in the urethra, prostate, and bladder. In contrast to the as-needed dosing for ED, tadalafil is taken daily for the indication of BPH with or without ED. Dosing adjustments are necessary for impaired renal function and use with strong CYP450 3A4 inhibitors. Concomitant alpha-blocker therapy is not recommended because of increased risk of hypotension; however, tadalafil may be combined with a 5-ARI in men with moderate-to-severe LUTS and a significantly enlarged prostate.

For more information on counseling, adverse drug effects, drug interactions, and monitoring parameters for tadalafil, see Section 39-3, Erectile Dysfunction.

Miscellaneous agents

Although phytotherapy, or plant-based therapy, is widely used by patients for BPH, the clinical evidence is conflicting and contradictory. Examples include saw palmetto (*Serenoa repens*), stinging nettle (*Urtica dioica*), African plum tree (*Pygeum africanum*), and pumpkin seed. The American Urological Association guideline for the management of BPH recommends against phytotherapy.

39-5   Hypogonadism

Disease Overview

Hypogonadism is a clinical syndrome caused by the disruption of 1 or more levels of the hypothalamic-pituitary-gonadal (HPG) axis resulting in androgen (testosterone) deficiency.

Pathophysiology and Etiology

In adult men, the incidence of symptomatic testosterone deficiency ranges from 2% to 6%. Hypogonadism is more prevalent in men with advanced age, obesity, and comorbidities such as diabetes.

The production of testosterone in men is dependent on a negative feedback mechanism within the HPG axis (Figure 39-3). Primary hypogonadism, the most common type, occurs at the level of the testes. Androgen deficiency resulting from secondary hypogonadism is the result of disruption at the level of the hypothalamus, the pituitary gland, or both. Certain illnesses, genetic defects, injuries, and medications (Table 39-5) can lead to hypogonadism. Testosterone produced in the testes is converted by 5-alpha-reductase to DHT and by aromatase to **estradiol**. DHT and **estradiol** bind to androgen and estrogen receptors, respectively, thereby exerting their biological effects, which include the development and maintenance of male sexual and reproductive function and promotion of muscle and bone strength. These effects begin in the perinatal period and continue at puberty.

Diagnosis Principles

Diagnosis is based on the presence of persistent signs and symptoms in the setting of consistently low testosterone levels. Signs and symptoms may include low libido, ED, decreased testicular size, fatigue, depressed mood, poor concentration and memory, decreased muscle mass and strength, increased body fat, gynecomastia, loss of body hair, anemia, and low bone mass. Because several symptoms are nonspecific to androgen deficiency, 1 or more symptoms must be present in addition to low total testosterone (TT) levels.

Serum testosterone levels are subject to several factors (e.g., temporal variation: age, season, time of day; obesity; illnesses: diabetes, cirrhosis, hyper- and hypothyroidism; and medications); therefore, a universally

FIGURE 39-3. Pathophysiology of Male Hypogonadism

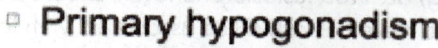

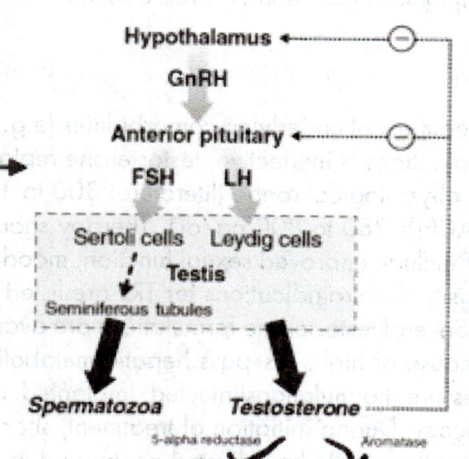

- Primary hypogonadism
  - Testicular dysfunction
    - ↓ Testosterone secretion
    - ↑ LH & FSH levels
- Secondary hypogonadism →
  - Pituitary dysfunction
    - ↓ Testosterone secretion
    - ↓ LH & FSH secretion
  - Hypothalamus dysfunction
    - ↓ Testosterone secretion
    - ↓ GnRH secretion

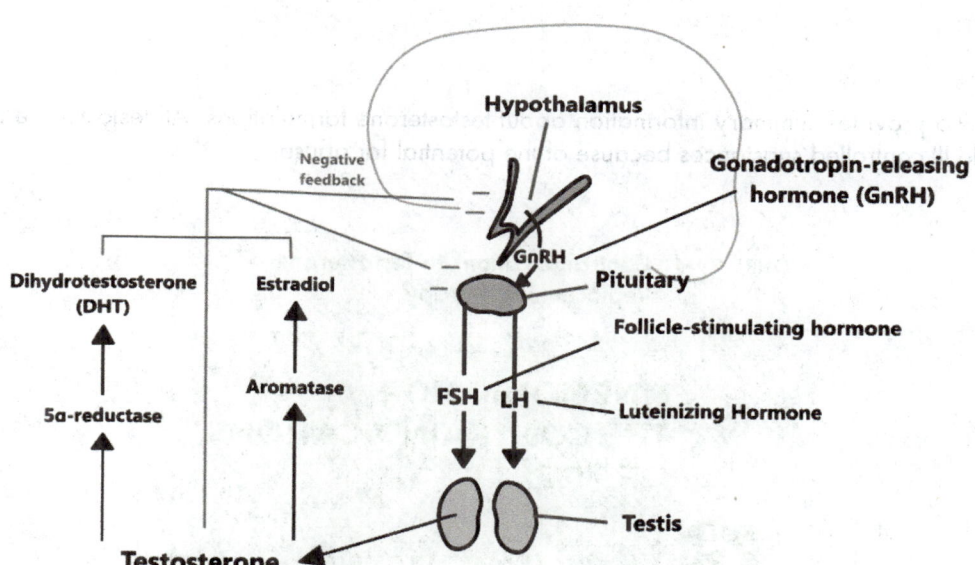

TABLE 39-5. Medications Causing Hypogonadism

Corticosteroids

Long-acting opioids

Anti-androgens (e.g., **spironolactone**, ketoconazole, cimetidine)

Gonadotropin-releasing hormone agonists (e.g., leuprolide, goserelin)

Chemotherapy

Metoclopramide

Psychoactives (e.g., antidepressants, antipsychotics, sedative-hypnotics)

Boldface indicates one of top 100 drugs for 2020 by prescription volume.

accepted definition of testosterone deficiency has not been reached. Testosterone levels should be obtained in the morning when testosterone is highest. Health care providers should retest the level after 1 month, because levels vary over time and more than 30% have normal levels when the test is repeated. Low testosterone is diagnosed when the TT is less than 280 to 300 ng/dL. Free testosterone levels should be considered in symptomatic men with TT levels close to normal or who have comorbidities associated with low testosterone.

Treatment Principles

If treatment of underlying comorbidities (e.g., sleep apnea, diabetes, obesity) and elimination of offending medications is ineffective, testosterone replacement therapy (TRT) can restore testosterone levels to within the physiological range (literature: 300 to 1000 ng/dL; American Association of Clinical Endocrinology [AACE]: 280 to 800 ng/dL). Therapy should aim to increase TT levels to mid-normal range. Benefits of TRT include improved sexual function, mood, cognition, lean muscle mass and strength, and bone mineral density. Contraindications for TRT are listed in Figure 39-4.

Several testosterone formulations are available in the United States. Oral tablets are not commonly used because of high, first-pass hepatic metabolism, increased risk of hepatotoxicity, and increases in blood pressure. Formulations injected, implanted, and applied topically avoid first-pass metabolism and improve efficacy. During initiation of treatment, short-acting formulations are preferred over long-acting agents to allow therapy to be adjusted or stopped in the case of adverse effects.

Drug Therapy

Testosterone

Table 39-6 provides summary information about testosterone formulations. All testosterone products are schedule III controlled substances because of the potential for abuse.

FIGURE 39-4. Contraindications to Testosterone Replacement Therapy

MNEMONIC FOR THE CONTRAINDICATIONS OF TRT

C — Cancers (breast, prostate)

O — Obstructive sleep apnea

U — Uncontrolled HF, untreated BPH

P — Prolactinemia, PSA elevated

E — Erythrocytosis

TABLE 39-6. Testosterone Formulations Available in the United States

Trade name	Available strengths	Initial dosing in hypogonadism	Comments
Long-acting injections			
Testosterone cypionate (Depo-Testosterone)	100 mg/mL, 200 mg/mL	50 to 400 mg I.M. every 2 to 4 weeks	Administer as deep gluteal muscle injection.
Testosterone enanthate (Delatestryl)	200 mg/mL	50 to 400 mg I.M. every 2 to 4 weeks	Administer as deep gluteal muscle injection.
Testosterone undecanoate (Aveed)	750 mg/3 mL	750 mg I.M. once, followed by repeat injections at 4 weeks and 10 weeks	Administer as deep gluteal muscle injection. REMS program medication—must be observed for 30 minutes to monitor for anaphylaxis or POME.
Transdermal patch			
Androderm	2 mg or 4 mg/24 hours	4 mg/24 h patch applied every evening to upper back, abdomen, upper arms, or thighs	Skin irritation is common and can be treated with a low-potency steroid cream.
Transdermal gels			
Androgel	20.25 mg and 40.5 mg per pump actuation or packet	40.5 mg once daily in the morning applied to shoulders or upper arm	
Fortesta	10 mg per pump actuation	40 mg once daily in the morning applied to thighs	
Testim	50 mg per gel tube	50 mg once daily in the morning applied to shoulders or upper arms	
Vogelxo	12.5 mg of testosterone in 1.25 g of gel per pump actuation, 50 mg of testosterone in 5 g of gel per tube/packet	50 mg once daily in the morning applied to shoulders or upper arms	
Pellet			
Testopel	75 mg pellet	150 to 450 mg implanted subcutaneously in the buttocks, lower abdomen, or thigh every 3 to 4 months, sometimes up to 6 months	Pellet is implanted aseptically by a health care provider under local anesthesia. Approximately ⅓ of drug is absorbed in the first month, ¼ in the second month, and ⅙ in the third month.
Nasal gel			
Natesto	5.5 mg per pump actuation	11 mg (1 pump in each nostril) 3 times per day	

I.M., intramuscular; REMS, Risk Evaluation and Mitigation Strategy; POME, pulmonary oil microembolism.

Mechanism of action

Testosterone is used to replace diminished levels of endogenous androgen hormones in symptomatic patients.

Patient instructions and counseling

- Do not apply to genitals.
- Skin irritation may occur at the application or injection site.
- Gels and solutions may be transferred to another person by skin-to-skin contact with the application site. To reduce secondary exposure, wash hands, cover the application site with clothing (once gel or solution has dried), and launder towels and linens that may have come into contact with the drug.
- Avoid flames, fire, or smoking until alcohol-based gels and solutions are dry, because they are flammable.
- Gel and solution applicators require priming before the first use. Refer to the package instructions for the recommended number of actuations for proper priming and discarding. Testosterone axillary topical solution should be applied after applying roll-on or stick antiperspirant or deodorant.
- Aveed ⚠ is available only through the Risk Evaluation and Mitigation Strategy (REMS) program. It requires a 30-minute observation period after injection because of the risk of pulmonary oil microembolism (POME).
- Intranasal spray: Blow your nose before administering 1 pump actuation per nostril. Aim at the lateral wall of the nostril, spray once, and then press on the nostrils and lightly massage. Do not blow your nose or sniff for 1 hour. Nasal irritation or nosebleeds may occur.
- Testosterone has been subject to abuse and dependence, typically at higher doses than recommended and in combination with other anabolic androgenic steroids. Abuse is associated with several adverse effects including heart attack, heart failure, stroke, depression, hostility, aggression, and male infertility.

Adverse drug effects

The following adverse effects may occur: erythrocytosis (discontinue TRT if hematocrit is > 54%), acne, male pattern baldness, gynecomastia, sleep apnea, induction or worsening of BPH symptoms, increased PSA levels, hepatotoxicity, infertility, and progression of hormone-dependent prostate and breast cancer. Increased risk of heart attacks and stroke is possible with testosterone use.

FDA boxed warnings

- Testosterone undecanoate injection may cause POME and anaphylaxis.
- Secondary exposure to testosterone gels and solutions have been reported to cause virilization in children.

Drug interactions

Avoid concomitant use with dehydroepiandrosterone (DHEA) supplements. Corticosteroids (systemic) may increase testosterone levels in patients on TRT.

 Aveed *FDA BOXED WARNING*

Serious pulmonary oil microembolism (POME) reactions can occur during or immediately after administration. Symptoms may include urge to cough, chest pain, dyspnea, and tightening of throat. Patients should be observed in a health care setting for 30 minutes after medication administration.

Monitoring parameters

Monitor testosterone level (baseline and repeat at 3 to 6 months), hematocrit (screen for erythrocytosis), PSA, digital rectal exam, blood pressure, and liver function tests. Bone mineral density testing is conducted after 1 to 2 years of TRT in men with osteoporosis or low trauma fracture.

39-6   Male Contraception

Disease Overview

Contraception is the prevention of pregnancy as a consequence of sexual intercourse by 1 of 2 methods: inhibiting contact of viable sperm with a mature ovum or preventing implantation of a fertilized ovum in the endometrium. Approximately half of pregnancies in the United States are unintended.

Treatment Principles

The selection of contraception method for males is based on effectiveness, cost, accessibility, reversibility, and ability to prevent HIV and other STIs. Options available include abstinence, withdrawal, fertility-based awareness, reversible contraception with barriers, and irreversible contraception with vasectomy. Abstinence is the most effective method for preventing unintended pregnancy, HIV, and STIs.

Male contraception options generally are less effective than hormonal contraceptive treatment in women. Several methods depend on consistent and correct use and, therefore, may have a wide range of effectiveness. Condoms and spermicide are 2 relatively inexpensive barrier methods that are widely available without a prescription. Barrier methods prevent a man's sperm from reaching a woman's egg. Failure rates for barrier methods are 18% to 28%. Success rates improve when latex condoms and spermicide are used together. The fertility-based awareness method and withdrawal (coitus interruptus) method have high unintended pregnancy rates as well (22% to 24%). Men using methods with high failure rates should be counseled on proper use as well as educated about emergency contraception options for women, discussed in Chapter 37, Women's Health: Menopause and Contraception. Vasectomy is a highly effective permanent sterilization procedure with a 0.15% risk of unintended pregnancy. Some men who undergo vasectomy, however, desire reversal.

Drug Therapy

Spermicide

Most spermicides contain nonoxynol-9, a surfactant that destroys sperm cell walls and acts as a barrier between the sperm and the cervix. Spermicide does not protect against viruses, including HIV, and may increase the risk of HIV transmission from a partner. Spermicide is available in foams, gels, creams, and suppositories. The drug is inserted into the vagina and requires a waiting period of 10 to 15 minutes to become effective. A spermicide is effective for 1 hour and must be reapplied before each episode of sexual intercourse. Adverse effects include vaginal burning and itching and allergic reaction.

Nondrug Therapy

Male condoms

A condom is a physical barrier that prevents the sperm from entering the uterus and reaching the ovum. The male condom is a thin sheath of material that is worn over an erect penis. Male condoms have a 2% failure rate with perfect use and 15% with typical use. Most condoms are made of latex, which is impermeable to viruses and protects both parties from HIV and STIs. If a man or his partner is allergic to latex, one of them may use condoms made from synthetic material (polyurethane) or lamb cecum (intestine). However, lamb cecum condoms are porous and do not protect against viruses. Oil-based lubricants, lotions, and medication creams can cause latex to break down; therefore, water-soluble or silicone-based lubricants are preferred. Avoid using a male condom with a female condom, because the combination can stick together, create friction, and ultimately break.

Withdrawal (coitus interruptus)

Withdrawal is a method in which the man removes his penis from the vagina and away from the external genitalia of the woman before he ejaculates. Withdrawal involves no barrier method and, therefore, no economical cost. This method, however, has a 22% failure rate and does not protect against STIs.

Fertility-based awareness (FBA) method

The FBA method involves identification of the fertile days of the menstrual cycle either by monitoring cycle days (calendar based) or observing for fertility signs (symptoms based). Intercourse is avoided (abstinence) or a barrier method is used during the period of fertility. This method has a 24% failure rate and does not protect against STIs.

Vasectomy

Vasectomy is a permanent and highly effective method. The vas deferens is tied, cut, clipped, or sealed to prevent release of sperm. Another form of contraception must be used for 2 to 4 months while the semen becomes totally free of sperm. Vasectomy does not prevent transmission of STIs.

39-7   Pharmacist's Role

Pharmacists can have an impact on men's health by identifying men with ED, BPH, and hypogonadism through medication review and counseling them on proper use of the drug to maximize effectiveness and minimize adverse effects. Community practice pharmacists are also uniquely positioned to counsel men on effective methods of contraception. Pharmacists working in the ambulatory care setting can screen men with conditions that contribute to ED (e.g., diabetes) to identify patients who are candidates for drug therapy, to navigate drug interactions, and to troubleshoot treatment failures.

NAPLEX Competency Statements

The questions in this chapter cover the following 2021 NAPLEX Competency Statements: **AREA 1:** 1.2; 1.3; 1.4; 1.5 **AREA 2:** 2.1; 2.2; 2.3 **AREA 3:** 3.1; 3.2; 3.3; 3.4; 3.5; 3.6; 3.7; 3.8; 3.10; 3.11; 3.12 **AREA 5:** 5.1.

39-8 Questions

1. A 58-year-old male is taking sildenafil for erectile dysfunction. He presents to the emergency department with a prolonged erection lasting more than 4 hours. Five days ago, he started treatment for *Helicobacter pylori* infection. Which of the following medications increases serum concentrations of sildenafil?

   A. Omeprazole
   B. Clarithromycin
   C. Chlorthalidone
   D. Amoxicillin
   E. Metformin

2. Which of the following statements about alprostadil administration is true?

   A. It is available as an oral formulation.
   B. Repeat the dose if no erection occurs in 1 hour.
   C. Fatty meals may impair absorption.
   D. It is administered as an intracavernosal injection.
   E. Avoid administration with nitrates.

3. A 62-year-old man with newly diagnosed ED was given samples of Stendra by his physician. He complains that the medication is not working. The most appropriate action is to verify that the patient was instructed on proper medication use. Which of the following counseling points for Stendra is correct? (Mark all that apply.)

   A. Take with or without food.
   B. Dissolve the tablet on the tongue.
   C. Administer 15 minutes before sexual intercourse.
   D. Inject 5 to 10 minutes before sexual intercourse.
   E. Insert suppository after urination.

4. A patient asks which of his medications could cause ED. A review of his medication list reveals that his ED symptoms are most likely caused by which of the following?

   A. Metoprolol
   B. Docusate
   C. Amiodarone
   D. Atorvastatin
   E. Enalapril

Use Patient Profile 39-1 to answer Question 5.

PATIENT PROFILE 39-1

Patient name: Charles Jones
Age: 56
Sex: Male
Diagnosis:
    Stable angina
    Dyspepsia
    Erectile dysfunction

Height: 5'10"
Weight: 150 lb
Allergies: NKA

Laboratory and diagnostic tests
Blood Pressure: 130/74 mmHg
Heart rate: 70 bpm

Medication Record

Famotidine 20 mg by mouth once daily as needed

Isosorbide mononitrate sustained-acting 30 mg by mouth once daily

5. The primary care physician wants to start treatment for Mr. Jones's erectile dysfunction. The patient is afraid of needles. Which of the following medications would be the best treatment option for Mr. Jones?

   A. Cialis
   B. MUSE
   C. Viagra
   D. Caverject
   E. Levitra

6. Which one of the following is responsible for the conversion of testosterone to dihydrotestosterone?

   A. PSA
   B. Aromatase
   C. 5-alpha-reductase
   D. PDE-5
   E. Nitric oxide

7. Which one of the following statements about dutasteride is correct?

   A. It is pregnancy category X.
   B. An adequate trial is 6 weeks.
   C. Do not administer with nitrates.
   D. It relaxes the detrusor muscle.
   E. It causes changes in vision.

8. What is the brand name of doxazosin?

A. Enablex
B. Levitra
C. Hytrin
D. Avodart
E. Cardura

9. Which of the following is can treat both erectile dysfunction and benign prostatic hyperplasia?

A. Avanafil
B. Finasteride
C. Silodosin
D. Tadalafil
E. Tamsulosin

10. Which one of the following medications can cause or worsen lower urinary tract symptoms of BPH?

A. Olmesartan
B. Furosemide
C. Metformin
D. Lansoprazole
E. Metoprolol

11. Which one of the following strategies is recommended to minimize orthostatic hypotension attributable to Cardura?

A. Advise the patient to take the medication with food.
B. Prescribe that the dose be taken in the morning.
C. Divide the target dose into twice-daily dosing.
D. Add an alpha-receptor agonist.
E. Start low, and slowly titrate to the target dose.

12. Which of the following drugs or drug classes is associated with androgen deficiency?

A. Opioids
B. Insulin
C. Nonsteroidal anti-inflammatory agents
D. Beta blockers
E. Laxatives

13. Testosterone replacement therapy should be discontinued in which one of the following patients?

A. 62-year-old male with a hemoglobin A1C of 9.2%
B. 77-year-old male with a blood pressure of 162/88 mmHg
C. 50-year-old male with a hematocrit level of 57%
D. 69-year-old male with a prostate-specific antigen level of 2 ng/mL
E. 56-year-old male with a body mass index of 30

14. Which one of the following counseling points is correct about Fortesta administration for testosterone deficiency?

A. Apply topically to the armpit (axilla).
B. Apply topically to the thigh.
C. Spray 1 actuation per nostril.
D. Apply topically to the shoulders and upper arms.
E. Apply topically to the scrotum.

15. A 65-year-old male has started Androgel 1.62% for his testosterone deficiency. Which one of the following statements about Androgel is true?

A. Cover the injection site to avoid secondary exposure.
B. Irritation of the gums has been reported.
C. Temporarily discontinue the medication with severe rhinitis.
D. Avoid open flames, fire, or smoking until the gel is dry.
E. Inject deep into the gluteal muscle.

16. Which of the following signs and symptoms are associated with hypogonadism? (Mark all that apply.)

A. Osteoporosis
B. Excess body hair
C. Fatigue
D. Decreased body fat
E. Erectile dysfunction

17. A man approaches your pharmacy seeking advice on contraception. Which of the following recommendations is the best choice for preventing unintended pregnancy and transmission of sexually transmitted diseases and human immunodeficiency virus?

    A. Latex condom and water-based lubricant
    B. Latex condom and oil-based lubricant
    C. Lamb cecum condom and spermicide
    D. Lamb cecum condom and water-based lubricant
    E. Lamb cecum condom and oil-based lubricant

18. Which of the following is the active ingredient in spermicide?

    A. Misoprostol
    B. Levonorgestrel
    C. Ulipristal
    D. Clomiphene
    E. Nonoxynol-9

19. Which of the following statements is correct regarding spermicide?

    A. Do not repeat spermicide application within 24 hours.
    B. Spermicide does not prevent transmission of HIV.
    C. Avoid spermicide use with a condom.
    D. Apply 1 hour before intercourse.
    E. Spermicide is available by prescription only.

20. Which of the following is the most effective method of male contraception?

    A. Spermicide
    B. Condoms
    C. Withdrawal
    D. Vasectomy
    E. Fertility-based awareness

 **39-9   Answers**

1. **B.** Clarithromycin is a CYP450 3A4 inhibitor, which increases serum concentrations of sildenafil, a CYP450 3A4 substrate. Elevated levels may result in enhanced adverse effects, such as priapism.

2. **D.** Alprostadil is available only as an intracavernosal injection and an intraurethral suppository. Administration is limited to 1 dose in 24 hours for the injection and 2 doses per 24 hours (maximum of 3 doses per week) for the suppository. Alprostadil can be taken regardless of concomitant nitrates or food.

3. **A, C.** Stendra, a PDE-5 inhibitor, should be taken orally 15 minutes before sexual activity regardless of meals. Stendra is not available as an orally disintegrating tablet, injection, or suppository.

4. **A.** Beta blockers are associated with symptoms of erectile dysfunction.

5. **B.** MUSE is the brand name of intraurethral alprostadil. The suppository is inserted into the urethra 5 to 10 minutes before sexual activity. MUSE is not contraindicated with nitrates, unlike PDE-5 inhibitors.

6. **C.** Testosterone is converted to DHT by 5-alpha-reductase.

7. **A.** Dutasteride is pregnancy category X. Women of childbearing age or those who are pregnant should not take or handle a 5-alpha-reductase inhibitor because of the toxic effects the drug could have on a male fetus. An adequate trial of a 5-ARI is 6 months.

8. **E.** The brand name of doxazosin is Cardura. The other options listed have the following generic (trade) names: darifenacin (Enablex), vardenafil (Levitra), terazosin (Hytrin), dutasteride (Avodart).

9. **D.** Once-daily tadalafil (Cialis) is approved for the treatment of symptoms of BPH and ED. Alpha blockers and 5-alpha-reductase inhibitors are prescribed to improve symptoms of BPH; however, they can cause sexual dysfunction.

10. **B.** Lower urinary tract symptoms, such as increased urinary frequency, can develop as a result of rapid refilling of the bladder. Diuretics, such as furosemide, cause rapid refilling of the bladder and increase urinary frequency, which can further worsen symptoms in a patient with BPH.

11. **E.** To avoid hypotension with nonselective alpha blockers, start with a low dose at bedtime and titrate slowly to the target dose. Cardura could also be switched to a selective alpha blocker, such as tamsulosin, which is less likely to cause adverse cardiovascular effects.

12. **A.** Treatment of chronic pain with long-acting opioids (such as morphine, oxycodone, methadone, or fentanyl) may result in opioid-associated androgen deficiency.

13. C. Testosterone therapy may cause erythrocytosis, which increases the risk of hyperviscosity and thrombosis. Therefore, testosterone should be discontinued in patients with a hematocrit level >54%.

14. B. Fortesta is a topical gel that is applied to the clean, dry, intact skin of the thigh at the same time every morning. Fortesta should never be applied to the scrotum.

15. D. Androgel 1.62% is a topical gel that is applied topically to the clean, dry, intact skin of the shoulders and upper arms at the same time every morning. After the gel has dried, the area should be covered to avoid secondary exposure.

16. A, C, E. Hypogonadism is characterized by several signs and symptoms such as low bone mass or osteoporosis, fatigue, depression, low libido, ED, decreased muscle mass, increased adiposity, and loss of body hair.

17. A. When used correctly and consistently, latex and polyurethane condoms have low unintended pregnancy rates and protect against STIs and HIV. Lamb cecum condoms do not protect against STIs or HIV. Unlike water-based lubricants, oil-based lubricants can break down latex and compromise protection from STIs. Spermicide alone does not protect against STIs and may increase the risk of HIV transmission from a partner.

18. E. Nonoxynol-9 is the active ingredient in spermicide.

19. B. Spermicide alone does not protect against viruses and may increase the risk of HIV transmission from a partner. Spermicide should be applied 10 to 15 minutes before each episode of sexual intercourse and is effective for 1 hour.

20. D. Of 100 women per year, less than 1 (0.15%) will have an unintended pregnancy with a man who has had a vasectomy and uses no other form of contraception. Other mentioned male contraception methods, except abstinence, have a failure rate of 18% or higher.

 **39-10 Additional Resources**

Erectile Dysfunction

Burnet AL. Nehra A, Breau RH, et al. Erectile Dysfunction: AUA Guideline. *J Urol.* 2018;200:633–641.

Lee M, Sharif R. Erectile dysfunction. In: DiPiro JT, Yee GC, Posey ML, et al., eds. *Pharmacotherapy: A Pathophysiologic Approach.* 11th ed. New York, NY: McGraw-Hill; 2020:1382–1410.

Benign Prostatic Hyperplasia

Lee M, Sharif R. Benign prostatic hyperplasia. In: DiPiro JT, Yee GC, Posey ML, et al., eds. *Pharmacotherapy: A Pathophysiologic Approach.* 11th ed. New York, NY: McGraw-Hill; 2020:1411–1420.

McVary KT, Roehrborn CG, Avins AL, et al. American Urological Association guideline: management of benign prostatic hyperplasia. Published 2010; reviewed and validity confirmed 2014. Available at: https://www.auanet.org /guidelines/benign-prostatic-hyperplasia-(bph)-guideline/benign-prostatic-hyperplasia-(2010-reviewed-and-validity -confirmed-2014). Accessed May 18, 2021.

Hypogonadism

Bhasin S, Brito JP, Cunningham GR, et al. Testosterone therapy in men with hypogonadism: an endocrine society clinical practice guideline. *J Clin Endocrinol Metab.* 2018;103(5):1715–1744.

Snyder PJ. Androgens and the Male Reproductive Tract. In: Brunton LL, Hilal-Dandan R, Knollmann BC, eds. *Goodman & Gilman's: The Pharmacological Basis of Therapeutics.* 13th ed. New York, NY: McGraw-Hill; 2018:833–844.

Contraception

Centers for Disease Control and Prevention. U.S. medical eligibility criteria for contraceptive use, 2016. *MMWR Recomm Rep.* 2016;65(3):1–104.

El-Ibiary SY, Shrader SP, Ragucci KR. Contraception. In: DiPiro JT, Yee GC, Posey ML, et al., eds. *Pharmacotherapy: A Pathophysiologic Approach.* 11th ed. New York, NY: McGraw-Hill; 2020:41–60.

Nonprescription Medications

KENNETH C. HOHMEIER   TYLER M. KILES

40-1 KEY POINTS

- The most common conditions treated with nonprescription medications are pain, cough and cold, allergy, heartburn, constipation and diarrhea, minor infections, and skin problems.
- Cough and cold products should not be used in children <4 years of age due to lack of safety and efficacy.
- Nonprescription drug treatment for the common cold includes symptomatic management using decongestants (nasal congestion), first-generation antihistamines (excess nasal discharge), analgesics (headache), and local anesthetic lozenges or sprays (pharyngitis).
- Nonprescription treatment of allergies includes systemic antihistamines (sedating or nonsedating), ocular antihistamines, decongestants, and intranasal steroids.
- Cough can be relieved by a product containing a cough suppressant (dextromethorphan). An expectorant (guaifenesin) should be recommended to enhance clearance of mucus.
- Bulk-forming laxatives and stool softeners are the safest products to prevent and treat constipation and can be used chronically. Stimulant laxatives should be used only occasionally because of laxative dependence or other complications. An exception to this rule is the scheduled use of stimulant laxatives with chronic opioid treatment.
- Loperamide or bismuth subsalicylate may be recommended to treat diarrhea.
- Nonprescription treatment options for nausea and vomiting include antihistamines (meclizine, dimenhydrinate) and phosphorated carbohydrate solution.
- Histamine-2–receptor antagonists (famotidine, **ranitidine**); antacids; or bismuth subsalicylate may relieve gastric discomfort or indigestion.
- Pain and fever may be treated with **aspirin** and other salicylates, nonsteroidal anti-inflammatory drugs (NSAIDs), or **acetaminophen**.
- **Aspirin** and NSAIDs inhibit platelet aggregation. Nonacetylated salicylates have little antiplatelet activity, and **acetaminophen** does not have antiplatelet activity.
- Salicylates and NSAIDs can cause gastropathy, including gastritis, gastric ulcers, and gastric bleeding. They may decrease the effectiveness of some antihypertensives and may have deleterious effects on kidney function.
- **Acetaminophen** does not have anti-inflammatory activity.
- First-line nonprescription agents for pharmacotherapy in smoking cessation are nicotine gum, nicotine lozenge, and nicotine patch. These products should be avoided 2 weeks after myocardial infarction, with serious arrhythmias, or with serious or worsening angina.
- Dietary supplements that should be stopped 7 to 10 days before surgery include ginkgo biloba, garlic, and ginseng.

40-2 STUDY GUIDE CHECKLIST

The following topics may guide your study of this subject area:

- ☐ Conditions that are self-treatable with nonprescription drugs.
- ☐ Nonprescription treatment appropriate in special populations (children, pregnant women, lactating women, etc.).
- ☐ First-line treatments for each self-treatable condition.
- ☐ Common or severe adverse effects of nonprescription drug classes.
- ☐ Drug–drug interactions between nonprescription and prescription drugs.
- ☐ Legal and regulatory considerations in nonprescription treatment.

40-3 Cough, Cold, and Allergy

Cough

Pathophysiology

A cough is an important defense mechanism to rid the airways of mucus and foreign bodies. A cough may be acute (<3 weeks duration) or chronic (>3 weeks duration). Coughs may be productive (mucus secretions easily expelled) or nonproductive (dry, hacking without expelled mucus secretions). Generally, productive coughs should not be suppressed using nonprescription therapies unless the potential benefit outweighs the risk.

Nonprescription Treatment

Cough suppressants

Cough suppressants (antitussives) may be narcotic or nonnarcotic. Table 40-1 shows selected examples of nonprescription cough products.

Codeine

Codeine, a narcotic, is the gold standard of antitussives.

- **Availability:** Without prescription in some states
- **Mechanism of action:** Centrally mediated suppression of cough
- **Adult dose:** 10 to 20 mg every 4 to 6 hours (120 mg/d maximum)
- **Role in therapy:** Primarily for night cough; contraindicated in children <12 years of age
- **Side effects:** Sedation, nausea, constipation; avoid during lactation

Dextromethorphan

- **Mechanism of action:** Centrally mediated suppression of cough
- **Adult dosage:** 10 to 30 mg every 4 to 8 hours (120 mg/d maximum)
- **Role in therapy:** Nonproductive cough

TABLE 40-1. Selected Examples of Nonprescription Cough Products

Type of product	Generic name	Action	Trade name
Expectorant	Guaifenesin	Immediate release	Robitussin Chest Congestion Syrup (100 mg/5 mL)
		Extended release	Mucinex tablets (600 mg)
Cough suppressant	Dextromethorphan HBr	Immediate release	Vicks DayQuil Cough (15 mg/15 mL)
	Dextromethorphan polistirex	Extended release	Delsym suspension (30 mg/5 mL)
Combination expectorant and cough suppressant	Guaifenesin and dextromethorphan HBr	Immediate release	Robitussin Cough + Chest Congestion DM (100 mg/10 mg per 5 mL)
		Extended release	Mucinex DM (600 mg/30 mg, 1200 mg/60 mg tablets)
		Immediate release	Alka-Seltzer Plus Max Cough, Mucus, and Congestion 200 mg/10 mg capsules
Combination expectorant, cough suppressant, and decongestant	Guaifenesin, dextromethorphan HBr, and phenylephrine HCl	Immediate release	Robitussin Multi-Symptom Cold (100 mg/10 mg/5 mg per 5 mL)

- *Side effects:* Drowsiness, gastrointestinal (GI) effects
- *Drug interactions:* Monoamine oxidase (MAO) inhibitors

Diphenhydramine

- *Mechanism of action:* Centrally mediated suppression of cough center and anticholinergic
- *Adult dosage:* 25 mg every 4 hours (75 mg/d maximum)

Expectorant

Guaifenesin

- *Mechanism of action:* Thinning of mucus to enhance clearance
- *Adult dosage:*
  - Immediate-release: 200 to 400 mg every 4 hours (maximum 2400 mg/d)
  - Extended-release: 600 to 1200 mg every 12 hours (maximum 2400 mg/d)
- *Role in therapy:* Productive cough
- *Side effects:* GI discomfort
- *Patient education:* Increase fluid intake

Topical antitussives

Of the volatile oils, only camphor and menthol are approved by the U.S. Food and Drug Administration (FDA).

- *Mechanism of action:* Local anesthetic effect in nasal mucosa
- *Product availability:* Lozenge, ointment, steam inhalation
- *Patient education:* Ointment and solution are toxic if ingested

Sore throat remedies

- Saline gargle
- Sprays and lozenges:
  - *Benzocaine:* Chloraseptic and Cepacol lozenges
  - *Dyclonine:* Sucrets Maximum Strength lozenges
  - *Phenol:* Chloraseptic spray
  - *Menthol:* Vicks VapoDrops

Special Patient Populations

Pregnancy

Dextromethorphan is viewed as probably safe.

Lactation

- Dextromethorphan, guaifenesin, and topical anesthetics are all low risk.
- Avoid codeine and diphenhydramine because of risk of excessive sedation leading to breathing problems, possibly fatal, in infants and difficulty with breastfeeding.

Common Cold

Clinical presentation

- Sore throat, nasal symptoms, watery eyes, sneezing, cough, malaise, low-grade fever
- Gradual onset with slow progression
- Duration of 1 to 2 weeks

Nonpharmacologic treatment

- Humidifiers
- Increased fluid intake

- Rest
- Head propped upright
- Rubber bulb nasal syringe for children <4 years of age
- Irrigation of nose with saline drops or mist

Nonprescription medication treatment (symptomatic)

- Decongestants for nasal congestion
- First-generation antihistamines used in combination with a decongestant for excess nasal discharge (not as effective as monotherapy for treatment of colds)
- Analgesics for related pain or headaches
- Local anesthetic lozenges or sprays for sore throat (pharyngitis)

Allergic Rhinitis

Clinical presentation

- *Nasal:* Congestion, rhinorrhea, nasal pruritus, sneezing, postnasal drip
- *Ocular:* Itching, lacrimation, redness, irritation
- *General:* Headache, malaise, mood swings, irritability

Nonprescription Treatment of the Common Cold and Allergies

Selected products for treating the common cold and allergies are shown in Tables 40-2, 40-3, and 40-4.

Antihistamines

Selected antihistamines are described in Table 40-2.

Pharmacology

- Antihistamines are histamine-1–receptor antagonists.
- First-generation antihistamines are nonselective and sedating.
- Second-generation antihistamines are peripherally selective and have a low incidence of sedation.

TABLE 40-2. Selected Nonprescription Antihistamine Products

Generic name	Trade name	Adult dosage (maximum daily dose)
Chlorpheniramine maleate	Chlor-Trimeton	4 mg every 4 to 6 hours (24 mg)
Diphenhydramine HCl	Benadryl	25 to 50 mg every 4 to 6 hours (300 mg)
Fexofenadine HCl	Allegra, Mucinex Allergy	60 mg every 12 hours or 180 mg daily (180 mg)
Loratadine	Claritin, Alavert	10 mg daily
Cetirizine HCl	Zyrtec	10 mg daily
Levocetirizine dihydrochloride	Xyzal	5 mg daily in evening

Boldface indicates one of top 100 drugs for 2020 by prescription volume.

TABLE 40-3. Selected Nonprescription Oral Decongestant Products

Generic name	Products	Comments	Adult dosage (maximum daily dose)
Phenylephrine HCl	Sudafed PE	Weakest oral decongestant	10 mg every 4 hours (60 mg)
Pseudoephedrine HCl	Sudafed	Less central nervous system stimulation	60 mg every 4 to 6 hours (240 mg)

TABLE 40-4. Selected Nonprescription Cold, Allergy, and Sinus Combination Products

Product	Trade name	Primary ingredients
Decongestant and analgesic	Aleve-D Sinus & Cold	Pseudoephedrine 120 mg + **naproxen** 220 mg
	Advil Cold and Sinus	Pseudoephedrine 30 mg + **ibuprofen** 200 mg
	Sudafed 12 Hour Pressure + Pain	Pseudoephedrine 120 mg + **naproxen** 220 mg
	Sudafed PE Pressure + Pain	Phenylephrine HCl 5 mg + **acetaminophen** 325 mg
	Advil Congestion Relief	Phenylephrine HCl 10 mg + **ibuprofen** 200 mg
Antihistamine, decongestant, and analgesic	Alka-Seltzer Plus Night Severe Cold, Cough and Flu	Diphenhydramine 25 mg + phenylephrine 10 mg + **acetaminophen** 650 mg per packet
	Advil Allergy and Congestion Relief	Chlorpheniramine maleate 4 mg + phenylephrine 10 mg + **ibuprofen** 200 mg
Decongestant, analgesic, and cough suppressant	Vicks Dayquil Cold and Flu LiquiCaps	Phenylephrine HCl 5 mg + **acetaminophen** 325 mg + dextromethorphan HBr 10 mg
	Alka-Seltzer Plus Cold and Cough Effervescent Tablets	Chlorpheniramine 4 mg + phenylephrine 15.6 mg + **aspirin** 650 mg + dextromethorphan 20 mg per dose
Antihistamine and decongestant	Dimetapp Cold and Allergy Syrup	Brompheniramine maleate 1 mg + phenylephrine HCl 2.5 mg per 5 mL
	Zyrtec D	**Cetirizine HCl** 5 mg + pseudoephedrine HCl 120 mg
	Claritin-D 12 Hour	**Loratadine** 5 mg + pseudoephedrine 120 mg
	Claritin-D 24 Hour	**Loratadine** 10 mg + pseudoephedrine sulfate 240 mg
	Allegra-D 12 Hour	Fexofenadine HCl 60 mg + pseudoephedrine HCl 120 mg

Boldface indicates one of top 100 drugs for 2020 by prescription volume.

Side effects
- Sedation (primarily with first-generation antihistamines)
- Anticholinergic effects
  - Dry mouth
  - Dry eyes
  - Urinary retention
  - Constipation
- Paradoxical stimulation in some children and elderly patients

Precautions and contraindications
- Do not drive or operate heavy machinery.
- Avoid use with alcohol.
- Prostatic hyperplasia can occur.
- Narrow-angle glaucoma is possible.

Intranasal corticosteroids

Triamcinolone acetonide (Nasacort Allergy 24HR), budesonide (Rhinocort Allergy Spray), fluticasone propionate (Flonase Allergy Relief, ClariSpray), fluticasone furoate (Flonase Sensimist)
- Decrease the influx of inflammatory cells and inhibit the release of cytokines, thereby reducing inflammation of the nasal mucosa
- Considered first-line therapy for moderate-to-severe allergic rhinitis
- More effective than antihistamines, especially for treatment of late allergic rhinitis symptoms such as nasal congestion

Dosing

- **Age 2 to 5 years:** Refer to primary care provider (PCP).
- **Age 6 to 12 years:** Increase dose to 2 sprays in each nostril daily.
- **Age ≥ 12 years:** Initiate at 2 sprays in each nostril daily (220 mcg/d).
  - Once symptoms are controlled, patient may be able to titrate down to 1 spray in each nostril daily.

Side effects

- Nasal irritation, dryness, or both
- Epistaxis
- Stinging, burning, or both
- Bitter taste

Precautions and contraindications

If a patient < 12 years of age plans on using an intranasal corticosteroid longer than 2 months per year, encourage the patient to see the PCP.

Oral decongestants

Selected oral decongestant products are described in Table 40-3.

Pharmacology

- Alpha-adrenergic agonists and vasoconstrictors
- Constriction of blood vessels to decrease blood supply to nasal mucosa and decrease mucosal edema
- No effect on histamine or allergy-mediated reaction

Regulation

The 2005 Combat Methamphetamine Epidemic Act has the following requirements:

- Pseudoephedrine must be kept either behind the sales counter or in a locked cabinet.
- Quantity is limited to 3.6 g/d and 9 g/mo per patient.

Side effects

These products are relatively safe with no dependence. They can be used long term, with the most common side effects as follows:

- Nervousness
- Irritability
- Restlessness
- Insomnia

Precautions and contraindications

- **Hypertension:** These agents are generally accepted with mild or well-controlled hypertension; they should not be used with uncontrolled hypertension.
- **Heart disease (arrhythmias and ischemic heart disease):** They increase the heart rate.
- **Diabetes:** They have a minimal effect on blood sugar level.
- **Hyperthyroidism:** This condition is more sensitive to sympathomimetics.
- **Enlarged prostate:** Benign prostatic hyperplasia is exacerbated by constricting smooth muscle of the bladder neck.
- **Narrow-angle glaucoma:** Dilation increases intraocular pressure.
- **Blood pressure:** Monoamine oxidase inhibitors (MAOIs) interact with decongestants to increase blood pressure.

Topical decongestants

Pharmacology

- Alpha-adrenergic agonists act locally as vasoconstrictors.
- These agents constrict blood vessels, decrease blood supply to the nose, and decrease mucosal edema.
- They have no effect on histamine or allergy-mediated reaction.

Side effects

Minimal systemic absorption results in few side effects. Local effects may include burning, nasal irritation, and sneezing.

Precautions and contraindications

Rhinitis medicamentosa (rebound congestion) may occur if duration of use is >3 to 5 days. The FDA recommends using these products no more than 3 days in duration.

Dosage forms of topical decongestants

Sprays

Sprays are the simplest dosage delivery and cover a large surface area. Imprecise dosing and contamination of the bottle are possible. Products include the following:

- **Short-acting:** Phenylephrine HCl (Neo-Synephrine)
- **Longest-acting:** Oxymetazoline HCl (Afrin, Vicks Sinex)

Nasal saline solution

This solution is very safe and is good for use in infants and children to remove dried, encrusted, or thick mucus from the nose while also moisturizing and soothing nasal passages. It can be used with oral decongestants. Products include the following:

- Saline drops (Ayr)
- Saline sprays (Ayr, Ocean Nasal Spray)
- Neti pot

Mast cell stabilizer

Cromolyn (Nasalcrom)

- **Pharmacology:** Prevention of the release of inflammatory mediators from mast cells
- **Dosage:** One spray per nostril every 4 to 6 hours
- **Onset of action:** Approximately 1 week; 2 to 4 weeks for maximal effect
- **Efficacy:** Not efficacious if taken as needed; must be taken on a scheduled basis and is more effective if started at least 1 week before symptom onset
- **Side effects:** Nasal irritation, nasal burning, stinging, sneezing, cough, unpleasant taste

Analgesics

Analgesics treat the pain, fever, and headaches associated with cold, flu, or allergies. Medications include the following:

- **Aspirin** (mostly replaced now by **acetaminophen** and nonsteroidal anti-inflammatory drugs [NSAIDs])
- **Acetaminophen** (N-acetyl-para-aminophenol [APAP])
- NSAIDs
- **Ibuprofen** (over-the-counter [OTC] form not approved for children <6 months of age)
- **Naproxen** (OTC form not approved for children <12 years of age)

Special populations

Children

- Do not use cough and cold products in children <4 years of age.
- All children <12 years of age are excluded from self-care of allergy unless they have been diagnosed by a health care provider and are approved for nonprescription therapy.
- Second-generation antihistamines and intranasal corticosteroids can be used for self-care in children <6 years of age (provided they have been diagnosed by a health care provider and approved for nonprescription treatment).

Pregnancy

- Avoid products containing pseudoephedrine in the first trimester.
- Oxymetazoline is the preferred topical decongestant.
- For allergy, cromolyn is considered first-line therapy, followed by the second-generation antihistamines: **loratadine** and **cetirizine**. Chlorpheniramine can also be used.

Lactation

- Avoid using the following topical decongestants: xylometazoline and naphazoline.
- All antihistamines can decrease milk production.
- For allergy, cromolyn is considered first-line therapy, followed by **loratadine** and chlorpheniramine.

40-4 Constipation

Clinical Presentation

- Patient has difficult or infrequent passage of stools.
- Patient may complain of abdominal or rectal fullness.

Etiology

Table 40-5 shows the common causes of constipation.

TABLE 40-5. Common Causes of Constipation

Daily habits	Diseases	Medications
Inadequate fluid intake	Parkinson's disease	Antacids containing Al or Ca
Inadequate fiber intake	Multiple sclerosis	Anticholinergics
Lack of physical exercise	Cerebrovascular disease	Phenothiazines
	Irritable bowel syndrome	Tricyclic antidepressants
	Hemorrhoids	Opiates
	Polyps and tumors	Antihistamines
	Diabetes	ACE inhibitors
	Hypothyroidism	Calcium channel blockers
		Sucralfate
		Iron

ACE, angiotensin-converting enzyme.

Nonpharmacologic Treatment

- Increase fluid intake.
- Increase dietary fiber.
- Exercise.
- Establish good bowel habits.

Nonprescription Medication Treatment

Bulk-forming laxatives

Selected bulk-forming laxative products are described in Table 40-6.

Mechanism of action

Natural or semisynthetic hydrophilic polysaccharide derivatives are present in bulk-forming laxatives. They absorb water to soften stool, increase bulk, and facilitate peristalsis and elimination. Onset of effect may not be seen for 2 to 3 days.

Role in therapy

Bulk-forming laxatives are the safest, most natural therapy for normal transit constipation. They are the most often recommended medication for chronic use. Use caution in patients with fluid restriction (i.e., renal dysfunction, heart failure), narcotic-associated dysmotility, and fecal impaction.

Drug interactions

- These laxatives may bind with digoxin, **warfarin**, and other drugs.
- Calcium complexes may bind with tetracycline, inhibiting its absorption.
- Recommend separating doses from other medications by 1 to 2 hours.

Side effects

- Dose should be increased gradually over several weeks to avoid bloating, flatulence, and abdominal pain.
- These laxatives can cause bowel obstruction if not taken with sufficient amounts of water.
- Caution patients with diabetes about sugar content of some products.

TABLE 40-6. Selected Nonprescription Treatments for Constipation

Medication class	Generic name	Brand name
Bulk-forming laxatives	Psyllium seed	Metamucil, Konsyl
	Methylcellulose	Citrucel
	Calcium polycarbophil	FiberCon
Emollient laxative	Docusate sodium	Colace
Saline laxatives	Magnesium hydroxide	Milk of Magnesia
	Magnesium citrate	Magnesium citrate
	Magnesium sulfate	Epsom salts
	Monobasic sodium phosphate	Fleets
Combination product	Senna + docusate sodium	Senokot-S

Emollient laxatives (stool softeners)

Emollient laxatives act as surfactants, absorbing water into the stool. Onset of effect may take 2 to 3 days. Emollient laxatives may cause systemic absorption of mineral oil; therefore, concurrent use is contraindicated.

Emollient laxatives are often used in combination products. They are useful in situations when straining should be avoided, such as following rectal surgery, during the postpartum time period, and following a recent myocardial infarction.

A selected emollient laxative product is described in Table 40-6.

Stimulant laxatives

Stimulant laxatives stimulate bowel motility through localized mucosal irritation. They increase secretion of fluids into the bowel. Impaired colon function occurs with chronic use.

Dangers of chronic stimulant laxative use include the following:

- Laxative habit
- Cathartic colon
- Melanosis coli
- Loss of fluids and electrolytes
- Cramping pains

Anthraquinones

Senna (Senokot and Ex-Lax) is an anthraquinone:

- *Pharmacology:* Anthraquinones are absorbed into the bloodstream with action on the large intestines. Onset of effects is 6 to 12 hours. This medication should be taken at bedtime.
- *Side effects:* Such effects include discoloration of urine, stimulant habituation, and melanosis coli (i.e., dark pigmentation of colonic mucosa).

Diphenylmethanes

Bisacodyl (Dulcolax tablets or suppositories) is a diphenylmethane. Minimal systemic absorption occurs with this drug. This medication is enteric coated; do not crush or take with antacids. The onset of effects varies with route of administration.

- *Oral:* 6 to 8 hours
- *Rectal:* 15 to 60 minutes

Stimulant oils

Castor oil acts on the small intestine. It is a strong cathartic and may induce fluid or electrolyte disturbances. Onset is rapid: 2 to 6 hours.

Hyperosmotic laxatives

Glycerin

Glycerin has an osmotic effect and is a local irritant that stimulates bowel movement. Onset of effect is usually within 30 minutes.

Products include Fleet Pedia-Lax Liquid Glycerin Suppository and Fleet Glycerin Suppository.

Polyethylene glycol 3350 (MiraLAX)

Polyethylene glycol (PEG) 3350 has a mechanism of action similar to that of glycerin. This agent is meant for short-term therapy for constipation. Onset of action is usually within 1 to 3 days. The adult dosage is 17 g of powder in 4 to 8 oz of water. Side effects are as follows:

- Bloating
- Abdominal discomfort
- Cramping
- Flatulence

Saline laxatives

With saline laxatives, nonabsorbable cations create osmotic gradient to pull water into the intestine. Onset varies depending on the route of administration:

- *Rectal:* 5 to 30 minutes
- *Oral:* 30 minutes to 4 hours

Twenty percent of magnesium may be absorbed systemically. Saline laxatives are contraindicated in patients with impaired renal function (magnesium- or phosphate-containing), congestive heart failure, or hypertension (sodium-containing). Selected saline laxative products are described in Table 40-6.

Enemas

Enemas include Fleet Enema (monobasic and dibasic sodium phosphates). They are typically used for acute treatment (fecal impaction), not for long-term management of constipation.

Lubricant laxatives

Selected lubricant laxative products are as follows:

- *Mineral oil:* Liquid petrolatum
- *Olive oil:* "Sweet oil"

Lubricant laxatives soften the feces by emulsifying the contents of the intestinal tract. Onset of action is 6 to 8 hours. Use in self-care is strongly discouraged because of high risk of adverse effects in children and the elderly. Do not administer with stool softeners.

Special Patient Populations

Children

- Mild constipation can be treated with increases in fluids and fruit juices containing sorbitol, such as apple, pear, prune, apricot, nectarine, or peach juice.
- Increase dietary fiber intake.
- For children 2 to 6 years of age, the following products are approved for use:
  - *Rectal:* Glycerin suppositories
  - *Oral:* Docusate sodium or magnesium hydroxide
- For children 6 to 12 years of age, the following products are approved for use:
  - *Rectal:* Glycerin or bisacodyl suppositories
  - *Oral:* Bulk-forming laxatives, docusate, and magnesium hydroxide are preferred; oral stimulants (senna, bisacodyl) should be reserved for when preferred treatments fail.
- For patients 6 to 17 years of age, one could apply off-label use of PEG 3350 at doses of 1 g/kg daily (not to exceed 17 g daily), but a health care provider must be involved with the care of these patients.
- For patients >17 years of age, PEG 3350 is FDA approved for use.

Pregnancy

- Attempt dietary changes first by incorporating more fiber via prunes or prune juice.
- If dietary changes do not work, use bulk-forming laxatives with sufficient amounts of water.
- For complaints of primarily dry, hard stools, use docusate.
- Senna or bisacodyl can be used safely short term and have more data supporting their use than does PEG 3350, but some experts use PEG 3350 as first-line treatment.
- Avoid castor oil (causes uterine contractions) and mineral oil (impairs maternal fat-soluble vitamin absorption).

Lactation

- Senna, bisacodyl, PEG 3350, and docusate are all compatible with breast-feeding.
- Avoid castor oil and mineral oil.

40-5 Diarrhea

Clinical Presentation

Diarrhea is the abnormal increase in frequency of stools and stool looseness. It may be acute (< 14 days) or chronic (> 4 weeks).

Etiology

Common causes of diarrhea are shown in Table 40-7.

Complications

- Dehydration (especially in infants and elderly patients)
- Electrolyte abnormalities

Nonpharmacologic Treatment

- Administer oral rehydration therapy, such as Pedialyte.
- Avoid fatty and spicy foods and foods with high sugar content.

Nonprescription Medication Treatment

Loperamide HCl (Imodium AD)

Loperamide is a synthetic opioid agonist that slows GI motility. The dosage is 4 mg initially and then 2 mg after each loose stool. For OTC use, maximum dose is 8 mg/d.

The medication is well tolerated, but typical side effects are as follows:

- Constipation
- Dizziness
- Dry mouth

Precautions and contraindications are as follows:

- Loperamide is not recommended for children <6 years of age without medical supervision.
- It should not be used if the patient has bloody or black stool; consult a health care provider before use if the patient has a fever, mucus in stool, or a history of liver disease.
- Antiperistaltic action could worsen effects of invasive or inflammatory bacterial infection.

TABLE 40-7. Common Causes of Diarrhea

Infection	Medications	Diet
Viral	Antibiotics	Allergies
Norwalk	Laxatives	Spicy foods
Rotavirus	Magnesium-containing antacids	High carbohydrate load
Bacterial	Cytotoxic agents	Lactose intolerance
Foodborne illness		
Contaminated water		
Traveler's diarrhea		
Protozoal		

Bismuth subsalicylate (Pepto-Bismol)

Bismuth subsalicylate reacts with stomach acid to form salicylic acid and bismuth oxychloride. It reduces frequency of diarrhea and improves stool consistency. It has a direct antimicrobial effect; therefore, it is effective in traveler's diarrhea.

Side effects include the following:

- Salicylate toxicity (tinnitus)
- Bismuth toxicity (neurotoxicity)
- Gray-black discoloration of tongue or stool

The medication is contraindicated in the following:

- **Aspirin** allergy
- Children and teens with viral illness (Reye's syndrome)
- Patients having a history of GI bleeding or using **warfarin**

40-6   Nausea and Vomiting

Physiology

Vomiting is coordinated by the vomiting center in the medulla. Stimuli from the peripheral nervous system and within the central nervous system (CNS) act on the vomiting center. Responding to these impulses, the vomiting center stimulates the abdominal muscles, stomach, and esophagus to induce vomiting.

Etiology

Common causes of nausea and vomiting are shown in Table 40-8.

TABLE 40-8. Common Causes of Nausea and Vomiting

Irritation of chemoreceptor trigger zone	Vestibular disorders	CNS disorders	GI disorders
Chemotherapy	Motion sickness	Psychogenic vomiting	Obstruction
Narcotics	Otitis interna	Migraines	Gastroparesis
Theophylline	Meniere's syndrome	Increased intracranial pressure	Gastroenteritis
Digoxin			Infection
Antibiotics			
Drug withdrawal			
Alcohol			
NSAIDs			
Antibiotics			
Ketoacidosis			
Uremia			
Pregnancy			
Electrolyte imbalances			

Complications

- Dehydration
- Electrolyte imbalance
- Aspiration
- Malnutrition
- Acid–base disturbances

Nonprescription Medication Treatment

In addition to the medications described in this section, Table 40-9 describes nonprescription drugs of choice for prevention of the nausea or vomiting associated with motion sickness.

Antihistamines

Antihistamines cross the blood-brain barrier to depress vestibular excitability.

Phosphorated carbohydrate solution (Emetrol)

This agent is a hyperosmolar solution of levulose (fructose), dextrose (glucose), and phosphoric acid. It is buffered to a pH of 1.5. It reduces gastric muscle contraction through an unknown direct effect. It must not be diluted (which raises the pH).

Bismuth subsalicylate (Pepto-Bismol)

Bismuth subsalicylate is available as nonprescription suspension, caplet, and chewable tablet. See Section 40-5 for additional information.

Histamine 2–receptor antagonists

Histamine 2–receptor antagonists may provide symptomatic relief by inhibiting gastric acid secretion. Potential drug interactions occur with cimetidine.
Side effects are as follows:

- Headache
- Constipation
- Diarrhea

TABLE 40-9. Nonprescription Drugs of Choice for Prevention of Motion Sickness

		Dosage		
Generic name	Trade name	Adults (maximum daily dose)	Children ages 6 to 12 years (maximum daily dose)	Children ages 2 to 6 years (maximum daily dose)
Dimenhydrinate	Dramamine	50 to 100 mg every 4 to 6 hours (400 mg)	25 to 50 mg every 6 to 8 hours (150 mg)	12.5 to 25 mg every 6 to 8 hours (75 mg)
Diphenhydramine	Benadryl	25 to 50 mg every 4 to 6 hours (300 mg)	12.5 to 25 mg every 4 hours (150 mg)	6.25 mg every 4 hours (25 mg)
Cyclizine	Marezine	50 mg every 4 to 6 hours (200 mg)	25 mg every 6 to 8 hours (75 mg)	Not recommended
Meclizine	Bonine	25 to 50 mg daily (50 mg)	Not recommended	Not recommended

Antacids

Antacids may treat nausea, dyspepsia, and stomach upset associated with excessive intake of food or drink. They are combinations of magnesium hydroxide, sodium salts, aluminum hydroxide, calcium carbonate, and magnesium carbonate. The usual adult dosage is 15 mL 30 minutes after meals and at bedtime.

Side effects include the following:

- Constipation
- Diarrhea
- Sodium overload

Antacids may decrease absorption of some medications; therefore, administer other medications 1 to 2 hours before or after antacids.

Special Patient Populations

Pregnancy

Especially during the first trimester, nonpharmacologic therapy is recommended.

- Ensure there is fresh air in the rooms where you sleep, prepare food, and eat.
- Eat small, frequent meals.
- Avoid rich, fatty foods.
- Before getting out of bed in the morning, eat several dry crackers and relax for 10 to 15 minutes.

Refer the patient to the health care provider if pharmacologic therapy is being considered. Once the health care provider is involved in care, the following medications are preferred for use in pregnancy:

- Antihistamines (meclizine, cyclizine, dimenhydrinate, diphenhydramine): All have a low risk of teratogenicity but should be reserved for those with severe symptoms unresponsive to non-pharmacologic measures.
- Pyridoxine (vitamin B_6): 10 to 25 mg 3 to 4 times daily
- Doxylamine succinate: 12.5 mg 3 to 4 times daily
- Calcium-containing antacids
- Ginger: There is evidence supporting its use in pregnancy (see Section 40-14 for herbal products).

40-7   Pain and Fever

Pathophysiology of Pain

Nociceptors are peripheral pain receptors. They send pain stimuli to the spinal cord through afferent, nociceptive nerves. Impulses then pass to the brain through dorsal root ganglia.

Pathophysiology of Fever

The core temperature is the temperature of the blood surrounding the hypothalamus. The thermoregulatory center in the anterior hypothalamus controls body temperature through physiologic and behavioral mechanisms. Pyrogens—fever-producing substances—increase the thermoregulatory set point, raising the body temperature.

Nonprescription Medication Treatment

Selected analgesic and antipyretic products are shown in Table 40-10.

TABLE 40-10. Selected Analgesic and Antipyretic Products

Generic name	Trade name	Dosage Adults (maximum daily dose)	Children (maximum daily dose)
Acetaminophen	Tylenol, FeverAll	325 to 1000 mg every 4 to 6 hours (4000 mg)ª	10 to 15 mg/kg every 4 to 6 hours (5 doses)
Aspirin	Bayer	650 to 1000 mg every 4 to 6 hours (4000 mg)	10 to 15 mg/kg every 4 to 6 hours (80 mg/kg)
Ibuprofen	Motrin, Advil	200 to 400 mg every 4 to 6 hours (1200 mg OTC)	5 to 10 mg/kg every 6 to 8 hours (40 mg/kg)
Naproxen sodium	Aleve	220 mg every 8 to 12 hours (660 mg)	Not recommended <12 years of age; ≥12 years of age: use adult dosage
Diclofenac gel	Voltaren	Lower extremities: Apply 4 g of 1% gel to affected area 4 times daily. Upper extremities: Apply 2 g of 1% gel to affected area 4 times daily.	Not recommended <18 years of age

Boldface indicates one of top 100 drugs for 2020 by prescription volume.
a. FDA maximum dose. See Section 40-7 in this chapter for McNeil product maximum doses for acetaminophen.

Acetaminophen

Acetaminophen exerts analgesic and antipyretic activity through central inhibition of prostaglandin synthesis. It does not have peripheral anti-inflammatory activity. **Acetaminophen** is generally well tolerated; however, hepatotoxicity is a possible side effect. In addition, the risk for severe liver injury increases when taking multiple products that contain **acetaminophen**.

Drug interactions can occur as follows:

- *Alcohol:* Drinking ≥3 alcoholic beverages a day increases the risk of hepatotoxicity.
- *Warfarin:* Higher doses (> 1.3 g for > 1 week) may enhance hypoprothrombinemic effect of **warfarin**.

Changes to McNeil (Tylenol brand) product labeling are as follows:

- Tylenol Extra Strength (500 mg tablets): Maximum dose is 3000 mg/d or 6 tablets/d.
- Tylenol Regular Strength (325 mg tablets): Maximum dose is 3250 mg/d or 10 tablets/d.
- These maximum doses are different than the official FDA-approved adult maximum daily dose of 4 g/day for generic **acetaminophen**.

Salicylates

Salicylates inhibit peripheral prostaglandin synthesis. They reduce pain, inflammation, and fever. Acetylated salicylates (e.g., **aspirin**) irreversibly inhibit platelet aggregation. Nonacetylated salicylates (e.g., prescription salsalate, magnesium subsalicylate) have reversible antiplatelet activity.

Side effects associated with salicylates include the following:

- Gastritis
- Gastric ulcers and bleeding
- Allergy and hypersensitivity:
  - Rare (<1%) in the general population
  - Higher risk in individuals with asthma and nasal polyps

■ Reye's syndrome, a potentially fatal illness associated with salicylate use in children and teens with concurrent viral illness (influenza, varicella-zoster)

Drug interactions may occur with the following:

■ *Alcohol:* GI toxicity is enhanced.
■ *Methotrexate:* Salicylates displace methotrexate from protein-binding sites.
■ *Warfarin:* Salicylates enhance hypoprothrombinemic effects of **warfarin**.

Patients should be aware of the following precautions and contraindications:

■ Bleeding disorders
■ Hemophilia
■ Peptic ulcer disease
■ Children or teenagers with viral illness (Reye's syndrome)
■ Gout

Nonsteroidal anti-inflammatory drugs

The FDA boxed warning for NSAIDs includes cautions about increased risks of (1) myocardial infarction and stroke, which can be fatal and may occur early in treatment and may increase with duration of use, and (2) bleeding, ulceration, and perforation of the stomach or intestines, which can be fatal and can occur at any time during use and without warning symptoms.

NSAIDs provide peripheral inhibition of prostaglandin synthesis. They offer analgesic, antipyretic, and anti-inflammatory activity.

Side effects include the following:

■ GI effects, including bleeding
■ Rash
■ Photosensitivity
■ High incidence of cross-reactivity in individuals with **aspirin** allergy

Drug interactions may occur as follows:

■ *Warfarin:* Increased bleeding risk
■ *Alcohol:* Increased risk of GI bleeding
■ *Methotrexate:* Decreased methotrexate clearance
■ *Antihypertensives:*
  ▪ Angiotensin-converting enzyme inhibitors: Decreased hypotensive effects, hyperkalemia
  ▪ Beta blockers: Decreased hypotensive effects
  ▪ Potassium-sparing diuretics: Hyperkalemia
■ *Digoxin:* Decreased renal clearance, risk of digoxin toxicity

Precautions and contraindications are as follows:

■ Renal impairment
■ Congestive heart failure

The following patients are at increased risk of severe stomach bleed with NSAID use:

■ >60 years of age
■ History of peptic ulcer disease
■ Concomitant use of **warfarin**, other NSAIDs, or alcohol
■ Duration of use longer than recommended

Special Patient Populations

Pregnancy and lactation

- **Acetaminophen** is preferred.
- **Ibuprofen** and **naproxen** are compatible with breast-feeding.
- Avoid NSAIDs in the third trimester of pregnancy because of increased risk of premature closure of the fetal ductus arteriosus.

40-8   Ophthalmic Disorders

Dry Eye

- *Definition:* Tear film instability caused by a deficiency of any component of the tear film
- *Clinical presentation:* Ocular discomfort, blurred vision, desire to rub the eyes, burning, or redness

Table 40-11 describes the pharmacologic treatment of dry eyes.

Redness Caused by Minor Irritation

Eye redness can be caused by airborne pollutants (gases or smoke), chlorinated water, infectious diseases, or glaucoma.

Nonprescription treatment

Ophthalmic vasoconstrictors, as described in Table 40-12, are used to treat eye redness.

The medications constrict blood vessels of the conjunctiva. Instill 1 to 2 drops in the affected eye up to 4 times daily. Minimize systemic absorption by closing the eye after instillation and occluding the tear duct with a finger (punctal occlusion).

These agents are contraindicated in patients with narrow-angle glaucoma because they cause mydriasis. Contact lens wearers also should avoid ophthalmic vasoconstrictors.

A rebound hyperemia can occur, especially with overuse. If agents are absorbed systemically, tachycardia and arrhythmias can occur.

Ocular decongestants should be avoided in patients with heart disease, high blood pressure, an enlarged prostate, or narrow-angle glaucoma.

TABLE 40-11. Pharmacologic Treatment of Dry Eyes

Product	Common preparations	Comments
Artificial tears[a]		
Cellulose derivatives (carboxymethylcellulose)	Bion Tears, Refresh Celluvisc, Clear Eyes CLR	Has enhanced duration compared to other products; tends to form dry crusts, which may be easily washed off with warm water
Polyvinyl alcohol (glycerin, propylene glycol, polyethylene glycols, polysorbate 80)	Hypo Tears, Murine Tears, Oasis Tears Plus	Has shorter duration; has no crust formation
Povidone and dextran 70	AquaSite	Can cause transient stinging or burning
Ocular emollients[b]		
Lanolin, mineral oil, petrolatum, white ointment, white wax, or yellow wax	Moisture Eyes PM, Lacri-Lube SOP, Refresh PM	

a. Artificial tears act as demulcents to mimic mucin. Use twice daily as suggested.
b. Ointments have longer contact and are more likely to cause blurred vision.

TABLE 40-12. Ophthalmic Vasoconstrictors

Product	Common preparations	Key points
Naphazoline	Clear Eyes, Clear Eyes Redness Relief, Allerest, All Clear, All Clear AR	Ocular decongestant of choice
Tetrahydrozoline	Visine, Vision Clear, Visine Maximum Redness Relief, OptiClear	Less likely to alter pupil size; possible stinging on instillation
Oxymetazoline	Visine LR	Relatively free of ocular or systemic side effects

Allergic Conjunctivitis

Symptoms

Symptoms include chronic and recurring itching. Eyes are slightly red and tear and burn, but they have little discharge.

Nonprescription treatment

Antihistamine and mast cell stabilizer

Ketotifen fumarate 0.025% (Zaditor, Alaway), an antihistamine and mast cell stabilizer, may be used to treat allergic conjunctivitis. Instill 1 drop every 8 to 12 hours in the affected eye. Use in patients ≥3 years of age. Olopatadine HCl is available in 2 strengths (Pataday 0.1% Twice Daily Relief and Pataday 0.2% Once Daily Relief). Instill 1 drop every 12 hours in the affected eye. Use in patients ≥2 years of age. Relief is provided within minutes, and effects may last up to 12 hours.

Topical decongestants

Naphazoline HCl 0.12% (Clear Eyes), phenylephrine HCl 0.12% (Refresh Redness Relief), tetrahydrozoline HCl 0.05% (Visine), and oxymetazoline HCl 0.25% (Visine L.R.) are topical decongestants for treatment of conjunctival swelling and redness. Instill 1 to 2 drops into affected eye(s) up to 4 times daily.

Combination products

The following combination products containing an ophthalmic vasoconstrictor and an ocular antihistamine may be used:

- Naphazoline + pheniramine (Naphcon A, Visine A, Opcon-A)
- Naphazoline + antazoline (Vasocon-A)

Instill 1 to 2 drops in the affected eye up to 4 times daily.

Combination products containing ocular decongestants should be avoided in patients with heart disease, high blood pressure, enlarged prostate, or narrow-angle glaucoma.

Conditions Requiring Referral to a Health Care Provider or Eye Care Specialist

Corneal edema

Symptoms

Symptoms include foggy vision, halos around lights, photophobia, irritation, sensation of a foreign body, and extreme pain.

Nonprescription treatment

After seeking medical care from a PCP, the patient can use sodium chloride (2% to 5%) to treat corneal edema. Instill 1 to 2 drops in the affected eye every 6 hours. If eye drops do not provide relief, add ointment to therapy.

Foreign body in the eye

Foreign bodies include metal shavings, wood splinters, and dust. Improper removal may lead to permanent eye damage.

Ocular trauma

Automobile accidents and sports injuries are common causes of ocular trauma.

Chemical exposure

If chemical exposure occurs, follow these steps:

- Remove contact lenses.
- Flush eye immediately with lukewarm water for at least 15 minutes.
- Do not place drops in the eyes.

40-9   Otic Disorders

Impacted Cerumen

Cerumen-softening agents are used as follows:

- Instill in ear.
- Follow with warm water irrigation using otic syringe.

Cerumen-softening agents

- *Carbamide peroxide 6.5% in anhydrous glycerin:* Products include Auro Ear Drops and Debrox Earwax Removal Aid Kit. This agent softens earwax and facilitates its removal.
- *Hydrogen peroxide and water:* A 1:1 solution of warm water and 3% hydrogen peroxide is used. This mixture is not an effective drying agent.
- *Glycerin:* This emollient and humectant may facilitate the removal of earwax.
- *Olive oil:* Sometimes called sweet oil, this agent can also be used.

Water-Clogged Ears

A solution of 95% isopropyl alcohol in 5% anhydrous glycerin (Swim Ear or Auro Dri Drops) may be used to treat water-clogged ears. This solution is the only FDA-approved ear-drying aid.

40-10   Smoking Cessation

Unless the patient has contraindications, pharmacotherapy should be offered to all patients attempting to quit smoking (Table 40-13).

First-line agents double long-term smoking abstinence rates. Nonprescription nicotine replacement therapy (NRT) comprises the following first-line agents:

- Nicotine gum (Nicorette, generic): OTC
- Nicotine patch (Nicotrol, NicoDerm CQ, generic): OTC
- Nicotine lozenge (Commit): OTC

TABLE 40-13. The "5 A's" Clinicians Should Use to Assist Patients in Smoking Cessation

Ask about tobacco use.	Identify and document tobacco use status for every patient at every visit.
Advise to quit.	In a clear, strong, and personalized manner, urge every tobacco user to quit.
Assess willingness to make a quit attempt.	Is the tobacco user willing to make a quit attempt at this time?
Assist in quit attempt.	For the patient willing to make a quit attempt, use counseling and pharmacotherapy to help him or her quit.
Arrange follow-up.	Schedule follow-up contact, preferably within the first week after the quit date.

Side Effects

NRT can have various side effects:

- Gum
  - Patients may experience an unpleasant taste, mouth irritation, jaw muscle soreness, hypersalivation, hiccups, and dyspepsia.
  - Warn patients against chewing the gum too fast and chewing more than 1 piece at a time.
- Lozenge
  - Mouth irritation, nausea, hiccups, cough, heartburn, headache, flatulence, and insomnia can occur.
  - Patients should not use more than 1 lozenge at a time.
- Patch
  - Local skin reactions (erythema, burning, pruritus) can occur. Treat by rotating sites or applying hydrocortisone or triamcinolone cream.
  - Vivid or abnormal dreams, insomnia, and headache can occur. These effects are more common in the 24-hour patch. Patients can minimize the effects by using the 16-hour patch or by removing the patch at night before bed.

Precautions and Contraindications

Cardiovascular disease is a contraindication to the use of NRT in the following cases:

- <2 weeks following myocardial infarction
- Serious arrhythmias
- Serious or worsening angina

NRT is also contraindicated in the following:

- Esophagitis (gum or lozenge form only)
- Peptic ulcer disease (gum or lozenge form only)

Patients on NRT should seek medical advice if they are pregnant women or lactating women. Patients should attempt to stop smoking before starting NRT, but it is not required.

40-11   Overweight and Obesity

Nonprescription Medication Treatment

Orlistat

Orlistat decreases the absorption of dietary fats and inhibits gastric and pancreatic lipases.

Indication

This agent is used in patients ≥18 years of age who are overweight (body mass index [BMI] ≥25) in conjunction with lifestyle modification.

Note: According to the 2013 AHA/ACC/TOS Guideline for the Management of Overweight and Obesity in Adults, pharmacologic therapy is not recommended as an adjunct to a comprehensive lifestyle intervention unless a patient has a BMI ≥30 or BMI ≥27 in addition to 1 obesity-related comorbidity.

Dose

Patients should take one 60 mg capsule before meals. They do not have to take the medication if the meal does not contain fat.

Side effects

Side effects include the following:

- Flatulence with oily spotting
- Loose and frequent stools
- Fatty stools
- Fecal urgency
- Incontinence

Decreasing the amount of ingested fat can minimize side effects. Effects generally resolve within a few weeks of initiating therapy.

Precautions

Counsel patients on the signs and symptoms associated with liver damage (anorexia, pruritus, jaundice, dark urine, light-colored stools, right upper quadrant pain).

Contraindications

Patients on cyclosporine and patients with malabsorption disorders should not use this medication. Patients with a history of thyroid disease, cholelithiasis, nephrolithiasis, or pancreatitis should consult a health care provider before use.

Interactions

Decreased absorption of fat-soluble vitamins (especially D and E) occurs. Take a multivitamin at bedtime or separate it from orlistat dose by at least 2 hours.

Concern exists over vitamin K absorption and possible effects on **warfarin**; therefore, recommend increased monitoring.

40-12 Overactive Bladder

Overactive bladder is often associated with detrusor instability, defined as the detrusor muscle squeezing too often or without warning and causing urinary incontinence or the sudden urge to urinate.

Nonprescription Medication Treatment

Oxytrol for Women (oxybutynin)

This transdermal delivery system (3.9 mg/d) is indicated in women ≥18 years of age. Clear patch must be changed every 4 days and is applied to the abdomen, hip, or buttock. The full benefit of this medication is seen in about 2 weeks. When the agent is combined with daily lifestyle modifications (timed urination, pelvic floor exercises, fluid management), studies show a reduction of urinary accidents by 75% with Oxytrol versus 50% with placebo.

Side effects

Anticholinergic effects may occur as follows:

- Dry mouth or eyes
- Constipation
- Itching, rash, or redness where patch was placed
- Sleepiness
- Dizziness
- Blurry vision

Precautions and contraindications

Oxybutynin is not for use in men, women < 18 years of age, or other types of urinary incontinence.

40-13 Home Monitoring and Testing Devices

Fertility Prediction Tests

Basal thermometry

Temperatures can be taken orally, rectally, and vaginally. Temperatures are taken every morning before rising.

Resting temperatures are usually below normal for the first part of the reproductive cycle. Temperatures are closer to normal after ovulation.

Temperature results are plotted graphically against time to assess spikes (ovulation). Tests are very user dependent.

Clearblue Easy Fertility Monitor

This test for luteinizing hormone (LH) and estrone-3-glucuronide is a monitoring device with strips that are inserted into a monitor. The user tests urine daily for 10 to 20 consecutive days. The results are listed as low, high, and peak fertility. It can identify up to 6 fertile days; however, it is expensive in comparison to ovulation prediction kits.

OV-Watch

This device is a watch worn while sleeping that measures chloride ions in perspiration every 30 minutes. It must be worn at least 6 hours each night. This device alerts the user 4 days before ovulation. It also is expensive in comparison to ovulation prediction kits.

Ovulation prediction kits

This test contains antibodies that bind to the LH in urine. An LH surge is detected by a difference in color or color intensity from one day to the next.

Early morning urine collection is recommended. The user must know the length of the past 3 cycles before using. Testing usually begins 2 to 4 days before ovulation (based on the average of the past 3 cycles).

Pregnancy Detection

Early testing is very important. Tests detect levels of human chorionic gonadotropin (hCG) in urine (within 1 to 2 weeks after conception). Antibodies designed to react with hCG form the shape of a straight line, check, or plus sign. If the user is a pregnant woman, color is produced.

TABLE 40-14. Causes of Error in Home Pregnancy Testing

False positives	False negatives
Miscarriage within previous 8 weeks	Test performed first day of a missed cycle
Childbirth within previous 8 weeks	Refrigerated urine not allowed to come to room temperature
Use of fertility medications (Pergonal, Profasi)	Wax cups or household containers with soap residues used for test

Pregnancy tests are 98% to 100% accurate; however, human error decreases that rate to 50% to 75% (Table 40-14).

Important tips for patients using pregnancy tests are as follows:

- Use of first morning urine to test is encouraged because hCG is more concentrated.
- If use of first morning urine is not possible, the patient should restrict fluids 4 to 6 hours before urine collection.
- Use only supplied collection devices.
- Try to test the sample immediately after collection. If this is not possible, allow refrigerated samples to come to room temperature.
- If the test is negative, wait 1 week and retest if the cycle has not yet started.
- If the test is positive, contact an obstetrician–gynecologist immediately and start prenatal vitamins.

Urinary Tract Infection Tests

AZO Test Strips

- Test for nitrites and leukocyte esterase
- Specific only for gram-negative organisms

Fecal Occult Blood Tests

Three categories are available:

- Toilet tests (EZ-Detect Stool Blood Test), which use biodegradable paper that is placed in the toilet bowl after a bowel movement
- Stool wipes (LifeGuard)
- Manual stool application tests (Colon-Test-Sensitive)

A colorimetric assay is used for hemoglobin. A blue-green color indicates a positive test.

Tests are more likely to detect lower GI problems. False-positive tests can occur with the ingestion of red meat or vitamin C.

Human Immunodeficiency Virus (HIV) Screening

OraQuick In-Home HIV Test screens for autoantibodies to HIV-1 and HIV-2. Patients should be aware that they need to wait for at least 3 months after exposure before testing.

The patient obtains an oral swab sample. Results show in the device window within 20 to 40 minutes. A positive result is indicated by a line present near the C and T on the device window. A negative result is indicated by a line near only the C on the device window. This test has a sensitivity of 92% and a specificity of 99.98%.

40-14 Dietary Supplements

Definition

According to the Dietary Supplement and Health Education Act (DSHEA) of 1994, a *dietary supplement* is "a product intended to supplement the diet that bears or contains one or more of the following dietary ingredients: a vitamin, mineral, herb or other botanical, amino acid; a dietary substance for use by man to supplement the diet by increasing the total daily intake; or a concentrate, metabolite, constituent, extract, or combination of these ingredients."

Regulation of Dietary Supplements

Dietary supplements are not regulated as closely as drugs. Table 40-15 provides a comparison. The following agencies are responsible for regulation:

- **U.S. Food and Drug Administration:** Regulates labeling, safety, and manufacturing
- **U.S. Federal Trade Commission:** Regulates advertising

Herbal Products

Asian ginseng (Panax ginseng)

Common uses

Asian ginseng is taken for enhancement of immunity and mental performance.

Side effects

Side effects are insomnia, headache, blood pressure changes, anorexia, rash, mastalgia, and menstrual abnormalities. Long-term use can cause a ginseng abuse syndrome.

Precautions

Caution is warranted in the following circumstances:

- Cardiovascular disease
- Hypertension with or without medical treatment
- Diabetes (specifically with patients receiving medications that may cause hypoglycemia or having a diagnosis of hypoglycemia unawareness)
- History of hypotension

Contraindications

- Renal failure
- Acute infection
- Pregnancy and lactation
- Active bleeding (peptic ulcer)

TABLE 40-15. Drugs versus Dietary Supplements

Drug	Dietary supplement
Active ingredient is identified.	Active ingredient may not be identified.
Safety and efficacy are proved by manufacturer.	No proof of efficacy is required; FDA must provide proof if unsafe.
Purity and contents are regulated.	No standards exist for quality or purity.
Claims to treat, cure, or prevent disease are made.	No claims to treat, cure, or prevent specific disease are made.

Interactions

- Stimulants (including caffeine)
- Antipsychotics

Coenzyme Q10 (Ubiquinone)

Common uses

Coenzyme Q10 (CoQ10) is commonly used for heart failure, hypertension, and statin-induced myopathy.

Side effects

Side effects include nausea, GI distress, headache, irritability, and dizziness.

Interactions

- CoQ10 has a similar structure to synthetic vitamin K, which may cause a decrease in international normalized ratio (INR) levels if used concomitantly with **warfarin**.
- HMG-CoA (3-hydroxy-3-methyl-glutaryl-coenzyme A) reductase inhibitors reduce serum levels of CoQ10.

Echinacea purpurea

Common uses

Echinacea purpurea is used for the treatment of upper respiratory tract infections.

Dosage

Dosing should begin at the onset of viral symptoms, and treatment should continue until 24 to 48 hours after symptoms abate. Typical use is 14-days duration. It is not recommended for cold prevention.

Side effects

Side effects include mild GI discomfort, tingling sensation of the tongue, and headache. Allergic reactions can occur.

Contraindications

This product should not be taken by patients with severe systemic illness (HIV/AIDS [acquired immune deficiency syndrome], multiple sclerosis, tuberculosis) or autoimmune disorders or by patients taking immunosuppressants. Avoid in patients with an allergy to Asteraceae (daisy) family of plants and in patients with severe allergy, allergic rhinitis, or atopy.

Interactions

There are no clinical interactions of importance.

Fish oil

Common uses

Fish oil often is taken to improve cardiovascular health. Patients with coronary artery disease, hypertension, hypertriglyceridemia, or rheumatoid arthritis also take fish oil.

Dosage

- Based on eicosapentaenoic acid/docosahexaenoic acid (EPA/DHA) content of capsules
- *General use:* 1 to 2 g daily
- *Hypertriglyceridemia:* 2 to 4 g daily

Side effects

Side effects include GI distress and fish burp, which may be avoided by using enteric-coated products, taking with meals, or storing the capsules in a refrigerator.

Interactions

At doses >4 g daily, increased bleeding risk is present; therefore, patients on anticoagulation or antiplatelet therapy should be limited to 3 g daily.

Garlic (Allium sativum)

Common uses

Garlic is taken to lower cholesterol and to prevent atherosclerosis and cardiovascular disease.

Side effects

Side effects include malodorous breath and smell of garlic that may permeate the skin, GI discomfort, heartburn, and gas.

Contraindications

Active bleeding (peptic ulcer) can occur. Garlic should be stopped 10 to 14 days before surgery to avoid potential bleeding complications.

Interactions

- ***Anticoagulants and antiplatelet agents:*** **Aspirin**, ticlopidine, **clopidogrel**, dipyridamole, **warfarin**, ginkgo, ginseng
- ***Saquinavir:*** 50% decrease in area under the curve (AUC) in healthy volunteers

Ginger

Common use

Ginger is used as an antiemetic.

Dosage

- ***Pregnancy-induced nausea or vomiting:*** Dried ginger 250 mg daily
- ***Motion sickness:*** Two 500 mg capsules taken 30 minutes before travel, followed by 1 to 2 more 500 mg capsules as needed every 4 hours

Side effects

Heartburn, belching, or dermatitis may occur.

Interactions

Ginger may increase the risk of hypoglycemia and alter platelet function at doses >1 g/day. Use with caution in patients receiving antiplatelet and anticoagulation therapy.

Ginkgo biloba

Common uses

Ginkgo biloba is used to enhance memory and concentration. Credible scientific evidence supports its use in the treatment of cerebral insufficiency, dementia, generalized anxiety disorder, and schizophrenia.

Side effects

- ***Mild:*** GI distress, headache, and dizziness can occur.
- ***Serious:*** Spontaneous bleeding has been reported (e.g., subdural hematomas, subarachnoid hemorrhage).

Contraindications

Ginkgo biloba should be stopped at least 7 days before surgery to avoid potential bleeding complications.

Interactions

This product may interact with both medications (**aspirin**, ticlopidine, **clopidogrel**, dipyridamole, **warfarin**) and herbs (garlic, ginseng). Interactions result from antiplatelet or anticoagulant activity.

Glucosamine and chondroitin sulfate

Common uses

Glucosamine and chondroitin sulfate products are used for osteoarthritis.

Dosage

- ■ *Glucosamine:* 500 mg 3 times daily (with meals) glucosamine sulfate
- ■ *Chondroitin:* 400 mg 3 times daily

These agents are often in a combination product. Full effects may not be seen for 4 to 6 months.

Side effects

Side effects include mild GI upset, nausea, heartburn, constipation, and diarrhea.

Contraindications

Patients with severe shellfish allergy should not take this product. Avoid in pregnancy and lactation.

Green tea

Common uses

Green tea is taken as a performance enhancer and as protection from the development of cardiovascular disease and cancer.

Side effects

GI irritation and both CNS and cardiac stimulation can occur because of caffeine content. Green tea can contain a range of 8 to 30 mg of caffeine per tea bag.

Drug interactions

Large doses may decrease INR levels, although brewing destroys most of the vitamin K content.

Melatonin

Common uses

Melatonin is commonly used to treat sleep disorders and to reset the sleep–wake cycle (jet lag).

Dosage

- ■ *Insomnia:* 0.3 to 5 mg 30 minutes before bedtime
- ■ *Jet lag:* 2 to 5 mg in the evening between 5:00 PM and 10:00 PM on the day of arrival and at bedtime for 2 to 5 days after arrival

Long-term administration is not recommended.

Side effects

Melatonin may worsen depression. Other side effects include headache and confusion. Melatonin is possibly an immune stimulant.

Interactions

When melatonin is taken with benzodiazepines, anxiolytic effects are enhanced.

Probiotics

Common uses

Probiotics are taken for antibiotic-induced diarrhea, GI disorders, and atopic dermatitis.

Side effects

Bloating, flatulence, and diarrhea may occur.

Contraindications

Because of reports of systemic infection, immunocompromised patients should avoid use. Systemic infection is more common with the use of probiotics containing *Saccharomyces boulardii*.

Interactions

Probiotics may decrease antibiotic absorption; therefore, antimicrobial agents should be administered several hours apart from taking probiotics.

Fenugreek

Common uses

Fenugreek is often used by women to stimulate breast milk production when lactating. It is also used for diabetes.

Dosage

The dosage is 2.5 g orally twice daily.

Side effects

Urine, sweat, and breast milk may have the odor of maple syrup.

Precautions and contraindications

Avoid in patients with an allergy to chickpeas. Avoid in pregnancy.

Interactions

Use with caution in patients receiving antiplatelet and anticoagulation therapy because of possible decrease in platelet aggregation caused by fenugreek.

Aloe vera

Common uses

Aloe vera is commonly used topically for burns or psoriasis and systemically for constipation.

Dosage

No clear optimal topical dosage exists. It is not recommended as a first-line agent for constipation, but the dose suggested in many sources is the minimum amount to maintain a soft stool.

Side effects

Abdominal cramps and diarrhea can occur with oral use.

Precautions and contraindications

Use caution if patients with diabetes are taking aloe vera orally and are on hypoglycemic medications.

Interactions

Interactions do not typically occur with topical application.

St. John's wort (Hypericum perforatum)

Common uses

St. John's wort is used to treat depression and somatoform disorders.

Proposed mechanisms

Active ingredients are hypericin and hyperforin. This product is thought to inhibit dopamine, serotonin, and norepinephrine reuptake and to decrease interleukin-6 (IL-6) concentrations.

Dosage

This product is standardized to 0.3% hypericin or 5% hyperforin. The recommended dose is 300 to 600 mg 3 times daily.

Side effects

The most commonly reported side effects are paresthesia, headache, nausea, dry mouth, agitation, decreased libido, and skin reactions. Photosensitivity can occur: recommend sun avoidance or sunscreen.

Precautions and contraindications

Avoid in patients with schizophrenia or bipolar disorder.

Interactions

Interactions are well documented and clinically significant.

Antidepressants (selective serotonin reuptake inhibitors [SSRIs] and tricyclic antidepressants [TCAs]) interact with this product because of a similar mechanism of action, which could result in serotonin syndrome.

St. John's wort is an inducer of CYP (cytochrome 450) 3A4, 1A2, 2C9, 2C19, and 2E1 and P-glycoprotein, causing decreased blood levels of medications and possibly resulting in reduced therapeutic effects. Medications affected include the following:

- Cyclosporine
- Indinavir
- Digoxin
- Oral contraceptives (**estradiol** component)

40-15 Homeopathic Products

Although beyond the scope of this textbook, APhA does recognize patient autonomy regarding the use of homeopathic products. Homeopathy is distinct from herbal medications and supplements and is based on the principle of "like cures like" (diseases can be cured by a substance that produces similar symptoms in healthy people) and "law of minimum dose" (the lower the dose the greater the effectiveness). Pharmacists should educate patients who choose to use homeopathic products. APhA supports the demonstration of safety and efficacy of homeopathic products from adequate, well-designed scientific studies before pharmacists advocate or sell homeopathic products.

40-16   Pharmacist's Role

Pharmacists play perhaps the largest role of any health care provider in the safe and appropriate use of nonprescription medications. As the most accessible health care provider, pharmacists have a vital role to triage care for those patients seeking self-care. When a patient presents to the pharmacy with a health complaint requiring a pharmacist consult, the pharmacist should collect pertinent patient information (e.g., medications, disease states, allergies, symptoms), assess the patient for eligibility for self-care, create a plan for either referring the patient if ineligible for self-care or identify the appropriate nonprescription medication and directions, and implement the recommendation by showing the patient exactly where they can find the appropriate medication. Importantly, in some patients self-care will not be a safe option. In these patients the pharmacist plays the critical role of triage and referral.

NAPLEX Competency Statements

The questions in this chapter cover the following 2021 NAPLEX Competency Statements: **AREA 1:** 1.2; 1.4; 1.5; 1.6; 1.7 **AREA 2:** 2.1; 2.2; 2.3; 2.4 **AREA 3:** 3.1; 3.2; 3.3; 3.4; 3.5; 3.6; 3.7; 3.8; 3.10; 3.11; 3.12 **AREA 4:** 4.1; 4.2; 4.5; 4.9 **AREA 5:** 5.1 **AREA 6:** 6.3; 6.4.

 40-17   Questions

1. Which of the following is the primary advantage of recommending dextromethorphan instead of codeine?

A. It is twice as effective as codeine in suppression of cough.
B. It has less dependence potential than codeine.
C. It has peripheral rather than the central action of codeine.
D. It is less expensive than codeine.
E. It is much longer acting than codeine.

2. Which of the following statements regarding guaifenesin is (are) correct? (Mark all that apply.)

A. It is the only OTC expectorant approved by the U.S. Food and Drug Administration.
B. It requires large amounts of water to be effective.
C. It is available OTC as Robitussin.
D. It may cause a decrease in platelet aggregation and an increase in bleeding time.
E. It is available in some prescription cough and cold formulations.

3. Which of the following statements regarding diphenhydramine is (are) correct? (Mark all that apply.)

A. It is less likely to cause drowsiness than other OTC antihistamines.
B. It is the active ingredient in some OTC products for insomnia.
C. It is available OTC under the trade name of Benadryl.
D. A small percentage of children may exhibit a paradoxical CNS stimulant effect.
E. Elderly patients may experience delirium or confusion with diphenhydramine.

4. Which of the following statements about the routine use of oral decongestants in treating the common cold is (are) true? (Mark all that apply.)

A. They cannot be used in patients on MAO inhibitor antidepressants.
B. They are relatively safe, with no dependence.
C. They are absolutely contraindicated in patients with controlled diabetes and mild hypertension.
D. The most common side effects are nervousness and insomnia.
E. Their purchase is much more regulated today than in the past.

5. When should a patient using OTC Nasacort Allergy 24HR with no symptom improvement be referred for further evaluation of sinus problems?

A. 1 week
B. 2 weeks
C. 1 month
D. 2 months
E. 6 months

6. A mother comes into the pharmacy looking for the most appropriate treatment for her 30-month-old son who has had 3 loose bowel movements this morning. He does not have a fever, is in good spirits, and is eating, drinking, and urinating appropriately. What should be recommended?

A. Refer her to a primary care provider.
B. Recommend loperamide 2 mg 2 caplets now and 1 caplet after each subsequent loose stool.
C. Recommend loperamide (Imodium A-D) liquid for children 15 mL now and 7.5 mL after subsequent loose stools.
D. Recommend milk of magnesia 15 to 30 mL at bedtime.
E. Recommend oral replacement with Pedialyte; offer solution as needed after loose bowel movements depending on fluid intake.

7. Which of the following is (are) an adverse effect of Pepto-Bismol? (Mark all that apply.)

A. Anticholinergic effects, dry mouth, and dry eyes
B. Tinnitus
C. Cross-sensitivity to aspirin allergy
D. Grayish-black tongue
E. Dark stools

8. Which of the following drugs exhibits analgesic and antipyretic properties, but not peripheral anti-inflammatory properties?

A. Ibuprofen
B. Sodium salicylate
C. Acetaminophen
D. Magnesium salicylate
E. Naproxen

9. What is the maximum daily dose of Tylenol Regular Strength?

A. 4000 mg/d or 6 tablets per 24-hour period
B. 3000 mg/d or 6 tablets per 24-hour period
C. 3250 mg/d or 10 tablets per 24-hour period
D. 3000 mg/d or 10 tablets per 24-hour period
E. 4550 mg/d or 14 tablets per 24-hour period

10. Mary is a 32-year-old female with asthma and serious aspirin sensitivity. She comes to the pharmacist seeking assistance in selecting a nonprescription product for aches and pains. Which of the following should the pharmacist recommend for Mary?

A. Ibuprofen
B. Naproxen
C. Acetaminophen
D. Oral aloe vera
E. Salicylate dissolvable powder

11. Nonprescription antiemetics are primarily useful for preventing which type of nausea?

A. Nausea caused by alterations in the vestibular apparatus
B. Nausea caused by drugs acting centrally on the chemoreceptor trigger zone
C. Nausea caused by visceral pain
D. Nausea caused by cortical stimulation from smells or sight
E. Nausea caused by afferent impulses from the GI tract

12. A mother requests advice for her 6-year-old child, who has been constipated for the past 2 days after beginning cereal feedings. Which of the following agents would be the best laxative agent to recommend?

A. Dulcolax
B. Fletcher's Castoria
C. Mineral oil
D. Glycerin suppositories
E. Milk of magnesia

13. Which of the following statements about stool softeners are correct? (Mark all that apply.)

   A. They are not safe to use in pregnancy.
   B. The onset of action is usually within 1 to 2 days.
   C. They are useful in patients with constipation who have hemorrhoids.
   D. Extra water helps their effectiveness.
   E. They often are combined with mild stimulant laxatives.

14. Which of the following statements about bisacodyl are correct? (Mark all that apply.)

   A. It should not be taken concurrently with antacids.
   B. It can be crushed or chewed if needed.
   C. It should not be recommended in pregnancy for long-term use.
   D. It is available in oral tablet and suppository dosage forms.
   E. It is the active ingredient in Dulcolax.

15. Which of the following counseling points regarding the use of Oxytrol for Women transdermal patch is the most appropriate?

   A. When used with lifestyle modifications, the patch can reduce urinary accidents by 10% more than by using lifestyle modifications alone.
   B. It will take up to 6 weeks to see the full benefit from the medication.
   C. The best place to apply the patch is on the upper arm.
   D. The patient must reapply the patch every 4 days.
   E. This product should not be used by women <65 years of age.

16. A 1-year-old child weighs 24 lb. He has a fever of 102°F, is irritable, seems uncomfortable, and is not sleeping well. His mother is confused by the assortment of fever relief products. You recommend acetaminophen. Which product and dosage do you recommend?

   A. Tylenol Infant Drops 80 mg/0.8 mL; give 1.6 mL every 4 to 6 hours.
   B. Tylenol Children's Liquid 160 mg/5 mL; give 2 tsp every 6 to 8 hours.
   C. Advil Infant Drops 50 mg/1.25 mL; give 1.25 mL every 4 to 6 hours.
   D. Motrin Children's Suspension 100 mg/5 mL; give 2.5 mL every 6 to 8 hours.
   E. Tylenol Infant Drops 80 mg/0.8 mL; give 3.2 mL every 4 to 6 hours.

17. A 1-year-old child weighs 24 lb. He has a fever of 102°F, is irritable, seems uncomfortable, and is not sleeping well. His mother is confused by the assortment of fever relief products. You recommend an appropriate acetaminophen product and the mother purchases this product. The next morning, the child's mother returns to your pharmacy. Her pediatrician recommended alternating the maximum dose of ibuprofen with the acetaminophen, and she is asking for help selecting an ibuprofen product and dosage. Which product and dosage do you recommend?

   A. Advil Infant Drops 50 mg/1.25 mL; give 0.625 mL every 8 hours.
   B. Motrin Children's Suspension 100 mg/5 mL; give 2 tsp every 4 hours.
   C. Motrin Infant Drops 50 mg/1.25 mL; give 2.5 mL every 6 hours.
   D. Advil Children's Chewable Tablet 50 mg; give 1 tablet every 8 hours.
   E. Advil Children's Chewable Tablet 50 mg; give 1/2 tablet every 4 hours.

18. A 35-year-old male requests guidance on the results of his OraQuick In-Home HIV Test. He thinks he was exposed to HIV about 1 year ago because of unprotected sex. He followed the package directions for use of the diagnostic tool correctly. The result window shows a line by the C and the T. How should this patient be counseled regarding his results?

   A. The test indicates a positive result, so refer the patient to a primary care provider for confirmation.
   B. The test indicates a negative result, so refer the patient to a primary care provider for confirmation.
   C. The test is inconclusive because of testing too early and must be repeated.
   D. The test indicates a positive result, and because of specificity of the product, confirmation is not needed.
   E. The test is inaccurate when taken more than 6 months after exposure to HIV, so refer him to his primary care provider.

19. What dietary supplement can cause a user's urine and sweat to smell of maple syrup?

   A. Ginseng
   B. Echinacea
   C. Fenugreek
   D. Garlic
   E. Black cohosh

20. Which of the following products should be discontinued before surgery?

A. Ginkgo biloba
B. Gentian root
C. Glutamine
D. Glucosamine
E. Folic acid

21. Cough and cold products are not to be used in children less than _____ years of age.

A. 2
B. 4
C. 6
D. 8
E. 12

22. When a patient is considering the use of nonprescription orlistat, which of the following vitamins may the patient need as additional supplementation because of decreased absorption?

A. B_{12}
B. B_6
C. D
D. C
E. B_1

 **40-18** **Answers**

1. B. Although limited recreational abuse of dextromethorphan has been reported, its potential for dependence and addiction is significantly less than that of codeine.

2. A, B, C, E. It is the only FDA-approved OTC expectorant, works better with increased fluid intake, is included in some prescription products, and is included in Robitussin products. Answer D is incorrect. Guaifenesin does not have any effects on platelet aggregation or bleeding time.

3. B, C, D, E. Only A is incorrect. Diphenhydramine, an ethanolamine, is the most sedating OTC antihistamine.

4. A, B, D, E. Only C is incorrect. Systemic decongestants are not recommended in individuals with uncontrolled diabetes or hypertension because of their sympathomimetic effects. They are contraindicated with MAO inhibitors and can commonly cause nervousness or insomnia.

5. D. The patient will not see the full benefit of Nasacort Allergy 24HR until about 2 to 4 weeks of treatment. If minimal to no improvement has been seen by 2 months, the patient should seek further evaluation by a primary care provider.

6. E. Referring this child to a primary care provider is not needed because the child is still taking fluids and no signs and symptoms of infection are present (i.e., fever). He can be treated at home with oral rehydration solutions, such as Pedialyte. Loperamide is not for use in children <6 years of age. Milk of magnesia would make the diarrhea worse and is not an appropriate choice of treatment for acute diarrhea.

7. B, C, D, E. Only A is incorrect. Common adverse effects of Pepto-Bismol include tinnitus and grayish-black tongue or stools. Pepto-Bismol does contain a salicylate and, therefore, should not be used in individuals with aspirin allergy.

8. C. Acetaminophen is a centrally acting antipyretic and analgesic, but it does not exhibit peripheral anti-inflammatory activity. Salicylates and other NSAIDs do.

9. C. McNeil manufactures Tylenol Regular Strength (325 mg tablets). Maximum dose is 3250 mg/d or 10 tablets/d. These maximum doses are different than the official FDA-approved adult maximum daily dose of 4 g for generic acetaminophen.

10. C. All NSAIDs and aspirin-containing products should be avoided in individuals with aspirin sensitivity. Acetaminophen can be recommended in this setting.

11. A. Nonprescription antiemetics are antihistamines that exert their effect by inhibiting histamine in neural centers controlling vomiting, salivation, and vestibular excitability, making them especially well suited for motion sickness.

12. D. Glycerin suppositories are safe for children 2 to 6 years of age. The other agents should not be used in this patient population.

13. B, C, D, E. Only A is incorrect. Stool softeners are safe to use in pregnancy and usually exert their effect within 1 to 2 days. Stool softeners are recommended for individuals in whom hard stools or straining could cause pain or complications (e.g., hemorrhoids, postoperative or postpartum time periods, or postmyocardial infarction). Increased fluid intake enhances their effectiveness. They are frequently used in combination products containing stimulant laxatives.

14. **A, C, D, E.** Only B is incorrect. Because bisacodyl is an enteric-coated product, it should not be taken with antacids or be crushed, chewed, or broken. It should not be used in pregnancy long term. It is available in both oral tablets and rectal suppositories.

15. **D.** The patient must reapply the Oxytrol for Women patch to the abdomen, hip, or buttock every 4 days. When the patch is used with lifestyle modifications, urinary accidents can be reduced by 25% more than by using lifestyle modifications alone. The full benefit from this medication will be seen in about 2 weeks.

16. **A.** The pediatric dosage of acetaminophen is 10 to 15 mg/kg every 4 to 6 hours:

24 lb × kg/2.2 lb = 10.9 kg × 10 to 15 mg/kg = 109 to 163.5 mg

Tylenol Infant Drops 80 mg/0.8 mL; 1.6 mL = 160 mg acetaminophen

17. **C.** The pediatric dosage of ibuprofen is 5 to 10 mg/kg every 4 to 6 hours:

24 lb × kg/2.2 lb = 10.9 kg × 5 to 10 mg/kg = 54.5 to 109 mg

Motrin Infant Drops 50 mg/1.25 mL; 2.5 mL = 100 mg ibuprofen

18. **A.** OraQuick In-Home HIV Test with a line present near the C and T in the result window indicates a positive result. Exposure over 3 months allows for appropriate use of this test in this individual. This test has a specificity of 99.98%, which means 1 false-positive can occur in every 5000 results in uninfected individuals. Therefore, a positive result does not mean that the person is definitely infected with HIV, but that additional testing by a primary care provider is required to confirm the results.

19. **C.** Fenugreek can cause the urine, sweat, and breast milk of the user to smell of maple syrup. This supplement is typically used as a galactagogue.

20. **A.** Ginkgo biloba has antiplatelet activity and should, therefore, be withheld before surgical procedures.

21. **B.** The Consumer Health Care Products Association announced in October 2008 that manufacturers were voluntarily updating all cough and cold products to state "do not use" in children under 4 years of age.

22. **C.** Vitamin D is a fat-soluble vitamin that may have decreased absorption with concomitant orlistat use despite multivitamin supplementation. A multivitamin is best taken at bedtime or separate from an orlistat dose by at least 2 hours.

40-19 Additional Resources

Eckel RH, Jakicic JM, Ard JD, et al. 2013 AHA/ACC guideline on lifestyle management to reduce cardiovascular risk: a report of the American College of Cardiology/American Heart Association Task Force on Practice Guidelines. *Circulation.* 2014;129(25 Suppl 2):S76–99.

Fiore MC, Bailey WC, Cohen SJ, et al. *Treating Tobacco Use and Dependence: Clinical Practice Guideline.* Rockville, MD: U.S. Department of Health and Human Services; 2008.

Jensen MD, Ryan DH, Apovian CM, et al. 2013 AHA/ACC/TOS guideline for the management of overweight and obesity in adults: a report of the American College of Cardiology/American Heart Association Task Force on Practice Guidelines and The Obesity Society. *J Am Coll Cardiol.* 2014;63(25):2985–3023.

Krinsky DL, Ferreri SP, Hemstreet B, et al., eds. *Handbook of Nonprescription Drugs: An Interactive Approach to Self-Care.* 20th ed. Washington, DC: American Pharmacists Association; 2020.

Natural Medicines. Available at: https://naturalmedicines.therapeuticresearch.com. Accessed April 24, 2021.

OraQuick In-Home HIV Test. Available at: http://www.oraquick.com. Accessed April 24, 2021.

OXYTROL-oxybutynin patch. U.S. National Library of Medicine. Available at: https://dailymed.nlm.nih.gov/dailymed/lookup.cfm?setid=20dee37f-1412-44ed-9e8b-f4379ce23eb0.

U.S. Department of Agriculture–U.S. Department of Health and Human Services. Dietary Guidelines for Americans 2020–2025. Available at: https://www.dietaryguidelines.gov.

U.S. Department of Health and Human Services, Office of Disease Prevention and Health Promotion. 2nd ed. 2018 Physical Activity Guidelines for Americans. https://www.health.gov/paguidelines. Accessed May 13, 2021.

Dermatologic Disorders

41

DANIEL R. MALCOM

41-1 KEY POINTS

ACNE (ACNE VULGARIS)

- Benzoyl peroxide, topical retinoids, and topical and oral antibiotics form the basis of therapy for mild and moderate acne.
- Oral isotretinoin is the drug of choice for severe, nodulocystic acne.
- Isotretinoin is contraindicated in pregnancy because of the risk of serious birth defects.

FUNGAL SKIN INFECTIONS (DERMATOPHYTOSIS)

- The most efficacious nonprescription topical antifungal is terbinafine (Lamisil).
- Systemic antifungal therapy is required for treatment of tinea capitis (scalp) and tinea unguium (toenails or fingernails).

HAIR LOSS (ALOPECIA)

- Androgenic alopecia—predominantly seen in males—is due to dihydrotestosterone, which binds to the hair follicles.
- Topical minoxidil (Rogaine) or oral **finasteride** (Propecia) can be effective treatments.

ALLERGIC CONTACT DERMATITIS

- Contact dermatitis is initially treated with topical corticosteroid products.
- Absorption and subsequent adverse systemic effects of topical corticosteroids are increased with high-potency agents, occlusion, and long-term use.

POISON IVY, POISON OAK, AND POISON SUMAC ALLERGIC DERMATITIS

- The most important initial treatment is removing the resin from the skin.
- Severe cases may require systemic corticosteroids to relieve symptoms.

DANDRUFF

- Zinc pyrithione (in Head and Shoulders) and selenium sulfide (in Selsun Blue) are effective in treating dandruff.

SEBORRHEA (SEBORRHEIC DERMATITIS)

- Seborrhea is a chronic, inflammatory, noncontagious skin disease characterized by yellowish, greasy scales and pruritis.
- Treatment includes topical corticosteroids as well as shampoos active against *Pityrosporum ovale*.

PLAQUE PSORIASIS

- Psoriasis is a chronic disease characterized by inflammation and plaque formation.
- Many patients can be treated with topical agents, but advanced psoriasis may require systemic medications for effective management.

HEAD LICE (PEDICULOSIS CAPITIS)

- Head lice is a common condition caused by infestation of *Pediculus humanus capitis* that occurs mostly in children during school months.
- Permethrin (Nix) is the nonprescription agent of choice for treatment.

WARTS

- Warts result from a localized infection of the human papillomavirus on the skin.
- They can be removed by surgery, cryotherapy, or application of caustics (e.g., salicylic acid).
- Self-treatment for warts with over-the-counter agents is not recommended for diabetic patients because of reduced sensation in their feet.

41-2 STUDY GUIDE CHECKLIST

The following topics may guide your study of this subject area:

- ☐ Classification and clinical presentation of acne, fungal skin infections (dermatophytosis), alopecia, dermatitis, poison ivy, poison oak, poison sumac, scaly dermatoses (dandruff, seborrhea, and psoriasis), pediculosis, and warts.
- ☐ Selection of appropriate therapy for all disease states.
- ☐ Important counseling points and adverse reactions for all therapies.
- ☐ Availability and patient instructions for topical acne formulations.
- ☐ Relative potency of topical corticosteroid preparations.

Editor's Note: This chapter is based on the 12th edition chapter written by Daniel R. Malcom.

Isotretinoin *FDA BOXED WARNING*

Use is associated with severe, life-threatening birth defects—use is contraindicated in pregnancy. Due to teratogenicity and to minimize fetal exposure risk, it is only approved for use under a restricted distribution program (iPledge).

41-3   Acne (Acne Vulgaris)

Acne is an inflammatory disorder of the pilosebaceous glands that occurs most commonly during puberty. It may reappear later or even begin in adulthood, more commonly in women than in men.

Pathophysiology

- Sebum production by androgenic hormones increases during puberty.
- Hair follicle openings are obstructed, producing closed comedones (whiteheads) that progress to open comedones (blackheads).
- Growth of *Propionibacterium acnes* (now referred to as *Cutibacterium acnes* or *C. acnes* by some) increases on skin and in sebaceous ducts.
- *C. acnes* causes inflammation, ultimately resulting in pustule formation.

Classification and Clinical Presentation

- *Mild:* Primarily noninflammatory lesions (open and closed comedones), relatively few superficial inflammatory lesions, and no scarring
- *Moderate:* Multiple papules (inflammatory and noninflammatory) on the face and trunk and minimal scarring
- *Severe:* Advanced form, with inflammatory lesions that can lead to scarring

Treatment Principles

Proper skin care is essential for all stages of therapy, including twice-daily use of a gentle cleanser. Combination topical therapy is common, especially in moderate or severe cases. Improvement in skin may take 1 to 2 months. All agents (topical and systemic) may cause redness, dryness, burning, itching, peeling, and swelling, and side effects may appear before benefits. Treatment may include a combination of benzoyl peroxide, oral antimicrobials, topical antimicrobials, and/or topical retinoids for mild, moderate, or severe acne. Table 41-1 contains guideline-recommended acne treatments.

Topical Therapy

Antimicrobial therapy

Topical antimicrobial therapy targeting *C. acnes* (one of the pathophysiologic mechanisms of acne vulgaris) is a mainstay of treatment for more severe mild or moderate disease. See Table 41-2 for more information about topical antimicrobial products.

Benzoyl peroxide

Benzoyl peroxide (BPO) is the most effective over-the-counter (OTC) agent and is available in 2.5% to 10% strengths. Examples of branded products include Clean and Clear Gel and Clearasil, but many generic formulations are available.

TABLE 41-1. Treatment Guide for Acne Vulgaris

	Mild	Moderate	Severe
First-line treatment	BPO or TR	BPO + TA	OA + BPO + TA**
	BPO + TA**	BPO + TR**	OA + BPO + TR**
	BPO + TR**	BPO + TR + TA**	OA + BPO + TR + TA**
	BPO + TR + TA**	BPO + OA + TR + TA**	Oral isotretinoin
Alternative treatment	Add BPO or TR (if not on already)	Consider alternative combination therapy	Consider change in OA
	Consider alternative TR	Consider change in OA	Add oral contraceptives or oral **spironolactone** (in females)
	Consider topical dapsone	Add oral contraceptives or oral **spironolactone** (in females)	
		Consider oral isotretinoin	

Boldface indicates one of top 100 drugs for 2020 by prescription volume.
BPO, benzoyl peroxide; OA, oral antimicrobials; TA, topical antimicrobials; TR, topical retinoids.
**Topical combination therapy.

Mechanism of action

BPO destroys the anaerobic *C. acnes* through the release of oxygen. Importantly, *C. acnes* does not become resistant to BPO; therefore, BPO can be used concurrently with topical antibiotics to prevent resistance.

Patient instructions and counseling

- Clinically visible improvements should occur by the third week of therapy.
- Maximum efficacy can be expected after approximately 8 to 12 weeks of use.
- Continuous use is normally required to maintain clinical response.
- Avoid unnecessary sun exposure and use sunscreen.

TABLE 41-2. Topical Acne Products

Generic name	Trade name	Strength and dosage forms available
Topical antimicrobials		
Benzoyl peroxide	Benzac AC, Panoxyl	2.5% to 10% cleansers, cream, gel, lotion, pads
Clindamycin	Cleocin T, Evoclin	1% foam, gel, lotion, pads, pledgets, solution
Dapsone	Aczone	5%, 7.5% gel
Erythromycin	Ery, Akne-mycin	2% gel, ointment, pads, pledgets, solution
Topical retinoids		
Adapalene	Differin	0.1% cream, gel, and lotion (0.1% gel OTC); 0.3% gel
Tazarotene	Tazorac	0.05%, 0.1% cream and gel; 0.1% foam
Tretinoin	Retin-A, Avita, Differin	0.025% to 0.1% cream; 0.01% to 0.025% gel, 0.05% liquid
Additional products		
Azelaic acid	Azelex, Finacea	15% foam and gel; 20% cream
Salicylic acid	Oxy, Stridex	0.5% to 2% cleansers, cream, foam, gel, pads, pledgets, soaps, solutions (OTC and prescription)

OTC, over-the-counter.

Adverse effects

- These agents may cause redness, dryness, burning, itching, peeling, and swelling.
- They may bleach hair or dyed fabrics (pillowcases, towels, clothing).

Clindamycin (topical)

Mechanism of action

Clindamycin suppresses growth of *C. acnes*. It may also directly reduce free fatty acid concentrations on the skin.

Patient instructions and counseling

- Improvement should be seen by 6 weeks.
- Discontinue medication and contact your health care provider if severe diarrhea or abdominal cramping or pain develops.

Adverse drug effects

- Hypersensitivity contact dermatitis

Dapsone (topical)

Mechanism of action

Dapsone has anti-inflammatory and antimicrobial properties and can be used to reduce the number of acne lesions in patients over 12 years old. It should be considered in patients unable to tolerate other topical acne medications.

Patient instructions and counseling

- The topical 5% formulation is applied twice daily, while the 7.5% is applied once daily.
- If sensitivity develops, discontinue use.
- Keep away from mouth, eyes, and mucous membranes.

Adverse drug effects

- Temporary yellow-orange skin discoloration has occurred when patients use BPO and topical dapsone simultaneously. Advise separating applications and washing face between use for patients using both.
- Patients taking oral dapsone who have a glucose-6-phosphate dehydrogenase (G6PD) deficiency have an increased risk of hemolytic anemia. With the topical formulation, however, no significant issues have been seen and no pretesting is required.

Erythromycin (topical)

Mechanism of action

Erythromycin suppresses growth of *C. acnes*.

Patient instructions and counseling

- Wait at least 1 hour before applying any other topical acne medication.
- Avoid contact with eyes, mouth, nose, and other mucous membranes.
- Although improvement is generally expected within 4 weeks, some patients do not respond for 8 to 12 weeks.

Adverse drug effects

- **More common:** Dry or scaly skin, irritation, itching
- **Less common:** Stinging sensation, peeling, redness

Topical retinoids

See Table 41-2 for more information about topical retinoid products.

Mechanism of action

- Retinoids are chemically related to vitamin A.
- Retinoids normalize follicular keratinization, heal comedones, decrease sebum production, and decrease inflammatory lesions.

Patient instructions and counseling

- Do not use astringents, drying agents, abrasive scrubs, or harsh soaps concurrently.
- Apply every other night for the first 2 weeks to adjust to drying effect.
- Apply nightly after 2 weeks.
- Expect that skin may take up to 2 to 3 months to improve.
- Use sunscreen on face daily and especially before sun exposure because of increased sensitivity.

Adverse drug effects

- These agents may irritate skin and cause redness, dryness, and scaling.
- Tazarotene is the most irritating retinoid.
- Adapalene (now available without a prescription in the 0.1% gel formulation) appears to be least irritating and is preferred for sensitive skin.

Alternative Therapy

See Table 41-2 for more information about additional topical products used in the treatment of acne.

Azelaic acid

Mechanism of action

Azelaic acid 20% is antibacterial and works for both inflammatory and noninflammatory lesions. It normalizes keratinization, leading to an anticomedonal effect. The 15% strength (gel) is only FDA-approved in the United States for the treatment of rosacea, though it is approved for the treatment of acne in many other countries.

Patient instructions and counseling

- If sensitivity develops, discontinue use.
- Keep away from mouth, eyes, and mucous membranes.
- Other topical medications must be used at different times during the day.

Adverse drug effects

- Temporary dryness and skin irritation (pruritus and burning) may occur on initiation.
- Hypopigmentation may occur (caution in dark-skinned individuals).

Salicylic acid

Salicylic acid 0.5% to 2% is useful for mild acne in patients with sensitive skin who may not be able to tolerate BPO.

Mechanism of action

It has an irritant effect, keratolytic action, and increases the turnover rate of epithelial cells. Examples of branded products include the following:

- Oxy Maximum Cleansing Pads
- Stridex products

Patient instructions and counseling
- It is usually applied once daily for initial therapy and can be increased to 2 to 3 times daily if needed.
- Frequency can be reduced to daily or every other day if dryness or peeling develops.

Adverse effects
- OTC preparations are limited to 2% maximum concentration. In 20% to 30% concentrations, salicylic acid can be used as a chemical peeling agent.
- It is irritating to the skin and often is formulated in drying hydroethanolic vehicles.

Combination Therapy

Combining topical retinoids with antimicrobials can result in improved efficacy with potentially improved adherence. Available coformulated products are shown in Table 41-3.

Systemic Therapy

Antimicrobials

Systemic antimicrobials are useful for moderate-to-severe acne, in conjunction with topical therapies. In the absence of contraindications (e.g., ≤ 8 years of age, allergy, pregnancy), tetracyclines are considered first-line therapy.

Mechanism of action

Antimicrobials suppress growth of *C. acnes* in sebaceous ducts. These agents also have an anti-inflammatory effect.

Dosing

See Table 41-4 for full dosing recommendations. Oral antibiotics should be used for the shortest duration possible to minimize development of resistance, ideally 3 to 4 months when used in combination with a topical retinoid. Monotherapy is not recommended.

Patient instructions and counseling, adverse drug effects, and drug–drug interactions

See Chapter 34 on anti-infective agents.

TABLE 41-3. Topical Combination Products

Products and strengths	Trade name
Benzoyl peroxide 5%, clindamycin 1%	BenzaClin
Benzoyl peroxide 5%, clindamycin 1.2%	Duac, Neuac
Benzoyl peroxide 2.5%, clindamycin 1.2%	Acanya
Benzoyl peroxide 3.75%, clindamycin 1.2%	Onexton
Benzoyl peroxide 5%, erythromycin 3%	Benzamycin
Benzoyl peroxide 2.5%, adapalene 0.1%	Epiduo
Benzoyl peroxide 2.5%, adapalene 0.3%	Epiduo Forte
Clindamycin 1.2%, tretinoin 0.025%	Veltin, Ziana

TABLE 41-4. Oral Antimicrobials

Generic name	Dosage and form
Doxycycline	50 to 100 mg twice daily or 100 mg once daily
	Delayed-release formulation (Doryx): 100 mg twice daily for 1 day, then 100 mg daily
	Delayed-release formulation, subantimicrobial dosing (Oracea): 20 mg twice daily or 40 mg daily
Erythromycin	500 mg twice daily (base)
Minocycline	50 mg daily to 3 times a day
	Extended-release formulation (CoreMino, Monoliro, Solodyn, Ximino): 1 mg/kg/d, round to nearest available strength (strengths range 45 to 135 mg)
Tetracycline	500 mg twice daily; when improvement occurs in 1 to 2 weeks, taper dose down to 125 to 500 mg daily

Isotretinoin

An isomer of retinoic acid, oral isotretinoin is useful for patients with severe recalcitrant nodular acne. It results in less production of sebum, fewer lesions, and decreased scarring, along with decreased anxiety and depression associated with the disease.

Mechanism of action

Isotretinoin reduces sebum production up to 90%. It decreases production of microcomedones, possibly by decreasing cohesiveness of follicular epithelial cells, and can have an anti-inflammatory effect.

Dosing

Isotretinoin is available in 10, 20, 30, and 40 mg capsules. Trade names include Absorica (which is not AB-rated to Accutane brand) and Claravis, Myorisan, Sotret, and Zenatane (all AB-rated with Accutane). Accutane brand has been discontinued by the manufacturer. Treatment may be initiated at 0.5 mg/kg/d for the first month, then increased to 1 mg/kg/d as tolerated.

Patient instructions and counseling

- Absorica can be taken with or without food, whereas generic products AB-rated to Accutane brand should be taken with food.
- Effects are gradual, and acne may worsen during the first month of therapy; however, improvement usually begins by the sixth week of therapy.

Adverse drug effects

Isotretinoin is teratogenic and contraindicated in pregnancy. Females of childbearing potential must take measures to avoid pregnancy during isotretinoin therapy.

Side effects and toxicity are as follows:

- Most common (90% to 100%):
  - Cheilitis (chapped lips)
  - Dry mouth
  - Dry skin
  - Pruritus
- Common (30% to 40%):
  - Dry nose, eyes
  - Muscular soreness or stiffness

- Less common (10% to 25%):
  - Headaches
  - Hyperlipidemia (primarily elevation of triglycerides, which may lead to pancreatitis)
- Rare (less than 5%):
  - Thinning of hair
  - Peeling of palms and soles
  - Skin rash and skin infections
- Very rare (< 1%):
  - Acute depression and mood changes (very rare, but reversible if detected early)
  - Pseudotumor cerebri (benign intracranial hypertension with visual disturbances)
- Treatment of most common side effects:
  - *Cheilitis:* Frequent use of lip balm
  - *Dry skin:* Skin lubrication with moisturizers
  - *Nosebleeds:* Lubrication of the nostrils with petrolatum, nasal saline spray
  - *Muscular soreness or stiffness:* Use of mild OTC analgesic and anti-inflammatory agents

Monitoring parameters

- *Lipid panel:* Serum cholesterol and triglycerides have been known to increase, though no definitive cardiovascular risk has been associated.
- *Liver function tests:* Elevations are common during initiation of therapy, but they usually return to normal during treatment.
- *Routine complete blood count:* Monitoring is no longer recommended.
- *Pregnancy testing:* Testing is recommended before initiation.

iPLEDGE program

iPLEDGE is the risk-management program approved by the U.S. Food and Drug Administration (FDA) for all isotretinoin products. It mandates registration of prescribers, patients, wholesalers, and pharmacies to further the goal of eliminating fetal exposure to isotretinoin.

The iPLEDGE program requires that all patients meet qualification criteria and monthly program requirements. Before the patient receives his or her isotretinoin prescription each month, the prescriber must counsel the patient about the risks of isotretinoin and document it in the iPLEDGE system.

Female patients should be tested for pregnancy before initiation of therapy and instructed to use 2 methods of contraception beginning at least 1 month before initiation of therapy and continuing for 1 month after discontinuation of therapy.

Hormonal therapy

Combined oral contraceptives

For female patients postmenarche, combined oral contraceptives (COCs) (containing both an estrogen and a progestin) may be considered in moderate-to-severe acne as adjunct therapy or in mild acne if topical agents fail. They can be used alone or in combination with other acne treatments. However, reduction of acne with COCs takes time; combination with other acne treatments, such as topical agents, may be beneficial for the first few months of treatment. See Chapter 38 for a full discussion of COCs.

Spironolactone (Aldactone)

Female patients with androgenization may benefit from the addition of **spironolactone**, an aldosterone antagonist that exhibits antiandrogen effects. Doses range from 25 to 200 mg daily, with many patients controlled on 50 mg daily.

Oral corticosteroids

An initial short course of oral corticosteroids may be beneficial in certain patients with severe disease. Systemic corticosteroids used continuously may actually cause or worsen acne, and topical corticosteroids have no value in acne treatment.

41-4   Fungal Skin Infections (Dermatophytoses)

Tinea are skin infections known as *dermatomytoses* caused by the fungi *Trichophyton, Microsporum,* and *Epidermophyton.*

Classification

- Tinea pedis ("athlete's foot")
- Tinea capitis (ringworm of the scalp)
- Tinea cruris ("jock itch")
- Tinea corporis (ringworm of the skin)
- Tinea unguium (onychomycosis: fungal infection of toenails and fingernails)

Pathophysiology

The fungi invade dead cells of the stratum corneum of skin, hair, and nails, digesting keratin.

Treatment Principles and Goals

- ***All dermatophyte infections:*** Avoid topical corticosteroids if dermatophyte infection is suspected. The immunosuppressive effect of steroids can worsen the infection and cause it to spread deeper into the skin.
- ***Tinea pedis, tinea cruris, tinea corporis:*** Self-treat initially with OTC agents topically; if ineffective, add oral agents.
- ***Tinea capitis, tinea unguium:*** Use oral systemic therapy initially.

Drug Therapy

OTC treatment

Table 41-5 lists OTC topical medications used in the treatment of fungal skin infections (dermatophytoses).

Prescription treatment

Table 41-6 lists prescription medications used in the treatment of fungal skin infections (dermatophytoses).

Topical treatments

Topical antifungals are typically applied once or twice daily, and therapy should be continued after symptoms resolve. Most OTC topical antifungals are available in generic form. Aerosol powders and solutions can be effective for large areas, but the propellants can cause skin reactions in some individuals. Terbinafine 1% is considered the most efficacious OTC topical antifungal agent.

TABLE 41-5. Over-the-Counter Topical Antifungal Agents

Generic name and strength	Trade name(s)	Dosage form(s)
Butenafine 1%	Lotrimin Ultra, Mentax	Cream
Clotrimazole 1%	Lotrimin AF	Cream, ointment, solution
Miconazole 2%	Micatin, Desenex	Aerosol (liquid, powder), cream, lotion, ointment, powder, solution
Terbinafine 1%	Lamisil AT	Aerosol liquid, cream, gel
Tolnaftate 1%	Tinactin	Aerosol (liquid, powder), cream, powder, solution

TABLE 41-6. Prescription Topical Antifungal Agents

Generic name	Trade name(s)	Strength(s) and dosage form(s)
Ciclopirox	Loprox, Penlac	0.77%: cream, gel, suspension
		1%: shampoo
		8%: solution
Econazole	Ecoza	1%: cream, foam
Luliconazole	Luzu	1%: cream
Naftifine	Naftin	1%: cream, gel
		2%: cream, gel
Oxiconazole	Oxistat	1%: cream, lotion
Sertaconazole	Ertaczo	2%: cream
Sulconazole	Exelderm	1%: cream, solution

Systemic therapy

Systemic therapy options include the following:

- Griseofulvin (Grifulvin V)
- Fluconazole (Diflucan)
- Itraconazole (Sporanox)
- Terbinafine (Lamisil)

See Chapter 34 on anti-infective agents for discussion of systemic antifungals.

Patient instructions and counseling

- Because fungi thrive in warm, moist environments, patients should be encouraged to wear loose-fitting garments (preferably cotton or moisture-wicking material).
- Socks should be cotton or have similar moisture-wicking properties.
- Dry the areas likely to be infected (groin, feet, etc.) thoroughly before covering with clothes.
- Avoid walking barefoot (particularly in high-risk areas such as dorm or gym showers) and sharing garments.

⚠ **Itraconazole (Sporanox)** *FDA BOXED WARNING*

May cause or exacerbate congestive heart failure (CHF). Do not administer for treatment of onychomycosis in patients with evidence of ventricular dysfunction. Significant number of drug–drug interactions and contraindications—see package insert for full list.

41-5 Hair Loss (Alopecia)

Male pattern baldness (androgenic alopecia) is the gradual and progressive loss of hair in males as they age.

Clinical Presentation

- Onset and progression vary greatly.
- A distinct pattern of progressive hair loss on the scalp develops in the frontotemporal areas and crown with sparing of the occiput.

Pathophysiology

Alopecia is primarily due to 2 factors: genetics (heredity) and the presence of testosterone. Testosterone is converted to dihydrotestosterone (DHT) by the enzyme 5-alpha-reductase, which binds preferentially to receptors in the hair follicles on the scalp and causes them to produce progressively thinner hair until the follicles eventually cease activity altogether.

Treatment Principles and Goals

Although androgenic alopecia has no cure, two drugs are available for its treatment:

- Minoxidil 2% to 5% (Rogaine); topical, available OTC
- **Finasteride** 1 mg (Propecia); systemic, by prescription only

In alopecia's early stages, topical minoxidil or oral **finasteride** may reverse the gradually decreasing diameter of the hair shaft.

Any hair growth stimulation is temporary and lasts only as long as therapy continues. If therapy is discontinued, new hair growth is lost within 1 year. Treatment is most likely to be effective in younger men who have only recently begun to lose hair.

Drug Therapy

Minoxidil

OTC trade names are Rogaine 2% and Rogaine Extra Strength 5%.

Mechanism of action

Minoxidil likely increases cutaneous blood flow directly to hair follicles because of its direct vasodilatory activity.

Patient instructions and counseling

- Minoxidil may be applied without shampooing hair.
- Use at least 4 hours before bedtime to avoid oil on pillows and bed linens.
- The drug is absorbed over a 4-hour period, so do not swim, shampoo, or walk in rain for 4 hours.
- Do not use on infected, irritated, inflamed, or sunburned skin.
- Discontinue use immediately and seek medical care if chest pain, increased heart rate, faintness, dizziness, or swollen hands or feet occur.
- Women should avoid 5% strength (which has no better results than 2%); they have greater incidence of increased growth of facial hair with the 5% solution.
- Generally, treatment takes 4 to 6 months before any benefit occurs.
- A lack of effects within 8 months for females and 12 months for males indicates therapeutic failure, and treatment should be discontinued.
- Patients must continue using minoxidil to maintain new hair growth.

Adverse drug effects

- Scalp dermatitis is common, producing dryness, pruritus, and flaking or scaling.
- Hypertrichosis (excessive hair growth) can occur on areas other than scalp (chest, forearms, ear rim, back, face, arms, and so forth).

■ Use is contraindicated in patients less than 18 years of age, or in women who are pregnant or breast-feeding.

Finasteride

Finasteride (Propecia) was originally developed for the treatment of benign prostatic hyperplasia in a 5 mg dose (Proscar). A 1 mg daily dose is approved for males only as prescription treatment for androgenic alopecia. Over a 2-year period, **finasteride** may halt the progressive hair loss caused by androgenic alopecia.

Mechanism of action

Finasteride inhibits the enzyme 5-alpha-reductase, which is responsible for the conversion of testosterone to DHT—the main androgen responsible for androgenic hair loss.

Patient instructions and counseling
■ Take for at least 3 months to see if the drug is effective.
■ Improvement lasts only as long as treatment continues. New hair will be lost within 1 year of stopping treatment.

Adverse drug effects
■ Decreased libido, erectile dysfunction, and ejaculatory dysfunction occur but are reversible when the drug is discontinued.
■ Gynecomastia (breast enlargement and tenderness) has been reported from 2 weeks to 2 years following initial therapy, but it is also usually reversible when therapy is discontinued.
■ Hypersensitivity (skin rash, swelling of lips) has been reported.
■ Use is contraindicated in females of childbearing age, because of abnormalities of the external genitalia in male fetuses. **Finasteride** is not effective in postmenopausal females.

41-6 Allergic Contact Dermatitis

Dermatitis is a nonspecific term describing a variety of inflammatory dermatologic conditions characterized by erythema. It is a general term describing any eczematous rash of unknown etiology that cannot be classified among the major endogenous dermatoses. *Eczema* and *dermatitis* are often used interchangeably.

Clinical Presentation

Allergic contact dermatitis is a process of sensitization with reaction on elicitation. More than 50% of all dermatitis is allergic contact dermatitis.

Examples of reactive elements include benzocaine, zinc pyrithione (ZPT), neomycin, sodium bisulfite, perfumes, many cosmetics, skin lubricants, antiseptic creams, rubber and epoxy glues, poison ivy and oak, and many other common substances.

Treatment Principles and Goals

Treat dermatitis by applying a corticosteroid, according to the following principles:

■ Choose the lowest potency agent to be used for the shortest duration possible to minimize adverse effects.
■ Ointments and creams are more lubricating than solutions, lotions, or gels.

- Lotions or gels should be recommended for a weeping, eczematous dermatitis.
- Lotions, solutions, and gels are easier to use in hairy areas of the body.
- Improvement should begin within 1 week.
- Avoid excess soap, and keep skin lubricated with moisturizers.
- Treat itching with camphor, menthol, phenol, or local anesthetics.
- In severe cases, patients may have to use systemic corticosteroids for 1 to 2 weeks.

Drug Therapy

Topical corticosteroids

Table 41-7 contains information about topical corticosteroids.

Adverse drug effects

- Striae may result in skin folds.
- Thinning of epidermis occurs where subcutaneous vessels become visible.
- The more potent types can cause or aggravate acne or rosacea on the face.
- Percutaneous absorption can lead to systemic effects (see Chapter 18 on endocrine drugs for complete list of systemic adverse effects) such as the following:
  - Hyperglycemia
  - Glycosuria

TABLE 41-7. Selected Topical Corticosteroids

Relative potency	Generic name and strength	Dosage form(s)	Trade name(s)
Low	Hydrocortisone 0.5%, 1%	Cream, lotion, ointment, solution, spray	Cortaid, Cortizone
Medium	Desonide 0.05%	Cream, foam, lotion	DesOwen
	Fluocinolone acetonide 0.01%	Cream, oil, shampoo, solution	Derma-Smoothe, Synalar
	Flurandrenolide 0.05%	Cream, lotion, ointment	Cordran
	Hydrocortisone butyrate 0.1%	Cream, lotion, ointment, spray	Coritzone-10, Locoid
	Hydrocortisone valerate 0.2%	Cream	Westcort
	Triamcinolone acetonide 0.025%, 0.1%	Cream, lotion, ointment	Aristocort, Kenalog
High	Betamethasone valerate 0.1%, 0.12%	Foam, ointment	Valisone, Luxiq
	Fluocinolone acetonide 0.025%	Cream, ointment	Synalar
	Triamcinolone acetonide 0.5%	Cream, ointment	Aristocort HP, Kenalog
Very high	Betamethasone dipropionate 0.05%	Cream, ointment	Diprosone
	Desoximetasone 0.25%	Cream, gel, ointment	Topicort
	Diflorasone diacetate 0.05%	Cream, emollient	ApexiCon
	Fluocinonide 0.05%	Cream, gel, ointment, solution	Lidex
	Halcinonide 0.1%	Cream, ointment	Halog
Ultrahigh	Betamethasone dipropionate, augmented 0.05%	Gel, lotion, ointment	Diprolene AF
	Clobetasol propionate 0.05%	Cream, foam, gel, lotion, ointment, shampoo, solution, spray	Temovate, Clobex, Olux
	Diflorasone diacetate 0.05%	Ointment	Psorcon
	Fluocinonide 0.1%	Cream	Vanos
	Halobetasol propionate 0.05%	Cream, ointment	Ultravate

- Hypothalamic–pituitary–adrenal axis suppression, which could pose a threat in case of surgery, systemic illness, trauma, or injury
- Percutaneous absorption leads to systemic effects most likely with the following:
  - Higher potency corticosteroids
  - Inflamed skin (also in infants and children)
  - Long-term use or use over a large area of the skin
  - *Caution:* Occlusion markedly increases absorption of topical corticosteroids and should therefore be used cautiously in limited areas and reserved for severe, resistant lesions.

Topical antipruritics

Topical antipruritics include the following:

- Local anesthetics (benzocaine up to 20%, pramoxine 1%)
- Benzyl alcohol
- Colloidal oatmeal (e.g., Aveeno)

Emollients

- Petrolatum
- Lanolin
- Mineral oil

Prescription topical immunomodulators

Topical immunomodulators (calcineurin inhibitors) are approved for atopic dermatitis. They inhibit activation of T-cells and release of certain inflammatory mediators (cytokines).

They are typically applied twice daily, with improvement expected in 1 to 3 weeks. Side effects include stinging, burning, pruritus, and rare flu-like symptoms. Patients should be cautioned to use sunscreen. Continuous long-term use should be avoided; rare cases of malignancy have been reported.

Products include

- Tacrolimus (Protopic) 0.03% and 0.1% ointment ⚠
- Pimecrolimus (Elidel) 1% cream ⚠

Oral corticosteroids

Corticosteroids are the only systemic anti-inflammatory agents that are effective.

Oral antihistamines

Oral antihistamines have very limited effectiveness but are possibly antipruritic.

 Tacrolimus (Protopic) 0.03% and 0.1% ointment, and Pimecrolimus (Elidel) 1% cream *FDA BOXED WARNINGS*

Safety related to long-term use has not been established. Continuous use over a prolonged time period is not recommended. Rare cases of skin malignancy have been reported. Avoid use in children less than 2 years of age.

41-7 ▶ Poison Ivy, Poison Oak, and Poison Sumac Allergic Dermatitis

Allergic reaction occurs to sap (urushiol) of some plants of the genus *Rhus* (poison ivy, poison oak, poison sumac). Direct contact with leaves, roots, or branches is not required to get a rash. Sap can reach skin indirectly from clothing, a pet, or burning (volatilization).

Clinical Presentation

Redness and intense pruritis are most common, followed by development of papules, plaques, or vesicles arranged in a pattern mimicking the way the plant came in contact with the skin. If the face or genitals are involved, edema can be significant. If the resin is left in contact with the skin for a prolonged period and allowed to oxidize, "black spot" dermatitis can develop and the resin cannot be washed off.

- Rash appears after a latent period that varies from 4 hours to 10 days, depending on an individual's sensitivity and the amount of plant contact.
- Fluid in blisters does not spread the rash.
- If more rash appears after treatment has begun, these are areas with a longer latent period.
- Symptoms may last from 5 to 21 days following initial rash.
- Secondary infections can occur if scratching excoriates the skin and the abrasions become infected.

Treatment Principles and Goals

The initial objective should be to remove from the skin—via mechanical or other physical means—the sap or resin that caused the reaction. Generally, the reaction is self-limited; mild cases will clear without treatment in 7 to 14 days.

Treatment is symptomatic, centered on preventing itching, excessive scratching, and possible secondary skin infections, as well as providing relief to the irritated skin. Avoid using topical antihistamines, topical anesthetics, topical antibiotics, and poison ivy extracts because these have their own potential to elicit immune responses.

Treatment options include the following:

- *Mild cases:* Use topical antipruritics, such as calamine, camphor, or menthol, to prevent itching, and topical hydrocortisone cream or ointment.
- *Moderate cases:* Use topical high-potency corticosteroids for small areas (except on the face).
- *Severe cases:* Use systemic corticosteroids daily up to 2 weeks. Severe rash needs systemic corticosteroids to ease the misery and disability. Systemic corticosteroids are usually needed during early severe stages because remedies applied to skin may not penetrate deeply enough.

OTC Topical Therapy

Symptomatic relief

Compresses, soaks, or wet dressings will dry the oozing, reduce the weeping, aid in removal of crusts, and soothe the skin. Hot showers may make the itching worse, but cool compresses or showers may help. Suggestions include the following:

- Aluminum acetate solution, 1:40 ratio (Burow's solution)
- Aluminum sulfate/calcium acetate powder (Domeboro)
- Calamine lotion
- Colloidal oatmeal (Aveeno)

Antipruritics

These products may contain benzocaine up to 20%, pramoxine 1%, and benzyl alcohol. They include Caladryl lotion (calamine and pramoxine 1%) and Ivarest cream (calamine, benzyl alcohol, and diphenhydramine 2%) among others.

Topical steroids

Topical corticosteroids are used to relieve itching symptoms and promote the drying of lesions. They are most effective when started early in treatment, before formation of vesicles, which are more difficult to treat. Avoid applying ointments on weeping lesions because they are occlusive and will impede healing. Hydrocortisone 1% cream may reduce weeping, so use only in mild cases.

Prescription Topical Therapy

Use topical medium-to-high-potency corticosteroids (see discussion in section on allergic contact dermatitis).

Prescription Systemic Therapy

Use of systemic corticosteroids (intramuscular or oral) is the only therapy that will actually reduce the severity and duration of the allergic response. See the discussion on allergic contact dermatitis in this chapter and the discussion on endocrine disorders in Chapter 18 for complete details.

Effects of oral corticosteroids are dramatic (patients can take up to 40 to 100 mg **prednisone** for 2 to 3 weeks if necessary); however, many cases clear up quickly with a corticosteroid dose pack (e.g., Decadron or Medrol Dosepak). Extremely severe cases or large-scale rash may require a parenteral dose of corticosteroid (100 mg **prednisone** equivalent).

Other Recommendations

- *Avoidance:* Identify and avoid causative plants. Long pants and long-sleeved shirts are recommended for those sensitive to the effects.
- *Removal:* Washing with soap and water within 10 to 15 minutes of exposure (removing the sap or resin) may reduce the extent and duration of dermatitis. Showering is recommended over bathing. Urushiol is not water soluble, but large volumes of water can help rinse it away. Products such as Tecnu and Zanfel are marketed as scrubs to assist in binding urushiol and removing it from the skin but degreasing soaps such as GOOP and dishwashing liquid are just as effective.
- *Bentoquatam 5% lotion:* Formerly marketed under the trade name IvyBlock, this lotion is an organoclay and the only barrier product approved by the FDA. It has been discontinued by the manufacturer, but patients may have stock available. Instructions are to apply the lotion 15 minutes before possible plant contact and reapply every 4 hours.

41-8   Scaly Dermatoses

The 3 common forms of scaly dermatoses are dandruff, seborrhea, and psoriasis.

Dandruff

Dandruff is a chronic, noninflammatory scalp condition resulting in excessive scaling of the scalp epidermis. It is a common condition affecting 20% of the population. Though not a serious disorder, dandruff can be cosmetically unsightly.

Clinical presentation

Scaling and pruritus occur, causing white flakes to accumulate on the scalp.

Pathophysiology

Increased epidermal cell turnover rate of approximately twice the normal rate (time reduced from 25 to 30 days to 13 to 15 days) prevents complete keratinization of desquamated cells caused by unknown processes. Dandruff may be related to increased *Pityrosporum ovale,* a fungal scalp organism.

Treatment

Routine shampooing with mild hypoallergenic shampoo is essential.

Cytostatic agents

Cytostatic agents suppress cell turnover. The goal is to reduce the epidermal rate of turnover of scalp cells. Agents and their mechanisms of action are as follows:

- **ZPT (0.3% to 2%):** Products include Denorex, Head and Shoulders, X-Seb T, and Zincon. ZPT has an antifungal effect and reduces cell turnover rate.
- **Selenium sulfide 1%:** Products include Head and Shoulders Clinical Strength Shampoo and Selsun Blue Medicated Formula. Selenium sulfide reduces the cell rate turnover and inhibits growth of *P. ovale.*
- **Coal tar:** Products include Denorex and Neutrogena-T. Coal tar reduces the number and size of epidermal cells.

Patients should be counseled that contact time with cytostatic agents is very important for effectiveness. Advise patients to rub shampoo in well and leave it in up to 5 minutes before rinsing it out.

Keratolytic agents

Keratolytic agents include the following:

- **Salicylic acid (1.8% to 3%):** Products include Ionil, Neutrogena, Scalpicin, and Sebucare. Salicylic acid can lower the pH of tissues, thereby increasing the water concentration of epidermal cells, which softens and destroys the stratum corneum. It causes the upper skin layer to become inflamed and soft, followed by desquamation. This keratolytic action removes dandruff scales.
- **Sulfur (2% to 5%):** Products include Sulfoam, Sul-Ray, and Exsel. Sulfur possibly exerts an antifungal effect. Sulfur is usually found in combination with salicylic acid.
- **Combination of sulfur and salicylic acid:** Products include Meted and Sebulex.

Antifungals

Antifungals include the following:

- Ketoconazole (1%) shampoo (Nizoral A-D)
- Ciclopirox 1% shampoo (Loprox)

Ciclopirox is active against *P. ovale.* Patients should be counseled to use it twice weekly or every 3 or 4 days. Stress adequate contact time for a minimum of 3 minutes. Adverse effects include itching, stinging, or irritation.

Seborrhea (Seborrheic Dermatitis)

Seborrhea is a noncontagious chronic inflammatory skin disease in areas of greatest sebaceous gland activity, including on the scalp and other hairy areas such as the face, trunk, armpits, and groin. It typically persists for life, but it can be controlled.

Clinical presentation

- Scaling rash accompanied by pruritus
- Yellowish, greasy scales unlike the dry scales of dandruff
- Inflammation, often accompanied by erythema
- Fluctuation in severity, characterized by exacerbations and remissions
- Most common on the face, eyebrows, and eyelashes, but not on the extremities

Pathophysiology

- Accelerated cell turnover rate is approximately 3 times the normal rate, probably as few as 9 to 10 days.
- Seborrhea has a higher cell turnover rate than dandruff, but less than psoriasis.
- *P. ovale* may be causative, but this theory is not universally accepted.

Treatment

Treatment is similar to that for dandruff, but seborrhea is more difficult to treat. Overuse of selenium can make the scalp oily and can exacerbate seborrhea.

Topical corticosteroids are used to control itching and inflammation (up to 7 days). Add the topical antifungal ketoconazole 1% shampoo (Nizoral AD) or ciclopirox 1% shampoo (Loprox). The combination is active against *P. ovale*. Patients should be counseled to use it twice weekly, every 3 or 4 days. Stress adequate contact time; leave it in for at least 3 minutes. Adverse effects include itching, stinging, and irritation.

Plaque Psoriasis

Disease overview

Plaque psoriasis (also known as *psoriasis vulgaris*) is a chronic, inflammatory, papulosquamous, erythematous skin disease, marked by the presence of silvery scales with sharply delineated edges (plaque). Lesions are usually localized but can gradually grow to cover large areas. Other types of psoriasis, including inverse, guttate, pustular, erythrodermic, and nail psoriasis, are less common clinical manifestations. Plaques affect 80% to 90% of all patients with psoriasis.

Classification

- *Mild/moderate (80% of patients):* Characterized by plaque affecting less than 5% to 10% of body surface area (BSA).
- *Severe (20% of patients):* More than 5% to 10% of BSA affected or lesions located in crucial body areas such as the hands, feet, face, or genitals.

Clinical presentation (Figure 41-1)

- Plaque is known also as *scales*—silvery on top and pink to red beneath. It may be found anywhere on the body but more likely on the scalp, sacral area, and extensor surfaces of knees and elbows (less common on face).
- Borders of plaque are sharp with inflammation surrounding the plaque.
- It is marked by spontaneous exacerbations and remissions over the course of the patient's life.

Pathophysiology

A hyperproliferative immune-modulated skin condition results from skin cell turnover rate of approximately 10 to 20 times the normal rate. Skin cells of psoriatic plaque reach the outermost layer in 3 to 4 days. A

FIGURE 41-1. Large Plaque Psoriasis Lesions on the Upper Extremities

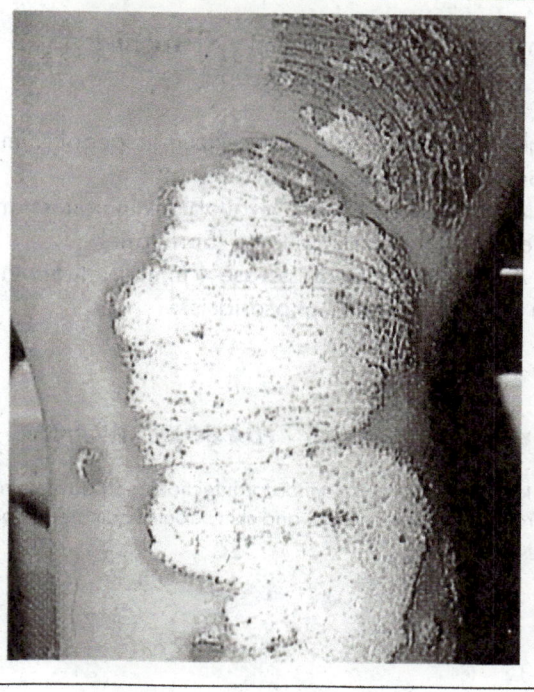

genetic predisposition contributes, as does exposure of the skin to trauma or triggering factors such as stressful incidents.

Treatment principles

Mild-to-moderate disease can generally be managed with topical therapies, while severe disease often requires systemic therapy. The advent of biologic therapies including monoclonal antibodies (MAbs) that target the immune system has revolutionized treatment of severe or refractory disease.

Drug Therapy

Topical treatments

Topical treatments include the following:

- Topical corticosteroids (see Table 40-5)
- Coal tar (contained in Denorex, Neutrogena T, Polytar)
- Keratolytics (salicylic acid, sulfur)
- Retinoids (See topical retinoids portion of Table 40-1)
- Anthralin (Anthraforte, Anthranol, Dritho-Scalp)
- Vitamin D_3 analogs: calcipotriene (Dovonex), calcitriol (Vectical)
  - *Caution:* If used in combination with phototherapy, typically PUVA (psoralen with ultraviolet A), calcipotriene should be applied after phototherapy, because PUVA inactivates this product.

Combinations of potent topical corticosteroids and calcipotriene, calcitriol, tazarotene, or phototherapy are commonly seen. Calcipotriene alone can be used continuously and the combination with potent corticosteroids used intermittently (such as on weekends) for maintenance. A combination product containing betamethasone dipropionate and calcipotriene (Taclonex) is available.

Systemic treatment

Systemic treatment may involve the following:

- Oral corticosteroids
- Antimetabolites, such as methotrexate and cyclosporine
- Psoralens (combined with ultraviolet light therapy)
- Biologics
    - *TNF-inhibitors:* Adalimumab (Humira) ⚠, certolizumab pegol (Cimzia) ⚠, etanercept (Enbrel) ⚠, golimumab (Simponi) ⚠, infliximab (Remicade) ⚠
    - *Interleukin (IL) inhibitors:* Table 41-8 lists available IL inhibitors and their targets
- Retinoids (vitamin A analogs), such as acitretin (Soriatane) ⚠
- Apremilast (Otezla): An oral phosphodiesterase-4 inhibitor that inhibits the production of multiple cytokines involved in the pathogenesis of psoriasis

 Methotrexate (oral formulation) *FDA BOXED WARNING*

Can cause severe or fatal toxicities—closely monitor for infections and adverse reactions of bone marrow, kidneys, liver, nervous system, gastrointestinal tract, lungs, and skin. Contraindicated in pregnancy for non-neoplastic diseases due to embryo-fetal toxicity.

 Cyclosporine *FDA BOXED WARNING*

Must be prescribed by physicians experienced in immunosuppressive therapy. Sandimmune® and Neoral® are not interchangeable. May increase susceptibility to infection and development of neoplasia. Increased risk of hypertension and nephrotoxicity, even at recommended therapeutic doses. Variable absorption—requires frequent monitoring. Psoriasis patients previously treated with psoralens plus ultraviolet A are at an increased risk of developing skin malignancies.

 Adalimumab (Humira) *FDA BOXED WARNING*

Increased risk of serious infections (e.g., tuberculosis, invasive fungal infections). Lymphoma and other malignancies have been reported in children and adolescent patients.

 Certolizumab Pegol (Cimzia) *FDA BOXED WARNING*

Increased risk of serious infections (e.g., tuberculosis, invasive fungal infections). Lymphoma and other malignancies have been reported in children and adolescent patients. Not indicated for use in pediatric patients.

 Etanercept (Enbrel) *FDA BOXED WARNING*

Increased risk of serious infections (e.g., tuberculosis, invasive fungal infections). Lymphoma and other malignancies have been reported in children and adolescent patients.

Golimumab (Simponi) *FDA BOXED WARNING*

Increased risk of serious infections (e.g., tuberculosis, invasive fungal infections). Lymphoma and other malignancies have been reported in children and adolescent patients.

 Infliximab (Remicade) *FDA BOXED WARNING*

Increased risk of serious infections (e.g., tuberculosis, invasive fungal infections). Lymphoma and other malignancies have been reported in children and adolescent patients.

 Acitretin (Soriatane) *FDA BOXED WARNING*

Highly teratogenic—contraindicated in pregnancy. Women receiving treatment should not become pregnant for at least 3 years after treatment ends. Only available through a specialized distribution and education program called "Do your P.A.R.T." Anyone (women and men) receiving therapy cannot donate blood during treatment or for at least 3 years after treatment ends. Increased risk of liver toxicity.

Methotrexate has been used for many years in an intermittent weekly low-dose regimen, like that for rheumatoid arthritis. The usual dose is 7.5 to 25 mg per week. In head-to-head studies, however, the efficacy of methotrexate appears to be less than with newer biologic agents.

Biologic therapies, specifically those targeting tumor necrosis factor alpha (TNF-α), as well as interleukins (IL) 12, 17, 23, and 39, have shown reliable safety and efficacy and are important treatment options for psoriasis. A meta-analysis including adalimumab, etanercept, infliximab, and ustekinumab showed infliximab as the most effective of these, with the highest likelihood for achieving 75% improvement in Psoriasis

TABLE 41-8. Interleukin (IL) Inhibitors for Treatment of Plaque Psoriasis

Generic name	Trade name	Target
Ustekinumab	Stelara	IL-12, IL-23
Secukinumab	Cosentyx	IL-17A
Ixekizumab	Taltz	IL-17A
Brodalumab ⚠	Siliq	IL-17 RA (receptor)
Guselkumab	Tremfya	IL-23, IL-39
Tildrakizumab	Illumya	IL-23
Risankizumab-rzaa	Skyrizi	IL-23(p19)

 Brodalumab *FDA BOXED WARNING*

Increased risk of suicidal ideation and behavior. Risks and benefits should be assessed before initiation of therapy. Close monitoring required. Only available through SILIQ REMS program.

Area and Severity Index (PASI 75) scores after 8 to 16 weeks of therapy. As these biologic therapies are very costly, coverage is a major issue in choosing the appropriate therapy.

Acitretin is used in severe and extensive psoriasis, including pustular and erythrodermic forms, as well as in human immunodeficiency virus (HIV)–associated psoriasis. When combined with ultraviolet (UV) light therapy, response rate is improved and less intense UV light may be used. Adverse effects include dry lips, dry skin, nail changes, dry eyes, hair loss, hyperlipidemia, pancreatitis, hepatotoxicity, myalgias, and arthralgias. Acitretin is highly teratogenic, and it is indicated only in persons of nonreproductive potential. Pregnancy and blood donation are contraindicated during therapy and for 3 years after discontinuing the drug.

41-9 Head Lice (Pediculosis Capitis)

Disease Overview

Head lice is a common condition caused by infestation of *Pediculus humanus capitis*. Lice are especially common in schoolchildren and affect individuals of all socioeconomic backgrounds. They are transmitted by direct contact with the head of an infected individual or through fomites (inanimate objects capable of transmitting disease, such as shared combs, brushes, hats, or scarves).

Pathophysiology and Life Cycle

A female louse lives about 1 month, laying 7 to 10 eggs per day. These "nits" are attached firmly to the base of a hair and hatch 7 to 8 days later. After hatching, the egg casings become white. Adult lice feed on blood from the scalp and can survive >48 hours without a host.

Clinical Presentation

- Pruritus, occurring as an allergic reaction to saliva injected by the lice during feeding, is the most common symptom. Sensitization can be delayed up to 4 to 6 weeks in a previously uninfected host, potentially delaying recognition of infection.
- Because lice infestation is usually symptomatic, diagnosis is made visually by seeing live lice.
- The flat, gray-brown adult lice are difficult to locate. Nits are more likely to be seen, indicating progression in the life cycle.
- Systematic combing of wet or dry hair with a nit comb (teeth 0.2 mm apart) is a better method for detecting both live lice and nits than visual inspection alone.

Drug Therapy

Pyrethroids (synergized pyrethrins, permethrin 1%)

Pyrethrins are naturally derived from chrysanthemum extract and are neurotoxic to lice. Products are often synergized by the addition of 2% to 4% piperonyl butoxide (petroleum derivative), which inhibits the breakdown of pyrethrins within the louse. Trade names for this OTC combination product include A-200, LiceMD, Licide, and RID.

Permethrin (Nix) is a synthetic pyrethroid that is more effective than the naturally derived pyrethrins. A 5% prescription version of permethrin (Elimite) is available but is no more effective for head lice than the 1% OTC preparation. Topical pyrethroids are first-line therapies and should be used before other topical therapies unless the patient cannot tolerate therapy or resistance develops.

Directions for use

Wash hair with conditioner-free shampoo, rinse with water, and towel dry before application. Apply enough product to fully saturate hair, scalp, and neck. Leave on for 10 minutes, then rinse off with warm water. Use a lice-nit comb to remove dead lice and nits following rinsing. Repeat treatment in 7 to 10 days, if indicated.

Patient instructions and counseling

- Treat all family members.
- Avoid contact with the eyes, mouth, and nose.
- Do not use on irritated or inflamed scalp.

Adverse drug effects

Adverse effects include irritation, erythema, and itching.

Malathion 0.5% (Ovide; prescription only)

Malathion is an organophosphate insecticide that irreversibly inhibits acetylcholinesterase, causing death in the insect. Initially FDA approved in the 1980s, it has seen increased use because of concern about resistance to pyrethroids. It is available in a topical lotion formulation.

Directions for use

Apply to dry hair and scalp, rubbing gently until thoroughly moistened. Allow hair to dry naturally, leaving uncovered. Wash hair with nonmedicated shampoo after 8 to 12 hours and use a nit-comb to remove dead lice and eggs.

Patient instructions and counseling

- Evaluate other close contacts of patient to determine if they should be treated.
- Avoid contact with eyes.
- Wash hands immediately after use.

Adverse drug effects

Adverse effects include skin irritation, drying (contains isopropyl alcohol), and stinging.

Benzyl alcohol 5% (Ulesfia; prescription only)

The mechanism of action involves asphyxiation of lice by combination of benzyl alcohol and mineral oil vehicle.

Directions for use

Apply to dry hair until saturated, leaving on for 10 minutes. Thoroughly rinse hair with water and allow to dry. Use a nit-comb to remove dead lice and nits. Repeat treatment after 7 days.

Patient instructions and counseling

- It is approved for use by patients 6 months of age or older.
- Benzyl alcohol kills lice but has no activity against ova.
- There is minimal absorption after application.

Adverse drug effects

Adverse effects include irritation and transient numbness of skin at site of application.

Spinosad 0.9% (Natroba; prescription only)

Spinosad acts as a nicotinic acetylcholine receptor agonist, causing insect motor excitation, paralysis, and death.

Directions for use

Shake well before use. Apply to dry scalp, covering it completely, then apply to dry hair. Leave on for 10 minutes (starting time after scalp and hair are covered), and then rinse hair with warm water. If live lice are seen after 7 days, repeat application. Nit combing is not required.

Patient instructions and counseling

- Spinosad is approved for use by patients 6 months of age or older.
- Wash hands after use.
- There is no detected absorption after application.

Adverse drug effects

Adverse effects include skin irritation, drying (contains isopropyl alcohol), and stinging.

Ivermectin 0.5% (Sklice; prescription only)

Ivermectin binds to glutamate- and gamma-aminobutyric acid (GABA)–gated channels in the nervous system, causing insect paralysis and death. It is available in topical lotion formulation.

Directions for use

Starting with dry scalp, apply outward from scalp toward ends of hair, completely covering scalp and hair. Leave on for 10 minutes, and then rinse thoroughly with warm water.

Patient instructions and counseling

- Ivermectin is approved for use by patients 6 months of age or older.
- Wash hands after use.
- Lotion is for 1-time use only; discard any unused portion.

Adverse drug effects

Adverse effects include skin irritation and burning.

Lindane (Kwell; prescription only)

First used in the 1950s, lindane is a GABA-receptor, chloride-channel complex inhibitor, causing insect neuronal hyperstimulation, paralysis, and death. It carries a boxed warning related to neurologic toxicity, including seizures, even at recommended doses.

Directions for use

Apply sufficient amount to dry scalp, covering it completely, and then apply to dry hair. Leave on for 10 minutes (starting time after scalp and hair are covered), and then rinse hair with warm water. If live lice are seen after 7 days, repeat application. Nit combing is not required.

Patient instructions and counseling

- Lindane should be used only by patients who cannot tolerate other therapies or when other therapies have failed.
- Use with caution by the elderly, very young children, patients with other skin conditions, or patients weighing <50 kg.

Adverse drug effects

Lindane is absorbed significantly through the skin and has been reported to have significant neurotoxic effects, especially in infants and children. Central nervous system effects reported include seizures, dizziness, lack of coordination, restlessness, and irritability. Other effects include rapid heartbeat, muscle cramps, and vomiting.

Nondrug Recommendations

- Change clothing daily.
- Treat infested clothes, and shower daily.
- All household contacts should be inspected and treated if necessary.
- All bed linens, clothes, hats, and towels should be dry-cleaned or washed in the hot water cycle and dried on hot.
- Wash hairbrushes, combs, and toys in hot water for at least 10 minutes.
- Treat surrounding environment (bedding, pillows, carpets, draperies, furniture) with A-200 Control Spray or RID Control Spray.

41-10 Warts

Warts (*verrucae*) are harmless skin growths caused by the human papillomavirus.

Classification

- Common warts (*verruca vulgaris*) occur on the fingers, hands, and knees.
- Plantar warts (*verruca plantaris*) occur on the soles of the feet.

Clinical Presentation

- Warts are contagious (even to another part of the patient's body) and are more common in children and immunocompromised patients.
- Warts occurring on pressure areas such as the bottom of the feet (plantar warts) grow inward from the pressure of standing and walking and are often painful.

Treatment Principles and Goals

Many warts will go away without treatment, though that may take up to several years in adults. In children, warts may spontaneously remit in as little as 2 years. Warts can be eliminated by the following:

- Direct application of caustics (e.g., salicylic acid)
- Freezing (cryotherapy) with liquid nitrogen or with dimethyl ether and propane
- Surgery

OTC Drug Therapy
Salicylic acid

Patient instructions and counseling:

- Use topical salicylic acid preparations daily until the wart is gone.
- Use special care in washing hands before and after treatment and use a separate towel for drying other parts of the body.

- Do not use salicylic acid on irritated, broken, or infected skin.
- If the wart remains after 12 weeks of continuous treatment, see a dermatologist or podiatrist.

Salicylic acid products are contraindicated in patients with diabetes and other patients with poor circulation because reduced sensation in the foot delays awareness of skin breakdown. Diabetic patients should see a physician or podiatrist for removal of warts.

OTC salicylic acid products include the following:

- *Salicylic acid 17% in flexible collodion vehicle:* Compound W gel and liquid, Dr. Scholl's Clear Away Fast-Acting Liquid
- *Salicylic acid 40% embedded in pads or discs:* Compound W One Step Pads, Dr. Scholl's Clear Away Medicated Discs. Duct tape can be used to securely attach salicylic acid pads to skin. If tape is used, pads and tape should be replaced every 48 hours.

Cryotherapy

Dimethyl ether and propane are FDA approved for OTC removal of common warts and plantar warts. Cryotherapy irritation leads the host to produce an immune response against the causative virus (similar to liquid nitrogen, which can be administered only by a health care provider). After about 10 days, the frozen skin and wart fall off, revealing newly formed skin underneath.

OTC cryotherapy products include the following:

- *Dimethyl ether and propane:* Dr. Scholl's Freeze Away Wart Remover and Wartner Cryogenic Wart Removal System are approved for removal of common warts.
- *Dimethyl ether, propane, and isobutane:* Compound W Freeze Off is approved for removal of common warts and plantar warts.

Patient instructions include

- Place the applicator in the spray can, which becomes very cold (−55°C).
- After the applicator is saturated, hold it on the wart for a product-specific time period to freeze the wart (20 seconds for Wartner; 40 seconds for Compound W).
- The process may be repeated after 10 days for persistent warts.
- *Caution:* Do not use on children under 4 years of age, diabetics, or pregnant or breast-feeding females; on the face, armpits, breasts, buttocks, or genitals; on irritated skin; or on mucous membranes (e.g., mouth, nose, anus).

41-11   Pharmacist's Role

Pharmacists have a direct role in helping patients recognize, diagnose, and treat many skin conditions, especially in the community and ambulatory settings. In some jurisdictions, pharmacists are also allowed to prescribe certain non-OTC topical treatments based on collaborative practice agreements or protocols. Patient education and counseling are vitally important to ensure optimal use of all agents used to treat dermatologic disorders. Many topical medications elicit adverse effects such as redness, burning, and itching prior to the therapeutic benefits (in some cases weeks before), so it is important that patients do not prematurely discontinue treatment. Additionally, pharmacists across practice settings can help monitor the effectiveness of treatments for dermatologic conditions and refer patients for more advanced care when appropriate.

NAPLEX Competency Statements

The questions in this chapter cover the following 2021 NAPLEX Competency Statements: **AREA 1:** 1.1; 1.5; 1.6 **AREA 2:** 2.1; 2.2; 2.4 **AREA 3:** 3.1; 3.2; 3.4; 3.5; 3.6; 3.7; 3.8.

 **41-12   Questions**

1. Which of the following initial treatment plans would be appropriate for a newly diagnosed 14-year-old male patient with mild acne?

   A. Topical benzoyl peroxide alone
   B. Combined oral contraceptive
   C. Oral doxycycline and topical adapalene
   D. Oral isotretinoin alone
   E. Oral tetracycline and topical clindamycin

2. Which of the following is the most appropriate therapy for a patient over 12 years of age with mild acne who is unable to tolerate topical retinoids?

   A. Oral tetracycline
   B. Topical dapsone
   C. Topical tazarotene
   D. Oral isotretinoin
   E. Oral doxycycline

3. J. L. is a 22-year-old male purchasing OTC adapalene at the pharmacy. What is an appropriate counseling point for this product?

   A. Use this product twice daily for the first 2 weeks.
   B. Expect rapid improvement within 2 or 3 days of starting therapy.
   C. Astringents should be used before using this product.
   D. Use sunblock before exposure to sunlight.
   E. Product works best if followed with aggressive exfoliating scrub.

4. Which of the following is the most common side effect of oral isotretinoin?

   A. Skin rash
   B. Acute depression
   C. Decreased night vision
   D. Insomnia
   E. Dry, chapped lips

5. Which of the following is an important contraindication and precaution to the use of isotretinoin?

   A. Hypertension
   B. Migraines
   C. Allergic rhinitis
   D. Pregnancy
   E. Asthma

6. Which of the following is the most efficacious nonprescription topical antifungal?

   A. Tolnaftate
   B. Terbinafine
   C. Miconazole
   D. Clotrimazole
   E. Butenafine

7. Using the image below, identify the site of infection of tinea capitis.

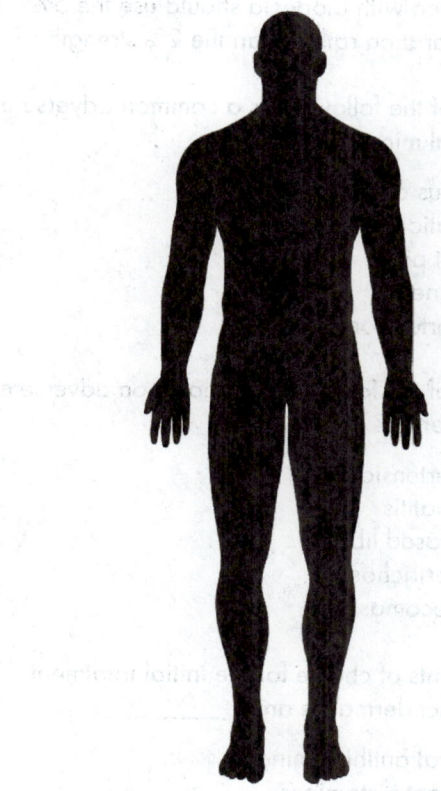

Source: https://openclipart.org/detail/314198/man-body-silhouette

8. Which of the following products is available without a prescription?

   A. Itraconazole (Sporanox)
   B. Fluconazole (Diflucan)
   C. Griseofulvin (Grifulvin V)
   D. Naftifine (Naftin)
   E. Tolnaftate (Tinactin)

9. Which of the following are appropriate patient instructions for the proper use of topical minoxidil? (Mark all that apply.)

   A. It should be applied on the scalp and left for 4 hours for maximum effect.
   B. The patient should not swim, shampoo, or walk in rain soon after the application of minoxidil.
   C. It should not be used on infected, irritated, inflamed, or sunburned skin.
   D. The patient must continue therapy to maintain effectiveness.
   E. Women with alopecia should use the 5% preparation rather than the 2% strength.

10. Which of the following is a common adverse effect of topical minoxidil?

   A. Pruritus of the scalp
   B. Hepatic damage
   C. Chest pain
   D. Dizziness
   E. Hypertension

11. Which of the following is a common adverse effect of finasteride?

   A. Hypertension
   B. Dermatitis
   C. Increased libido
   D. Hypertrichosis
   E. Gynecomastia

12. The agents of choice for the initial treatment of contact dermatitis are _____.

   A. topical antihistamines
   B. oral antihistamines
   C. topical corticosteroids
   D. local anesthetics
   E. coal tar products

13. Which topical corticosteroid may safely be used on infants and small children?

   A. Betamethasone valerate
   B. Desoximetasone
   C. Halcinonide
   D. Clobetasol propionate
   E. Desonide

14. The treatment of choice for severe or extensive cases of poison ivy or poison oak is _____.

   A. a local anesthetic such as benzocaine
   B. a camphor and menthol antipruritic
   C. colloidal oatmeal
   D. a systemic corticosteroid
   E. cool compresses without medication

15. Rank the following topical corticosteroids in order of *least* potent to *most* potent:

Unordered options	Ordered response
Triamcinolone acetonide 0.1%	
Clobetasol propionate 0.05%	
Hydrocortisone 1%	

16. Treatment of advanced psoriasis may require topical therapy combined with which of the following systemic agents? (Mark all that apply.)

   A. Prednisone
   B. Methotrexate
   C. Anthralin
   D. Apremilast
   E. Fluconazole

17. A patient presents to the clinic with a diagnosis of mild plaque psoriasis isolated to the face and inside of the patient's elbows. What is the best treatment option?

   A. Topical clobetasol propionate
   B. Topical tacrolimus
   C. Oral acitretin
   D. Injectable etanercept
   E. Oral methotrexate

18. Lindane is associated with which of the following toxicities?

   A. Pulmonary
   B. Neurologic
   C. Renal
   D. Hepatic
   E. Cardiovascular

19. Which of the following is the most effective nonprescription agent for treatment of head lice?

A. Permethrin
B. Synergized pyrethrins
C. Lindane
D. Ketoconazole
E. Malathion

20. Nonprescription products for the treatment of warts contain which of the following agents?

A. Salicylic acid
B. Ketoconazole
C. Lactic acid
D. Hydrocortisone
E. Permethrin

 **41-13   Answers**

1. **A.** For mild acne, it is recommended to start with topical benzoyl peroxide or topical retinoid. This patient is male and, therefore, would not be a candidate for oral contraceptives. Combination therapy and oral isotretinoin would be appropriate for moderate or severe acne.

2. **B.** Topical dapsone is a good option for patients who are unable to tolerate topical retinoids because it has anti-inflammatory and antimicrobial properties. Topical tazarotene is the most irritating retinoid. Systemic therapies such as oral antibiotics or isotretinoin would not be appropriate for mild acne.

3. **D.** Topical retinoid therapy will sensitize skin to ultraviolet light rays; therefore, patients should use sunblock before sun exposure. Topical retinoids should be used every other day for the first 2 weeks, then nightly. Patients using topical retinoids should use only mild soaps for cleansing the face and avoid astringents, drying agents, and abrasive soaps. Improvement will usually occur within 2 to 3 weeks after initiation of therapy.

4. **E.** Cheilitis (dry, chapped lips) together with dry skin and dry mouth are the most common side effects of isotretinoin therapy.

5. **D.** Isotretinoin is contraindicated in pregnancy because of the high incidence of serious birth defects.

6. **B.** Terbinafine (Lamisil) is the most effective nonprescription topical antifungal.

7. Tinea capitis is an infection of the scalp, so the correct location to highlight would be the area below.

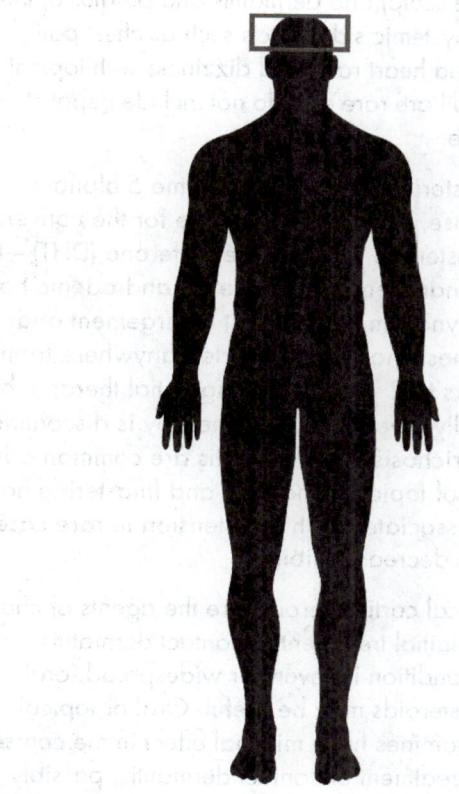

Source: https://openclipart.org/detail/314198/man-body-silhouette

8. **E.** Tolnaftate (Tinactin) is available without a prescription. Fluconazole (Diflucan), itraconazole (Sporanox), and griseofulvin (Grifulvin V) are prescription systemic antifungal agents, and naftifine (Naftin) is a prescription topical antifungal.

9. **A, B, C, D.** Minoxidil should be applied on the scalp and left for 4 hours for maximum effect. The patient should not swim, shampoo, or walk in rain soon after the application of minoxidil, and it should not be used on infected, irritated, inflamed, or sunburned skin. The patient must continue therapy to maintain effectiveness. However, women should use only the 2% strength preparation of minoxidil. Studies indicate that there is no greater degree of effectiveness with the

5% strength preparation, and the incidence of adverse effects (including increased growth of facial hair) is much greater in women using the 5% preparation.

10. A. Common adverse effects of minoxidil include hypertrichosis (increased hair growth in areas other than the scalp) and dermatitis and pruritus of the scalp. Systemic side effects such as chest pain, increased heart rate, and dizziness with topical minoxidil are rare and do not include hepatic damage.

11. E. Finasteride inhibits the enzyme 5-alpha-reductase, which is responsible for the conversion of testosterone to dihydrotestosterone (DHT)—the main androgen responsible for androgenic hair loss. Gynecomastia (breast enlargement and tenderness) has been reported anywhere from 2 weeks to 2 years following initial therapy, but it is usually reversible when therapy is discontinued. Hypertrichosis and dermatitis are common adverse effects of topical minoxidil, and finasteride has been associated with hypotension in rare cases as well as decreased libido.

12. C. Topical corticosteroids are the agents of choice for the initial treatment of contact dermatitis. If the condition is severe or widespread, oral corticosteroids may be useful. Oral or topical antihistamines have minimal effect in the course of the treatment of contact dermatitis, possibly producing some antipruritic effect but not affecting the course of the condition.

13. E. Desonide is a medium potency topical corticosteroid that may be used on infants and small children. The other choices are high, very high, and ultrahigh potency agents that should be avoided in this patient population. Topical corticosteroid systemic absorption is increased on infants' and children's skin. Systemic corticosteroids' adverse effects may be severe and include adrenocortical suppression.

14. D. Systemic corticosteroids are the treatment of choice for severe or extensive cases of poison ivy or poison oak. Topical agents are limited in effectiveness and do not alter the course of the condition. Cool compresses without medication are not appropriate for this condition.

15. Hydrocortisone 1% is classified as a low-potency agent, triamcinolone acetonide 0.1% is classified as medium potency, and clobetasol propionate 0.05% is classified as ultrahigh potency.

Unordered options	Ordered response
Triamcinolone acetonide 0.1%	Hydrocortisone 1%
Clobetasol propionate 0.05%	Triamcinolone acetonide 0.1%
Hydrocortisone 1%	Clobetasol propionate 0.05%

16. A, B, D. Treatment of advanced psoriasis may require topical therapy combined with either oral corticosteroids (like prednisone), antimetabolites like methotrexate, or apremilast.

17. B. Topical calcineurin inhibitors like tacrolimus and pimecrolimus are the treatment of choice for plaque psoriasis on the face, skin folds (e.g., elbows), and intertriginous (skin-touching-skin) areas in adults.

18. B. Lindane is absorbed significantly through the skin and has been reported to have significant neurotoxic effects, especially in infants and children. Central nervous system effects reported include seizures, dizziness, lack of coordination, restlessness, and irritability.

19. A. Permethrin (Nix) does not have to be repeated in 7 to 10 days as does the other available nonprescription pediculicidal agent, synergized pyrethrins (A-200). Lindane (Kwell) is not available over the counter, and significant neurologic toxicities have been reported with its use. Malathion (Ovide) also requires a prescription.

20. A. Nonprescription products for the treatment of warts contain salicylic acid as the active therapeutic agent.

41-14 Additional Resources

Arndt KA, Hsu JHS, Alam M, et al., eds. *Manual of Dermatologic Therapies: With Essentials of Diagnosis.* 8th ed. Philadelphia, PA: Lippincott Williams & Wilkins; 2014.

DiPiro JT, Talbert RL, Posey ML, et al., eds. *Pharmacotherapy: A Pathophysiologic Approach.* 11th ed. New York, NY: McGraw-Hill Medical; 2020.

Ely JW, Rosenfeld S, Stone MS. Diagnosis and management of tinea infections. *Am Fam Physician.* 2014;90(10):702–710.

Ference JD, Last AR. Choosing topical corticosteroids. *Am Fam Physician.* 2009;79(2):135–140.

Griffiths C, Barker J, Bleiker TO, et al., eds. *Rook's Textbook of Dermatology.* 9th ed. Oxford, UK: Wiley-Blackwell; 2016.

Jeon C, Sekhon S, Yan D, et al. Monoclonal antibodies inhibiting IL-12, -23, and -17 for the treatment of psoriasis. *Hum Vaccin Immunother.* 2017;13(10):2247–2259.

Krinsky, DL, Ferreri SP, Hemstreet BA, et al., eds. *Handbook of Nonprescription Drugs.* 19th ed. Washington, DC: American Pharmacists Association; 2017.

Menter A, Korman NJ, Elmets CA, et al. Guidelines of care for the management of psoriasis and psoriatic arthritis: Section 3. Guidelines of care for the management and treatment of psoriasis with topical therapies. *J Am Acad Dermatol.* 2009;60(4):643–659.

Menter A, Strober BE, Kaplan DH, et al. Joint AAD-NPF guidelines of care for the management and treatment of psoriasis with biologics. *J Am Acad Dermatol.* 2019;80(4):1029–1072.

Zaenglein AL, Pathy AL, Schlosser BJ, et al. Guidelines of care for the management of acne vulgaris. *J Am Acad Dermatol.* 2016;74(5):945–973.e33.

Solid Organ Transplantation

42

BENJAMIN T. DUHART, JR.

42-1 KEY POINTS

- The goal of solid organ transplantation is to improve patients' quality of life and survival by stabilizing or improving complications related to end-organ failure.
- The immune system is a highly intricate system with mechanisms for antigen recognition in a highly specific manner as well as in a nonspecific manner.
- Acute rejection may be T-cell– and/or B-cell–mediated and is a normal physiologic immune response to transplantation of donor antigens.
- The incidence of acute rejection is organ specific and depends on multiple pre- and posttransplant factors.
- Selection of the posttransplant immunosuppression regimen for prevention of acute rejection should be individualized on the basis of known risk and potential toxicity.
- Adjustment in the posttransplant immunosuppression regimen should focus on the balance between acute rejection, infection, and toxicity.
- Selection of the agent to be used to treat acute rejection is organ dependent and depends on the severity of acute rejection, as well as, institutional protocols.
- Immunosuppressive complications, both infectious and noninfectious, are an important cause of morbidity and mortality and require close management following transplantation.
- Clinician expertise in immunosuppressive therapeutic drug monitoring is required to optimize efficacy and reduce toxicity of immunosuppressants.
- Immunosuppressants have the potential for numerous pharmacokinetic and pharmacodynamic drug interactions.
  - Calcineurin inhibitors are considered the cornerstone of maintenance immunosuppression.
  - Use of induction therapy allows for either delayed initiation or slow dose escalation of calcineurin inhibitors.
  - Induction therapy is used primarily in patients with a high risk of rejection.
  - Immunosuppressants can increase the risk of infection and malignancies posttransplant.
- Advise patients of the following:
  - Avoid taking the morning dose of cyclosporine , everolimus, sirolimus, and tacrolimus on the day of therapeutic drug monitoring.
  - Because of the high risk for multiple drug–drug interactions that may decrease the safety and efficacy of immunosuppressants, avoid taking new prescriptions and over-the-counter medications (including herbals) without discussing with the pharmacist.
  - If mycophenolate is prescribed for women of childbearing age, a risk evaluation and mitigation strategy must be discussed before dispensing.
  - Because of suppression of the immune system by immunosuppressants, the efficacy of vaccinations may be compromised. Avoid live vaccinations posttransplant.

42-2 STUDY GUIDE CHECKLIST

The following topics may guide your study of this subject area:

- [ ] Factors that increase the risk for acute rejection.
- [ ] Selection of immunosuppressants for induction and maintenance therapy.
- [ ] Considerations for selection of immunosuppressants based on patient condition.
- [ ] Mechanism of actions of various categories of immunosuppressants.
- [ ] Available formulations of cyclosporine and tacrolimus (not interchangeable).
- [ ] Major adverse effects specific for selected immunosuppressants.
- [ ] Significant drug interactions for immunosuppressants.
- [ ] Unique counseling points for selected immunosuppressants.
- [ ] Selection of immunosuppressants to treat acute rejection.

Cyclosporine *FDA BOXED WARNING*

Must be prescribed by physicians experienced in immunosuppressive therapy. Sandimmune® and Neoral® are NOT interchangeable. Variable absorption-requires frequent monitoring.

 **42-3** **Overview of Organ Transplantation**

Definitions

- *Acute rejection:* A normal physiologic response by the immune system to donor antigens
- *Adaptive immunity:* Involves the stimulation of cells and soluble mediators in response to specific antigens with a markedly enhanced response on repeat exposure
- *Human leukocyte antigen (HLA):* Antigen-binding proteins that rescue protein fragments from intracellular catabolism (class I or II) or select antigens from the extracellular milieu that are then presented to lymphocytes (class II)
- *Induction:* Administration of short-term therapy before and during the initial transplant as prophylaxis for acute rejection in high-risk recipients
- *Innate immunity:* Involves the stimulation of cells and soluble mediators that nonspecifically recognize antigens and have no ability to alter response with repeat exposure
- *Panel reactive antibody (PRA):* A test that quantifies a patient's immunologic reactivity to a given pool of antigens
- *Phagocytosis:* A process by which recognized antigens are engulfed and subsequently undergo intracellular catabolism

Basic Immunology and Acute Rejection

Fundamental types of immunity

Innate immunity

The following are selected cellular components that contribute to rejection:

- *Macrophages and dendritic cells:* These are phagocytic cells found throughout the body that may function as antigen-presenting cells (APC).
- *Complement:* When activated, these proteins lead to formation of lipophilic complexes, called *membrane-attack complexes,* in the cell membrane of the target cell and result in osmotic leaks.

Adaptive immunity

The following are selected cellular components that contribute to rejection:

- *Thymus-derived lymphocytes (T-cells):* Mature T-cells become activated when they encounter an APC. T-cells do not recognize antigens directly.
  - CD4+ T-cells (*helper T-cells*) recognize HLA class II antigens presented via APC.
  - CD8+ T-cells (*cytotoxic T-cells*) recognize HLA class I antigens presented via APC.
- *Bone marrow–derived lymphocytes (B-cells):* B-cells encounter the antigen to which their surface immunoglobulin has specificity, either through its APC function or by interaction with an activated CD4+ T-cell.

FIGURE 42-1. Signals for Acute Rejection

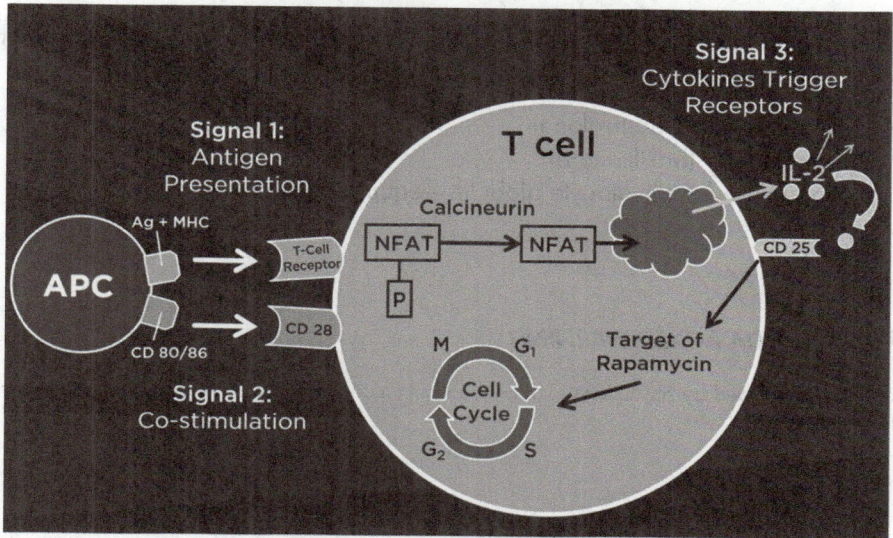

1. *Signal 1:* The foreign antigen is recognized via self- or non-self-recognition from the immune system, and the APC presents the foreign antigen to inactive CD4+ T-cells to create an antigen–T-cell receptor (TCR) complex.
2. *Signal 2:* Activation of the immune response depends on the subsequent binding of multiple proteins on the cell surface to produce a second signal or "costimulatory pathway." Subsequently, the active CD4+ T-cell produces and releases various lymphokines, particularly interleukin-2 (IL-2), which is important for activation and proliferation of numerous lymphocyte lineages.
3. *Signal 3:* The binding of IL-2 to the IL-2 receptor on the active CD4+ T-cell creates monoclonal expansion of the CD4+ T-cell as well as the production of multiple lymphokines that recruit multiple cell lineages of the immune system to cause antigen and tissue destruction.

Acute rejection

Pathophysiology

During transplantation, the recipient is exposed to donor antigens. As a result, acute rejection occurs. This response can be divided into 3 signals as shown in Figure 42-1.

Incidence

The incidence is organ specific and depends on many pre- and posttransplant factors. Several known factors increase risk (Box 42-1).

Immunosuppressive Strategies

Balance of immunosuppression

Selection of an immunosuppression regimen for the prevention of acute rejection should be individualized on the basis of known risk and potential for toxicity. Subsequent adjustment must focus on the balance of the triad: rejection, infection, and toxicity.

BOX 42-1. Factors Known to Increase the Risk of Auto Rejection

- High number of HLA mismatches
- Factors affecting previous sensitization (e.g., history of pregnancy, multiple blood transfusions, previous transplantation, previous rejection, PRA >20%, presence of donor-specific antibody)
- Ethnicity (i.e., Black recipients)

- Age (i.e., pediatric recipients)
- Donor source (i.e., deceased donor)
- Prolonged preservation time
- Nonadherence (i.e., medications, clinic visits)

Phases of preventive immunosuppression

Induction

The early phase is intended to provide highly potent, multifocal suppression of the immune system for several days to a few weeks. Commonly used agents include the following:

- Corticosteroids (methylprednisolone)
- Monoclonal antibody (basiliximab)
- Polyclonal antibody (antithymocyte globulin—equine or rabbit)

> ⚠ **Basiliximab** *FDA BOXED WARNING*
>
> Should only be prescribed by physicians experienced in immunosuppression therapy and management of organ transplantation patients.

> ⚠ **Antithymocyte globulin—equine or rabbit** *FDA BOXED WARNING*
>
> Should only be prescribed by physicians experienced in immunosuppression therapy and management of organ transplantation patients.

Maintenance

The immunosuppression regimen is designed to provide chronic, balanced immunodeficiency. Some commonly used regimens are listed in Box 42-2.

Phases of immunosuppression during treatment

Treatment

Selection of the agents is organ specific and depends on the severity of acute rejection, as well as, institutional protocol. Commonly used agents include the following:

- Corticosteroids
- Calcineurin inhibitor
  - Tacrolimus may be used as the primary treatment of acute rejection in liver recipients.
  - Tacrolimus may also have a role as adjuvant therapy in refractory acute rejection in various other solid organ recipients.
- Polyclonal antibody (antithymocyte globulin—equine or rabbit)

> **BOX 42-2. Common Immunosuppression Regimes**
>
> - Double therapy
>   - Calcineurin inhibitor + steroids
>   - Calcineurin inhibitor + antimetabolite
>   - Calcineurin inhibitor + mTOR (mammalian target of rapamycin) inhibitor
>
> - Triple therapy
>   - Calcineurin inhibitor + antimetabolite + steroids
>   - mTOR inhibitor + calcineurin inhibitor + steroids
>   - mTOR inhibitor + antimetabolite + steroids
>   - Costimulation blocker + antimetabolite + steroids

Maintenance reevaluation

The decision to heighten maintenance immunosuppression depends on the cause for and severity of rejection (i.e., failure of regimen versus noncompliance).

Immunosuppressive Complications

Infectious

Infectious complications are an important cause of early morbidity and mortality. The incidence is organ specific and is closely linked to the net degree of immunodeficiency. Prevention is a key management strategy following transplantation. For example, nystatin, valganciclovir, and sulfamethoxazole/trimethoprim are commonly used to prevent fungal, viral, and bacterial infections such as candidiasis, cytomegalovirus, and pneumocystis pneumonia.

Noninfectious

The noninfectious complications are specific to the agents included in the immunosuppressive regimen and may be an important contributor to the progression of cardiovascular disease.

42-4   Immunosuppressants

Calcineurin Inhibitors

Cyclosporine ⚠

Generic name	Trade name	Dosage form	Dose
Cyclosporine (nonmodified)	Sandimmune	Injection: 50 mg/mL; oral solution: 100 mg/mL; capsules: 25, 100 mg	Intravenous: 5 to 6 mg/kg/d; oral: 8 to 14 mg/kg/d divided every 12 hours; adjusted to desired trough concentration
Cyclosporine (modified)	Neoral	Oral solution: 100 mg/mL; capsules: 25, 100 mg	Oral: 5 to 10 mg/kg/d divided every 12 hours; adjusted to desired trough concentration

Mechanism of action

Cyclosporine binds to cyclophilin, forming a complex that inhibits calcineurin-dependent translocation of the cytosolic subunit of nuclear factor of activated T-cells (NFAT) into the nucleus, thereby inhibiting transcription and synthesis of IL-2.

Administration

- Intravenous (I.V.)
  - Administer 5 to 6 mg/kg/d divided every 12 hours or as a continuous infusion. Each milliliter of I.V. concentrate should be diluted in 20 to 100 mL of normal saline (NS) or 5% dextrose in water (D5W) in a glass container. The dose should be infused over 2 to 6 hours.

⚠ **Cyclosporine** *FDA BOXED WARNING*

Must be prescribed by physicians experienced in immunosuppressive therapy. Sandimmune® and Neoral® are NOT interchangeable. Variable absorption—requires frequent monitoring.

TABLE 42-1. Drug Interactions Leading to Altered Exposure of CYP450 3A Isoenzyme Substrates

CYP450 3A4 enzyme inducers[a]	CYP450 3A4 enzyme inhibitors[b]
Anticonvulsants: phenytoin, phenobarbital, carbamazepine	Antidepressants: nefazodone
Antimicrobial agents: rifampin, rifabutin	Antiviral agents: boceprevir, delavirdine, indinavir, nelfinavir, ritonavir, saquinavir, telaprevir
Antiviral agents: nevirapine, efavirenz	Azole antifungal agents: clotrimazole, fluconazole, itraconazole, ketoconazole, posaconazole, voriconazole
Herbal products: St. John's wort	Calcium channel blockers: **diltiazem**, nicardipine, verapamil
	Macrolide antimicrobial agents: clarithromycin, erythromycin
	Food–drug interaction: grapefruit juice

Boldface indicates one of top 100 drugs for 2020 by prescription volume.
The table shows examples only. Numerous other interactions are associated with CYP450 3A4 substrates. See current journals or drug interaction texts for a more detailed list.
a. Inducers result in increased metabolism of substrates of the same system.
b. Inhibitors result in decreased metabolism of substrates of the same system.

- Oral
  - *Capsules:* Administer the daily dose as 2 equally divided doses every 12 hours at consistent times with or without meals.
  - *Oral solution:* Administer the daily dose as 2 equally divided doses every 12 hours with meals. The solution may be diluted with chocolate milk or orange juice in a glass container. Additional diluent should be used to rinse the container to ensure administration of the total dose.

Drug–drug interactions

The drug is metabolized primarily via cytochrome P450 (CYP450) 3A isoenzymes. Substances known to alter functionality of these enzymes will alter bioavailability and elimination of this drug (Table 42-1). Drug interactions lead to altered exposure of other drugs by cyclosporine (Table 42-2).

TABLE 42-2. Select Drug Interactions Leading to Altered Exposure of Other Drugs by Cyclosporine[a]

Mechanism	Drug	Comment
CYP450 3A4 enzyme substrates	HMG-CoA reductase inhibitors: **lovastatin, simvastatin, atorvastatin**	Co-administration of these agents with CsA results in significant increases in HMG-CoA reductase inhibitor exposure and may place patients at increased risk of rhabdomyolysis.
CYP450 3A4 enzyme substrates	Sirolimus	Simultaneous administration increases C_{max} and area under the curve of sirolimus by 120% to 500% and 140% to 230%, respectively; administration 4 hours apart increases C_{max} and area under the curve of sirolimus by 30% to 40% and 35% to 80%, respectively.
Alteration in enterohepatic recycling	Mycophenolate mofetil	CsA co-administration inhibits MPAG excretion via hepatocytes, thus interfering with MPA enterohepatic recycling and leading to reduced exposure of the active metabolite, MPA.

Boldface indicates one of top 100 drugs for 2020 by prescription volume.
CsA, cyclosporine A; HMG-CoA, 3-hydroxy-3-methyglutaryl coenzyme A; MPA, mycophenolic acid; MPAG, phenolic glucuronide of MPA.

Drug–disease interactions

- **Altered biliary flow:** Diversion of biliary flow can significantly reduce adsorption. This more profoundly affects nonmodified cyclosporine than it does modified cyclosporine.
- **Diabetes mellitus:** Administration may worsen glycemic control in patients with preexisting diabetes.

Adverse drug effects

- **Central nervous system (CNS):** Seizure, hallucinations, insomnia, tremor, paresthesias
- **Head, ears, eyes, nose, and throat (HEENT):** Gingival hyperplasia
- **Cardiovascular (CV):** Hypertension
- **Gastrointestinal (GI):** Hepatotoxicity
- **Renal:** Nephrotoxicity
- **Endocrine and metabolic:** Hyperlipidemia, hyperuricemia, hyperkalemia, hypomagnesemia, new onset diabetes after transplant
- **Dermatologic:** Hirsutism, hypertrichosis, acne

Patient instructions

- Keep cyclosporine stored in its original container.
- Take the prescribed dose twice daily at consistent times with or without meals.
- After the monitoring is complete, take your morning medication immediately and then return to your original medication schedule.

Monitoring

- **C_0 (trough):** Goals depend on multifactorial risk assessment and assay type.
- **C2 (concentration 2 hours after dose):** Goals depend on multifactorial risk assessment and assay type.

Pharmacokinetics

- **Cyclosporine (nonmodified):** Highly lipoprotein bound
  - **Bioavailability:** Significant intra- and interpatient variability
  - **Mean bioavailability:** F = 30%, range 10% to 89%
  - **Elimination:** Half-life = 19 hours; range 10 to 27 hours (increased with hepatic dysfunction)
- **Cyclosporine (modified):** Highly lipoprotein bound
  - **Bioavailability:** Improved and more consistent absorption (23% to 50% greater than nonmodified formulation)
  - **Elimination:** Half-life = 8 hours; range 5 to 18 hours (increased with hepatic dysfunction)

Tacrolimus ⚠

Generic name	Trade name	Dosage form	Dose
Tacrolimus	Prograf	Injection: 5 mg ampules; capsules: 0.5, 1, 5 mg	Intravenous: 0.03 to 0.05 mg/kg/d as continuous infusion; oral: 0.1 to 0.2 mg/kg/d divided every 12 hours; adjusted to desired trough concentration
Tacrolimus–extended release	Astagraf XL	Capsules: 0.5, 1, 5 mg	Oral: 0.1 to 0.2 mg/kg/d every 12 hours; adjusted to desired trough concentration
	Envarsus XR	Tablets: 0.75, 1, 4 mg	Oral: 0.14 mg/kg/d every 24 hours; adjusted to desired trough concentration

Mechanism of action

Tacrolimus inhibits translocation of the cytosolic subunit of NFAT, the promoter gene for IL-2, into the nucleus via its binding with the protein FK506 binding protein (FKBP)–12 and a calcium-calmodulin-calcineurin complex, thereby inhibiting transcription and synthesis of IL-2.

Tacrolimus *FDA BOXED WARNING*

Increased risk of lymphoma and other malignancies. Increased susceptibility to bacterial, viral, fungal, and protozoal infections. Should only be prescribed by physicians experienced in immunosuppressive therapies.

Administration

- **Intravenous:** Dilute in NS or D5W to a concentration between 0.004 and 0.02 mg/mL, and administer as a continuous infusion via a container and tubing free of PVC (polyvinylchloride).
- **Oral:** Administer immediate-release product in 2 equally divided doses orally every 12 hours consistently, with or without food. Administer extended-release product orally once every 24 hours consistently, with or without food.

Drug–drug interactions

Because tacrolimus is metabolized primarily via CYP450 3A isoenzymes, substances known to alter functionality of these enzymes will alter bioavailability and elimination of this drug (Table 42-1).

Drug–disease interactions

- **Diabetes:** Administration worsens glycemic control in patients with preexisting diabetes.
- **Liver transplantation:** The extended-release formulation (Astagraf XL) has been associated with an increased risk of mortality in female liver transplant recipients.

Adverse drug effects

- **CNS:** Seizure, hallucinations, insomnia, tremor, depression, psychosis, anorexia
- **HEENT:** Alopecia
- **CV:** Hypertension, QT prolongation
- **GI:** Hepatotoxicity
- **Renal:** Nephrotoxicity
- **Endocrine and metabolic:** Hyperlipidemia, hyperkalemia, hypercalcemia, hypomagnesemia, hypophosphatemia, new onset diabetes after transplant
- **Hematologic:** Anemia
- **Other:** Malignancies, infection

Patient instructions

- Take the prescribed dose at a consistent time once or twice daily (extended-release or immediate-release formulations), with or without food, but always in the same way to maintain consistency.
- After the monitoring is complete, take your morning medication immediately and then return to your original medication schedule.

Monitoring

Monitor C_0. Goals depend on multifactorial risk assessment (in general, 5 to 15 ng/mL).

Pharmacokinetics

- **Tacrolimus:** Highly protein bound
- **Bioavailability:** F = 17% to 31%; ~50% greater for extended release formulation
- **Elimination:** Half-life = 8.7 to 37.9 hours (increased with hepatic dysfunction); ~37 hours for extended-release formulation

mTOR Inhibitors

Everolimus ⚠

Generic name	Trade name	Dosage form	Dose
Everolimus	Zortress	Tablets: 0.25, 0.5, and 0.75 mg	0.75 mg every 12 hours in combination with basiliximab induction, reduced dose cyclosporine, and corticosteroids adjusted to achieve desired trough level (3 to 8 ng/mL)

Mechanism of action

Everolimus binds to FKBP-12 to form a complex that binds and inhibits activation of its target protein, mTOR, a kinase that is critical in IL-2–mediated cell-cycle progression.

Administration

- Administer every 12 hours at the same time consistently with or without food.

Drug–drug interactions

Because everolimus is metabolized primarily via CYP450 3A isoenzymes, substances known to alter functionality of these enzymes will alter bioavailability and elimination of this drug (Table 42-1).

Additionally, the pharmacokinetic profile of everolimus is significantly altered by concomitant cyclosporine (Table 42-2).

Drug–disease interactions

- **Kidney transplantation:** Everolimus is associated with arterial and venous thrombosis of the kidney allograft and may cause proteinuria.
- **Heart transplantation:** Everolimus is associated with increased mortality when used within 3 months posttransplant.
- **Angioedema:** Everolimus has been associated with angioedema.
- **Edema:** Everolimus has been associated with peripheral edema and pleural and pericardial effusions.
- **Infertility:** Everolimus has been associated with male infertility.
- **Hepatic artery thrombosis:** mTOR inhibitors have been associated with hepatic artery thrombosis within 30 days posttransplant.
- **Hyperlipidemia:** Everolimus increases triglycerides and cholesterol.

Adverse drug effects

- **CNS:** Fatigue, headache
- **HEENT:** Oral ulcers
- **GI:** Anorexia, constipation, diarrhea, nausea
- **Renal:** Synergistic nephrotoxicity with calcineurin inhibitors, proteinuria
- **Endocrine and metabolic:** Hyperlipidemia, hypertension, hyperkalemia

 Everolimus *FDA BOXED WARNING*

Increased risk of lymphoma and other malignancies. Increased susceptibility to bacterial, viral, fungal, and protozoal infections. Increased risk of kidney arterial and venous thrombosis. Increased nephrotoxicity if used in combination with cyclosporine. Use is not recommended in heart transplantations due to increased risk of mortality. Should only be prescribed by physicians experienced in immunosuppressive therapies.

- **Dermatologic:** Rash, acne
- **Hematologic:** Anemia, leukopenia, thrombocytopenia, pancytopenia, thrombosis
- **Other:** Lymphocele, pneumonitis

Patient instructions

- Take the prescribed dose at a consistent time twice daily, with or without food.
- After the monitoring is complete, take morning medication immediately and then return to original medication schedule.

Monitoring

Monitor C_0. Goal depends on multifactorial risk assessment and assay type (in general, 3 to 8 ng/mL).

Pharmacokinetics

- **Bioavailability:** F = 30%
- **Elimination:** Half-life = 30 hours (increased with hepatic dysfunction)

Sirolimus ⚠

Generic name	Trade name	Dosage form	Dose
Sirolimus	Rapamune	Oral solution: 1 mg/mL; tablets: 0.5, 1, 2 mg tablets: 0.25, 0.5, and 0.75 mg	Initial: adults: 6 to 15 mg orally; pediatrics: ≥13 years of age and <40 kg, 3 mg/m²; ≥13 years of age and >40 kg, 6 mg orally Maintenance: adults: 2 to 5 mg orally daily; adjusted to desired trough concentration; pediatrics: ≥13 years of age and <40 kg, 1 mg/m² orally daily; ≥13 years of age and >40 kg, 2 mg orally daily

Mechanism of action

Sirolimus binds to FKBP-12 to form a complex that binds and inhibits activation of its target protein, mTOR, a kinase that is critical in IL-2-mediated cell-cycle progression.

Administration

- With tablets, administer by mouth every 24 hours consistently with or without food.
- With oral solution, mix the dose in 60 mL of water or orange juice, stir vigorously, and drink at once. Then refill container with 120 mL of water or orange juice, stir vigorously, and drink.

Drug–drug interactions

Because sirolimus is metabolized primarily via CYP450 3A isoenzymes, substances known to alter functionality of these enzymes will alter bioavailability and elimination of this drug (Table 42-1).

Additionally, the pharmacokinetic profile of sirolimus is significantly altered by concomitant cyclosporine (Table 42-2).

 Sirolimus *FDA BOXED WARNING*

Increased risk of infection. Increased risk of lymphoma. Use is not recommended in liver or lung transplants due to increased mortality.

Drug–disease interactions
- **Edema:** Sirolimus has been associated with peripheral edema and pleural and pericardial effusions.
- **Hyperlipidemia:** Sirolimus increases levels of triglycerides and cholesterol.
- **Kidney transplantation:** Sirolimus may delay recovery of graft function posttransplant and is associated with increased urinary protein excretion after conversion from calcineurin inhibitors.
- **Liver transplantation:** Sirolimus is associated with increased incidence of mortality, graft loss, and hepatic artery thrombosis in de novo liver transplant recipients.
- **Lung transplantation:** There have been cases of fatal bronchial anastomotic dehiscence in de novo lung transplant recipients.

Adverse drug effects
- **CNS:** Anorexia
- **HEENT:** Oral ulcers
- **GI:** Diarrhea, esophagitis, gastritis, gastroenteritis, hepatotoxicity, hepatic artery thrombosis in de novo liver transplant recipients
- **Renal:** Synergistic nephrotoxicity with calcineurin inhibitors, proteinuria
- **Endocrine and metabolic:** Hyperlipidemia, hypertension, hyperkalemia
- **Dermatologic:** Rash, acne
- **Hematologic:** Leukopenia, thrombocytopenia, pancytopenia, thrombosis
- **Other:** Arthralgia, lymphocele, pneumonitis, bronchial anastomotic dehiscence in de novo lung transplant recipients

Patient instructions
- Take the prescribed dose at a consistent time once daily, with or without food, but in the same way to maintain consistency.
- After the monitoring is complete, take your morning medication immediately and then return to your original medication schedule.

Monitoring
Monitor C_0. Goal depends on multifactorial risk assessment and assay type (in general, 5 to 15 ng/mL).

Pharmacokinetics
- **Bioavailability:** F = 14% (oral solution), 27% greater for tablets
- **Elimination:** Half-life = 61 to 71 hours (increased with hepatic dysfunction)

Selective T-Cell Costimulation Blocker

Belatacept ⚠

Generic name	Trade name	Dosage form	Dose
Belatacept	Nulojix	Injection: 250 mg vials	Initial: 10 mg/kg I.V. on day 1 (day of transplant, before transplantation), day 5, and end of weeks 2, 4, 8, and 12
			Maintenance: 5 mg/kg end of week 16 and every 4 weeks thereafter given in combination with basiliximab induction, mycophenolate mofetil, and corticosteroids

Mechanism of action
Belatacept binds to costimulation proteins CD80 and CD86 on the APC to prevent binding to the T-cell proteins (i.e., CD28) necessary for activation of the T-cell.

Belatacept *FDA BOXED WARNING*

Increased risk of infection and malignancies. Increased risk of developing post-transplant lymphoproliferative disorder. Should only be prescribed by physicians who have experience with patients with kidney transplants and immunosuppressive therapies. Use in liver transplant patients is not recommended due to increased mortality.

Administration

Intravenous: Reconstitute contents with 10.5 mL of sterile water for injection, NS, or D5W. Calculate total volume of reconstituted solution necessary for prescribed dose. The reconstituted solution is diluted with NS or D5W to a final concentration of 2 to 10 mg/mL Administer peripherally or centrally over 30 minutes with a 0.1 to 1.2 μm low-protein-binding filter.

Drug–drug interactions

Avoid administration of belatacept within 12 hours of an equine or rabbit antithymocyte globulin infusion.

Drug–disease interactions

- *Liver transplantation:* In a clinical trial with more frequent administration than noted above, belatacept was associated with increased graft loss and mortality.
- *Posttransplant lymphoproliferative disease (PTLD):* Belatacept is associated with an increased risk of PTLD involving the central nervous system and, thus, is avoided in patients that are seronegative for Epstein-Barr virus or have unknown status.
- *Tuberculosis:* An increased incidence of tuberculosis has been reported with belatacept; thus, patients should be evaluated for latent tuberculosis infection before administering belatacept.

Adverse drug effects

- *CNS:* Headache, insomnia, anxiety, PTLD
- *CV:* Hypertension
- *GI:* Diarrhea, constipation, nausea, vomiting, abdominal pain
- *Hematologic:* Anemia, leukopenia
- *Renal:* Hematuria, proteinuria, dysuria
- *Endocrine and metabolic:* Hypocalcemia, hypo- or hyperkalemia, hypophosphatemia, dyslipidemia, hyperglycemia
- *Dermatologic:* Acne
- *Other:* Urinary tract infection, peripheral edema, upper respiratory infection, progressive multi-focal leukoencephalopathy, polyomavirus nephropathy

Patient instructions

Report any adverse drug effects to a health care provider immediately.

Monitoring

Patients should be monitored closely for signs and symptoms of infection or PTLD (i.e., behavioral changes).

Pharmacokinetics

- *Dosing:* Based on actual body weight
- *Linear pharmacokinetics:* First-order elimination
- *Elimination:* Half-life = ~ 10 days

Antiproliferative Agents

Azathioprine ⚠

Generic name	Trade name	Dosage form	Dose
Azathioprine	Imuran	Injection: 100 mg vials; tablets: 50 mg	Initial: 3 to 5 mg/kg I.V. or orally
			Maintenance: 1 to 3 mg/kg I.V. or orally daily

Mechanism of action

Azathioprine is a purine analogue prodrug, which is cleaved to 6-mercaptopurine; 6-mercaptopurine is activated intracellularly to several active metabolites, which can be incorporated directly into deoxyribonucleic acid (DNA) and inhibit further replication.

Administration

- **Intravenous:** Dilute dose in NS or D5W, and administer I.V. infusion over 30 to 60 minutes.
- **Oral:** Administer oral dose once a day.

Drug–drug interactions

Xanthine oxidase is responsible for the elimination of the active metabolites of azathioprine. Concomitant use of **allopurinol** with azathioprine results in significantly increased azathioprine-induced toxicity. Reduce dose of azathioprine by 65% to 75%. Avoid concurrent use with febuxostat.

Drug–disease interactions

- **Renal insufficiency:** Bioavailability is significantly reduced in uremic patients.
- **Thiopurine S-methyltransferase (TPMT) deficiency:** Increased risk of toxicity occurs, and substantial dose reduction may be necessary.

Adverse drug effects

- **HEENT:** Retinopathy
- **GI:** Nausea, vomiting, diarrhea, anorexia, pancreatitis, hepatotoxicity
- **Dermatologic:** Rash, skin cancer
- **Hematologic:** Leukopenia, thrombocytopenia, pancytopenia

Patient instructions

Take the prescribed dose at a consistent time once daily, with or without food.

Monitoring

Pharmacokinetic monitoring is not required.

Pharmacokinetics

- **Bioavailability:** F ≥ 47%
- **Elimination:** half-life 5 to 8 hours

 Azathioprine *FDA BOXED WARNING*

Increased risk of malignancy.

Mycophenolate mofetil ⚠

Generic name	Trade name	Dosage form	Dose
Mycophenolate mofetil	Cellcept	Injection: 500 mg vials; oral suspension: 200 mg/mL; capsules: 250 mg; tablets: 500 mg	Initial and maintenance: adults: 2 to 3 g/d divided every 8 to 12 hours I.V. or orally; pediatrics: ≥3 months of age, 600 mg/m^2 oral suspension twice daily (maximum dose of 2 g/d); if BSA = 1.25 to 1.5 m^2, 750 mg twice daily; if BSA > 1.5 m^2, 1000 mg twice daily

Mechanism of action

Mycophenolate mofetil is metabolized to mycophenolic acid (MPA), which causes noncompetitive, reversible inhibition of inosine monophosphate dehydrogenase, a critical enzyme in the de novo pathway of purine synthesis, which results in the inhibition of B- and T-lymphocyte proliferation.

Administration

- **Intravenous:** Dilute in D5W to a concentration of 6 mg/mL, and infuse over at least 2 hours.
- **Oral:** Administer as equally divided oral doses every 8 to 12 hours consistently with or without food.

Drug–drug interactions

- **Cyclosporine:** See Table 42-2.
- **Cholestyramine:** Because of the interruption of enterohepatic recirculation, administration can decrease MPA exposure.
- **Colestipol and colesevelam:** Simultaneous administration can decrease MPA exposure.
- **Antacids:** Simultaneous administration with magnesium- or aluminum-containing antacids reduces absorption and decreases MPA exposure.

Note: Efficacy of oral contraceptives may decrease with therapy. Additional birth control methods are recommended.

Drug–disease interactions

- **Pregnancy:** Mycophenolate has been shown to increase risks of first trimester birth loss and congenital malformations. Provide counseling on a risk evaluation mitigation strategy before dispensing to patients of childbearing age. Abstinence or contraception must be used during as well as 6 weeks after discontinuation.
- **Severe renal impairment:** Mycophenolate mofetil reduces protein binding of MPA.

Adverse drug effects

- **GI:** Nausea, vomiting, diarrhea, abdominal pain
- **Hematologic:** Leukopenia, thrombocytopenia, anemia, pancytopenia

Patient instructions

- Take the prescribed dose at consistent times during the day, with or without food.
- Do not take the medication before therapeutic drug monitoring (if necessary).

 Mycophenolate mofetil *FDA BOXED WARNING*

Increased risk of first trimester pregnancy loss and congenital malformations if used during pregnancy. Increased risk of lymphoma and other malignancies. Increased risk of bacterial, viral, fungal, and protozoa infections.

Monitoring

Pharmacokinetic monitoring is not required.

Pharmacokinetics

- **MPA:** Highly protein bound
- **Bioavailability:** F = 94%
- **Elimination:** Half-life = 16 to 18 hours

Mycophenolate sodium ⚠

Generic name	Trade name	Dosage form	Dose
Mycophenolate sodium	Myfortic	Tablets: 180, 360 mg	Initial and maintenance: adults: 720 mg orally every 12 hours; pediatrics: 400 mg/m² orally every 12 hours (maximum dose of 720 mg orally every 12 hours); if BSA = 1.19 to 1.58 m², 540 mg orally twice daily (1080 mg daily); if BSA < 1.19 m², cannot be accurately administered

BSA, body surface area.

Mechanism of action

Delayed-release tablets deliver MPA, which causes noncompetitive, reversible inhibition of inosine mono-phosphate dehydrogenase, a critical enzyme in the de novo pathway of purine synthesis, which results in the inhibition of B- and T-lymphocyte proliferation.

Administration

Administer as equally divided doses by mouth every 12 hours consistently with or without food.

Drug–drug interactions

- **Cholestyramine:** Administration interrupts enterohepatic recirculation and decreases MPA exposure.
- **Antacids:** Simultaneous administration with magnesium- or aluminum-containing antacids reduces absorption and decreases MPA exposure.

Note: Efficacy of oral contraceptives may decrease with therapy. Additional birth control methods are recommended.

Drug–disease interactions

- **Pregnancy:** Mycophenolate has been shown to increase risks of first trimester birth loss and congenital malformations. Provide counseling on a risk evaluation mitigation strategy before dispensing to patients of childbearing age.
- **Severe renal impairment:** Reduced protein binding of MPA leads to increased exposure, and dose reduction may be necessary.

Adverse drug effects

- **GI:** Nausea, vomiting, diarrhea, abdominal pain
- **Hematologic:** Leukopenia, thrombocytopenia, anemia, pancytopenia

---

 Mycophenolate sodium *FDA BOXED WARNING*

Increased risk of first trimester pregnancy loss and congenital malformations if used during pregnancy. Increased risk of lymphoma and other malignancies. Increased risk of bacterial, viral, fungal, and protozoal infections.

Patient instructions

- Take the prescribed dose with or without food at consistent times during the day.
- Do not take the medication before therapeutic drug monitoring (if necessary).

Monitoring

Pharmacokinetic monitoring is not required.

Pharmacokinetics

- **MPA:** Highly protein bound
- **Bioavailability:** F = 72% to 92%
- **Elimination:** Half-life = 8 to 16 hours

Corticosteroids

Selection of agent

Selection of the corticosteroid used is based on the ratio of glucocorticoid to mineralocorticoid potency. Common I.V. agents are methylprednisolone and dexamethasone. Common oral agents are **prednisone**, prednisolone, and dexamethasone.

Mechanism of action

Corticosteroids bind to cytosolic glucocorticoid receptors, which translocate to the nucleus, where the complexes bind to regulatory DNA sequences, glucocorticoid-responsive elements within the promoter section of various genes. Activation of these glucocorticoid-responsive elements modifies activities of promoter genes such as NFAT, AP-1, and NF-κB, which results in downregulation of expression of HLA and numerous cell adhesion molecules, as well as decreased synthesis of numerous lymphokines responsible for activation, proliferation, and migration (i.e., IL-1, IL-2, IL-6, IL-8, IFN-γ, TNF-α).

Administration

Administration depends on the individual agent.

Drug–drug interactions

Because corticosteroids are metabolized primarily via CYP450 3A isoenzymes, substances known to alter functionality of these enzymes will alter bioavailability and elimination of these drugs (Table 42-1).

Drug–disease interactions

- **Diabetes:** Administration worsens glycemic control in patients with preexisting diabetes.
- **Osteopenia and osteoporosis:** Administration alters calcium and phosphate absorption and excretion, as well as osteoblast activity, resulting in progression of bone loss that is common in metabolic diseases such as end-stage kidney disease and liver failure.

Adverse drug effects

The incidence and extent of most adverse drug effects with corticosteroids depend on the ratio of glucocorticoid to mineralocorticoid potency. Adverse drug effects include the following:

- **CNS:** Seizure, psychosis, delirium, hallucinations, mood swings, insomnia, pseudotumor cerebri
- **HEENT:** Cataracts, glaucoma
- **CV:** Hypertension, cardiomyopathy

- **GI:** Increased appetite, gastroesophageal reflux disease, peptic ulcer disease, pancreatitis
- **Renal:** Edema, alkalosis, hyperkalemia
- **Endocrine and metabolic:** Hyperlipidemia, hypothalamic-pituitary-adrenal axis suppression, growth suppression, new onset diabetes after transplant
- **Dermatologic:** Hirsutism, acne, skin atrophy, impaired wound healing
- **Hematologic:** Transient leukocytosis
- **Musculoskeletal:** Arthralgia, myopathy, osteoporosis, avascular necrosis

Patient instructions
When taking orally, take daily dose in the morning with food.

Monitoring
Pharmacokinetic monitoring is not required.

Pharmacokinetics
Pharmacokinetics depend on the individual agent.

Monoclonal Antibodies

Basiliximab ⚠

Generic name	Trade name	Dosage form	Dose
Basiliximab	Simulect	Injection: 10, 20 mg vials	Induction: adults and pediatrics >35 kg: 20 mg I.V. on day 0 and day 4; pediatrics <35 kg: 10 mg I.V. on day 0 and day 4

Mechanism of action
Chimeric (murine or human), monoclonal immunoglobulin G (IgG) specifically binds to the subunit, CD25, of the IL-2 receptor, which is expressed on activated lymphocytes resulting in the competitive inhibition of IL-2 and subsequent elimination of activated lymphocytes.

Administration
Dilute to a concentration of 0.4 mg/mL in NS or D5W. Administer peripherally or centrally as a bolus or continuous infusion over 20 to 30 minutes.

Drug–drug and drug–disease interactions
No clinically significant drug–drug or drug–disease interactions occur.

Adverse drug effects
Severe acute hypersensitivity, including anaphylaxis, may occur within the 24 hours following administration of the initial dose or on repeat exposure.

 Basiliximab *FDA BOXED WARNING*

Should only be prescribed by physicians experienced in immunosuppression therapy and management of organ transplantation patients.

Patient instructions

Report any shortness of breath, palpitations, light-headedness, or itching to a health care provider immediately.

Monitoring

Pharmacokinetic monitoring is not required.

Pharmacokinetics

- **Adults** (following a 20 mg I.V. infusion over 20 minutes)**:**
  - Mean $C_{max} = 7.1 \pm 5.1$ mg/L
  - Mean half-life $= 7.2 \pm 3.2$ days
- **Children:** Mean half-life $= 11.5 \pm 6.3$ days

Pharmacodynamics

- **Adults:** CD25 saturation is at or above serum concentration of 0.2 mcg/mL. Mean duration of saturation depends on concomitant immunosuppressive regimen.
- **Children:** CD25 saturation is similar to that seen in adults.

Polyclonal Antibodies

Antithymocyte globulin (equine) ⚠

Generic name	Trade name	Dosage form	Dose
Antithymocyte globulin (equine)	ATGAM	Injection: 50 mg vials	Induction: 10 to 15 mg/kg I.V. daily × 14 days; acute rejection: 15 mg/kg I.V. once daily × 14 days, then every other day if necessary for a total of 21 doses

Mechanism of action

This antithymocyte globulin is purified, sterile, polyclonal IgG harvested from horses immunized with human thymocytes. The preparation includes IgG directed against multiple cell surface markers, targeting multiple phases of immunity, including T-cell activation.

Administration

- Premedication:
  - **Dose 1:** Giving I.V. steroids, **acetaminophen**, and antihistamines 1 hour before the dose is strongly recommended to modify first-dose reactions.
  - **Subsequent doses:** Give **acetaminophen** and antihistamines 30 to 60 minutes before the dose. Steroids may be necessary if infusion reactions occur.
- Dosing:
  - Dilute the dose to a concentration not to exceed 4 mg/mL in ½ NS or D5W.
  - Administer centrally over 4 to 6 hours.

Drug–drug and drug–disease interactions

No clinically significant drug–drug or drug–disease interactions occur.

 Antithymocyte globulin (equine) *FDA BOXED WARNING*

Should only be prescribed by physicians experienced in immunosuppression therapy and management of organ transplantation patients.

Adverse drug effects

Most adverse drug effects with antithymocyte globulin (equine) are infusion-related reactions (i.e., fever, chills, dyspnea); leukopenia; thrombocytopenia; or rash.

Patient instructions

Report any shortness of breath, palpitations, light-headedness, tremor, fever, or itching to a health care provider immediately.

Monitoring

The goal for treatment of acute rejection is suppression of CD3 lineage to <50 cells/mm³.

Pharmacokinetics

For elimination, half-life = ~5.7 days.

Antithymocyte globulin (rabbit) ⚠

Generic name	Trade name	Dosage form	Dose
Antithymocyte globulin (rabbit)	Thymoglobulin	Injection: 25 mg vials	Induction: 1.5 mg/kg I.V. once daily × 3 to 7 days; acute rejection: 1.5 mg/kg I.V. once daily × 7 to 14 days

Mechanism of action

This antithymocyte globulin is purified, pasteurized, polyclonal IgG harvested from pathogen-free rabbits immunized with human thymocytes. This preparation includes IgG directed against multiple cell surface markers, targeting multiple phases of immunity, including T-cell activation.

Administration

- Premedication:
  - *Dose 1:* Giving I.V. steroids, **acetaminophen**, and antihistamines 1 hour before the dose is strongly recommended to modify first-dose reactions.
  - *Subsequent doses:* Give **acetaminophen** and antihistamines 30 to 60 minutes before the dose and steroids as needed for infusion reactions.
- Dose:
  - Dilute dose to a concentration of 0.5 mg/mL in NS or D5W.
  - Administer centrally over 4 to 6 hours through 0.22-micron in-line filter.

Drug–drug and drug–disease interactions

No clinically significant drug–drug or drug–disease interactions occur.

Adverse drug effects

Most adverse drug effects with antithymocyte globulin (rabbit) are infusion-related reactions (i.e., fever, chills, dyspnea); leukopenia; thrombocytopenia; or rash.

 Antithymocyte globulin (rabbit) *FDA BOXED WARNING*

Should only be prescribed by physicians experienced in immunosuppression therapy and management of organ transplantation patients.

Patient instructions

Report any shortness of breath, palpitations, light-headedness, tremor, fever, or itching to a health care provider immediately.

Monitoring

The goal for treatment of acute rejection is suppression of CD3 lineage to <50 cells/mm³.

Pharmacokinetics

A 2-compartment model is used. For terminal elimination, half-life = 2 to 3 days for first dose; range = 14 to 45 days with multiple doses.

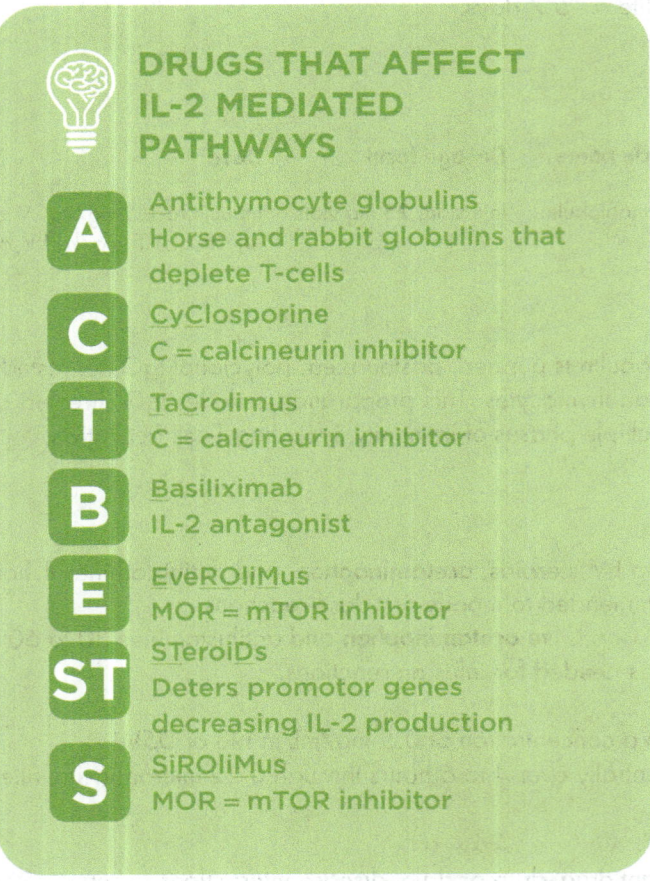

DRUGS THAT AFFECT IL-2 MEDIATED PATHWAYS

A Antithymocyte globulins
Horse and rabbit globulins that deplete T-cells

C CyClosporine
C = calcineurin inhibitor

T TaCrolimus
C = calcineurin inhibitor

B Basiliximab
IL-2 antagonist

E EveROliMus
MOR = mTOR inhibitor

ST STeroiDs
Deters promotor genes decreasing IL-2 production

S SiROliMus
MOR = mTOR inhibitor

42-5 Pharmacist's Role

Transplant pharmacists are integral members of the transplant team. As a result, transplant centers are required by the United Network for Organ Sharing (UNOS) and Center for Medicare and Medicaid Services (CMS) to document participation of a transplant pharmacist on multidisciplinary patient rounds. Clinical responsibilities occur among multiple phases of the transplant process, which include pretransplant, perioperative, and posttransplant. Some of the duties of a transplant pharmacist may include the following: assessment of pharmacologic and nonpharmacologic consideration and medication adherence

DRUGS THAT ARE INDICATED FOR MAINTENANCE IMMUNOSUPPRESSION

M Mycophenolate mofetil and MycoPhenolate soDium
IMPD = inhibits ionosine monophosphate dehydrogenase affecting B and T cell production

C CyClosporine
C = calcineurin inhibitor

B BelataCept
CB = costimulatory blocker

E EveROliMus
MOR = mTOR inhibitor

A AzathioPrine
PA = purine analog that inhibits DNA synthesis

T TaCrolimus
C = calcineurin inhibitor

ST STeroiDs
Deters promotor genes decreasing IL-2 production

S SiROliMus
MOR = mTOR inhibitor

for transplant candidates, assisting with the development and implementation of protocols, and providing drug information and recommendations for medication selection, dosing, and monitoring.

In summary, a transplant pharmacist has a vast range of responsibilities and challenges to fulfill for each stage of the transplant process. Currently, a pharmacy practice residency (PGY1) and a specialized transplant pharmacy practice residency (PGY2) is recommended for the opportunity to practice as a transplant pharmacist.

NAPLEX Competency Statements

The questions in this chapter cover the following 2021 NAPLEX Competency Statements: **AREA 1:** 1.1; 1.6 **AREA 2:** 2.1; 2.2 **AREA 3:** 3.2; 3.4; 3.5; 3.6; 3.7; 3.8.

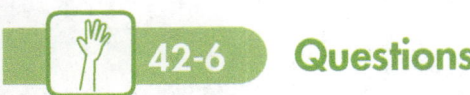

42-6   Questions

Please use the following patient profile for the Questions 1 to 4:

PATIENT PROFILE

Patient Name: Maxwell House

Age: 52

Sex: Male   **Ethnicity:** White

PMH: type 2 diabetes, s/p kidney transplant last month

SHx: Never smoker, No EtOH

FHx: Noncontributory

Height: 5'9"

Weight: 185 lb

Allergies: NKDA

Current medications:
Tacrolimus 3 mg orally twice daily
Mycophenolate mofetil 500 mg orally twice daily
Azathioprine 50 mg orally daily
Prednisone 5 mg orally daily
Dapsone 50 mg orally daily
Valganciclovir 450 mg orally daily
Fluconazole 200 mg orally daily
Glimepiride 2 mg orally daily
Enteric coated aspirin 81 mg orally daily

Vital signs:
BP 135/80 mmHg
Pulse 80 bpm

Labs:
HbA1c 6.4%
K 5.6, BUN 15, Scr 1, FBG 110

---

1. After your medication interview, you discovered that the patient was allergic to sulfonamides and developed a severe rash with hives. Which of the following medications should be given with caution after transplant because of the patient's sulfonamide allergy?

A. Furosemide
B. Fluconazole
C. Azathioprine
D. Valganciclovir
E. Tacrolimus

2. Which of the following combinations of drugs from the medication profile represents a therapeutic duplication?

A. Tacrolimus and azathioprine
B. Azathioprine and mycophenolate mofetil
C. Dapsone and valganciclovir
D. Glimepiride and tacrolimus
E. Prednisone and mycophenolate mofetil

3. Which of the following combinations of drugs from the medication profile interact?

A. Fluconazole and tacrolimus
B. Fluconazole and valganciclovir
C. Dapsone and furosemide
D. Valcyte and prednisone
E. Valganciclovir and ECASA

4. Which medication from the profile may be associated with drug-induced hyperkalemia?

A. Mycophenolate mofetil
B. Furosemide
C. Prednisone
D. Tacrolimus
E. Aspirin

5. Which of the following medications is classified as a calcineurin inhibitor?

A. Sirolimus
B. Everolimus
C. Belatacept
D. Azathioprine
E. Cyclosporine

6. Which of the following medications may cause myelosuppression? (Mark all that apply.)

A. Sirolimus
B. Mycophenolate mofetil
C. Prednisone
D. Cyclosporine
E. Basiliximab

7. Which of the following medications requires bile for emulsification and absorption?

A. Azathioprine
B. Cyclosporine
C. Tacrolimus
D. Prednisone
E. All of the above

8. Which of the following are known adverse effects of cyclosporine? (Mark all that apply.)

A. Hirsutism
B. Nephrotoxicity
C. Oral ulceration
D. Gingival hyperplasia
E. Hyperlipidemia

9. Which of the following are contraindications or precautions associated with sirolimus? (Mark all that apply.)

A. De novo lung transplant recipient
B. Hyperlipidemia
C. Diabetes mellitus
D. De novo liver transplant recipient
E. Hypertension

10. What is the generic name for Imuran?

A. Mycophenolate mofetil
B. Azathioprine
C. Cyclosporine
D. Tacrolimus
E. Prednisone

11. Which of the following immunosuppressive medications may cause new onset diabetes after transplant?

A. Antithymocyte globulin (equine)
B. Azathioprine
C. Mycophenolate mofetil
D. Basiliximab
E. Tacrolimus

12. Which of the following medications requires therapeutic drug monitoring via trough concentrations?

A. Belatacept
B. Tacrolimus
C. Daclizumab
D. Basiliximab
E. Azathioprine

13. Which of the following medications is a monoclonal antibody that inhibits signal 3 by binding to the CD25 subunit of the IL-2 receptor?

A. Antithymocyte globulin (rabbit)
B. Antithymocyte globulin (equine)
C. Basiliximab
D. Everolimus
E. Belatacept

14. Which of the following medications produces a significant pharmacokinetic interaction when administered with azathioprine?

A. Allopurinol
B. Fluconazole
C. Sirolimus
D. Probenecid
E. Tacrolimus

15. Which of the following conditions alters the pharmacokinetic profile of cyclosporine? (Mark all that apply.)

A. Biliary obstruction
B. Hyperglycemia
C. Obesity
D. Hepatotoxicity
E. End stage renal disease

16. Which of the following medications interacts with everolimus?

A. Erythromycin
B. Metoprolol
C. Furosemide
D. Nifedipine
E. Gentamicin

17. Which of the following immunosuppressants should *not* be administered at the same time secondary to an interaction related to timing of doses?

A. Tacrolimus and azathioprine
B. Sirolimus and cyclosporine
C. Cyclosporine and azathioprine
D. Sirolimus and tacrolimus
E. Sirolimus and mycophenolate mofetil

18. On binding of antigen displayed by the antigen-presenting cell to the T-cell receptor complex, what additional step is required for T-helper-cell activation?

A. Binding of the costimulatory pathway
B. Activation of the promoter gene NFAT
C. Transcription of the IL-2 gene
D. No additional step required
E. Translation of IL-2

19. According to the figure below, which cytokine released by activated CD4+ lymphocytes plays a major role in the subsequent activation of numerous lymphocyte lineages?

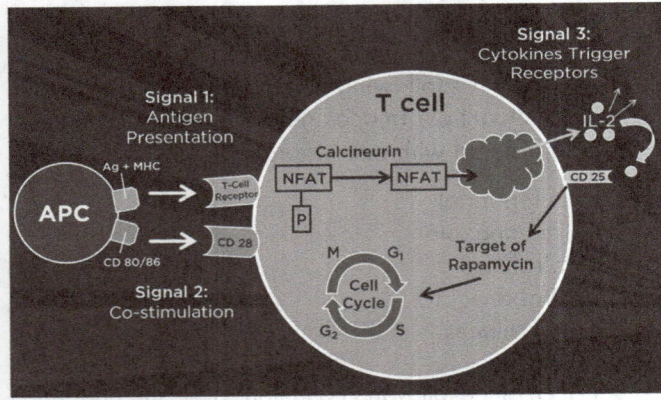

20. Which of the following medications should be avoided in female liver transplant recipients?

A. Tacrolimus extended release
B. Cyclosporine
C. Mycophenolate sodium
D. Azathioprine
E. Tacrolimus

21. Which of the following medications is a polyclonal antibody?

A. Belatacept
B. Basiliximab
C. Mycophenolate sodium
D. Antithymocyte globulin (rabbit)
E. Sirolimus

 **42-7** **Answers**

1. **A.** Furosemide (Lasix) is structurally similar to sulfonamides and would be expected to elicit a similar allergic response.

2. **B.** Both azathioprine (Imuran) and mycophenolate mofetil (CellCept) are classified as antiproliferative agents. Both agents inhibit purine biosynthesis and would not act synergistically.

3. **A.** Fluconazole (Diflucan) is an inhibitor of CYP450 3A isoenzymes, which is the enzyme system that is responsible for metabolism of tacrolimus.

4. **D.** Hyperkalemia (incidence 20% to 40%) is a well-documented adverse drug reaction with tacrolimus (Prograf).

5. **E.** Cyclosporine is a calcineurin inhibitor.

6. **A, B.** Sirolimus and mycophenolate mofetil can cause myelosuppression.

7. **B.** Cyclosporine is highly lipophilic and requires bile for emulsification and absorption.

8. **A, B, D, E.** Hirsutism, nephrotoxicity, gingival hyperplasia, and hyperlipidemia are known adverse effects of cyclosporine.

9. **A, B, D.** The use of sirolimus in de novo lung and liver transplant recipients is contraindicated because of an increased incidence of fatal adverse drug effects. Additionally, use of sirolimus in patients with uncontrolled hyperlipidemia is strongly discouraged because of its profound effects on lipid biosynthesis and catabolism.

10. **B.** Azathioprine is the generic name for Imuran.

11. **E.** Tacrolimus may cause new onset diabetes after transplant.

12. **B.** Tacrolimus requires therapeutic drug monitoring via trough concentrations to obtain desired therapeutic effects.

13. C. Basiliximab selects for destruction of activated lymphocytes by binding to the CD25 subunit of the high-affinity IL-2 receptor.

14. A. Xanthine oxidase is responsible for the elimination of the active metabolites of azathioprine. Concomitant use of allopurinol with azathioprine results in significantly increased azathioprine-induced toxicity. Reduce the dose of azathioprine by 65% to 75%.

15. A, D. Biliary obstruction and hepatotoxicity would change the pharmacokinetic profile of cyclosporine. Cyclosporine requires bile for emulsification and absorption. If bile flow is obstructed, then the bioavailability is significantly decreased. Additionally, cyclosporine is metabolized by enzymes in the liver, and changes in liver function may decrease elimination.

16. A. Erythromycin inhibits CYP450 3A isoenzymes, which is the enzyme system that is responsible for sirolimus metabolism.

17. B. Simultaneous administration of sirolimus and cyclosporine increases C_{max} and the area under the curve of sirolimus by 120% to 500% and 140% to 230%, respectively. Administration 4 hours apart increases C_{max} and the area under the curve of sirolimus by 30% to 40% and 35% to 80%, respectively.

18. A. Activation is dependent on antigen–HLA binding to the T-cell receptor complex and the subsequent binding of a second signal or "costimulatory pathway."

19. Active CD4+ T-cells produce and release various lymphokines, particularly IL-2, which is important for activation and proliferation of numerous lymphocyte lineages.

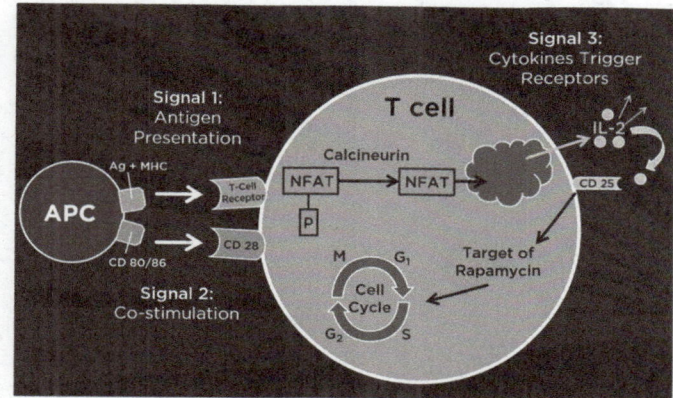

20. A. Tacrolimus extended release (Astagraf XL) is associated with increased mortality in female liver transplant recipients.

21. D. Antithymocyte globulin (rabbit) is a polyclonal antibody with an FDA-approved indication for prevention and treatment of acute rejection.

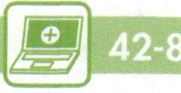 **42-8   Additional Resources**

Alloway RR, Dupuis R, Garbardi S, et al. Evolution of the role of the transplant pharmacist on the multidisciplinary transplant team. *Am J of Transpl.* 2011;11:1576–1583.

Costanzo MR, Dipchand A, Starling R, et al. The International Society of Heart and Lung Transplantation guidelines for the care of heart transplant recipients. *J Heart Lung Transplant.* 2010;29(8):914–956.

Kasiske BL, Zeier MG, Chapman JR, et al. KDIGO clinical practice guideline for the care of kidney transplant recipients: a summary. *Kidney Int.* 2010;77(4):299–311.

Lucey MR, Terrault N, Ojo L, et al. Long-term management of the successful adult liver transplant: 2012 Practice Guideline by the American Association for the Study of Liver Diseases and the American Society of Transplantation. *Liver Transpl.* 2013;19(1):3–26.

Maldonado A, Hall RC, Pilch NA, et al. ASHP guidelines on pharmacy services in solid organ transplantation. *Am J Health Syst Pharm.* 2020;77:222–232.

Nankivell BJ, Alexander SI. Rejection of kidney allograft. *N Engl J Med.* 2010;363:1451–1462.

Substance Misuse and Toxicology

43

BRIAN L. WINBIGLER   PETER A. CHYKA

43-1 KEY POINTS

- Medications are the most common cause of poisoning morbidity and mortality. Any chemical can become toxic if too much is taken in relation to body weight and physiologic capacity.
- Substance misuse often leads to acute and chronic toxicity from a variety of medications, commercial products, and illicit agents. The management of acute toxicity from substance misuse typically follows the same general approaches as those for poisoning and overdose. A challenge faced in many acute drug overdoses is determining the agents taken and possible adulterants or contaminants. Chronic misuse can lead to dependence, tolerance, withdrawal, and addiction.
- Substance use disorder is a maladaptive pattern of substance use leading to clinically significant impairment or distress within a 12-month period. It is a disease that typically starts with drug experimentation and escalates to physiologic, behavioral, and mental changes.
- A comprehensive treatment plan for substance use disorder involves a variety of approaches including medication-assisted therapy with long-term use of drug-substitution, -aversion, and -antagonist therapy.
- Several approaches can minimize the risk of unintentional childhood poisonings (e.g., use of safety latches, proper storage of poisonous substances, adherence to label instructions), but the proper use of child-resistant containers (safety caps) is one of the most effective means.
- Immediate first aid for a poison exposure can minimize potential toxic effects and involves water and fresh air, depending on the route of exposure. Contact a poison control center immediately through the nationwide access number (1-800-222-1222) to determine whether first aid should be administered or whether a poisoning emergency exists.
- Hospital-based therapies include supportive and symptomatic care, single or multiple doses of activated charcoal (to reduce absorption or to enhance systemic elimination, respectively), whole bowel irrigation (to evacuate the intestinal tract), hemodialysis (to enhance systemic elimination), and use of antidotes (to antagonize or reverse toxic effects).
- Few antidotes are available relative to the large number of potential poisons. The use of an antidote is usually an adjunct to conventional and supportive therapies. Commonly used antidotes include acetylcysteine, atropine, pralidoxime, digoxin immune Fab, and naloxone.

43-2 STUDY GUIDE CHECKLIST

The following topics may guide your study of this subject area:

- ☐ Recognition of typical effects of common serious poisonings and drug overdoses.
- ☐ Basic first-aid and general treatment measures for a poison exposure.
- ☐ Poison prevention measures for patient counseling.
- ☐ Matching of antidotes or the medication-assisted therapy for substance misuse with the offending agent.
- ☐ The mechanism of action of common antidotes and medication-assisted therapy for substance use disorders.
- ☐ The route of administration of common antidotes and medication-assisted therapy for substance use disorders.
- ☐ Contraindications and warnings for common medication-assisted therapy for substance use disorder.
- ☐ Approaches to reducing drug-related overdose deaths.

43-3   Substance Misuse

Substance misuse often leads to acute and chronic toxicity. For those having an illicit drug use disorder, the most common were for marijuana (4.4 million) and misuse of prescription pain medication (1.7 million). Management of the acute condition generally follows the same guidelines as those for management of poisonings and overdoses as described in the following section on poisoning. A challenge in treating patients with an acute drug overdose is determining the possible agents taken and the possible bulking agents, adulterants, or contaminants (e.g., talc, strychnine, fentanyl and other drugs, or illicitly manufactured substances). Chronic substance misuse can lead to both physical and psychological dependence and, in extreme cases, addiction. All drugs have the potential to be misused. Select drugs and commonly misused substances and their effects are described in Table 43-1.

> ⚠ **Fentanyl** *FDA BOXED WARNING*
>
> Potential for misuse, abuse, and addiction. Potential for life-threatening respiratory depression, especially if used concomitantly with benzodiazepines. Monitor interactions with medications metabolized by CYP3A4. Avoid use in pregnant women due to risk of neonatal opioid withdrawal. Exposure to heat (e.g., heating pads, electric blankets) may increase fentanyl levels when using patch formulation. Risk of accidental exposure to children resulting in fatal overdose when using patch formulation.

TABLE 43-1. Select Drugs and Misused Substances

Substance (slang names)	Methods of misuse	Major or unique health effects
Androgenic anabolic steroids (Arnolds, juice, Gym Candy, Pumpers, Roids) C-III By enacting the Anabolic Steroid Control Acts of 1990 and 2004, Congress placed a total of 59 anabolic steroids in Schedule III of the Controlled Substances Act. The salts, esters, and ethers of these 59 anabolic steroids are also controlled. Congress provided a definition to administratively classify additional steroids as Schedule III anabolic steroids.	Taken orally, applied topically, or injected, in patterns lasting weeks to months ("cycling"). During cycles users may take 2 or more different anabolic steroids, usually mixing oral and injectable types ("stacking"). Other drugs and supplements are commonly used to counteract side effects (e.g., tamoxifen for gynecomastia).	Anabolic steroids are synthetic derivatives of testosterone. Misuse can lead to serious health problems. *Men:* Shrunken testicles, reduced sperm count, baldness, gynecomastia, testicular cancer *Women:* Growth of facial hair, male-pattern baldness, changes in or cessation of the menstrual cycle, enlargement of the clitoris, decreased breast size, and deepened voice *Adolescents:* Stunted growth and accelerated puberty Other major side effects include severe acne, peliosis hepatis, and jaundice. Major mood disorders such as mania, hypomania, violence, and depression.
Cocaine (blow, bump, coke, crack [name for cocaine freebase for smoking]). C-II	The water-soluble hydrochloride form of cocaine is snorted, rubbed on the gums, or injected. All mucous membranes readily absorb cocaine. The water-insoluble base form (crack) is smoked and makes a "crackling" sound when heated. Intravenous and intramuscular injections, snorting, and smoking are the common routes of administration.	A strong CNS stimulant, cocaine causes short-term euphoria (hypersensitivity to light, sound, and touch), increased energy, alertness, dilated pupils, hyperthermia, tachycardia, and hypertension. Long-term nasal use can cause problems with swallowing, loss of sense of smell, nosebleeds, and permanent damage to the nasal septum. Cocaine-related deaths often result from cardiac arrest, seizures, and stroke. Tolerance develops and depression, fatigue, and insomnia are common withdrawal symptoms.

TABLE 43-1. Select Drugs and Misused Substances *(Continued)*

Substance (slang names)	Methods of misuse	Major or unique health effects
Dextromethorphan (DXM, robotripping, skittles, triple C's) Some states limit sales to minors.	Most commonly taken orally by drinking dextromethorphan-containing cold and cough syrups. Tablets are crushed and snorted.	Dextromethorphan is an antitussive with a chemical structure similar to ketamine and PCP and produces a dissociative "out of body" state at supratherapeutic doses. Symptoms of acute toxicity include euphoria, inappropriate laughing, psychosis, tachycardia, dilated pupils, and excessive sweating. Misused most commonly by adolescents and young adults who report a heightened sense of perceptual awareness, altered time perception, and hallucinations. There are more than 140 products worldwide that contain dextromethorphan. DXM may cause a false-positive test result with some urine immunoassays for PCP.
Ethanol (various names [hooch, liquid courage, sauce] and alcoholic drinks) Sales and consumption restricted to persons 21 years of age and older.	Typically ingested and commonly used or given together with other sedating drugs to potentiate their effects.	Ethanol is a CNS depressant that can lower inhibitions at low doses and create an excited feeling. High doses and mixing with other CNS depressants increase the risks for injury, motor vehicle accident, respiratory depression, and sexual assault. Acute intoxication leads to ataxia, slurred speech, emesis, and sedation. Chronic misuse leads to hepatic failure with ascites and esophageal varices. Ethanol related digestive issues and malnutrition contribute to thiamine deficiency and Wernicke–Korsakoff syndrome. Tolerance, dependence, withdrawal, and addiction develop with chronic use.
Gamma-hydroxybutyrate (GHB) (date rape, liquid ecstasy, easy lay, Georgia home boy, somatomax, salty dog, scoop, vita-G) C-I; C-III for sodium oxybate (Xyrem) ⚠. Though Xyrem is a Schedule III controlled substance, trafficking of Xyrem is subject to Schedule I penalties.	Produced in either an odorless, colorless liquid form (Xyrem) or as a white powdered material. It is taken orally, typically combined with a liquid mixer such as a soft drink, water, or sports drink. GHB usually has a salty taste. This saltiness can be masked if it is mixed with a sweet drink, increasing the risk of accidental ingestion. The drug can be slipped into a drink without the recipient's knowledge and has been involved in date rapes.	GHB is a CNS depressant originally used as a growth hormone stimulator. Misused by teens and young adults at all-night parties and "raves" for enhanced sexual experiences. Depending on the dose, effects can range from euphoria, intoxication, muscle relaxation, and hallucinations to dizziness, nausea, vomiting, respiratory depression, seizures, confusion, amnesia, unconsciousness, coma, and even death. Currently, there is no antidote available for GHB overdose. Chronic abuse of GHB produces a withdrawal syndrome characterized by insomnia, anxiety, tremors, marked autonomic activation (i.e., increased heart rate and blood pressure) and occasional psychotic thoughts.
Heroin (black tar [name given to impure heroin, dark in color], china white, dope, H, smack) C-I	Pure heroin, white in color, can be snorted, smoked, or injected. Black tar heroin, sticky like tar or hard like coal, is typically dissolved, diluted, and injected. Increasingly adulterated with fentanyl and highly potent fentanyl analogs, contributing to overdose death rates.	Heroin is a fat-soluble opioid and whether injected, sniffed, or snorted, exerts effects on the brain quickly. Users feel an almost immediate rush, or "smack" of euphoria, especially when the drug is injected. Chronic heroin use leads to scarred and collapsed veins, bacterial infections of the blood vessels and heart valves, boils, a variety of soft-tissue infections, infectious diseases (see "Injected drugs" below), kidney problems, liver disease, and fatal overdose. Heroin is often combined with other drugs such as illicit fentanyl + carfentanil + U-47700 ("Gray Death"); **alprazolam** ("Chocolate bars"); cocaine ("Speedball"); methamphetamine ("Screwball"); crack ("Dragon rock"); LSD + PCP ("LBJ"), leading to multiple drug toxicities.

(continued)

TABLE 43-1. Select Drugs and Misused Substances *(Continued)*

Substance (slang names)	Methods of misuse	Major or unique health effects
Inhalants (various names) Some states limit sales to minors.	Volatile substances that produce chemical vapors that are sniffed, snorted, inhaled, or huffed.	Most inhalants depress the CNS and produce effects similar to those produced by ethanol ingestion. Compulsive use and a mild withdrawal syndrome can occur with long-term inhalant misuse.
Injected drugs (various names)	Such drugs are injected, which is referred to as "shooting up," "skin-popping," or "mainlining."	Drug users who inject are at risk for transmitting or acquiring HIV/AIDS, hepatitis, bacterial infections, and fungal infections if needles or other injection equipment are shared. Chronic users may develop collapsed veins, infection of the heart lining and valves (endocarditis), skin abscesses, cellulitis, and liver disease. Many substances need to be dissolved to be injected. Emboli can form from insoluble adulterants used to cut drugs or insoluble tablet materials.
Ketamine (K, special K, cat, Valium, vitamin K) C-III	Ketamine as a clear liquid is injected, ingested, snorted, or smoked (liquid or powder added to tobacco or marijuana cigarettes).	Ketamine is approved for both human and animal use as an injectable anesthetic and is obtained via diversion, frequently from veterinary office theft. Hallucinations ("K-land" or "K-state") are the desired effect. Users report feeling a nonlocalized numbness and falling into a dream-like state that produces feelings of detachment and introversion along with blurred vision, muffled or distorted hearing, and a floating sensation. High-dose toxicity ("K-hole") includes delirium, amnesia, convulsions, hypertension, and potentially fatal respiratory depression.
Lysergic acid diethylamide (LSD) (acid, blotters, cubes, dots, lucy, microdots, sugar, trip, windowpanes). C-I Its 2 precursors, lysergic acid and lysergic acid amide, are both schedule III substances under the CSA. The LSD precursors, ergotamine and ergonovine, are DEA List I chemicals (chemicals designated as those that are used in the manufacture of controlled substances).	LSD is a clear or white odorless material that is ingested. The crystalline form can be formed into tablets ("microdots") or thin squares of gelatin ("windowpanes") and dissolved in the mouth. It is more commonly dissolved with water or alcohol and added to absorbent paper and divided into small squares ("blotters") or placed on dot-like candy ("dots") or sugar cubes ("cubes," "sugar").	LSD is a potent mood and perception altering hallucinogenic drug. Physical effects include hypertension, tachycardia, increased temperature, dizziness, loss of appetite, tremors, and mydriasis. LSD induces a heightened awareness of sensory input that is accompanied by an enhanced sense of clarity but reduced ability to control what is experienced. Hallucinogenic effects are unpredictable and depend in part by the user's personality, mood, and surroundings. The user may report "hearing colors" or "seeing sounds." Users can experience enjoyable sensations on some "trips" and terrifying anxiety, paranoia, and despair on others. Chronic use is associated with psychosis and hallucinogen persisting perception disorder ("flashbacks"). Flashbacks typically involve bright flashes, auras, halos, or trails attached to moving objects after the "trip" has ended.

TABLE 43-1. Select Drugs and Misused Substances (Continued)

Substance (slang names)	Methods of misuse	Major or unique health effects
Marijuana (pot, bud, grass, ganja, herb, weed, and many others) C-I	Marijuana is smoked as a cigarette ("joint"), in a pipe ("bong"), or in hollowed out cigar ("blunt"). It can also be ingested when mixed in food substances and is available in countless consumable products. Butane hash oil (BHO) and other THC concentrates are inhaled by "dabbing."	The main psychoactive chemical in marijuana is delta-9-tetrahydrocannabinol (THC). Heightened sensations of music and light, relaxation, increased appetite ("the munchies"), and diminished physical activity ("stoned"). Short-term effects also include slowed reaction time, problems with learning and memory, ataxia, anxiety, and paranoia. Smoking marijuana carries the same risks as cigarette smoking. Long-term daily use can cause a rare condition, cannabinoid hyperemesis syndrome that leads to repeated and severe bouts of vomiting.
3,4-methylenedioxy-methamphetamine (MDMA) (Ecstasy, Adam, disco biscuits, E, molly, scooby snacks, XTC) C-I	MDMA is ingested, snorted, injected, or used in suppository form ("plugging").	MDMA is a synthetic psychoactive drug with stimulant and hallucinogenic properties. It increases pulse and blood pressure and heightens sensations, particularly those having to do with happiness and intimacy. In high doses it can cause malignant hyperthermia and rhabdomyolysis (muscle breakdown with kidney and cardiovascular system failure). Drinking large amounts of water to overcome overheating and dehydration can cause hyponatremia and life-threatening brain swelling and seizures. Psychological symptoms of depression, drug craving, impaired attention and memory, anxiety, aggression, and irritability can occur following use and can last for weeks. Physical symptoms include involuntary jaw clenching, lack of appetite, restless legs, nausea, hot flashes or chills, headache, and muscle or joint stiffness.
Methamphetamine (blue, crank, crystal, ice, meth, speed) C-II	Methamphetamine can be ingested, snorted, injected, and smoked. The clear glassy or shiny blue-white chunks resembling ice can be smoked and are referred to as "ice," "crystal," and "glass."	Methamphetamine is a highly addictive CNS stimulant. It produces euphoria, increased wakefulness and physical activity, decreased appetite, tachycardia, hypertension, hyperthermia, and arrhythmias. High doses can lead to stroke, cardiovascular collapse, and death. Severe hyperthermia and convulsion can also result in death. Long-term use results in extreme paranoia with hallucinations, anorexia, dental problems ("meth mouth"), and intense itching leading to skin lesions. Methamphetamine can be made at home by combining pseudoephedrine (found in decongestants), a lithium battery, and household items ("shake and bake"), but most is made in illicit laboratories and imported into the United States. Both methods produce product that may contain harmful contaminants and byproducts.

(continued)

TABLE 43-1. Select Drugs and Misused Substances *(Continued)*

Substance (slang names)	Methods of misuse	Major or unique health effects
Opioids (various names) ⚠ C-II, C-III, or C-IV	Opioids are ingested, injected, snorted, and smoked.	Natural opioids (referred to as opiates) include opium and morphine (MS Contin). Synthetic opioids include codeine, **oxycodone** (OxyContin, Percocet), hydrocodone (Norco), hydromorphone (Dilaudid), memthadone (Dolophine), meperidine (Demerol), and fentanyl (Duragesic, Abstral, Actiq, Fentora, Lazanda, Sublimaze, Subsys). See "heroin." Physical dependence develops rapidly relative to dose and duration of use, and persons can experience withdrawal after a few days of use. Avoidance of withdrawal can lead to continued use beyond therapeutic need. Tolerance and the lack of a ceiling effect facilitate the need for escalating does increasing the risk of misuse and overdose. Typical overdose effects include hypotension, miosis, respiratory depression, coma, seizures, and death. Mixing with other CNS depressants, particularly benzodiazepines, increases the risk of overdose and death. Chronic use produces physical dependence, tolerance, withdrawal symptoms, and addiction. Every age group has been affected by the relative ease of opioid availability and the perceived safety of these products by medical prescribers. Sometimes viewed as a "white collar" addiction, hydrocodone misuse has increased among all ethnic and economic groups.
Phencyclidine (PCP) (angel dust, ozone, rocket fuel; killer joints, supergrass, or wets when combined with marijuana) C-II	PCP is ingested, injected, smoked, and snorted. Commonly applied to leafy material (mint, oregano, parsley, or marijuana) and smoked in a pipe or cigarette form. Commercial cigarettes are dipped in a PCP solution.	PCP is a synthetic hallucinogen with sedative and stimulant properties no longer produced or used for medical purposes in the United States. Use was discontinued due to the high incidence of patients experiencing postoperative delirium with hallucinations. Users frequently exhibit delusions of grandeur, feel little to no pain, lose physical and mental control, and become violent injuring themselves and others. Low doses elicit stimulant-like effects including hypertension, tachycardia, profuse sweating, flushing, and numbness in hands and feet. High doses produce sedative effects. Users can experience hypotension, bradycardia, respiratory depression, nausea, vomiting, drooling, seizures, coma, and death (death is often secondary to accidental injury or suicide during PCP intoxication). PCP mimics the full range of symptoms of schizophrenia, and users frequently experience delusions, paranoia, and impaired judgment.

TABLE 43-1. Select Drugs and Misused Substances (Continued)

Substance (slang names)	Methods of misuse	Major or unique health effects
Sedatives Barbiturates: pentobarbital (Nembutal), phenobarbital C-II Benzodiazepines ⚠: **alprazolam** (Xanax), diazepam (Valium), **lorazepam** (Ativan), triazolam (Halcion), **clonazepam** (Klonopin) C-II Sleep medications: eszopiclone (Lunesta) ⚠, Suvorexant (Belsomra) zaleplon (Sonata) ⚠, **zolpidem** (Ambien) ⚠ C-IV	Barbiturates, benzodiazepines, and sleep medications can be ingested, injected, or snorted. They are often used or given together with other sedating drugs such as opioids, alcohol, and skeletal muscle relaxants, which increases the risks for accidental injury, motor vehicle accident, life-threatening overdose, and drug-assisted sexual assault.	Toxic effects: Drowsiness, sedation; slurred speech, confusion, ataxia; clammy skin; impaired judgment, coordination, and memory; lowered blood pressure; slowed breathing; coma and death Dangerous bradycardia and respiratory distress lead to unresponsiveness; respiratory arrest, sometimes complicated by pulmonary aspiration; and death—unlikely with ingestion of benzodiazepines alone. Sleep medications and benzodiazepines are sometimes used as date rape drugs typically placed in alcoholic drinks. Flunitrazepam (Rohypnol), a benzodiazepine smuggled into the United States, is another drug used for drug-assisted sexual assault. These drugs interact pharmacodynamically with alcohol and opioids to increase CNS depression and the risk of life-threatening effects, including death. Some drugs with sedating properties, such as carisoprodol (Soma; C-IV) and **gabapentin** (Neurontin), are also used to heighten the effects of opioids and sedatives.
Stimulants, amphetamines, and related compounds (speed, dexies, uppers) C-II	These drugs are typically ingested, but tablets can also be crushed and snorted or injected.	These substances are CNS stimulants that increase alertness, attention, and energy, as well as increase blood pressure, pulse, and respiration. High doses can lead to arrhythmias, hypertension, hyperthermia, and potential for cardiovascular failure, stroke, or lethal seizures. Taking high doses of some stimulants repeatedly over a short period of time can lead to hostility or feelings of paranoia. Stimulants such as **dextroamphetamine** (Dexedrine) ⚠, **amphetamine/dextroamphetamine** (Adderall) ⚠, atomoxetine (Strattera), **lisdexamfetamine** (Vyvanse), and **methylphenidate** (Ritalin, Concerta) can be addictive when misused and are abused as "studying aids," "cognitive enhancers," and "smart drugs" by high school and college students.
Tianeptine (Tiannaa, stablon, coaxil). Not controlled under the CSA but was added to Michigan's list of C-II controlled substances in 2018.	Tianeptine as a powder is typically ingested, snorted, injected, or smoked. It is commonly found pressed into counterfeit pills mimicking hydrocodone or **oxycodone** and in individual bags commonly used to distribute heroin.	Similar in structure to tricyclic-antidepressants, tianeptine acts an agonist at the mu opioid receptor and produces euphoric properties similar to other opioids. Physical toxicity include agitation, nausea, vomiting, tachycardia, hypertension, and diaphoresis. Severe adverse health effects, including respiratory depression, severe sedation, and death.

Boldface indicates one of top 100 drugs for 2020 by prescription volume.

C-I, C-II, C-III, and C-IV are the schedules within the Controlled Substances Act that are used to classify drugs on the basis of their abuse potential, medical applications, and safety; CNS, central nervous system; FDA, U.S. Food and Drug Administration; HIV/AIDS, human immunodeficiency virus/acquired immune deficiency syndrome.

FDA BOXED WARNINGS

Sodium Oxybate (Xyrem)
Risk of significant respiratory depression. Risk of respiratory depression, decreased consciousness, coma, and death when misused or abused. Required REMS program due to risks of CNS depression, misuse, and abuse.

Opioids (various names)
Potential for misuse, abuse, and addiction. Potential for life-threatening respiratory depression, especially if used concomitantly with benzodiazepines. Monitor interactions with medications metabolized by CYP enzymes.

Benzodiazepines
Concomitant use with opioids increases risk of sedation, respiratory depression, coma, and death. Risk of misuse, dependence, addiction, and withdrawal reactions.

Eszopiclone (Lunesta)
Risk of complex sleep behaviors (e.g., sleep-walking, sleep-driving). Discontinue immediately if complex sleep behaviors occur.

Zaleplon (Sonata)
Risk of complex sleep behaviors (e.g., sleep-walking, sleep-driving). Discontinue immediately if complex sleep behaviors occur.

Zolpidem (Ambien)
Risk of complex sleep behaviors (e.g., sleep-walking, sleep-driving). Discontinue immediately if complex sleep behaviors occur.

Dextroamphetamine (Dexedrine)
High potential for misuse and dependence. Misuse may cause sudden death and serious cardiovascular events.

Amphetamine/Dextroamphetamine (Adderall)
High potential for misuse and dependence. Misuse may cause sudden death and serious cardiovascular events.

Nature of Substance Abuse

Substance use disorder (SUD) is a maladaptive pattern of substance use leading to clinically significant impairment or distress within a 12-month period. It is a neurobiological disease with genetic, psychosocial, and environmental factors that typically start with life-style choices that lead to physiologic, behavioral, and mental changes. The spectrum of substance use disorders spans a wide variety of problems encompassing 11 different assessment criteria (Table 43-2) and generally follows an order of stages: initiation of substance misuse by experimentation, regular substance abuse, addiction, and recovery. The first 3 stages produce harmful health, behavioral, and societal effects with increasing intensity. These stages are associated with symptoms that drive repeated use: rewarding or pleasurable effects, avoidance of substance withdrawal, and substance-seeking behavior. The cycle becomes more severe as a person continues illicit drug use and produces changes affecting specific regions of the brain (basal ganglia, prefrontal cortex, and extended amygdala). These changes impact motivation and behavior, creating intense cravings that increase the likelihood of repeated and continued use.

The following terms are related to substance abuse:

- *Drug misuse:* Use of a drug for a nontherapeutic effect to alter mood, emotion, or state of consciousness (e.g., alcohol use by minors, use of illicit drug, and misuse of pharmaceuticals in a manner other than prescribed or directed)
- *Tolerance:* The body's physical adaptation to a drug where greater amounts are required over time to achieve the initial desired effect or continued use of the same amount produces markedly diminished effect
- *Dependence:* A physical state that develops during regular drug use in which a withdrawal syndrome results upon drug cessation or tolerance

TABLE 43-2. DSM-V Substance Use Disorder Assessment

Criteria	Scoring system (2 out of 11 criteria clustering in a 12-month period are needed to meet disorder threshold)
Recurrent substance use in situations where it is physically hazardous	Mild = 2 to 3
Recurrent substance use resulting in a failure to fulfill major role obligations at work, school, or home	Moderate = 4 to 5
Continued substance use despite having persistent or recurrent social or interpersonal problems caused or exacerbated by the effects of the substance	Severe = 6+
Craving or a strong desire or urge to use the substance	
Substance is taken in larger amounts or over a longer period than was intended	
There is a persistent desire or unsuccessful efforts to cut down or control substance use	
A great deal of time is spent in activities necessary to obtain the substance, use the substance, or recover from its effects	
Important social, occupational, or recreational activities are given up or reduced because of substance use	
Substance use is continued despite knowledge of having a persistent or recurrent physical or psychological problem that is likely to have been caused or exacerbated by substance use	
Tolerance, as defined by either (1) a need for markedly increased amounts of substance to achieve intoxication or desired effect or (2) a markedly diminished effect with continued use of the same amount of the substance	
Withdrawal, as manifested by either (1) the characteristic withdrawal syndrome for the substance or (2) the substance (or a closely related substance) is taken to relieve or avoid withdrawal symptoms	

Note: This criterion is not considered met for those taking opioids, sedatives, hypnotics or anxiolytics, or stimulant medications solely under appropriate medical supervision.

■ *Withdrawal:* Unpleasant symptoms after abrupt cessation, rapid dose reduction, decreasing drug concentrations, or administration of an antagonist (also known as abstinence syndrome)
■ *Addiction:* A primary, chronic, neurobiological disease with genetic, psychosocial, and environmental factors influencing its development and manifestations; characterized by impaired control over substance use, compulsive use, craving, and continued use despite adverse social, psychological, and physical consequences
■ *Recovery:* A process of change through which individuals improve their health and wellness, live self-directed lives, and strive to reach their full potential. Although abstinence from all substance misuse is a cardinal feature of a recovery lifestyle, patients taking FDA-approved medication to treat SUD can be considered in recovery.
■ *Drug overdose:* Intentional or unintentional acute consumption of an excessive (supratherapeutic) amount of a drug (similar to the definition of poisoning)
■ *Unintentional drug overdose death:* Drug overdoses of 1 or more misused drugs resulting in death (frequently the result of combining CNS depressants or using opioids unknowingly mixed with fentanyl or fentanyl analogs)

Treatment Options for Substance Use Disorder

Effective treatment (Box 43-1) addresses multiple needs of the individual beyond drug use or misuse and needs to be readily available. The choice of treatment depends on the assessment, urgency, resources, substances misused, presence of co-occurring mental disorders, and a variety of other individual circumstances.

> **BOX 43-1. Comprehensive Treatment Plans Include Several Options**

- Screening, assessment, and diagnosis of substance use disorder
- Testing for HIV/AIDS, hepatitis B and C, tuberculosis, and other infectious diseases, risk-reduction counseling, and links to appropriate treatment
- Individual counseling and monitoring use

- Acute detoxification, withdrawal, and stabilization
- Residential and outpatient rehabilitation programs
- Support groups and recovery programs
- Long-term drug-substitution, -aversion, and -antagonist therapy (medication-assisted therapy)

In 2018, 21.1 million people aged 12 or older were identified as needing substance use treatment with only 3.7 million receiving any substance use treatment. Remaining in treatment for an adequate period of time is crucial and SUD treatment often requires continuing treatment rather than episodic, acute-care treatment approaches. Treatment plans should be assessed regularly and adjusted as needed to fit each individual's changing needs.

43-4   Selected Medication-Assisted Therapies

Medication-assisted therapy (MAT) for substance use disorder is the use of FDA-approved medications in combination with counseling and behavioral therapies generally indicated for patients who are motivated to adhere to a treatment plan and who have no contraindications to the drug therapy. Three phases of treatment typically include the following:

- The person has abstained from using the problem substance (e.g., 12 to 24 hours for many opioids) and is in the early stages of withdrawal (induction).
- The person has discontinued or greatly reduced misuse of the problem substance, no longer has cravings, and experiences few side effects so that the dose of the MAT drug can be adjusted (stabilization).
- The patient is doing well on a steady dose of the MAT drug (maintenance).

Buprenorphine ⚠

Buprenorphine is indicated for treatment of opioid use disorder and is available in several forms such as sublingual (SL) tablets and buccal films without naloxone (Subutex and generic) and SL tablets and buccal

 Buprenorphine FDA BOXED WARNING

Serious, life-threatening respiratory depression, overdose, and death may occur with buprenorphine use. Concomitant use with benzodiazepines increases risk for severe CNS depression. The drug exposes patients and other users to the risks of opioid misuse and addiction. Use during pregnancy can result in neonatal opioid withdrawal syndrome. A REMS program is in place to evaluate risk vs benefit and also a REMS specific to subdermal buprenorphine implants (Probuphine) due to risk of implant migration, protrusion, and expulsion.

Potential for misuse, abuse, and addiction. Potential for life-threatening respiratory depression, especially if used concomitantly with benzodiazepines. Avoid use in pregnant women due to risk of neonatal opioid withdrawal. Accidental exposure to even one dose by children can result in a fatal overdose. Risk of serious harm or death with extended-release injection.

films with naloxone (Suboxone, Zubsolv, Bunavail, Cassipa). It is also available as an intradermal implant (Probuphine) and extended-release injection (Sublocade). Buprenorphine is a schedule III (C-III) drug under the drug classification schedules of the Controlled Substance Act.

Uses

Under the Drug Addiction Treatment Act of 2000 (DATA 2000), qualified U.S. physicians, and mid-level practitioners with an X-license can offer buprenorphine for opioid dependency in various settings, including in an office (physicians only), community hospital, health department, or correctional facility (midlevel practitioners). It can be dispensed by any pharmacy. Probuphine is available only through a restricted program called the Probuphine REMS Program requiring live training on implant insertion and removal. Health care settings and pharmacies must get a Sublocade REMS Program certification to dispense the medication for direct subcutaneous administration by a health care provider; intravenous (I.V.) self-injection by patients can cause death.

Mechanism of action

Buprenorphine is a partial opioid antagonist used to treat opioid dependence by lowering the potential for misuse and diminishing the effects of physical dependency to opioids, such as withdrawal symptoms and craving. Like other opioids, it can produce euphoria and respiratory depression, but the effects are weaker than with other opioids (e.g., heroin, methadone).

Buprenorphine's opioid effects increase with each dose until leveling off creating a *ceiling effect* (Figure 43-1). The effectiveness and sedation or respiratory effects do not increase after a certain dosing level, even if more is taken, lowering the risk of misuse, dependency, and side effects. Buprenorphine is a long-acting (24 to 72 hours) opioid that produces less respiratory depression at high doses than other opioids. Like other opioids, buprenorphine can produce significant euphoria and is misused by various routes of administration (sublingual, intranasal, and injection) gaining popularity as a heroin substitute and as a primary drug of misuse. Most of the oral products include naloxone to decrease the likelihood of diversion and misuse by injection. When buprenorphine/naloxone is taken as a SL tablet or buccal film, buprenorphine's opioid effects dominate and mitigate opioid withdrawal. If the SL tablets or buccal

FIGURE 43-1. Time versus Mu-Receptor Activation

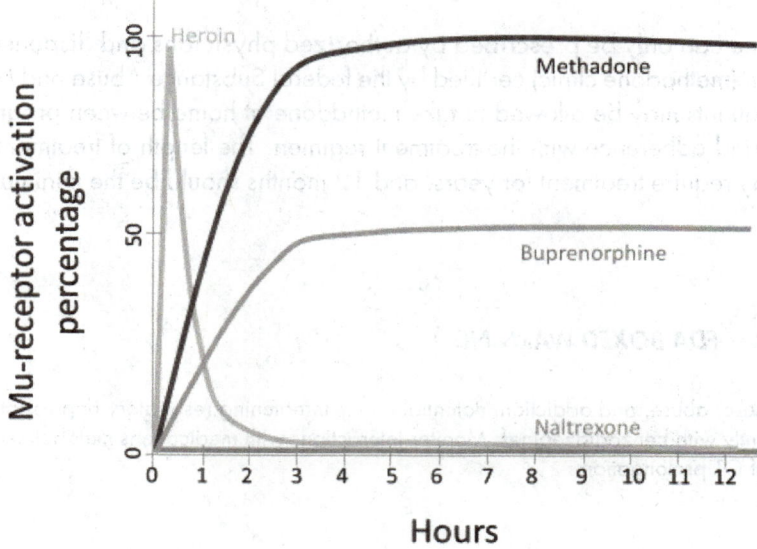

films are dissolved and injected, the naloxone effect dominates, blocking the euphoric effect, and can potentially bring on opioid withdrawal symptoms.

Adverse effects

Common adverse effects are related to its opioid actions and include nausea, vomiting, and constipation; sleepiness; muscle aches and cramps; cravings; and irritability. The implant and injection may cause implantation or injection site pain, itchiness, and redness. A lump may be present following the Sublocade injection that will gradually diminish over several weeks.

Cautions and warnings

- Use with caution in patients with polysubstance use and in those who have severe hepatic impairment, compromised respiratory function, or head injury.
- Significant respiratory depression and death have occurred particularly when misused intravenously or in combination with benzodiazepines or other CNS depressants including alcohol or other drugs that slow breathing.
- Buprenorphine may precipitate withdrawal if initiated before the patient is in opioid withdrawal, particularly in patients being transferred from methadone.
- Insertion and removal of Probuphine is associated with the risk of implant migration where pieces can move into blood vessels causing pulmonary embolism and death. Protrusion, expulsion, and nerve damage can also result from the procedure.

Dosage schedule

Oral buprenorphine is typically taken once daily, every other day, or 3 times a week in the maintenance phase on the basis of response. The subcutaneous injection releases buprenorphine for 1 month and the intradermal implant actively releases buprenorphine for 6 months.

Methadone ⚠

Methadone is the most studied pharmacotherapy for opioid use disorder and is available in several oral forms including liquid concentrate or solution (Methadose) and tablet (Dolophine). It is a schedule II (C-II) drug under the drug classification schedules of the Controlled Substance Act.

Uses

By law, methadone can only be prescribed by authorized physicians and dispensed through an opioid treatment program (methadone clinic) certified by the federal Substance Abuse and Mental Health Services Administration. Patients may be allowed to take methadone at home between program visits on the basis of their progress and adherence with the treatment regimen. The length of treatment varies by individual. Some patients may require treatment for years, and 12 months should be the minimum length of treatment.

 Methadone *FDA BOXED WARNING*

Potential for misuse, abuse, and addiction. Potential for life-threatening respiratory depression, especially if used concomitantly with benzodiazepines. Monitor interactions with medications metabolized by CYP enzymes. Increased risk of QT prolongation.

(*Note:* methadone dispensed from a pharmacy with the sole purpose of short-term opioid analgesia does not require special certification.)

Mechanism of action

Methadone is a long-acting full mu-opioid receptor agonist that is used for initial detoxification then as a maintenance treatment for opioid dependence. By serving as an opioid-substitute, methadone lessens the distressing symptoms of opioid withdrawal, blocks the euphoric effects of opioids, and allows people to manage their disorder by improving the ability to function emotionally and socially.

Adverse effects

Methadone has a complex pharmacokinetic profile exhibiting accumulation in the body until a stable maintenance dose is achieved. Patient specific half-lives can range from 8 to 59 hours and taking more methadone, other opioids, or CNS depressants can cause unintentional life-threatening overdose symptoms. Signs of potential opioid overdose are listed in Figure 43-2. Typical opioid adverse effects such as constipation and sleepiness may occur during methadone treatment.

FIGURE 43-2. Recognizing Opioid Overdose

SIGNS OF POTENTIAL OPIOID OVERDOSE

P Pulse slow or erratic

U Unconscious

U Unresponsive

L Limp body

L Loud snoring or gurgling noises

S Shallow, slow, or no breathing

S Skin pale/gray, clammy

E Evaluate eyes, lips, and fingertips (miosis, lips/fingertips cyanotic/bluish)

Cautions and warnings

Methadone is contraindicated in patients with respiratory depression, acute bronchial asthma, or hypercarbia and those suspected of having a paralytic ileus. If a patient wants to stop methadone treatment, it must be stopped gradually to prevent withdrawal and under a physician's supervision.

Several important drug interactions are known to occur, and many involve cytochrome P450 (CYP) isoenzymes.

- Increased methadone concentrations from CYP inhibition: **amitriptyline** ⚠, **fluoxetine** ⚠, fluvoxamine ⚠, **paroxetine** ⚠, **sertraline** ⚠, ciprofloxacin ⚠, clarithromycin, erythromycin, fluconazole, itraconazole ⚠, ketoconazole ⚠
- Decreased methadone concentrations with CYP inducement: Amprenavir, efavirenz, nelfinavir, ritonavir ⚠, phenytoin ⚠, phenobarbital, rifampin, carbamazepine ⚠, St. John's wort
- Increased risk of serotonin syndrome: Monoamine oxidase inhibitors (e.g., selegiline ⚠ inhibits serotonin metabolism while methadone increases serotonin release)

 Amitriptyline *FDA BOXED WARNING*

Increased risk of suicidality, particularly in people under 24 years old. Not approved for pediatric use.

 Fluoxetine *FDA BOXED WARNING*

Increased risk of suicidality, particularly in people under 24 years old. Not approved for use under 7 years of age.

 Fluvoxamine *FDA BOXED WARNING*

Increased risk of suicidality, particularly in people under 24 years old.

 Paroxetine *FDA BOXED WARNING*

Increased risk of suicidality, particularly in pediatric and young adults.

 Sertraline *FDA BOXED WARNING*

Increased risk of suicidality, particularly in people under 24 years old.

Ciprofloxacin *FDA BOXED WARNING*

Risk of serious adverse reactions including tendinitis, tendon rupture, peripheral neuropathy, central nervous effects, and exacerbation of myasthenia gravis.

 Itraconazole *FDA BOXED WARNING*

May cause or exacerbate congestive heart failure (CHF). Do not administer for treatment of onychomycosis in patients with evidence of ventricular dysfunction. Significant number of drug–drug interactions and contraindications—see package insert for full list.

 Ketoconazole *FDA BOXED WARNING*

Risk of serious hepatotoxicity when taken orally. Use is contraindicated with methadone and other certain QT prolonging drugs due to risk of torsades de pointes.

 Ritonavir *FDA BOXED WARNING*

Coadministration with several classes of drugs (sedative hypnotics, antiarrhythmics, ergot alkaloids) may result in severe adverse reactions.

 Phenytoin *FDA BOXED WARNING*

Rate of intravenous infusion should not exceed 50 mg/minute in adults and 1 to 3 mg/kg/minute due to risk of severe hypotension and cardiac arrhythmias.

 Carbamazepine *FDA BOXED WARNING*

Increased risk of serious dermatologic reactions, including toxic epidermal necrolysis and Stevens-Johnson syndrome. Increased risk of aplastic anemia and agranulocytosis.

 Selegiline *FDA BOXED WARNING*

Increased risk of suicidality, particularly in pediatric and young adults.

FDA boxed warnings

- Respiratory depression, including fatal cases, have been reported during initiation and conversion of patients to methadone and even when the drug has been used as recommended and not misused or abused. Monitor for respiratory depression, especially during initiation of methadone or following a dose increase.
- Concomitant use of opioids with benzodiazepines or other CNS depressants, including alcohol, is a risk factor for respiratory depression and death. If the patient is visibly sedated, evaluate the cause of sedation and consider delaying or omitting daily methadone dosing.
- Accidental ingestion of methadone, especially in children, can result in fatal overdose of methadone.
- QT-interval prolongation and serious arrhythmias (torsades de pointes) have occurred during treatment with methadone.
- Neonatal opioid withdrawal syndrome is an expected and treatable outcome of use of methadone during pregnancy and may be life-threatening if not recognized and treated in the neonate.
- Methadone exposes patients and other users to the risks of misuse, abuse, and addiction, which can lead to overdose and death requiring assessment of each patient's risk prior to prescribing. Monitor all patients regularly for development of these behaviors and conditions.
- The concomitant use of methadone with all cytochrome P450 (CYP450) 3A4, 2B6, 2C19, 2C9, or 2D6 inhibitors may result in an increase in methadone plasma concentrations, which could cause potentially fatal respiratory depression, and discontinuation of concomitantly used CYP450 3A4, 2B6, 2C19, or 2C9 inducers may also result in an increase in methadone plasma concentration. Follow patients closely for respiratory depression and sedation and consider dosage reduction with any changes of concomitant medications that can result in an increase in methadone levels.

Dosage schedule

Methadone is typically administered once a day. Switching from one liquid formulation of methadone to another liquid formulation at the same dose may elicit withdrawal symptoms, leading to nonadherence and problematic substance use. Substitutions should be avoided if possible.

Naltrexone

Naltrexone is FDA approved to treat opioid use disorder and alcohol use disorder. It is available as a tablet (ReVia) and an intramuscular (I.M.) injectable extended-release form (Vivitrol). It is not a controlled substance.

Uses

For opioid use disorder, naltrexone is used to prevent relapse following opioid detoxification and is appropriate for patients who have been detoxified from opioids for 7 to 10 days. Injectable naltrexone may be beneficial to patients who have not responded to other pharmacological and behavioral treatments for opioid use disorder and alcohol use disorder, particularly those with poor medication adherence. Any licensed prescriber can prescribe naltrexone. The injectable form is administered by a health care provider and is available through specialty pharmacies only.

Mechanism of action

Naltrexone is competitive mu-opioid receptor antagonist with strong receptor affinity that blocks the actions of opioids and may reduce craving in patients with opioid use disorder. Its action for alcohol use disorder is not well understood, but it appears to reduce the rewarding, pleasurable effects of alcohol (reduces heavy drinking) and the craving for it (helps abstention).

Adverse effects

Common adverse effects include gastric distress or vomiting, diarrhea, headache and nervousness, sleep problems, and joint or muscle pain. Typically, these effects are mild and subside with continued use. The symptoms of protracted alcohol withdrawal (e.g., sleep disturbance) may overlap with the side effects of naltrexone. Naltrexone may cause liver injury and lead to weakness or tiredness, jaundice, or right upper quadrant abdominal pain. Injection site reactions such as pain or redness may occur from injectable naltrexone.

Cautions and warnings (Boxes 43-2 and 43-3)

Naltrexone can precipitate severe, acute opioid withdrawal symptoms if used by persons who have not completely cleared all opioids from their body. Patients must be opioid free for 7 to 10 days or at least 14 days for patients who have been taking methadone for more than 3 to 4 weeks. Patients who have been treated with extended-release injectable naltrexone will have reduced tolerance to opioids. Subsequent exposure to previously tolerated or even smaller amounts of opioids may result in life-threatening overdose. No significant drug interactions are known except for naltrexone's effects on opioids.

Dosage schedule

Injectable naltrexone is administered monthly, and the tablet form is administered once a day. Long-term naltrexone therapy extending beyond 3 months appears to be most effective, and it can be used indefinitely. No tapering is required when discontinued.

BOX 43-2. When to Use Caution in Prescribing Naltrexone

- For patients with active liver disease, monitor liver function.
- For patients with moderate to severe renal impairment, monitor renal function.

- For pregnant and nursing women, do not use unless potential benefits outweigh risks.
- For women of childbearing age, encourage use of effective birth control methods.

BOX 43-3. Naltrexone Contraindications and Warnings

Contraindications include the following:

- Patients currently using opioids (as indicated by self-report or a positive drug screen)
- Patients on buprenorphine or methadone maintenance therapy for opioid dependence
- Patients currently undergoing opioid withdrawal
- Patients with acute hepatitis or liver failure
- Patients who need to use opioid analgesics within 7 days or who are receiving long-term opioid therapy
- Patients sensitive to naltrexone, structurally similar compounds (e.g., naloxone, nalmefene), or an inactive ingredient in the tablet or injectable solution
- Patients with lean body mass that precludes IM injection with a 2-inch needle in the gluteal muscle; severe injection site reactions can occur from inadvertent subcutaneous injection

FDA boxed warnings

- Naltrexone has the capacity to cause hepatocellular injury when given in excessive doses.
- Naltrexone is contraindicated in acute hepatitis or liver failure, and its use in patients with active liver disease must be carefully considered in light of its hepatotoxic effects.
- Patients should be warned of the risk of hepatic injury and advised to stop the use of naltrexone and seek medical attention if they experience symptoms of acute hepatitis.

Acamprosate

Acamprosate (Campral) is FDA approved for the treatment of alcohol use disorder and is available as a delayed-release tablet. This drug is not covered by the Controlled Substance Act.

Uses

Acamprosate is most effective for patients who are motivated to achieve complete abstinence from alcohol and avoid drinking rather than decrease drinking. It is typically started on the fifth day of abstinence, reaching full effectiveness in 5 to 8 days and should be continued even if the patient relapses. When the patient has achieved stable abstinence or is not adherent to therapy, acamprosate can be discontinued without tapering. It can be prescribed by any licensed prescriber and dispensed by any pharmacy for outpatient use.

Mechanism of action

Acamprosate's mechanism of action has not been clearly established, but it may restore the balance of neuronal excitation and inhibition from chronic alcohol use by acting on the glutamate neurotransmitter system, counteracting the imbalance between glutamatergic and gamma-aminobutyric acid-ergic (GABAergic) systems. It appears to normalize alcohol-related changes in brain activity and efficacy is primarily due to its ability to reduce the negative symptoms associated with the period immediately following alcohol withdrawal such as disturbances in sleep and mood that may trigger a relapse. Acamprosate does not exhibit tolerance or dependence, can be taken with opioids and alcohol safely, has no apparent misuse potential, has no clinically significant drug interactions, and is not metabolized by the liver.

Adverse effects

The most common adverse effect is mild and transient diarrhea that typically resolves within the first initial weeks of treatment. Less common effects include intestinal cramps, flatulence, nausea, headache, increased or decreased libido, insomnia, anxiety, muscle weakness, itchiness, and dizziness.

Cautions and warnings

Acamprosate is contraindicated in patients with severe renal impairment (creatinine clearance [CrCl] <30 mL/min), and dosage should be reduced with moderate renal impairment.

Suicidal ideation is closely linked with substance use disorders, with or without acamprosate use, but suicidal ideation and suicide attempts are uncommon with acamprosate use.

Dosage schedule

Two acamprosate delayed-release tablets are typically taken 3 times per day. Patients with moderate renal impairment (CrCl 30 to 50 mL/min) take 1 tablet 3 times a day. Tablets must be swallowed whole, not crushed or broken.

Disulfiram ⚠

Disulfiram (Antabuse) is FDA approved for the treatment of alcohol use disorder, is available as a tablet, and is not a controlled substance.

Uses

Disulfiram is an alcohol-aversive agent and causes acute, unpleasant-to-serious physical reactions such as nausea/vomiting, flushing, and heart palpitations when a patient drinks or applies alcohol. Disulfiram

Disulfiram *FDA BOXED WARNING*

Disulfiram should never be administered to a patient when they are in a state of alcohol intoxication, or without their full knowledge.

may not reduce the urge to drink alcohol, but the knowledge that such reactions are likely if alcohol is consumed acts as a deterrent to drinking and may motivate patients to remain abstinent. It can be prescribed by any licensed prescriber and dispensed by any pharmacy. The use of disulfiram has declined with the availability of other treatments and several manufacturers have stopped production. Disulfiram is suggested for patients who want to abstain from alcohol and either prefer disulfiram or are unable to tolerate or are unresponsive to naltrexone and acamprosate.

Mechanism of action

Disulfiram blocks the oxidation of alcohol at the acetaldehyde stage by inhibiting aldehyde dehydrogenase. This inhibition increases serum acetaldehyde levels, causing a reaction of flushing, vertigo, sweating, nausea, and tachycardia when alcohol is ingested.

Adverse effects

The following adverse effects can occur during the first 2 weeks and decrease spontaneously or after a decrease in dosage: acneiform eruptions, allergic dermatitis, drowsiness, fatigue, headache, impotence, and bitter (garlic) or metallic aftertaste.

Cautions and warnings

- *FDA boxed warning:* Disulfiram should never be administered to a patient when he or she is in a state of alcohol intoxication or without his or her full knowledge. The health care provider should instruct relatives accordingly.
- *Contraindications:* Disulfiram is contraindicated in patients with severe myocardial disease or coronary occlusion, psychoses, and hypersensitivity to disulfiram or to other thiuram derivatives used in pesticides and rubber vulcanization.

The disulfiram–alcohol interaction can produce life-threatening effects that are generally proportional to the amounts of disulfiram and alcohol ingested. Effects typically start 10 to 30 minutes after alcohol use and last 30 to 60 minutes to several hours or as long as alcohol is in the body. The effects can occur up to 14 days after the last dose of disulfiram and patients should avoid alcohol consumption for at least 12 hours before taking disulfiram.

The following substances must be out of the body before starting disulfiram: alcohol or alcohol-containing preparations (e.g., cough syrups, elixirs, tonics), alcohol in disguised forms (sauces, vinegars, aftershave lotions, sunscreens), **metronidazole** ⚠ (CNS and psychosis risk), and ethylene dibromide or its vapors (found in some paint, paint thinner, varnish, and shellac).

 Metronidazole *FDA BOXED WARNING*

Shown to be carcinogenic in mice and rats. Reserve use only for indicated conditions.

Disulfiram should be avoided or used with caution in patients who have cardiac disease, diabetes, hypothyroidism, epilepsy, cerebral damage, chronic or acute nephritis, hepatitis C, or are pregnant or nursing.

Dosage schedule

One tablet is taken once a day. Therapy may continue for months or years until the patient has established long-term alcohol abstinence.

43-5   Overview of Poisoning and Toxicology

Poisoning in America

Poison exposures and drug overdoses affect more than 2.2 million people annually. A large number of poisonings occur in young children (< 1% of deaths are in preschool-age children), but most fatalities occur in adults.

Most poisonings in preschool-age children are unintentional or accidental. Unintentional poisonings can also occur in adolescents and adults. Intentional (suicide and drug abuse) poisonings and overdoses, however, are common.

Toxicology is the study of the adverse effects of chemicals and other xenobiotics on living organisms. Any chemical can become toxic (Box 43-4) if the exposure is too great in relation to body weight and physiologic capacity. Medications are the most common cause of poisoning morbidity and mortality.

Poison Prevention Approaches and Pharmacy

Poison Prevention Packaging Act of 1970: Safety caps

The Poison Prevention Packaging Act of 1970 was enacted to prevent preschool-age children from opening packaging and ingesting harmful substances or to delay the opening of packaging containing such substances (to limit the amount of harmful substance that may be ingested within a reasonable amount of time).

Drugs requiring safety caps include **aspirin, ibuprofen** ⚠, **acetaminophen** ⚠, and oral prescription drugs with certain exceptions (e.g., birth control pills and nitroglycerin).

Use of poison control centers

A poison control center determines if a true poisoning exists, recommends first aid, refers poisoning victims to health care facilities for further evaluation and treatment, monitors the progress and outcome of each poisoning case, and documents poisoning experiences. Programs and materials on poison prevention are also available (Box 43-5).

Nationwide access is available by calling 1-800-222-1222 for 24-hour poison control center services for the area from which the call is placed in the United States.

BOX 43-4. Mechanisms by Which a Chemical Can Produce Toxicity

- Exaggeration of pharmacologic effects
- Formation of reactive toxic metabolites
- Formation of intracellular free radicals
- Interference with enzyme action
- Interference with DNA (deoxyribonucleic acid) or RNA (ribonucleic acid) synthesis
- Inactivation of biochemical cofactors
- Initiation of premature cell aging (apoptosis)
- Tissue destruction on contact

Ibuprofen *FDA BOXED WARNING*

Increased risk of cardiovascular thrombotic events. Increased risk of serious gastrointestinal adverse events (e.g., stomach bleed, ulcers).

 Acetaminophen *FDA BOXED WARNING*

Increased risk of hepatotoxicity.

BOX 43-5. Poison Prevention Tips for Consumers

- Store all drugs and chemicals out of the reach of children.
- Never put chemicals in food containers.
- Choose products with safety caps when there is a choice, and use them properly.

- Read and follow all label directions carefully.
- Never call medication "candy."
- Use cabinet safety latches where medications, cleaning supplies, and toxic products are stored.

43-6 General Treatment of Poisonings

Emergency Actions

First aid for poisoning emergencies should be administered, if applicable. Figure 43-3 describes first-aid techniques.

Other considerations

- Try to decrease contact immediately.
- Early initiation of first aid leads to the best possible outcome. Immediately call 911 or an ambulance if the person is not breathing, has had a seizure, or is unresponsive.
- For other situations, contact a poison control center immediately (1-800-222-1222) to determine whether first aid should be used or whether a poisoning emergency exists.

Hospital-based Management

The goals of treatment are to support vital organ function, treat symptoms as needed, decrease absorption, enhance elimination, and antagonize the effects with antidotes. During the past 3 decades, the practice and means of using drugs to decrease the absorption of other drugs from the gastrointestinal tract has declined. Current recommendations, as well as basic information about the drugs and procedures used to decontaminate the gastrointestinal tract, are described in this section.

Current recommendations

Ipecac syrup (an emetic) has questionable effectiveness, and its use is now generally avoided at home and in health care facilities.

FIGURE 43-3. First Aid for Poison Exposures

Inhaled Poison

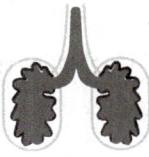

- Immediately get the person to fresh air.
- Avoid breathing fumes.
- Open doors and windows wide.
- If victim not breathing, start artificial respiration, call 911.

Poison on the Skin

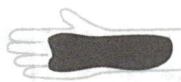

- Remove contaminated clothing and flood skin with water for 10 minutes.
- Wash gently with soap and water and rinse.
- Avoid self-contamination.

Poison in the Eye

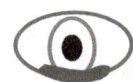

- Flood the eye with lukewarm or cool water poured from a glass 2 or 3 inches from the eye.
- Repeat for 15 minutes.
- Keep eye open, but do not force the eyelid open.
- Remove contact lenses.
- Do not instill vasoconstrictor eye drops.

Swallowed Poison

- Unless the patient is
  - unconscious,
  - having convulsions, or
  - cannot swallow

  give 2-4 ounces of water immediately.
- Contact a poison control center for further advice.

Things To Avoid In A Suspected Poisoning

- Don't panic
- Don't delay first aid if needed
- Don't waste time looking for home "antidotes"
- Don't delay getting advice from a poison control center
- Don't wait until a person is sick to get help
- Don't use ipecac syrup or activated charcoal at home
- Don't use home remedies, e.g., salt water, raw eggs, mustard powder, hydrogen peroxide, cooking grease, or gagging

---

Gastric lavage involves placing a tube into the stomach through a nostril or the mouth and repetitively washing out the stomach contents with water or a saline solution. This method of gastric decontamination is of questionable effectiveness, particularly if it is performed more than 1 hour after ingestion of toxin.

Cathartics such as magnesium citrate are no longer routinely used.

Activated charcoal given orally is often the only treatment necessary if the toxin is adsorbed to it.

Whole bowel irrigation with products like GoLYTLEY or CoLyte can be considered if the toxin is poorly or slowly adsorbed and its presence in the gastrointestinal tract is likely.

Table 43-3 lists general treatment approaches for acute poisonings.

Activated charcoal

Indications and dosage

This agent adsorbs poisons in an alert or comatose patient. Administer as a slurry by mouth in alert patients or through a gastric lavage tube.

- *Children:* 25 to 50 g
- *Adults:* 25 to 100 g

> **TABLE 43-3. General Approaches for Acute Poisonings**
>
> - Monitor and maintain vital signs
> - Supportive and symptomatic care
> - Minimize absorption
>   - Topical decontamination
>   - Activated charcoal, single-dose
>   - Gastric lavage or no evacuation
>   - Whole bowel irrigation
> - Enhance elimination
>   - Multiple doses of activated charcoal
>   - Extracorporeal removal, when indicated
> - Administer antidote, if available and indicated

Contraindications

- Ingestions of aliphatic hydrocarbons and caustics
- Absence of bowel sounds
- Ingestions of heavy metals (lithium, iron, or lead) or simple alcohols (activated charcoal is not used because of the poor adsorption of these agents)

Adverse effects

- **Uncommon:** Tracheal aspiration, pneumonitis
- **Common:** Emesis, soiling of clothes and furnishings

Advantages and disadvantages

- **Advantages:** Rapid onset of action, nonspecific action for a wide variety of chemicals, reasonable effectiveness within 1 to 2 hours of ingestion of the toxin. It can be effective up to 4 hours after ingestion of slow release medications or when gastrointestinal motility is slowed due to drugs such as opioids and anticholinergics.
- **Disadvantages:** Messy and difficult administration, possible removal of beneficial drugs together with the toxin

Whole bowel irrigation

Indications and technique

Whole bowel irrigation is generally used to wash out the gastrointestinal tract when using charcoal may be inappropriate (e.g., if iron or lithium was ingested) and when the toxin is suspected to be present in the gastrointestinal tract (e.g., when drugs are sustained-release formulations or when the patient ingested illicit drugs packed in condoms). It is not routinely used to treat poisonings except in these unique circumstances.

Larger volumes of polyethylene glycol electrolyte solutions (e.g., CoLyte, GoLYTELY) are used compared to the amounts conventionally used for bowel preparation. Administer by mouth or through a gastric or duodenal tube for treatment of poisoning.

- **Children:** 25 mL/kg/h (approximately 500 mL/h) up to 2 to 5 L
- **Adults:** 2 L/h up to 5 to 10 L

Contraindications

- Ingestion of caustics or hydrocarbons
- Patients with absent bowel sounds or gastrointestinal tract obstruction/perforation

Adverse effects

Few adverse effects have been reported such as nausea, vomiting, and intestinal cramping.

Advantages and disadvantages

- **Advantages:** Prompt whole bowel evacuation within 2 to 8 hours
- **Disadvantages:** Messy procedure because of rectal effluent

Other hospital-based therapies

These therapies include supportive and symptomatic care, multiple doses of activated charcoal (to enhance systemic elimination when appropriate), hemodialysis (to enhance systemic elimination when appropriate), and use of antidotes (to antagonize or reverse toxic effects when indicated).

43-7 Antidotes

Role of Antidotes

An antidote counteracts or changes the nature of a poison. Few antidotes are available relative to the large number of potential poisons. Table 43-4 lists antidotes that are commonly used in the treatment of a patient with a poisoning or an overdose.

Selected Antidotes

Acetylcysteine

Acetylcysteine is available under the trade names Mucomyst (10% oral solution), and Acetadote (20% for injection).

Uses

Acetylcysteine is used to treat acute **acetaminophen** overdose.

Mechanism of action

Acetylcysteine protects the liver from the toxic effects of an **acetaminophen** metabolite by supplying a surrogate for glutathione to aid in the metabolism of the reactive metabolite. Other mechanisms are also proposed, which include providing sulfate for **acetaminophen** metabolism and minimizing the formation of free radicals.

This agent may be useful in minimizing hepatotoxic injury once it has begun. It also may aid in cases of fulminant hepatic failure.

Indications

Acute overdoses of **acetaminophen** produce a reactive metabolite that leads to hepatotoxicity (jaundice, coagulopathy, hypoglycemia, hepatic failure, hepatic encephalopathy, hepatorenal failure). Symptoms become evident 1 to 2 days after ingestion.

Acetylcysteine can prevent or minimize hepatic injury if given early. For best results, administer within 10 hours of ingestion of **acetaminophen** overdose. It is minimally effective when started 24 hours after ingestion for most patients.

The need for therapy is determined by obtaining a serum concentration of **acetaminophen** at least 4 hours after ingestion (and within 24 hours) and plotting it on the **acetaminophen** nomogram to determine whether there is a risk for hepatotoxicity.

Contraindications

Use of acetylcysteine is contraindicated if there is a known hypersensitivity to the drug.

TABLE 43-4. Some Common Antidotes for Poisonings

Toxin	Antidote (trade name)	Route of administration[a]
Acetaminophen	Acetylcysteine (Mucomyst)	Oral loading and maintenance doses
	Acetylcysteine (Acetadote)	I.V. infusion
Anticholinergics	Physostigmine salicylate	Slow I.V. infusion over 3 to 5 minutes
Benzodiazepines	Flumazenil (Romazicon)[b]	I.V. bolus
β-blockers	Glucagon (GlucaGen)[c]	I.V. bolus followed by I.V. infusion
Calcium channel blockers	Calcium chloride 10%[c]	I.V. bolus followed by I.V. infusion
	Regular insulin and dextrose[c]	I.V. infusion
Cyanide	Sodium nitrite 3% and sodium thiosulfate 25% (Nithiodote)	Slow I.V. infusion
	Hydroxocobalamin (CyanoKit)	I.V. infusion over 15 minutes
Digoxin	Digoxin immune Fab (DigiFab)	I.V. bolus
Ethylene glycol, methanol	Ethanol 10%[c]	I.V. infusion or orally followed by maintenance doses
	Fomepizole (Antizol)	I.V. bolus
Iron	Deferoxamine (Desferal)	I.V. infusion
Lead[d]	Succimer (Chemet)	Oral
	Dimercaprol (BAL in Oil)	I.M.
	Calcium disodium ethylenediaminetetraacetic acid (Calcium Disodium Versenate)	I.V. infusion over 12 to 24 hours
Methemoglobinemia	Methylene blue	Slow I.V. infusion
Opioids	Naloxone for injection	I.V. bolus or I.M.
	Naloxone autoinjector (Evzio)	I.M.
	Naloxone nasal spray (Narcan, Kloxxado)	Spray into nostrils
Organophosphates	Atropine	I.V. bolus
	Pralidoxime (Protopam)	Slow I.V. infusion, followed by continuous infusion
Sulfonylurea drugs	Dextrose 50%	I.V. infusion
	Octreotide (Sandostatin)[c]	Subcutaneous or I.V.

Boldface indicates one of top 100 drugs for 2020 by prescription volume.

I.V., intravenous; I.M., intramuscular.

a. This table lists some common antidotes that are used for patients presenting with acute toxic exposures and overdoses. Consult the package insert or appropriate references for doses, dosage regimens, adverse effects, and preparation of the parenteral solution when indicated.

b. In acute overdose situations of unknown drugs and for persons dependent on benzodiazepines or taking tricyclic antidepressants, the risk of causing seizures with flumazenil use in these situations may exceed benefit.

c. Off-label indication for use.

d. Lead poisoning typically occurs from chronic exposures (weeks to years).

 Flumazenil (Romazicon) *FDA BOXED WARNING*

Increased risk of seizures.

Adverse effects

With oral administration, nausea and vomiting are common.

With intravenous (I.V.) administration, anaphylactoid reactions (rash, hypotension, wheezing, dyspnea) and vomiting have been reported. Acute flushing and erythema may occur during the first hour of infusion and typically resolve spontaneously.

Atropine

Uses

Atropine is used in cases of organophosphate (including chemical warfare and terrorism nerve agents) and carbamate anticholinesterase insecticide poisoning.

Mechanism of action

Atropine is an anticholinergic agent that competitively inhibits acetylcholine at muscarinic receptors. It has little effect on nicotinic receptors in cases of organophosphate insecticide poisoning.

Indications

- For control of pulmonary hypersecretion, atropine is given in repeated I.V. doses until secretions have decreased. Atropinization may have to be maintained for hours to days.
- For control of bradycardia, atropine is given until the heart rate increases to an acceptable rate or until a need for alternatives is indicated.

Contraindications

There are no contraindications in cases of insecticide poisoning.

Adverse effects

Exaggeration of anticholinergic effects (e.g., tachycardia, hypertension, sedation, hallucinations, mydriasis, changes in intraocular pressure, warm red skin, dry mouth, urinary retention, ileus, dysrhythmias, seizures) can occur.

When large doses of atropine are used, the agent should be free of preservatives because agents such as benzyl alcohol or chlorobutanol can produce their own toxicity. The doses of atropine for organophosphate are much higher than those routinely used for other indications, such as sinus bradycardia in advanced cardiac life support and anesthesia premedication.

Digoxin immune Fab (DigiFab)

Uses

Digoxin immune Fab is used to treat life-threatening acute or chronic digoxin poisoning.

Some cross-reactivity with digitoxin and other digoxin-like compounds (digitalis, foxglove, lily of the valley, and bufadienolide from cane frogs) can occur.

Mechanism of action

Digoxin immune Fab binds digoxin in plasma, promotes redistribution from tissues, and enhances elimination in the urine. The digoxin bound to digoxin immune Fab is inactive. Each 40 mg (1 vial) binds 0.6 mg of digoxin.

Digoxin immune Fab is a monovalent, digoxin-specific, antigen-binding fragment (Fab) that is produced in healthy sheep.

Indications

Chronic digoxin toxicity typically begins with nausea, vomiting, diarrhea, fatigue, confusion, blurred vision, diplopia, and the observation of white borders or halos around dark objects. Deterioration of renal function, hypokalemia, or drug interactions often leads to toxicity.

Acute digoxin poisoning has early symptoms similar to those of chronic poisoning, but the onset is more abrupt. Nausea and vomiting are common, and the serum potassium concentration is typically normal or dangerously elevated.

A wide variety of arrhythmias occur with acute or chronic digoxin poisoning.

Digoxin immune Fab is reserved for life-threatening symptoms such as bradycardia, second- and third-degree heart block that is unresponsive to atropine, ventricular arrhythmias, and hyperkalemia (typically in excess of 5 mEq/L).

Contraindications

Digoxin immune Fab is relatively contraindicated in patients with hypersensitivity to sheep.

Adverse effects

Common adverse effects include hypokalemia, allergic reactions (1% of patients), and hypotension. For patients on maintenance digoxin therapy, the abrupt binding of digoxin will lead to loss of therapeutic effect and a prompt decrease in potassium concentrations.

Flumazenil (Romazicon)

Uses

Flumazenil is used for reversal of conscious sedation and general anesthesia from benzodiazepines. To avoid adverse effects, its use for poisoning and acute drug overdose is limited to situations when no other drugs are involved and the patient is not a chronic user of benzodiazepines. Because these situations are often difficult to determine, flumazenil is rarely used for acute drug overdoses.

Mechanism of action

Flumazenil is a competitive antagonist of the benzodiazepine receptor in the central nervous system (CNS).

Indications

Flumazenil should be used adjunctively with supportive care. Sedation can recur following ingestion of a benzodiazepine with a long half-life, requiring additional doses of flumazenil. In a suicidal overdose, it is rarely used because of the risk of potential co-ingestants. If no response occurs to a 5 mg cumulative dose, the sedation is probably not related to a benzodiazepine.

Contraindications

Flumazenil is contraindicated in patients with known hypersensitivity to it.

Co-ingestion of tricyclic antidepressants may precipitate ventricular dysrhythmias or seizures. Other mixed overdoses can decrease the seizure threshold (e.g., haloperidol, **bupropion**, lithium, stimulants).

Abrupt benzodiazepine withdrawal following flumazenil use in patients on maintenance benzodiazepine therapy, such as for treatment of epilepsy, can precipitate seizures.

Flumazenil is contraindicated in patients with increased intracranial pressure because the antidote may potentially alter cerebral blood flow.

It can produce withdrawal in the benzodiazepine-dependent patient.

Adverse effects

Flumazenil has a wide margin of safety when not contraindicated.

Adverse effects include agitation, sweating, headache, abnormal vision, dizziness, and pain at the administration site. Rarely reported adverse effects include bradycardia, tachycardia, hypotension, and hypertension.

Naloxone

Naloxone is available in several dosage forms: 0.4 mg/mL and 1 mg/mL for injection, 2 mg/0.4 mL intramuscular (I.M.) autoinjectors (Evzio), 4 mg/0.1 mL nasal spray (Narcan Nasal Spray), and 8 mg/mL nasal spray (Kloxxado).

Uses

Naloxone is used in the following cases:

- Reversal of opioid anesthesia
- Respiratory or CNS depression related to opioid overdose
- Empiric administration in patients with altered mental status of unknown etiology

Mechanism of action

Naloxone is an opioid antagonist. It competes at several CNS opioid receptors (mu, kappa, delta) and reverses the depressive opioid effects. Because it has no agonist activity, naloxone will not worsen respiratory depression.

Indications

Opioids cause sedation, respiratory depression, hypotension, miosis, and analgesia. The goal of therapy is to restore adequate spontaneous respirations.

When administering naloxone, monitor a patient for respiratory rate changes and for opioid withdrawal symptoms (anxiety, hypertension, tachycardia, diarrhea, seizure). To avoid withdrawal, use the lowest possible dose that maintains proper spontaneous ventilation. The patient should be observed for respiratory depression once naloxone therapy is discontinued because the duration of naloxone is typically shorter than most opioids. If a patient is not responsive to 10 to 15 mg of naloxone, it is doubtful that an opioid is the primary or sole cause of respiratory depression.

Contraindications

Avoid in patients with a known hypersensitivity to the drug.

Adverse effects

Reversal of an opioid overdose may cause confusion, agitation, and vomiting. Use in an opioid-dependent patient can precipitate withdrawal. Withdrawal convulsions in a neonate can be life threatening.

Hypertension and dysrhythmias occur more often with opioid reversal in postoperative patients who have underlying cardiac and pulmonary complications.

Pralidoxime (Protopam, 2-PAM)

Uses

Pralidoxime is used in cases of severe poisoning by an organophosphate anticholinesterase insecticide or chemical terrorism nerve agent.

Mechanism of action

Pralidoxime regenerates acetylcholinesterase activity by dephosphorylating the anticholinesterase agent's binding to acetylcholinesterase.

Indications

Pralidoxime is indicated in severe organophosphate or nerve agent poisoning, in combination with atropine, to resolve nicotinic (muscle and diaphragmatic weakness, fasciculations, muscle cramps) and central (coma, seizures) cholinergic manifestations.

Contraindications

Pralidoxime should not be used in patients who are hypersensitive to the drug.

Adverse effects

- Tachycardia, dizziness, hyperventilation, and laryngospasm associated with rapid I.V. infusion
- Blurred vision and diplopia
- Possible neuromuscular blockade (weakness) with high levels or in patients with myasthenia gravis

43-8 Pharmacist's Role

To reduce deaths and harm from illicit drug use, several approaches have been initiated that pharmacists should promote, incorporate in their practice, and include in patient counseling.

- Drug take-back, drop-box, and disposal programs (see Chapter 2) to help reduce the diversion and misuse of unused, unwanted, and/or expired medications
- Promoting use of overdose-reversing rescue drugs like naloxone to patients at risk and by family, friends, active bystanders, emergency medical services, and police
- Provide persons who inject drugs access to sterile supplies to reduce the transmission of blood borne infection or refer them to a Syringe Services Program
- Recommend innovative drug products with deterrents to misuse when appropriate (see Chapter 4)
- Use prescription drug monitoring programs (also known as controlled substances monitoring databases) to help identify overutilization, doctor shopping, and other red flags that could indicate an emerging or current SUD.
- Employ risk evaluation and mitigation strategies (see Chapter 2)
- Utilize a perpetual inventory system to deter and detect diversion in pharmacies, all health care facilities, and verify shipments of controlled substances immediately upon receipt
- Promote health and behavioral care for substance use disorders, rehabilitation, and co-occurring mental illness (see Chapter 29) and incorporate screening tools into workflow to assess and identify at-risk patients
- During patient counseling, promote poison prevention measures such as child-resistant closures, secure medicine cabinets/storage, appropriate product usage, and poison control center access (1-800-222-1222)

NAPLEX Competency Statements

The questions in this chapter cover the following 2021 NAPLEX Competency Statements: **AREA 1:** 1.2; 1.5 **AREA 2:** 2.1; 2.2 **AREA 3:** 3.2; 3.3; 3.4; 3.5; 3.6; 3.7 **AREA 6:** 6.3; 6.4.

43-9 Questions

1. Flumazenil is contraindicated in which of the following? (Mark all that apply.)

   A. A patient with QRS widening with a known ingestion of amitriptyline (Elavil)
   B. A patient who was previously given flumazenil last month and who now complains of abnormal vision and dizziness
   C. A patient with known use of cocaine before arrival of emergency medical services
   D. A patient who ingested ethanol
   E. A patient with severe dental problems indicative of "meth mouth"

2. At the emergency department, a patient is experiencing CNS and respiratory depression, which are suspected to be related to ingestion of MS Contin (morphine). Together with supportive care, which of the following drugs is indicated?

   A. Flumazenil
   B. Naloxone
   C. Lorazepam
   D. Flumazenil and naloxone
   E. Naltrexone injection

3. FDA-approved medications for substance use disorder include which of the following? (Mark all that apply.)

   A. Buprenorphine
   B. Methadone
   C. Naloxone
   D. Naltrexone
   E. Pralidoxime

4. Which of the following, when clustered in a 12-month period, contribute to a substance use disorder diagnosis? (Mark all that apply.)

A. Substance is taken in larger amounts or over a longer period than was intended
B. Recurrent substance use in situations where it is physically hazardous
C. There is a persistent desire or unsuccessful efforts to cut down or control substance use
D. Withdrawal manifested by taking opioids, sedatives, hypnotics or anxiolytics, or stimulant medications solely under appropriate medical supervision
E. Substance use is continued without knowledge of having a persistent or recurrent physical or psychological problem that is likely to have been caused or exacerbated by substance use

5. Which medication can be prescribed by any licensed provider to treat opioid use disorder and is available as a tablet and I.M. injection?

A. Buprenorphine
B. Naltrexone
C. Methadone
D. Naloxone
E. Disulfiram

6. Which drug does not exhibit tolerance or dependence, has no clinically significant drug interactions, and can lessen the negative symptoms associated with alcohol withdrawal?

A. MDMA
B. Ketamine
C. Acamprosate
D. Disulfiram
E. Naloxone

7. QT-interval prolongation and serious arrhythmias (torsades de pointes) can occur during treatment with which of the following medications?

A. Acamprosate
B. Methadone
C. Disulfiram
D. Acetylcysteine
E. Naltrexone

8. Some states limit sales of certain products to minors and include which of the following products? (Mark all that apply.)

A. Dextromethorphan
B. Ketamine
C. Inhalants
D. Phencyclidine
E. Naproxen

9. A cab driver presents to the emergency department with vomiting, diarrhea, sweating, salivation, moist rales, bradycardia, muscle tremor, and weakness. He reports inhaling a mist dropped from a low-flying plane several hours earlier. Miosis is present, and his respiratory difficulty is increasing rapidly. Which of the following is the likely mechanism of toxicity of the poison?

A. Inhibition of protein synthesis
B. Binding of the agent to cytochrome oxidase
C. Inhibition of acetylcholinesterase
D. An alkylating agent that cross-links DNA strands
E. Inhibiting aldehyde dehydrogenase

10. Which of the following drugs is indicated for the initial management of muscarinic symptoms from an organophosphate poisoning?

A. Sodium bicarbonate
B. Disulfiram
C. Succimer
D. Pralidoxime
E. Atropine

11. For which of the following conditions or situations is ipecac syrup routinely administered?

A. Ingestion of a plant leaf
B. Not routinely administered for any situation
C. Unresponsiveness to verbal commands
D. Ingestion of a corrosive agent
E. Reversal of opioid induced respiratory depression

12. Which of the following is an effect of activated charcoal? (Mark all that apply.)

A. Minimizes drug absorption from the gastrointestinal tract
B. Increases urinary flow
C. Enhances systemic elimination of certain drugs
D. Decreases intestinal blood flow
E. Increases elimination half-life of certain drugs

13. Which of the following drugs is useful in the treatment of acetaminophen poisoning?

A. Acetylcysteine
B. Dimercaprol
C. Pralidoxime
D. Atropine
E. Flumazenil

14. You are working as a pharmacist in a retail setting when a regular patient approaches the counter with a prescription for a controlled substance he picks up monthly. It is 10 days early, and you explain that you cannot fill the CII prescription and ask the patient about the need for the early fill. The patient explains that he has needed more tablets daily and just does not feel right when taking the prescribed dose. He explains that he has been out for 2 days and has missed work and important social events because he feels terrible without the medication. From the information the patient provided, which of the following accurately describes the patient's Substance Use Disorder Assessment?

A. Low 0 to 1
B. Mild 2 to 3
C. Moderate 4 to 5
D. Severe 6+
E. None

15. Hyperemesis syndrome is associated with chronic use of which of the following?

A. Heroin
B. Marijuana
C. Methamphetamine
D. Suvorexant
E. Ethanol

16. Which of the following mechanisms is associated with the production of hepatic injury from an acute overdose of acetaminophen?

A. Interference with RNA synthesis
B. Interference with transaminase enzyme activity
C. Direct toxic effect of acetaminophen
D. Formation of a toxic metabolite of acetaminophen
E. Binding of the agent to cytochrome oxidase

17. Which of the following signs or symptoms is characteristic of an overdose from the ingestion of a benzodiazepine?

A. Salivation and runny nose
B. Ataxia
C. Muscle rigidity
D. Shock
E. Hyperemesis syndrome

18. When used concomitantly with benzodiazepines, these substances increase the risk of respiratory depression and death. (Mark all that apply.)

A. Methadone
B. Buprenorphine
C. Naltrexone
D. Gamma-hydroxybutyrate
E. Methamphetamine

19. Which of the following represents the appropriate place to administer Narcan?

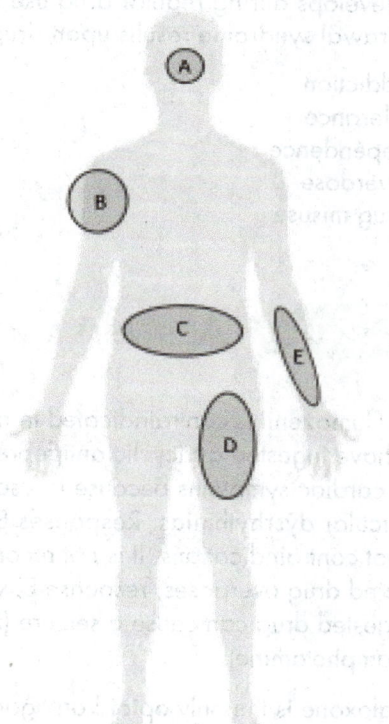

A.
B.
C.
D.
E.

20. A patient misusing multiple substances, primarily prescription opioids and alcohol, who has failed to cutback use on his own would receive the most potential benefit from which of the following treatment options?

A. Disulfiram
B. Counseling and buprenorphine
C. Counseling and Naltrexone
D. Abstinence based support group
E. Acute detoxification

21. Acute hepatitis is a contraindication to starting or continuing to receive which of the following medications?

A. Acamprosate
B. Buprenorphine
C. Naltrexone
D. Methadone
E. Disulfiram

22. Which of the following refers to a physical state that develops during regular drug use in which a withdrawal syndrome results upon drug cessation?

A. Addiction
B. Tolerance
C. Dependence
D. Overdose
E. Drug misuse

 **43-10   Answers**

1. **A, C.** Flumazenil is contraindicated in all patients who have ingested a tricyclic antidepressant and have cardiac symptoms because its use could cause ventricular dysrhythmias. Responses B and D are not contraindications. It is not recommended in mixed drug overdoses, response E, where the co-ingested drug can cause a seizure (i.e., cocaine, methamphetamine).

2. **B.** Naloxone is the only opioid antagonist on the list. The combination of naloxone and flumazenil offers no additional benefit and may increase the risk of seizures if other drugs have been taken.

3. **A, B, D.** Naloxone is a rescue drug that reverses acute episodes of opioid-induced respiratory depression. Pralidoxime is indicated in severe organophosphate or nerve agent poisoning.

4. **A, B, C.** Tolerance developed while taking opioids, sedatives, hypnotics or anxiolytics, or stimulant medications as directed under appropriate medical supervision is not one of the 11 diagnostic criteria for SUD, choice D. Only when substance use is continued "with" knowledge of having a persistent or recurrent physical or psychological problem that is likely to have been caused or exacerbated by substance use, is it included.

5. **B.** Naltrexone is FDA approved to treat opioid use disorder and alcohol use disorder and can be prescribed by any licensed prescriber. An X-license is required to prescribe buprenorphine to treat OUD. Methadone can only be prescribed by authorized physicians and dispensed through an opioid treatment program (methadone clinic) certified by the federal Substance Misuse and Mental Health Services Administration. Naloxone is used to reverse opioid induced respiratory depression. Disulfiram is used in the treatment of alcohol use disorder.

6. **C.** Acamprosate does not exhibit tolerance or dependence, can be taken with opioids and alcohol safely, has no apparent misuse potential, has no clinically significant drug interactions, and is not metabolized by the liver. MDMA is a synthetic psychoactive drug with stimulant and hallucinogenic properties that in high doses can cause malignant hyperthermia and rhabdomyolysis. Ketamine is approved for both human and animal use as an injectable anesthetic and is obtained via diversion, frequently from veterinary office theft. Disulfiram is approved for alcohol use disorder and the disulfiram–alcohol interaction can produce life-threatening effects that are generally proportional to the amounts of disulfiram and alcohol ingested. Survorexant is a sleep medication that, along with benzodiazepines, is sometimes used as a date rape drug typically placed in alcoholic drinks. Ethanol is a CNS depressant and tolerance, dependence, withdrawal, and addiction develop with chronic use.

7. **B.** Methadone has been associated with QT-interval prolongation, particularly when other drugs are present that have the same risk, such as disopyramide, dofetilide, ibutilide, procainamide, quinidine, sotalol, and many more cardiac and noncardiac drugs. Acamprosate is contraindicated in patients with severe renal impairment. Disulfiram should never be administered to a person in a state of alcohol intoxication or without his or her full knowledge. Acetylcysteine is contraindicated if there is a known hypersensitivity to the drug. Naltrexone is associated with hepatocellular injury.

8. **A, C.** Ketamine is prescription only but is sometimes diverted from veterinary offices and misused for its hallucinogenic properties. Phencyclidine (PCP) is a "dissociative" drug and induces distortion of sight and sound, producing feelings of detachment. Naproxen is an over-the-counter, anti-inflammatory pain reliever.

9. **C.** The symptoms exhibited are classically cholinergic, and the likely chemical agents causing these symptoms are organophosphates such as chemical warfare nerve agents or commercial insecticides. Both can be spread by low-flying planes.

10. **E.** Atropine is used to treat the organophosphate-induced muscarinic symptoms (miosis, nausea and vomiting, diarrhea, urination, bradycardia, and excessive bronchial, lacrimal, dermal, nasal, and salivary secretions). Pralidoxime is used with atropine to resolve severe organophosphate symptoms (such as those from exposure to nerve agents), including nicotinic symptoms of muscle weakness and cramps, fasciculations, and tachycardia and CNS symptoms such as coma and seizures. Succimer is used for lead poisoning. Sodium bicarbonate has several uses including the treatment of tricyclic antidepressant toxicity. Neither succimer nor sodium bicarbonate has a role for the muscarinic effects.

11. **B.** Ipecac syrup is no longer used to cause vomiting after the ingestion of a suspected toxin.

12. **A, C.** Activated charcoal adsorbs chemicals on contact and prevents their absorption into the bloodstream. For certain drugs (e.g., phenobarbital, theophylline), multiple doses of activated charcoal can promote the back diffusion of drugs across the intestinal capillary bed into the lumen of the gut, trap it there, and promote its elimination. The elimination half-life can be decreased by as much as one-half.

13. **A.** Acetylcysteine prevents the development of liver injury from acetaminophen if given early after ingestion and, in some cases, may help minimize the effects of hepatotoxicity after it has occurred. The other drugs do not prevent or treat acetaminophen toxicity.

14. **B.** This patient displays 3 of the DSM-V Substance Use Disorder Assessment criteria. Important social,

occupational, or recreational activities are given up or reduced because of substance use. Tolerance, as defined by either (1) a need for markedly increased amounts of substance to achieve intoxication or desired effect or (2) a markedly diminished effect with continued use of the same amount of the substance. Withdrawal, as manifested by either (1) the characteristic withdrawal syndrome for the substance or (2) the substance (or a closely related substance) is taken to relieve or avoid withdrawal symptoms.

15. **B.** Marijuana is the only drug listed that with long-term daily use contributes to a rare condition, cannabinoid hyperemesis syndrome, leading to repeated and severe bouts of vomiting.

16. **D.** Acetaminophen forms a toxic metabolite that has a direct toxic effect within the hepatocyte. It has other proposed mechanisms, but this mechanism is thought to be the inciting event.

17. **B.** Ataxia is a common effect of excessive benzodiazepines. It also can cause sedation but rarely unresponsiveness and respiratory distress unless taken with other CNS depressants or quickly injected intravenously. The other symptoms are not observed.

18. **A, B, D.** Combining CNS depressants increases the risk of respiratory depression and death. Naltrexone is an opioid antagonist that blocks or reverses CNS depressant effects of opioids. Methamphetamine is a CNS stimulant.

19. **A.** Narcan nasal spray should be administered nasally. I.M. forms of naloxone can be given in the deltoid (B) or anterior lateral thigh (D). E represents I.V. administration. C is a subcutaneous injection region and not appropriate for naloxone administration.

20. **C.** Naltrexone is approved to treat both opioid and alcohol use disorders. Disulfiram is only approved for the treatment of alcohol use disorder. Buprenorphine is approved to treat opioid use disorder. Multimodal treatment is more effective than any single treatment alone.

21. **C.** Naltrexone has the capacity to cause hepatocellular injury when given in excessive doses, is contraindicated in acute hepatitis or liver failure, and its use in patients with active liver disease must be carefully considered due to its hepatotoxic effects.

22. C. Addiction is primary, chronic, neurobiological disease with genetic, psychosocial, and environmental factors influencing its development and manifestations. Tolerance is the body's physical adaptation to a drug where greater amounts are required over time to achieve the initial desired effect or continued use of the same amount produces markedly diminished effect. Overdose is an intentional or unintentional acute consumption of an excessive (supratherapeutic) amount of a drug (similar to the definition of poisoning). Use of a drug for a nontherapeutic effect to alter mood, emotion, or state of consciousness is drug misuse.

43-11   Additional Resources

Substance Misuse

Substance Abuse and Mental Health Services Administration. *Medications for Opioid Use Disorder*. Treatment Improvement Protocol (TIP) Series 63. Publication No. PEP20-02-01-006. Rockville, MD: Substance Abuse and Mental Health Services Administration; 2021. https://store.samhsa.gov/product/TIP-63-Medications-for-Opioid-Use-Disorder-Full-Document/PEP21-02-01-002.

Substance Abuse and Mental Health Services Administration. *Key substance use and mental health indicators in the United States: Results from the 2018 National Survey on Drug Use and Health* (HHS Publication No. PEP19-5068, NSDUH Series H-54). Rockville, MD: Center for Behavioral Health Statistics and Quality, Substance Abuse and Mental Health Services Administration; 2020. https://www.samhsa.gov/data/sites/default/files/reports/rpt29393/2019NSDUHFFRPDFWHTML/2019NSDUHFFR090120.htm.

United States Drug Enforcement Administration: Diversion Control Division. *Drug & Chemical Evaluation Section*. Available at: https://www.deadiversion.usdoj.gov/drug_chem_info/index.html. Accessed May 22, 2020.

General Toxicology

Hayes BD, Chyka PA. Clinical toxicology. In: DiPiro JT, Yee GC, Posey ML, et al., eds. *Pharmacotherapy: A Pathophysiologic Approach*. 11th ed. New York, NY: McGraw-Hill; 2019:e19–e20.

Olson KR, ed. *Poisoning and Drug Overdose*. 7th ed. New York, NY: Lange/McGraw-Hill; 2018.

Sheinhait I, Zhou S. Managing drug overdoses and poisonings. In: Zeind CS, Carvalho MG, eds. *Applied Therapeutics: The Clinical Use of Drugs*. 11th ed. Philadelphia, PA: Wolters Kluwer, 2018:62–82.

Appendix A: FDA Boxed Warnings

Drug	Boxed warning
Abacavir	Patients who carry the HLA-B*5701 allele are at a higher risk of a hypersensitivity reaction to abacavir.
Abaloparatide	Dose-dependent increase in incidence of osteosarcoma observed in rats. Use is not recommended in patients at increased risk of osteosarcoma. Cumulative use of this medication should not exceed 2 years.
ACE Inhibitors	All drugs that act directly on the renin-angiotensin system can cause injury and death to the developing fetus. When pregnancy is detected, all ACE inhibitors should be discontinued as soon as possible, particularly during the second and third trimesters.
Acetaminophen (Tylenol)	Acetaminophen has been associated with cases of acute liver failure that may result in death or require liver transplant. The risk of liver injury is greater with doses that exceed the maximum daily limits as well as when taking more than one acetaminophen-containing product.
	Acetaminophen injection carries to potential for dosing errors that could result in accidental overdose and death. Ensure the following: the dose in milligrams and milliliters is not confused; the dosing is based on weight for patients less than 50 kg; infusion pumps are properly programmed; and the total daily dose of acetaminophen from all sources does not exceed maximum daily limits.
Acitretin (Soriatane)	Highly teratogenic—contraindicated in pregnancy. Women receiving treatment should not become pregnant for at least 3 years after treatment ends. Only available through a specialized distribution and education program called "Do your P.A.R.T." Anyone (women and men) receiving therapy cannot donate blood during treatment or for at least 3 years after treatment ends. Increased risk of liver toxicity.
Adalimumab (Humira)	Increased risk of serious infections (e.g., tuberculosis, invasive fungal infections). Lymphoma and other malignancies have been reported in children and adolescent patients.

(continued)

Drug	Boxed warning
Ado-trastuzumab Emtansine	Cardiotoxicity, hepatotoxicity, teratogenicity
Albiglutide	Albiglutide is contraindicated in patients with a personal or family history of medullary thyroid carcinoma or in patients with multiple endocrine neoplasia type 2 (MEN2).
Aldesleukin (IL-2)	Use aldesleukin with extreme caution in patients who have a history of cardiac or pulmonary disease. Withhold aldesleukin administration in patients developing moderate-to-severe lethargy or somnolence. Aldesleukin treatment is associated with an increased risk of disseminated infection, including sepsis and bacterial endocarditis. Aldesleukin administration has been associated with capillary leak syndrome. Administer aldesleukin in a hospital setting under the supervision of a qualified physician experienced in the use of anticancer agents.
Alemtuzumab	Serious, including fatal, pancytopenia/marrow hypoplasia, autoimmune idiopathic thrombocytopenia, and autoimmune hemolytic anemia can occur in patients receiving alemtuzumab. Alemtuzumab causes serious and life-threatening infusion reactions. Alemtuzumab may cause an increased risk of stroke, serious, including fatal, bacterial, viral, fungal, and protozoan infections, and malignancies, including thyroid cancer, melanoma, and lymphoproliferative disorders. Lemtrada has a REMS program.
Alosetron	Infrequent but serious gastrointestinal adverse reactions have been reported with the use of alosetron hydrochloride. These events, including ischemic colitis and serious complications of constipation, have resulted in hospitalization, and rarely, blood transfusion, surgery, and death.
Alpha Blockers	Abrupt withdrawal is not advised in patients with angina pectoris, coronary artery disease (CAD), or ischemic heart disease. Severe exacerbation of angina and the occurrence of MI and ventricular arrhythmias have been reported in angina patients following abrupt discontinuation. When discontinuation of these drugs is planned, patients should be observed carefully and advised to limit physical activity to a minimum. If the angina worsens or acute coronary insufficiency develops, promptly reinstituting atenolol, at least temporarily, is recommended. Because CAD is common and unrecognized, the prudent approach may be not to discontinue atenolol/nadolol/metoprolol therapy abruptly in patients treated only for hypertension and in patients considered at risk of having occult atherosclerotic heart disease who are given propranolol for other reasons. Gradually reduce dosage over at least 1 to 2 weeks. If angina markedly worsens or acute coronary insufficiency develops on drug withdrawal, reinstate therapy, at least temporarily. Advise the patient against cessation or interruption of therapy without the advice of a physician.
Alprazolam	Concomitant use of benzodiazepines and opioids may result in profound respiratory depression, coma, and death. Reserve combination for patients without other treatment options. Limit dosages and durations to the minimum required and follow patients for signs and symptoms of respiratory depression. Risk of abuse, misuse, addiction, physical dependence, and withdrawal reactions.
Amikacin	Close monitoring of serum concentrations, renal function, and toxicities required due to risk of renal toxicity, neurotoxicity, and ototoxicity. Avoid concomitant use of other nephrotoxic and neurotoxic medications.
Amiloride	Like other potassium-conserving agents, amiloride may cause hyperkalemia (serum potassium levels greater than 5.5 mEq per liter) which, if uncorrected, is potentially fatal. Hyperkalemia occurs commonly (about 10%) when amiloride is used without a kaliuretic diuretic. This incidence is greater in patients with renal impairment, diabetes mellitus (with or without recognized renal insufficiency), and in the elderly. When amiloride hydrochloride is used concomitantly with a thiazide diuretic in patients without these complications, the risk of hyperkalemia is reduced to about 1 to 2 percent. It is thus essential to monitor serum potassium levels carefully in any patient receiving amiloride, particularly when it is first introduced, at the time of diuretic dosage adjustments, and during any illness that could affect renal function.
Aminoglycosides	Close monitoring of serum concentrations, renal function, and toxicities required due to risk of renal toxicity, neurotoxicity, and ototoxicity. Avoid concomitant use of other nephrotoxic and neurotoxic medications. Risk of fetal harm—avoid use in pregnancy.
Amiodarone	May cause potentially fatal toxicities, including pulmonary toxicity, hepatotoxicity, liver injury and worsened arrhythmia. Intended for use only in patients with life-threatening arrhythmias when other treatments ineffective or not tolerated.

Drug	Boxed warning
Amitriptyline	Increased risk of suicidality, particularly in people under 24 years old. Not approved for pediatric use.
Amphetamine	Amphetamines have a high potential for abuse and dependence. Access to drug supply should be limited as there is a potential for non-therapeutic use or distribution to others. Misuse of amphetamines may cause sudden death and serious cardiovascular adverse reactions.
Amphetamine/ Dextroamphetamine (Adderall)	High potential for misuse and dependence. Misuse may cause sudden death and serious cardiovascular events.
Amphotericin B	Only use in patients with progressive and potentially life-threatening fungal infections—should not be used to treat noninvasive fungal infections. Should not be given in doses greater than 1.5 mg/kg.
Androgen	SECONDARY EXPOSURE TO TESTOSTERONE: Virilization has been reported in children who were secondarily exposed to testosterone gel. Children should avoid contact with unwashed or unclothed application sites in men using testosterone gel. Health care providers should advise patients to strictly adhere to recommended instructions for use.
Antithymocyte globulin—equine or rabbit	Should only be prescribed by physicians experienced in immunosuppression therapy and management of organ transplantation patients.
Apixaban (Eliquis)	Increased risk of thrombotic events when discontinued prematurely. Risk of epidural or spinal hematoma if receiving neuraxial anesthesia or undergoing spinal puncture.
ARBs	When used in pregnancy, all ARBs can cause injury and even death to the developing fetus. When pregnancy is detected, these agents should be discontinued as soon as possible.
Aripiprazole	Increased risk of death in elderly patients with dementia related psychosis. Increased risk of suicidal thinking and behaviors in children and young adults under the age of 24.
Asenapine	Increased risk of death in elderly patients with dementia-related psychosis.
Atenolol	Cessation of therapy Myocardial infarction and exacerbations of angina pectoris have occurred following abrupt discontinuation of therapy with beta-blockers. Avoid abrupt discontinuation of therapy. Abrupt discontinuation increases risk of cardiac events.
Atomoxetine	Atomoxetine increased the risk of suicidal ideation in short-term studies in children or adolescents with attention deficit hyperactivity disorder (ADHD).
Auranofin	Contains gold—risk of gold toxicity.
Aveed	Serious pulmonary oil microembolism (POME) reactions can occur during or immediately after administration. Symptoms may include urge to cough, chest pain, dyspnea, and tightening of throat. Patients should be observed in a health care setting for 30 minutes after medication administration.
Azathioprine	Increased risk of malignancy.
Baraclude (entecavir)	Risk of severe acute exacerbations of hepatitis B in patients who discontinue treatment-continue to monitor hepatic function for several months after treatment. Patients who have HIV/HBV coinfections should also be receiving antiretroviral therapy for HIV (entecavir alone could promote resistance to nucleoside reverse transcriptase inhibitors). Risk of lactic acidosis and severe hepatomegaly with steatosis.
Baricitinib	Serious infections leading to hospitalization or death, including tuberculosis and bacterial, invasive fungal, viral, and other opportunistic infections have occurred. Lymphoma and other malignancies have been observed. Thrombosis, including deep venous thrombosis, pulmonary embolism, and arterial thrombosis have occurred.
Basiliximab	Should only be prescribed by physicians experienced in immunosuppression therapy and management of organ transplantation patients.
Belatacept	Increased risk of infection and malignancies. Increased risk of developing post-transplant lymphoproliferative disorder. Should only be prescribed by physicians who have experience with patients with kidney transplants and immunosuppressive therapies. Use in liver transplant patients is not recommended due to increased mortality.

(continued)

Drug	Boxed warning
Benzodiazepines	Concomitant use with opioids increases risk of sedation, respiratory depression, coma, and death. Risk of misuse, dependence, addiction, and withdrawal reactions.
Bleomycin	Idiosyncratic reaction, pulmonary toxicity (with increased risk with cumulative dose > 400 units)
Blinatumomab	Cytokine release syndrome (CRS) and neurological toxicities, which may be life-threatening or fatal, occurred in patients receiving blinatumomab.
Brentuximab Vedotin	Progressive multifocal leukoencephalopathy
Brexpiprazole	Increased risk of death in elderly patients with dementia-related psychosis. Increased risk of suicidal thinking and behaviors in children and young adults under the age of 24.
Brodalumab	Increased risk of suicidal ideation and behavior. Risks and benefits should be assessed before initiation of therapy. Close monitoring required. Only available through SILIQ REMS program.
Buprenorphine	Serious, life-threatening respiratory depression, overdose, and death may occur with buprenorphine use. Concomitant use with benzodiazepines increases risk for severe CNS depression. The drug exposes patients and other users to the risks of opioid misuse and addiction. Use during pregnancy can result in neonatal opioid withdrawal syndrome. A REMS program is in place to evaluate risk vs benefit and also a REMS specific to subdermal buprenorphine implants (Probuphine) due to risk of implant migration, protrusion, and expulsion. Potential for misuse, abuse, and addiction. Potential for life-threatening respiratory depression, especially if used concomitantly with benzodiazepines. Avoid use in pregnant women due to risk of neonatal opioid withdrawal. Accidental exposure to even one dose by children can result in a fatal overdose. Risk of serious harm or death with extended-release injection.
Busulfan	Busulfan is a potent drug. Busulfan oral tablets should not be used unless a diagnosis of chronic myelogenous leukemia (CML) has been adequately established and the responsible health care provider is knowledgeable in assessing response to chemotherapy. (2) Busulfan tablets can induce severe bone marrow hypoplasia. Reduce or discontinue the dosage of oral busulfan immediately at the first sign of any unusual depression of bone marrow function as reflected by an abnormal decrease in any of the formed elements of the blood. A bone marrow examination should be performed if the bone marrow status is uncertain. Busulfan injection causes severe and prolonged myelosuppression at the recommended dosage. Hematopoietic progenitor cell transplantation is required to prevent potentially fatal complications of the prolonged myelosuppression.
Cabazitaxel	Hypersensitivity, neutropenia
Capecitabine	Warfarin interaction
Carbamazepine	Carbamazepine has been reported to be associated with aplastic anemia and agranulocytosis. In addition, Stevens-Johnson syndrome and toxic epidermal necrolysis have been reported, especially with HLA-B*1502 allele.
Carboplatin	Bone marrow suppression, hypersensitivity reactions, vomiting
Cariprazine	Increased risk of death in elderly patients with dementia-related psychosis.
Carmustine	Bone marrow suppression, pulmonary toxicity (with increased risk at cumulative doses > 1400 mg/m^2)
Celecoxib	Serious cardiovascular risk and serious gastrointestinal risk. Nonsteroidal anti-inflammatory drugs (NSAIDs) have an increased risk of serious cardiovascular events including myocardial infarction and stroke. NSAIDs also cause an increased risk of serious gastrointestinal adverse events including bleeding, ulceration, and perforation of the stomach or intestines. Increased risk of cardiovascular thrombotic events. Increased risk of serious gastrointestinal adverse events (ex: stomach bleed, ulcers).
Certolizumab Pegol (Cimzia)	Increased risk of serious infections (e.g., tuberculosis, invasive fungal infections). Lymphoma and other malignancies have been reported in children and adolescent patients. Not indicated for use in pediatric patients.
Cetuximab	Cetuximab may cause serious and fatal infusion reactions. Cardiopulmonary arrest or sudden death occurred in patients with squamous cell carcinoma of the head and neck receiving cetuximab.
Chlorambucil	Bone marrow suppression, teratogenicity

Drug	Boxed warning
Chlorpromazine	Increased risk of death in elderly patients with dementia-related psychosis.
Cilostazol	Cilostazol is contraindicated in patients with congestive heart failure of any severity.
Ciprofloxacin	Risk of serious adverse reactions including tendinitis, tendon rupture, peripheral neuropathy, central nervous effects, and exacerbation of myasthenia gravis.
Cisplatin	Myelosuppression, nausea and vomiting, nephrotoxicity, peripheral neuropathy
Citalopram	Increased risk of suicidality, particularly in people under 24 years old. Not approved for pediatric use.
Cladribine	Bone marrow suppression, malignancy, nephrotoxicity, neurotoxicity, teratogenicity
Clindamycin (Cleocin)	Clindamycin has been associated with severe Clostridioides (formerly Clostridium) difficile-associated diarrhea (CDAD) which may result in death. Do not use clindamycin for nonbacterial infections, such as most upper respiratory infections.
Clomipramine	Increased risk of suicidality, particularly in people under 24 years old. Not approved for pediatric use.
Clopidogrel	Consider the use of another platelet inhibitor in patients identified as poor CYP2C19 metabolizers.
Clorazepate	Increased risk of profound sedation if use concomitantly with opioids. Risk of abuse, misuse, addiction, physical dependence, and withdrawal reactions.
Clozapine	May cause severe neutropenia, which can lead to serious and fatal infections. Patients initiating and continuing treatment with clozapine must have a baseline blood absolute neutrophil count (ANC) measured before treatment initiation and regular ANC monitoring during treatment. Orthostatic hypotension, bradycardia, and syncope: risk is dose related. Starting dose is 12.5 mg. Titrate gradually and use divided dosages. Seizure: Risk is dose-related. Titrate gradually and use divided doses. Use with caution in patients with history of seizure or risk factors for seizure. Myocarditis, cardiomyopathy, and mitral valve Incompetence: Can be fatal. Discontinue and obtain cardiac evaluation if findings suggest these cardiac reactions. Increased mortality in Elderly patients with dementia-related psychosis.
Clozapine	Risk of severe neutropenia, orthostatic hypotension, bradycardia, syncope, seizure, myocarditis, and cardiomyopathy. Increased mortality in elderly patients with dementia-related psychosis.
Codeine	Codeine has a REMS program to ensure that the benefits of opioid analgesics outweigh the risks of addiction, abuse, and misuse. Prolonged use of codeine during pregnancy can result in neonatal opioid withdrawal syndrome. Serious, life-threatening, or fatal respiratory depression may occur with use of codeine. Concomitant use of opioids with benzodiazepines or other CNS depressants, including alcohol, may result in profound sedation, respiratory depression, coma, and death. Use of cytochrome P450 3A4 inducers, 3A4 inhibitors, or 2D6 inhibitors with codeine requires careful consideration of the effects on the parent drug, codeine, and the active metabolite morphine. CYP2D6 ultra-rapid metabolism and other risk factors for life-threatening respiratory depression may occur in children who receive codeine.
Cyclophosphamide	Increased risk of first trimester pregnancy loss and congenital malformations. Increased risk of lymphomas and other malignancies. Increased risk of serious infections.
Cyclosporine	Must be prescribed by physicians experienced in immunosuppressive therapy. Sandimmune® and Neoral® are NOT interchangeable. May increase susceptibility to infection and development of neoplasia. Increased risk of hypertension and nephrotoxicity, even at recommended therapeutic doses. Variable absorption—requires frequent monitoring. Psoriasis patients previously treated with psoralens plus ultraviolet A are at an increased risk of developing skin malignancies.
Cytarabine, Liposomal	Chemical arachnoiditis
Dabigatran (Pradaxa)	Increased risk of thrombotic events when discontinued prematurely. Risk of epidural or spinal hematoma if receiving neuraxial anesthesia or undergoing spinal puncture.
Dacarbazine	Bone marrow suppression, hepatic necrosis, teratogenicity
Daklinza (daclatasvir + sofosbuvir)	Risk of reactivation of hepatitis B-patients should be tested for evidence of current or prior hepatitis B infection before initiation of treatment.
Darbepoetin alfa	Erythropoiesis-stimulating agents (ESAs) increase the risk of death, myocardial infarction (MI), stroke, venous thromboembolism, and thrombosis of vascular access. Use the lowest effective dose.

(continued)

Drug	Boxed warning
Daunorubicin, Conventional	Bone marrow suppression, cardiomyopathy (with increased risk at cumulative doses > 400 to 550 mg/m^2), extravasation, hepatic impairment, renal impairment
Daunorubicin, Liposomal	Bone marrow suppression, hepatic impairment, infusion reactions, myocardial toxicity
Daytrana	Daytrana should be given cautiously to patients with a history of drug dependence or alcoholism. Long term abusive use may lead to psychological dependence, abnormal behavior, and psychotic episodes. During withdrawal from abusive use, severe depression may occur.

Use cautiously in patients with history of drug dependence of alcoholism. Long term abusive use may lead to psychological dependence, abnormal behavior, and psychotic episodes. |
Depo-Provera	Risk of significant bone mineral density loss which may not be completely reversible. Unknown if use in adolescence or early adulthood increases risk of osteoporotic fracture later in life. Avoid use for longer than 2 years.
Depo-SubQ Provera 104	Risk of significant bone mineral density loss which may not be completely reversible. Unknown if use in adolescence or early adulthood increases risk of osteoporotic fracture later in life. Avoid use for longer than 2 years.
Desipramine	Suicidality and antidepressants. Antidepressants including desipramine increased the risk of suicidal thinking and behaviors in children and young adults under the age of 24. Patients of all ages starting desipramine should be monitored for suicidality and unusual changes in behavior. Increased risk of suicidality.
Desvenlafaxine	Increased risk of suicidality, particularly in people under 24 years old.
Dexmethylphenidate	CNS stimulants, including dexmethylphenidate, methylphenidate-containing products, and amphetamines, have a high potential for abuse and dependence.

High potential for abuse and dependence. |
Dextroamphetamine (Dexedrine)	High potential for misuse and dependence. Misuse may cause sudden death and serious cardiovascular events.
Diazepam	Increased risk of profound sedation if use concomitantly with opioids. Risk of abuse, misuse, addiction, physical dependence, and withdrawal reactions.
Diclofenac	Serious cardiovascular risk and serious gastrointestinal risk. Nonsteroidal anti-inflammatory drugs (NSAIDs) have an increased risk of serious cardiovascular events including myocardial infarction and stroke. NSAIDs also cause an increased risk of serious gastrointestinal adverse events including bleeding, ulceration, and perforation of the stomach or intestines. Increased risk of cardiovascular thrombotic events. Increased risk of serious gastrointestinal adverse events (ex: stomach bleed, ulcers).
Dihydroergotamine	Concurrent drug therapy. Serious or life-threatening peripheral ischemia has been associated with co-administration of dihydroergotamine with potent CYP3A4 inhibitors.

Co-administration of potent CYP3A4 inhibitors increases risk of severe peripheral ischemia. |
Dinutuximab	Neurotoxicities and serious and potentially life-threatening infusion reactions can occur in patients treated with dinutuximab.
Direct Renin Inhibitor	When pregnancy is detected, these drugs should be discontinued as soon as possible. Drugs that act directly on the renin-angiotensin system can cause injury and death to a developing fetus.
Disulfiram	Disulfiram should never be administered to a patient when they are in a state of alcohol intoxication, or without their full knowledge.
Divalproex Sodium	Valproic acid and its derivatives have FDA boxed warnings for hepatotoxicity, pancreatitis, fetal risk, and are contraindicated in patients with mitochondrial disease. Children under 2 years of age are at a considerably increased risk of hepatotoxicity.

Valproate is contraindicated in patients with known mitochondrial disorders and in children younger than two who are clinically suspected to have a mitochondrial disorder. In addition, valproate can cause neural tube defects, and is contraindicated in women of childbearing potential who are not using effective contraception. Increased risk of hepatotoxicity. Increased risk of pancreatitis. Use in pregnant women is contraindicated due to increased risk of congenital malformations. |

Drug	Boxed warning
Docetaxel	Fluid retention, hepatic function impairment, hypersensitivity, increased mortality, neutropenia
Dofetilide	To minimize the risk of induced arrhythmia, patients initiated or re-initiated on dofetilide should be placed for a minimum of 3 days in a facility that can provide calculations of creatinine clearance, continuous ECG monitoring, and cardiac resuscitation.
Doxepin	Increased risk of suicidality, particularly in people under 24 years old. Not approved for pediatric use.
Doxorubicin, Conventional	Cardiomyopathy (increased risk at cumulative doses > 450 mg/m^2), extravasation, secondary malignancy, myelosuppression
Doxorubicin, Liposomal	Cardiomyopathy (increased risk at cumulative doses > 450 mg/m^2), infusion-related reactions
Dronedarone	Increased risk of death, stroke, and heart failure in patients with decompensated heart failure or permanent atrial fibrillation. In patients with symptomatic heart failure and recent decompensation requiring hospitalization or NYHA Class IV heart failure, dronedarone hydrochloride doubles the risk of death. Dronedarone hydrochloride is contraindicated in patients with symptomatic heart failure with recent de-compensation requiring hospitalization or NYHA Class IV heart failure. In patients with permanent atrial fibrillation, dronedarone hydrochloride doubles the risk of death, stroke, and hospitalization for heart failure. Dronedarone hydrochloride is contraindicated in patients in atrial fibrillation (AF) who will not or cannot be cardioverted into normal sinus rhythm.
Duavee	Increased risk of endometrial cancer in a woman with a uterus who uses unopposed estrogens. Do not use for the prevention of cardiovascular disease or dementia. Do not use concurrently with any other estrogen therapy. Use should be limited to lowest dose and least amount of time necessary.
Dulaglutide	Dulaglutide is contraindicated in patients with a personal or family history of medullary thyroid carcinoma and in patients with multiple endocrine neoplasia syndrome type 2 (MEN 2).
Duloxetine	Increased risk of suicidal thoughts and behavior in patients less than 24 years old.
Dyanavel XR	CNS stimulants, including DYANAVEL XR, other amphetamine-containing products, and methylphenidate, have a high potential for abuse and dependence. High potential for abuse and dependence.
Eculizumab	Life-threatening and fatal meningococcal infections have occurred in patients treated with eculizumab. Eculizumab is available only through a restricted program under a Risk Evaluation and Mitigation Strategy (REMS).
Edoxaban (Savaysa)	Reduced efficacy in nonvalvular atrial fibrillation if creatinine clearance is greater than 95 ml/min. Increased risk of thrombotic events when discontinued prematurely. Risk of epidural or spinal hematoma if receiving neuraxial anesthesia or undergoing spinal puncture.
Emtriva (emtricitabine)	Risk of severe acute exacerbations of hepatitis B in patients who discontinue treatment-continue to monitor hepatic function for several months after treatment.
Enalaprilat	When used in pregnancy during the second and third trimesters, ACE inhibitors can cause injury and even death to the developing fetus. When pregnancy is detected, enalaprilat injection should be discontinued as soon as possible.
Enoxaparin, Fodaparinux	Spinal or epidural hematoma Patients receiving neuraxial anesthesia or undergoing spinal puncture are at risk for the development of epidural or spinal hematomas, which may result in long-term or permanent paralysis. Risk factors include the use of indwelling epidural catheters, the concomitant use of medications that increase the risk of bleeding (NSAIDs, antiplatelet agents, other anticoagulants), a history of traumatic or repeated spinal or epidural punctures, and a history of spinal surgery or deformity.
Epclusa (sofosbuvir/velpatasvir)	Risk of reactivation of hepatitis B-patients should be tested for evidence of current or prior hepatitis B infection before initiation of treatment.
Epirubicin	Bone marrow suppression, cardiac toxicity (increased risk after cumulative dose of 550 mg/m^2), extravasation and tissue necrosis, secondary malignancy

(continued)

Drug	Boxed warning
Epivir (lamivudine)	Risk of severe acute exacerbations of hepatitis B in patients who discontinue treatment-continue to monitor hepatic function for several months after treatment. Risk of HIV-1 resistance if used in patients with unrecognized or untreated HIV-1. Important to note that HIV-1 and HBV formulations have different doses and should not be interchanged.
Epoetin alfa	Erythropoiesis-stimulating agents (ESAs) increase the risk of death, myocardial infarction (MI), stroke, venous thromboembolism, and thrombosis of vascular access. Use the lowest effective dose.
Ergotamine	Concurrent drug therapy. Serious or life-threatening peripheral ischemia has been associated with co-administration of ergotamine with potent CYP3A4 inhibitors. Co-administration of potent CYP3A4 inhibitors increases risk of severe peripheral ischemia.
Erythropoiesis-Stimulating Agents (ESAs)	**Cardiovascular events** Erythropoiesis-stimulating agents (ESAs) increase the risk of death, MI, stroke, venous thromboembolism, thrombosis of vascular access. **Chronic kidney disease** In controlled trials, patients experienced greater risks for death, serious adverse cardiovascular reactions, and stroke when administered ESAs to target a hemoglobin level > 11 g/dL. No trial has identified a hemoglobin target level, ESA dose, or dosing strategy that does not increase these risks. Use the lowest ESA dose sufficient to reduce the need for red blood cell (RBC) transfusions.
Escitalopram	Increased risk of suicidality, particular in pediatric and young adult patients. Not approved for use under 12 years of age.
Esketamine (Spravato)	Risk of sedation, dissociation, abuse/misuse, and suicidality. Patients must be monitored in-clinic for at least 2 hours after administration.
Estrogen-Containing Contraceptive Products	Cigarette smoking increases risk of serious cardiovascular effects including myocardial infarction, thromboembolism, and stroke. Avoid use in women over 35 years old who smoke.
Eszopiclone	Risk of complex sleep behaviors (e.g., sleepwalking, sleep-driving). Discontinue immediately if complex sleep behaviors occur.
Etanercept	Increased risk of serious infections (ex: tuberculosis, invasive fungal infections, other opportunistic infections). Lymphoma and other malignancies have been reported in children and adolescent patients. Certolizumab pegol not indicated for use in pediatric patients.
Etoposide	Bone marrow suppression
Everolimus	Increased risk of lymphoma and other malignancies. Increased susceptibility to bacterial, viral, fungal, and protozoal infections. Increased risk of kidney arterial and venous thrombosis. Increased nephrotoxicity if used in combination with cyclosporine. Use is not recommended in heart transplantations due to increased risk of mortality. Should only be prescribed by physicians experienced in immunosuppressive therapies.
Exenatide	Exenatide extended release (ER) causes an increased incidence in thyroid C-cell tumors in animal studies.
Factor VII	Serious arterial and venous thrombotic events following administration of Factor VIIa (recombinant) have been reported.
Febuxostat	Increased risk of cardiovascular (CV) death in patients with established CV disease.
Felbamate	Felbamate has been reported to be associated with aplastic anemia and acute liver failure.
Fentanyl	Potential for misuse, abuse, and addiction. Potential for life-threatening respiratory depression, especially if used concomitantly with benzodiazepines. Monitor interactions with medications metabolized by CYP3A4. Avoid use in pregnant women due to risk of neonatal opioid withdrawal. Exposure to heat (e.g., heating pads, electric blankets) may increase fentanyl levels when using patch formulation. Risk of accidental exposure to children resulting in fatal overdose when using patch formulation.
Ferumoxytol (Feraheme)	Fatal and serious hypersensitivity reactions including anaphylaxis have occurred in patients receiving ferumoxytol.

Drug	Boxed warning
Flecainide	Increased mortality and nonfatal cardiac arrest in patients with non-life-threatening ventricular arrhythmias and structural heart disease; consider avoiding flecainide in these patients. Flecainide is not recommended for use in patients with chronic atrial fibrillation.
Flucytosine	Use with extreme caution in patients with renal impairment. Requires close monitoring of hematologic, renal, and hepatic status.
Fludarabine	Autoimmune effects, bone marrow suppression, neurotoxicity, pulmonary toxicity (in combination with pentostatin)
Flumazenil (Romazicon)	Increased risk of seizures.
Fluoroquinolones	Risk of serious adverse reactions including tendinitis, tendon rupture, peripheral neuropathy, central nervous effects, and exacerbation of myasthenia gravis.
Fluorouracil	Hematologic risk
Fluoxetine	Antidepressants increased the risk of suicidal thinking and behavior in children, adolescents, and young adults with major depressive disorder (MDD) and other psychiatric disorders. Closely monitor patients being started on antidepressants for suicidal ideation or other changes in behavior. Fluoxetine is approved for use in children with MDD (aged 8 years and older) and obsessive-compulsive disorder (OCD; aged 7 years and older). Sarafem is not approved for use in children.
Fluphenazine	Increased risk of death in elderly patients with dementia-related psychosis.
Flurazepam	Increased risk of profound sedation if use concomitantly with opioids. Risk of abuse, misuse, addiction, physical dependence, and withdrawal reactions.
Flutamide	Hepatic injury
Fluvoxamine	Increased risk of suicidality, particularly in people under 24 years old.
Fosphenytoin	Both fosphenytoin and phenytoin are associated with a boxed warning for the risk of severe hypotension and cardiac arrhythmias with rapid intravenous infusions.
Furosemide	Furosemide is a potent diuretic which, if given in excessive amounts, can lead to a profound diuresis with water and electrolyte depletion. Therefore, careful medical supervision is required, and dose and dosage interval must be adjusted to the individual patient's needs.
Gentamicin	Close monitoring of serum concentrations and toxicities required due to risk of renal toxicity, neurotoxicity, and ototoxicity. Avoid concomitant use of other nephrotoxic and neurotoxic medications. Risk of fetal harm—avoid use in pregnancy.
Glasdegib	Glasdegib can cause embryo-fetal death or severe birth defects when administered to a pregnant woman. Glasdegib is embryotoxic, fetotoxic, and teratogenic in animals. Conduct pregnancy testing in females of reproductive potential prior to initiation of glasdegib treatment. Advise females of reproductive potential to use effective contraception during treatment with glasdegib and for at least 30 days after the last dose. Advise males of the potential risk of glasdegib exposure through semen and to use condoms with a pregnant partner or a female partner of reproductive potential during treatment with glasdegib and for at least 30 days after the last dose to avoid potential drug exposure.
Glucagon-Like Peptide-1 Agonists	Dulaglutide, Exenatide extended release, Liraglutide, Semaglutide (subcutaneous injection and oral tablet). Animal models demonstrated increased risk of thyroid C-cell tumors. It is not currently known if these agents cause thyroid C-cell tumors (e.g., medullary thyroid carcinoma) in humans. These agents are contraindicated for use in patients with a personal or family history of medullary thyroid carcinoma and patients with history of multiple endocrine neoplasia type 2.
Golimumab	Increased risk of serious infections (ex: tuberculosis, invasive fungal infections, other opportunistic infections). Lymphoma and other malignancies have been reported in children and adolescent patients. Certolizumab pegol not indicated for use in pediatric patients.
Haloperidol	Increased risk of death in elderly patients with dementia-related psychosis.

(continued)

Drug	Boxed warning
Hepsera (adefovir)	Risk of severe acute exacerbations of hepatitis B in patients who discontinue treatment-continue to monitor hepatic function for several months after treatment. Risk of HIV-1 resistance if used in patients with unrecognized or untreated HIV-1. Risk of nephrotoxicity, lactic acidosis, and severe hepatomegaly with steatosis.
Hormone Therapy – Oral Products	Estrogen-Alone Therapy: Increased risk of endometrial cancer if woman still has a uterus. Do not use for the prevention of cardiovascular disease or dementia. Should be used at lowest dose possible for the least amount of time that is necessary.
	Estrogen plus Progestin Therapy: Do not use for the prevention of cardiovascular disease or dementia. Increased risk of DVT, PE, and MI in postmenopausal women. Increased risk of invasive breast cancer. Should be used at lowest dose possible for the least amount of time that is necessary.
Hormone Therapy – Transdermal Products	Estrogen-Alone Therapy: Increased risk of endometrial cancer if woman still has a uterus. Do not use for the prevention of cardiovascular disease or dementia. Should be used at lowest dose possible for the least amount of time that is necessary.
	Estrogen plus Progestin Therapy: Do not use for the prevention of cardiovascular disease or dementia. Increased risk of DVT, PE, and MI in postmenopausal women. Increased risk of invasive breast cancer. Should be used at lowest dose possible for the least amount of time that is necessary.
	Evamist: Breast budding and breast masses in prepubertal females and gynecomastia and breast masses in prepubertal males have been reported following unintentional secondary exposure. Ensure that children do not come into contact with application sites.
Hormone Therapy – Vaginal Products	Estrogen-Alone Therapy: Increased risk of endometrial cancer if woman still has a uterus. Do not use for the prevention of cardiovascular disease or dementia. Use should be limited to lowest dose and least amount of time necessary.
	Estrogen plus Progestin Therapy: Do not use for the prevention of cardiovascular disease or dementia. Increased risk of DVT, PE, and MI in postmenopausal women. Increased risk of invasive breast cancer. Use should be limited to lowest dose and least amount of time necessary.
Hydroxyurea	Bone marrow suppression, secondary malignancy
Ibritumomab tiuxetan	Serious infusion reactions, prolonged and severe cytopenias, and severe cutaneous and mucocutaneous reactions have been reported.
Ibuprofen (Motrin)	Ibuprofen use is associated with increased risk of serious cardiovascular thrombotic events including myocardial infarction and stroke. It is contraindicated in patients undergoing coronary artery bypass graft surgery. Ibuprofen is also associated with increased risk of gastrointestinal (GI) bleeding, ulcerations, and perforation during any time of use which may result in death. Elderly patients and those with a prior history of peptic ulcer disease or GI bleed are at greater risk for serious GI complications.
Ibutilide	Ibutilide fumarate can cause potentially fatal arrhythmias, particularly sustained polymorphic ventricular tachycardia, usually in association with QT prolongation (torsades de pointes), but sometimes without documented QT prolongation.
	These arrhythmias can be reversed if treated promptly. It is essential that ibutilide fumarate injection be administered in a setting of continuous ECG monitoring and by personnel trained in identification and treatment of acute ventricular arrhythmias, particularly polymorphic ventricular tachycardia. Patients with atrial fibrillation of more than 2 to 3 days' duration must be adequately anticoagulated, generally for at least 2 weeks. Patients with chronic atrial fibrillation have a strong tendency to revert after conversion to sinus rhythm and treatments to maintain sinus rhythm carry risks. Patients to be treated with ibutilide fumarate injection, therefore, should be carefully selected such that the expected benefits of maintaining sinus rhythm outweigh the immediate risks of ibutilide fumarate injection, and the risks of maintenance therapy, and are likely to offer an advantage compared with alternative management.
Idarubicin	Bone marrow suppression, cardiomyopathy, extravasation, hepatic impairment, renal impairment
Ifosfamide	Bone marrow suppression, CNS toxicity, hemorrhagic cystitis, nephrotoxicity
Iloperidone	Increased risk of death in elderly patients with dementia-related psychosis.

Drug	Boxed warning
Imipramine	Antidepressant use has been associated with an increased risk of suicidal thinking and behavior in children, adolescents, and young adults. Short-term studies did not show an increase in the risk of suicidality with antidepressants compared with placebo in adults beyond age 24, and there was a reduction in risk with antidepressants compared with placebo in adults aged 65 or older.
Infliximab	Increased risk of serious infections (ex: tuberculosis, invasive fungal infections, other opportunistic infections). Lymphoma and other malignancies have been reported in children and adolescent patients. Certolizumab pegol not indicated for use in pediatric patients.
Inhaled Insulin	Acute bronchospasms have been observed in patients with asthma and COPD who are using inhaled insulin. Prior to initiation of therapy with inhaled insulin, patients should have pulmonary function testing to identify undiagnosed chronic lung disease.
Interferon alfa-2b	Alpha interferons, including interferon alfa-2b, cause or aggravate fatal or life-threatening neuropsychiatric, autoimmune, ischemic, and infectious disorders.
Ipilimumab	Immune-mediated adverse reactions
Irinotecan, Conventional	Bone marrow suppression, diarrhea
Iron Dextran	Anaphylactic-type reactions, including fatalities, have followed the parenteral administration of iron dextran injection.
Isoniazid	Risk of severe or fatal hepatitis. Risk increases with age as well as alcohol consumption.
Isotretinoin	Use is associated with severe, life-threatening birth defects—use is contraindicated in pregnancy. Due to teratogenicity and to minimize fetal exposure risk, it is only approved for use under a restricted distribution program (iPledge).
Itraconazole	May cause or exacerbate congestive heart failure (CHF). Do not administer for treatment of onychomycosis in patients with evidence of ventricular dysfunction. Significant number of drug–drug interactions and contraindications—see package insert for full list.
Ixabepilone	Hepatic impairment
Ketoconazole	Ketoconazole is associated with serious hepatotoxicity that may result in liver transplantation or death. Due to serious adverse effects, ketoconazole tablets are not indicated for the treatment of onychomycosis, cutaneous dermatophyte infections, or Candida infections. Use ketoconazole only when other effective antifungal therapy is not available or tolerated and the potential benefits are considered to outweigh the potential risks. Ketoconazole is contraindicated with the following drugs: dofetilide, quinidine, pimozide, cisapride, methadone, disopyramide, dronedarone, and ranolazine. Ketoconazole can cause elevated plasma concentrations of these drugs and may prolong QT intervals, sometimes resulting in life-threatening ventricular dysrhythmias, such as torsades de pointes.
Ketoprofen	NSAIDs cause an increased risk of serious cardiovascular thrombotic events, including myocardial infarction and stroke, which can be fatal. Can cause peptic ulcers, gastrointestinal bleeding and/or perforation of the stomach or intestines, which can be fatal. **Contraindications** ■ treatment of perioperative pain in the setting of coronary artery bypass graft (CABG) ■ patients with advanced renal impairment and in patients at risk for renal failure due to volume depletion ■ patients with suspected or confirmed cerebrovascular bleeding, patients with hemorrhagic diathesis, incomplete hemostasis and those at high risk of bleeding ■ prophylactic analgesic before any major surgery ■ labor and delivery ■ nursing mothers ■ patients currently receiving aspirin or NSAIDs because of the cumulative risk of inducing serious NSAID-related side effects **Special Populations** ■ dosage should be adjusted for patients 65 years or older, for patients under 50 kilograms (110 pounds) of body weight and for patients with moderately elevated serum creatinine.

(continued)

Drug	Boxed warning
Lamotrigine	Risk of serious skin rashes (e.g., Stevens-Johnson syndrome, toxic epidermal necrolysis).
Lapatinib	Hepatotoxicity
Leflunomide	Contraindicated in pregnant women. Contraindicated in patients with hepatic impairment.
Lenalidomide	Fetal risk, hematologic toxicity, venous and arterial thromboembolism
Leukotriene modifiers	Risk of serious neuropsychiatric events (e.g., agitation, aggression, depression, sleep disturbances, suicidal thoughts). Risk versus benefit should be assessed prior to initiation of therapy.
Levofloxacin	Risk of serious adverse reactions including tendinitis, tendon rupture, peripheral neuropathy, central nervous effects, and exacerbation of myasthenia gravis.
Levomilnacipran	Increased risk of suicidality, particularly in people under 24 years old. Not approved for use in pediatric patients.
Levorphanol	Levorphanol has FDA boxed warnings for addiction, abuse, and misuse, life-threatening respiratory depression, accidental ingestion, neonatal opioid withdrawal syndrome, and risks from concomitant use with benzodiazepines or other CNS depressants. Levorphanol also has an opioid analgesic risk evaluation and mitigation strategy (REMS) to ensure the benefits of therapy outweigh the risks. Potential for addiction, abuse, and misuse. Potential for life-threatening respiratory depression, especially if used concomitantly with benzodiazepines. Avoid use in pregnant women due to risk of neonatal opioid withdrawal.
Linaclotide	Contraindicated in pediatric patients up less than 6 years of age; in nonclinical studies in neonatal mice, administration of a single, clinically relevant adult oral dose of linaclotide caused deaths due to dehydration. Avoid use of linaclotide in pediatric patients 6 to less than 18 years of age. The safety and efficacy of linaclotide has not been established in pediatric patients under 18 years of age
Lisdexamfetamine (Vyvanse)	High potential for abuse and dependence.
Lithium	Risk of lithium toxicity—monitor levels regularly.
LMWHs	Risk of life-threatening epidural or spinal hematoma if patient is receiving neuraxial anesthesia or undergoing a spinal puncture. Risk increases if patient has an indwelling epidural catheter, is taking other medications that affect hemostasis (e.g., NSAIDs, anticoagulants), has a history of traumatic or repeated epidural or spinal punctures, or has a history of spinal deformity or spinal surgery.
Lomitapide	Lomitapide can cause elevations in transaminases.
Long-Acting Beta-2 Agonist (LABA)	Long-acting beta-2 agonists (LABAs) increase the risk of asthma-related death when used as monotherapy.
Loperamide	Cases of torsades de pointes, cardiac arrest, and death have been reported with the use of a higher than recommended dosages of loperamide hydrochloride. Loperamide hydrochloride is contraindicated in pediatric patients less than 2 years of age. Avoid loperamide hydrochloride dosages higher than recommended in adults and pediatric patients 2 years of age and older due to the risk of serious cardiac adverse reactions.
Lorazepam	Concomitant use of benzodiazepines and opioids may result in profound sedation, respiratory depression, coma, and death. Limit doses and durations to the minimum required. Use of benzodiazepines expose users to risks of abuse, misuse, and addiction, which can lead to overdose and death. Continued use of benzodiazepines for several days to weeks may led to significant physical dependence.
Lumateperone	Increased risk of death in elderly patients with dementia-related psychosis.
Lurasidone	Increased risk of death in elderly patients with dementia-related psychosis.
Maprotiline	Antidepressants increased the risk of suicidal thinking in children, adolescents, and young adults in short-term studies of major depressive disorder and other psychiatric disorders. No increased risk beyond age 24, and there was a reduction in risk with antidepressants compared to placebo in adults aged 65 and older.
Medroxyprogesterone acetate	Estrogen plus Progestin Therapy: Do not use for the prevention of cardiovascular disease or dementia. Increased risk of DVT, PE, and MI in postmenopausal women. Increased risk of invasive breast cancer. Should be used at lowest dose possible for the least amount of time that is necessary.

Drug	Boxed warning
Melphalan	Bone marrow suppression, hypersensitivity, secondary malignancy
Mesoridazine	Mesoridazine has been shown to prolong the QTc interval in a dose related manner, and drugs with this potential have been associated with torsades de pointes–type arrhythmias and sudden death.
Metadate CD	Metadate CD should be given cautiously to patients with a history of drug dependence or alcoholism. Long term abusive use may lead to psychological dependence, abnormal behavior, and psychotic episodes. During withdrawal from abusive use, severe depression may occur.
	Use cautiously in emotionally unstable patients (ex: history of drug dependence or alcohol). Long term abusive use may lead to psychological dependence, abnormal behavior, and psychotic episodes.
Metformin	Lactic acidosis has been associated with metformin use in patients with renal impairment, age $\geq$ 65 years, recent use of contrast for a radiologic study, surgery, hypoxemia, excessive alcohol consumption, hepatic impairment, and when used with carbonic anhydrase inhibitors (e.g., Topiramate).
Methadone	Potential for misuse, abuse, and addiction. Potential for life-threatening respiratory depression, especially if used concomitantly with benzodiazepines. Monitor interactions with medications metabolized by CYP enzymes. Increased risk of QT prolongation.
Methotrexate	Can cause severe or fatal toxicities—closely monitor for infections and adverse reactions of bone marrow, kidneys, liver, nervous system, gastrointestinal tract, lungs, and skin. Contraindicated in pregnancy for non-neoplastic diseases due to embryo-fetal toxicity.
Methylin	Methylin should be given cautiously to emotionally unstable patients, such as those with a history of drug dependence or alcoholism, because such patients may increase dosage on their own initiative. Long term abusive use may lead to psychological dependence, abnormal behavior, and psychotic episodes. During withdrawal from abusive use, severe depression as well as the effects of chronic overactivity may occur.
	Use cautiously in emotionally unstable patients (e.g., history of drug dependence or alcohol). Long term abusive use may lead to psychological dependence, abnormal behavior, and psychotic episodes.
Methylphenidate	CNS stimulants, including methylphenidate-containing products and amphetamines, have a high potential for abuse and dependence. Long term abusive use may lead to psychotic episodes.
Metoclopramide	Risk of tardive dyskinesia. Avoid treatment greater than 12 weeks.
Metoprolol	Ischemic heart disease. Avoid abrupt discontinuation as it is associated with exacerbations of angina pectoris and myocardial infarction.
Metronidazole	Shown to be carcinogenic in mice and rats. Reserve use only for indicated conditions.
Minoxidil	Minoxidil can cause pericardial effusion, occasionally progressing to tamponade, and angina pectoris may be exacerbated. Minoxidil should be reserved for hypertensive patients who do not respond adequately to maximum therapeutic doses of a diuretic and two other antihypertensive agents. Minoxidil must be administered under close supervision, usually concomitantly with therapeutic doses of a beta-adrenergic blocking agent to prevent tachycardia and increased myocardial workload. It must also usually be given with a diuretic, frequently one acting in the ascending limb of the loop of Henle, to prevent serious fluid accumulation. Patients with malignant hypertension and those already receiving guanethidine should be hospitalized when minoxidil is first administered so that they can be monitored to avoid too rapid, or large orthostatic, decreases in blood pressure.
Mipomersen	Mipomersen sodium can cause elevations in transaminases and increases hepatic fat (with or without concomitant increases in transaminases).
Mirtazapine (Remeron and Remeron SolTab)	Increased risk of suicidality. Not approved for use in pediatric patients.
Misoprostol	Avoid use in women of child-bearing age. Should not be used by pregnant women—increased risk of abortion, premature birth, and birth defects.

(continued)

Drug	Boxed warning
Mitomycin	Bone marrow suppression, hemolytic uremic syndrome
Mitotane	In patients taking mitotane, adrenal crisis occurs in the setting of shock or severe trauma and response to shock is impaired. Administer hydrocortisone, monitor for escalating signs of shock, and discontinue mitotane until recovery.
Mitoxantrone	Appropriate administration (I.V. only), bone marrow suppression, cardiotoxicity (increased risk with cumulative doses > 140 mg/m^2), secondary leukemia
Morphine	Serious, life-threatening, or fatal respiratory depression has occurred with use of morphine especially with concomitant use of benzodiazepines or other CNS depressants. Prolonged use of morphine during pregnancy can result in neonatal opioid withdrawal syndrome. Ensure accuracy when prescribing, dispensing, and administering morphine oral solution. To ensure that the benefits of opioid analgesics outweigh the risks of addiction, abuse, and misuse, the FDA has required a REMS for morphine. Because of the risk of severe adverse effects when the epidural or intrathecal route of administration is employed, patients must be observed in a fully equipped and staffed environment for at least 24 hours after the initial dose.
Moxifloxacin	Risk of serious adverse reactions including tendinitis, tendon rupture, peripheral neuropathy, central nervous effects, and exacerbation of myasthenia gravis.
Mycophenolate	Increased risk of first trimester pregnancy loss and congenital malformations. Increased risk of lymphomas and other malignancies. Increased risk of serious infections.
Nadolol	Exacerbation of cardiac ischemia following abrupt withdrawal. Myocardial infarction and exacerbations of angina pectoris have occurred following abrupt discontinuation of therapy with beta-blockers. When discontinuing chronically administered nadolol, gradually reduce the dose over 1 to 2 weeks. Avoid abrupt discontinuation of therapy. Abrupt discontinuation increases risk of cardiac events.
Naproxen	Serious cardiovascular risk and serious gastrointestinal risk. Nonsteroidal anti-inflammatory drugs (NSAIDs) have an increased risk of serious cardiovascular events including myocardial infarction and stroke. NSAIDs also cause an increased risk of serious gastrointestinal adverse events including bleeding, ulceration, and perforation of the stomach or intestines. Increased risk of cardiovascular thrombotic events. Increased risk of serious gastrointestinal adverse events (ex: stomach bleed, ulcers).
Natalizumab	Natalizumab increases the risk of progressive multifocal leukoencephalopathy (PML), an opportunistic viral infection of the brain that usually leads to death or severe disability. Because of the risk of PML, natalizumab is available only through a restricted distribution program called the TOUCH® Prescribing Program.
Nelarabine	Severe neurologic adverse reactions have been reported with the use of nelarabine. These reactions have included altered mental states, including severe somnolence; CNS effects, including convulsions; and peripheral neuropathy, ranging from numbness and paresthesias to motor weakness and paralysis. There have also been reports of adverse reactions associated with demyelination and ascending peripheral neuropathies similar in appearance to Guillain-Barré syndrome. Full recovery from these reactions has not always occurred with cessation of therapy with nelarabine. Monitor frequently for signs and symptoms of neurologic toxicity during treatment with nelarabine. Discontinue nelarabine for neurologic reactions of National Cancer Institute (NCI) Common Toxicity Criteria for Adverse Events (CTCAE) grade 2 or greater.
Nilotinib	QT prolongation and sudden deaths
Nilutamide	Interstitial pneumonitis
Nimodipine	Do not administer nimodipine intravenously or by other parenteral routes. Death and serious, life-threatening adverse events have occurred when the contents of nimodipine capsules have been injected parenterally.
Nortriptyline	Increased risk of suicidality, particularly in people under 24 years old. Not approved for pediatric use.

Drug	Boxed warning
Novel oral anticoagulants (NOACs)	■ Premature discontinuation of dabigatran, apixaban, rivaroxaban, and edoxaban increases the risk of thromboembolic events. ■ Spinal and epidural hematoma may occur when receiving neuraxial anesthesia or undergoing spinal procedures. ■ With edoxaban, there is reduced efficacy in nonvalvular atrial fibrillation patients with creatinine clearance greater than 95 mL/min.
Nonsteroidal Anti-inflammatory Drugs (NSAIDs)	Increased risk of cardiovascular thrombotic events (e.g., MI, stroke). Increased risk of gastrointestinal (GI) adverse events (e.g., bleeding, ulceration).
Nucleoside Reverse Transcriptase Inhibitors (NRTIs)	NRTIs have increased risk of lactic acidosis and severe hepatomegaly with steatosis.
NuvaRing	Cigarette smoking increases risk of serious cardiovascular effects including myocardial infarction, thromboembolism, and stroke. Avoid use in women over 35 years old who smoke.
Obinutuzumab	Hepatitis B virus reactivation, progressive multifocal leukoencephalopathy
Ofatumumab	Hepatitis B virus reactivation, progressive multifocal leukoencephalopathy
Olanzapine	Increased risk of death in elderly patients with dementia-related psychosis.
Omalizumab (Xolair)	Risk of anaphylaxis (e.g., bronchospasm, hypotension, syncope, urticaria, and/or angioedema of throat or tongue). Anaphylaxis may occur at first dose but has also occurred beyond 1 year after regularly administered doses. First dose should be given in a health care setting.
OnabotulinumtoxinA	Spread of toxin effect. The effects of all onabotulinum toxin products may spread from the area of injection to product symptoms consistent with botulinum toxin effects. These can include asthenia, generalized muscle weakness, diplopia, ptosis, dysphagia, dysphonia, incontinence, and breathing difficulties. Risk of botulinum toxin spreading from injection area.
Opioids	Potential for addiction, abuse, and misuse. Potential for life-threatening respiratory depression, especially if used concomitantly with benzodiazepines. Monitor interactions with medications metabolized by CYP enzymes. Avoid use in pregnant women due to risk of neonatal opioid withdrawal. All immediate release (IR) and Extended-Release and Long-Acting (ER/LA) Opioid Analgesics are subject to the FDA's Risk Evaluation and Mitigation Strategy (REMS) to ensure that the benefits of opioid analgesics used in the outpatient setting outweigh the risks. Butorphonal has an accidental exposure (intranasal) warning. Fentanyl patches have warnings specific to exposure to heat (ex: heating pads, electric blankets) may increase fentanyl levels. Risk of accidental exposure to children resulting in fatal overdose when using patch formulation. Methadone has conditions for distribution and use of methadone products for the treatment of opioid addiction and Increased risk of QT prolongation. Morphine's extended-release capsules have a warning with ethanol use, the oral solution has a risk of medication errors warning, and the brand names Infumorph, Duramorph, and Mitigo have risks with neuraxial administration. Meperidine should not be used concomitantly with MAOIs. The oral solution has a risk of medication errors. Tapentadol's extended-release formulation has a warning for interaction with alcohol. Tramadol has warnings of accidental ingestion, ultra-rapid metabolism of tramadol and other risk factors for life threatening respiratory depression in children.
Ospemifene	Increased risk of endometrial cancer if used concurrently with unopposed estrogens by a woman with a uterus. Increased risk of thromboembolic and hemorrhagic stroke. Use should be limited to lowest dose and least amount of time necessary.
Oxaliplatin	Hypersensitivity/anaphylactic reactions

(continued)

Drug	Boxed warning
Oxazepam	Concomitant use of benzodiazepines and opioids may result in profound sedation, respiratory depression, coma, and death. Limit doses and durations to the minimum required. Use of benzodiazepines expose users to risks of abuse, misuse, and addiction, which can lead to overdose and death. Continued use of benzodiazepines for several days to weeks may led to significant physical dependence.
Paclitaxel	Bone marrow suppression, hypersensitivity reactions (premedication regimen required)
Paclitaxel, Protein-bound	Do not interchange, neutropenia
Paliperidone	Increased risk of death in elderly patients with dementia-related psychosis.
Panitumumab	Dermatologic toxicity
Parathyroid hormone	In male and female rats, parathyroid hormone caused an increase in the incidence of osteosarcoma. Natpara has a REMS Program.
Paroxetine	Increased risk of suicidality, particularly in people under 24 years old.
Pazopanib	Hepatotoxicity
Peginterferon (Peg-IFN)	May cause or aggravate fatal or life-threatening neuropsychiatric, autoimmune, ischemic, and infectious disorders.
Peginterferon alfa-2a	Peginterferon alfa-2a may cause or aggravate fatal or life-threatening neuropsychiatric, autoimmune, ischemic, and infectious disorders.
Peginterferon alfa-2b	Alpha interferons, including peginterferon alfa-2b, cause or aggravate fatal or life-threatening neuropsychiatric, autoimmune, ischemic, and infectious disorders.
Pegloticase	Risk of anaphylaxis and infusion reactions. Should be administered in health care setting and pretreated with antihistamines and corticosteroids. Do not administer to patients with G6PD deficiency.
Pentazocine	Pentazocine has FDA boxed warnings for addiction, abuse, misuse, life-threatening respiratory depression, neonatal opioid withdrawal syndrome, and risks from concomitant use with benzodiazepines and other CNS depressants. Potential for addiction, abuse, and misuse.
	Potential for life-threatening respiratory depression, especially if used concomitantly with benzodiazepines. Avoid use in pregnant women due to risk of neonatal opioid withdrawal.
Perampanel	Perampanel has a boxed warning for serious psychiatric and behavior reactions with its use.
Perphenazine	Increased risk of death in elderly patients with dementia-related psychosis.
Pertuzumab	Cardiotoxicity, pregnancy
Phenelzine	Increased risk of suicidality, particularly in people under 24 years old. Not approved for pediatric use.
Phenytoin	The rate of intravenous phenytoin administration should not exceed 50 mg/minute in adults and 1 to 3 mg/kg/minute (or 50 mg/minute, whichever is slower) in pediatric patients because of the risk of severe hypotension and cardiac arrhythmias. Careful cardiac monitoring is needed during and after administering intravenous phenytoin.
Pimavanserin	Elderly patients with dementia-related psychosis treated with antipsychotics are at an increased risk of death.
Polymyxin B	Risk of nephrotoxicity and neurotoxicity—avoid concomitant use with other nephrotoxic or neurotoxic agents. Must be administered in a hospital setting for continuous monitoring. Do not use in pregnancy—safety has not been determined.
Pomalidomide	Pregnancy, thromboembolic events
Ponatinib	Arterial occlusion, heart failure, hepatotoxicity, venous thromboembolism (VTE)
Pramlintide	Hypoglycemia. Pramlintide increases the risk of severe hypoglycemia, especially in patients with type 1 diabetes. Severe hypoglycemia is typically observed within 3 hours of pramlintide administration. To prevent risk of severe hypoglycemia, mealtime (bolus) insulin dose should be reduced.

Drug	Boxed warning
Prasugrel	Prasugrel can cause significant and sometimes fatal bleeding. Do not use prasugrel in patients with active pathological bleeding or a history of transient ischemic attack or stroke. Risk factors for bleeding include body weight of less than 60 kg, propensity to bleed, and concomitant use of medications that increase the risk of bleeding (e.g., warfarin, heparin, fibrinolytics, chronic use of NSAIDs). Prasugrel is not recommended in patients 75 years of age or older, except for high-risk situations (diabetes, history of prior myocardial infarction). Do not start prasugrel in patients likely to undergo urgent CABG and discontinue at least 7 days prior to any surgery. If possible, manage bleeding without discontinuing prasugrel, as discontinuation in the first few weeks after ACS may increase risk for subsequent cardiovascular events.
Procainamide	The prolonged administration of procainamide often leads to the development of a positive antinuclear antibody (ANA) test. Agranulocytosis, bone marrow depression, neutropenia, hypoplastic anemia, and thrombocytopenia in patients receiving procainamide. Due to the proarrhythmic properties of procainamide, it should be reserved for patients with life-threatening ventricular arrhythmias.
Prochlorperazine	Increased risk of death in elderly patients with dementia-related psychosis.
Promethazine	Respiratory depression in pediatrics. Promethazine should not be used in pediatric patients younger than 2 years. Promethazine also has a boxed warning for severe tissue injury including gangrene with the injection formulation, causing severe chemical irritation. The preferred route is deep intramuscular injection, subcutaneous injection is contraindicated. Do not use in patients less than 2 years old—potential for fatal respiratory depression.
Propafenone	Given the lack of any evidence that these drugs improve survival, antiarrhythmic agents should generally be avoided in patients with non-life-threatening ventricular arrhythmias, even if the patients are experiencing unpleasant, but not life-threatening, symptoms or signs.
Propranolol	Cardiac ischemia after abrupt discontinuation with brand names Inderal LA, Inderal XL, and Innopral XL. Myocardial infarction and exacerbations of angina pectoris have occurred following abrupt discontinuation of therapy with beta-blockers. Avoid abrupt discontinuation due to increased risk of cardiac adverse events.
Propylthiouracil	Severe liver injury and acute liver failure, in some cases fatal, have been reported in patients treated with propylthiouracil. These reports of hepatic reactions include cases requiring liver transplantation in adult and pediatric patients. Propylthiouracil should be reserved for patients who cannot tolerate methimazole and in whom radioactive iodine therapy or surgery are not appropriate treatments for the management of hyperthyroidism. Propylthiouracil may be the treatment of choice when an antithyroid drug is indicated during or just prior to the first trimester of pregnancy.
Quetiapine	Increased risk of death in elderly patients with dementia-related psychosis.
Quillivant XR	CNS stimulants, including Quillivant XR, other methylphenidate-containing products, and amphetamines, have a high potential for abuse and dependence. High potential for abuse and dependence.
Quinidine	Increased risk of mortality when compared to other antiarrhythmics.
Raloxifene	Increased risk of deep vein thrombosis (DVT) and pulmonary embolism (PE). Avoid use in patients with current or history of venous thromboembolic disorders. Increased risk of stroke in postmenopausal women with history of coronary heart disease.
Rasburicase	Risk of serious and fatal hypersensitivity reactions and methemoglobinemia. Contraindicated in patients with G6PD deficiency due to risk of hemolysis.
Rebetol (ribavirin)	Monotherapy is not effective for treatment of chronic hepatitis C virus. Risk of hemolytic anemia which may result in worsening of cardiac disease. Teratogenic and embryocidal effects have been demonstrated in animal species contraindicated in pregnancy. Due to long half-life, pregnancy should be avoided for at least 6 months after completion of treatment.
Regorafenib	Hepatotoxicity

(continued)

Drug	Boxed warning
Reslizumab (Cinqair)	Risk of anaphylaxis. Patients should be observed after infusion.
Risperidone	Increased risk of death in elderly patients with dementia-related psychosis.
Ritalin LA	CNS stimulants, including Ritalin LA, other methylphenidate-containing products, and amphetamines, have a high potential for abuse and dependence. High potential for abuse and dependence.
Ritonavir	Coadministration with several classes of drugs (sedative hypnotics, antiarrhythmics, ergot alkaloids) may result in severe adverse reactions.
Rituximab	Hepatitis B virus reactivation, infusion-related reactions, mucocutaneous reactions, progressive multifocal leukoencephalopathy
Rivaroxaban (Xarelto)	Increased risk of thrombotic events when discontinued prematurely. Risk of epidural or spinal hematoma if receiving neuraxial anesthesia or undergoing spinal puncture.
Romosozumab-aqqg	May increase risk of MI, stroke, and cardiovascular death. Do not initiate therapy for patients who have had a MI or stroke within the preceding year.
Sarilumab	Increased risk of serious infections (e.g., tuberculosis, invasive fungal infections, opportunistic infections).
Selegiline	Increased risk of suicidality, particularly in people under 24 years old. Not approved for pediatric use.
Sertraline	Increased risk of suicidality, particularly in people under 24 years old.
Sirolimus	Increased risk of infection. Increased risk of lymphoma. Use is not recommended in liver or lung transplants due to increased mortality.
Sodium nitroprusside	Sodium nitroprusside may cause precipitous decreases in blood pressure and may lead to irreversible ischemic injuries or death. Continuous blood pressure monitoring is required. Sodium nitroprusside metabolism produces dose-related cyanide and may be lethal. Limit infusions at the maximum rate (10 mcg/kg/min) to the shortest duration possible as patient's ability to buffer cyanide will be exceeded in less than 1 hour at this rate.
Sodium Oxybate (Xyrem)	Risk of significant respiratory depression. Risk of respiratory depression, decreased consciousness, coma, and death when misused or abused. Required REMS program due to risks of CNS depression, misuse, and abuse.
Sonidegib	Sonidegib can cause embryo-fetal death or severe birth defects when administered to a pregnant woman. Sonidegib is embryotoxic, fetotoxic, and teratogenic in animals. Verify the pregnancy status of females of reproductive potential prior to initiating therapy. Advise females of reproductive potential to use effective contraception during treatment with sonidegib and for at least 20 months after the last dose. Advise males of the potential risk of exposure through semen and to use condoms with a pregnant partner or a female partner of reproductive potential during treatment with sonidegib and for at least 8 months after the last dose.
Sotalol	Sotalol can cause life threatening ventricular tachycardia associated with QT interval prolongation. To minimize the risk of drug-induced arrhythmia, initiate or reinitiate oral sotalol in a facility that can provide cardiac resuscitation and continuous electrocardiographic monitoring. Sotalol can cause life threatening ventricular tachycardia associated with QT interval prolongation. If the QT interval prolongs to 500 msec or greater, reduce the dose, lengthen the dosing interval, or discontinue the drug. Calculate creatinine clearance to determine appropriate dosing.
Spironolactone	Abnormal elevation of serum potassium levels (greater than or equal to 5.5 mEq/L (5.5 mmol/L)) can occur with all potassium-sparing diuretic combinations, including hydrochlorothiazide/triamterene capsules. Hyperkalemia is more likely to occur in patients with renal impairment and diabetes (even without evidence of renal impairment), and in the elderly or severely ill. Since uncorrected hyperkalemia may be fatal, serum potassium levels must be monitored at frequent intervals, especially in patients first receiving hydrochlorothiazide/triamterene capsules, when dosages are changed or with any illness that may influence renal function.

Drug	Boxed warning
Streptozocin	<ul><li>Streptozocin should be administered under the supervision of a physician experienced in the use of cancer chemotherapeutic agents. A patient need not be hospitalized but should have access to a facility with a laboratory and supportive resources sufficient to monitor drug tolerance and to protect and maintain a patient compromised by drug toxicity. The physician must judge the possible benefit to the patient against the known toxic effects of this drug in considering the advisability of therapy with streptozocin. The physician should be familiar with the following text before making a judgment and beginning treatment.</li><li>Renal toxicity is dose-related and cumulative and may be severe or fatal. Other major toxicities are nausea and vomiting, which may be severe and at times treatment-limiting. In addition, liver dysfunction, diarrhea and hematological changes have been observed in some patients.</li><li>Streptozocin is mutagenic. When administered parenterally, it has been found to be tumorigenic or carcinogenic in some rodents.</li></ul>
Sunitinib	Hepatotoxicity
Tacrolimus	Increased risk of lymphoma and other malignancies. Increased susceptibility to bacterial, viral, fungal, and protozoal infections. Should only be prescribed by physicians experienced in immunosuppressive therapies.
Tacrolimus (Protopic) 0.03% and 0.1% ointment and Pimecrolimus (Elidel) 1% cream	Safety related to long-term use has not been established. Continuous use over a prolonged period is not recommended. Rare cases of skin malignancy have been reported. Avoid use in children less than 2 years of age.
Tamoxifen	Uterine malignancies and thromboembolic events
Telavancin	Moderate to severe renal impairment, nephrotoxicity, and embryofetal toxicity. Avoid use in patients with CrCl less than 50 ml/min unless benefit outweighs risk. Monitor renal function in all patients.
Temazepam	Concomitant use of benzodiazepines and opioids may result in profound sedation, respiratory depression, coma, and death. Limit dosages and durations to the minimum required in patients who must receive the combination. The use of benzodiazepines exposes users to risks of abuse, misuse, and addiction. The continued use of benzodiazepines may lead to clinically significant physical dependence.
Temly (tenofovir alafenamide)	Risk of severe acute exacerbations of hepatitis B in patients who discontinue treatment-continue to monitor hepatic function for several months after treatment.
Teriparatide	In rats, teriparatide caused an increase in the incidence of osteosarcoma. Teriparatide should be used only for patients for whom potential benefits outweigh potential risk. It should not be prescribed for patients at increased baseline risk for osteosarcoma.
Testosterone undecanoate	Testosterone undecanoate and testosterone enanthate can cause blood pressure (BP) increases that can increase the risk of major adverse cardiovascular events. Virilization has been reported in children who were secondarily exposed to topical testosterone gel and solution. Because of the risks of serious POME reactions and anaphylaxis, testosterone undecanoate is available only through a restricted program under a risk evaluation and mitigation strategy (REMS) called the Aveed REMS Program.
Tetrabenazine	Tetrabenazine can increase the risk of depression and suicidal thoughts and behavior (suicidality) in patients with Huntington disease.
Thalidomide	Pregnancy, thromboembolic events
Thiazolidinediones (TZDs)	Congestive heart failure. Rosiglitazone and pioglitazone have been shown to cause or exacerbate congestive heart failure in some patients. Rosiglitazone and pioglitazone are contraindicated in patients with NHYA class III or IV heart failure.
Thioridazine	May prolong the QT interval in a dose-related manner, and drugs with this potential have been associated with torsades de pointes–type arrhythmias and sudden death. Elderly patients with dementia-related psychosis treated with antipsychotic drugs are at an increased risk of death.
Thyroid Hormones	Though thyroid hormone medications can cause weight loss, a U.S. Food and Drug Administration (FDA) boxed warning states that these medications should not be used for treatment of obesity or for weight loss.

(continued)

Drug	Boxed warning
Ticagrelor	Ticagrelor can cause significant, sometimes fatal, bleeding. Do not use in patients with active pathological bleeding or history of intracranial hemorrhage. Do not start in patients undergoing urgent CABG. If possible, manage bleeding without discontinuing ticagrelor. Stopping ticagrelor increases the risk of subsequent cardiovascular events. Maintenance doses of aspirin above 100 mg in patients with ACS reduce the effectiveness of ticagrelor and should be avoided.
Tigecycline	Increase in all-cause mortality observed in a meta-analysis of phase 3 and 4 clinical trials—reserve for use in patients where alternative treatment is not suitable.
Timolol	Exacerbation of ischemic heart disease following abrupt withdrawal. Myocardial infarction and exacerbations of angina pectoris have occurred following abrupt discontinuation of therapy with beta-blockers. When discontinuing chronically administered timolol, gradually reduce the dose over 1 to 2 weeks. Increased risk of ischemic heart disease exacerbation with abrupt withdrawal.
Tobramycin	Close monitoring of serum concentrations, renal function, and toxicities required due to risk of renal toxicity, neurotoxicity, and ototoxicity. Avoid concomitant use of other nephrotoxic and neurotoxic medications. Risk of fetal harm—avoid use in pregnancy.
Tocilizumab	Increased risk of serious infections (e.g., tuberculosis, invasive fungal infections, opportunistic infections).
Tofacitinib	Increased risk of serious infections (e.g., tuberculosis, invasive fungal infections, other opportunistic infections, other opportunistic infections), thrombosis, lymphoma, and other malignancies. Increased risk of mortality in patients with rheumatoid arthritis taking 10 mg twice daily. Patients who have undergone a kidney transplant have an increased risk of Epstein-Barr virus-associated lymphoproliferative disorder.
Tolcapone	Potentially fatal, acute fulminant hepatic failure risk; reserve for patients on levodopa-carbidopa with symptom fluctuations who are not candidates or not responding to alternative adjunct treatment. Discontinue treatment if no substantial benefit after 3 weeks.
Topotecan	Bone marrow suppression
Toremifene	Toremifene has been shown to prolong the QTc interval in a dose- and concentration-related manner. Prolongation of the QT interval can result in a type of ventricular tachycardia called torsades de pointes, which may result in syncope, seizure, and/or death. Toremifene should not be prescribed to patients with congenital/acquired QT prolongation, uncorrected hypokalemia, or uncorrected hypomagnesemia. Avoid drugs known to prolong the QT interval and strong CYP3A4 inhibitors.
Tramadol	Potential for addiction, abuse, and misuse. Potential for life-threatening respiratory depression, especially if used concomitantly with benzodiazepines or if ultra-rapid metabolizer. Monitor interactions with medications metabolized by CYP3A4 and CPY2D6. Avoid use in pregnant women due to risk of neonatal opioid withdrawal.
Tranylcypromine	Increased risk of suicidality, particularly in people under 24 years old. Not approved for pediatric use. Avoid tyramine-containing foods due to risk of hypertensive crisis.
Trastuzumab	Trastuzumab product administration can result in subclinical and clinical cardiac failure. Trastuzumab product administration can result in serious and fatal infusion reactions and pulmonary toxicity. Exposure to trastuzumab products during pregnancy can result in oligohydramnios and oligohydramnios sequence manifesting as pulmonary hypoplasia, skeletal abnormalities, and neonatal death.
Trazodone	Increased risk of suicidality. Not approved for use in pediatric patients.
Triamterene	May cause hyperkalemia, which if uncorrected, is potentially fatal. Hyperkalemia is more likely to occur in patients with renal impairment, diabetes mellitus (with or without recognized renal insufficiency), and in the elderly or severely ill. Monitor serum potassium levels carefully in any patient receiving triamterene.
Trimipramine	Antidepressants increased the risk of suicidal thoughts and behaviors in pediatric and young adult patients in short-term studies. These studies did not show any increased risk of suicidality with antidepressants compared to placebo in adults beyond age 24; there was a reduction in risk with antidepressants compared to placebo in adults aged 65 and older.

Drug	Boxed warning
Tyzeka (telbivudine)	Risk of severe acute exacerbations of hepatitis B in patients who discontinue treatment-continue to monitor hepatic function for several months after treatment.
Upadacitinib	Serious infections leading to hospitalization or death, including tuberculosis and bacterial, invasive fungal, viral, and other opportunistic infections have occurred. Lymphoma and other malignancies have been observed. Thrombosis, including deep venous thrombosis, pulmonary embolism, and arterial thrombosis have occurred.
Vaccinia (smallpox)	Injection (Powder for Solution)
	Suspected cases of myocarditis and/or pericarditis have been observed in healthy adult primary vaccinees (at an approximate rate of 5.7 per 1000, 95% confidence interval (CI): 1.9 to 13.3) receiving ACAM2000™ (smallpox (vaccinia) vaccine, live).
	Encephalitis, encephalomyelitis, encephalopathy, progressive vaccinia, generalized vaccinia, severe vaccinial skin infections, and erythema multiforme major (including Stevens-Johnson Syndrome) and eczema vaccinatum resulting in permanent sequelae or death, ocular complications, blindness, and fetal death have occurred following either primary vaccination or revaccination with smallpox vaccines.
	Risk of encephalitis, encephalomyelitis, encephalopathy, progressive vaccinia, generalized vaccinia, and severe skin infections or reactions. Suspected cases of myocarditis and/or pericarditis have been observed in healthy adults. Risk of smallpox transmission to people with close contact with vaccinated individual.
Valproic Acid	Valproate is associated with liver failure resulting in death. Children < 2 years of age are at increased risk of fatal hepatotoxicity and this risk is compounded in patients on multiple anticonvulsants, those with congenital metabolic disorders, severe seizures accompanied by mental retardation, and organic brain disease. There is an increased risk of liver failure and death in patients with mitochondrial disorders caused by POLG mutations and children < 2 years of age suspected of having a mitochondrial disorder.
	Valproate should not be used in pregnant women or women of child-bearing potential due to the risk of major congenital malformations, particularly neural tube defects and decreased IQ scores and neurodevelopmental disorders. If therapy is necessary, contraception should be used.
	Cases of life-threatening pancreatitis have been reported in both children and adults receiving valproate.
Venlafaxine	Increased risk of suicidality, particularly in people under 24 years old.
Viekira (paritaprevir/ritonavir/ombitasvir/dasabuvir)	Risk of reactivation of hepatitis B-patients should be tested for evidence of current or prior hepatitis B infection before initiation of treatment.
Vigabatrin	Vigabatrin has been associated with permanent vision loss and is only available through a risk evaluation and mitigation strategy (REMS) program.
Vilazodone (Viibryd)	Increased risk of suicidality. Not approved for use in pediatric patients.
Vinblastine	Appropriate administration (I.V. only), extravasation
Vincristine	Appropriate administration (I.V. only), extravasation
Vinorelbine	Bone marrow suppression
Viread (tenofovir disoproxil fumarate)	Risk of severe acute exacerbations of hepatitis B in patients who discontinue treatment-continue to monitor hepatic function for several months after treatment.
Vismodegib	Vismodegib can cause embryofetal death or severe birth defects when administered to a pregnant woman. Vismodegib is embryotoxic, fetotoxic, and teratogenic in animals. Teratogenic effects included severe midline defects, missing digits, and other irreversible malformations. Verify pregnancy status of females of reproductive potential within 7 days prior to initiating vismodegib. Advise pregnant women of the potential risks to a fetus. Advise females of reproductive potential to use effective contraception during and after vismodegib. Advise males of the potential risk of vismodegib exposure through semen and to use condoms with a pregnant partner or a female partner of reproductive potential.

(continued)

Drug	Boxed warning
Vorapaxar	Antiplatelet agents increase the risk of bleeding, including intracranial hemorrhage (ICH) and fatal bleeding. Do not use vorapaxar in patients with active pathological bleeding or a history of stroke, TIA, or ICH.
Vortioxetine (Trintellix)	Increased risk of suicidality. Not approved for use in pediatric patients.
Warfarin	Warfarin is associated with major or fatal bleeding. Regular monitoring of international normalized ratio (INR) and patient education should be performed.
Xulane	Cigarette smoking increases risk of serious cardiovascular effects including myocardial infarction, thromboembolism, and stroke. Avoid use in women over 35 years old who smoke. Contraindicated in women with a BMI greater than or equal to 30 due to increased risk of VTE.
Zaleplon	Risk of complex sleep behaviors (e.g., sleepwalking, sleep-driving). Discontinue immediately if complex sleep behaviors occur.
Zepatier (elbasvir/ grazoprevir)	Risk of reactivation of hepatitis B-patients should be tested for evidence of current or prior hepatitis B infection before initiation of treatment.
Ziprasidone	Increased risk of death in elderly patients with dementia-related psychosis.
Ziv-aflibercept	Compromised wound healing, GI perforation, hemorrhage
Zolpidem (Ambien)	Risk of complex sleep behaviors (e.g., sleepwalking, sleep-driving). Discontinue immediately if complex sleep behaviors occur.

Appendix B: Top 100 Drugs

Top 100 Drugs by Prescription Volume

Provided by the ClinCalc DrugStats Database
https://clincalc.com/DrugStats/Top200Drugs.aspx

1	Lisinopril	26	Citalopram
2	Atorvastatin	27	Dextroamphetamine; Amphetamine
3	Levothyroxine	28	Ibuprofen
4	Metformin	29	Carvedilol
5	Amlodipine	30	Trazodone
6	Metoprolol	31	Fluoxetine
7	Omeprazole	32	Tramadol
8	Simvastatin	33	Insulin Glargine
9	Losartan	34	Clonazepam
10	Albuterol	35	Tamsulosin
11	Gabapentin	36	Atenolol
12	Hydrochlorothiazide	37	Potassium
13	Acetaminophen + Hydrocodone	38	Meloxicam
14	Sertraline	39	Rosuvastatin
15	Fluticasone	40	Clopidogrel
16	Montelukast	41	Propranolol
17	Furosemide	42	Aspirin
18	Amoxicillin	43	Cyclobenzaprine
19	Pantoprazole	44	Lisinopril + Hydrochlorothiazide
20	Escitalopram	45	Glipizide
21	Alprazolam	46	Duloxetine
22	Prednisone	47	Methylphenidate
23	Bupropion	48	Ranitidine
24	Pravastatin	49	Venlafaxine
25	Acetaminophen	50	Zolpidem

(continued)

Top 100 Drugs by Prescription Volume (Continued)

51	Warfarin	76	Quetiapine
52	Oxycodone	77	Topiramate
53	Ethinyl Estradiol + Norethindrone	78	Bacitracin + Neomycin + Polymyxin B
54	Allopurinol	79	Clonidine
55	Ergocalciferol	80	Buspirone
56	Insulin Aspart	81	Latanoprost
57	Azithromycin	82	Tiotropium
58	Metronidazole	83	Ondansetron
59	Loratadine	84	Lovastatin
60	Lorazepam	85	Valsartan
61	Estradiol	86	Finasteride
62	Ethinyl Estradiol; Norgestimate	87	Amitriptyline
63	Lamotrigine	88	Esomeprazole
64	Glimepiride	89	Tizanidine
65	Fluticasone; Salmeterol	90	Alendronate
66	Cetirizine	91	Lisdexamfetamine Dimesylate
67	Losartan + Hydrochlorothiazide	92	Ferrous Sulfate
68	Paroxetine	93	Apixaban
69	Spironolactone	94	Diclofenac
70	Fenofibrate	95	Sitagliptin
71	Naproxen	96	Folic Acid
72	Pregabalin	97	Sumatriptan
73	Insulin Human	98	Drospirenone; Ethinyl Estradiol
74	Budesonide + Formoterol	99	Hydroxyzine
75	Diltiazem	100	Oxybutynin

Note: The data source (MEPS prescribed medicines file) is released annually by the U.S. Government. This data release represents survey data from two years prior. The ClinCalc DrugStats Database sanitizes and standardizes this data, and is typically released within a few months of the MEPS release. There is an inherent delay in collecting the survey data (e.g., in the 2018 calendar year), MEPS releasing the data from patients (August 2020), and the ClinCalc DrugStats release (a few months later, classified as the 2021 drug list).

Index

Note: Page numbers followed by *b, f, or t* indicate material in boxes, figures, or tables, respectively. Page numbers in italics refer to entries in the appendices.